Acute Care Surgery and Trauma

"Remember, the critical questions in the field of Surgery never change, just the answers!"

J. Bradley Aust, MD, 1926–2010

Acute Care Surgery and Trauma: Evidence-Based Practice discusses important surgical management approaches and clinical decision-making based on scientific evidence found in the published literature.

Updated and fully revised, this new edition continues to support clinicians by providing the most up-to-date information and evidence on which to base their decisions across a wide range of topics in acute care surgery and trauma, thus optimizing the decision-making process for the care of individual patients.

What can be better for the busy clinician than having all the answers to complex questions extensively researched by experts in the field and readily available without requiring further intensive literature searches?

Featuring chapters written by specialists in acute care, trauma, and emergency surgery, with extensive references throughout, the text features tables summarizing key evidence and clinical recommendations for quick reference and easy interpretation. This is an invaluable resource for all acute care surgery and trauma practitioners.

Acute Care Surgery and Trauma

Evidence-Based Practice

Third edition

Edited by

Stephen M. Cohn, MD, FACS
Saint Barnabas Hospital
New York, New York

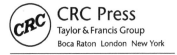

CRC Press
Taylor & Francis Group
Boca Raton London New York

CRC Press is an imprint of the
Taylor & Francis Group, an **informa** business

Cover images courtesy of Dr. Stephen M. Cohn

Third edition published 2024
by CRC Press
6000 Broken Sound Parkway NW, Suite 300, Boca Raton, FL 33487-2742

and by CRC Press
4 Park Square, Milton Park, Abingdon, Oxon, OX14 4RN

CRC Press is an imprint of Taylor & Francis Group, LLC

© 2024 Taylor & Francis Group, LLC

Library of Congress Cataloging-in-Publication Data

Names: Cohn, Stephen M, editor.
Title: Acute care surgery and trauma : evidence-based practice / edited by Stephen M Cohn.
Description: Third edition. | Boca Raton : CRC Press, 2024. | Includes bibliographical references and index.
Identifiers: LCCN 2023009087 | ISBN 9781032326986 (paperback) | ISBN 9781032328034 (hardcover) | ISBN 9781003316800 (ebook)
Subjects: MESH: Wounds and Injuries--surgery | Surgical Procedures, Operative--methods | Evidence-Based Emergency Medicine | Emergencies
Classification: LCC RD51.5 | NLM WO 750 | DDC 617.9/19--dc23/eng/20230626
LC record available at https://lccn.loc.gov/2023009087

ISBN: 9781032328034 (hbk)
ISBN: 9781032326986 (pbk)
ISBN: 9781003316800 (ebk)

DOI: 10.1201/9781003316800

Typeset in Times LT Std
by KnowledgeWorks Global Ltd.

This textbook is dedicated to my wife, Miryame, for her unwavering love and support.

Contents

Foreword by Basil A. Pruitt[1]

Evidence-based medicine (EBM), as defined by Sackett et al., is "the conscientious, explicit, and judicious use of current best evidence in making decisions about the care of individual patients" [1]. In the assessment of medical evidence, a systematic review (SR) of randomized controlled trials (RCTs) and RTCs per se are considered to provide the highest levels of medical evidence, i.e., Ia and Ib, respectively [2]. RCTs are widely and relatively readily conducted in the evaluation of various drugs and medical treatments but are more difficult to apply in comparative evaluations of surgical procedures. The relative rarity of class I citations in the tables presented with the various chapters in this book, particularly those related to operative procedures, attests to that difficulty.

Specific limitations affecting the usefulness and validity of an RCT comparing surgical procedures include ethical concerns about sham operations and, conversely, the variable influence of the placebo effect in the absence of a sham operation. Other limitations include variations in the operating surgeons' technical skills and experience (minimized by specific training before starting the trial), the evolution of surgical procedures across time, and differences in postoperative care among surgeons and institutions. Difficulty in blinding both patients and surgeons is also of concern if the effect on symptoms or quality of life is the outcome of interest. That potential for bias can be reduced by the use of independent investigators for outcome evaluation. Other limitations in the application of RCTs to address surgical questions include excessive limitation of eligibility criteria that can compromise external validity and generalizability of the results. Conversely, in less restricted nonrandom studies, the selection of treatment based on surgical preference can bias the results. Finally, there are few, if any, readily accessible funding sources for surgical clinical studies or the evaluation of an operative innovation [2–4].

In recognition of those limitations, it was reported in the late 1990s that although roughly comparable percentages of medical treatments and surgical practice were evidence-based, i.e., 82% and 95%, respectively, 53% of medical treatments were based on Level I data but only 25% of surgical practice was supported by RCTs [2]. Despite the difficulties in applying RCTs to address surgical questions, more and more surgical studies have generated higher levels of evidence that have been utilized to develop treatment guidelines. In 2011, it was claimed that surgical practice had been revolutionized by the application of the results of RCTs [5]. Changes in the treatment of breast cancer are cited as particular examples of the benefits of evidence-based surgery, but more than half of the published surgical RCTs have compared medical therapies in surgical patients, and less than half have compared surgical procedures

per se [2, 5]. The relative scarcity of PTCs for surgical procedures is considered by some to represent an imbalance, if not a waste of research effort, which should be addressed by the conduct of more RCTs comparing operations, the results of which can be used to define evidence-based surgery [6, 7].

Groups of research methodologists and clinicians have formed to advance the use of evidence-based surgery and promote the conduct of RCTs to compare operative interventions. Members of the Surgical Outcomes Research Centre (SOURCE) at McMaster University, representing "various subspecialties," have produced articles focused on clinically relevant surgical issues to transfer to the surgical community the skills needed "to critically appraise evidence" [8]. Similar organizations, the BALLIOL Collaboration and its successor, the IDEAL Collaboration, have proposed a five-stage process by which innovative surgical procedures can be developed and evaluated, i.e., innovation (Stage 1), development (Stage 2a), exploration (Stage 2b), assessment (Stage 3), and long-term study (Stage 4) [9].

At each stage of the development of a surgical procedure, reports regarding that procedure become progressively more demanding and scientifically rigorous. At Stage 1, innovation, in which proof of concept is the goal, reports are commonly structured as case reports. In Stage 2a, development, the studies of patients from whom ethical approval is required should be reported as consecutive cases in prospective development studies. At Stage 2b, exploration, studies should be prospective, with data collected systematically and reported as prospective uncontrolled studies or, if controlled, as feasibility or exploratory RCTs. At Stage 3, assessment, in which the innovation is compared with the current standard to determine which is best, reporting takes the form of an RCT. At Stage 4, long-term studies, the procedure is monitored for rare outcomes and long-term effects, with the results used to form a registry [10, 11]. When assessing the strength of evidence in evaluating an innovative procedure or comparing two established procedures, one should, as the authors of this text have done, grade the strength of the supporting evidence about the location of the procedure of interest in the *ideal* framework for developing surgical procedures. The successful transit of an operative procedure or surgical innovation through the early stages of this process delivers a relatively mature product to the doorstep of an RTC. Such a preparation decreases the high risk of RTC failure of operative procedures without such staging [12].

Fortunately, evidence-based surgery (EBS) is not captive to the RTC and can be predicated on well-designed prospective observational research. Observational studies may also have limitations that include systematic overestimation of treatment

---

[1] *Note:* Dr. Pruitt sadly died in 2019 after a long and illustrious career. This Foreword has been minimally modified by the Editor.

effect, confounding, and bias that can be reduced or eliminated by patient matching, cohort selection, use of sophisticated statistical techniques, and standardized data collection [5]. Those limitations should influence the grading and acceptance of evidence generated by observational studies.

The ultimate goal of EBS is the development of practical guidelines for decision support and patient education. To that end, the American College of Surgeons has produced "clinical guideline summaries" to formulate "evidence-based decisions in surgery," which offer recommendations for the diagnosis and treatment of, at present, 35 surgical conditions [13]. The grading of the evidence supporting the recommendations by the American College of Surgeon members considered to be "experts" is generic and ranges from "weak" to "strong" without the granularity of evidence level grading provided in this text by the authors, who have used the levels of evidence defined by the National Health Services Research and Development, Centre for Evidence-Based Medicine [2].

The increased use of EBS in the development of clinical guidelines has led to many improvements in care, but flaws and misuse of the process have become apparent to such an extent that EBM has been questioned as "a movement in crisis" [14]. Specific concerns include misattribution of clinical significance to statistically significant benefits; shift from patient-centered care to system-driven care by the imposition of inflexible rules; difficulty in managing an excessive number of clinical guidelines; uncertain application of guidelines to patients, particularly the elderly, with multiple comorbid conditions; and abuse of the process by commercial and other special interests. The identification of those problems, which both authors and readers should have in mind when grading evidence, has prompted a call for "a return to real evidence-based medicine" in which care of individual patients based on studies focused on clinical usefulness and free of commercial interference and bias is enlightened by clinical expertise. The editors and authors of this book have provided rigorous grading of the papers supporting their recommendations for diagnosis and treatment, which have been tempered by invited comments of recognized clinical experts to realize the goal of scientifically based, resource-conserving, patient-oriented EBS.

Acute Care Surgery and Trauma: Evidence-Based Practice confirms the fact that EBS is not, to paraphrase Sackett, "cookbook surgery" [1] but is a perpetually evolving process. The differences between EBM and EBS suggest that clinical reality and the intrinsic characteristics of surgery that limit the application of RCTs support affixing the word "best" to the term "evidence-based surgery." The inclusion of EBM in the medical education process and EBS in surgical education has been justified by the increasing emphasis on EBM in clinical practice [15]. This book, the 3rd edition, which promotes that trend, should be in the library of every medical school, every department of surgery, and with all surgeons.

REFERENCES

1. Sackett DL, Rosenberg WMC, Gray JAM, Haynes RB, Richardson WS. Evidence based medicine: What it is and what it isn't. *BMJ* 1996;*312*:71–72.
2. Wente MN, Seiler CM, Uhl W, Büchler MV. Perspectives of evidence-based surgery. *Digestive Surgery* 2003;*20*: 263–269.
3. Johnson J, Rogers W, Lotz M, Townley C, Meyerson D, Tomassy G. Ethical challenges of innovative surgery: A response to the IDEAL recommendations. *The Lancet* 2010;*376*:1113–1115.
4. Cook JA. The challenges faced in the design, conduct and analysis of surgical randomised controlled trials. *Trials* 2009;*10*:9.
5. Merkow RP, Ko CY. Evidence-based medicine in surgery. The importance of both experimental and observational study designs. *JAMA* 2011;*306(4)*:436–437.
6. Students 4 Best Evidence, Evidence-based surgery: What sets it apart? Available at http://www.students4bestevidence.net/evidence-based-surgery/. Accessed January 14, 2015.
7. Ioannidis J. Editorial. Clinical trials: What a waste. *BMJ* 2014;*349*;g7089.
8. McMaster University, Surgical Outcomes Research Centre (SOURCE), EBS. Evidence based surgery.
9. McCulloch P, Altman DG, Campbell WB, Flum DR, Glasziou P, Marshall JC, Nicholl J, for the Balliol Collaboration. Surgical Innovation and Evaluation 3. No surgical innovation without evaluation: The IDEAL recommendations. *The Lancet* 2009;*374*:1105–1112.
10. The IDEAL Collaboration. Stages of innovation in surgery.
11. Köckerling F. The need for registries in the early scientific evaluation of surgical innovations. *Frontiers in Surgery* 2014;*1*:12.
12. McColloch PG. Editorial. Re: Clinical trials: What a waste. Available at http://www.bmj.com/content/349/bmj.g7089. Accessed March 3, 2015.
13. American College of Surgeons. Evidence-based decisions in surgery (Based on Practice Guidelines), Chicago, IL. Available at https://www.facs.org/education/resources/ebds-guidelines. Accessed February 17, 2015.
14. Greenhalgh T, Howick J, Maskrey N, for the Evidence Based Medicine Renaissance Group. Evidence based medicine: A movement in crisis? *BMJ* 2014;*348*:g3725.
15. Kwaan MR, Melton GB. Evidence-based medicine in surgical education. *Clinics in Colon and Rectal Surgery* 2012;*25*:151–155.

Author Biography

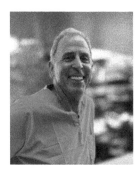

Stephen M. Cohn, MD, FACS

I am a native of Oakland, California, and attended Baylor College of Medicine after completing a biochemistry degree at the University of California, Santa Barbara. I completed my general surgical training and trauma/critical care fellowship at Boston University. I joined Yale University School of Medicine as the Chief of the Trauma Service, but within a few months I was called to serve with the U.S. Army Medical Corps in Desert Storm. Upon my return to New Haven, I was asked to assume the position of Division Chief of Trauma and Surgical Critical Care, where I built a successful ACS Level 1 trauma center and a surgical critical care fellowship. In addition, I started an active research program utilizing animal models of trauma. I later assumed the role of medical director of the Ryder Trauma Center, as the Robert Zeppa Endowed Professor of Surgery at the University of Miami, and ran the Divisions of Trauma and Surgical Critical Care. We also started the Army training center for forward surgical teams at that time. Subsequently, I served as the chairman of the Department of Surgery at the University of Texas Health Science Center in San Antonio. I currently live in New York City and continue to operate, educate, and be an active researcher.

I have produced more than 300 publications, have completed my eighth textbook, have had extensive funded research, am a member of many professional organizations, and serve as a reviewer for numerous journals, among many other activities. My academic and research interests are in the areas of trauma and combat casualty care and surgical infections. I have been the recipient of several teaching awards, including the Teacher of the Year awards at Boston University, University of Massachusetts, Yale, University of Miami, and Northwell Health. I am most proud, professionally, of the large number (>100) of ICU, trauma, and research fellows and numerous residents and students I have had the pleasure to help educate.

Contributors

Suresh K. Agarwal
Department of Surgery
Duke University Medical Center
Durham, North Carolina

Abdul Q. Alarhayem
Department of Surgery
Texas Tech Health Science Center
Odessa, Texas

Zaid Alirhayim

Jordyn Baldwin
Department of Surgery
Henry Ford Macomb
Clinton Township, Michigan

Stephen W. Behrman
Department of Surgery
Baptist Health Sciences University
Memphis, Tennessee

Elizabeth Benjamin
Department of Surgery
Emory School of Medicine
Grady Health System
Atlanta, Georgia

John K. Bini
Department of Surgery
University of Texas Health Science Center
San Antonio, Texas

Steven Blau
Department of Surgery
Saint Barnabas
Bronx, New York

Daniel J. Bonville
Department of Surgery
Baylor College of Medicine
University of Houston
Houston, Texas

Susan Brien

Garrett W. Britton
Department of Surgery
US Army Institute for Surgical Research
Brooke Army Medical Center
San Antonio, Texas

Steven Brower
Department of Surgery
Icahn School of Medicine
Englewood, New Jersey

Horeb Cano-Gonzalez
Department of Surgery
University of Houston
Houston, Texas

Josh Cassedy

Clarence E. Clark
Department of Surgery
Dignity Health Medical Group
Chandler, Arizona

Mark Cockburn
Department of Surgery
Florida Medical Center
Ft. Lauderdale, Florida

Panna A. Codner

Danielle Collins
Department of Surgery
Henry Ford Macomb
Clinton Township, Michigan

Abigail Coots
Department of Surgery
Reading Hospital
Reading, Pennsylvania

Moti Cordoba
Division of trauma and
    critical care surgery
Sheba medical center
Tel Hashomer, Israel

Morgan Crigger
Department of Surgery
University of Arizona College of Medicine
Phoenix, Arizona

Bruce A. Crookes
Department of Surgery
Medical University of South Carolina
Charleston, South Carolina

Marc A. de Moya
Department of Surgery
Medical College of Wisconsin
Milwaukee, Wisconsin

Linda C. Degutis
Department of Chronic Disease Epidemiology
Yale School of Public Health
New Haven, Connecticut

Tara DiNitto
Department of Trauma and Critical Care Surgery
Trident Medical Center
North Charleston, South Carolina

Matthew O. Dolich
Division of Trauma, Critical Care, Burns,
    and Acute Care Surgery
University of California, Irvine Medical Center
Orange, California

Brian J. Eastridge
Department of Surgery
University of Texas Health Science Center San Antonio
San Antonio, Texas

Sara B. Edwards

Sebastian R. Eid
Department of Surgery
Hackensack University Medical Center
Hackensack, New Jersey

Akpofure Peter Ekeh
Department of Surgery
Miami Valley Hospital
Dayton, Ohio

Ara J. Feinstein
Department of Surgery
University of Arizona College of Medicine
Phoenix, Arizona

Jared S. Folwell
Department of Surgery
Burn Surgeons US Army Institute for Surgical Research
Brook Army Medical Center
San Antonio, Texas

Alexander Fortgang
Department of General Surgery
Hackensack Meridian Health at Palisades
North Bergen, New Jersey

Eliza Fox
Department of Surgery
Augusta University Medical Center
Augusta, Georgia

Gregory J. Gallina
Department of General Surgery
Hackensack Meridian Health at Palisades
North Bergen, New Jersey

Megan Gilchrist
Department of Surgery
HCA/USF Morsani College of Medicine
Tampa, Florida

Adam Lee Goldstein
Department of Trauma Surgery
Wolfson Medical Center
Holon, Israel

Gerald Gollin
Department of Surgery
University of California
and
Rady Children's Hospital
San Diego, California

Zoe Guzman
Department of Surgery
Hackensack University Medical Center
Hackensack, New Jersey

Fahim Habib
Department of Surgery
Allegheny Health Network
Pittsburgh, Pennsylvania

S. Morad Hameed
Department of Surgery
University of British Columbia
Vancouver, British Columbia, Canada

Samuel Hawkins
Department of Surgery
NYU–Brooklyn
Brooklyn, New York

Connor Hogan
Department of Surgery
University of Houston
Houston, Texas

David Holzer
Department of Surgery
Thomas Jefferson Medical College
Philadelphia, Pennsylvania

John J. Hong
Department of Surgery
Lehigh Valley Health Network
Allentown, Pennsylvania

Kenji Inaba
Department of Surgery
University of Southern California
Los Angeles, California

Katherine R. Iverson
Department of Surgery
Medical College of Wisconsin
Milwaukee, Wisconsin

Erin Jennings
Department of Ophthalmology
NYU Grossman School of Medicine
New York City, New York

Danby Kang
Department of Surgery
University of Pittsburgh Medical Center
Pittsburgh, Pennsylvania

Benjamin Keller
Department of Surgery
San Diego School of Medicine
University of California
Rady Children's Hospital
San Diego, California

Emily A. Kerby
Department of Transplant Surgery
Henry Ford Hospital
Detroit, Michigan

Natasha Keric
Department of Surgery
Banner-University Medical Center
Phoenix, Arizona

Mustafa Tamim Alam Khan
Division of Plastic Surgery and
    Department of Surgery
University of Texas Health Science Center
San Antonio, Texas

Jennie S. Kim
Division of Trauma & Acute Care Surgery
Los Angeles General Medical Center
Los Angeles, California

Ki Won Kim
Department of Surgery
Englewood Health
Hackensack Meridian School of Medicine
Nutley, New Jersey

David R. King
Department of Surgery
Massachusetts General Hospital
Boston, Massachusetts

Yoram Klein
Division of Trauma and Critical Care Surgery
Sheba Medical Center
Tel Hashomer, Israel

Varun Krishnan
Department of Surgery
Morristown Medical Center
Morristown, New Jersey

Vishal Kumar

Marc LaFonte
Department of Acute Care Surgery
Rutgers Health/Robert Wood Johnson
    Medical School
New Brunswick, New Jersey

Andrew Lawson
Department of Surgery
Augusta University Medical Center
Augusta, Georgia

Alex Lee

Ethan Levitch
Department of Surgery
University of Queensland-Ochsner
    Medical Program
Brisbane, Australia

Sungho Lim

David H. Livingston
Department of Surgery
Rutgers-New Jersey Medical School
Newark, New Jersey

Peter P. Lopez
Department of Surgery
Henry Forb Macomb
Clinton Township, Michigan

Jose Lopez-Vera
Department of Surgery
University of Houston
Houston, Texas

Joseph Love
Department of Surgery
HCA/USF Morsani College of Medicine
Tampa, Florida

Stephanie Lumpkin
Department of Surgery
Duke University Medical Center
Durham, North Carolina

George Mazpule
Department of Surgery
Hackensack University Medical Center
Hackensack, New Jersey

Yasha Modi
Department of Ophthalmology
NYU Grossman School of Medicine
New York City, New York

Deborah L. Mueller
Department of Surgery
University of Texas Health Sciences
    Center San Antonio
San Antonio, Texas

David O'Connor
Department of Surgery
Hackensack University Medical Center
Hackensack, New Jersey

Terence O'Keeffe
Department of Surgery
Augusta University Medical Center
Augusta, Georgia

Adatee Okonkwo
Department of Surgery
Dignity Health Medical Group
Chandler, Arizona

Adrian W. Ong
Department of Surgery
Reading Hospital
Reading, Pennsylvania

Jakob Oury
Department of Surgery
University of Queensland-Ochsner
    Medical Program
Brisbane, Australia

Harsimran Panesar
Department of Surgery
Morristown Medical Center
Morristown, New Jersey

Leah M. Pearl
Department of Surgery
Henry Ford Macomb
Clinton Township, Michigan

Andrew B. Peitzman
Department of Surgery
University of Pittsburgh School of Medicine
UPMC-Presbyterian
Pittsburgh, Pennsylvania

J. Martin Perez
Department of Surgery–Trauma and Surgical
    Critical Care
Berkshire Medical Center
Pittsfield, Massachusetts

Edgar J. Pierre
Department of Surgery
Critical Care Medicine South
    Miami Hospital
Miami, Florida

Brad H. Pollock
Department of Public Health Sciences
Davis School of Medicine
University of California
Davis, California

Aashish Rajesh
Division of Plastic Surgery and
    Department of Surgery
University of Texas Health Science Center
San Antonio, Texas

Juliet J. Ray

Christopher R. Reed
Duke University Medical Center
Durham, North Carolina

Peter M. Rhee
Department of Surgery
Saint Barnabas Hospital
Bronx, New York

Paolo Rigor
Department of Surgery
Dartmouth, Hitchcock Medical Center
Geisel School of Medicine
Dartmouth College
Lebanon, New Hampshire

Valerie G. Sams
Department of Surgery
University of Cincinnati
Cincinnati, Ohio

Steven Satterly
Department of Surgery
Duke University
Durham, North Caroline

Stephanie A. Savage

Mark D. Sawyer
Mayo Clinic
Rochester, Minnesota

Carl I. Schulman
Department of Surgery
University of Miami
School of Medicine
Miami, Florida

Steven D. Schwaitzberg
Department of Surgery
Jacobs School of Medicine and Biomedical Sciences
University at Buffalo
Buffalo, New York

Brian I. Shaw
Department of Surgery
Duke University
Durham, North Caroline

Joseph H. Shin
Department of Surgery
Dartmouth, Hitchcock Medical Center
Geisel School of Medicine
Hanover, New Hampshire

Gregory Simonian
Davis School of Medicine
Hackensack University Medical Center
Hackensack, New Jersey

Dror Soffer
Division of Trauma Unit
Ichilov Medical Center
Tel Aviv, Israel

Kenneth Stahl

Zachary E. Stiles
Roswell Park Comprehensive Cancer Center
Buffalo, New York

Mary Stuever

Pedro G.R. Teixeira
Department of Surgery and Perioperative
   Care
Dell Medical School
University of Texas at Austin
Austin, Texas

Christopher S. Thomas
Davis School of Medicine
Medical University of South Carolina
South Carolina, Texas

Tabitha Threatt
Department of Surgery
University of Texas Health Science Center
San Antonio, Texas

Boulos Toursarkissian
Division of Vascular Surgery
University of Texas Health Sciences Center
San Antonio, Texas

Alexandre Tran

George C. Velmahos
Department of Surgery
Massachusetts General Hospital
Boston, Massachusetts

Howard T. Wang
Division of Plastic Surgery and
   Department of Surgery
Department of Otolaryngology
University of Texas Health Science Center
San Antonio, Texas

Jessica Wassef
Department of General Surgery
Hackensack Meridian Health at Palisades
North Bergen, New Jersey

Yinglun Wu
Department of Surgery
Dartmouth, Hitchcock Medical Center
Geisel School of Medicine
Dartmouth College
Lebanon, New Hampshire

Bardiya Zangbar
Department of Surgery
Westchester Medical Center
New York Medical College (NYMC)
Valhalla, New York

Introduction

Brad H. Pollock

Important questions about surgical management approaches are posed in this textbook. The answers are informed by scientific evidence from the published literature. But how is such evidence gathered and used? In this introduction, a description of the attributes of clinical (or patient-oriented) research studies and how their results may be combined is provided to guide clinical decision-making. Evidence-based medicine (EBM) helps make informed decisions by integrating individual clinical expertise with the best available external clinical evidence. Doing so optimizes decision-making to improve the care and outcome of individual patients [1]. Patient-oriented research studies can address a broad array of goals—ascertaining the etiology of a health problem, evaluating the accuracy and utility of new tests including biomarkers, determining the most efficacious interventions, identifying prognostic factors, etc. The most common application of EBM is assessment of the safety and efficacy of new treatments and rehabilitative or preventive interventions. Evidence gathered from multiple studies is often combined to make more accurate clinical inferences to inform the selection of the most appropriate treatment plan for individual patients.

Strength of Evidence from Clinical Research Studies

Four attributes define the strength of evidence provided by clinical research study: (1) Level of the evidence—dictated by the type of study design used; (2) quality of evidence—directly related to minimization of bias; (3) statistical precision—the degree to which true effects can be distinguished from spurious effects due to random chance alone; and (4) selection of study endpoints to measure effect—an endpoint's appropriateness to accurately represent a clinically meaningful outcome—along with the magnitude of the observed effect. For practical reasons, the selection of study subjects almost always is less than ideal, so the degree to which a chosen study population represents an intended target population also impacts the strength of evidence provided by that investigation.

Study Design

Different types of study designs are used in clinical research, each with their own profile of relative advantages and limitations due to biases. Case reports and case series can provide novel descriptions of the effects of an intervention or clinical course from an individual patient or very small groups of patients. However, these are subject to selection bias (i.e., cherry-picking cases), they often include subjective outcome assessments, and they are imprecise due to very small samples. In addition, case reports and case series have no comparison control groups.

Cross-sectional studies, where both exposure and outcome information are collected simultaneously, are not used often in clinical research. These studies are usually limited to assessing prevalent rather than acute or episodic conditions and cannot directly address cause-and-effect temporal relationships.

Case-control studies include subjects who have already developed the outcome of interest (cases) and a group of unaffected subjects (controls) and can be performed in a timelier and often much less expensive manner than other types of studies. A temporal relationship between cause and effect can only be inferred and not directly observed because of the retrospective nature of this design. Case-control studies are subject to the biased recall of antecedent events and exposures and to selection bias, most often related to the selection of unrepresentative control groups, and are most often used for very rare outcomes or when there is a long latency between exposure and the subsequent effect.

Prospective cohort studies recruit subjects who do not have the outcome of interest. All subjects are then actively followed over time for the occurrence of the outcomes. Recruitment may be restrictive based on accruing an equal number of subjects into preselected exposure categories; matching on other factors is possible to reduce confounding and improve the precision of comparisons across exposure groups. Alternatively, prospective cohort study recruitment need not be based on predetermined categories of exposure, but rather more representative of a general population using random selection—more common when there are multiple exposures of equal interest. A related design is the historical or retrospective cohort study where previously collected information, often from comprehensive clinical databases, is used to retrospectively classify exposure status and clinical outcomes. Prospective cohort studies are typically more expensive than retrospective study designs. However, because exposure status is not randomly assigned, cohort studies are more subject to confounding bias than are randomized controlled trials (RCTs). This happens because exposure status may be correlated with extraneous factors (*confounders*) that are unaccounted for. For example, a cohort study comparing a new less invasive surgical procedure with an established more invasive procedure may selectively enroll older, more frail patients to one group; this would introduce confounding bias. There are methods to minimize this type of bias (described later), but they do not address unknown or unmeasurable confounders. Prospective studies are typically more resource-intensive and time-consuming than retrospective designs but provide a clear picture of the temporal relationship between a cause and an effect. Cross-sectional, case-control, and cohort studies are all observational designs where the exposure or treatment of interest is merely observed and not assigned.

Compared to other study designs, RCTs provide the greatest weight of evidence. RCTs allocate subjects to one or more exposures of interest for the sole purpose of obtaining unbiased estimates of treatment effects; thus they are experimental in nature. Their key advantage is a much lower likelihood of confounding bias from *unknown* or *unmeasurable* factors. RCTs and other designs can all use techniques that account for potential confounding—these include eligibility restriction, stratified block design, or statistical adjustment. However, randomized allocation of subjects in RCTs to treatment groups tends to even out the distribution of confounders between groups, especially unknown or unmeasurable potential confounders. RCTs can also be masked (or blinded) so that the exposure status is unknown to observers. Typically, RCTs are more expensive to conduct and recruitment of subjects can be more challenging as potential subjects may decline being "experimented" on. However, they represent the "gold standard" for clinical research; they provide the strongest weight of evidence for causal inference compared to other designs.

Crossover designs are studies in which all subjects serve as their own controls. For a typical simple crossover study, half the study population is randomly assigned to receive the primary treatment first and then crosses over to receive the second treatment; the other half receives the treatments in reverse order. The primary advantage of these studies is that because each subject serves as their own control, person-to-person variability is eliminated, thus substantially reducing sample size requirements. A major assumption in crossover studies is that the residual effects of a treatment disappear by the time the groups are crossed over. This is not applicable for many interventions, especially surgical interventions, where a subject's condition is permanently altered by the therapy (e.g., limb amputation), or for certain pharmaceutical trials, where the washout period for the new drug is too long or of unknown duration. Factorial trial designs attempt to evaluate the impact of two or more factors more efficiently in the separate trials, but only realize efficiencies (primarily lower sample size requirements) when there is likely to be no or minimal interaction between the factors being evaluated.

Study Validity

The quality of a clinical research study depends on internal and external factors. Studies have internal validity when, apart from random error (dependent on sample size), the resulting differences between compared exposure groups can only be attributed to the exposure under study. Internal validity factors include selection bias and information bias. These manifest themselves in different ways and degrees for alternative study designs. Statistical precision also impacts internal validity. In contrast, external validity refers to the generalizability of a study and addresses the issue of whether study results derived from the assessment of a specific study population (usually a subset or sample of a target population) can be extrapolated to another population of interest. If a study is not internally valid, one need not consider whether it is externally valid; biased and/or imprecise study results should never be extrapolated to another population.

Selection bias results when an unrepresentative sample of subjects is included in a study. For case-control studies, selection bias can skew the main measures of effect; biased selection of controls is particularly important. For prospective studies, selection bias is more likely to compromise the study's generalizability. Measurement bias is inaccuracy related to the method of measuring values for a study. Examples include miscalibrated blood pressure readings, inaccurate height measurements, and flawed laboratory methods that give erroneous values. Observer bias is inaccuracy related to measuring a study outcome and can occur when an observer knows the subject's intervention group assignment. It is also more likely to occur when outcome measures are subjective: e.g., assessment of symptoms or toxicities, patient self-report measures, and interpretations of physical examination findings. If observers know which treatment a patient received, their outcome assessments may be biased. Blinding (also referred to as masking) is used to reduce observer bias. Double blinding is where neither the observer nor the patient knows the treatment assignment. However, for many surgical interventions, such as total limb vs. partial limb amputation, or regimens with very idiosyncratic symptoms or toxicity profiles, blinding may be impractical or impossible. Confounding bias is the mixing up of effects so that the primary effect under study cannot be separated from the influence of extraneous factors. For example, failing to account for preoperative disease severity in a study comparing two surgical approaches might lead to confounding if sicker patients are preferentially included in one of the groups. While the likelihood of this is much greater in prospective cohort studies, even RCTs should be appropriately designed to minimize such confounding.

Statistical precision refers to the ability to distinguish real effects from those due to random chance, i.e., chance associations. For example, with just six subjects (three in each group) in an RCT comparing a new postsurgical antibiotic regimen to a conventional regimen for sepsis prophylaxis, an extreme finding could likely be attributed to random chance alone, not to a true biological drug effect. Chance errors are less likely to occur with larger sample sizes. Trials are always planned to limit the likelihood of chance errors; acceptable levels of error (for type 1 and type 2 statistical errors) are selected and the target minimum detectable effect size is chosen. Sample size/power calculations are performed in the design phase to ensure adequate statistical precision. Other designs that may offer more efficiencies (e.g., lower sample sizes) such as adaptive trials are increasingly being used in clinical research.

External validity refers to the ability to generalize a study's results to the population of interest. Determining whether the study population possess unique characteristics that might modify the effect of an intervention in a way that would render it ineffective in some other group is critical. There is a tendency for published surgical and nonsurgical intervention studies to enroll subjects at larger academic institutions that may not be representative of patients seen at smaller nonacademic centers. Large multicenter trials conducted from geographically diverse locations may also improve generalizability.

Strength of Evidence

Study design, precision, and validity affect a study's weight of evidence for causal inference. For practical reasons, the investigator who is designing a new study is always confronted with trade-offs between these factors and cost. For example, including only sicker patients with high expected mortality to gain statistical precision (higher event rate) would come at the cost of generalizability. Likewise, recruiting only males into a trial would eliminate sex as a confounding factor but at the expense of generalizability (and equity). Selecting *death* instead of *death plus sepsis* as a study endpoint for an antibiotic trial may decrease observer bias at the expense of statistical precision of the outcome assessment (fewer events). Investigators are faced with many challenges when designing intervention studies, and compromises must be made for practical reasons; however, the overriding goal is to produce the strongest level of evidence to impact clinical care.

Literature Reviews

Reviews of published studies can take multiple forms. Single studies may be sufficient for medical decision-making when based on a very large, highly valid RCT. Alternatively, narrative reviews or systematic reviews evaluate multiple publications.

Narrative reviews can address a broad set of clinical questions and be less focused on a specific question; they tend to be more qualitative and less quantitative. In contrast, systematic reviews are usually focused on a specific clinical issue, incorporate objective criteria for the selection of published studies, include an evaluation of quality and worthiness, and often use a quantitative summary to synthesize combined results.

Narrative reviews may be one of the first academic endeavors that young physicians complete during their training. The subjective nature of narrative reviews increases the likelihood that inferences are affected by imprecision and bias. For example, some reports merely tally the number of included studies supporting and the number of studies refuting a particular issue, then declare a winner. For narrative reviews, little consideration of study attributes may be given for study design, statistical precision, and other elements of validity or the likelihood that studies with null results may be published (publication bias).

Systematic Reviews

Systematic reviews are a staple of EBM [2]. They provide the best means to combine evidence from multiple studies and follow a defined protocol to identify, summarize, and combine information. Systematic reviews may restrict the inclusion of studies to specific study designs, such as RCTs or include a broader set of study designs. These reviews can be very labor-intensive, costly, and may include attempts to collect unpublished information. Combining evidence across different study designs as well as studies that used very different methodological approaches or different endpoint measures is challenging.

A protocol for a systematic review should include a strict set of guidelines for selecting and amalgamating information from the literature. Cochrane Collaboration [3] guidelines for developing systematic review protocols require the following: A background section explaining the context and rationale for the review, objectives, and clearly defined inclusion and exclusion criteria. Inclusion criteria can be based on study designs, study populations, types of interventions, and outcome measures. The search strategy for the systematic review as well as methods for combining data from each study should be fully described. Data synthesis in a systematic review includes how the results or outcomes from individual studies are combined and analyzed and include statistical considerations such as choice of summary effect measures, assessment of heterogeneity of effect across studies, prespecification of subgroup analyses, use of random or fixed effects statistical models, and assessment of publication bias.

The existence and conduct of many clinical studies is often not reflected by resultant publications in the medical literature. The U.S. Food and Drug Administration initiated a public registry and results database of privately and publicly funded clinical studies—ClinicalTrials.gov. This has become an important source to identify trials not reported in the medical literature. The U.S. Department of Health and Human Services issued a Final Rule for Clinical Trials Registration and Results Information Submission (42 CFR Part 11) describing the regulatory registration and results submission [4].

Meta-Analysis

Systematic reviews often, but not always, include a meta-analysis. The goals of meta-analysis are to combine data from independent studies of the same topic. Potentially they can provide a more precise summary estimate of the effect and determine if the effect is both robust and combinable across a range of populations and studies [5]. Meta-analyses include data extracted from each individual study that may be used to calculate a point estimate of effect along with a measure of uncertainty, e.g., the 95% confidence interval. This is repeated for individual studies included in the meta-analysis. Then a decision is made about whether the results can be pooled to calculate a summary effect estimate across all studies. While meta-analyses can combine data from several studies, they are most typically used for RCTs, but can be used to combine weaker observational studies. Combining a few very large, well-conducted RCTs in a meta-analysis may provide much stronger evidence than combining numerous smaller observational studies in a meta-analysis.

The decision to numerically combine or not combine studies is made by assessing the heterogeneity of effect across studies. A large magnitude of statistical heterogeneity suggests the true underlying treatment effects in the trials are not identical, i.e., the observed treatment effects have a greater difference than one should expect due to random error alone. Importantly, uncovering heterogeneity and attributing it to one or more factors may be the primary goal of a meta-analysis. Analysis of heterogeneity may elucidate previously unrecognized differences between studies. Only in the absence of significant heterogeneity is it valid to numerically calculate a summary measure of effect. Calculation of a summary measure of effect relies on a mathematical process that attributes additional weight to the results from studies that provide more information (usually those with larger study populations) or have higher quality. Often, data for all included studies are plotted on a graph known as a "forest plot," which includes a graphical representation of the magnitude of effect and degree of uncertainty for each study (plotted as confidence intervals). Meta-analysis can reveal the impact of potential confounders on the treatment effect.

Publication Bias

All studies are statistically subject to type I errors, where evidence is found to reject a null hypothesis of no effect, or type II errors, where evidence is found failing to reject the null hypothesis when a true effect exists. Studies with statistically significant results ("positive" studies) are more likely to be accepted for publication in the medical literature than studies without statistically significant results ("negative" studies). Such negative studies, even if adequately powered with very low type II error rates, are less likely to be accepted for publication than smaller positive studies. A single very large negative study may provide definitive evidence against adopting a new treatment or intervention but because of publication bias may not impact clinical practice.

Levels of Evidence and Grades of Recommendations

All reviews evaluate historical information and are therefore subject to systematic bias and random error. While a number of approaches have been used to rate levels of evidence for clinical question, for different study objectives (e.g., determining the impact of a therapeutic or preventive intervention), the Oxford Centre for Evidence-Based Medicine Levels of Evidence [6] has provided a framework to evaluate the level of evidence based on a review of the literature, study design, and quality. The highest level of evidence for therapeutic intervention is provided by systematic reviews of *multiple* large, methodologically valid RCTs that show homogeneity of effect across trials (Level Ia). The next highest is for an *individual* RCT with a narrow confidence interval (Level Ib); this is followed by an all-or-none effect related to the introduction of a treatment (Level Ic). The level of evidence decreases with weaker study designs such as cohort studies (Level II) followed by case-control studies (Level III), case series (Level IV), and, at the lowest level, expert opinion (Level V). Grades of recommendations are based on the consistency of higher-level

studies: an "A" grade shows consistency across Level I studies; a "B" grade shows consistency across Level II or III studies or extrapolations from Level I studies; a "C" grade shows consistency across Level IV studies or extrapolations from Level II or III studies; and a "D" grade shows Level V evidence or inconsistency across studies of any level. Meta-analyses can be used to combine results for different study types, but the design and quality of the included studies determine the level of evidence. The Grading of Recommendations Assessment, Development and Evaluation (GRADE) framework has been adopted by Cochrane for assessing the evidence with a scale, including high, moderate, low, and very low [3].

Clinical Research Infrastructure

A major shift in past decades has been the evolution of clinical research performed by isolated researchers in individual clinics toward larger team science multi-institutional studies. This transition began in select areas of clinical research such as oncology with the initiation of the National Cancer Institute–sponsored clinical trials cooperative groups some 66 years ago and has progressed over time with the formation of the NIH Clinical Translational Research Award Consortium in 2006 and to other large team science transdisciplinary research consortia in other biomedical research domains. The core goal of these consortia is to provide research infrastructure to efficiently address important clinical and translational research hypotheses that lead to improved clinical practice. Commonly, these groups rely on a clinical research infrastructure emphasizing study population inclusiveness; quality control; harmonized research information technology resources; adherence to best statistical practices for planning, monitoring, and analysis; and rapid dissemination of knowledge for discoveries. Increasingly, clinical discoveries and research results are being efficiently disseminated to nonacademic health providers with a growing emphasis on implementing and sustaining evidence-based healthcare interventions in the general population (dissemination and implementation science). The continuum of biomedical research from the laboratory bench to the patient bedside to the community feeds back to the design of research investigations at all stages [7].

In contrast to many clinical trials, which are often conducted in highly structured research environments, pragmatic trials tend to be conducted in real-world clinical practice settings with clinicians who may or may not have research backgrounds and include study subjects who are more broadly representative of the general population; i.e., those who receive healthcare at places other than research-intensive academic health centers. Clinical research data sources are broadening data collected from a research protocol to include information from electronic health records, product and disease registries, administrative claims databases, patient-generated data from mobile devices, and social media.

Trials conducted using data derived from clinical care settings, in contrast to data generated in specialized research environments from formal research investigations, are likely to play an increasing role in clinical research; these are called point-of-care trials [8]. The FDA defines real-world evidence as clinical evidence regarding the usage and potential benefits, or risks, of a medical product derived from analysis of real-world data. Real-world evidence can come from not only formal RCTs but other types of studies, including pragmatic trials and observational studies (prospective and/or retrospective). It is expected that the role of real-world data and real-world evidence will grow.

Summary

EBM used in surgical practice need not be limited to the evaluation of RCTs and formal meta-analyses. A broader range of external evidence, including information from other study designs, can be used to address clinical questions. However, appropriate consideration of strength of evidence needs to drive what will eventually become the basis for changes in clinical practice. Practice guidelines developed using EBM can have a positive impact on patient outcomes. EBM guidelines have reduced mortality from myocardial infarctions, improved care for persons with diabetes, increased cancer survival, and improved surgical outcomes. EBM supplements physicians' judgments that might otherwise be based solely on anecdotal clinical experience. Ultimately, developing and incorporating faster and more efficient decision support tools (including model-based and machine learning–based tools) to improve prediction and guide treatment at the bedside are the goals of clinical research. EBM provides a framework to improve the quality of surgical practice and ultimately surgical outcomes.

REFERENCES

1. Sackett DL, Rosenberg WMC, Gray JAM, Haynes RB, Richardson WS. Evidence based medicine: What it is and what it isn't. *BMJ.* 1996;312:71–72.
2. Egger M, Davey Smith G, Altman D. *Systematic Reviews in Health Care: Meta-Analysis in Context*, *3rd* Edition. BMJ Books; 2022:608.
3. Cochrane. Cochrane. Accessed 2/2/2023, 2023. https://www.cochrane.org/
4. National Institutes of Health DoHaHS. Clinical Trials Registration and Results Information Submission. U.S. National Archives. Accessed 2/5/2023, 2023. https://www.federalregister.gov/documents/2016/09/21/2016-22129/clinical-trials-registration-and-results-information-submission
5. Borenstein M, Hedges L, Higgins J, Rothstein H. *Introduction to Meta-Analysis, 2nd* Edition. Wiley; 2021:544.
6. Medicine OCfE-B. Centre for Evidence-Based Medicine. Accessed 2/5/2023, 2023. https://www.cebm.ox.ac.uk/
7. Mehta TG, Mahoney J, Leppin AL, et al. Integrating dissemination and implementation sciences within Clinical and Translational Science Award programs to advance translational research: Recommendations to national and local leaders. *J Clin Transl Sci.* 2021;5(1):e151. doi:10.1017/cts.2021.815
8. Califf RM, Cavazzoni P, Woodcock J. Benefits of streamlined point-of-care trial designs: Lessons learned from the UK recovery study. *JAMA Intern Med.* Dec 1 2022;182(12):1243–1244. doi:10.1001/jamainternmed.2022.4810

1

Patient Safety in the Care of Trauma Patients

J. Martin Perez, Kenneth Stahl, and Susan Brien

1.1 Introduction

Trauma care aims to save the lives of injured patients and prevent further organ damage from the metabolic and phythemologic derangements caused by their injuries. To achieve this goal, a critical judgment affecting a trauma patient's survival is required every 72 seconds during the first hours of the patient's care [1]. Despite the best efforts from the trauma team, the urgency and accuracy required for this decision-making process are conducive to producing errors. The circumstances likely to result in errors are unstable patients, fatigued operators, incomplete clinical information, delayed decisions, multiple concurrent tasks involving complex teams, transportation of unstable patients, and multiple hand-offs of patients' care. Due to these factors, the management of trauma patients poses significant challenges and creates a "perfect storm for medical errors" [2].

1.2 Incidence

Adverse outcomes and error reporting in healthcare are sporadic at best [3]. For this reason, the actual number of errors that occur in the care of trauma victims is difficult to accurately assess. However, adverse outcomes as a result of errors in patient care do occur, and some patients are seriously and sometimes fatally harmed [4]. Preventable deaths secondary to human and system errors account for up to 10% of fatalities in patients with otherwise survivable injuries treated at Level I trauma centers [5–7]. This number of unintended deaths equates to as many as 15,000 lost lives per year in the United States, or almost 2 lives lost every hour [8]. This is two to four times higher than deaths due to errors reported in the general hospital patient population [9].

1.3 Mechanisms of Errors

In-hospital errors in the management of trauma patients that ultimately lead to adverse outcomes can occur at any time during their management and begin on admission. The primary survey is a rapid assessment and concurrent stabilization of the patient and is usually complete within the first 30 minutes of the resuscitative phase of trauma care. During this period, 2.5 errors per patient (760 errors in 300 patients) have been observed [1]. Patients with a low Glasgow Coma Score,

psychiatric history, or drug and alcohol use provide trauma teams with additional challenges. Older patients, who already pose diagnostic challenges due to concurrent diseases, have an increased risk of adverse events [10].

Life-threatening errors include inadequate airway management, missed tension pneumothorax, underestimates of the severity of bleeding, and failure to manage acute shock states [11]. Delay in the diagnosis or mishandling of any of these conditions during the initial resuscitation will lead to failure of the trauma team to rescue the patient. Studies indicate that 16% of preventable trauma deaths are due to failure of airway management, 28% to failure to identify or control hemorrhage, 14.5% to errors in diagnosis, and 11.8% to missed diagnosis during the primary survey [12]. Errors in the triage of hemodynamically precarious patients in need of prompt operative intervention can lead to hemodynamic collapse and avoidable cardiac arrest in the radiology suite or observation area. One of the difficulties in identifying patients "in shock" is that our diagnostic studies (heart rate, blood pressure, base deficit) fail to identify hypoperfusion approximately 20% of the time [49].

A diagnostic peritoneal lavage may be required to make the correct decision for the disposition of the patient to the operating room for immediate surgery or radiology for further evaluation [13]. A recent meta-analysis of errors in trauma resuscitation identified 39 unique error types, which were divided into nine categories: emergency medical services handover, airway, assessment of injuries, patient monitoring and access, transfusion-related, management of injuries, team communication/dynamics, procedure error, and disposition. Systems processes that were utilized to identify errors included morbidity and mortality conference, tertiary review, radiology review, and deviation from a guideline. Most of the error types are situated in the resuscitative phase of trauma care. The findings of the meta-analysis confirm the findings that the resuscitative phase of trauma care encompasses the majority of errors in trauma. Unfortunately, there is no accepted classification scheme for trauma resuscitation errors [50] (Table 1.1).

The secondary survey begins when the primary survey is completed, resuscitation efforts are well established, and vital signs are stabilized. The secondary survey is a head-to-toe evaluation of the trauma patient, including a complete history and physical examination as the clinical circumstances allow. In addition, a careful reassessment of the patient's response to the initial resuscitation and a search for more subtle injuries are carried out. Injuries can be missed during the secondary survey and lead to significant morbidity or mortality that

DOI: 10.1201/9781003316800-1

TABLE 1.1

Common Errors in Trauma and Error-Producing Conditions

Common Errors in Trauma Care	Error-Producing Conditions	Solutions
Resuscitation		
Airway management	• High-risk/low-frequency event Information overload • One-way decision gate	Simulation training, procedural checklists, algorithms
Missed injuries on surveys	• Poor information transfer • Time pressure • Information overload • Low signal-to-noise ratio • Volume overload and task saturation	Checklist use, adherence to established standard procedures, mass casualty simulation, drills
Inappropriate triage	• Time pressure • Task overload • Faulty risk assessment • Normalization of deviance	Diminish reliance on "normal vitals and X-rays," high-level supervision
Operative		
Delayed surgery	• Time pressure • High-risk/low-frequency event • Task overload • Poor information transfer • Faulty risk assessment	Adherence to standards of care, teamwork decision-making, communication skills training
Prolonged surgery	• Fatigue • Faulty risk assessment • Time pressure	Situational awareness strategies, team training and empowerment, HRO mindset adoption
Critical care		
Missed diagnosis	• Poor information transfer • High-risk/low-frequency event	Cognitive bias prevention strategies, simulation training
Prophylaxis	• Lack of standardization • Faulty risk assessment • Inaccurate communication	Standardized orders, team training, communication skills training

occurs in up to 8.1% of trauma patients. Seventeen percent of these missed injuries are abdominal, 16.3% intrathoracic, and 40.8% extremity injuries [14]. This same study demonstrated that 65.1% of injuries were missed due to inadequate or incorrect primary or secondary surveys, with 34.9% due to radiographic misinterpretations and 34.1% due to delayed surgeries. The tertiary survey (TTS) follows the secondary survey and is a comprehensive general physical re-examination and review of all investigations, laboratory results, and diagnostic imaging reports within the last 24 hours [51]. The TTS is expected to reduce missed injuries and therefore improve the care of the trauma patient.

1.4 Errors in the Operative Phase of Trauma Care

The surgical procedure itself has been the subject of numerous safety analyses, and avoiding technical mishaps in the surgical management of individual injuries and organ systems is detailed elsewhere in this text. As a general principle, the trauma surgeon needs to understand that, regardless of the patient's injuries, excellent surgical outcomes depend on expeditious and skilled surgical procedures and meticulous attention to the cognitive and physiological aspects of the operation. Failure of the surgeon to maintain constant awareness of the physiological condition of the patient, including fluid and transfusion requirements, coagulation state, acid/base balance, and core temperature, leads to prolonged operations and increases the mortality of patients with otherwise survivable injuries [15]. This is the concept of damage-control surgery that has been well established by a recent meta-analysis [16]. The trauma surgeon needs the cognitive discipline and judgment to abort complex and timely organ repairs and defer to damage control surgery when the patient's condition demands this for survival. Persistence in an operation that is compromised by the bigger picture of the patient's deteriorating physiology is known as "cognitive anchoring bias" [17] and must be avoided by knowing and staying within the boundaries of the trauma safety box (see Section 1.7).

Additionally, the environment in the operating room needs to be managed by the trauma surgeon. This is necessary to ensure accurate communication of critical patient information and minimize distractions to avoid adverse outcomes [18]. The maintenance of situational awareness (the "big picture") and crew resource management skills are equally important [19]. This is best exemplified in the actively hemorrhaging patient in the operating room with deranged physiology (hypothermia, acidosis, and coagulopathy), where timely and appropriate management decisions are made by not just the surgical team. Key clinical decisions in this setting require interdisciplinary communication by trauma surgery and anesthesiology.

A constant open dialogue promotes good team functioning and is another essential element of optimizing surgical outcomes and patient safety efforts [20].

1.5 Errors in the Intensive Care Unit and Postoperative Phases of Trauma Care

The risk of error during the intensive care unit (ICU) management of trauma patients is in the range of 1.7 adverse events per patient per day, of which 13% are life-threatening or fatal [21]. Forty-five percent of these errors were judged to have been preventable. Level II evidence-based studies indicate that the presence of at least one adverse event increased the odds ratio of mortality as much as 17-fold over matched controls with hemorrhaging events [21]. Errors such as failure to recognize the development of abdominal or limb compartment syndrome [22], failure to recognize occult bleeding, and delayed onset of shock and respiratory failure are potentially avoidable events that contribute to adverse outcomes [7]. Medication errors that may occur at any phase of the care of the trauma patient are also an area of potential improvement in safety; however, few studies have been identified specifically addressing medication error in trauma patients [52].

1.6 Result of Errors in Trauma Care

The actual rate of adverse events leading to death in trauma patients may be higher than reported if autopsy statistics are included. Studies that included autopsy findings document that mortality due to errors ranges between 15% and 28% [24]. In a retrospective observational analysis of admissions to a Level I center, 1032 avoidable errors were found in the care of 893 (4%) patients. These errors contributed to 76 preventable or potentially preventable deaths. This same study found that 5.6% of fatalities over the study period could have been prevented. This study also indicated that errors occur in all three phases of the management of trauma victims. Thirty-six percent of errors led to a fatality in the resuscitative phase, 14% in the operative phase, and 50% in the ICU phase [25].

1.7 Methods to Reduce Errors in Trauma Care

The nature of human and system errors that lead to adverse outcomes has been investigated in complex systems such as the commercial aviation industry and the nuclear power industry, environments that closely mimic trauma care. Organizations such as these are collectively known as "high-reliability organizations" (HROs); detailed descriptions can be found in the safety literature [2]. HROs are defined as high-risk, error-intolerant systems that repeatedly carry out potentially dangerous procedures with minimal actual error. HROs understand circumstances that are likely to lead to adverse events known as "error-producing conditions" (EPCs). Sets of these conditions have been arrived at after careful analysis of accidents and near-miss incidents with the use of mathematical modeling of contributing factors [26, 27]. The most

important EPCs that affect trauma patient care are fatigue; high-risk, low-frequency events; time pressure; normalization of deviancy; poor supervision; faulty risk (injury severity) perception; and task overload.

High-reliability safety theories have generated strategies to avoid both individual and organizational errors. The application of these error-management strategies can reduce adverse outcomes in trauma care [2]. Safety in trauma care can be achieved by understanding and anticipating chances for errors and thus effectively trapping these small missteps before major adverse events take place [28]. Several safety methods of HROs have led to this kind of consistent error trapping and reductions in adverse outcomes, which can be emulated by trauma systems. These include a preoccupation with studying and recognizing error patterns with root cause analysis, a reluctance to simplify interpretations of critical situations, attention to system operations, developing resiliency to recover from unexpected events, and deference to expertise. The HRO safety literature has described the successful adoption of these principles as culminating in a state of "collective HRO mindfulness" that enhances team function [29].

In addition to this safety mindfulness, there are important sets of specific and teachable team skills that can be added to bring an overarching system for patient safety in trauma care. These HRO safety skills are divided into six broad categories: crew resource management (CRM), situational awareness (SA), time-critical decision-making (DM), team leadership and supervision, communication skills, and human factors (HFs). These skills are closely interrelated and combine the central principles of teamwork and communication capabilities with individual performance. Level II evidence-based studies indicate that these methods can be utilized to enhance and improve surgical outcomes [30, 31].

Combining these concepts of mental preparedness and error avoidance with team competencies can enhance safety outcomes in the management of trauma victims. This will result in an overarching "high-reliability mindset" [32] incorporating error awareness theories of HROs with error avoidance strategies for personal and team behaviors. This is an effective error mitigation strategy given that trauma centers operate in an environment demanding perfection without an HRO-like system safety net [33]. However, at present, there are no studies specifically examining the role of HRO principles in the setting of trauma.

The concept of a "high-reliability mindset" has already transitioned into HRO and aviation safety with "scenario-based training" (SBT) that stresses advanced risk awareness and management and decision-making skills. Threat and error management is not new, and using this knowledge to create "mindset training" has received broad HRO industry acceptance [34]. This mindset, as it applies to trauma training and practice, includes the understanding of the specific conditions that define times when an error is more likely to occur and thus predict unsafe circumstances to which patients may be exposed [35].

Derived from this understanding of inherently risk-producing conditions is the final component of the "high-reliability mindset," which is the concept of operating within the confines of a theoretical "box" that has specific safety boundaries and provides a safety net. James Reason's reference to this as the "safety space" offers a useful mental model of a three-dimensional area within which safe operations are assured [36]. The trauma safety box has sides defined by patient physiology, individual skills and currency of the primary surgeon, surgical team training, and human and environmental factors. To assure safe outcomes, trauma surgeons must mentally define this box, and all team members must understand the safety boundaries as they exist in any clinical situation. Operating "outside the box" is sometimes required due to variances in the condition of trauma patients, but it is essential to understand when such events occur. During these times, additional error-producing conditions may exist and dominate the environment. Therefore, a heightened level of individual vigilance and team performance is needed to prevent complications, as the greatest risk to the patient is when the surgeon and the team are outside this safety box but are not aware they are there.

The conceptual model of the "high-reliability mindset" combines concepts of error avoidance by understanding circumstances when an error is more likely to occur and strategies to manage these risks. The HRO mindset encompasses a global awareness of the "safety space," including a central "safety box" that defines the boundaries of safe operations with minimal risks of adverse outcomes. The areas outside the box are also part of the overall safety mindset and predict the increased risk of error and conditions that make these errors more likely to occur. Best outcomes in the management of trauma victims come with the knowledge of the boundaries of the safety box, understanding the risks of operating outside these boundaries, awareness of when the trauma surgeon and patient are outside the safety box, and a treatment strategy for returning inside the safety envelope.

The "high-reliability mindset" ingrains in the adopter a sense of enhanced vigilance during such times when an increased risk of error exists. The importance of the individual surgeon adopting this mindset in trauma care is emphasized by Helmreich, who showed that, although individual error occurs infrequently, it leads to a high risk of fatal or near-fatal outcomes [36]. This has critical implications in trauma care because of the role of human factors such as fatigue on individual performance.

1.7.1 Teamwork

Another integral part of the high-reliability mindset is teamwork. In every aspect of healthcare, teamwork is more effective than non-team care [38]. Studies of high-performance, trained healthcare teams show a reduction in relative risk for major complications, a reduction in relative risk of postoperative death, and a reduction in postoperative length of stay [39]. Observational studies in the operating room have consistently demonstrated that training clinicians in teamwork skills provides important safety benefits [40–42].

Advanced teamwork skills include precise communication with "read-backs" and acknowledgments of understanding with "hear-backs" by team members to avoid errors while exchanging critical patient information. This also reduces the risk of adverse events occurring during the transfer of care and hand-offs to other trauma teams [43]. Failure to carry out precise communications led to serious adverse patient consequences in over one-third of cases evaluated in a study of surgical information transfer within surgical teams [44]. A communication adjunct for high-reliability team skills is the use of aviation-style checklists to prevent team members from losing critical information. Published data document that checklists designed in a style that has been perfected in the cockpit can be adopted for team care of critically ill surgical patients with excellent results [45].

Another important team function is to define the roles and duties of each member of the trauma team. Key components of this training model have been taught as a curriculum known as "crew resource management" and emphasize organizing workloads and task assignments, clinical task planning, and review and critique strategies with preprocedure briefs and postprocedure debriefs. Level II evidence-based data support the conclusion that these skills enhance the performance of the operating team, leading to improved patient outcomes [16]. No specific trauma studies, however, have demonstrated that any element of CRM, debriefs, or checklists reduce errors in the trauma population.

1.7.2 Simulation

HRO- and aviation-style simulation, both high and low fidelity, can be used to train and practice these key elements of the high-reliability mindset. Simulation training can be used for teaching safe trauma care because specific team actions as well as surgical tasks can be taught, practiced, and perfected in a simulated environment. A prospective observational study of trauma resuscitations demonstrated significant improvements in outcomes after aviation-style simulation practice sessions in study teams caring for multiple injured patients [46].

An innovative approach to teach safety in laparoscopic cholecystectomy designed to reduce the risk of common bile duct injury has been proposed, which is based on the aviation training principles of situational awareness and spatial disorientation [47]. This is an excellent demonstration of the cross-applicability of the two training methods and shows that simulated presentations of uncommon but critical scenarios that require immediate recognition and attention can be programmed and practiced for both pattern recognition and technical management skills [48]. Video recording of trauma resuscitation, which is employed at some trauma centers, may also allow for post hoc analysis of teamwork, communication, and other elements of optimal teamwork

1.8 Conclusions and Algorithm

Errors that lead to serious adverse outcomes in trauma management occur at a significant rate and can cause death in patients who might otherwise have survived their injuries. An understanding of the circumstances that make the occurrence of errors more likely is necessary to avoid adverse outcomes. Aviation and HRO safety theory can be used to teach individual skills and team behaviors that lead to enhanced trauma patient safety. These safety skills can coalesce into a useful "high-reliability safety mindset" that forms overarching principles for the safe management of trauma patients.

A successful adaption of these skills for use in our trauma practice and current curriculum training has been demonstrated [49]. Incorporation of this error understanding and avoidance strategy will help reduce the risks or unintended outcomes that trauma patients are exposed to during their hospital care (Table 1.1).

Editor's Note

Trauma patients present as a mystery. We, healthcare providers, have little knowledge of the actual time from injury, the true mechanism of injury, or the forces experienced. Therefore, we have a poor understanding of the type of injuries sustained. This is a fertile environment for medical error. Using standardized protocols, we methodically march through the steps of resuscitation, recognizing that even patients with the most severe injuries, with concomitant hypoperfusion, may not manifest altered vital signs or acidosis in 20% of cases. Continual reassessment of the trauma patient is thus essential to look for subtle changes in patient status.

Patients with severe injuries are uncommon at most trauma centers, and those with occult hypoperfusion are even rarer. But it is these patients who represent the biggest challenge to clinicians to avoid preventable deaths. Filming trauma resuscitations for later educational training has been quite valuable in my experience in improving the conduct of the providers.

The second major arena where trauma patients sustain avoidable medical errors is in the operating theater. As the unstable trauma patient requiring emergent laparotomy or thoracotomy is very unusual at most trauma centers, there is less experience among the operating room team with deteriorating trauma victims. The anesthesiologists and their team may be quite accomplished but may not know the surgeons and vice versa. Communication between the operators and the anesthesiologists is essential for optimal outcomes.

Medical error in trauma patients is a challenging problem to correct. One possible solution is the further regionalization of trauma care to fewer, higher-volume centers. The problem then is the time that may be required to transport unstable patients to these facilities. The nature of trauma is that it requires rapid transport to a trauma center for immediate, accurate diagnosis and optimal, errorless resuscitation and operation to salvage the small subset of catastrophically injured patients. Unfortunately, safety, by its very nature, is difficult to study prospectively, as clinical equipoise is very hard to establish. Thus, there is little high-quality evidence to guide us in reducing medical errors. Much of what we do to improve the safety of our patients appears to be borrowed from other industries such as aviation.

REFERENCES

1. Fitzgerald M, Cameron P, Mackenzie C, et al. Trauma resuscitation errors and computer-assisted decision support. *Arch Surg.* 2011;*146(2)*:218–225.
2. Stahl KD, Brien SB. Reducing patient errors in trauma care. In: Cohn S, ed. *Acute Care Surgery: Evidenced-Based Practice.* Informa Healthcare USA Inc.: New York, pp. 276–287, 2009.
3. Pietro DA, Shyavitz LJ, Smith RA, et al. Detecting and reporting medical errors; why the dilemma? *Br Med J.* 2000;*320*:794–798.
4. Weingart SN, Wison RM, Gibberd RW, et al. Epidemiology of medical error. *Br Med J.* 2000;*320*:774–777.
5. Ivatury RR, Guilford K, Malhotra AK, et al. Patient safety in trauma: Maximal impact management errors at a Level I trauma center. *J Trauma.* 2008;*64*:265–272.
6. Gruen RL, Jurkovich GJ, McIntyre LK, et al. Patterns of errors contributing to trauma mortality: Lessons learned from 2594 deaths. *Ann Surg.* 2006;*244*:371–380.
7. Teixeira PG, Inaba K, Hadjizacharia P, et al. Preventable or potentially preventable mortality at a mature trauma center. *J Trauma.* 2007;*63*:1338–1346.
8. Miniño AM, Anderson RN, Fingerhut LA, et al. Deaths: Injuries, 2002. In: *National Vital Statistics Reports.* Vol. 54, *No. 10.* National Center for Health Statistics: Hyattsville, MD, pp. 32–37, 2006.
9. Institute of Medicine. *To Err Is Human: Building a Safer Health System.* National Academy Press: Washington, DC, 2000.
10. Ackroyd-Stolarz S, Read Guerney J, MacKinnon NJ, et al. The association between a prolonged stay in the emergency department and adverse events in older patients admitted to hospital: A retrospective cohort study. *BMJ Qual Saf.* 2011;*20*:564–569.
11. Mackersie MC. Pitfalls in the evaluation and resuscitation of the trauma patient. *Emerg Med Clin N Am.* 2010;*28*: 1–27.
12. Houshin S, Larse MS, Holm C. Missed injuries in a Level I trauma center. *J Trauma.* 2002;*52*:715–719.
13. Gonzalez RP, Icker J, Gachassin P. Complementary roles of diagnostic peritoneal lavage and computed tomography in the evaluation of blunt abdominal trauma. *J Trauma.* December 2001;*51(6)*:1128–1134.
14. Budhan G, McRitchie D. Missed injuries in patients with multiple trauma. *J Trauma.* 2000;*49*:600–605.
15. Jonson J, Gracias V, Schwab C, et al. Evolution in damage control for exsanguinating penetrating abdominal injury. *J Trauma.* 2001;*51*:261–271.
16. Ciocchi R, Montedori A. Damage control surgery for abdominal trauma. *Cochrane Database Syst Rev.* March 28, 2013;*(3)*:1–14.
17. Epley N, Gilovich T. Putting adjustment back in the anchoring and adjustment heuristic: Differential processing of self-generated and experimenter-provided anchors. *Psychol Sci.* 2001;*12(5)*:391–396. McCarthyCathy D, Blumenthal D. *Committed to safety: Ten case studies on reducing harm to patients.* The Commonwealth Fund, New York, April 2006.
18. Hurert S, Garrett J. Improving operating room safety. *Patient Saf Surg.* 2009;*3*:25.
19. Pronovost P, Freischlag JA. Improving teamwork to reduce surgical mortality. *JAMA.* 2010;*304(15)*:1721–1722.
20. Rothchildchld JM, Lanrian CP, Cronin JW, et al. The critical care safety study: The incidence and nature of adverse events and serious medical errors in intensive care. *Crit Care Med.* 2005;*33(8)*:1694–1700.
21. Orgeas MG, Timit JF, So L, et al. Impact of adverse events on outcomes in intensive care unit patients. *Crit Care Med.* 2008;*36(7)*:2041–2047.

22. Maxell RA, Faian TC, Croce M. Secondary abdominal compartment syndrome: An underappreciated manifestation of severe hemorrhagic shock. *J Trauma*. December 1999;*47(6)*:995.

23. Lau G. Perioperative deaths: A further comparative review of coroner's autopsies with particular reference to the occurrence of fatal iatrogenic injury. *Ann Acad Med Singapore*. July 2000;*29(4)*:486–487.

24. Davis W, Hoyt DB, McArdle MS, et al. An analysis of errors causing morbidity and mortality in a trauma system: A guide for quality improvement. *J Trauma*. 1992;*32*:660–666.

25. Williams JC. A data-based method for assessing and reducing human error to improve operational performance. In: *Fourth IEEE Conference on Human Factors in Nuclear Power Plants*, Monterey, CA, pp. 436–450, June 6–9, 1988.

26. Hendy K. Defense R&D Canada—Toronto technical report DRDC Toronto TR 2002-057, March 2003.

27. Sundt TM, Brow JP, Uhlig PN, STS Workforce on Patient Advocacy, Communications, and Safety. Focus on patient safety: Good news for the practicing surgeon. *Ann Thorac Surg*. 2005;*79*:11–15.

28. Weck KE, Sutclife KM, Obstfeld D. Organizing for high reliability: Processes of collective mindfulness. *Crisis Manage*. 2008;*3*:31–37.

29. Shojnia KG, Dunan BW, McDonald KM et al. Making health care safer: A critical analysis of patient safety practices. Evidence Report/Technology Assessment No. 43 (Prepared by the University of California at San Francisco–Stanford Evidence-based Practice Center under Contract No. 290-97-0013), AHRQ Publication No. 01-E058. Agency for Healthcare Research and Quality: Rockville, MD, July 2001.

30. Riser DT, Rice MM, Salisbury ML, et al. The potential for improved teamwork to reduce medical errors in the emergency department. The MedTeams research consortium. *Ann Emerg Med*. 1999;*34*:373–383.

31. Stahl K. Doctors don't die, pilots do (sometimes), and parachutes work. The patient safety initiative blog, http://www.thepatientsafetyinitiative.com/2011/04. Accessed November 3, 2014.

32. Stahl K, Brien S. Patient safety in surgical care. In: S. Cohn, editor. 2nd ed. *Surgery Evidenced-Based Practice*. People's Medical Publishing House: Shelton, Connecticut, pp. 14–22, 2012.

33. Wright R. Training's future. *Aviat Saf*. 2011;*31(1)*:8–11.

34. Hollnagel E. *Barriers and Accident Prevention*. Ashgate Publishing Limited: Hampshire, U.K., 2004.

35. Reason J. *The Human Contribution*. Ashgate Publishing Ltd.: Farnham, England, pp. 265–279, 2008.

36. Helmreich R. On error management: Lessons from aviation. *BMJ*. 2000;*320*:781–785.

37. Jeffcott SA, MacKenzie CF. Measuring team performance in healthcare: Review of research and implications for patient safety. *J Crit Care*. 2008;*23*:188–196.

38. Beomo R, Goldsith S, Uchino J, et al. Prospective controlled trial of the effect of the medical emergency team on postoperative morbidity and mortality rates. *Crit Care Med*. 2004;*32(4)*:916–921.

39. Heley AN, Undre S, Vinent CA. Defining the technical skills of teamwork in surgery. *Qual Saf HealthCare*. 2004;*15*:231–234.

40. Awad SS, Faga SP, Bello C, et al. Bridging the communication gap in the operating room with medical team training. *Am J Surg*. November 2005;*190(5)*:770–774.

41. Lingard L, Epsin S, Whyte S, et al. Communication failures in the operating room: An observational classification of recurrent types and effects. *Qual Saf Health*. 2004;*13*:330–334.

42. Arora V, Johnon J, Lovinger D, et al. Communication failures in patient sign-out and suggestions for improvement: A critical incident analysis. *Qual Saf Health Care*. 2005;*14*:401–407.

43. Williams RG, Silerman R, Schwind C, et al. Surgeon information transfer and communication: Factors affecting quality and efficiency of inpatient care. *Ann Surg*. 2007;*245*:159–169.

44. Stahl K, Palileo A, Schulman C, et al. Enhancing patient safety in the trauma/surgical intensive care unit. *J Trauma*. 2009;*67*:430–435.

45. Holcomb JB, Dumie RD, Cormme JW, et al. Evaluation of trauma team performance using an advanced human patient simulator for resuscitation training. *J Trauma*. 2002; *52*:1078–1086.

46. Hugh TB. New strategies to prevent laparoscopic bile duct injury—Surgeons can learn from pilots. *Surgery*. 2002;*132(5)*:826–835.

47. Gaba DM. Anesthesiology as a model for patient safety in healthcare. *BMJ*. 2000;*320*:785–788.

48. Stahl K, Augenstein J, Schulman C, et al. Assessing the impact of teaching patient safety principles to medical students during surgical clerkship. *J Surg Res*. 2011:e1–e12.

49. Cohn SM, Nathens AB, Moore FA, Rhee P, et al. Tissue oxygen saturation predicts the development of organ dysfunction during traumatic shock resuscitation. *J Trauma*. January 2007;*62(1)*:44–54; discussion 54-5. DOI: 10.1097/TA.0b013e31802eb817.PMID: 17215732

50. Nikouline A, Quirion A, Jung JJ, et al. Errors in adult trauma resuscitation: a systematic review. *Can J Emerg Med*. 2021;*23*:537–546.

51. Biffl WL, Harrington DT, Cioffi WG. Implementation of a tertiary trauma survey decreases missed injuries. *J Trauma*. 2003;*54*:38–44. [Janjua KJ, Sugrue M, Deane SA. Prospective evaluation of early missed injuries and the role of tertiary trauma survey. J Trauma. 1998;44:1000-7.]

52. De Antonio JH, Nguyen T, Chenault G. Medications and patient safety in the trauma setting: A systematic review. *World J Emerg Surg*. 2019;*14*:5.

2

Injury Prevention Strategies

Linda C. Degutis

2.1 Introduction

In 2020, 278,345 people in the United States died of injuries, with injuries continuing to be the leading cause of death for people ages 1–44 years. Injuries are the leading cause of potential years of life lost before age 65 [1]. The impact of nonfatal injuries includes hospitalizations and emergency department visits as well as short-term and long-term disability, work loss, family structure disruption, and health care and economic costs. In 2019, injuries in the United States accounted for $4.2 trillion, including $327 billion in medical care, $69 billion in work loss, and $3.8 trillion in value of statistical life and quality-of-life losses. More than one-half of the cost ($2.4 trillion) was among working-aged adults (aged 25–64 years) [2]. The prevention of injury morbidity and mortality requires multiple strategies and collaboration to develop, research, and implement evidence-based interventions at the primary, secondary, and tertiary prevention levels. The foundation of the prevention strategies encompasses ongoing surveillance data, engagement of the community, research, and evaluation, as well as consideration of the factors that affect the occurrence of injury events. Bill Haddon, a physician and engineer, developed a conceptual framework for injury prevention as well as a description of 10 strategies (Figure 2.1) for the prevention and mitigation of the transfer of energy to human tissues [3]. Using Haddon's strategies and conceptual framework, Haddon's matrix (Table 2.1) makes it possible to examine primary, secondary, and tertiary prevention of injuries and explore interventions along

Haddon's 10 strategies

1. Prevent the creation of the hazard in the first place.
2. Reduce the number of hazards brought into being.
3. Prevent the release of a hazard that already exists.
4. Modify the rate or spatial distribution of the release of a hazard from its source.
5. Separate in time and space the hazard and that which is to be protected.
6. Separate the hazard and that which is to be protected by the interposition of a material barrier.
7. Modify the relevant basic qualities of the hazard.
8. Make what is to be protected more resistant to the hazard.
9. Begin to counter damage already done by the hazard.
10. Stabilize, repair, and rehabilitate the object of damage.

FIGURE 2.1 Haddon's 10 strategies for injury prevention.

various points in the trajectory of injury prevention. In this chapter, the focus will be on primary and secondary prevention, as tertiary prevention focuses on the interventions that occur after an injury event, and these are described in detail in other chapters in this book.

In addition to its role in caring for the patient who has been injured, the trauma team can play an integral part in primary and secondary prevention to decrease the burden of injury in the population. Starting in 2007, the American College of Surgeons established a requirement for trauma centers to engage in injury prevention as part of the trauma center verification process. This requirement was strengthened in 2015 [4].

TABLE 2.1

Haddon's Matrix

	Human Factors	**Agent Factors**	**Physical Environment**	**Sociocultural Environment**
Pre-event phase	Age, sex, race/ethnicity, body habitus, preexisting disease, alcohol or other drug use, mental health issues, protective device use	Condition of tires, air bags, muzzle velocity of firearm	Weather, road surface condition, railings on staircase	Community norms
Event phase	Location in a motor vehicle, height of fall, and landing surface	Vehicle speed, air bag deployment, type of ammunition, type of knife blade	Time of day, weather, lighting	
Post-event phase	Injury severity, blood loss	Recovery of weapon		Trauma system, EMS response time, rehabilitation services, insurance coverage

DOI: 10.1201/9781003316800-2

TABLE 2.2

Injury Prevention Strategies

Individual	Population
Policy – laws, regulations	Policy – laws, regulations
Extreme risk protection orders (ERPOs), restraining orders	DWI laws, firearm background checks
Counseling	Product design
SBIRT, trauma-informed care	Motor vehicle safety requirements
Protective devices without requirements for use	Protective devices with requirements for use
Environment	Environment
Shower grab bars, wheelchair ramp	Road design, pedestrian crossings
Referral to mental health resources	Universal screening for risks
	Intimate partner violence screening, adverse childhood experiences screening (ACEs)

Prevention interventions may be individually based or population-based, with each of these involving consideration of the factors that place persons at risk for specific types of injury events. Table 2.2 provides examples of types of individual and population-based strategies.

2.2 Foundational Components of Injury Prevention Strategies

2.2.1 Data

To truly understand the prevention needs of the community as well as the broader population that is served by any institution, it is important to have and understand data that is as timely as possible and to identify trends in the epidemiology of various types of injury events and the morbidity and mortality resulting from them. In addition, understanding common and specific risk factors that contribute to injury is a key component of the foundational data for the population served. This includes an understanding of the physical and sociocultural environments of the community, the demographics of the general population, and the persons who present to the trauma center with injuries or who die in the field.

Trauma registry data can provide an informative picture, while additional data from public health surveillance, medical examiners and coroners, emergency medical services, rehabilitation services, local hospitals, law enforcement, and transportation agencies can round out the picture of injuries and injury-related deaths and can add information about the contributions of family violence, intimate partner violence, criminal activities and alcohol, and drug involvement. All of these are important aspects of the risks to be considered in implementing prevention strategies.

2.2.2 Community Engagement

Engagement of members of the community that is affected can also inform and prioritize prevention efforts. Community members contribute their knowledge of what happens daily and also contribute their perspectives on what is needed to improve the health of the community through injury prevention and may provide information about what has or has not worked in the past and why. They may also aid in developing collaborative approaches to prevention through the engagement of community-based organizations that are interested in the health and welfare of the population.

2.2.3 Research and Evidence

Prevention programming is dependent on evidence that a specific intervention works. In reviewing evidence for specific strategies, important considerations are examining the setting in which the intervention took place and its similarity to or difference from the community in which program implementation is planned. For some interventions, such as screening for risky alcohol use, a professional organization that sets practice standards may recommend a specific strategy. This is an effective way to have a successful intervention implemented broadly, as is the case with the American College of Surgeons' requirement for alcohol use screening [5]. The recommendation is based on strong evidence that screening and identification of risky alcohol consumption (screening, brief intervention, and referral to treatment [SBIRT]) can lead to interventions such as motivational interviewing for risky use and referral to treatment for persons who screen positive for heavy drinking or alcohol addiction [6–8].

Identifying an emerging issue in the context of injury forms the basis for research into what might be done to prevent injuries or mitigate the problem. Examples of this are the work that has been done to describe the risk of completed suicide when someone uses a firearm, a lethal means [9]. After work was done that identified this risk, researchers worked with owners of gun shops to determine whether there was an opportunity for the shop owners and employees to intervene to prevent the purchase of a firearm that was intended to be used in a suicide attempt. Researchers educated the gun shop owners and employees on the signs that indicated that someone might be thinking of firearm suicide. There is evidence that this prevention strategy is effective in restricting access to a firearm [10]. This example demonstrates the importance of data in identifying an injury problem and testing an intervention to prevent it.

2.2.4 Evaluation

It may seem that the evaluation of a particular strategy or intervention may not be necessary, as it has already been demonstrated to be effective. A study was done to look at the effectiveness of the Interrupters program, which was an effective community-based intervention in Chicago. The program was implemented in four neighborhoods in Baltimore, Maryland, and was evaluated. It was demonstrated to have an effect in decreasing firearm violence in three of the four neighborhoods. When the researchers evaluated the program, they determined that it was likely that the failure was due to a difference in the community structure in the neighborhood in which it failed [11].

2.2.5 Collaboration

Not one person, group, or organization alone can implement effective prevention strategies, although each contributes to prevention. Individually targeted strategies may be implemented in clinical as well as other settings such as schools, community centers, and governmental and nongovernmental agencies and range from actions such as universal screening for alcohol and other drug use or family violence to actions such as counseling about fall prevention that are based on demographic factors such as age, gender, functional status, cognitive and sensory functions, preexisting physical and mental health conditions, or the use of medications.

Population-based strategies, which include legislation and regulation; governmental and institutional policies; product design, distribution, or access regulations and requirements; or passive and active protection systems, may be initiated or implemented by governmental or nongovernmental organizations within the health sector or other sectors that impact the population at large. As with individually based strategies, effective population-based strategies require a foundation of data and research to determine their effectiveness in achieving the outcomes of decreasing injuries and injury-related deaths.

The collaborations that contribute to the success of both individual and population-based strategies require the engagement of stakeholders to provide the services necessary to act upon issues that are identified in screening processes; to identify technological approaches for modifications of product design to make consumer products safer; to evaluate the success of new interventions as well as the implementation of interventions that have been demonstrated to be effective; to engage community members who can provide knowledge and understanding of individual and community norms; and to involve lawmakers who create policy, criminal justice, and law enforcement agencies, health educators and communicators, and public health agencies.

Trauma surgeons and other members of the trauma team, as well as trauma center staff, have a crucial role to play in both types of interventions, some of which can be incorporated into clinical practice, while others may take place in community settings and policy strategies that are based in legislative and institutional jurisdictions. The specific expertise of trauma team members and trauma researchers that is invaluable in prevention includes knowledge of risk factors for injury morbidity and mortality, understanding of the data related to injuries and violence in the local community, and its relationship to other health issues [12].

Several organizations engage in highlighting injury prevention strategies in institutional as well as community settings. Engagement with, and involvement in, these types of organizations aid in providing opportunities for sharing effective prevention strategies as well as learning about the impact and effectiveness of strategies occurring in other locales. These are in addition to the presentations and discussions that occur at meetings of the American College of Surgeons (ACS), the American Association for the Surgery of Trauma (AAST), the Eastern Association for the Surgery of Trauma (EAST), and the Western Trauma Association (WTA). They include but are not limited to the Health Alliance for Violence Intervention (HAVI), the Society for Violence and Injury Research (SAVIR), the American Public Health Association (APHA), the American Trauma Society (ATS), and The Injury Free Coalition for Kids (IFCK) [13].

2.3 Prevention Strategies

The following sections describe both individually based and population based injury prevention strategies. Prevention strategies evolve, so that a strategy that is identified as being effective at one point in time may be modified for improvement or eliminated as it becomes clear that another strategy is more effective or the initial strategy is no longer working. An example of this is what occurred with automatic seatbelts in the front seats of passenger cars in the 1980s and early 1990s. The concept was that a shoulder harness strap would automatically fit into place as the car door was closed and the engine started. The passenger would then be required to lock the lap belt to complete the restraint system. If the seatbelt was not in place, the car would not start and a warning would sound. Car owners found ways to circumvent the system, and some found ways to disconnect it. In addition, a study done by the University of North Carolina found that only 28.6% of people put the lap belt in place. The use of the shoulder harness alone placed passengers at risk of injuries from the shoulder belt. As it became clear that this was not an effective approach to passenger restraints, the design feature was discontinued [14].

2.3.1 Road Traffic Safety

A great deal of progress has been made in the area of road traffic safety by addressing human, agent, and environmental factors that contribute to injury. Federal legislation has required specific provisions for drivers with a blood alcohol concentration of about a legal limit of 0.08 mg%. Also, all states raised the minimum legal drinking age to 21 years, and federal legislation set disincentives for states that did not pass zero-tolerance laws for drivers under the age of 21. The National Highway Traffic Safety Administration (NHTSA) commissioned a report by the National Academy of Medicine on how to further decrease alcohol-related motor vehicle crashes, injuries, and deaths that was released in 2018 [15]. Other initiatives have focused on graduated licensure laws for newly licensed young drivers. These are state-level laws that are effective in decreasing crashes and subsequent injuries and deaths in young, inexperienced drivers. The laws differ from state to state but focus on the initial age for a permit to drive, the age at which a license may be obtained, restrictions on hours of vehicle operation during the first several months of driving, and passenger restrictions for young drivers.

Road design has impacted the occurrence of crashes as well as pedestrian injuries and fatalities. Jersey barriers on multilane highways, elimination of toll booths, and energy-absorbing objects placed in front of structures such as overpasses have all contributed to decreases in crash risk. Motor vehicle design has also had an impact, although it takes longer for these changes to have their full impact, as vehicles remain in service for longer than a year or two, so not all vehicles that are on the road include the safety improvements. These include modifications to crumple zones and steering columns to improve energy absorption, elimination of sharp objects on control panels to prevent injury risk, head restraints that absorb energy in collisions, front and side airbags, active safety features that include various cameras, and sensors that link to braking and steering systems.

Strategy – Screen for seatbelt use and counsel regarding the importance of use in conjunction with other vehicle protection systems (airbags). Discuss appropriate head restraint adjustment.

Discuss the importance of seatbelt use for both front and rear passengers

2.3.1.1 Child and Infant Safety Seats

In the United States, all 50 states now have seatbelt laws, as well as laws requiring that children within a specific age range be restrained in child safety seats or booster seats [16]. A portion of the strategy related to the use of child safety seats is the use of safety seat checks by persons who have been trained to perform the checks and to teach children's caretakers how to ensure that a child safety seat is properly installed and that the child is properly restrained. Some trauma centers sponsor safety checks, while some also have instituted programs that include staff from pediatrics or maternity services to ensure that newborns, as well as other children being discharged from the hospital, go home in a vehicle in which they are secured in an infant or child safety seat. In addition, if a family does not have the resources to purchase an infant or child safety seat, the hospital may provide one of the appropriate sizes for the infant or child who is discharged.

Strategy – Screen for infant and child safety seat use and proper installation.

- Hold infant and child safety seat inspection events.
- Provide infant and child safety seats or access to them for caregivers who do not have them.

2.3.1.2 Front and Side Airbags

There is a current requirement for passenger vehicles to have a prescribed set of airbags installed during the manufacturing process. The technology that is used deploys the airbag if the vehicle is in a collision at a relatively low speed. Airbags have been demonstrated to be effective at preventing a restrained passenger's head and face from striking the dashboard or steering wheel in the front seat of the vehicle, and side impact airbags prevent a passenger or driver from striking the side of the vehicle structure.

The airbags deploy at a relatively high speed, and research has found that this deployment poses a threat to a child who is restrained in the front seat. Because of this, the NHTSA recommends that children under the age of 12 be restrained in the rear seat of a passenger vehicle in an appropriate restraint [17].

Strategy – The physician and other members of the trauma team can provide counseling for parents and other caregivers to inform them about both the safety and the risks of passenger airbags as related to a child's size.

2.3.1.3 Falls

Falls are a leading contributor to morbidity and mortality in older adults, and there are effective interventions that have been demonstrated to be effective in preventing falls. Risk factors for falls include impaired mobility, decreased balance, medications that may cause dizziness or lightheadedness, ill-fitting footwear, objects that obstruct stairways as well as lack of railings on stairways, decreased vision, poor lighting, throw rugs that create a trip hazard, and chronic diseases that impact motor function such as Parkinson's disease. An awareness of the risk factors on an individual level can inform interventions and counseling about preventing falls. In addition, research has demonstrated that there are prevention strategies that are effective in decreasing fall risk. In addition to maintaining exercise routines, programs that aid in improving balance, such as tai chi, are effective in decreasing fall risk in older adults. The Centers for Disease Control and Prevention (CDC) has developed a program known as STEADI (Stopping Elderly Accidents, Deaths, and Injuries) that guides practitioners, caregivers, and their patients in decreasing fall and subsequent injury risk [18].

Strategy – Screen for fall risk in older adults, including review of medications that may increase the risk of dizziness or syncope. Use the STEADI program to inform screening and intervention to decrease fall risk and falls in older adults.

Young children are also at risk for injuries related to falls. Because of their innate curiosity, they may climb onto furniture and objects that put them at risk of a fall from a height. Young children also do not understand the risk of falling and may attempt to jump through a window that is not covered by protection or may climb on a balcony railing. Some cities and towns have implemented construction and housing requirements that are focused on preventing falls through a requirement for bars on windows that are at a height that poses a risk, as well as requirements for specific spacing of railing balusters on stairs as well as balcony spaces [19]. One of the early programs that addressed this issue in New York City was the "Kids Can't Fly" program that was developed and implemented by Dr. Barbara Barlow, a pediatric surgeon at Harlem Children's Hospital. Playgrounds and playground equipment may also pose a risk of serious falls, dependent on both the height of the piece of equipment and the type of surface on the ground. These factors may be addressed by providing a ground surface that is energy absorbing and ensuring that equipment is in good repair. Children are also at risk of falling and being injured in the process of playing various sports, as well as falling down stairs [20, 21].

Strategy – Counsel parents and caregivers on the risks of falls.

Screen for risks in the home environment.

2.3.1.4 Intimate Partner Violence

Approximately one in four women and one in seven men in the United States have experienced some form of intimate partner violence (IPV) in their lifetime, according to the National Intimate Partner and Sexual Violence Survey (NISVS), an ongoing survey conducted by the CDC [22]. The general pattern of IPV when it occurs in a relationship is that it evolves with a trajectory that can lead to life-threatening injuries and death, with severity risk increasing over time, and being greatest when a partner decides to leave the relationship. Research has demonstrated that universal screening for IPV can be effective in identifying its occurrence and in decreasing the risk of injury and death [23].

Strategy – Screen all patients for IPV using screening tools that have been demonstrated to be effective; refer persons involved in a violent relationship to treatment resources.

2.3.1.5 Firearm Violence

Firearm violence–related deaths continue to increase in the United States and began to exceed deaths from motor vehicle crashes in 2017. Approximately 60% of firearm violence deaths are firearm suicide deaths, while 35% are homicides, 5% unintentional, and the remainder due to law enforcement intervention or unclassified. While the events that lead to firearm deaths differ in origin, some strategies can have an impact on decreasing firearm-related injuries and deaths regardless of the type of event. Restricting access to firearms for persons who are at risk for suicide due to a crisis or for persons who are at risk of harming others may be done using several strategies. For example, safe storage of firearms, in which a firearm is stored in a locked compartment and unloaded, can prevent access for someone who may be in crisis, a child whose curiosity would lead to him or her handling a firearm, or someone who plans to use a firearm to injure another person. Extreme risk protection orders or red flag laws may aid in decreasing the risk of the use of a firearm in IPV or a suicide attempt. Background checks can identify people who have a history of violence.

In addition to policy, technology may aid in the prevention of firearm violence through such strategies as creating an identification process so that only the owner can fire the weapon or microstamping bullets that identify the firearm from which a piece of ammunition has been fired.

Strategy – Screen for firearm ownership and storage practices and counsel patients on safe storage to prevent harm.

2.3.2 Policy as Prevention

There are multiple areas of policy that have had impacts on injury morbidity and mortality, with traffic safety being one of the areas in which there has been a great deal of success. Road safety policy continues to evolve as traffic fatalities continue to occur, and some specific aspects of the traffic safety risk are continuing to evolve. Firearm violence prevention policy has not reached the degree of success that road safety policy has, but there is evidence that certain policies are effective in decreasing firearm violence and its related injuries and deaths. Other policy areas that trauma surgeons can directly impact include sports policy, with specific reference to traumatic brain injury.

One of the challenges in moving injury prevention policy forward is to ensure that the policymakers, their staff, and the public, as well as other stakeholders, understand the impact of the issues that are being addressed. There is a need to both bring the data forward in a way that is understandable and accessible and to put a face on the data, to highlight the human impact of the problem. The trauma surgeon and other members of the team, who have knowledge of the data and what it means and who are trusted members of the community, can be instrumental in explaining the data, describing its human impact, or partnering with affected community members to put the human face on it so that policymakers can visualize what it means in human terms. The trauma team can also identify emerging trends in injury and violence and bring them forward.

Strategy – Provide oral or written testimony and use local data to illustrate the impact of injuries and injury-related fatalities. Work with community organizations to aid them in understanding the data and putting a face on the data.

2.4 Summary

While this is not a comprehensive description of injury prevention strategies for every type of injury event that might occur, it presents the general set of concepts and information about collaborative relationships that may aid in the implementation of successful interventions. Data, evidence, ongoing research, community engagement, evaluation, and communication with the public are key, and the trauma team plays a critical role in each aspect of prevention.

Successful programs will be science-based and evidence-informed, with continued evaluation and modification to ensure their continued effectiveness in achieving the goal of injury and violence morbidity and mortality prevention.

Editor's Note

This is an excellent review of the topic of injury prevention strategies. It might be helpful to the reader to understand an example of how this might be employed. The following story is representative.

Some years ago, shortly after arriving in Miami, it was obvious that the trauma center was swamped with a huge number of severely injured pedestrians struck by vehicles. This was unique. The providers felt that this was business as usual. We decided to compile our data from the prior three years and we found over 1,000 pedestrians were struck and about half were grade school–age children. The mortality of the elderly was over 30% and 5% of the children died.

We decided to review the world's literature on injury prevention for pediatric pedestrians struck. We found that most of these programs were highly successful in reducing the incidence of this injury, but the programs disappeared after either the supporting grant ended or the local funding dried up. We endeavored to establish a program (WalkSafe) that was essential without cost and sustainable. We joined educators, law enforcement, engineers, and parent organizations together and put forth a combined educational program and simple redesign of some of the elementary school properties in an attempt to improve safety. We initiated this in just two of four high-risk grade schools and noted that it seemed to be effective, with an apparent reduction in injuries. Ultimately this program was utilized in the Miami-Metro Dade school system (over 100,000 children), lowering the death rate from pedestrian injuries from about 23 to 2. Then it was adopted statewide, where I am told it remains in place. This is the type of injury prevention program that is highly successful because there was a recognition of the problem by all and a high level of collaboration.

REFERENCES

1. National Center for Injury Prevention and Control. WISQARS https://www.cdc.gov/injury/wisqars/ accessed 9.30.2022.
2. Peterson C, Miller GF, Barnett SB, Florence C. Economic Cost of Injury—United States, 2019. MMWR Morb Mortal Wkly Rep 2021;70:1655–1659. DOI: http://dx.doi.org/10.15585/mmwr.mm7048a1
3. Haddon W Jr. On the escape of tigers: An ecologic note. Am J Public Health Nations Health. 1970 Dec;60(12): 2229–2234. DOI: 10.2105/ajph.60.12.2229-b. PMID: 5530409; PMCID: PMC1349282.
4. Committee on Trauma American College of Surgeons. Resources for Optimal Care of the Injured Patient. American College of Surgeons: Chicago, IL, 2014.
5. American College of Surgeons. Statement on Insurance, Alcohol-Related Injuries, and Trauma Centers https://www.facs.org/about-acs/statements/insurance-alcohol-related-injuries-and-trauma-centers/ accessed 9.30.2022
6. Babor TF, Kadden RM. Screening and interventions for alcohol and drug problems in medical settings: What works? J Trauma Injury Infect Crit Care. 2005;59(3):S80–S87.
7. Ewing JA. Detecting alcohol: The CAGE questionnaire. JAMA. 1984;252(14):1905–1907.
8. Gentilello LM, Ebel BE, Wickizer TM, et al. Alcohol interventions for trauma patients treated in emergency departments and hospitals: A cost benefit analysis. Ann Surg. 2005;241(4):541–550.
9. Runyan CW, Brooks-Russell A, Betz ME. Points of influence for lethal means counseling and safe gun storage practices. J Public Health Manag Pract. 2019 Jan/Feb;25(1):86–89. DOI: 10.1097/PHH.0000000000000801. PMID: 29889177; PMCID: PMC6279463.
10. Polzer E, Brandspigel S, Kelly T, Betz M. 'Gun shop projects' for suicide prevention in the USA: current state and future directions. Inj Prev. 2021 Apr;27(2):150–154. DOI: 10.1136/injuryprev-2020-043648. Epub 2020 Mar 25. PMID: 32213533.
11. Webster DW, Whitehill JM, Vernick JS, Curriero FC. Effects of Baltimore's safe streets program on gun violence: A replication of Chicago's ceasefire program. J Urban Health. 2013 Feb;90(1):27–40. DOI: 10.1007/s11524-012-9731-5. PMID: 22696175; PMCID: PMC3579298.
12. Sleet DA, Dahlberg LL, Basavaraju SV, Mercy JA, McGuire LC, Greenspan A. Injury prevention, violence prevention, and trauma care: Building the scientific base. MMWR Surveill Summ. 2011;60(suppl):78–85.
13. Pressley JC, Barlow B, Durkin M, Jacko SA, Dominguez DR, Johnson L. A national program for injury prevention in children and adolescents: the injury-free coalition for kids. J Urban Health. 2005 Sep;82(3):389–402. DOI: 10.1093/jurban/jti078. Epub 2005 Jun 15. PMID: 15958785; PMCID: PMC3456057.
14. Reinfurt DW, St Cyr CL, Hunter WW. Usage patterns and misuse rates of automatic seat belts by system type. Accid Anal Prev. 1991 Dec;23(6):521–530. DOI: 10.1016/0001-4575(91)90017-y. PMID: 1772554.
15. National Academies of Sciences, Engineering, and Medicine. Getting to Zero Alcohol-Impaired Driving Fatalities: A Comprehensive Approach to a Persistent Problem. The National Academies Press: Washington, DC, 2018. https://doi.org/10.17226/24951.
16. Governors Highway Safety Administration. All States Have Child Safety Seat Laws. https://www.ghsa.org/state-laws/issues/child%20passenger%20safety#:~:text=All%20states%20and%20territories%20require,on%20age%2C%20weight%20and%20height.
17. Children's Hospital of Pennsylvania. https://www.chop.edu/video/air-bag-safety-infants-toddlers-and-children#:~:text=Airbags%20have%20been%20improved%20since,ride%20in%20the%20front%20seat accessed 9.30.2022
18. National Center for Injury Prevention and Control. Stopping Elderly Accidents Deaths and Injuries. https://www.cdc.gov/steadi/ accessed 9.30.2022
19. Freyne B, Doyle J, McNamara R, Nicholson AJ. Epidemiology of high falls from windows in children. Ir Med J. 2014 Feb;107(2):57–59. PMID: 24654490.
20. Britton JW. Kids can't fly: Preventing fall injuries in children. WMJ. 2005 Jan;104(1):33–36. PMID: 15779722;
21. Khambalia A, Joshi P, Brussoni M, Raina P, Morrongiello B, Macarthur C. Risk factors for unintentional injuries due to falls in children aged 0–6 years: A systematic review. Inj Prev. 2006 Dec;12(6):378–381. DOI: 10.1136/ip.2006.012161. PMID: 17170185; PMCID: PMC2564414.
22. National Center for Injury Prevention and Control. National Intimate Partner and Sexual Violence Survey. https://www.cdc.gov/violenceprevention/datasources/nisvs/index.html accessed 9.30.2022.
23. O'Doherty L, Hegarty K, Ramsay J, Davidson LL, Feder G, Taft A. Screening women for intimate partner violence in healthcare settings. Cochrane Database Syst Rev. 2015 Jul 22;2015(7):CD007007. DOI: 10.1002/14651858.CD007007.pub3. PMID: 26200817; PMCID: PMC6599831.

3

Trauma Systems: A Dynamic Public Health Strategy for Injury Control

Alex Lee, Alexandre Tran, and S. Morad Hameed

3.1 The Global Phenomenon of Trauma Systems

The evolution and future opportunities for trauma systems are illustrated in diverse examples.

> *ORLANDO: At 0157 hour on Sunday, June 12, 2016, a gunman entered the Pulse nightclub in Orlando, Florida, and opened fire on a dance party attended by over 300 people. At 0200 hour, the Orlando Fire Department notified the operator at Orlando Medical Center (ORMC), the only Level 1 trauma center in Central Florida, that an active shooter event was in progress in the vicinity of the hospital* [1].

> *CHICAGO: At 0800 hour on May 1, 2018, the doors of a new adult Level 1 trauma center opened in Chicago's South Side, in the midst of a trauma desert, after years of advocacy from surrounding communities that have faced socioeconomic trauma, including epidemics of violence that have claimed thousands of lives, for generations* [2]. *The University of Chicago Medicine Trauma Center carries the hope of addressing the consequences and causes of long-standing structural inequality* [3].

3.2 A Defining Challenge in Public Health

The injury epidemic is global, with low- and middle-income countries shouldering 90% of the burden of injury [4]. Risk of injury is highly influenced by the interplay of social, economic, environmental, and even geographic factors, and outcome is highly influenced by our ability to rapidly interrupt shock and its downstream consequences and restore cognitive and musculoskeletal integrity and function. To be effective, injury control must begin even before the moment of impact, must be prepared to efficiently integrate and apply multidisciplinary knowledge to acute, lifesaving care, and end only when risk is eliminated and patients return to their places in society.

Modern trauma systems are dynamic networks that span cities and remote environments, collecting data to prevent injury, and, when injuries do occur, facilitating quick and seamless transfers of patients to optimal, state-of-the-art trauma care. Trauma systems have evolved both as a strategy to deliver coordinated, acute care when it is most urgently needed and as a comprehensive response to one of the greatest public health challenges of our time (Figure 3.1). But despite the successes of trauma systems, the burden of injury is evidence that proven strategies must be scaled and new innovations must be developed and rapidly advanced.

3.3 Trauma Systems: The Evolution of a Public Health Response

In recent years, surgeons have taken critical roles in the development of a comprehensive approach to injury control. In 1922, the American College of Surgeons (ACS) established the Committee on Trauma (ACS-COT) to provide surgical leadership in trauma care. Since its publication in 1976, the ACS-COT *Resources for Optimal Care of the Injured Patient* has set the standards for trauma care, and each new edition has been broader in scope and more influential than the last [5].

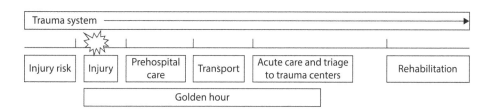

FIGURE 3.1 Integrated trauma systems span the continuum of trauma care. Trauma systems represent society's most complete and multimodal responses to injury, from prevention to prompt and effective acute care and to rehabilitation and reintegration into society.

DOI: 10.1201/9781003316800-3

13

The ACS-COT considers injury control to be most effectively accomplished in a public health framework that includes approaches to prevention, optimization of access to acute care, acute care itself, rehabilitation, and research. In each of these areas, the ACS-COT promotes a public health approach that includes ongoing *assessment* of injury data and the epidemiology of injury, evidence-based *policy development*, and ongoing *assurance* of efficacy of processes [5]. These core functions are driven by the systematic collection and analysis of injury data in ACS-COT–mandated trauma registries.

A *trauma system* is defined as an organized and comprehensive public health response to injury within a specified geographic area that includes injury prevention, prehospital care, triage and transport, acute medical and surgical care, rehabilitation, education, and research. This chapter summarizes the best recent evidence on the impact of trauma systems on injury prevention and trauma care, outlines areas where more data are required, and briefly describes the exciting threshold to which trauma system development has brought us.

3.4 Injury Prevention: Can Trauma Systems Prevent Injury?

Traumatic deaths occur in a trimodal distribution, with 45% of deaths occurring within 1 hour of injury, 34% occurring within 1–4 hours, and 20% occurring after a week [6]. Although streamlined trauma systems and improvements in acute trauma care reduce the risk of delayed deaths, even the fastest and best acute care cannot address the high proportion of immediate deaths at the scene, which are often due to devastating central nervous system and cardiovascular injuries. This first mortality peak is thought to be more amenable to injury prevention efforts than to advances in acute care. The magnitude of this peak is so great that some investigators believe that the most significant advances in injury control in the future will come mainly from prevention initiatives [7].

Most injuries can be found to result from a combination of potentially modifiable personal, mechanical, and environmental risk factors. An understanding of the elements of this combination of risks is fundamental to the development of effective countermeasures that reduce risk and prevent injury. In 1970, William Haddon developed an elegant framework to deconstruct the complex determinants of injury. The Haddon Matrix considers three phases of injury: *Pre-event* (which is a focus for primary prevention efforts), *event* (a focus for secondary prevention efforts), and *post-event* (a focus for tertiary prevention efforts). Within each phase, the risk or impact of injury is determined by the interplay of four types of factors: *Host factors* (individual characteristics or behaviors that increase susceptibility to injury), *agent factors* (characteristics of the objects or vectors that inflict energy transfer and injury), *physical environment factors* (characteristics of the built environment that may predispose populations to injury), and *social environment factors* (the social, economic, and political milieu that influence the risk of injury) [8]. Haddon's phase-factor matrix has become the basis for thought and action in modern injury prevention.

The biggest gains in injury control will likely result from the identification of populations that remain vulnerable to injury, followed by thoughtful and comprehensive approaches to the modification of risk factors within each phase of injury in these groups. Primary prevention efforts, which take place before an injury occurs (pre-event) in the effort to prevent it completely, have addressed host factors (graduated licensing has reduced motor vehicle crashes among inexperienced drivers by 28%), agent factors (restrictions of motorcycle engine size for young riders has decreased casualties in this group by 25%), physical environment factors (bicycle lanes have reduced casualties among cyclists by 35%), and social environment factors (legislation on motor vehicle speeding law enforcement and driver alcohol consumption have reduced injury mortality substantially) [9]. Perhaps the best evidence of the promise of trauma center–based injury prevention is provided by a prospective randomized controlled trial of a brief intervention for alcohol abuse, which demonstrated substantial reductions in alcohol consumption (22 vs. 7 drinks per week) and reinjury risk (47%) [10]. As with primary prevention, secondary prevention efforts, which diminish the risk of injury once an event has occurred (seatbelts, airbags) [11], and tertiary prevention efforts, which seek to minimize the consequences of established injury (prehospital care, acute trauma care, rehabilitation), have also been shown to substantially reduce the burden and impact of injury.

However, a comprehensive survey of American trauma centers revealed that, despite a strong interest in injury prevention, less than 20% of them have dedicated coordinators, and more than two-thirds have no specific funding for injury prevention programs [12]. Even where evidence exists for the cost-effectiveness of hospital-based injury prevention strategies, as is the case with the alcohol screening and brief intervention initiative [13], resource limitations and competing priorities resulted in its adoption by only half of surveyed trauma centers.

RECOMMENDATION

Trauma systems have a key role in primary, secondary, and tertiary injury prevention.

Grade of recommendation: A

3.5 Clinical Trauma Care

Over the years, the focus of trauma systems has widened from trauma center–based injury care to multidimensional approaches to injury control that include public policy, prevention, prehospital care, acute medical care, and rehabilitation. All of these areas have grown up together, and it is difficult to examine their progress and effects in isolation. Still, some insights into their value and potential can result from this approach.

3.5.1 Prehospital Care: Scoop and Run or Stay and Play?

Prompt control of injuries, including achievement of hemostasis and reversal of shock, is the basis of the golden hour concept of trauma care [14] and has become a first principle of trauma systems. The exact logistics of the delivery of lifesaving care in the

3

Trauma Systems: A Dynamic Public Health Strategy for Injury Control

Alex Lee, Alexandre Tran, and S. Morad Hameed

3.1 The Global Phenomenon of Trauma Systems

The evolution and future opportunities for trauma systems are illustrated in diverse examples.

> *ORLANDO: At 0157 hour on Sunday, June 12, 2016, a gunman entered the Pulse nightclub in Orlando, Florida, and opened fire on a dance party attended by over 300 people. At 0200 hour, the Orlando Fire Department notified the operator at Orlando Medical Center (ORMC), the only Level 1 trauma center in Central Florida, that an active shooter event was in progress in the vicinity of the hospital* [1].

> *CHICAGO: At 0800 hour on May 1, 2018, the doors of a new adult Level 1 trauma center opened in Chicago's South Side, in the midst of a trauma desert, after years of advocacy from surrounding communities that have faced socioeconomic trauma, including epidemics of violence that have claimed thousands of lives, for generations* [2]. *The University of Chicago Medicine Trauma Center carries the hope of addressing the consequences and causes of long-standing structural inequality* [3].

3.2 A Defining Challenge in Public Health

The injury epidemic is global, with low- and middle-income countries shouldering 90% of the burden of injury [4]. Risk of injury is highly influenced by the interplay of social, economic, environmental, and even geographic factors, and outcome is highly influenced by our ability to rapidly interrupt shock and its downstream consequences and restore cognitive and musculoskeletal integrity and function. To be effective, injury control must begin even before the moment of impact, must be prepared to efficiently integrate and apply multidisciplinary knowledge to acute, lifesaving care, and end only when risk is eliminated and patients return to their places in society.

Modern trauma systems are dynamic networks that span cities and remote environments, collecting data to prevent injury, and, when injuries do occur, facilitating quick and seamless transfers of patients to optimal, state-of-the-art trauma care. Trauma systems have evolved both as a strategy to deliver coordinated, acute care when it is most urgently needed and as a comprehensive response to one of the greatest public health challenges of our time (Figure 3.1). But despite the successes of trauma systems, the burden of injury is evidence that proven strategies must be scaled and new innovations must be developed and rapidly advanced.

3.3 Trauma Systems: The Evolution of a Public Health Response

In recent years, surgeons have taken critical roles in the development of a comprehensive approach to injury control. In 1922, the American College of Surgeons (ACS) established the Committee on Trauma (ACS-COT) to provide surgical leadership in trauma care. Since its publication in 1976, the ACS-COT *Resources for Optimal Care of the Injured Patient* has set the standards for trauma care, and each new edition has been broader in scope and more influential than the last [5].

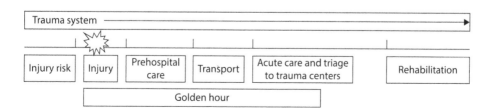

FIGURE 3.1 Integrated trauma systems span the continuum of trauma care. Trauma systems represent society's most complete and multimodal responses to injury, from prevention to prompt and effective acute care and to rehabilitation and reintegration into society.

DOI: 10.1201/9781003316800-3

The ACS-COT considers injury control to be most effectively accomplished in a public health framework that includes approaches to prevention, optimization of access to acute care, acute care itself, rehabilitation, and research. In each of these areas, the ACS-COT promotes a public health approach that includes ongoing *assessment* of injury data and the epidemiology of injury, evidence-based *policy development*, and ongoing *assurance* of efficacy of processes [5]. These core functions are driven by the systematic collection and analysis of injury data in ACS-COT–mandated trauma registries.

A *trauma system* is defined as an organized and comprehensive public health response to injury within a specified geographic area that includes injury prevention, prehospital care, triage and transport, acute medical and surgical care, rehabilitation, education, and research. This chapter summarizes the best recent evidence on the impact of trauma systems on injury prevention and trauma care, outlines areas where more data are required, and briefly describes the exciting threshold to which trauma system development has brought us.

3.4 Injury Prevention: Can Trauma Systems Prevent Injury?

Traumatic deaths occur in a trimodal distribution, with 45% of deaths occurring within 1 hour of injury, 34% occurring within 1–4 hours, and 20% occurring after a week [6]. Although streamlined trauma systems and improvements in acute trauma care reduce the risk of delayed deaths, even the fastest and best acute care cannot address the high proportion of immediate deaths at the scene, which are often due to devastating central nervous system and cardiovascular injuries. This first mortality peak is thought to be more amenable to injury prevention efforts than to advances in acute care. The magnitude of this peak is so great that some investigators believe that the most significant advances in injury control in the future will come mainly from prevention initiatives [7].

Most injuries can be found to result from a combination of potentially modifiable personal, mechanical, and environmental risk factors. An understanding of the elements of this combination of risks is fundamental to the development of effective countermeasures that reduce risk and prevent injury. In 1970, William Haddon developed an elegant framework to deconstruct the complex determinants of injury. The Haddon Matrix considers three phases of injury: *Pre-event* (which is a focus for primary prevention efforts), *event* (a focus for secondary prevention efforts), and *post-event* (a focus for tertiary prevention efforts). Within each phase, the risk or impact of injury is determined by the interplay of four types of factors: *Host factors* (individual characteristics or behaviors that increase susceptibility to injury), *agent factors* (characteristics of the objects or vectors that inflict energy transfer and injury), *physical environment factors* (characteristics of the built environment that may predispose populations to injury), and *social environment factors* (the social, economic, and political milieu that influence the risk of injury) [8]. Haddon's phase-factor matrix has become the basis for thought and action in modern injury prevention.

The biggest gains in injury control will likely result from the identification of populations that remain vulnerable to injury, followed by thoughtful and comprehensive approaches to the modification of risk factors within each phase of injury in these groups. Primary prevention efforts, which take place before an injury occurs (pre-event) in the effort to prevent it completely, have addressed host factors (graduated licensing has reduced motor vehicle crashes among inexperienced drivers by 28%), agent factors (restrictions of motorcycle engine size for young riders has decreased casualties in this group by 25%), physical environment factors (bicycle lanes have reduced casualties among cyclists by 35%), and social environment factors (legislation on motor vehicle speeding law enforcement and driver alcohol consumption have reduced injury mortality substantially) [9]. Perhaps the best evidence of the promise of trauma center–based injury prevention is provided by a prospective randomized controlled trial of a brief intervention for alcohol abuse, which demonstrated substantial reductions in alcohol consumption (22 vs. 7 drinks per week) and reinjury risk (47%) [10]. As with primary prevention, secondary prevention efforts, which diminish the risk of injury once an event has occurred (seatbelts, airbags) [11], and tertiary prevention efforts, which seek to minimize the consequences of established injury (prehospital care, acute trauma care, rehabilitation), have also been shown to substantially reduce the burden and impact of injury.

However, a comprehensive survey of American trauma centers revealed that, despite a strong interest in injury prevention, less than 20% of them have dedicated coordinators, and more than two-thirds have no specific funding for injury prevention programs [12]. Even where evidence exists for the cost-effectiveness of hospital-based injury prevention strategies, as is the case with the alcohol screening and brief intervention initiative [13], resource limitations and competing priorities resulted in its adoption by only half of surveyed trauma centers.

RECOMMENDATION

Trauma systems have a key role in primary, secondary, and tertiary injury prevention.

Grade of recommendation: A

3.5 Clinical Trauma Care

Over the years, the focus of trauma systems has widened from trauma center–based injury care to multidimensional approaches to injury control that include public policy, prevention, prehospital care, acute medical care, and rehabilitation. All of these areas have grown up together, and it is difficult to examine their progress and effects in isolation. Still, some insights into their value and potential can result from this approach.

3.5.1 Prehospital Care: Scoop and Run or Stay and Play?

Prompt control of injuries, including achievement of hemostasis and reversal of shock, is the basis of the golden hour concept of trauma care [14] and has become a first principle of trauma systems. The exact logistics of the delivery of lifesaving care in the critical first hours after injury, including in the prehospital setting, are a central focus of injury research with practical policy implications. There is evidence that a less invasive approach to initial fluid resuscitation may be beneficial. A prospective, alternate-day trial of penetrating trauma in an urban environment, suggested that survival increases if paramedics defer intravenous fluid resuscitation in patients sustaining penetrating torso trauma until a time when surgical hemostasis has been achieved [15]. The conclusions from these early studies have favoured the notion that a "scoop and run" prehospital strategy, minimizing potentially harmful on-site interventions and prolonged scene times, may improve outcomes after severe injury.

Prehospital care issues were re-examined in one of the largest and most comprehensive studies of prehospital care to date. Stiell et al. investigated the effect of a system-wide introduction of advanced life support skills for paramedics on survival after severe injury in 2,867 patients. This before–after controlled clinical trial suggested that augmentation of paramedic skills was not associated with improved survival and was associated with *worse* survival in the subset of patients (*n* = 598) with Glasgow Coma Scale score of less than 9. Intubation in the field was associated with increased mortality (odds ratio [OR] 2.8) [16].

The reasons for failure of advanced paramedic training to make a significant impact on trauma outcomes are not well understood. Recent studies of jurisdictions that place a strong emphasis on prehospital care were not able to show a difference between field resuscitation versus rapid transport approaches [17]. It is possible that a combination of technical factors leading to inadvertent hypoxia or hyperoxia, aspiration, hypocapnea, hypotension, or intracranial hypertension during intubation can compound or exacerbate the primary injury and compromise recovery [18]. Until these factors are better characterized individually, it is reasonable to apply advanced life support measures in the prehospital setting selectively and cautiously and to continue to expedite patients' transfer to definitive care.

This brings us to the issue of mode of transport. As trauma systems have been designed to minimize time to definitive care, considerable attention has been focused on the role and value of helicopters in modern trauma systems. In general, ground ambulance transport (GAT) is widely available and can be readily dispatched. Air medical transport (AMT) by helicopter may, in some jurisdictions, take longer to dispatch, but often has more sophisticated medical capability (advanced paramedics or physicians) and is faster once launched. Geographic analyses have suggested that distance thresholds from trauma centers to injury locations exist: Beyond certain distances AMT is consistently faster than GAT [19]. For trauma patients living at considerable distance from trauma centers, AMT is considered to be potentially lifesaving.

RECOMMENDATION

Prehospital care should attempt to minimize scene time and prioritize immediate lifesaving measures only, with rapid and efficient transfer to the most appropriate trauma center for resuscitation and definitive care.

Grade of recommendation: B

3.5.2 Trauma Centers: Are They Accessible?

At the heart of trauma systems, trauma centers focus expertise and resources to bring high-quality care to patients with severe and complex injuries and take the lead in their communities on prevention and quality improvement initiatives and scientific research. Between 1991 and 2002, the number of trauma centers in the United States more than doubled from 471 to 1,154 [20]. Unfortunately, nearly 50 million Americans, mostly in rural areas, still cannot get to Level 1 or Level 2 care within 1 hour of injury. The observation that injuries sustained in rural environments have higher injury severity–adjusted mortality than those in urban environments [21] may, in part, be attributable to the poor reach of trauma systems into these areas. Promotion of policies, such as the Emergency Medical Treatment and Active Labor Act, which require trauma centers to receive severely injured patients if capacity exists, may help to establish access as an entrenched and fundamental property of trauma systems [22], but more work remains to be done.

RECOMMENDATION

Rural and remote communities shoulder a heavy burden of injury and do not have ready access to urban trauma systems. Reappraisal of access to trauma systems in these environments and new ideas to reduce early mortality in these populations are urgently needed.

Grade of recommendation: B

3.5.3 Do Trauma Systems Save Lives?

The *structure* of trauma centers might include the presence of in-house trauma-attending and multidisciplinary trauma teams, well-equipped trauma bays, ready access to operating theaters, the presence of clinical protocols and educational curricula, research capacity and injury prevention activity, and participation in external review and designation. Studies have suggested that the presence of trauma-attending in-house and other structural interventions reduce time to definitive treatment, cost, and even mortality [23], prompting organizations such as the ACS-COT and the Trauma Association of Canada to provide trauma surgeon response time guidelines. *Process* in trauma systems is assessed using measures of function: How fast does the team respond, how long do patients spend in the emergency department, how long to get to the operating room? Implementation of trauma systems has been shown to improve processes of care [24]. Finally, and most importantly, *outcome* of trauma patients, including mortality, length of stay, and functional measures, may all provide insights into how well a trauma center is fulfilling its mandate.

The trauma systems literature is dominated by this outcome bottom line, and particularly by mortality, as it has been most consistently measured. *Analyses of preventable deaths* by expert panels provided the earliest justification for the regionalization of trauma care in dedicated centers. In a striking example, West et al. compared the proportion of preventable in-hospital trauma deaths in San Francisco County, where trauma care was regionalized to a single trauma center, to that in Orange County, where over 40 centers participated in trauma care. They found only 1% of deaths in San Francisco to be preventable, while a staggering 73% of deaths would have been preventable in Orange County with access to high-quality trauma care [25]. Four years later, after the implementation of regionalized trauma care in Orange County, the proportion of preventable deaths fell to an eighth of its previous level [26]. Other early trauma center studies have involved *comparisons of trauma center patient outcomes to national norms* (using Trauma and Injury Severity Score methodology and comparisons with reference data from the Major Trauma Outcomes Study) [27] and use of *population-based methods* to examine populations with and without access to trauma systems. Each of these strategies provided early evidence in favor of trauma centers and systems [28].

In one of the most widely cited population-based studies of trauma system effectiveness, investigators from the University of Washington led by Nathens examined the effect of trauma systems on motor vehicle crash mortality in 22 states using the national Fatality Analysis Reporting System database. The study found that an 8% mortality reduction attributable to trauma systems was evident by 15 years following trauma system implementation [29]. Celso et al. recently published another landmark study [30] of the effectiveness of trauma systems. Their review of the literature and meta-analysis examined 14 population-based studies, comparing mortality rates before and after implementation of trauma systems or comparing mortality in jurisdictions with and without trauma systems. Improved odds of survival were noted in 8 of the 14 studies, and a meta-analysis including 6 of the studies demonstrated a 15% reduction in mortality where trauma systems were present. In another landmark trial, Mackenzie et al. used data from the National Study on the Costs and Outcomes of Trauma (NSCOT) to compare mortality between Level 1 trauma centers and large nontrauma centers in metropolitan areas of 14 states. The authors found that in-hospital and 1-year mortality were significantly lower for trauma centers (risk ratio [RR] 0.80 and 0.75, respectively) and that this effect was more pronounced in younger patients with more severe injuries [31].

Trauma centers have also shown promise in the management of pediatric injuries [32]. Based on observed improved traumatic brain injury outcomes in high-level pediatric trauma centers, the ACS has recommended that children with such injuries be managed at these facilities. However, a recent study of six U.S. states suggests that almost one-third of children do not get to high-level care. Access for children is an important research priority.

RECOMMENDATION

Trauma systems improve injury survival and should be widely implemented based on this evidence alone.

Grade of recommendation: B

3.5.4 What Features of Trauma Systems Make a Difference?

The rapid evolution of trauma systems has depended on (and will continue to depend on) close and ongoing evaluation of their structure and processes. In Quebec, such evaluation and evidence-based and context-specific evolution have resulted in a decline in mortality from severe injury from 51.8% in 1992 to 8.6% in 2002 [33]. In a study of over 72,000 patients, investigators probed the specific strengths of trauma systems and demonstrated that mortality following severe injury is strongly affected by structural and process issues such as advance notification of trauma centers by prehospital crews (OR 6.1), by the presence of hospital-based performance improvement programs (OR 0.44), and by trauma center experience (OR 0.98) and tertiary designation (OR 0.68) [34].

The effects of experience and trauma center designation have also received attention from other trauma research groups. To define the experience effect, Nathens et al. compared outcomes in trauma patients treated at 31 university-affiliated Level 1 and Level 2 trauma centers. They observed that as trauma center volumes increase, hospital lengths of stay decrease, reflecting, perhaps, more rapid recovery in more experienced centers. This relationship descends to a plateau once injury admissions exceeded 600 (Injury Severity Score >15) per year. Also, odds of death from severe injuries relative to the smallest centers were shown to start decreasing above the 600 admissions threshold, again suggesting that about 600–650 major trauma admissions per year might be the boundary between low- and high-volume trauma centers. Nathens' group found significantly lower mortality among patients presenting to high-volume trauma centers with penetrating abdominal trauma and hypotension (OR 0.02) and with multisystem injuries with low Glasgow Coma Score (GCS) (OR 0.49) [35]. However, an analysis of 12,254 patients from the National Trauma Data Bank, focusing on a slightly different population of severely injured patients and using different volume thresholds, found ACS-COT trauma center *designation* level (i.e., degree of preparedness and resources for trauma care) to be more predictive of outcome than patient volume [36]. Disability at discharge (20.3 vs. 33.8%) and mortality (25.3 vs. 29.3) were significantly lower in Level 1 than in Level 2 centers, but trauma volumes were not associated with outcome differences. Both studies suggest that care provided in dedicated trauma centers, either because of experience or preparedness, has the potential to reduce morbidity and save lives.

It is difficult to know how exactly high-volume or trauma center designation influence patient outcome, but education, experience, and attention to process likely play significant roles. Trauma center designation is associated with formalized approaches to performance improvement (e.g., through the ACS Trauma Quality Improvement Program [TQIP]), and research, implementation of education, and quality programs reflect a deeper institutional commitment to trauma care and injury control, which likely have a collective impact on outcomes.

> ### RECOMMENDATION
>
> Specific structure and process features of trauma systems, including integrated prehospital care, trauma center volumes, verification/accreditation by external expert agencies such as the ACS-COT, and ongoing dedication to leadership and quality, influence trauma system performance. These features of trauma systems should be ongoing areas of focus and optimization.
>
> Grade of recommendation: B

3.5.5 Beyond Saving Lives: What Are the Long-Term Outcomes of Trauma Systems?

As mortality from multisystem trauma has fallen both in military and civilian settings, many survivors are returning home to their communities and to productive life. Unfortunately, data on the long-term functional outcomes after traumatic conditions such as shock, multiorgan failure, traumatic brain injury, and pelvic and long bone fractures are expensive and not routinely collected. Recently, Moore et al. validated trauma center readmission rates as a key indicator of trauma system performance. This is a welcome measure that will assist trauma systems in the optimization of intermediate-term outcomes [37]. In the longer term, Gabbe et al. found that 6 months after major trauma, only 42% of patients had returned to work and only 32% characterized their recovery as good [38]. Outcome measures at the time of hospital discharge such as the modified Functional Independence Measure and the Glasgow Outcome Score, which are often used as indicators of functional recovery, were not found to be reliably predictive of long-term outcomes, emphasizing how little insight we get from hospital data on ultimate outcomes. These findings, and others by this group, highlight the urgency of data collection, continued research, and action in this area (Table 3.1).

TABLE 3.1

Evidence and Recommendations

Statement	Evidence	Recommendation
Injury prevention		
Trauma systems prevent injury recidivism associated with alcohol abuse.	1b	A
Trauma system implementation has been associated with reductions in mortality from motor vehicle crashes.	2c	B
Trauma systems should play a more active role in injury prevention.	2c	B
Prehospital care		
Prehospital intubation in traumatic brain injury should be selective and attempted with caution.	2b	B
Prehospital fluid resuscitation should be limited in patients with penetrating mechanisms in urban environments.	1b	B
Scene time and interventions in trauma should be minimized until more is known about the effects of specific interventions.	2a	B
Local analyses should be done to determine trauma center catchments that may be more rapidly served by AMT.	2b	B
Accessibility		
Systems of trauma care in rural, low-resource environments require a thorough reappraisal and new ideas on how to address the disproportionate burden of early mortality in these settings.	2c	B
Survival		
Trauma systems increase survival.	2c	B
Features of trauma systems		
Trauma center volume influences outcome.	2c	B
Trauma center verification influences outcome.	2c	B
Trauma center education programs influence outcomes.	2b	B
Trauma center quality improvement programs influence outcomes.	2b	B
Long-term outcomes		
Long-term outcomes in severe trauma are poor.	2b	—
Trauma systems should collect and account for long-term outcome data. Broad consensus on specific indicators or benchmarks of long-term trauma outcomes is required.	—	—
Integrated systems of trauma care		
A systematic approach to trauma care improves survival.	2a	B
Inclusive trauma systems improve survival.	2c	B
Inclusive trauma systems may improve survival in mass casualty and multicasualty situations.	Needed	
Trauma systems are cost-effective.	2b	B
Global health		
Trauma systems reduce morbidity and mortality in low-income settings.	Needed	—

RECOMMENDATION

Long-term outcomes after severe injury are poor and poorly understood. Consensus on specific indicators of long-term outcomes and systematic measurement of these outcomes are essential to inform the ongoing evolution of trauma systems.

Grade of recommendation: B

3.6 Future Directions

3.6.1 Integrated Systems of Trauma Care

In recent years, the concept of trauma systems has transitioned from regionalization of trauma care in (often single) specialized high-volume trauma centers, to a more holistic and multidisciplinary or *systems* approach, to injury control that starts with injury prevention and emphasizes a wider response to trauma, including prehospital and posthospital care. Nathens' studies of the effect of trauma systems on motor vehicle crash survival have suggested that successful injury control may depend on a broad-based, systematic, and coordinated approach that includes seatbelt legislation, helmet use, and established speed limits, in addition to the presence of trauma centers [29, 39]. It is becoming increasingly evident that the observed successes of trauma systems cannot be attributed to any one component or measure, but rather to a systematic approach to injury control.

Trauma investigators have speculated that a more participatory or *inclusive* approach to trauma care, which involves all of a region's acute hospitals (to the extent that their resources permit), could streamline the triage and early care of injured patients and extend the reach of trauma systems beyond the catchments of large, urban trauma centers to more rural and remote regions. A recent comparison of American states with the traditional single trauma center–based exclusive trauma systems with states with inclusive trauma systems used administrative discharge data from 24 states to demonstrate that states with the highest levels of inclusiveness (38%–100% of hospitals designated as Levels 1–5 trauma centers) had the lowest odds of mortality (OR 0.77) after adjustment for factors such as injury mechanism and trauma system maturity. The authors of this study speculated that early care of patients in inclusive systems at local trauma centers, and more efficient transfers to higher levels of trauma care when needed, may have been responsible for the observed advantage of inclusive systems [40]. These conclusions about sharing the work in inclusive trauma systems may seem to be at odds with other studies documenting the importance of the volume–outcome relationship in severe trauma [35]. It is true that increasing the profile of Level 1 and Level 2 trauma centers decreases trauma volumes at nearby Level 1 trauma centers, but it may do so without decreasing injury severity at the Level 1 centers and while reducing mortality [41]. Although the ACS-COT is moving toward a more inclusive approach to trauma system design, the designation of new Levels 2, 3, and 4 centers within a given health-care ecosystem must be thoughtful; must carefully account for a population's needs; and must preserve the critical clinical, education, and research activities of regional Level 1 centers.

Inclusive trauma systems depend on great attention to triage, or the sorting and movement of patients, both from the scene and between hospitals, and the networks that include emergency medical systems and all levels of trauma systems must be evidence-driven, responsive, and dynamic. The need for rapid and accurate assessment of patient needs and accurate triage to appropriate facilities is underscored in a report by Sampalis et al. in Montreal [42], who found that severely injured patients initially taken to less specialized hospitals and then transferred to trauma centers had almost twice the mortality of those transferred directly to trauma centers.

The interesting challenge of modern trauma systems will be to reconcile observations about volume–outcome relationships, benefits of inclusive systems, and challenges of triage and transport. Trauma systems will be increasingly customized to match local needs. What seems clear is that this effort is not confined to a single agency, center, or discipline, but requires an integrated approach. Germany initiated a process to build a nationwide trauma program in 2006. By 2014, a system of 44 regional trauma networks, with an average of 14.5 trauma centers each, covering 90% of the country, and supported by an integrated national trauma registry, was in place. This was a large-scale effort that has laid the foundation for the optimization of trauma care and injury prevention on a national scale and could serve as a template for other countries [43].

3.6.2 Vulnerability and Access

Ensuring universal access to excellent trauma care is a core principle of trauma systems development and has been discussed on a broad level in this chapter. In order to continue to achieve meaningful advances in injury control, the architects of modern trauma systems must remain aware of vulnerable populations at high risk of injury or with low access to definitive trauma care. Socioeconomic status, age, race, and insurance status, as well as geography, have been associated with vulnerability to injury or poor access to care [44, 45]. One great area of concern is trauma among the elderly, which is an impending epidemic. Trauma systems must remain sensitive to the risk and implications of injury among the elderly and focus their care on the preservation of functional independence [46]. The ongoing optimization of trauma systems will require new strategies to understand vulnerability and risk and new ways to extend the reach of systems, including inclusive systems, education and outreach, telehealth, and applications of web-based technologies.

3.6.3 Economic Considerations

A survey of the additional capabilities and costs associated with 24-hour trauma system preparedness in 10 trauma centers in Florida suggested that the annual costs of such preparedness is $2.7 million per center. Most of these costs were attributed to physician on-call coverage. The authors note that these costs of preparedness may not translate to billable patient care and are therefore not recouped [47]. The financial benefits of preparedness in terms of reductions in morbidity and mortality, however, are difficult to accurately quantify and are probably undervalued. A more global economic evaluation of trauma care examined the cost per quality-adjusted life year (cost/QALY) gained by treatment at a tertiary trauma center in Ottawa, Canada. The investigators found that the increase in cost/QALY for treatment at a tertiary trauma center compared with a non-trauma center ($4,303) compared favorably with other established health-care interventions [48]. Another analysis of the Florida trauma system confirmed that although care at trauma centers was more expensive, it was associated with a reduction in mortality of 18%, resulting in a cost of $35,000 per life saved at trauma centers. Again, when restored productivity was considered, the authors concluded that trauma center care compared very favorably with other established medical interventions.

RECOMMENDATION

The creation of more integrated systems of trauma care that balance inclusivity with trauma center performance, that continue to address issues of vulnerability and poor access, and that remain focused on the economic value of injury prevention and effective trauma care are key future directions in the ongoing evolution of trauma systems.

Grade of recommendation: B

3.6.4 Global Health: Can Trauma Systems Save Lives in Low-Resource Settings?

Low- and middle-income countries, with stretched health-care and public health budgets, shoulder an immense burden of injury. But a lack of resources should not be a deterrent to the pursuit of advances in trauma care; millions of lives stand to be improved or even saved if trauma systems can find more universal applications [4, 49]. Trauma systems prevent injury and improve outcomes in part because they are successful in reorganizing scarce resources and focusing them on achieving high standards of injury control.

Recognizing the promise of a public health/trauma systems approach to injury control in low-resource settings, the International Association for Trauma and Surgical Intensive Care and the World Health Organization, along with a number of prominent trauma organizations from around the world, set out to identify fundamental priorities for trauma care that must be achieved regardless of the level of individual or societal wealth. The results of their deliberations were published in 2004 in the document *Guidelines for Essential Trauma Care* [50]. These guidelines are the low-resource counterpart to the ACS-COT *Resources for Optimal Care of the Injured Patients*. They are geared to economies that spend as little as $3–4 per capita per year on health, are rallying points for advocacy, create tangible goals, and can be modified to fit local circumstances. They represent the starting point for action on injury control at the global level.

A key first step in the development of trauma systems is the collection and analysis of high-quality injury data or injury surveillance. Data collection is a necessary prerequisite for the improvement of clinical care, for the allocation of finite resources to acute care and rehabilitation, and for evidence-based injury prevention. While North American trauma systems have been built on a foundation of injury surveillance in

the form of hospital-based trauma registries, in lower-resource settings, the costs of data collection and analysis have often proven to be prohibitive [51]. However, early initiatives in this area have suggested that trauma registries may be feasible and would play an important role, with trauma registries beginning to flourish in low- and middle-income settings [52, 53]. The widespread availability and computational power of mobile information technology tools are poised to change injury surveillance and the ways in which data are applied to guide global trauma systems development. For example, a mobile, point-of-care electronic health record for trauma care [54] helped frontline physicians document 10,000 consecutive trauma admissions (including resuscitation, operative, and discharge notes) in its first 10 months of implementation at a busy South African trauma center. Data from these records wirelessly populated an electronic trauma registry in real time with an estimated 3.5 million data points, providing unprecedented insights in an environment without formal data collection.

To advance the equitability and performance of trauma systems, the increased capacity to collect data must be matched with the thoughtful selection of data fields. Many efforts have been made to create universal, minimal, and interoperable datasets for trauma, but the drive to standardize data collection should be balanced against the need to collect context-specific data elements with the capability to drive context-specific change [55, 56].

RECOMMENDATION

The ongoing development of trauma systems is a global public health priority. Injury surveillance and the application of data to addressing issues in injury control are feasible in low- and middle-income countries (LMICs) and should be major areas of thought and action in an ambitious global trauma systems agenda.

Grade of recommendation: E

3.6.5 Innovation to Extend the Reach of Trauma Systems

The capabilities of multidisciplinary trauma teams can be enhanced and extended through innovative uses of simulation and team training. For example, the Rural Trauma Team Development Course (RTDC), which, building on the ATLS program, trains teams in resource-limited environments in the resuscitation and stabilization of trauma patients, has been shown to significantly reduce emergency department wait times in referring hospitals functioning in inclusive trauma systems [57]. Operative trauma courses (Advanced Trauma Operative Management, Definitive Surgical Trauma Care) similarly provide trauma teams in rural or remote areas with knowledge, experience, and confidence to navigate high-acuity, low-occurrence trauma situations.

Advances in communication technology and the increasing reach of broadband Internet (e.g., Starlink) are creating unprecedented opportunities for trauma systems to serve vulnerable populations in austere settings, effectively extending the reach of trauma systems. Telementoring, including the use of augmented reality, has been shown to be of benefit in trauma diagnostics and resuscitation [58] and lifesaving procedures such as cricothyroidotomy [59].

These innovations and their infinite applications place modern trauma systems at an inflection point, poised to increase the effectiveness, reach, and scale of their activities. New paradigms such as task sharing and task shifting, when combined with new ways to train and communicate, will create even more inclusive systems of trauma care, with increased potential to alter the curve of the global burden of trauma.

3.7 Summary

ORLANDO: At 0210 hour, the first casualty arrived at ORMC with a gunshot wound to the abdomen. The trauma service and the hospital escalated their response to match the waves of incoming patients, mobilizing skilled personnel, the emergency department, operating rooms, and critical care environments, while coordinating seamlessly with the fire and police departments to keep the hospital functional and secure and communicating compassionately with families and the public. Forty-nine critically injured patients were evaluated and treated. Twenty-nine operations were performed within the first 24 hours, and 54 surgical procedures had been performed within the first week. All 40 patients who arrived at ORMC with perfusing vital signs survived. In one of the worst mass shootings in U.S. history, a well-prepared, constantly practicing, and seamlessly integrated trauma system moved patients rapidly to safety, saved lives, and though still not perfect, averted unquantifiable tragedies.

CHICAGO: The new UChicago Medicine Trauma Service, built by its founders on generations of surgical and public health knowledge, has begun to shorten prehospital times, integrate with its communities to provide wrap-around comprehensive care for the survivors of trauma, and advocate at the highest levels for health policy to treat gun violence as a public health issue with modifiable determinants that are rooted in the strengthening of individual purpose and collective relationships within strong communities.

In recent years, the value of trauma systems has been confirmed by a wealth of Level 2 data (population-based cohort and ecological studies) in civilian and military [60] contexts, and trauma systems have become an important feature of the public health landscape. They illustrate that comprehensive public health approaches can make a difference in diseases with complex determinants and severe consequences. But gaps in the trauma systems literature and the persistence of injury as a major public health issue in North America and around the world mean that the work is still far from accomplished. More studies are needed, including economic evaluations so that long-term benefits can be accounted for and so that trauma systems remain efficient. Innovative analyses of access to trauma systems are needed so that their reach might be extended further into our rural, remote, and global communities. Finally, local successes have global implications. In the era of mobile information technology, surgeons working in trauma systems around the world will have unprecedented power to collect and share data, thereby broadening their reach and amplifying their potential impact on public health.

Editor's Note

This fine chapter underscores the fact that trauma care is delivered in diverse ways across the globe. In countries such as Germany, trauma centers are strategically located to serve the population centers and address geography, attempting to place the populace within a reasonable distance by helicopter from a receiving hospital. In the United States, it seems to be more of a random distribution. In states such as Maryland (with over 6 million inhabitants), significant trauma victims are flown to one of two adult or the solitary pediatric Level I trauma centers in Baltimore. The state also has four Level II adult trauma centers. This seems to be an ideal concentration of resources. In Boston, there are seven Level I and one Level II adult trauma centers for a population of under 700,000 in the city proper and 8.5 million in the metro area. In other places, like the state of New York, there appears to be no grand plan, and for many years it seemed that any hospital could declare itself a trauma center and receive injury victims. Perhaps regionalization of trauma care in the United States with fewer, higher-quality centers would lead to better outcomes.

REFERENCES

1. Cheatham ML, Smith CP, Ibrahim JA, Havron WS, Lube MW, Levy MS, Ono SK (2016) Orlando regional medical center responds to pulse nightclub shooting. Bull Am Coll Surg 101:12–19
2. Gross DA (2018) Chicago's South Side finally has an adult trauma center again. New Yorker
3. Heher A (2018) UChicago Medicine gets approval to be Level 1 adult trauma center. UChicago News
4. Mock C, Joshipura M, Goosen J, Lormand JD, Maier R (2005) Strengthening trauma systems globally: The essential trauma care project. J Trauma Acute Care Surg 59:1243–1246
5. American College of Surgeons (2014) Resources for the optimal care of the injured patient. https://www.facs. org/~/media/files/qualityprograms/trauma/vrcresources/ resourcesforoptimalcare2014v11.ashx. Accessed 18 Dec 2022
6. Trunkey DD (1983) Trauma. Accidental and intentional injuries account for more years of life lost in the U.S. than cancer and heart disease. Among the prescribed remedies are improved preventive efforts, speedier surgery and further research. Sci Am 249:28–35
7. Stewart RM, Myers JG, Dent DL, Ermis P, Gray GA, Villarreal R, Blow O, Woods B, McFarland M, Garavaglia J, Root HD, Pruitt BAJ (2003) Seven hundred fifty-three consecutive deaths in a Level I trauma center: the argument for injury prevention. J Trauma 54:61–66. https://doi. org/10.1097/00005373-200301000-00009
8. Runyan CW (2003) Introduction: back to the future–revisiting Haddon's conceptualization of injury epidemiology and prevention. Epidemiol Rev 25:60–64. https://doi.org/ 10.1093/epirev/mxg005
9. Ameratunga S, Hijar M, Norton R (2006) Road-traffic injuries: confronting disparities to address a global-health problem. Lancet (London, England) 367:1533–1540. https://doi. org/10.1016/S0140-6736(06)68654-6

10. Gentilello LM, Rivara FP, Donovan DM, Jurkovich GJ, Daranciang E, Dunn CW, Villaveces A, Copass M, Ries RR (1999) Alcohol interventions in a trauma center as a means of reducing the risk of injury recurrence. Ann Surg 230:473. https://doi.org/10.1097/00000658-199910000-00003

11. McGwin GJ, Metzger J, Alonso JE, Rue LW 3rd (2003) The association between occupant restraint systems and risk of injury in frontal motor vehicle collisions. J Trauma 54: 1182–1187. https://doi.org/10.1097/01.TA.0000056165.49112.F4

12. McDonald EM, MacKenzie EJ, Teitelbaum SD, Carlini AR, Teter HJ, Valenziano CP (2007) Injury prevention activities in U.S. trauma centres: are we doing enough? Injury 38:538–547. https://doi.org/10.1016/j.injury.2006.11.020

13. Gentilello LM, Ebel BE, Wickizer TM, Salkever DS, Rivara FP (2005) Alcohol interventions for trauma patients treated in emergency departments and hospitals: A cost benefit analysis. Ann Surg 241:541–550. https://doi.org/10.1097/01.sla.0000157133.80396.1c

14. Cowley RA, Hudson F, Scanlan E, Gill W, Lally RJ, Long W, Kuhn AO (1973) An economical and proved helicopter program for transporting the emergency critically ill and injured patient in Maryland. J Trauma 13:1029–1038. https://doi.org/10.1097/00005373-197312000-00001

15. Bickell WH, Wall MJJ, Pepe PE, Martin RR, Ginger VF, Allen MK, Mattox KL (1994) Immediate versus delayed fluid resuscitation for hypotensive patients with penetrating torso injuries. N Engl J Med 331:1105–1109. https://doi.org/10.1056/NEJM199410273311701

16. Stiell IG, Nesbitt LP, Pickett W, Munkley D, Spaite DW, Banek J, Field B, Luinstra-Toohey L, Maloney J, Dreyer J, Lyver M, Campeau T, Wells GA (2008) The OPALS major trauma study: impact of advanced life-support on survival and morbidity. C Can Med Assoc J/J l'Association Medicale Can 178:1141–1152. https://doi.org/10.1503/cmaj.071154

17. Liberman M, Mulder D, Lavoie A, Denis R, Sampalis JS (2003) Multicenter Canadian study of prehospital trauma care. Ann Surg 237:153–160. https://doi.org/10.1097/01.SLA.0000048374.46952.10

18. Davis DP (2008) Should invasive airway management be done in the field? C Can Med Assoc J/J l'Association Medicale Can 178:1171–1173. https://doi.org/10.1503/cmaj.080234

19. Karanicolas PJ, Bhatia P, Williamson J, Malthaner RA, Parry NG, Girotti MJ, Gray DK (2006) The fastest route between two points is not always a straight line: an analysis of air and land transfer of nonpenetrating trauma patients. J Trauma 61:396–403. https://doi.org/10.1097/01.ta.0000222974.31728.2a

20. MacKenzie EJ, Hoyt DB, Sacra JC, Jurkovich GJ, Carlini AR, Teitelbaum SD, Teter HJ (2003) National inventory of hospital trauma centers. JAMA 289:1515–1522. https://doi.org/10.1001/jama.289.12.1515

21. Muelleman RL, Wadman MC, Tran TP, Ullrich F, Anderson JR (2007) Rural motor vehicle crash risk of death is higher after controlling for injury severity. J Trauma 62:221–226. https://doi.org/10.1097/01.ta.0000231696.65548.06

22. Spain DA, Bellino M, Kopelman A, Chang J, Park J, Gregg DL, Brundage SI (2007) Requests for 692 transfers to an academic Level I trauma center: implications of the emergency medical treatment and active labor act. J Trauma 62:63–68. https://doi.org/10.1097/TA.0b013e31802d9716

23. Luchette F, Kelly B, Davis K, Johanningman J, Heink N, James L, Ottaway M, Hurst J (1997) Impact of the in-house trauma surgeon on initial patient care, outcome, and cost. J Trauma 42:490–497. https://doi.org/10.1097/00005373-199703000-00017

24. Cornwell EE 3rd, Chang DC, Phillips J, Campbell KA (2003) Enhanced trauma program commitment at a Level I trauma center: effect on the process and outcome of care. Arch Surg 138:838–843. https://doi.org/10.1001/archsurg.138.8.838

25. West JG, Trunkey DD, Lim RC (1979) Systems of trauma care. A study of two counties. Arch Surg 114:455–460. https://doi.org/10.1001/archsurg.1979.01370280109016

26. West JG, Cales RH, Gazzaniga AB (1983) Impact of regionalization. The orange county experience. Arch Surg 118:740–744. https://doi.org/10.1001/archsurg.1983.01390060058013

27. Champion HR, Copes WS, Sacco WJ, Lawnick MM, Keast SL, Bain LWJ, Flanagan ME, Frey CF (1990) The major trauma outcome study: establishing national norms for trauma care. J Trauma 30:1356–1365

28. Mullins RJ, Mann NC (1999) Population-based research assessing the effectiveness of trauma systems. J Trauma 47:S59–S66. https://doi.org/10.1097/00005373-199909001-00013

29. Nathens AB, Jurkovich GJ, Cummings P, Rivara FP, Maier RV (2000) The effect of organized systems of trauma care on motor vehicle crash mortality. JAMA 283:1990–1994. https://doi.org/10.1001/jama.283.15.1990

30. Celso B, Tepas J, Langland-Orban B, Pracht E, Papa L, Lottenberg L, Flint L (2006) A systematic review and meta-analysis comparing outcome of severely injured patients treated in trauma centers following the establishment of trauma systems. J Trauma 60:371–378; discussion 378. https://doi.org/10.1097/01.ta.0000197916.99629.eb

31. MacKenzie EJ, Rivara FP, Jurkovich GJ, Nathens AB, Frey KP, Egleston BL, Salkever DS, Scharfstein DO (2006) A national evaluation of the effect of trauma-center care on mortality. N Engl J Med 354:366–378. https://doi.org/10.1056/NEJMsa052049

32. Wang NE, Saynina O, Vogel LD, Newgard CD, Bhattacharya J, Phibbs CS (2013) The effect of trauma center care on pediatric injury mortality in California, 1999 to 2011. J Trauma Acute Care Surg 75:704–716. https://doi.org/10.1097/TA.0b013e31829a0a65

33. Liberman M, Mulder DS, Lavoie A, Sampalis JS (2004) Implementation of a trauma care system: evolution through evaluation. J Trauma 56:1330–1335. https://doi.org/10.1097/01.ta.0000071297.76727.8b

34. Liberman M, Mulder DS, Jurkovich GJ, Sampalis JS (2005) The association between trauma system and trauma center components and outcome in a mature regionalized trauma system. Surgery 137:647–658. https://doi.org/10.1016/j.surg.2005.03.011

35. Nathens AB, Jurkovich GJ, Maier R V, Grossman DC, MacKenzie EJ, Moore M, Rivara FP (2001) Relationship between trauma center volume and outcomes. JAMA 285:1164–1171. https://doi.org/10.1001/jama.285.9.1164

36. Demetriades D, Martin M, Salim A, Rhee P, Brown C, Chan L (2005) The effect of trauma center designation and trauma volume on outcome in specific severe injuries. Ann Surg 242:512–519. https://doi.org/10.1097/01.sla.0000184169.73614.09

37. Moore L, Stelfox HT, Turgeon AF, Nathens AB, Lavoie A, Bourgeois G, Lapointe J (2014) Derivation and validation of a quality indicator for 30-day unplanned hospital readmission to evaluate trauma care. J Trauma Acute Care Surg 76:1310–1316. https://doi.org/10.1097/TA.0000000000000202

38. Gabbe BJ, Simpson PM, Sutherland AM, Williamson OD, Judson R, Kossmann T, Cameron PA (2008) Functional measures at discharge: are they useful predictors of longer term outcomes for trauma registries? Ann Surg 247:854–859. https://doi.org/10.1097/SLA.0b013e3181656d1e

39. Shafi S, Nathens AB, Elliott AC, Gentilello L (2006) Effect of trauma systems on motor vehicle occupant mortality: a comparison between states with and without a formal system. J Trauma 61:1374–1379. https://doi.org/10.1097/01.ta.0000246698.07125.c0

40. Utter GH, Maier R V, Rivara FP, Mock CN, Jurkovich GJ, Nathens AB (2006) Inclusive trauma systems: do they improve triage or outcomes of the severely injured? J Trauma 60:529–537. https://doi.org/10.1097/01.ta.0000204022.36214.9e

41. Carr BG, Geiger J, McWilliams N, Reilly PM, Wiebe DJ (2014) Impact of adding Level II and III trauma centers on volume and disease severity at a nearby Level I trauma center. J Trauma Acute Care Surg 77:764–768. https://doi.org/10.1097/TA.0000000000000430

42. Sampalis JS, Denis R, Fréchette P, Brown R, Fleiszer D, Mulder D (1997) Direct transport to tertiary trauma centers versus transfer from lower level facilities: impact on mortality and morbidity among patients with major trauma. J Trauma 43:286–288. https://doi.org/10.1097/00005373-199708000-00014

43. Ruchholtz S, Lefering R, Lewan U, Debus F, Mand C, Siebert H, Kühne CA (2014) Implementation of a nationwide trauma network for the care of severely injured patients. J Trauma Acute Care Surg 76:1456–1461. https://doi.org/10.1097/TA.0000000000000245

44. Delgado MK, Yokell MA, Staudenmayer KL, Spain DA, Hernandez-Boussard T, Wang NE (2014) Factors associated with the disposition of severely injured patients initially seen at non–trauma center emergency departments: disparities by insurance status. JAMA Surg 149:422–430. https://doi.org/10.1001/jamasurg.2013.4398

45. Schuurman N, Hameed SM, Fiedler R, Bell N, Simons RK (2008) The spatial epidemiology of trauma: the potential of geographic information science to organize data and reveal patterns of injury and services. Can J Surg 51:389–395

46. Ang D, Norwood S, Barquist E, McKenney M, Kurek S, Kimbrell B, Garcia A, Walsh CB, Liu H, Ziglar M, Hurst J (2014) Geriatric outcomes for trauma patients in the state of Florida after the advent of a large trauma network. J Trauma Acute Care Surg 77:155–160; discussion 160. https://doi.org/10.1097/TA.0000000000000272

47. Taheri PA, Butz DA, Lottenberg L, Clawson A, Flint LM (2004) The cost of trauma center readiness. Am J Surg 187:7–13. https://doi.org/10.1016/j.amjsurg.2003.06.002

48. Séguin J, Garber BG, Coyle D, Hébert PC (1999) An economic evaluation of trauma care in a Canadian lead trauma hospital. J Trauma 47:S99–103. https://doi.org/10.1097/00005373-199909001-00022

49. Mock C, Joshipura M, Arreola-Risa C, Quansah R (2012) An estimate of the number of lives that could be saved through improvements in trauma care globally. World J Surg 36:959–963. https://doi.org/10.1007/s00268-012-1459-6

50. Mock C (2004) Guidelines for essential trauma care. World Health Organization

51. O'Reilly GM, Joshipura M, Cameron PA, Gruen R (2013) Trauma registries in developing countries: a review of the published experience. Injury 44:713–721

52. Schultz CR, Ford HR, Cassidy LD, Shultz BL, Blanc C, King-Schultz LW, Perry HB (2007) Development of a hospital-based trauma registry in Haiti: an approach for improving injury surveillance in developing and resource-poor settings. J Trauma 63:1143–1154. https://doi.org/10.1097/TA.0b013e31815688e3

53. Rosenkrantz L, Schuurman N, Hameed M (2019) Trauma registry implementation and operation in low and middle income countries: a scoping review. Glob Public Health 14:1884–1897. https://doi.org/10.1080/17441692.2019.1622761

54. Zargaran E, Schuurman N, Nicol AJ, Matzopoulos R, Cinnamon J, Taulu T, Ricker B, Garbutt Brown DR, Navsaria P, Hameed SM (2014) The electronic trauma health record: design and usability of a novel tablet-based tool for trauma care and injury surveillance in low resource settings. J Am Coll Surg 218:41–50. https://doi.org/10.1016/j.jamcollsurg.2013.10.001

55. Conrick KM, Mills B, Mohamed K, Bulger EM, Arbabi S, Vil CS, Dotolo D, Solano E, Vavilala MS, Rowhani-Rahbar A, Moore M (2022) Improving data collection and abstraction to assess health equity in trauma care. J Med Syst 46:21. https://doi.org/10.1007/s10916-022-01804-4

56. Zargaran E, Adolph L, Schuurman N, Roux L, Ramsey D, Simons R, Spence R, Nicol AJ, Navsaria P, Puyana JC, Parry N, Moore L, Aboutanos M, Yanchar N, Razek T, Ball CG, Hameed SM (2016) A global agenda for electronic injury surveillance: consensus statement from the Trauma Association of Canada, the Trauma Society of South Africa, and the Pan-American Trauma Society. J Trauma Acute Care Surg 80:168–170. https://doi.org/10.1097/TA.0000000000000880

57. Dennis BM, Vella MA, Gunter OL, Smith MD, Wilson CS, Patel MB, Nunez TC, Guillamondegui OD (2016) Rural trauma team development course decreases time to transfer for trauma patients. J Trauma Acute Care Surg 81(4):632–637. doi:10.1097/TA.0000000000001188

58. Kirkpatrick AW (2019) Point-of-care resuscitation research: from extreme to mainstream: Trauma Association of Canada Fraser Gurd Lecture 2019. J Trauma Acute Care Surg 87:571–581

59. Rojas-Muñoz E, Lin C, Sanchez-Tamayo N, Cabrera ME, Andersen D, Popescu V, Barragan JA, Zarzaur B, Murphy P, Anderson K, Douglas T, Griffis C, McKee J, Kirkpatrick AW, Wachs JP (2020) Evaluation of an augmented reality platform for austere surgical telementoring: a randomized controlled crossover study in cricothyroidotomies. NPJ Digit Med 3:75. https://doi.org/10.1038/s41746-020-0284-9

60. Eastridge BJ, Jenkins D, Flaherty S, Schiller H, Holcomb JB (2006) Trauma system development in a theater of war: experiences from operation Iraqi freedom and operation enduring freedom. J Trauma 61:1363–1366. https://doi.org/10.1097/01.ta.0000245894.78941.90

4

Military Injury Outcomes

Brian J. Eastridge and John K. Bini

4.1 Introduction

The development of trauma care has been a synergistic relationship between the military and civilian medical environments and has paralleled the history of war for the past several centuries [1, 2]. "He who would become a surgeon should join an army and follow it for war is the only proper school for a surgeon." In the sixteenth century, Ambrose Pare conceptualized novel methods for the management of gunshot wounds as well as the ligation of large vessels, particularly during amputation. Jean Dominique Larrey, as surgeon-in-chief of the Napoleonic armies, introduced the concepts of triage and battlefield evacuation with his "ambulance volante," or flying ambulance, during the French conflicts of the late eighteenth and early nineteenth centuries. During the Civil War, military physicians realized the utility of prompt attention to the wounded, early debridement and amputation to mitigate the effects of tissue injury and infection, and evacuation of the casualty from the battlefield. World War I saw further advances in the concept of evacuation, topical antisepsis, and the development of echelons of medical care. With World War II, antibiotics, blood transfusion, and resuscitative fluids, including plasma, were widely introduced into the combat environment, and surgical practice was improved to care for wounded soldiers. From his World War II experiences, Dr Michael DeBakey, the surgical consultant to the Army Surgeon General, noted that wars have always promoted advances in trauma care due to the concentrated exposure of military hospitals to large numbers. Wartime medical experience fostered a fundamental drive to improve outcomes by improving practice [3]. Technological advances in aviation and medicine at the beginning of the Korean conflict led to the increase in deployed surgical capability, helicopters for patient evacuation from the locations where injuries occur, and primary repair and grafting for vascular injury. In Vietnam, more highly trained medics at the location of the wounded and more prompt aeromedical evacuation decreased the battlefield mortality rate even further [4]. In addition, concerted efforts to gather combat injury data led to increased insights into the management of injury and improvements in trauma care in the United States [5–7].

The impact of military outcome improvement has important civilian trauma implications. The impact of DeBakey's seminal paper is a prime example. The most significant impact of this work was the author's recognition that improvements in care could only take place with robust data collection and analysis. With this recognition, they established the first formal vascular injury registry and in doing so, established a heritage of military vascular surgeons who built upon their work, collected data, and improved the care of trauma patients in the combat and civilian environments. Carl Hughes captured Korean War vascular injury data as we progressed from routine ligation to vascular repair. Norman Rich created the Viet Nam Vascular Registry. These lessons learned were carried forward to the recent conflicts in Iraq and Afghanistan. Todd Rasmussen's development of the Balad Vascular Registry in Iraq led to the Global War on Terror Vascular Initiative and contributed significantly to the establishment of the Joint Theatre Trauma Registry, which is now the Department of Defense (DoD) Trauma Registry. In an attempt to bring these lessons learned to civilian vascular trauma, Joe Dubose and Todd Rasmussen have partnered with the American Association for the Surgery of Trauma (AAST) to establish the PROspective Observational Vascular Injury Treatment (PROOVIT) database to prospectively collect robust data on civilian vascular trauma. This process has proven to be the cornerstone of modern trauma system development and process improvement and historically validates the importance of the American College of Surgeons (ACS) trauma verification process.

4.2 What Is the Role of a Trauma System in Combat Injury Outcomes?

Trauma centers and trauma systems in the United States have had a remarkable impact on improving the outcomes of injured patients [1, 4, 8–20], reducing mortality by up to 15% in evolved systems. With the onset of the conflicts in Iraq and Afghanistan, a military trauma system was developed and modeled after the successes of civilian systems, but modified to address the realities of combat. The system implementation mandated emplacement of infrastructure elements, including a trauma registry, performance improvement capability, and research. Data derived from the trauma registry were responsible for the development of 40 evidence-based clinical practice guidelines utilized to optimize combat casualty care. The joint trauma system improved information dissemination and performance enhancement along the continuum of care from battlefield wounding through the entire evacuation process, resulting in the lowest fatality rate (10.4%) in the history of warfare [21]. Development of the trauma system has also minimized postinjury complications such as hypothermia and compartment syndrome [22].

DOI: 10.1201/9781003316800-4

Telecommunication and technology advances since the Vietnam War have enabled access to robust and improved battlefield combat casualty care data. Based on the military conflicts of antiquity, the epidemiology of combat injury has largely been documented by individuals, collated from medical administrative data, or by post hoc evaluation of data sources such as the Wound and Munitions Effectiveness Team data from Vietnam [23]. One central tenet evaluated by these previous data sets was the notion of combat survivability, and it noted that in the past century, 90% of battlefield casualties happened on the battlefield before ever reaching medical care. Data derived from these sources were consistently based on Level 4 and 5 evidence. However, this evidence alluded to the fact that prehospital injury care was a critical and perhaps underappreciated aspect of the trauma system [24–26]. Following the recent conflicts in Southeast Asia, collaborative investigations linking combat casualty care outcomes to postmortem evaluations have resulted in a large amount of detailed data. From an analysis of 558 combat casualties in a military medical treatment facility, 51.4% were considered to have potentially survivable injury, whereas 48.6% had nonsurvivable injury. The majority of the nonsurvivable injuries were related to traumatic brain injury. In those casualties with potentially survivable injury, the primary pathology resulting in death was hemorrhage (80%) [27]. In a successive review, 87% of combat casualty mortality occurred before reaching a medical treatment facility. Of this prehospital casualty mortality number, 24% was potentially survivable, the majority of which (90%) died due to secondary hemorrhage [28]. The value of such analyses is based on their potential to justify allocation of resources and training with a specific focus.

Perhaps the most important contribution of trauma systems is the impact on standardization of care. Howard and colleagues conducted a retrospective analysis of all available data compiled from DoD databases on all 56,763 U.S. military casualties injured in battle in Afghanistan and Iraq from October 1, 2001, through December 31, 2017 [29]. They analyzed trends in overall combat casualty statistics to assess interventions and to simulate how mortality rates would have changed had the interventions not occurred. They found that case fatality rate (CFR) decreased in Afghanistan (20.0% to 8.6%) and Iraq (20.4% to 10.1%) from early stages to later stages of the conflicts. Survival for critically injured casualties (Injury Severity Score, 25–75 [critical]) increased from 2.2% to 39.9% in Afghanistan and from 8.9% to 32.9% in Iraq. Simulations showed that without interventions assessed, CFR would likely have been higher in Afghanistan (15.6% estimated vs. 8.6% observed) and Iraq (16.3% estimated vs. 10.1% observed), equating to 3,672 additional deaths [29]. Systematic responses to changes in injury patterns facilitated the increased use of tourniquets. Trauma system maturation and development were directly responsible for the forward availability of blood component therapy. Systematic restructuring and standardization of casualty evacuation to the most appropriate facility significantly decreased transport times. Of these additional deaths, 1,623 (44.2%) were associated with the interventions studied: 474 deaths (12.9%) associated with the use of tourniquets, 873 (23.8%) with blood transfusion, and 275 (7.5%) with prehospital transport times <60 minutes [29].

RECOMMENDATIONS

1. Trauma systems are responsible for improvements in outcomes following combat injury and should be a key element of the battlefield medical system.
2. Most combat casualty death occurs prehospital. Hemorrhage is the most substantial etiology of potentially survivable battlefield injury death that validates prehospital care as a key entity in combat casualty care continuum.

Grade of recommendations: 1. B; 2. B.

4.3 What Are the Impacts of Damage Control Measures on the Morbidity and Mortality of Combat Injury?

The concept of damage control resuscitation provides for hemostatic and hypotensive resuscitation strategies in order to manage hemorrhage and coagulopathy after combat injury. This resuscitative principle was predicated upon the equally balanced ratio of packed red blood cells (PRBCs) to plasma, and later platelets. The ability to recognize patients who require damage control resuscitation has improved due to analysis of DOD trauma system data. Cap reported that in patients with serious injuries, the presence of three of the four features listed next indicates a 70% predicted risk of MT and 85% risk if all four are present:

- Systolic blood pressure <110 mmHg
- Heart rate >105 bpm
- Hematocrit <32%
- pH <7.25 [Cap]

Other risk factors associated with MT, or at least a need for aggressive resuscitation, include:

- Injury pattern (above-the-knee traumatic amputation especially if pelvic injury is present, multiamputation, clinically obvious penetrating injury to chest or abdomen)
- More than two regions positive on focused assessment with sonography for trauma (FAST) scan
- Lactate concentration on admission >2.5
- Admission international normalized ration (INR) ≥1.2–1.4
- BD >6 mEq/L [Cap]

In casualties requiring massive transfusion, Borgman et al. demonstrated a decrease in mortality from 60% to approximately 20% after combat injury [30]. Subsequent studies from the military injury population, including a more recent performance improvement analysis of the outcomes of damage control resuscitation techniques, have established that the evolution of the balanced ratio resuscitation principle has further reduced the battlefield mortality of casualties requiring massive transfusion to approximately 15% [31–33].

Damage control surgery techniques have dramatically altered the outcomes of troops injured on the battlefield. In the Vietnam War, in several case series, it was observed that temporizing surgical procedures demonstrated a survival advantage when compared to definitive surgical therapy [5]. A number of authors have also described the expansion of this lifesaving surgical practice to include thoracic, vascular, orthopedic, and neurosurgical procedures [34–38]. In one of the largest studies of damage control surgery in combat, prospective data were collected between April 2003 and January 2009 on 170 patients who underwent an exploratory laparotomy for injury sustained on the battlefield. Damage control laparotomy, defined as an abbreviated exploratory laparotomy resulting in an open abdomen, was performed on 86 (51%) patients. Analyses revealed blood transfusion as the most significant risk factor for damage control. Patients after damage control surgery had increased complications when compared to the non–damage control cohort, but despite this fact, survival between the groups was the same [39]. In a related study by Edens et al., 12,536 trauma admissions yielded 101 resuscitative thoracotomies (0.01%). In patients undergoing thoracotomy, penetrating trauma accounted for the majority of injuries (93%). There were no survivors after emergency department thoracotomy for blunt trauma ($N = 7$). Expanding the indication for resuscitative thoracotomy to abdomen (30%) and extremities (22%), 12% (12/101) of all patients requiring thoracotomy survived [40].

RECOMMENDATIONS

1. Damage control resuscitation has proven effective in minimizing mortality in high-acuity combat casualties and should be the resuscitative strategy of choice in casualties at risk for massive transfusion with the understanding that risk of complications may increase.

2. Damage control surgery techniques, including extraabdominal procedures, should be followed for severe battlefield injury with unstable physiology.

3. The indication for resuscitative thoracotomy should be considered in all patients in extremis, excluding isolated brain injury.

Grade of recommendations: 1. B; 2. C; 3. C.

4.4 What Are the Contemporary Techniques and Outcomes of Colon Surgery Performed on the Battlefield?

The practice of colon repair after injury has been intimately related to the lessons learned on the battlefield. In World War II,

the propensity for complications and attributable mortality from failed primary colon repair led to a mandate from the British Surgeon General to exteriorize all colon injuries [41]. This paradigm was pervasive for the subsequent 50 years of surgical history. Civilian trauma surgeons in the 1990s challenged the veracity of this dogmatic approach and found that primary repair of colon injury was both safe and effective [42–45]. However, there remains a controversy as to whether the ballistic energy of the combat injury makes this type of enteric injury a different entity from that of the civilian environment. Duncan et al. demonstrated an overall complication rate of 48% and a leak rate of 30% in a small population of combat injured marines with colon injury managed by primary repair [46]. In a separate analysis of casualties from contemporary contingency operations, diversion was compared to primary repair/primary anastomosis. Primary repair was associated with a leak rate of only 10%, but once again, there was an attendant bias to divert colon injuries distal to the splenic flexure and repair those that occurred more proximally in the colon. Diversion was associated with a significantly lower incidence of complication. However, despite the differences in complication between the treatment modalities, there was no attributable increase in sepsis or mortality in the patient population with complications [47]. In a series of 65 patients with colon injury, Vertrees et al. noted that primary repair was attempted in right-sided ($n = 18$, 60%), transverse ($n = 11$, 85%), and left-sided ($n = 9$, 38%) colon injuries. Delayed definitive treatment of colon injuries occurred in 42% of patients after damage control celiotomy. Failure of colon repair occurred in 16% of patients and was more likely with concomitant pancreatic, stomach, or renal injury. The associated complication rate for diversion was 30% but increased dramatically to 75% in patients with primary repair or delayed definitive reconstruction failure [48]. A more contemporary analysis of military casualties with colorectal injuries was notable for a colostomy rate of 37%. The diversion rate for rectal injuries was 56%, whereas left-sided and right-sided injuries were diverted at rates of 41% and 20%, respectively. ISS ≥16 and the requirement for a damage control surgical intervention were likewise associated with higher diversion rates [49].

RECOMMENDATIONS

1. In the combat environment, colon diversion should be strongly considered in patients with high-energy colon injury who would not tolerate complications such as anastomotic leak.

2. Reconstruction with resection and anastomosis may be considered at a higher echelon of care after an initial damage control procedure when there is no progression of injury beyond the previously resected margins in a fully resuscitated patient.

Grade of recommendation: 1. B; 2. B.

4.5 What Are the Contemporary Techniques and Outcomes of Vascular Surgery Performed on the Battlefield?

Advances in vascular surgery have been made in times of war. Although conceptualized for over two centuries, the first successful arterial repair for injury was done in 1896 by Murphy [50]. During World War I, German surgeons reported repair of more than 100 arterial injuries and pioneered autogenous reconstruction of injured vessels. However, the proclivity for mass casualty, significant soft tissue injury, and protracted transport times made routine reconstruction impractical, and subsequently ligation of vessels became the standard practice [50]. DeBakey reported 2,471 arterial injuries treated by ligation in World War II with a 49% amputation rate [50]. Hughes in Korea reported arterial repair as a standard of practice with a 13% amputation rate [51]. Similar success was demonstrated by Rich et al. from the conflict in Vietnam [6, 7, 50].

Improvements in the paradigm of casualty resuscitation during the current conflict have dramatically affected the capability of deployed surgeons to effectively perform vascular repair after injury on the battlefield. Damage control surgery techniques available to surgeons include temporary vascular shunts. Rasmussen et al. demonstrated that 57% of casualties had shunts placed at forward surgical facilities and 86% of proximal shunts were patent on admission to the combat support hospital. This patency of flow allowed for ongoing resuscitation in the context of a perfused extremity [52]. In two separate analyses, Fox et al. showed that damage control resuscitation and damage control surgery techniques applied in the context of vascular injury were associated with the ability to perform prolonged complex limb revascularizations with limb salvage rates of 95% [53, 54]. Clouse et al., Sohn et al., and Fox et al. independently demonstrated acute limb salvage rates for revascularization in theater of 92%–95% [55–57]. Late complications associated with revascularization included thrombosis, infection, and compartment syndrome [55]. The factor most significantly associated with post-revascularization morbidity was the use of prosthetic graft implants. In this population, the incidence of graft loss was 80% [55, 58].

The management of venous injuries on the battlefield included ligation in 63% and repair in 37%. All patients developed postoperative edema. Thrombosis of the repair was demonstrated in 16% of the repaired veins. There was no acute limb loss associated with venous ligation or venous graft failure [59]. In a study of 111 U.S. military casualties with limb salvage for extremity vascular injuries, 25% were revascularized by a primary repair or end anastomosis, 72% were revascularized by saphenovenous reconstruction, and 3% revascularized with prosthetic conduit. With a mean follow-up of 347 days, 86% of the vascular reconstructions remained patent, and the remaining 14% required a delayed amputation. Of this group, casualties with popliteal arterial injuries had the highest rate of amputation manifested by an amputation rate of 30% (7/23). The authors concluded that definitive vascular surgical intervention procedures performed at battlefield medical treatment facilities had excellent limb salvage results [60].

Proximity injury in the civilian penetrating extremity trauma population has been classically managed expectantly after studies by Thal and Frykberg and colleagues demonstrated no increased incidence of vascular lesions requiring surgical therapy [61–63]. However, the high-energy nature of combat wounds has led investigators to reevaluate this diagnostic/management paradigm in the proximity combat penetrating extremity population. In a study of 99 patients who underwent angiography after evacuation for wound proximity, 47% had vascular abnormalities noted on angiography. Two-thirds of this group had a normal physical examination. Of this population with an abnormal angiogram, 52% required operative intervention [64]. In a similar analysis by Fox et al., a similar study of cervical vascular proximity by computerized tomographic angiography detected occult injury in 30% of studies, of which 50% required interventional or surgical management [65].

RECOMMENDATIONS

1. Damage control techniques, including shunting, should be utilized to optimize survival and revascularization outcomes.

2. In the combat environment, arterial reconstruction can be performed with good long-term outcomes. Autogenous tissue optimizes outcome benefit potential.

3. In the context of battlefield venous injury, venous ligation is a safe and effective option for the management of venous vascular injury.

4. In the combat environment, proximity extremity injury should be evaluated by angiography to mitigate the risk of occult vascular injury.

Grade of recommendations: 1. B; 2. B; 3. B; 4. C.

4.6 What Are the Contemporary Techniques and Outcomes of Burn Surgery Performed on the Battlefield?

The complexity of burn management in the combat environment is manifest across the spectrum of medical care from point of injury through resuscitation, intensive care through the continuum, and ultimately definitive surgical care. Contemporary data from the battlefield demonstrate that 52%–63% of burn injuries are battle injuries [66, 67]. The majority of these burns are associated with explosive etiology. Early surgical care for burn injury is limited to escharotomy and debridement of devitalized tissue. The most challenging phase of the battlefield burn casualty is the intensive care evacuation process performed by the U.S. Air Force Critical Care Air Transport Team and the U.S. Army Burn Flight Team. Classically, burn resuscitation has been practiced on a paradigm based on weight and body surface area burned, according to the guidelines developed at the Parkland Memorial

Hospital and the Brooke Army Burn Center. Ennis et al. reported that a urine output–based resuscitation paradigm tracked by a flow sheet resulted in a decrease in the rate of resuscitation-associated abdominal compartment syndrome from 16% to 5% with an attendant decrease in mortality [68]. In a separate study of burn injuries from combat versus the civilian environment, Wolf and colleagues showed that the most important effectors of burn-related mortality were total body surface area (TBSA) burned, age ≥40 years, and the presence of inhalation injury [67]. The conflict in Southwest Asia presents an opportunity to develop contemporary resource requirements to manage combat-related burn injury. Military burn surgeons discovered a relationship of approximately one acute operative intervention required per 5% TBSA burn consisting of all operations performed during the acute and convalescent/reconstructive phases of care. Truncal burn involvement was demonstrated to be a significant determinant of acute surgical therapy, whereas upper extremity burns were a significant determinant of reconstruction surgical necessity [69].

RECOMMENDATIONS

1. Burn casualties should be resuscitated based on urine output.
2. Combat burn mortality is related to TBSA burn, age >40 years, and the presence of inhalation injury.
3. Combat burn surgical requirements can be predicted based on TBSA burn as well as burn location.

Grade of recommendations: 1. B; 2. B; 3. B.

4.7 What Are the Contemporary Techniques and Outcomes of Severe Brain Injury Sustained on the Battlefield?

The management of severe traumatic brain injury on the battlefield demonstrates many unique complexities in addition to the inherent difficulty of managing this severely injured patient population. In cases where the primary brain injury has already occurred and the injured tissue is not amenable to repair, and thus unrecoverable, the focus of managing these patients is directed toward minimizing secondary brain injury. Multiple circumstances, including a medically austere environment, limited critical care resources, and prolonged aeromedical evacuation, prompted a more aggressive surgical approach to limit secondary brain injury in severe traumatic brain injury incurred on the battlefield. DuBose et al. evaluated a cohort of isolated severe traumatic brain injury patients garnered from the Joint Theater Trauma Registry and compared with a case-matched cohort of like patients from the National Trauma Data Bank [70]. From this analysis, the cohort of military patients had a greater propensity to have surgical intervention (27.0%), including operative cranial decompression, lobectomy, or debridement. Most prominently, the data demonstrated substantial differences in intracranial pressure monitoring (13.8% military vs. 1.7% civilian) and craniectomy (8.8% military vs. 0.6% civilian). Most importantly, the survival was also significantly better among military casualties overall (92.3% military vs. 79% civilian), particularly after penetrating mechanisms of injury (94.4% military vs. 52.1% civilian). The survival benefit was even more pronounced with increasing severity of traumatic brain injury from Abbreviated Injury Scale (AIS) 3 to AIS 5 (Table 4.1).

TABLE 4.1

Summary of Evidence and Recommendations

Question	Answer	Level of Evidence	Grade of Recommendation	References
Do trauma systems improve outcome after combat injury?	Trauma systems are responsible for improvements in outcome after combat injury and should be a key element of the battlefield medical system.	2b	B	[8–23]
Where do combat casualty deaths occur?	Most combat casualty death occurs prehospital. Hemorrhage is the most substantial etiology of potentially survivable battlefield injury death, which validates prehospital care as a key entity in the combat casualty care continuum.	2c	B	[23–28]
Is damage control resuscitation effective in severely injured patients?	Damage control resuscitation has proven to be effective at minimizing mortality in high-acuity combat casualties and should be the resuscitative strategy of choice in casualties at risk for massive transfusion.	2b	B	[33–39]
When is fecal diversion necessary for colon injury incurred on the battlefield?	Colon diversion should be performed in patients with high-energy colon injury that would not tolerate complications.	2b	C	[42–49]
Is arterial reconstruction after combat vascular injury safe and effective?	In the combat environment, arterial reconstruction should be performed with good long-term outcomes. Autogenous tissue optimizes outcome benefit potential.	2b	B	[50–55]
Should diagnostic studies be done for vascular proximity?	Proximity is an indication for vascular interrogation, secondary to the high-energy mechanism and associated increase in vascular injury.	2b	C	[63–65]
How should burn casualties be resuscitated?	Urine output	2b	B	[66–67]
Is surgical management of battlefield brain injury warranted?	Aggressive surgical management of severe traumatic brain injury in combat improves mortality and is indicated after severe traumatic brain injury.	2b	C	[70]

RECOMMENDATIONS

1. Aggressive surgical management of severe traumatic brain injury in combat improves mortality.
2. Prompt and aggressive surgical management of traumatic brain injury is indicated.

Grade of recommendations: 1. C; 2. C.

Commentary on Military Injury Outcomes

Following WWII and the Korean conflict, surgical care focused on the treatment of shock, wounds, and the physiology of organ failure. During the conflict in Korea, a major problem was the high incidence of acute tubular necrosis due to shock. There was not much that could be done since dialysis was in the embryonic stages of providing support to the patient post injury. During the Vietnam War, patients were given excess amounts of fluid, which put them into acute respiratory distress syndrome (ARDS). During the next conflict, Desert Storm, multiple problems were identified. This led to meetings with the General Accounting Office. They documented some of the medical problems, including full medical army capability was not achieved. Additionally, the General Accounting Office stated there was needed improvement required in the Navy's wartime medical care program. The other problems involved the Air Force, particularly medical readiness. They also stated the readiness system used to regulate movement of patients did not function adequately. They documented a poor system of forming teams, which was problematic. Troop morale was a problem, and there were numerous units, after-action lessons learned, documented problems submitted had no action, or minimal action taken.

As the war progressed in Afghanistan, excellence in wound care was the norm. DuBose et al. did an excellent study on traumatic brain injuries sustained in combat operations. They compared the mortality outcomes and the lessons to be learned in contrast to civilian counterparts. The authors had access to the Joint Trauma Theater Registry (JTTR) and National Trauma Database (NTDB). There were 181 matched patients from the JTTR and an equal amount from the NTDB. They looked at any operative intervention, the number of patients that had intracranial pressure (ICP) monitoring, craniotomy, craniectomy, brain lobectomy, other brain incision, skull debridement, and brain debridement. The number of patients in the JTTR was impressive, and 39 patients had operative intervention, 25 patients had ICP monitoring, 12 had craniotomy, 16 had craniectomy, 4 had brain lobectomy, 2 had brain incisions, 14 had skull debridement, and 9 had brain debridement. The operative intervention in ICP monitoring received a p-value of less than 0.001. Craniectomy was done in 16 patients in the JTTR and only 1 in the NTDB.

Another table shows the comparison of mortality in JTTR and NTDB matched patients. The JTTR patients had an overall mortality of 7.7%, or 14 patients out of 181. The NTDB had a 21% mortality rate, or 38 out of 181 patients. The p-value was 0.001. The mortality of penetrating trauma was 5.6% in the JTTR and 38.1% in the NTDB. The p-value was 0.001. The most remarkable number is the mortality in the patients who had AIS Head 5, which was 68.6% in the NTDB and only 5.7% in the JTTR registry. The p-value was 0.001.

There are other issues of civilian neurosurgery, including manpower. There are approximately 3,000 neurosurgeons in the United States. There are 130–140 new trainees each year; however, this has increased slightly. About 250 neurosurgeons retire each year. Approximately 8 years is required to start new programs. Neurosurgeons limit their practice. Among these, 57% have eliminated pediatrics, 13% no longer do trauma, 11% no longer do craniotomies, and many neurosurgeons limit their practice to back surgery. During the 1996 match in neurosurgery, there were 140 residents, and in 2006, there were 165 residents.

Another issue is on-call pay in trauma hospitals. Neurosurgeons require \$4,000–\$7,000 a night, orthopedists get \$2,000–\$4,000 a night, and general surgeons get \$1,000–\$2,000 a night. Specialty surgeons operative cases per annum in level 1 hospital for neurosurgeon and orthopedics. In neurosurgery, there are 45 centers with an average of 33 patients during the year, with the range running from 0 to 105. Orthopedics has 33 centers. Their operative cases are 256 on average. The range is 12–754.

REFERENCES

1. Trunkey DD. History and development of trauma care in the United States. *Clin Orthop Relat Res.* 2000;*374*:36–46.
2. Trunkey DD. In search of solutions. *J Trauma.* 2002; *53(6)*:1189–1191.
3. DeBakey ME. History, the torch that illuminates: Lessons from military medicine. *Mil Med.* 1996;*161(12)*:711–716.
4. Hoff WS, Schwab CW. Trauma system development in North America. *Clin Orthop Relat Res.* 2004;*422*:17–22.
5. Rich NM. Vietnam missile wounds evaluated in 750 patients. *Mil Med.* 1968;*133(1)*:9–22.
6. Rich NM, Baugh JH, Hughes CW. Acute arterial injuries in Vietnam: 1,000 cases. *J Trauma.* 1970;*10(5)*:359–369.
7. Rich NM, Hughes CW. Vietnam vascular registry: A preliminary report. *Surgery.* 1969;*65(1)*:218–226.
8. Demetriades D, Kimbrell B, Salim A et al. Trauma deaths in a mature urban trauma system: Is "trimodal" distribution a valid concept? *J Am Coll Surg.* 2005;*201(3)*:343–348.
9. Jurkovich GJ, Mock C. Systematic review of trauma system effectiveness based on registry comparisons. *J Trauma.* 1999;*47(3 Suppl)*:S46–S55.
10. Mann NC. Assessing the effectiveness and optimal structure of trauma systems: A consensus among experts. *J Trauma.* 1999;*47(3 Suppl)*:S69–S74.
11. Mann NC, Mullins RJ. Research recommendations and proposed action items to facilitate trauma system implementation and evaluation. *J Trauma.* 1999;*47(3 Suppl)*: S75–S78.

12. Mann NC, Mullins RJ, MacKenzie Ef et al. Systematic review of published evidence regarding trauma system effectiveness. *J Trauma.* 1999;*47(3 Suppl)*:S25–S33.

13. Mullins RJ. A historical perspective of trauma system development in the United States. *J Trauma.* 1999;*47(3 Suppl)*: S8–S14.

14. Mullins RJ, Mann NC. Population-based research assessing the effectiveness of trauma systems. *J Trauma.* 1999; *47(3 Suppl)*:S59–S66.

15. Mullins RJ, Mann NC. Introduction to the academic symposium to evaluate evidence regarding the efficacy of trauma systems. *J Trauma.* 1999;*47(3 Suppl)*:S3–S7.

16. Mullins RJ, Veum-Stone J, Hedges JR et al. Influence of a statewide trauma system on location of hospitalization and outcome of injured patients. *J Trauma.* 1996;*40(4)*:536–545; discussion 545–546.

17. Nathens AB, Jurkovich GJ, Rivara FP et al. Effectiveness of state trauma systems in reducing injury-related mortality: A national evaluation. *J Trauma.* 2000;*48(1)*:25–30; discussion 30–31.

18. O'Keefe GE, Jurkovich GJ, Copass M et al. Ten-year trend in survival and resource utilization at a Level I trauma center. *Ann Surg.* 1999;*229(3)*:409–415.

19. Trunkey DD. Trauma care systems. *Emerg Med Clin North Am.* 1984;*2(4)*:913–922.

20. West JG, Williams MJ, Trunkey DD et al. Trauma systems: Current status—Future challenges. *JAMA.* 1988;*259(24)*: 3597–3600.

21. Eastridge BJ, Jenkins D, Flaherty S et al. Trauma system development in a theater of war: Experiences from Operation Iraqi Freedom and Operation Enduring Freedom. *J Trauma.* 2006;*61(6)*:1366–1372; discussion 1372–1373.

22. Palm K, Apodaca A, Spencer D, Costanzo G, Bailey J, Fortuna G, Blackbourne LH, Spott MA, Eastridge BJ. Evaluation of military trauma system practices related to complications after injury. *J Trauma Acute Care Surg.* December 2012;*73(6 Suppl 5)*:S465–S471.

23. Carey ME. Learning from traditional combat mortality and morbidity data used in the evaluation of combat medical care. *Mil Med.* 1987;*152(1)*:6–13.

24. Bellamy RF, Maningas PA, Vayer JS. Epidemiology of trauma: Military experience. *Ann Emerg Med.* 1986;*15(12)*: 1384–1388.

25. Bellamy RF. The causes of death in conventional land warfare: Imply cations for combat casualty care research. *Mil Med.* 1984;*149(2)*:55–62.

26. Champion HR, Holcomb JB, Lawnick MM et al. Improved characterization of combat injury. *J Trauma.* 2010;*68(5)*: 1139–1150.

27. Eastridge BJ, Hardin M, Cantrell J et al. Died of Wounds (DOW): Cause of death after battlefield injury. *J Trauma.* July 2011;*71*:S4–S8.

28. Eastridge BJ, Mabry RL, Seguin P et al. Death on the battlefield (2001–2011): Implications for the future of combat casualty care. *J Trauma Acute Care Surg.* December 2012; *73(6 Suppl 5)*:S431–S437.

29. Howard JT, Kotwal RS, Stern CA et al. Use of combat casualty care data to assess the US Military trauma system during Afghanistan and Iraq conflicts, 2001–2017. *JAMA Surg.* March 2019;*154(7)*:600–608.

30. Borgman MA, Spinella PC, Perkins JG, Grathwohl KW, Repine T, Beekley AC, Sebesta J, Jenkins D, Wade CE, Holcomb JB. The ratio of blood products transfused affects mortality in patients receiving massive transfusions at a combat support hospital. *J Trauma.* October 2007;*63(4)*:805–813.

31. Spinella PC, Perkins JG, Grathwohl KW et al. Effect of plasma and red blood cell transfusions on survival in patients with combat related traumatic injuries. *J Trauma.* 2008;*64(2 Suppl)*:S69–S77; discussion S77–S78.

32. Palm K, Apodaca A, Spencer D, Costanzo G, Bailey J, Blackbourne LH, Spott MA, Eastridge BJ. Evaluation of military trauma system practices related to damage control resuscitation. *J Trauma Acute Care Surg.* December 2012;*73(6 Suppl 5)*:S459–S464.

33. Langan NR, Eckert M, Martin MJ. Changing patterns of in hospital deaths following implementation of damage control resuscitation practices in US forward military treatment facilities. *JAMA Surg.* September 2014;*149(9)*:904–912.

34. Johnson JW, Gracias VH, Reilly PM et al. Evolution in damage control for exsanguinating penetrating abdominal injury. *J Trauma.* 2001;*51(2)*:261–269; discussion 269–271.

35. Rotondo MF, Bard MR. Damage control surgery for thoracic injuries. *Injury.* 2004;*35(7)*:649–654.

36. Rotondo MF, Schwab CW, McGonigal MD et al. 'Damage control': An approach for improved survival in exsanguinating penetrating abdominal injury. *J Trauma.* 1993;*35(3)*:375–382; discussion 382–383.

37. Rotondo MF, Zonies DH. The damage control sequence and underlying logic. *Surg Clin North Am.* 1997;*77(4)*:761–777.

38. Shapiro MB, Jenkins DH, Schwab CW et al. Damage control: Collective review. *J Trauma.* 2000;*49(5)*:969–978.

39. Bograd B, Rodriguez C, Amdur R et al. Use of damage control and the open abdomen in combat. *Am Surg.* August 2013;*79(8)*:747–753.

40. Edens J, Beekley A, Chung KK et al. Long-term outcomes after combat casualty emergency department thoracotomy. *J Am Coll Surg.* August 2009;*209(2)*:188–197.

41. Imes PR. The emergency management of abdominal trauma. *Surg Clin North Am.* 1956:1289–1294.

42. George SM, Jr, Fabian TC, Mangiante EC. Colon trauma: Further support for primary repair. *Am J Surg.* 1988;*156(1)*:16–20.

43. Fabian TC. Infection in penetrating abdominal trauma: Risk factors and preventive antibiotics. *Am Surg.* 2002;*68(1)*:29–35.

44. Stone HH, Fabian TC. Management of perforating colon trauma: Randomization between primary closure and exteriorization. *Ann Surg.* 1979;*190(4)*:430–436.

45. Croce MA, Fabian TC, Mangiante EC. Penetrating colon trauma. *J Tenn Med Assoc.* 1986;*79(11)*:706–707.

46. Duncan JE, Corwin CH, Sweeney WB et al. Management of colorectal injuries during Operation Iraqi Freedom: Patterns of stoma usage. *J Trauma.* 2008;*64(4)*:1043–1047.

47. Steele SR, Wolcott KE, Mullenix PS et al. Colon and rectal injuries during operation Iraqi Freedom: Are there any changing trends in management or outcome? *Dis Colon Rectum.* 2007;*50(6)*:870–877.

48. Vertrees A, Wakefield M, Pickett C et al. Outcomes of primary repair and primary anastomosis in war-related colon injuries. *J Trauma.* May 2009;*66(5)*:1286–1291; discussion 1291–1293.

49. Watson JD, Aden JK, Engel JE, Rasmussen TE, Glasgow SC. Risk factors for colostomy in military colorectal trauma: A review of 867 patients. *Surgery*. June 2014;*155(6)*: 1052–1061.

50. Rich NM, Rhee P. An historical tour of vascular injury management: From its inception to the new millennium. *Surg Clin North Am*. 2001;*81(6)*:1199–1215.

51. Hughes CW. The primary repair of wounds of major arteries; an analysis of experience in Korea in 1953. *Ann Surg*. 1955;*141(3)*:297–303.

52. Rasmussen TE, Clouse WD, Jenkins DH et al. The use of temporary vascular shunts as a damage control adjunct in the management of wartime vascular injury. *J Trauma*. 2006;*61(1)*:8–12; discussion 12–15.

53. Fox CJ, Gillespie DL, Cox ED et al. Damage control resuscitation for vascular surgery in a combat support hospital. *J Trauma*. 2008;*65(1)*:1–9.

54. Fox CJ, Gillespie DL, Cox ED et al. The effectiveness of a damage control resuscitation strategy for vascular injury in a combat support hospital: Results of a case control study. *J Trauma*. 2008;*64(2 Suppl)*:S99–S106; discussion S106–S107.

55. Fox CJ, Gillespie DL, O'Donnell SD et al. Contemporary management of wartime vascular trauma. *J Vasc Surg*. 2005;*41(4)*:638–644.

56. Clouse WD, Rasmussen TE, Peck MA et al. In-theater management of vascular injury: 2 years of the Balad vascular registry. *J Am Coll Surg*. 2007;*204(4)*:625–632.

57. Sohn VY, Arthurs ZM, Herbert GS et al. Demographics, treatment, and early outcomes in penetrating vascular combat trauma. *Arch Surg*. 2008;*143(8)*:783–787.

58. Rasmussen TE, Clouse WD, Jenkins DH et al. Echelons of care and the management of wartime vascular injury: A report from the 332nd EMDG/Air Force Theater Hospital, Balad Air Base, Iraq. *Perspect Vasc Surg Endovasc Ther*. 2006;*18(2)*:91–99.

59. Quan RW, Gillespie DL, Stuart RP et al. The effect of vein repair on the risk of venous thromboembolic events: A review of more than 100 traumatic military venous injuries. *J Vasc Surg*. 2008;*47(3)*:571–577.

60. Dua A, Patel B, Kragh JF, Jr, Holcomb JB, Fox CJ. Long-term follow-up and amputation-free survival in 497 casualties with combat-related vascular injuries and damage-control resuscitation. *J Trauma Acute Care Surg*. December 2012;*73(6)*:1517–1524.

61. Dennis JW, Frykberg ER, Crump JM et al. New perspectives on the management of penetrating trauma in proximity to major limb arteries. *J Vasc Surg*. 1990;*11(1)*:84–92; discussion 92–93.

62. Frykberg ER, Crump JM, Vines FS et al. A reassessment of the role of arteriography in penetrating proximity extremity trauma: A prospective study. *J Trauma*. 1989;*29(8)*: 1041–1050; discussion 1050–1052.

63. Francis H 3rd, Thal ER, Weigelt JA et al. Vascular proximity: Is it a valid indication for arteriography in asymptomatic patients? *J Trauma*. 1991;*31(4)*:512–514.

64. Johnson ON 3rd, Fox CJ, White P et al. Physical exam and occult post-traumatic vascular lesions: Implications for the evaluation and management of arterial injuries in modern warfare in the endovascular era. *J Cardiovasc Surg (Torino)*. 2007;*48(5)*:581–586.

65. Fox CJ, Gillespie DL, Neber MA et al. Delayed evaluation of combat-related penetrating neck trauma. *J Vasc Surg*. 2006;*44(1)*:86–93.

66. Kauvar DS, Wolf SE, Wade CE et al. Burns sustained in combat explosions in Operations Iraqi and Enduring Freedom (OIF/OEF explosion burns). *Burns*. 2006;*32(7)*: 853–857.

67. Wolf SE, Wolf SE, Wade CE et al. Comparison between civilian burns and combat burns from Operation Iraqi Freedom and Operation Enduring Freedom. *Ann Surg*. 2006;*243(6)*:786–792; discussion 792–795.

68. Ennis JL, Chung KK, Renz EM et al. Joint theater trauma system implementation of burn resuscitation guidelines improves outcomes in severely burned military casualties. *J Trauma*. 2008;*64(2 Suppl)*:S146–S151; discussion S151–S152.

69. Chan RK, Aden J Wu, Hale RG, Renz EM, Wolf SE. Operative utilization following severe combat-related burns. *J Burn Care Res*. 2015 March–April;*36(2)*:287–296.

70. DuBose JJ, Barmparas G, Inaba K, Stein DM, Scalea T, Cancio LC, Cole J, Eastridge B, Blackbourne L. Isolated severe traumatic brain injuries sustained during combat operations: Demographics, mortality outcomes, and lessons to be learned from contrasts to civilian counterparts. *J Trauma*. January 2011;*70(1)*:11–16; discussion 16–18.

5

Traumatized Airway

Edgar J. Pierre, Ethan Levitch, Jakob Oury, and David Holzer

5.1 Introduction

Airway management is of paramount importance in caring for the trauma patient. The primary goals of airway intervention are to relieve or prevent airway obstruction, secure the unprotected airway from aspiration, provide adequate gas exchange, and maintain cervical spine stabilization. Acute airway trauma is a rare yet potentially lethal injury that is often difficult to diagnose. The recent literature estimates the incidence of airway trauma is less than 0.1% of all trauma patients; however, the mortality of these injuries is high—up to 20% for blunt trauma and up to 40% for penetrating trauma [1, 2]. Long-term outcomes are usually favorable if the patient is treated within 24 hours of presentation, but more than 60% of patients have other associated injuries, making diagnosis and management problematic [1, 3, 4].

Gaining control of the traumatized airway is the ultimate test of the provider's adeptness and clinical acumen. When the airway is secured, it is important to complete a diagnostic workup to determine the severity of the injury, as structures that can potentially be damaged after trauma to the face and neck include the upper airway, vascular structures, cervical spine, and aerodigestive tract [1]. Once the extent of the injury is determined, the choice remains whether to treat the injury conservatively or surgically.

Presented first are some of the key questions a provider must understand to properly manage the airway of these patients. Addressed next is a discussion directed at successfully navigating the challenge of airway management in the presence of acute airway trauma.

5.2 What Is the Optimal Prehospital Airway?

Endotracheal intubation remains the gold standard for securing the airway in a trauma patient. However, endotracheal intubation is not without its risks, and therefore should be performed in controlled settings by the most experienced personnel if possible [2]. Intubation in the prehospital setting, however, can rarely be performed under these conditions.

Prehospital intubation (PHI) has failed to show mortality benefits in several studies [5–8]. This also holds for additional advanced airway devices. Though not specific to trauma patients, several studies involving patients with cardiac emergencies have documented worse neurologic outcomes and worse survival rates when advanced airway management was employed in the prehospital setting compared to bag-valve-mask ventilation [9, 10]. A meta-analysis comparing PHI and emergency department intubation in trauma patients found significantly increased mortality in cases where PHI was performed [11]. This, combined with the high heterogeneity of training in advanced airway management among prehospital providers and the variation of usage of prehospital neuromuscular blockade, suggests that the optimal prehospital airway is effective ventilation with a bag-valve-mask. Only if ventilation with a bag-valve-mask is unsuccessful should attempts at endotracheal intubation or placement of advanced airway devices be made.

> **RECOMMENDATION**
>
> The optimal prehospital airway is effective ventilation with a bag-valve-mask.
>
> Grade of recommendation: B.

5.3 What Is the Role of Prehospital Intubation?

Data in the literature regarding the safety and efficacy of PHI are almost entirely derived from retrospective and descriptive studies, as randomization and standardization of such an intervention are nearly impossible to achieve. Studies from the United States suggest a success rate of prehospital endotracheal intubation of 86–90%, but it can be as low as 50% when performed by rescuers who don't often perform the procedure [7]. Additionally, PHI has largely not been shown to improve outcomes in the literature: In a prospective observational study at a large Level 1 trauma center study by Cobas et al., there was a 31% incidence of failed PHI and no difference in mortality between patients who were properly intubated and those who were not [7]. Furthermore, PHI has been associated with increased mortality both in patients with traumatic brain injury and in patients with penetrating trauma [5, 6]. In another retrospective study by Stockinger et al., trauma patients who underwent PHI had increased mortality compared to those ventilated with a bag-valve-mask.

> **RECOMMENDATION**
>
> Prehospital endotracheal intubation in the United States should be limited to experienced providers only if ventilation with a bag-valve-mask is unsuccessful.
>
> Grade of recommendation: B.

DOI: 10.1201/9781003316800-5

5.4 What Is the Optimal Size Endotracheal Tube?

In 1928, Magill recommended the placement of "the largest endotracheal tube which the larynx will comfortably accommodate" [12]. As recently as the 1980s, it was common to place 9- or even 10-mm tubes for men and 8-mm tubes for women [13]. Over recent years there has been a trend to place increasingly smaller tubes, primarily because of data correlating larger tube sizes with increased incidence of sore throat as well as more serious, though rare complications like airway stenosis [14, 15]. As such, major anesthesiology textbooks now recommend the placement of an 8- to 9-mm tube for men and a 7- to 8- mm tube for women [16, 17]. Still, there are no widely accepted evidence-based guidelines for endotracheal tube size selection in adults. In a prospective cross-sectional study by Coordes et al., they evaluated tracheal morphometry of patients by CT scan and subsequently made the recommendation of an 8-mm tube for an average-height man and a 7-mm tube for an average-height woman [18]. Growing evidence also suggests the need for uniform tube labeling based on biometric data like height and BMI [19, 20].

In trauma patients, providers may be quick to select a smaller tube, as visualization of the larynx while using a smaller tube is often described as subjectively better [21]. However, an important consideration should be given to trauma patients often having prolonged ICU stays. In this regard, a larger tube size may be beneficial for two important reasons: First, it allows for decreased work of breathing and potential resultant ease with which to wean from a ventilator [22]. Second, a larger tube size allows for better pulmonary toilet and easier insertion of a fiberoptic bronchoscope, both critical aspects of the care of trauma and burn patients [13]. For this reason, the authors recommend that a half-size increase in tube size be considered for trauma patients for whom a prolonged ICU stay is anticipated.

In children, the selection of endotracheal tube size is far more complex but equally lacking in evidence-based guidelines. It is often taught that the internal diameter of the appropriately sized endotracheal tube will roughly approximate the size of the child's little finger, but this estimation is frequently difficult and unreliable [23]. Age-based formulas are frequently utilized, but endotracheal tube size selection is more reliably based on a child's body length, and length-based resuscitation tapes (like the Broselow tape) are helpful for children up to 35 kg [24]. Uncuffed endotracheal tubes were advised over cuffed tubes at one time, yet cuffed tubes are equally safe for infants beyond the newborn period and in children [25, 26].

RECOMMENDATION

The optimal-sized endotracheal tube varies based on experience and convention, ranging from an 8-mm to 9-mm tube for men, a 7-mm to 8-mm tube for women, and a length-based size selection for children.

Grade of recommendation: C.

5.5 What Medications Should Be Used for Rapid Sequence Intubation?

Rapid sequence intubation (RSI) is the procedure of choice for securing the airway in trauma patients. In the Guidelines for Emergency Tracheal Intubation Immediately after Traumatic Injury by Dunham et al., it is recommended that if orotracheal intubation is required and the patient's jaws are not flaccid, a drug regimen should be administered to accomplish the following objectives: Neuromuscular paralysis, sedation as needed, maintain hemodynamic stability, prevent intracranial hypertension, prevent vomiting, and prevent intraocular content extrusion [27]. The specific drug regimen selected, however, is highly dependent on the patient's particular injuries and clinical condition and remains a topic of continued debate.

Commonly selected induction agents for trauma patients included etomidate and ketamine for their favorable hemodynamic effects. In a randomized controlled trial by Jabre et al., there was no difference in mortality found between the use of etomidate and ketamine for intubation of acutely ill patients [28]. The main concern with the usage of etomidate is that it can produce adrenal insufficiency; however, studies have failed to conclusively prove that this increases morbidity or mortality [28–30]. Ketamine has generally been avoided in patients with suspected traumatic brain injury due to concern that it increases intracranial pressure, but that fact remains controversial, and some newer data suggest ketamine may even be neuroprotective [31].

Commonly selected paralytic agents include rocuronium and succinylcholine due to their rapid onset of action. In a systematic review by Tran et al., succinylcholine was found to be clinically superior as it produced excellent intubating conditions with a slightly faster onset of action [32]. However, important contraindications to succinylcholine include severe burn or *crush* injuries beyond 48 hours, ocular injury, and spinal cord injury.

RECOMMENDATION

For RSI, a drug regimen should be administered to accomplish the following objectives: Neuromuscular paralysis, sedation as needed, maintaining hemodynamic stability, preventing intracranial hypertension, preventing vomiting, and preventing intraocular content extrusion.

Grade of recommendation: C.

5.6 What Airway Adjuncts Should Be Considered If Unable to Intubate?

As per the American Society of Anesthesiologists Practice Guidelines for the Management of a Difficult Airway, if a patient cannot be intubated (and cannot be adequately ventilated by a face mask), a supraglottic airway (SGA) is indicated [33]. The best-studied and most often utilized is the laryngeal mask airway (LMA). If ventilation with the LMA is adequate, the provider has time and options to consider alternative methods of intubation, including but not limited to intubating stylets/exchange catheters, utilizing SGAs as a conduit to intubation, light wands, or fiberoptic intubation. If ventilation with the LMA is inadequate, this places a provider on the emergency arm of the pathway. In a suggested modified algorithm for the trauma patient, additional adjuncts to be considered if ventilation with an LMA is inadequate include assisted laryngoscopy, alternative laryngoscope blades, combined techniques, intubating SGA, flexible bronchoscopy, introducer, and lighted stylet or light wand [33]. Selection between these methods of emergency noninvasive ventilation is far more controversial, and if these methods fail, steps must be taken to obtain an emergency invasive airway. Emergency invasive airway techniques include surgical cricothyrotomy, needle cricothyrotomy with a pressure-regulated device, large-bore cannula cricothyrotomy, or surgical tracheostomy [33].

RECOMMENDATION

If unable to intubate, a supraglottic airway should be placed.

Grade of recommendation: C.

5.7 What Is the Role of Video Laryngoscopy?

Compared with direct laryngoscopy, video laryngoscopy has been associated with improved laryngeal views, a higher frequency of successful intubations, fewer intubation maneuvers, reduced rates of hypoxemic events, and a higher frequency of first-attempt intubations. There was no difference in time to intubation, airway trauma, lip/gum trauma, or dental trauma. In randomized control trials, no significant differences were found comparing channel-guided to non-channel-guided video laryngoscopes as well as hyperangulated to nonangulated video laryngoscopes. As such, video laryngoscopy should be considered a useful initial approach to intubation in a predicted difficult airway or as an adjunct if an initial intubation attempt by direct laryngoscopy is unsuccessful [33, 34].

RECOMMENDATION

Video laryngoscopy likely provides a safer risk profile compared to direct laryngoscopy and can be considered a useful approach to intubation in a predicted difficult airway or as an adjunct if an initial trial intubation attempt by direct laryngoscopy fails.

Grade of recommendation: B.

5.8 What Is the Role of Cricothyroidotomy?

When assessing difficult airway scenarios, it is essential to have a systematic approach to avoid significant morbidity and mortality. The American Society of Anesthesiologists has provided the framework in their algorithm to manage the unanticipated difficult airway [33]. As one progresses to the end of the algorithm, the "can't intubate can't ventilate" scenario recommends the use of invasive airway access via cricothyroidotomy. However, the incidence of this scenario has decreased due to the improvements made in noninvasive emergency airway techniques [35].

To determine the best methodology to obtain airway access invasively, several studies have required the use of cadaver models to assess the efficacy, complications, overall ease, and procedural speed when comparing surgical vs. percutaneous techniques [36]. In a study comparing the surgical method, percutaneous Seldinger, and percutaneous trocar methods, the success rate for surgical cricothyrotomy (95%) was greater than that of the Seldinger (50%) and trocar (55%) cricothyrotomy methods. Percutaneous methods are often associated with bloody airways that make for a bad view. One study was able to show that the use of ultrasound guidance in percutaneous cricothyrotomy significantly increased success rates. However, it did increase the time of the procedure (>3 minutes), which might prove unfeasible in emergency management. It is worth noting that both preceding studies were performed with inexperienced subjects following training. In another study comparing the percutaneous vs. open technique among emergency room attending and resident physicians, the results showed no significant differences other than the attending's ability to perform both procedures more quickly than the residents. The complication rates, ease of performance, and times were not significantly different [37]. Ultimately, an individual provider's level of experience with a given technique has shown to be the determining factor as to the speed and efficacy at which airway access is secured.

RECOMMENDATION

If a patient cannot be intubated or ventilated by other measures, surgical airway access is indicated via cricothyroidotomy.

Grade of recommendation: B.

5.9 What Is the Best Strategy for Establishing an Emergency Airway in Children?

In the assessment of the emergency airway in children, it is vital to be aware of the unique challenges present in pediatric patients. A prominent occiput leaves the neck in a slightly flexed position when supine. Additionally, the presence of a large, floppy epiglottis; large tonsils; and large tongue relative to the size of the oral cavity impedes the visualization of the deeper airway during direct laryngoscopy [38]. The position of the larynx in children is also more cephalad and anterior when compared to adults, causing a more acute angle between the epiglottis and the base of the tongue. Once the trachea and vocal cords have been visualized and the endotracheal tube has been placed, it is imperative to recognize that children's tracheas are narrow and short compared to adults, leading to a greater risk of endobronchial intubations or inadvertent extubations [39].

From a physiologic standpoint, children have faster respiratory rates, which reduces the time available to complete RSI and avoid hypoxemia. Considering the oxyhemoglobin dissociation curve, it is ideal to achieve 100% oxyhemoglobin saturation during the preoxygenation phase to maximize the time to perform laryngoscopy. Efforts should be halted after saturation declines to 90% to avoid a falloff in the steep range of the oxyhemoglobin dissociation curve, which would result in critical desaturation [40, 41].

RECOMMENDATION

The best strategy for emergency airway management in children is RSI.

Grade of recommendation: B.

5.10 How Should One Evaluate for Airway Injury?

The most sensitive way to diagnose airway injury is by history and physical exam. Signs and symptoms vary widely and often do not manifest for hours, particularly in blunt trauma [42]. In a study by Randall et al., the most common signs and symptoms found in laryngotracheal trauma include airway obstruction, subcutaneous emphysema, stridor, hoarseness, and odynophagia [1]. In the case of penetrating trauma, blood and wounds will be visible. It is worth noting, however, that 15% of patients had no presenting indicator of airway injury, thus making diagnosis more difficult [43]. Undetected blunt trauma can acutely result in pneumomediastinum or pneumothorax, while later complications may include pneumonitis, atelectasis, and tracheoesophageal fistula [44]. If the patient is stable and tracheal injury is suspected, the airway should be evaluated with a fiberoptic bronchoscope to identify the extent of the injury. In addition, CT is a useful diagnostic tool in a patient with severe blunt force trauma to the anterior neck, unknown extent of injury, or physical exam findings obscuring examination (such as hematoma or edema) [1].

In a patient who presents with impending respiratory collapse, securing the airway is the priority. After the airway is secured (generally defined as a tube present in the trachea with the cuff inflated distal to the injury), further diagnostic workup can be initiated [43]. Other than the aforementioned flexible fiberoptic bronchoscopy and CT, other diagnostic modalities include chest and lateral neck radiographs initially, then esophagogastroduodenoscopy, and barium swallow to evaluate for aerodigestive injuries [45, 46]. CT with angiography protocol (CTA) can provide information regarding the spine, airway, soft tissue of the neck, and most importantly, the proximity of injury to vascular structures, identifying with about a 99% sensitivity the presence of dissection, pseudoaneurysm, occlusion, and transection.

RECOMMENDATION

History and physical exam are the first step in the evaluation of a traumatic airway, but should be used in conjunction with imaging studies, as some patients present with an injury out of proportion to their symptoms.

Grade of recommendation: C.

5.11 How Does One Secure the Airway in the Setting of Airway Trauma?

Securing the airway in the face of airway trauma poses an enormous challenge and may vary greatly depending on the type of injury. Injuries that may compromise the airway include maxillofacial trauma, penetrating neck injuries, and blunt neck injuries, though there is often considerable overlap [46]. Patients who have sustained airway injury often prefer to take the sitting position, as it is easier for the patients to maintain a patent airway seated as opposed to the supine position. Assuming no absolute contraindications to this position exist, these patients should be allowed and encouraged to remain seated until the trauma team is ready to manage their airways definitively.

Facial trauma tends to be obvious, most often presenting with noticeable bleeding or facial distortion. However, sometimes mild-appearing soft tissue injuries will mask more severe internal injuries [45]. In fact, even a patient able to speak requires regular reassessment, as the status can deteriorate quickly [47]. Complex facial injuries pose an incredible risk for airway obstruction, posttraumatic hemorrhage, and edema. Therefore, immediate intubation is recommended to avoid unpredictable loss of the airway. In most trauma cases, endotracheal intubation is ideal. However, it is contraindicated in maxillofacial trauma due to interference with surgical repair. In the case of lower facial fracture, laryngopharynx obstruction, or failure to perform endotracheal intubation, an emergency tracheostomy is recommended [48]. Cricothyroidotomy is more rapid than a tracheostomy and can be performed in prehospital settings if necessary.

Penetrating neck injuries provide their challenges. In one study by Bhojani et al., the most common causes of penetrating trauma to the airway were gunshot wounds and stab wounds. About half of the patients in this study required emergency airways, about 0.1% of which were surgical airways [46]. Due to the extreme urgency of many penetrating neck injuries, assessment of the airway should be almost entirely clinical. Common findings include cervical ecchymoses or hematomas, stridor, wheezing, and hemoptysis. RSI with direct laryngoscopy and manual in-line stabilization remains the intubation method of choice, often utilized with the aid of a fiberoptic bronchoscope to evaluate the airway for signs of injury [2]. Sometimes it is easier and safer to intubate through an already existing neck wound, rather than creating another incision. However, due to the potential for creating or worsening a false lumen, confirmation of tracheal placement with fiberoptic bronchoscopy is mandatory after this maneuver. The caveat is that a prolonged struggle to intubate may be a misuse of the Golden Hour, compromising the patient's respiratory status and elevating intracranial pressure. Cricothyroidotomy is a useful alternative that Pierre et al. suggest would result in improved outcomes due to less hypoxia.

In contrast, motor vehicle collisions remain the most common cause of blunt airway injury. Blunt force trauma injuries to the trachea are less common, due in part to the flexibility of the tracheal cartilage and protection by the surrounding bony structures. However, many vital structures are associated with the trachea, so injuries present in this area are often severe. Common symptoms of pending respiratory compromise from blunt trauma include pain when swallowing or rotating the neck, subcutaneous emphysema, severe bruising of the chest and neck, hemoptysis, dyspnea that worsens with neck extension, and hoarseness. Signs and symptoms indicative of a vascular injury include a bruit or thrill, an expanding or pulsatile hematoma or hemorrhage, and a lack of a pulse. These symptoms should prompt immediate definitive diagnostic testing. Additionally, multiple injuries may obscure the presentation of airway injuries, as about 95% of patients with blunt vascular injuries of the neck have a concomitant major thoracic injury or a Glasgow Coma Score (GCS) score less than 9 [49]. If there is any symptomatology of respiratory distress, the patient can deteriorate quickly as the injury progresses, so it is important to secure the airway early. Orotracheal intubation may be problematic in laryngeal fractures, as the endotracheal tube could extend the injury, create a false passage, or disrupt what little anatomy remains intact [45]. In addition, laryngoscopy can be hindered by the presence of a cervical collar in the setting of a suspected spine injury, but this difficulty can be attenuated with manual in-line stabilization. In one study, about 50% of patients who suffered blunt airway injury required a surgical airway, so a surgical airway may be required in these patients [43]. Once the airway is secured and the patient is stable, the patient can undergo diagnostic tests to determine the extent of the injury, and decisions can be made regarding management. Unstable patients are taken directly to the operating room for surgical exploration of their injuries.

RECOMMENDATION

Oral intubation, tracheostomy, or cricothyroidotomy should be performed early in patients with airway trauma. Stable patients should be evaluated with imaging studies to determine the extent of the injury, while unstable patients should be taken immediately to the operating room for surgical exploration.

Grade of recommendation: D.

5.12 Summary

In addition to mastery of basic airway management, the key to improving outcomes in traumatic airway injury is early recognition and intervention, which is complicated by the scarcity of these injuries at most medical centers. Unstable patients should have their airways secured by the most experienced airway personnel available, with surgical backup immediately available in case a surgical airway is needed. Stable patients should have their airways secured and undergo a diagnostic evaluation to determine the safest definitive treatment, which is surgical the majority of the time.

Question	Answer	Levels of Evidence	Strength of Recommendation	References
What is the optimal prehospital airway?	The optimal prehospital airway is effective ventilation with a bag-valve-mask.	IIb	B	[2, 5–11]
What is the role of prehospital intubation?	Prehospital endotracheal intubation in the United States should be limited to experienced providers only if ventilation with a bag-valve-mask is unsuccessful.	IIc	B	[5–7]
What is the optimal-sized endotracheal tube?	The optimal-sized endotracheal tube varies based on experience and convention, ranging from an 8-mm to 9-mm tube for men, a 7-mm to 8-mm tube for women, and a length-based size selection for children.	IIIb, IV	C	[12–26]
What medications should be used for rapid sequence intubation?	For rapid sequence intubation, a drug regimen should be administered to accomplish the following objectives: Neuromuscular paralysis, sedation as needed, maintaining hemodynamic stability, preventing intracranial hypertension, preventing vomiting, and preventing intraocular content extrusion.	IIIa	C	[27–32]
What airway adjuncts should be considered if unable to intubate?	If unable to intubate, a supraglottic airway should be placed.	IIIa	C	[33]
What is the role of video laryngoscopy?	Compared with direct laryngoscopy, video laryngoscopy has been associated with improved laryngeal views, a higher frequency of successful intubations, and a higher frequency of first-attempt intubations.	IIb	B	[33–34]
What is the role of cricothyroidotomy?	If a patient cannot be intubated or ventilated, surgical airway access via cricothyroidotomy is indicated.	IIb	B	[33, 35–37]
What is the best strategy for establishing an emergency airway in children?	The best strategy for establishing an emergency airway in children is rapid sequence intubation.	IIc	B	[38–41]
How should one evaluate for airway injury?	History and physical exams are the first step in the evaluation of a traumatic airway but should be used in conjunction with imaging studies.	IIIb	C	[1, 42–46]
How does one secure the airway in the setting of airway trauma?	Oral intubation or cricothyroidotomy should be performed early in patients with airway trauma. Unstable patients should be taken immediately to the operating room for exploration, but stable patients should be evaluated with imaging studies to determine the extent of the damage.	V	D	[2, 43, 45–49]

Editor's Note

There is little in the way of high-level evidence supporting what we do in managing the traumatized airway. The type of airway control recommended in this chapter for loss of airway in the field on a trauma patient is a bag-valve-mask. This is based upon the "scoop and run" prehospital transport philosophy popular in North America. As endotracheal intubation requires both expertise and time, it is typically limited to patients with respiratory failure or those with expected long transports to the trauma center. The data supporting this approach is low quality and retrospective in nature. The optimal endotracheal tube size is unknown, and use is based on experience and convention.

The drug choices for rapid sequence intubation are numerous and are based on effectiveness (specifically, rapidity of onset), adverse effects, and finally cost. Etomidate and ketamine are common sedatives and are typically followed by succinylcholine or rocuronium for paralysis. The data to support the use of these various drugs is quite limited. (I like to use 100 mg of ketamine and 100 mg of succinylcholine on essentially all adults as an easy-to-remember and inexpensive regimen.)

Surgical airway (cricothyroidotomy on patients over 13 years of age) is indicated in the rare circumstance that endotracheal intubation is not possible in the setting of acute respiratory failure. This concept is based only on clinical experience. Direct airway injury after trauma is rare and can be suspected when stridor and respiratory distress accompany the presence of subcutaneous air or pneumothorax. Airway control with oral endotracheal intubation or surgical airway usually precedes CT imaging for confirmation. Again, this management scheme is based on clinical experience, as data is limited. As a trauma surgeon (not an anesthesiologist), I feel it is essential that a capable clinician prepare the neck for a surgical airway before attempts at intubation in a high-risk trauma patient.

REFERENCES

1. Randall DR, Rudmik LR, Ball CG, Bosch JD. External laryngotracheal trauma: Incidence, airway control, and outcomes in a large Canadian center. *Laryngoscope*. 2014; 124(4):E123–E133.
2. Pierre EJ, McNeer RR, Shamir MY. Early management of the traumatized airway. *Anesthesiol Clin*. 2007;25(1):1–11.
3. Farzanegan R, Alijanipour P, Akbarshahi H, et al. Major airways trauma, management, and long term results. *Ann Thorac Cardiovasc Surg*. 2011;17(6):544–551.
4. Mussi A, Ambrogi MC, Ribechini A, Lucchi M, Menoni F, Angeletti CA. Acute major airway injuries: Clinical features and management. *Eur J Cardiothorac Surg*. 2001;20(1):46–51, discussion 51–2.
5. Taghavi S, Vora HP, Jayarajan SN, et al. Prehospital intubation does not decrease complications in the penetrating trauma patient. *Am Surg*. 2014;80(1):9–14.
6. Davis DP, Peay J, Sise MJ, et al. The impact of prehospital endotracheal intubation on outcome in moderate to severe traumatic brain injury. *J Trauma*. 2005;58(5):933–939.
7. Cobas MA, De la Pena MA, Manning R, Candiotti K, Varon AJ. Prehospital intubations and mortality: A level 1 trauma center perspective. *Anesth Analg*. 2009;109(2):489–493.
8. Lecky F, Bryden D, Little R, Tong N, Moulton C. Emergency intubation for acutely ill and injured patients. *Cochrane Database Syst Rev*. 2008;(2):CD001429.
9. Hasegawa K, Hiraide A, Chang Y, Brown DF. Association of prehospital advanced airway management with neurologic outcome and survival in patients with out-of-hospital cardiac arrest. *JAMA*. 2013;309(3):257–266.
10. Lupton JR, Schmicker RH, Stephens S, et al. Outcomes with the use of bag–valve–mask ventilation during out-of-hospital cardiac arrest in the pragmatic airway resuscitation trial. *Acad Emerg Med*. 2020;27(3):366–374.
11. Fevang E, Perkins Z, Lockey D, Jeppesen E, Lossius HM. A systematic review and meta-analysis comparing mortality in pre-hospital tracheal intubation to emergency department intubation in trauma patients. *Critical Care*. 2017;21(7):1–14.
12. Magill IW. Technique in endotracheal anesthesia. *Br Med J*. 1930;2(3645):817–819.
13. Farrow S, Farrow C, Soni N. Size matters: Choosing the right tracheal tube. *Anesthesia*. 2012;67(8):815–819.
14. Hu B, Bao R, Wang X, Liu S, Tao T, et al. The size of the endotracheal tube and sore throat after surgery: A systematic review and meta-analysis. *PLoS One*. 2013;8(10):e74467.
15. Halum SL, Ting JY, Plowman EK, et al. A multi-institutional analysis of tracheotomy complications. *Laryngoscope*. 2012;122(1):38–45.
16. Barash PG, Cullen BF, Stoelting RK, Cahalan MK, Stock MC, Ortega R, eds. *Clinical anesthesia*. 7th ed. Lippincott Williams & Williams; 2013.
17. Miller RD, Eriksson LI, Fleischer L, Wiener-Kronish JP, Young WL, eds. *Miller's anesthesia*. 7th ed. Churchill Livingstone; 2009.
18. Coordes A, Rademacher G, Knopke S, et al. Selection and placement of oral ventilation tubes based on tracheal morphometry. *Laryngoscope*. 2011;121(6):1225–1230.
19. Karmakar A, Pate MB, Solowski NL, Postma GN, Weinberger PM. Tracheal size variability is associated with sex: Implications for endotracheal tube selection. *Ann Otol Rhinol Laryngol*. 2015;124(10):132–136.
20. D'Anza B, Knight J, Greene JS. Does body mass index predict tracheal airway size? *Laryngoscope*. 2015;125(9):1093–1097.
21. Asai T, Shingu K. Difficulty in advancing a tracheal tube over a fiberoptic bronchoscope: Incidence, causes, and solutions. *Br J Anaesth*. 2004;92:870–871.
22. Bersten AD, Rutten AJ, Vedig AE, Skowronski GA. Additional work of breathing imposed by endotracheal tubes, breathing circuits, and intensive care ventilators. *Crit Care Med*. 1989;17(7):671–677.
23. Van den Berg AA, Mphanza T. Choice of tracheal tube size for children: Finger size or age-related formula? *Anesthesia*. 2004;52(1):701–703.
24. Hofer CK, Ganter M, Tucci M, et al. How reliable is the length-based determination of body weight and tracheal tube size in the pediatric age group? The Broselow tape was reconsidered. *Br J Anaesth*. 2002;88(2):283–285.

25. King BR, Baker MD, Braitman LE, Seidl-Friedman J, Schreiner MS. Endotracheal tube selection in children: A comparison of four methods. *Ann Emerg Med.* 1993; 22(3):530–534.

26. Topjian AA, Raymond TT, Atkins D, Chan M, Duff JP, Joyner BL Jr, et al. Pediatric basic and advanced life support collaborators. Part 4: Pediatric basic and advanced life support: 2020 American Heart Association guidelines for cardiopulmonary resuscitation and emergency cardiovascular care. *Circulation.* 2020;142:S469–S523.

27. Dunham CM, Barraco RD, Clark DE, et al. Guidelines for emergency tracheal intubation immediately after traumatic injury. *J Trauma.* 2003;55(1):162–179.

28. Jabre P, Combes X, Lapostolle F, et al. Etomidate versus ketamine for rapid sequence intubation in acutely ill patients: A multicentre randomized controlled trial. *Lancet.* 2009;374(9686):293–300.

29. de Jong FH, Mallios C, Jansen C, Scheck PA, Lamberts SW. Etomidate suppresses adrenocortical function by inhibition of 11 beta-hydroxylation. *J Clin Endocrinol Metab.* 1984;59(6):1143–1147.

30. Upchurch CP, Grijalva CG, Russ S, et al. Comparison of etomidate and ketamine for induction during rapid sequence intubation of adult trauma patients. *Ann Emerg Med.* 2017;69(1):24–33.

31. Morris C, Perris A, Klein J, Mahoney P. Anaesthesia in hemodynamically compromised emergency patients: Does ketamine represent the best choice of induction agent? *Anesthesia.* 2009;64(5):532–539.

32. Tran, DTT, Newton, EK, Mount, VAH, Lee, JS, Mansour, C, Wells, GA, Perry, JJ. Rocuronium vs. succinylcholine for rapid sequence intubation: A Cochrane systematic review. *Anaesthesia.* 2017;72(6):765–777.

33. Apfelbaum JL, Hagberg CA, Connis RT, et al. 2022 American society of anesthesiologists practice guidelines for management of the difficult airway. *Anesthesiology.* 2022;136(1):31–81.

34. Hansel J, Rogers AM, Lewis SR, et al. Video laryngoscopy versus direct laryngoscopy for adults undergoing tracheal intubation. *Cochrane Database Syst Rev.* 2022;4(4): 1465–1858.

35. Wong DT, Lai K, Chung FF, Ho RY. Cannot intubate-cannot ventilate and difficult intubation strategies: Results of a Canadian national survey. *Anesth Analg.* 2005;100(5): 1439–1446.

36. Heymans F, Feigl G, Graber S, et al. Emergency cricothyrotomy performed by surgical airway-naive medical personnel: A randomized crossover study in Cadavers comparing three commonly used techniques. *Anesthesiology.* 2016;125(8):295–303.

37. Kocurek D, Seaberg D, McCabe J. Percutaneous versus open methods in cricothyroidotomy and thoracostomy. *Am J Emerg Med.* 1995;13(6):681.

38. Mandal A., Kabra SK, Lodha R. Upper airway obstruction in children. *Indian J Pediatr.* 2015;82(8):737–744.

39. Litman RS, Weissend EE, Shibata D, Westesson PL. Developmental changes of laryngeal dimensions in unparalyzed, sedated children. *Anesthesiology.* 2003;98(1):41–45.

40. Maier P, et al. Three-dimensional printed realistic pediatric static and dynamic airway models for bronchoscopy and foreign body removal training. *Pediatr Pulmonol.* 2021;56(5):2654–2659.

41. Mittiga MR, et al. A modern and practical review of rapid-sequence intubation in pediatric emergencies. *Clin Pediatr Emerg Med.* 2015;16(9):172–185.

42. Schaefer SD. Management of acute blunt and penetrating external laryngeal trauma. *Laryngoscope.* 2014;124(1):233–244.

43. Kummer C, Netto FS, Rizoli S, Yee D. A review of traumatic airway injuries: Potential implications for airway assessment and management. *Injury.* 2007;38(1):27–33.

44. Chhabra, A, Rudigwa, P, Selvam, SRP. Pathophysiology and management of airway trauma. *Trends Anaesth Crit Care.* 2013;3:216–219.

45. Rathlev NK, Medzon R, Bracken ME. Evaluation and management of neck trauma. *Emerg Med Clin North Am.* 2007;25(3):679–694.

46. Bhojani RA, Rosenbaum DH, Dikmen E, et al. Contemporary assessment of laryngotracheal trauma. *J Thorac Cardiovasc Surg.* 2005;130(2):426–432.

47. Tuckett JW, Lynham A, Lee GA, Perry M, Harrington U. Maxillofacial trauma in the emergency department: A review. *Surgeon.* 2014;12(2):106–114.

48. Bagga B, Kumar A, Chahal A, Gamanagatti S, Kumar S. "Traumatic airway injuries: Role of imaging." *Curr Probl Diagn Radiol.* 2020;49(1):48–53.

49. Ye D, Shen Z, Zhang Y, Qiu S, Kang C. Clinical features and management of closed injury of the cervical trachea due to blunt trauma. *Scand J Trauma Resusc Emerg Med.* 2013 Dec; 21(1):1–7.

6

Monitoring of the Trauma Patient

Abdul Q. Alarhayem, Zaid Alirhayim, and Natasha Keric

Traumatic injuries are the third leading cause of death among all age groups and the leading cause of death among Americans aged 44 years and younger. To improve outcomes, life-threatening injuries must be diagnosed and treated expeditiously. The trauma surgeon must decide what type of monitoring will ensure an accurate diagnosis of shock, adequate and timely resuscitation, and early identification of potential complications.

6.1 Are Heart Rate and Blood Pressure Adequate Indicators of Shock?

Shock is defined as a multisystem derangement caused by the body's inability to maintain the organ perfusion necessary to sustain aerobic metabolism [1]. In the trauma setting, the adage "All shock is hemorrhagic until proven otherwise" holds. Hemorrhage is still the most common cause of preventable death in both military and civilian settings [2]. Improving our ability to recognize, temporize, or definitively control hemorrhage in a timely fashion before the onset of shock represents a perpetual major challenge in reducing trauma mortality [3, 4]. Early detection of hemorrhage can be challenging. The use of traditional vital signs such as heart rate (HR) and systolic blood pressure (SBP) has the advantage of simplicity; however, numerous articles have displayed varying correlations between vital signs and major hemorrhage. More so, compensatory mechanisms allow for significant reductions in circulating blood volume well before changes in arterial blood pressure (BP) occur. Unrecognized volume loss during the early compensatory phase of hemorrhage leads to poor perfusion and progressive acidosis and delays intervention, with the potential for sudden catastrophic decompensation [5, 6].

Clinicians routinely refer to hypotension as an SBP <90 mmHg; however, this often marks the beginning of circulatory decompensation rather than compromise, and mortality rates in these patients may approach 50%. Trauma patients with an SBP <90 mmHg are twice as likely to die during hospitalization and three times more likely to require emergency thoracic or abdominal surgery [5]. A recent large review found an SBP of 110 mmHg to be a more clinically relevant definition of hypotension such that mortality was 4.8% greater for every 10 mmHg decrement in SBP [7]. Similar findings were reported in a large prospective European cohort study [8]. Although it may seem appropriate to expand current trauma triage criteria to include patients with SBP between 90 and 110 mmHg, this may result in an unacceptably high degree of overtriage.

Multiple studies have found that tachycardia does not reflect clinical reality accurately [9]. In a study of more than 10,000 patients, it was found that HR was neither sensitive nor specific in determining the need for emergent intervention or packed red blood cell transfusion in the first 24 hours of severe injury [10].

RECOMMENDATION

HR and BP are not adequate indicators of shock. Trauma patients with significant blood loss may present in compensated shock with normal vital signs. Other data in addition to HR and BP must be determined to detect occult hypoperfusion.

Grade of recommendation: B.

6.2 Do Local Tissue Perfusion Measures Improve Our Ability to Diagnose Shock? Does Their Use Improve Outcomes?

Oxygen delivery–consumption mismatch with resultant tissue malperfusion is the hallmark of shock. Monitoring tissue perfusion biomarkers may aid in identifying patients in compensated shock, i.e., before the onset of hemodynamic compromise. Such biomarkers assess the adequacy of tissue nutrient delivery and extraction either at the global level or within less vital organ beds (skin, gastrointestinal tract, etc.) [11]. Oxygen delivery (DO_2) far exceeds consumption during normal metabolism. As systemic perfusion decreases, tissue beds compensate by increasing oxygen extraction from arterial blood (with a resultant decrease in oxygen saturation of venous hemoglobin). Once oxygen delivery falls below a critical level, blood flow to the most vulnerable organs (brain and heart) is maintained at the expense of other organs (skin, muscle, and intestines). Anaerobic metabolism ensues, and its metabolites accumulate in these tissue beds. Systemically this is manifest as an increase in serum lactate. At the cellular level, changes in hydrogen ion concentration may be measured through gastric intramucosal pH and sublingual pCO_2.

Serum lactate: See Section 6.4.

Oxygen saturation of venous hemoglobin: Oxygen saturation of venous hemoglobin is measured readily in the pulmonary artery (SvO_2) or superior vena cava ($ScvO_2$) with acceptable correlation [12]. A low SvO_2 (<65%) is highly

DOI: 10.1201/9781003316800-6

suggestive of tissue hypoperfusion. In patients with traumatic brain injury, $ScvO_2$ values <65% in the first 24 hours have been associated with higher mortality [13].

Near-infrared spectroscopy (NIRS) is a monitoring strategy that enables direct measurement of oxygen saturation of hemoglobin found in peripheral muscle tissue or subcutaneous tissue (StO_2). Early studies suggest that StO_2 reflects global perfusion and may be as good as the base deficit (BD) for detecting shock [14]. Following a severe traumatic injury, patients with StO_2 >75% are highly unlikely to develop organ dysfunction and death [15]. Another study reported a threefold increase in mortality with every 10% decrease in StO_2 [16]. StO_2 has also been an independent predictor of blood transfusions and lifesaving interventions [17, 18].

Gastric tonometry is an indirect measurement of gastric intramucosal pH (pHim), which is an indicator of splanchnic tissue ischemia [19]. A nasogastric tube is placed in the mid-gastric position with a silicone balloon that is permeable to intraluminal CO_2, which is used to approximate intracellular pCO_2 and, thus, the degree of anaerobic metabolism. Although it can predict outcomes based on early low pHim, a meta-analysis demonstrated that therapeutic interventions guided by gastric tonometry were able to improve survival [24]. Follow-up randomized studies failed to show that pHim-directed resuscitation improved individual patient outcomes [20]. Gastric tonometry is also logistically difficult, and this might be a significant factor inhibiting the widespread use of this technology [21].

Sublingual PCO₂ (PslCO₂) is technically more easily applied than gastric tonometry. Although the internal carotid artery provides lingual blood flow, blood flow to the tongue and splanchnic beds fall similarly in response to global hypoperfusion [22]. Initial studies show that $PslCO_2$ is equivalent to lactic acid levels and BD in predicting the severity of shock and, more importantly, survival in hypotensive trauma patients. The $PslCO_2$ gap is also a useful prognosticator; patients with an initial $PslCO_2$ gap of >25 mmHg had higher mortality rates than those with a gap of <25 mmHg [23]. Further studies are required to determine the clinical utility of $PslCO_2$ as an endpoint guiding resuscitation.

RECOMMENDATIONS

Current local perfusion measures such as NIRS, gastric intramucosal pH, and sublingual capnography may help identify occult hypoperfusion; however, their lack of sensitivity limits their ability to guide resuscitation. Evidence suggesting they improve outcomes is lacking.

Grade of recommendation: B.

6.3 Does Hemodynamic Monitoring with a Pulmonary Artery Catheter Improve Outcomes?

One may argue that no monitoring device, no matter how insightful, will improve outcomes unless coupled with a treatment that itself improves outcomes. Although there is no debate about the measurements a pulmonary artery catheter (PAC) can offer, there is much controversy surrounding the benefits of this device [24, 25].

Static measures of preload, such as central venous pressure and pulmonary capillary wedge pressure, are limited by significant interpatient and intrapatient variability. In addition, these parameters do not correlate with intravascular volume status. However, the physiologic phenomenon of respiratory variability in preload can be used to assess fluid responsiveness. Large pulse pressure variation, systolic pressure variation, and stroke volume variation (SVV) are all dynamic measures and indicative of volume depletion. Although having consistently outperformed static measurements in predicting an increase in cardiac output in response to volume expansion, dynamic parameters have not been shown to improve outcomes, and thus their routine use is not recommended [11]. A recent meta-analysis that included all randomized controlled trials evaluating the use of a PAC failed to show any associated benefit. The Cochrane review shows that of the 12 studies included to evaluate the validity of the use of a PAC, there was no difference in mortality, complication rate, morbidity, cost, or length of stay with or without a PAC [26].

In severely injured trauma patients, Velmahos et al. found that there was no difference in mortality or organ failure even with goal-directed resuscitation [27]. The ESCAPE trial, a randomized controlled trial in patients with severe symptomatic heart failure, found no mortality benefit in patients assigned to clinical assessment–guided therapy versus those receiving PAC and clinical assessment–driven therapy [28]. In addition, some complications may arise directly from the use of a PAC; a study of 70 critically ill patients demonstrated that 4% died from complications related to the PAC and 20–30% had major complications [29].

As a result, the routine use of PAC in the intensive care unit (ICU) has been decreasing. Between 1993 and 2004, PAC use decreased by 65% from 5.66 to 1.99 per 1,000 medical admissions, with a similar trend for surgical patients [30]. With the advent of none or minimally invasive devices that can provide accurate hemodynamic assessments, the use of PAC is all but extinct, except in very select circumstances (combined shock states, discordant ventricular heart failure, and pulmonary hypertension).

RECOMMENDATIONS

PACs have not been shown to improve outcomes; routine use should be discouraged.

Grade of recommendation: A.

Routine use of dynamic measures of fluid responsiveness (e.g., pulse pressure variation [PPV], SVV) is not recommended.

Grade of recommendation: B.

Routine measurement of cardiac output for patients with shock is not recommended.

Grade of recommendation: B.

6.4 Is There a Biochemical Parameter that Best Identifies Shock and Guides Resuscitation?

Inadequate tissue O_2 delivery leads to anaerobic metabolism. Lactic acid and hydrogen ions, the two primary by-products of anaerobiosis, may serve as adjuncts in identifying "occult hypoperfusion." Lactate levels in the blood are a function of the balance between lactate production and clearance, with a normal value of less than 2.5 mg/dL. Both the initial lactate level and time to normalization of lactate correlate with the risk of multiple organ dysfunction syndrome and death [41]. Odom et al. demonstrated a dose-response relationship, with higher mortality seen in patients with higher lactate levels. Patient mortality was found to be 5.4% when the lactate level was <2.5 mg/dL but approached 20% in patients with a lactate level >4.0 mg/dL. Lactate clearance at 6 hours also independently predicted mortality; the adjusted odds ratio for death was 1.0, 3.5, and 4.3 for patients with clearances of ≥60%, 30–59%, and <30%, respectively [31]. Abramson also found prolonged lactate clearance to be a predictor of increased mortality in severely injured trauma patients; those who did not normalize by 48 hours had an 86% mortality rate, compared to a 100% survival rate in those who had normalized lactate levels at 24 hours [32].

A multicenter randomized controlled trial found lactate-guided therapy (aiming to decrease lactate levels by 20% or more per 2 hours for the initial 8 hours of ICU stay) significantly reduced hospital mortality when adjusting for predefined risk factors (hazard ratio [HR] 0.61). Lactate as an endpoint of resuscitation also allowed inotropes to be stopped earlier, and patients were weaned from mechanical ventilation and discharged from the ICU earlier [33]. Importantly, lactic acidosis may not correlate with tissue hypoperfusion in patients with malignancy, liver failure, and diabetic ketoacidosis and those taking certain drugs and even following heavy exercise.

BD is calculated from arterial blood gas and is the amount of base required to return the pH of 1 L of blood to a normal level. Thus, BD is a measure of uncompensated metabolic acidosis. Elevation of the BD beyond –3 correlates with the presence and severity of shock [34, 35].

Trauma patients with an abnormal BD on admission or those who fail to normalize their BDs have a higher incidence of mortality and poor outcomes, such as acute lung injury, multiple organ failure, and a greater need for blood transfusion [36–38]. Also, a BD that increases (becomes more negative) with ongoing resuscitation may suggest the presence of uncontrolled hemorrhage [34]. Importantly, large-volume saline resuscitation results in a non–anion gap, hyperchloremic, metabolic acidosis, and, hence, a persistently elevated BD despite normalization of perfusion. BD levels may also be confounded by alcohol intoxication, renal failure, chronic obstructive pulmonary disease, and other causes. Also, all measurements of BDs are rendered inaccurate in the setting of exogenous bicarbonate administration.

The serum bicarbonate concentration measurement may be used as a surrogate for the BD with reasonable correlation and does not require an arterial sample. Arterial pH is generally not useful because of the body's compensatory mechanisms.

RECOMMENDATIONS

In the absence of hypotension, abnormal serum lactate, arterial pH, bicarbonate, and BD suggest occult hypoperfusion. Failure to normalize these parameters correlates with poor outcomes. Lactate may be the best biochemical parameter to follow over time; using it as an endpoint of resuscitation has been found to reduce hospital mortality.

Grade of recommendation: B.

6.5 Should the Geriatric Trauma Patient Have More Invasive Monitoring?

Trauma in the elderly (≥65 years) is associated with higher mortality and complication rates compared with younger patients even after controlling for the degree of injury [39, 40]. Yet elderly patients are consistently undertriaged to major trauma centers, possibly due to difficulty in accurately identifying the severity of injury due to comorbidities and age-related differences in physiology. Following significant blood loss secondary to trauma, many elderly patients cannot appropriately augment their cardiac output, and therefore systemic vascular resistance is increased to maintain perfusion. As a result, elderly patients may demonstrate a normal BP while having severely depressed and compromised cardiac function, leading to overall poor systemic perfusion. In addition, older patients frequently have preexisting conditions that diminish physiologic reserve and take medications that mask signs of injury or hasten bleeding.

Adequacy of resuscitation and the oxygen debt and tissue perfusion can be monitored by BD measurements: A BD of –6 mmol/L indicates significant mortality risk, especially in patients older than 55 years. Normalizing lactate and BD levels can guide the adequacy of hemodynamic resuscitation [41] (Table 6.1).

RECOMMENDATION

Transfer to a designated trauma center and ICU admission should be considered in elderly patients with one or more severe anatomic injuries (i.e., one or more body system Abbreviated Injury Scale [AIS] score of ≥3) or an initial BD of –6 mEq/L or less. Indiscriminate hemodynamic monitoring solely based on age is not recommended.

Grade of recommendation: B.

TABLE 6.1

Monitoring of the Trauma Patient: Evidence and Grades of Recommendation

Question	Answer	Level of Evidence	Grade	References
Are HR and BP adequate indicators of shock?	• HR and BP are not adequate indicators of shock. • Trauma patients with significant blood loss may present in compensated shock with normal vital signs. • Other data in addition to HR and BP must be determined to detect occult hypoperfusion.	IIB, IIC	B	[2–10]
Do local tissue perfusion measures improve our ability to diagnose shock? Does their use improve outcomes?	• Routine use of dynamic measures of fluid responsiveness (e.g., PVV, SVV) and CO is not recommended. • Current local perfusion measures may help identify occult hypoperfusion. • Their lack of sensitivity limits their ability to guide resuscitation. Evidence suggesting, they improve outcomes is lacking.	IB	B	[11–13]
Does hemodynamic monitoring with a pulmonary artery catheter improve outcomes?	• The use of pulmonary artery catheters (PACs) has not been shown to improve outcomes. • Routine use should be discouraged.	IA	A	[24–26]
Is there a biochemical parameter that best identifies shock and guides resuscitation?	• In the absence of hypotension, abnormal serum lactate, arterial pH, bicarbonate, and base deficit suggest occult hypoperfusion. • Failure to normalize these parameters correlates with poor outcomes. • Lactate may be the best biochemical parameter to follow over time, using it as an endpoint of resuscitation has been found to significantly reduce hospital mortality.	IB	B	[31–37]
Should geriatric trauma patients have more invasive monitoring?	• Transfer to a designated trauma center and ICU admission should be considered in elderly patients with one or more severe anatomic injuries (i.e., one or more body system AIS score ≥3) or an initial BD of –6 mEq/L or less. • The indiscriminate use of pulmonary artery catheters in this population is not advocated.	IIB	B	[39–41]
What is the best noninvasive cardiac monitor available today?	• Continuous monitoring of stroke volume variation using minimally invasive technologies based on the analysis of the arterial pressure tracings reliably determines intravascular volume status and/or responsiveness to fluid therapy.	IB	B	

6.6 What Is the Best Noninvasive Cardiac Monitor Available Today?

Numerous minimally invasive technologies have been introduced over the last couple of decades that allow the continuous monitoring of cardiac output and stroke volume.

Studies have not found static volume measures (i.e., central venous pressure [CVP]) to be useful in predicting intravascular volume status or responsiveness to fluid therapy.

SVV has repeatedly been shown to predict fluid responsiveness well in various clinical settings. SVV is based on the phenomenon noted in mechanically ventilated patients where inspiration results in a rise in intrathoracic and intraarterial pressure (opposite during spontaneous breathing). It is calculated from percentage changes in stroke volume (SV) during the ventilatory cycle. In patients whose SVV is low (<12%), volume loading does not result in a significant increase in SVV. In patients with a high SVV (>12%), volume loading significantly increases SV. Several invasive and noninvasive technologies have been developed to measure CO, SVV, and PVV using pulse contour analysis or bioreactance.

Importantly, fluid responsiveness does not equate with "need for fluid." This should be determined clinically (hypotension, oliguria, elevated creatinine, lactic acidosis, etc.).

RECOMMENDATION

Continuous monitoring of SVV using minimally invasive technologies based on the analysis of the arterial pressure tracings reliably determines intravascular volume status and/or responsiveness to fluid therapy.

Grade of recommendation: B.

Editor's Note

A few years ago, a man was transported in extremis to our facility after sustaining a gunshot wound to the groin. Despite receiving four units of blood during his 90-minute helicopter ride, he arrived with no detectable blood pressure and only a faint carotid pulse. We rushed him to the operating room for the repair of a severed iliac artery. Three days later, he was recovering nicely on the floor and was discharged soon after without complications. While everyone would agree that this individual experienced profound hypoperfusion, or "shock," upon arrival, the fact that he developed no organ dysfunction suggests otherwise from a research perspective (meaning he would not have been considered to have had shock in the absence of organ dysfunction by the definition utilized in clinical trials).

One of the fundamental problems in the monitoring of trauma patients is the lack of a gold standard for the diagnosis of shock in the clinical setting. In a recent study, we prospectively evaluated our ability to detect hypoperfusion using a variety of routine parameters such as systolic blood pressure (<90 mmHg), pulse (>100 beats/min), base deficit (>5 mEq/L), and added tissue oxygen saturation (NIRS StO_2 < 75%) [14]. Investigators from seven major trauma centers agreed that it was critical to use the development of organ dysfunction as essential in our definition of "shock." Another difficulty encountered in making the diagnosis of hypoperfusion in the trauma patient are confounders that alter "normal" values. Pain, anxiety, drugs, and alcohol can alter patient presentation. Preexisting medical problems (COPD, CHF, renal dysfunction, cirrhosis) and medications (i.e., beta-blockers, antiplatelet drugs) may lead to baseline organ dysfunction and change the physiologic response of the trauma victim. The paucity of Level I data on this subject presented underscores the difficulty in conducting quality clinical trials in this field (where a waiver of informed consent is required, as severely injured subjects are unable to approve participation in studies), as well as problems deriving meaningful data from this highly heterogeneous population.

During "shock," heart rate elevation or diminished blood pressure is present only about 80% of the time and therefore 20% of the time is falsely normal in the setting of hypoperfusion leading to organ dysfunction. Changing our threshold for concern to include those people, for example, with systolic pressures less than 110 mmHg, rather than 90 mmHg, will improve the test sensitivity while making the endpoint less specific. Unlike decades ago, we are better informed as to our ignorance in the interpretation of vital signs, and we utilize biochemical markers today while continuing to investigate novel local tissue perfusion measures to assist us. A myriad of monitoring tools have been employed in an attempt to help us identify and intervene earlier in the setting of hypoperfusion. Cardiac monitoring, blood and tissue oxygen saturation assessment, gastric tonometry, and sublingual capnometry are but a few examples. None of these technologies have been shown to produce data that consistently identify patients with occult hypoperfusion or lead to superior clinical outcomes.

Another issue is that most of our trauma patients do extremely well, with only a very small subset of patients developing organ dysfunction or death. These folks are not usually hard to identify, as they are usually quite obviously severely injured and physiologically deranged. The challenge is to produce an inexpensive, safe, continuous, noninvasive monitor that can be used to diagnose hypoperfusion in key organ beds and inform us when to initiate and terminate resuscitation, ultimately leading to lower morbidity and mortality.

In the 1980s, patients were admitted to the ICU before major elective cases or after major trauma for placement of a pulmonary artery (PA) catheter. Aggressive fluid resuscitation was performed to facilitate the plotting of a Starling curve, and then the patients underwent crystalloid infusion, blood transfusion, and inotropic support to optimize oxygen delivery and consumption. Thankfully, this management scheme has been disproven, and tremendous resources are no longer consumed in this fashion. The use of PA catheters does not appear to convey benefits in clinical trials and may increase the risk of pulmonary embolism. The measure of central venous pressure does not correlate with volume status and should not be performed. The gold standard for hypovolemia today is failure to demonstrate a 10% increase in cardiac output (measured by noninvasive cardiac monitors) following a fluid challenge (usually 250 cc normal saline over 15 minutes).

Lactate and base deficit have been employed for several years and provide another valuable method of estimating hypoperfusion. While several conditions can make interpretation of these two markers difficult (liver and renal dysfunction, for example), they appear to be as accurate as heart rate and systolic blood pressure for identifying hypoperfusion. The magnitude of elevation in base deficit correlates with rising mortality. Normalization of lactate or base deficit is typically associated with improved outcomes. How well these markers can be used to guide resuscitation is uncertain, particularly in the elderly and in patients with preexisting medical problems.

In summary, we are not much better at making the diagnosis of shock or guiding our management than we were 40 years ago. The major advances in resuscitation have been related to earlier infusion of blood products and avoiding massive volumes of crystalloids; the use of angioembolization to terminate bleeding in inaccessible regions; and the abbreviation of operative procedures in patients who are failing to respond to routine measures and have become hemodynamically unstable, hypothermic, or coagulopathic.

REFERENCES

1. Vincent J, De. Backer D. Circulatory shock. The New England Journal of Medicine. 2013;369:1726–34.
2. Eastridge BJ, Mabry RL, Seguin P, Cantrell J, Tops T, Uribe P, et al. Death on the battlefield (2001–2011): implications for the future of combat casualty care. Journal of Trauma and Acute Care Surgery. 2012;73(6):S431–S7.
3. Johnson MC, Alarhayem A, Convertino V, Carter R III, Chung K, Stewart R, et al. Comparison of compensatory reserve and arterial lactate as markers of shock and resuscitation. Journal of Trauma and Acute Care Surgery. 2017;83(4):603–8.
4. Heckbert SR, Vedder NB, Hoffman W, Winn RK, Hudson LD, Jurkovich GJ, et al. Outcome after hemorrhagic shock in trauma patients. Journal of Trauma and Acute Care Surgery. 1998;45(3):545–49.
5. Lipsky AM, Gausche-Hill M, Henneman PL, Loffredo AJ, Eckhardt PB, Cryer HG, et al. Prehospital hypotension is a predictor of the need for an emergent, therapeutic operation in trauma patients with normal systolic blood pressure in the emergency department. Journal of Trauma and Acute Care Surgery. 2006;61(5):1228–33.

6. Moulton SL, Mulligan J, Grudic GZ, Convertino VA. Running on empty? The compensatory reserve index. Journal of Trauma and Acute Care Surgery. 2013;75(6):1053–59.

7. Eastridge BJ, Salinas J, McManus JG, Blackburn L, Bugler EM, Cooke WH, et al. Hypotension begins at 110 mm Hg: redefining "hypotension" with data. Journal of Trauma and Acute Care Surgery. 2007;63(2):291–99.

8. Hasler RM, Nüesch E, Jüni P, Bouamra O, Exadaktylos AK, Lecky F. Systolic blood pressure below 110 mmHg is associated with increased mortality in penetrating major trauma patients: multicentre cohort study. Resuscitation. 2012;83(4):476–81.

9. Mutschler M, Nienaber U, Brockamp T, Wafaisade A, Wyen H, Peiniger S, et al. A critical reappraisal of the ATLS classification of hypovolaemic shock: does it reflect clinical reality? Resuscitation. 2013;84(3):309–13.

10. Brasel KJ, Guse C, Gentilello LM, Nirula R. Heart rate: is it truly a vital sign? Journal of Trauma and Acute Care Surgery. 2007;62(4):812–17.

11. Antonelli M, Levy M, Andrews PJ, Chastre J, Hudson LD, Manthous C, et al. Hemodynamic monitoring in shock and implications for management. Intensive Care Medicine. 2007;33(4):575–90.

12. Ladakis C, Myrianthefs P, Karabinis A, Karatzas G, Dosios T, Fildissis G, et al. Central venous and mixed venous oxygen saturation in critically ill patients. Respiration. 2001;68(3):279–85.

13. Di Filippo A, Gonnelli C, Perretta L, Zagli G, Spina R, Chiostri M, et al. Low central venous saturation predicts poor outcome in patients with brain injury after major trauma: a prospective observational study. Scandinavian Journal of Trauma, Resuscitation and Emergency Medicine. 2009;17(1):1–7.

14. Cohn SM, Nathens AB, Moore FA, Rhee P, Puyana JC, Moore EE, et al. Tissue oxygen saturation predicts the development of organ dysfunction during traumatic shock resuscitation. Journal of Trauma and Acute Care Surgery. 2007;62(1):44–55.

15. Crookes BA, Cohn SM, Bloch S, Amortegui J, Manning R, Li P, et al. Can near-infrared spectroscopy identify the severity of shock in trauma patients? Journal of Trauma and Acute Care Surgery. 2005;58(4):806–16.

16. Sagraves SG, Newell MA, Bard MR, Watkins FR, Corcoran KJ, McMullen PD, et al. Tissue oxygenation monitoring in the field: a new EMS vital sign. Journal of Trauma and Acute Care Surgery. 2009;67(3):441–44.

17. Beekley AC, Martin MJ, Nelson T, Grathwohl KW, Griffith M, Beilman G, et al. Continuous noninvasive tissue oximetry in the early evaluation of the combat casualty: a prospective study. Journal of Trauma and Acute Care Surgery. 2010;69(1):S14–S25.

18. Moore FA, Nelson T, McKinley BA, Moore EE, Nathens AB, Rhee P, et al. Massive transfusion in trauma patients: tissue hemoglobin oxygen saturation predicts poor outcome. Journal of Trauma and Acute Care Surgery. 2008; 64(4):1010–23.

19. Costello WT. Gastric tonometry. Monitoring Technologies in Acute Care Environments: Springer; 2014. p. 317–20.

20. Gomersall CD, Joynt GM, Freebairn RC, Hung V, Buckley TA, Oh TE. Resuscitation of critically ill patients based on the results of gastric tonometry: a prospective, randomized, controlled trial. Critical Care Medicine. 2000;28(3):607–14.

21. Ivatury RR, Simon RJ, Islam S, Fueg A, Rohman M, Stahl WM. A prospective randomized study of end points of resuscitation after major trauma: global oxygen transport indices versus organ-specific gastric mucosal pH. Journal of the American College of Surgeons. 1996;183(2): 145–54.

22. Jin X, Weil MH, Sun S, Tang W, Bisera J, Mason EJ. Decreases in organ blood flows are associated with increases in sublingual pco_2 during hemorrhagic shock. Journal of Applied Physiology. 1998;85(6):2360–64.

23. Marik PE, Bankov A. Sublingual capnometry versus traditional markers of tissue oxygenation in critically ill patients. Critical Care Medicine. 2003;31(3):818–22.

24. Zhang X, Xuan W, Yin P, Wang L, Wu X, Wu Q. (2015). Gastric tonometry guided therapy in critical care patients: a systematic review and meta-analysis. Critical Care, 19, 1–11.

25. Shah MR, Hasselblad V, Stevenson LW, Binanay C, O'Connor CM, Sopko G, et al. Impact of the pulmonary artery catheter in critically ill patients: a meta-analysis of randomized clinical trials. JAMA. 2005;294(13):1664–70.

26. Rajaram SS, Desai NK, Kalra A, Gajera M, Cavanaugh SK, Brampton W, et al. Pulmonary artery catheters for adult patients in intensive care. Cochrane Database of Systematic Reviews. 2013(2). https://doi.org/10.1002/14651858.CD003408.pub3.

27. Velmahos GC, Demetriades D, Shoemaker WC, Chan LS, Tatevossian R, Wo CC, et al. Endpoints of resuscitation of critically injured patients: normal or supranormal?: a prospective randomized trial. Annals of Surgery. 2000; 232(3):409.

28. Binanay C, Califf RM, Hasselblad V, O'Connor CM, Shah MR, Sopko G, et al. Evaluation study of congestive heart failure and pulmonary artery catheterization effectiveness: the ESCAPE trial. JAMA. 2005;294(13):1625–33.

29. Fein AM, Goldberg SK, Walkenstein MD, Dershaw B, Braitman L, Lippmann ML. Is pulmonary artery catheterization necessary for the diagnosis of pulmonary edema? American Review of Respiratory Disease. 1984;129(6): 1006–9.

30. Wiener RS, Welch HG. Trends in the use of the pulmonary artery catheter in the United States, 1993–2004. JAMA. 2007;298(4):423–29.

31. Odom SR, Howell MD, Silva GS, Nielsen VM, Gupta A, Shapiro NI, et al. Lactate clearance as a predictor of mortality in trauma patients. Journal of Trauma and Acute Care Surgery. 2013;74(4):999–1004.

32. Abramson D, Scalea TM, Hitchcock R, Trooskin SZ, Henry SM, Greenspan J. Lactate clearance and survival following injury. The Journal of Trauma. 1993;35(4):584–88; discussion 8.

33. Jansen TC, van Bommel J, Schoonderbeek FJ, Sleeswijk Visser SJ, van der Klooster JM, Lima AP, et al. Early lactate-guided therapy in intensive care unit patients: a multicenter, open-label, randomized controlled trial. American Journal of Respiratory and Critical Care Medicine. 2010;182(6):752–61.

34. Davis JW, Shackford SR, Mackersie RC, Hoyt DB. Base deficit as a guide to volume resuscitation. The Journal of Trauma. 1988;28(10):1464–67.

35. Rutherford EJ, Morris JA, Jr, Reed GW, Hall KS. Base deficit stratifies mortality and determines therapy. The Journal of Trauma. 1992;33(3):417–23.

36. Davis JW, Parks SN, Kaups KL, Gladen HE, O'Donnell-Nicol S. Admission base deficit predicts transfusion requirements and risk of complications. Journal of Trauma and Acute Care Surgery. 1996;41(5):769–74.

37. Randolph LC, Takacs M, Davis KA. Resuscitation in the pediatric trauma population: admission base deficit remains an important prognostic indicator. Journal of Trauma and Acute Care Surgery. 2002;53(5):838–42.

38. Eberhard LW, Morabito DJ, Matthay MA, Mackersie RC, Campbell AR, Marks JD, et al. Initial severity of metabolic acidosis predicts the development of acute lung injury in severely traumatized patients. Critical Care Medicine. 2000; 28(1):125–31.

39. Broos P, D'Hoore A, Vanderschot P, Rommens P, Stappaerts K. Multiple trauma in elderly patients. Factors influencing outcome: the importance of aggressive care. Injury. 1993;24(6):365–8.

40. Champion HR, Copes WS, Buyer D, Flanagan ME, Bain L, Sacco WJ. Major trauma in geriatric patients. American Journal of Public Health. 1989;79(9):1278–82.

41. McNelis J, Marini CP, Jurkiewicz A, Szomstein S, Simms HH, Ritter G, et al. Prolonged lactate clearance is associated with increased mortality in the surgical intensive care unit. The American Journal of Surgery. 2001;182(5): 481–5.

7

Resuscitation of the Trauma Patient

David R. King

7.1 Introduction

The Edwin Smith Papyrus (1600 BC) described administering fluid by mouth following traumatic injury [1]. This may represent the earliest description of fluid resuscitation. Later, Cannon warned of the potential perils of aggressive fluid resuscitation, including exacerbating hemorrhage by (possibly) raising blood pressure and disrupting soft clots [2]. Indeed, the debates surrounding fluid resuscitation seem to predate this evidence-based textbook by centuries.

This chapter will address several fundamental questions related to the resuscitation of the trauma patient within an evidence-based construct. The particular questions are important; however, they do not represent all possible resuscitation-related dilemmas that may confront the surgeon or clinician. The goal, therefore, is to demonstrate and differentiate those maneuvers that are based on scientific evidence and discriminate them from those based solely on historical opinion. This is not to say that our surgical forefathers were wrong in their approaches (because in many cases, they were right on target), but to simply articulate those therapies that have a scientific basis from those whose basis should be questioned and improved upon if shown to be false.

7.2 Methods

An OVID Medline search was performed for all articles from 1950 to October 2022 using the terms "resuscitation" and "trauma." The search was limited to clinical trials and randomized controlled trials (RCTs) on human subjects. Multiple languages were accepted if there was an English language translation available. Manuscripts were screened for appropriateness to the topics listed, and article references were examined for relevant similar articles using PubMed. A review was also performed of the Cochrane library using similar key terms. Manuscripts were discarded if there were significant methodological flaws or if the papers represented multiple case reports.

Several important questions were posed, and evidence was evaluated to address each question. Each question's level of evidence was classified using the classification system of the Oxford Center for Evidence-Based Medicine.

7.3 Question Results

7.3.1 What Type of Fluid Should Be Used for Acute Resuscitation of the Trauma Patient?

Despite the trauma surgeon's historical fascination with lactated Ringer's solution, no evidence exists to suggest that this crystalloid solution has any survival benefit over others. Nearly every clinical trial demonstrates the equivalence of a variety of resuscitation fluids, including lactated Ringer's solution, normal saline, 3% or 7.5% hypertonic saline, hetastarch/pentastarch solutions, and gelatins [3–24]. A Cochrane systematic review of RCTs in critically ill patients with trauma, burns, or following surgery failed to show any difference in mortality between patients resuscitated with colloids (including albumin or plasma protein fraction, hydroxyethyl starch, modified gelatin or dextran) versus crystalloids. The results suggested a possible increase in mortality associated with hydroxyethyl starch [25].

Newer-generation hetastarch with improved C2/C6 ratios, 1:20 branching, and 0.75 degrees of substitution has no demonstrable effect on the coagulation system in small doses [14]. Although the use of hetastarch and gelatins has no proven morbidity or mortality advantage, less volume of these fluids is required to achieve similar resuscitation endpoints [4, 10–14, 16]. While this advantage may be of little significance in a resource-abundant civilian trauma center, there may be significant logistical advantages for the military, especially in far-forward units where supplies are limited by cubic and weight. Colloids, however, are dramatically more expensive than crystalloid solutions, and this is important in all environments [9, 24]. Colloids should be avoided if a traumatic brain injury is suspected and limited to small volumes of infusion to avoid coagulation and renal insults [8–10, 14, 25].

The use of 7.5% hypertonic saline has some theoretical advantages (potential for sodium to act as an osmotic dehydrating agent in the injured brain and prevent edema formation) over isotonic fluid resuscitation in the multitraumatized patient with a concurrent brain injury; however, results from multiple clinical trials are mixed, with the majority of studies demonstrating equivalence with isotonic fluid resuscitation [4–6, 12, 13, 18–20, 26]. Resuscitation with normal saline may result in hyperchloremic metabolic acidosis; however, the presence of said acidosis has never been convincingly demonstrated to worsen outcomes [8, 9]. The use of hypotonic fluids for trauma resuscitation has never been studied; therefore, a specific analysis of this type of fluid cannot be generated.

The use of hemoglobin-based oxygen carriers for trauma resuscitation remains a research interest only. Despite convincing animal studies demonstrating survival advantages, all trauma-related clinical trials with these agents result in higher mortality rates [15, 27–29]. There is currently not enough data to support their general use in trauma, although hemoglobin-based oxygen carriers remain the theoretical ideal resuscitation fluid.

RECOMMENDATION

Acute-phase trauma resuscitation may be conducted safely with any isotonic crystalloid, as well as hypertonic saline, but not colloids. In general, crystalloid solutions remain preferred because of their low cost and similar outcomes compared to colloids. The use of blood and blood products as an initial resuscitation fluid for the severely injured patient may also offer some mortality advantage over crystalloid solutions [30–34].

Level of evidence: 1a. Grade of recommendation: A.

7.3.2 How Does One Determine Whether a Traumatized Patient Requires Fluid Resuscitation?

Shock is generally defined as inadequate tissue perfusion. In trauma, this condition is often recognized based on vital signs and mental status. Shock should generally be regarded as present if any trauma patient presents with a systolic blood pressure (SBP) less than 110 mmHg and a heart rate greater than 100 beats/min [12, 35, 36]. This is a significant departure from earlier classical teaching, where blood pressure below 80 or 90 mmHg and heart rates above 120 beats/min were regarded as a reliable threshold for determination of shock. Altered mental status should also be regarded as a sign of shock until proven otherwise. If any of these parameters are present, fluid resuscitation and a hemostatic intervention (surgery, application of a tourniquet, angioembolization, etc.) should be immediately considered. One must understand that these parameters are meant for overtriaged trauma patients such that few or no patients in hemorrhagic shock are inappropriately excluded from fluid resuscitation efforts.

RECOMMENDATION

Following trauma, any patient with a heart rate above 100 beats/min or SBP less than 110 mmHg indicates shock and should trigger fluid resuscitation efforts combined with an aggressive hemorrhage control maneuver.

Level of evidence: 2c. Grade of recommendation: C.

7.3.3 What Are the Endpoints for the Termination of Fluid Resuscitation?

Reliable and well-defined endpoints for resuscitation remain elusive. Multiple strategies have been proposed and tested, and none have proven to be better than a clinical judgment based on vital signs, urine output, and simple laboratory tests such as arterial base deficit and lactate [30, 32, 33]. Oxygen delivery–based therapy and endpoints determined with a pulmonary artery catheter have excellent theoretical advantages; however, multiple clinical trials have shown no significant morbidity or mortality advantage [35, 37]. Tissue-level near-infrared spectroscopy, as well as intramuscular polarographic Clark-type electrode-tissue pO_2 monitoring, is useful in animal studies; however, their role as resuscitation endpoints in humans remains no better than clinical judgment [39–41]. The available data suggest that resuscitation endpoints would be more usefully conceptualized as a resuscitation spectrum, where fluid administration is not suddenly terminated once a specific criterion or point is reached, but rather slowly de-escalated as the patient's clinical condition improves. Certain exceptions to ongoing resuscitation endpoints exist in the setting of penetrating torso trauma; however, this will be addressed separately. One should also be aware that overresuscitation may equally be as deleterious as underresuscitation: recent evidence from retrospective cohorts suggests that aggressive early crystalloid resuscitation is associated with a substantial dose-dependent increase in morbidity, intensive care unit (ICU), and hospital length of stay in blunt trauma patients [43]. Limiting the volume and rate of fluid administration while prioritizing hemorrhage control is advised. The surgeon should constantly re-evaluate the trauma patient to prevent the overuse of resuscitation fluid and the consequences associated with this practice.

RECOMMENDATION

Clinical judgment combined with simple laboratory testing remains the best approach to deciding when to de-escalate fluid resuscitation. This should be approached as a continuum rather than a static point in care.

Level of evidence: 2b. Grade of recommendation: B.

7.3.4 Does the Concept of Hypotensive (Delayed) Resuscitation Have a Role in Trauma Care?

Hypotensive resuscitation, or delayed fluid resuscitation, is a concept whereby fluid administration is intentionally withheld, slowed, or halted at some point before the standard endpoints of resuscitation are achieved. This technique has consistently been associated with a lower risk of death in RCTs of fluid resuscitation in animal models of severe hemorrhage [43]. There is evidence of survival benefit with the use of a delayed resuscitation paradigm following penetrating torso injury [45], although no conclusive data exist for blunt or extremity injuries [45]. Patients with a penetrating injury should have intravenous access established and fluid administered withheld until surgical intervention is available. A plethora of expert opinions have been generated from the battlefields of the War on Terror in Iraq and Afghanistan. Most experts generally suggest that hypotensive resuscitation is appropriate for patients in shock until definitive surgical intervention is available. This opinion, however, remains unstudied in a randomized controlled fashion. Special considerations while caring for patients with traumatic brain injury or elderly trauma patients who may have coronary or carotid artery disease include their relative intolerance to hypotensive resuscitation and concurrent susceptibility to fluid overload–related complications [46].

RECOMMENDATION

Hypotensive or delayed fluid resuscitation should be considered following penetrating torso injuries. Some evidence exists to support that this strategy may be considered for patients suffering from shock after blunt trauma as well as extremity injuries.

Level of evidence: 1b. Grade of recommendation: A.

7.3.5 Should Blood or Blood Products Be Used as an Initial Resuscitation Fluid, When Available?

Some surgeons propose that in the setting of acute hemorrhage, one should replace lost intravascular volume with fresh whole blood or packed red blood cells (PRBCs). Unfortunately, capillary refill across the interstitial space occurs rapidly, and this interstitial free water deficit must be restored to return the patient to fluid equilibrium. Additionally, although many patients present with acute blood loss, most will be successfully managed without blood transfusion. The use of blood and blood products also exposes the patient to risks associated with communicable diseases and transfusion reactions. No evidence exists demonstrating any clinical advantage to this practice, as prehospital randomization of patients to crystalloid or red blood cells is logistically difficult. Some evidence exists in the early hospital-based resuscitation environment, suggesting that patients who have a large vascular injury and will require massive transfusion may benefit from early administration of blood and blood products [47–49]. Even in these series, however, the initial fluid of choice was the crystalloid solution before switching to blood. Patients with penetrating torso injury have retrospectively been reported to have lower mortality rates when managed with damage control resuscitation—defined as an SBP of 90 mmHg maintained using early resuscitation with fresh-frozen plasma and PRBCs in a high ratio—combined with a restrictive rather than standard crystalloid resuscitation strategy [50].

RECOMMENDATION

Initial fluid resuscitation should begin with a crystalloid solution. There is not sufficient evidence to support initial resuscitation with blood products.

Level of evidence: 2c. Grade of recommendation: C.

7.3.6 Do Vasoactive Drugs Play a Role in Early Resuscitation of the Trauma Patient?

The use of vasopressors in the acute resuscitation of trauma patients has regained substantial interest in recent years. Although multiple animal studies demonstrate dramatic survival advantages associated with early vasopressor use in trauma resuscitation, the clinical trial data squarely dispute these findings [51, 52]. The available clinical data suggest no morbidity or mortality advantage [53], and one multicenter trial demonstrated significantly greater mortality in the vasopressor group [51] (Table 7.1).

RECOMMENDATION

Although the early use of vasopressors after trauma remains an intense research interest, this practice is not currently supported by the existing body of clinical data. Hypotensive trauma patients should be managed with careful hypotensive fluid resuscitation, with a focus on the identification of the source of hemorrhage and rapid hemostatic intervention.

Level of evidence: 2c. Grade of recommendation: C.

TABLE 7.1

Evidence Table

Question	Answer	Grade of Recommendation	References
What type of fluid should be used for acute resuscitation of the trauma patient?	Isotonic crystalloids or blood products	A	[3–25, 27, 29]
How does one determine whether a traumatized patient requires fluid resuscitation?	Blood pressure less than 110 mmHg on presentation	C	[35, 36]
What are the endpoints for termination of fluid resuscitation?	Clinical judgment	B	[35, 37–41]
Does the concept of hypotensive (delayed) resuscitation have a role in trauma care?	Yes	A	[43–45]
Should blood or blood products be used as an initial resuscitation fluid, when available?	No	C	[47–49]
Do vasoactive drugs play a role in the early resuscitation of the trauma patient?	No	C	[51–53]

7.4 Closing Comments

The practice of evidence-based medicine allows the surgeon to make decisions based on the best science possible. By definition, evidence applies to populations of patients who share common characteristics. It would implore you, when your patient is failing to respond to conventional therapy, to reevaluate how that patient is *different* from the evidence-based study population. Often, what is good therapy for the population may not be entirely appropriate for a specific individual or group of individuals who make up a subset of the population. Lastly, we must be careful not to conflate resuscitation with hemorrhage control. The two may sometimes occur simultaneously, but should not be confused with each other and remain independent functions in the care of the acutely injured [54].

Editor's Note

This chapter has nicely summarized the current state of resuscitation in the trauma patient. There has been a huge amount of animal and clinical work investigating this topic, but many questions remain unanswered. It is clear that crystalloid resuscitation of hemorrhagic shock is equivalent to colloid. The potential advantage of a colloid (or hypertonic saline for that matter) lies in a smaller volume required to achieve the same endpoints of resuscitation. This, as stated earlier, is valuable in austere environments and in those where the fluids must be transported by healthcare personnel, such as in the combat zone.

The endpoint of resuscitation is hotly debated, and it appears, based on clinical observation and some clinical trials, that elevating the patient's blood pressure before obtaining control of the source of bleeding (i.e., removing the lacerated spleen) leads to worse outcomes. A variety of resuscitation endpoints have all demonstrated some value as identifiers of hemorrhagic shock, but each of them (heart rate, blood pressure, base deficit, lactate, tissue oxygen saturation, etc.) misses about 20% of these patients. When to terminate resuscitation is still controversial, but currently, it is a clinical decision based on the resolution of hemodynamic instability, normalization of metabolic acidosis, and correction of coagulopathy.

Finally, the use of vasoactive drugs to support blood pressure in unstable patients with hemorrhagic shock should be condemned, as the bulk of basic science and clinical studies support the notion that this practice increases morbidity and mortality.

REFERENCES

1. Rutkow IM. *Surgery: An Illustrated History.* Mosby: St. Louis, MO; *Medicine* 1991;84:554–557.
2. Cannon W, Fraser J, Cowell E. Preventive treatment of wound shock. *JAMA.* 1918;70:618–621.
3. Vassar MJ, Perry CA, Gannaway WL, Holcroft JW. 7.5% sodium chloride/dextran for resuscitation of trauma patients undergoing helicopter transport. *Arch Surg.* September 1991;126(9):1065–1072.
4. Vassar MJ, Fischer RP, O'Brien PE, Bachulis BL, Chambers JA, Hoyt DB, Holcroft JW. A multicenter trial for resuscitation of injured patients with 7.5% sodium chloride. The effect of added dextran 70. The multicenter group for the study of hypertonic saline in trauma patients. *Arch Surg.* September 1993;128(9):1003–1011; discussion 1011–1013.
5. Mattox KL, Maningas PA, Moore EE, Mateer JR, Marx JA, Aprahamian C, Burch JM, Pepe PE. Prehospital hypertonic saline/dextran infusion for post-traumatic hypotension. The U.S.A. multicenter trial. *Ann Surg.* May 1991;213(5):482–491.
6. Wade CE, Grady JJ, Kramer GC. Efficacy of hypertonic saline dextran fluid resuscitation for patients with hypotension from penetrating trauma. *J Trauma.* May 2003;54(5 Suppl):S144–S148.
7. Tranbaugh RF, Lewis FR. Crystalloid versus colloid for fluid resuscitation of hypovolemic patients. *Adv Shock Res.* 1983;9:203–216.
8. SAFE Study Investigators; Australian and New Zealand Intensive Care Society Clinical Trials Group; Australian Red Cross Blood Service; George Institute for International Health, Myburgh J, Cooper DJ, Finfer S, Bellomo R, Norton R, Bishop N, Kai Lo S, Vallance S. Saline or albumin for fluid resuscitation in patients with traumatic brain injury. *N Engl J Med.* August 2007;357(9):874–884.
9. Finfer S, Bellomo R, Boyce N, French J, Myburgh J, Norton R; SAFES Study Investigators. A comparison of albumin and saline for fluid resuscitation in the intensive care unit. *N Engl J Med.* May 27, 2004;350(22):2247–2256.
10. Shatney CH, Deepika K, Militello PR, Majerus TC, Dawson RB. Efficacy of hetastarch in the resuscitation of patients with multisystem trauma and shock. *Arch Surg.* July 1983;118(7):804–809.
11. Bulger EM, Jurkovich CJ, Nathens AB, et al. Hypertonic resuscitation of hypovolemic shock after blunt trauma: A randomized controlled trial. *Arch Surg.* February 2008; 143(2):139–148; discussion 149.
12. Rizoli SB, Rhind SG, Shek PN, Inaba K, Filips D, Tien H, Brenneman F, Rotstein O. The immunomodulatory effects of hypertonic saline resuscitation in patients sustaining traumatic hemorrhagic shock: A randomized, controlled, double-blinded trial. *Ann Surg.* January 2006;243(1):47–57.
13. Cooper DJ, Myles PS, McDermott FT, Murray LJ, Laidlaw J, Cooper G, Tremayne AB, Bernard SS, Ponsford J; HTS Study Investigators. Prehospital hypertonic saline resuscitation of patients with hypotension and severe traumatic brain injury: A randomized controlled trial. *JAMA.* March 2004;291(11):1350–1357.
14. Allison KP, Gosling P, Jones S, Pallister I, Porter KM. Randomizer trial of hydroxyethyl starch versus gelatine for trauma resuscitation. *J Trauma.* December 1999;47(6):1114–1121.
15. Sloan EP, Koenigsberg M, Gens D, Cipolle M, Runge J, Mallory MN, Rodman G, Jr. Diaspirin cross-linked hemoglobin (DCLHb) in the treatment of severe traumatic hemorrhagic shock: A randomized controlled efficacy trial. *JAMA.* November 1999;282(19):1857–1864.
16. Younes RN, Yin KC, Amino CJ, Itinoshe M, Rocha e Silva M, Birolini D. Use of pentastarch solution in the treatment of patients with hemorrhagic hypovolemia: Randomized phase II study in the emergency room. *World J Surg.* January 1998;22(1):2–5.

17. Nagy KK, Davis J, Duda J, Fildes J, Roberts R, Barrett J. A comparison of pentastarch and lactated Ringer's solution in the resuscitation of patients with hemorrhagic shock. *Circ Shock*. August 1993;*40(4)*:289–294.

18. Vassar MJ, Perry CA, Holcroft JW. Prehospital resuscitation of hypotensive trauma patients with 7.5% NaCl versus 7.5% NaCl with added dextran: A controlled trial. *J Trauma*. May 1993;*34(5)*:622–632; discussion 632–633.

19. Younes RN, Aun F, Accioly CQ, Casale LP, Szajnbok I, Birolini D. Hypertonic solutions in the treatment of hypovolemic shock: A prospective, randomized study in patients admitted to the emergency room. *Surgery*. April 1992;*111(4)*:380–385.

20. Holcroft JW, Vassar MJ, Turner JE, Derlet RW, Kramer GC. 3% NaCl and 7.5% NaCl/dextran 70 in the resuscitation of severely injured patients. *Ann Surg*. September 1987;*206(3)*:279–288.

21. Modig J. Advantages of dextran 70 over Ringer acetate solution in shock treatment and prevention of adult respiratory distress syndrome. A randomized study in man after traumatic-haemorrhagic shock. *Resuscitation*. August 1983;*10(4)*:219–226.

22. Moss GS, Lowe RJ, Jilek J, Levine HD. Colloid or crystalloid in the resuscitation of hemorrhagic shock: A controlled clinical trial. *Surgery*. April 1981;*89(4)*:434–438.

23. Lowe RJ, Moss GS, Jilek J, Levine HD. Crystalloid versus colloid in the etiology of pulmonary failure after trauma—A randomized trial in man. *Crit Care Med*. March 1979;*7(3)*:107–112.

24. Wu JJ, Huang MS, Tang GJ, Kao WF, Shih HC, Su CH, Lee CH. Hemodynamic response of modified fluid gelatin compared with lactated ringer's solution for volume expansion in emergency resuscitation of hypovolemic shock patients: Preliminary report of a prospective, randomized trial. *World J Surg*. May 2001;*25(5)*:598–602.

25. Perel P, Roberts I, Ker K. Colloids versus crystalloids for fluid resuscitation in critically ill patients. *Cochrane Database Syst Rev*. February 2013;*2*:CD000567.

26. York J, Arrillaga A, Graham R, Miller R. Fluid resuscitation of patients with multiple injuries and severe closed head injury: Experience with an aggressive fluid resuscitation strategy. *J Trauma*. March 2000;*48(3)*:376–379; discussion 379–380.

27. Moore EE, Cheng AM, Moore HB, Masuno T, Johnson JL. Hemoglobin based oxygen carriers in trauma care: Scientific rationale for the US multicenter prehospital trial. *World J Surg*. July 2006;*30(7)*:1247–1257.

28. Natanson C, Kern SJ, Lurie P, Banks SM, Wolfe SM. Well-bred hemoglobin-based blood substitutes and risk of myocardial infarction and death: A meta-analysis. *JAMA*. May 2008;*299(19)*:2304–2312.

29. Transcripts: Safety of hemoglobin-based oxygen carriers (Hbocs), April 29–30, 2008. Center for Biologics Evaluation and Research, FDA, The National Heart, Lung, and Blood Institute, NIH and Office of the Secretary and Office of Public Health and Science, DHHS, NIH Campus: Bethesda, Maryland. Updated April 9, 2013.

30. Velmahos GC, Demetriades D, Shoemaker WC et al. Endpoints of resuscitation of critically injured patients: Normal or supranormal? A prospective randomized trial. *Ann Surg*. September 2000;*232(3)*:409–418.

31. Guyette FX, Sperry JL, Peitzman AB, Billiar TR, Daley BJ, Miller RS, Harbrecht BG, Claridge JA, Putnam T, Duane TM, Phelan HA, Brown JB. Prehospital blood product and crystalloid resuscitation in the severely injured patient: A secondary analysis of the prehospital air medical plasma trial. *Ann Surg*. February 1, 2021;*273(2)*:358–364.

32. Kemp Bohan PM, McCarthy PM, Wall ME, Adams AM, Chick RC, Forcum JE, Radowsky JS, How RA, Sams VG. Safety and efficacy of low-titer O whole blood resuscitation in a civilian level I trauma center. *J Trauma Acute Care Surg*. August 1, 2021;*91(2S Suppl 2)*:S162–S168.

33. Sperry JL, Guyette FX, Brown JB, Yazer MH, Triulzi DJ, Early-Young BJ, Adams PW, Daley BJ, Miller RS, Harbrecht BG, Claridge JA, Phelan HA, Witham WR, Putnam AT, Duane TM, Alarcon LH, Callaway CW, Zuckerbraun BS, Neal MD, Rosengart MR, Forsythe RM, Billiar TR, Yealy DM, Peitzman AB, Zenati MS; PAMPer Study Group. Prehospital plasma during air medical transport in trauma patients at risk for hemorrhagic shock. *N Engl J Med*. July 26, 2018;*379(4)*:315–326.

34. Hazelton JP, Ssentongo AE, Oh JS, Ssentongo P, Seamon MJ, Byrne JP, Armento IG, Jenkins DH, Braverman MA, Mentzer C, Leonard GC, Perea LL, Docherty CK, Dunn JA, Smoot B, Martin MJ, Badiee J, Luis AJ, Murray JL, Noorbakhsh MR, Babowice JE, Mains C, Madayag RM, Kaafarani HMA, Mokhtari AK, Moore SA, Madden K, Tanner A 2nd, Redmond D, Millia DJ, Brandolino A, Nguyen U, Chinchilli V, Armen SB, Porter JM. Use of cold-stored whole blood is associated with improved mortality in hemostatic resuscitation of major bleeding: A multicenter study. *Ann Surg*. October 1, 2022;*276(4)*:579–588.

35. Holcomb JB, Tilley BC, Baraniuk S, Fox EE, Wade CE, Podbielski JM, del Junco DJ, Brasel KJ, Bulger EM, Callcut RA, Cohen MJ, Cotton BA, Fabian TC, Inaba K, Kerby JD, Muskat P, O'Keeffe T, Rizoli S, Robinson BR, Scalea TM, Schreiber MA, Stein DM, Weinberg JA, Callum JL, Hess JR, Matijevic N, Miller CN, Pittet JF, Hoyt DB, Pearson GD, Leroux B, van Belle G; PROPPR Study Group. Transfusion of plasma, platelets, and red blood cells in a 1:1:1 vs a 1:1:2 ratio and mortality in patients with severe trauma: The PROPPR randomized clinical trial. *JAMA*. February 3, 2015;*313(5)*:471–482.

36. Eastridge BJ, Salinas J, McManus JG, Blackburn L, Bugler EM, Cooke WH, Concertino VA, Wade CE, Holcomb JB. Hypotension begins at 110 mmHg: Redefining "hypotension" with data. *J Trauma*. August 2007;*63(2)*:291–297; discussion 297–299.

37. Miller PR, Meredith JW, Chang MC. Randomized, prospective comparison of increased preload versus inotropes in the resuscitation of trauma patients: Effects on cardiopulmonary function and visceral perfusion. *J Trauma*. January 1998;*44(1)*:107–113.

38. Durham RM, Neunaber K, Mazuski JE, Shapiro MJ, Baue AE. The use of oxygen consumption and delivery as endpoints for resuscitation in critically ill patients. *J Trauma*. July 1996;*41(1)*:32–39; discussion 39–40.

39. McKinley BA, Marvin RG, Cocanour CS, Moore FA. Tissue hemoglobin O_2 saturation during resuscitation of traumatic shock was monitored using near-infrared spectrometry. *J Trauma*. April 2000;*48(4)*:637–642.

40. Crookes BA, Cohn SM, Burton EA, et al. Can near-infrared spectroscopy identify the severity of shock in trauma patients? *J Trauma*. April 2005;*58(4)*:806–813; discussion 813–816.

41. Ikossi DG, Knudson MM, Morabito DJ, Cohen MJ, Wan JJ, Khaw L, Stewart CJ, Hemphill C, Manley GT. Continuous muscle tissue oxygenation in critically injured patients: A prospective observational study. *J Trauma*. October 2006;*61(4)*:780–788; discussion 788–790.

42. Kasotakis G, Sideris A, Chang Y, De Moya M, Alam H, King DR, Tompkins R, Velmahos G. Aggressive early crystalloid resuscitation adversely affects outcomes in adult blunt trauma patients: An analysis of the glue grant database. *J Trauma Acute Care Surg*. May 2013;*74(5)*:1215–1222.

43. Mapstone J, Roberts I, Evans P. Fluid resuscitation strategies: A systematic review of animal trials. *J Trauma*. 2003;*55*:571–589.

44. Bickell WH, Wall MJ, Jr, Pepe PE, Martin RR, Ginger VF, Allen MK, Mattox KL. Immediate versus delayed fluid resuscitation for hypotensive patients with penetrating torso injuries. *N Engl J Med*. October 1994;*331(17)*:1105–1109.

45. Dutton RP, Mackenzie CF, Scalea TM. Hypotensive resuscitation during active hemorrhage: Impact on in-hospital mortality. *J Trauma*. June 2002;*52(6)*:1141–1146.

46. Alam HB, Velmahos GC. New trends in resuscitation. *Curr Prob Surg*. August 2011;*48(8)*:531–564.

47. Spinella PC, Perkins JG, Grathwohl KW, Beekley AC, Niles SE, McLaughlin DF, Wade CE, Holcomb JB. Effect of plasma and red blood cell transfusions on survival in patients with combat-related traumatic injuries. *J Trauma*. February 2008;*64(2 Suppl)*:S69–S77; discussion S77–S78.

48. Stinger HK, Spinella PC, Perkins JG et al. The ratio of fibrinogen to red cells transfused affects survival in casualties receiving massive transfusions at an army combat support hospital. *J Trauma*. February 2008;*64(2 Suppl)*:S79–S85; discussion S85.

49. Borgman MA, Spinella PC, Perkins JG, Grathwohl KW, Repine T, Beekley AC, Sebesta J, Jenkins D, Wade CE, Holcomb JB. The ratio of blood products transfused affects mortality in patients receiving massive transfusions at a combat support hospital. *J Trauma*. October 2007;*63(4)*:805–813.

50. Duke MD, Guidry C, Guice J, Stuke L, Marr AB, Hunt JP, Meade P, McSwain NE, Jr, Duchesne JC. Restrictive fluid resuscitation in combination with damage control resuscitation: Time for adaptation. *J Trauma Acute Care Surg*. September 2012;*73(3)*:674–678.

51. Sperry JL, Minei JP, Frankel HL, West MA, Harbrecht BG, Moore EE, Maier RV, Nirula R. Early use of vasopressors after injury: Caution before constriction. *J Trauma*. January 2008;*64(1)*:9–14.

52. Lienhart HG, Wenzel V, Braun J et al. Vasopressin for therapy of persistent traumatic hemorrhagic shock: The VITRIS at study. *Anaesthesist*. February 2007;*56(2)*:145–148, 150.

53. Cohn SM, McCarthy J, Stewart RM, Jonas RB, Dent DL, Michalek JE. Impact of low-dose vasopressin on trauma outcome: Prospective randomized study. *World J Surg*. February 2011;*35(2)*:430–439.

54. King DR. Initial care of the severely injured patient. *N Engl J Med*. February 21 2019;*380(8)*:763–770.

8

Diagnosis of Injury in the Trauma Patient

Jennie S. Kim, Elizabeth Benjamin, Pedro G.R. Teixeira, and Kenji Inaba

8.1 Introduction

Diagnostic imaging remains critical to the management of acutely injured trauma patients, especially in the era of selective nonoperative management of many traumatic injuries. As diagnostic technology evolves, constant reassessment is required to ensure that the sensitivity and specificity parameters of any diagnostic test are well-understood and that the target population is well-defined to minimize cost, radiation burden, patient movement, and time. For unstable trauma patients, operative exploration maintains a central role in diagnosis and management. These patients often have ongoing hemorrhage and shock, and although simple radiologic procedures can be used as adjuncts to operative decision-making, the core principles of trauma surgery that mandate operative management of the unstable patient remain unchanged. For the stable trauma patient, however, rapid assessment and cataloging of injury burden are essential for optimal outcomes, and radiologic imaging plays a central role in data acquisition. Two main pathways result in the deterioration of the initially stable trauma patient. First, ongoing blood loss or underestimation of injury burden results in the conversion of the initially stable to the subsequently unstable patient. Hemorrhage remains a major cause of early death after trauma and the primary cause of preventable and potentially preventable death in both civilian and military populations [1]. Imaging is essential to identify areas of ongoing blood loss or potential hemorrhage in the otherwise stable patient. Second, missed injuries are a major component of potentially preventable morbidity and mortality. Delay in diagnosis can result in delayed treatment, increased infection risk, or failure of early mobilization.

Ultrasonography and computed tomography (CT) are widely available imaging modalities that have been fully incorporated into the armamentarium of the trauma surgeon and are essential components of trauma management algorithms. This chapter will review the evidence base to support the use of these modalities for the initial assessment of the injured patient (Table 8.1).

8.2 Focused Abdominal Sonography for Trauma

Focused abdominal sonography for trauma (FAST) is a standardized ultrasound examination that aims to identify the presence of free fluid in the pericardium and peritoneal cavity.

As an initial diagnostic adjunct, ultrasound has several advantages: It is noninvasive, repeatable, accessible, portable, rapid, and cost-effective. Reliance on ultrasound has, however, been tempered by interoperator variability and several patient-related factors such as subcutaneous emphysema, morbid obesity, and severe chest wall injury that can impair image acquisition. FAST was not designed to diagnose specific injuries, but instead was designed as a screening assessment tool. In unstable polytrauma patients, intraabdominal fluid in the setting of a normal chest radiograph may influence operative planning. Alternatively, a positive abdominal FAST examination in a stable, asymptomatic blunt trauma patient may influence the decision to obtain further definitive imaging. FAST is not intended as an isolated study, but instead is most effective when utilized in combination with additional imaging modalities and clinical presentation. The ability to perform a FAST should continue to be part of a surgeon's skill set, as its use beyond the emergency department such as in the intensive care unit or operating room can provide valuable information on the changing hemodynamic status of a trauma patient.

8.3 What Is the Role of FAST in the Initial Assessment of the Hemodynamically Stable Blunt Trauma Patient?

Physical examination alone is unreliable for the diagnosis of intraabdominal injuries in patients who have sustained blunt abdominal trauma. Diagnostic imaging is therefore relied on to diagnose or rule out intraabdominal injuries. The ideal screening examination for intraabdominal injuries has a high degree of sensitivity, which would allow for the safe exclusion of significant injuries while still maintaining an acceptable specificity, effectively decreasing the number of patients requiring definitive imaging.

Although early reports on abdominal FAST for the identification of intraabdominal injury after blunt trauma were encouraging [2], more recent studies suggest that this modality may lack sufficient sensitivity to consistently be used as a reliable screening test. In the hemodynamically stable blunt trauma patient, FAST has several limitations. Data suggest that a negative FAST is not sufficient to rule out intraabdominal injury, and conversely, a positive scan in a stable patient does not mandate immediate operation [3, 4]. In a well-designed prospective study with a uniform application of CT scan as the standard reference, Miller et al. found that FAST had a 42% sensitivity for intraperitoneal fluid in hemodynamically stable patients [5]. They concluded that ultrasound should not be the sole screening method for the evaluation of blunt abdominal trauma. These results were supported by a 7-year single-center review of FAST in the stable blunt trauma patient, which defined the sensitivity and specificity of FAST at 41% and 99%, respectively, with the authors concluding that FAST did not add value to the initial assessment of the stable blunt trauma patient [6].

A Cochrane review analyzing the use of ultrasound-based treatment algorithms suggested that the utilization of ultrasound in the evaluation of trauma patients had minimal impact on management decisions [7]. It has been demonstrated that 18–26% of patients with intraabdominal injuries have no detectable free intraperitoneal fluid and that up to 29% of abdominal injuries may be missed if ultrasound is the only diagnostic adjunct utilized in blunt trauma patients [3, 4]. In 2016, the National Institute for Health and Care Excellence (NICE) in England recommended immediate CT imaging and bypassing FAST in major trauma patients who are hemodynamically normal or responding to resuscitation for the evaluation of suspected hemorrhage [8]. Although there is some evidence suggesting that repeat imaging may improve the sensitivity of FAST [9], there is insufficient evidence to support the use of a negative FAST as the sole modality to rule out intraabdominal injury.

In contrast, in the setting of a positive FAST, there has been some evidence quantifying the intraabdominal fluid seen on ultrasound and developing an ultrasound hemoperitoneum score to help determine the need for a therapeutic laparotomy. McKenney et al.'s study of 100 blunt trauma patients with free intraperitoneal fluid identified on FAST showed that 40 of 46 patients with a score ≥3 (87%) required a therapeutic laparotomy while 46 of 54 patients with a score <3 (85%) did not need operative intervention. The sensitivity of sonography was 83% compared to systolic blood pressure (28%) and base deficit (49%) in determining the need for therapeutic operation [10].

However, in the era of selective nonoperative management of solid organ injuries, a positive FAST in the hemodynamically stable blunt trauma patient is still not sufficient to warrant operative intervention, and further definitive imaging is often indicated.

> **RECOMMENDATION**
>
> FAST should not be used as the only diagnostic modality to exclude significant intraabdominal injury in the initial assessment of the blunt trauma patient (Grade B). Patients with suspected intraabdominal injury should undergo clinical observation or further investigation, irrespective of the ultrasound findings (Grade B).

8.4 What Is the Role of FAST in the Initial Assessment of the Hemodynamically Unstable Blunt Trauma Patient?

In the hemodynamically unstable blunt trauma patient, FAST as a diagnostic adjunct is significantly more important. In this patient population, FAST has largely supplanted diagnostic peritoneal lavage as the primary diagnostic adjunct for the identification of free intraabdominal fluid. A positive FAST in the setting of hemodynamic instability mandates immediate surgical intervention to rule out intraabdominal bleeding as a source of instability. A positive FAST in hemodynamically unstable blunt-injured patients correlates to a therapeutic laparotomy in 83% of the cases [11]. A delay in operative intervention for additional imaging has been associated with increased mortality [12].

A negative FAST in the unstable blunt trauma patient, however, similar to a negative study in the hemodynamically stable patient, is of less value, with a significant number of false-negative results, especially in retroperitoneal injury and pelvic fracture [13, 14]. Lee et al. demonstrated that 37% of the patients with a negative FAST on initial investigation required therapeutic laparotomy [11], and in a multi-institutional review, Rowell et al. showed similar results with a 32% false-negative rate of FAST examinations in this population [15]. Holmes found that 32% of the unstable patients with a negative ultrasound had intraabdominal injuries [16]. A meta-analysis by Netherton et al. reviewed 75 studies and a subgroup analysis for the detection of intraabdominal free fluid in hypotensive patients showed a pooled sensitivity of 74% and specificity of 95% [17]. Even in the hands of a radiologist, a negative initial FAST is insufficient to rule out an intraabdominal injury with sensitivity, specificity and positive and negative predictive values of 62%, 96%, 84%, and 89%, respectively [18].

> **RECOMMENDATION**
>
> A positive FAST warrants laparotomy in hemodynamically unstable patients (Grade B). Negative FAST in a hemodynamically unstable patient is insufficient to rule out intraabdominal injury (Grade B).

8.5 What Is the Role of Ultrasound in the Initial Assessment of Penetrating Trauma Patients? Cardiac View and Abdominal View

Time is of the essence in the management of cardiac injuries. Early diagnosis and treatment are critical factors for survival. Physical examination, however, is inaccurate for the diagnosis of cardiac injury, as 25% of patients are completely asymptomatic.

The cardiac component of FAST, designed to assess the pericardial sac for the presence of fluid, is an immediately available, repeatable, and noninvasive diagnostic option. In a well-designed prospective study, Rozycki et al. investigated the role of ultrasound as the primary imaging modality used to determine the need for surgical intervention in patients with suspected cardiac injuries [19]. In this study, the ultrasound was 100% accurate in detecting hemopericardium, with no false-positive or false-negative results. This was followed by a prospective multicenter study including five Level I trauma centers confirming the reliability of ultrasound in identifying penetrating cardiac injuries with 100% sensitivity and 97% specificity [20]. Similar results were described in a prospective observational analysis of 130 patients with penetrating torso injury in which the cardiac FAST exam had a sensitivity and specificity of 100% for the detection of cardiac injury [21]. A positive cardiac FAST, however, relies on the presence of fluid trapped in the pericardial space. The potential decompression of blood into the left chest with a concurrent cardiac and pericardial injury has been described as a potential source of the false-negative exam. In a retrospective analysis of 228 patients, five false-negative pericardial FAST exams were identified, all of which were secondary to left chest penetrating injuries with associated hemothorax [22].

The pericardial FAST can be rapidly performed and has been shown to provide reliable information to influence clinical course. A negative exam in a hypotensive patient in the absence of hemothorax may direct attention to a noncardiac etiology, while a positive exam in a patient with multiple truncal and precordial wounds may reflect a cardiac injury, thus influencing operative incision order and choice [23].

As the role of nonoperative management in penetrating abdominal trauma expands, the utility of the abdominal windows of FAST in penetrating injuries is less clear. The decision for operative intervention is based less on peritoneal penetration or intraabdominal fluid and more on clinical presentation, patient reliability, and wound trajectory [24]. In a stable patient with penetrating injury, a positive FAST may represent solid organ injury and may not require operative intervention. Conversely, an unstable patient with penetrating abdominal trauma and peritonitis will undergo laparotomy regardless of ultrasound results. Although some reports of high sensitivity and specificity of FAST exist [21], the majority of the literature supports that this modality is insufficient to diagnose or rule out the intraabdominal injury that will require operative intervention in the stable trauma patient after penetrating injury. In a Western Trauma Association multicenter trial of 134 stable patients with penetrating abdominal trauma, the sensitivity of FAST was 21%, with a positive predictive value of 50% [25]. Similar results have been reported from the military experience, with a reported FAST sensitivity of 56% in a largely penetrating injury population [26]. These results support previous prospective analyses that established the low sensitivity of abdominal FAST (46–67%) to detect clinically significant penetrating abdominal injury [27–29]. In a study by Soffer et al. that included an analysis of clinical indications for operative intervention, the abdominal FAST results changed management in only 1.7% of patients [27]. Although the reported specificity of the abdominal FAST after penetrating trauma is

more compelling, reported at 94–100%, the negative predictive value ranges from 60% to 90% [20, 25–29]. The possibility of hollow viscus injury (HVI) causing a sonographically undetectable volume of abdominal fluid precludes the current FAST from acting as the sole indicator to rule out abdominal injury after penetrating trauma.

RECOMMENDATION

Ultrasound should be the initial diagnostic modality for patients with penetrating precordial wounds (Grade A), and a positive ultrasound for fluid in the pericardial sac warrants immediate surgical intervention (Grade A). FAST is not a reliable imaging modality in penetrating trauma for ruling out significant intraabdominal injury (Grade B).

8.6 What Is the Current Evidence to Support the Use of Ultrasound for the Diagnosis of Pneumothorax in the Resuscitation Area?

Traditionally, the diagnosis of pneumothorax in acute trauma is established using plain radiography. CT is a highly sensitive and specific method for the detection of pneumothorax and is considered the gold-standard imaging modality for this injury.

Plain radiography has several limitations for the detection of pneumothorax. Because air accumulates preferentially in the anteromedial and subpulmonic region in patients in the supine position, radiographic images obtained in supine trauma patients may miss pneumothoraces, although the clinical significance of these occult pneumothoraces is questionable. The process of obtaining the plain radiographs is time-consuming, involves radiation, and there is a delay in obtaining the images—all issues that may be obviated with the advantages of ultrasound.

eFAST, or extended FAST, has been widely applied as a simple, rapid, and noninvasive adjunct in most civilian and military trauma patients. Rowan et al. demonstrated in a small prospective study that ultrasound was more sensitive and accurate than plain chest radiograph in the detection of pneumothorax and had a sensitivity comparable to a CT scan [30]. Further prospective studies using CT scan as a reference standard confirmed the higher sensitivity for ultrasound (92–95%) compared to plain chest radiograph (52–79%) [31, 32]. Zhang et al. demonstrated in a prospective study that ultrasound outperformed plain radiograph for the detection of pneumothorax (86% vs. 28%, $p < 0.001$), allowing significantly faster detection of pneumothorax (2.3 ± 2.9 vs. 19.9 ± 10.3, $p < 0.001$), and had a stronger agreement with CT scan findings [33]. The meta-analysis by Netherton et al. included 17 studies examining the use of eFAST for the identification of pneumothorax, and the pooled sensitivity was 0.694 (95% confidence interval [CI] 0.660–0.727) while the specificity remained high at 0.99 (95% CI 0.99–0.99) [17]. Although thoracic ultrasound for trauma to identify pneumothorax has not been formally incorporated into national protocols, many centers rely heavily on this information for patient procedures and triage [34]. Trauma patients who present hemodynamically unstable may have bilateral chest tubes inserted empirically to exclude tension pneumothorax regardless of eFAST results; however, there is not yet evidence to support the benefit of chest tube insertion solely based on the absence of lung sliding in a stable patient. The clinical significance of the often occult pneumothorax identified on ultrasound remains unclear.

RECOMMENDATION

Ultrasound can be as sensitive as or more sensitive than plain chest radiography and can be utilized to diagnose (but not rule out) pneumothorax in injured patients (Grade B).

8.7 What Is the Role of CT Scan in the Assessment of Hollow Viscus Injury after Blunt Abdominal Trauma?

Traditionally, abdominal CT is thought to be a poor predictor of blunt HVI, with normal imaging identified in 13% of patients with known injury [35]. CT scan is more sensitive and specific than a clinical exam alone [36], but no single imaging modality has been shown to reliably rule in or out HVI [35]. With the advances in multidetector CT (MDCT) and reformatting software, however, the ability to detect HVI with CT imaging is again under investigation [37].

Intuitively, the presence of free air on a CT scan should correlate with HVI; however, this is often not the case after blunt abdominal trauma. In a single-center retrospective study, the presence of intraperitoneal free air on CT was benign in 60% of patients, often likely due to barotrauma [38]. The authors identified seatbelt signs, free fluid, and radiographic signs of bowel trauma to be predictors of clinically significant free air on CT scans. In a retrospective review, the presence of free intraperitoneal air had a sensitivity of only 50% and a positive predictive value of 9.5% for HVI [39]. Extraluminal free air in the presence of bowel wall discontinuity has also been shown to lack sensitivity but has high specificity and positive predictive value for bowel injury [40].

The significance of free fluid on CT scans, especially in the absence of solid organ injury, has also been the topic of much debate. In a review of 122 patients with free fluid on CT scan after blunt abdominal trauma in the absence of solid organ injury, small bowel injury was found in only 12 patients [41]. Conversely, in a review of 68 patients with blunt bowel and mesenteric injuries, all patients had free fluid present on CT imaging [42]. Gonser-Hafertepen et al. categorized the amount of free fluid to determine the predictive value for identifying HVI [43]. They found that no patient with trace free fluid required operation but that moderate to large amounts of fluid was an independent predictor of therapeutic laparotomy (odds rato [OR] 66, *p* < 0.001).

Aside from free fluid and pneumoperitoneum, several additional signs of potential injury have been described. Bowel wall thickening or increased contrast enhancement of the bowel wall can be a nonspecific finding after trauma when diffusely present, but focal enhancement or thickening has been described as a specific indicator of HVI [44, 45]. The accuracy of HVI detection is also thought to be higher in the stomach and duodenum when compared to the colon and remaining small bowel [46].

While some signs have high sensitivity and low specificity, others have low sensitivity but high specificity. No one sign has emerged as the sole indicator of injury; however, especially with the advances in MDCT, the overall combination of radiologic findings, in conjunction with physical examination, remains an important adjunct in the diagnosis of blunt HVI. A study by Firetto et al. showed high positive predictive values for blunt bowel and mesenteric trauma in patients with abdominal guarding (100%) along with bowel wall discontinuity and extraluminal gas (83.3%) [47]. Finally, with current technology, patients with blunt HVI are unlikely to have a completely negative preoperative CT scan [42, 48–50]. In a prospective study of 620 patients with blunt abdominal trauma, no patients with a completely negative CT scan were found to have HVI after observation, regardless of the presence of external signs of trauma [49]. A prospective study by Delaplain et al., evaluating only patients with an abdominal seatbelt sign, demonstrated that a completely negative CT scan is associated with the absence of an HVI (*p* = 0.014), suggesting there may even be a subset of patients with a seatbelt sign who do not need to be observed and can be safely discharged from the emergency department [50].

Despite better recognition of patterns of radiologic findings that suggest HVI, CT may still be inaccurate at identifying the viscous injury, and so clinical correlation with physical examination is essential. In an unexaminable patient, exploratory laparoscopy or laparotomy may be required to rule out HVI.

RECOMMENDATION

CT scan alone cannot be used to reliably rule in or rule out the presence of HVI after blunt abdominal trauma (Grade B). Using MDCT, pneumoperitoneum, free fluid, focal bowel wall thickening or enhancement, and bowel wall discontinuity are all signs suggestive of HVI, especially when present in combination (Grade B). In the presence of a completely negative CT scan, blunt HVI is unlikely (Grade B).

8.8 Can CT Scan Be Utilized to Diagnose or Rule Out Penetrating Diaphragmatic Injury?

The identification of diaphragmatic injury after penetrating trauma can be challenging. In the era of abdominal exploration for all penetrating abdominal injuries, the presence of diaphragmatic injury could be directly visualized. More recently, however, selective nonoperative management of penetrating torso trauma in the stable, evaluable patient has become widely accepted [24]. In this population, a CT scan is often used as a diagnostic adjunct to identify missile trajectory and injuries sustained. The utility of CT scan imaging to identify occult diaphragmatic injury, however, has been questioned. Diaphragmatic injuries occur in approximately 7–24% of patients after left thoracoabdominal penetrating trauma [51, 52]. Although small diaphragmatic injuries rarely cause immediate symptoms, they can expand over time and create a source of potential incarceration or strangulation of herniated abdominal contents. In contemporary practice, after a period of observation with serial abdominal exams to monitor for other indications requiring operative intervention, thoracoscopy or laparoscopy may be used as a diagnostic modality to identify occult diaphragmatic injury after penetrating left thoracoabdominal trauma before patient discharge [51, 53].

Although traditionally thought to lack sensitivity, new MDCT technology, with thinner cuts and advanced reconstruction, has shown promising results in the identification of diaphragmatic injury after penetrating thoracoabdominal trauma [54]. In a retrospective review using intraoperative injury identification as the gold standard, 64-slice MDCT had a sensitivity ranging from 71% to 100% and a specificity of 50–92% for the identification of diaphragmatic injury [55]. In addition, visualization of transdiaphragmatic trajectory and contiguous injury improves the sensitivity and specificity of CT scans [54, 56]. In a retrospective analysis of 136 patients with penetrating trauma and injury trajectory in the vicinity of the diaphragm, radiologists blinded to the operative findings reviewed the images [57]. The authors reported the sensitivity and specificity of MDCT as 87.2% and 72.4%, respectively, increasing to 88% and 82%, respectively, when a contiguous injury was identified.

RECOMMENDATION

MDCT can be used as a diagnostic adjunct to identify occult diaphragmatic injury after penetrating trauma and has improved sensitivity and specificity with the visualization of a transdiaphragmatic trajectory or contiguous injury (Grade B).

TABLE 8.1

Summary Points with Recommendations Including Level of Evidence and Grade of Recommendations

	Question	Answer	Levels of Evidence	Grade of Recommendation	References
1	What is the role of FAST in the initial assessment of the hemodynamically stable blunt trauma patient?	FAST should not be used as the only diagnostic modality to exclude significant intraabdominal injury in the initial assessment of the blunt trauma patient.	IIb, IIIa	B	[6–9]
	Should patients with suspected intraabdominal injury undergo clinical observation or further investigation, irrespective of the ultrasound findings?	Yes	IIb, IIIa	B	[7–9]
2	What is the role of FAST in the initial assessment of the hemodynamically unstable blunt trauma patient?	A positive FAST warrants laparotomy in hemodynamically unstable patients.	Ib, IIb	B	[4, 11]
	Is a negative FAST in a hemodynamically unstable patient insufficient to rule out intraabdominal injury?	Yes	IIIb	B	[13–15]
3	What is the role of ultrasound in the initial assessment of penetrating trauma patients: Cardiac view and abdominal view?	Ultrasound should be the initial diagnostic modality for patients with penetrating precordial wounds.	Ib, IIb	A	[4, 16, 17]
	Does a positive ultrasound for fluid in the pericardial sac warrant immediate surgical intervention?	Yes	Ib, IIb	A	[4, 16, 17]
	Is FAST a reliable imaging modality in penetrating trauma for ruling out significant intraabdominal injury?	No	Ib, IIb	B	[21, 22, 24]
4	What is the current evidence to support the use of ultrasound for the diagnosis of pneumothorax in the resuscitation area?	Ultrasound can be as sensitive as or more sensitive than plain chest radiography and can be utilized to diagnose pneumothorax in injured patients.	Ib	A	[29, 31]
5	What is the role of a CT scan in the assessment of hollow viscus injury after blunt abdominal trauma?	CT alone cannot be used to reliably rule in or rule out the presence of HVI after blunt abdominal trauma.	IIb	B	[32]

(Continued)

TABLE 8.1 (Continued)

Summary Points with Recommendations Including Level of Evidence and Grade of Recommendations

	Question	Answer	Levels of Evidence	Grade of Recommendation	References
	Is MDCT used, along with pneumoperitoneum, free fluid, focal bowel wall thickening or enhancement, and bowel wall discontinuity, to detect signs suggestive of HVI, especially when present in combination?	Yes	IIb, IIIb	B	[33, 35–37, 40, 44]
	In the presence of a completely negative CT scan, is blunt HVI unlikely?	Yes	IIb, IIIb	B	[39, 40, 44]
6	Can a CT scan be utilized to diagnose or rule out penetrating diaphragmatic injury?	MDCT can be used as a diagnostic adjunct to identify occult diaphragmatic injury after penetrating trauma and has improved sensitivity and specificity with visualization of a transdiaphragmatic trajectory or contiguous injury.	IIIb	B	[48–50]
		Diagnostic laparoscopy can be used to identify or rule out occult diaphragmatic injury.	IIb	B	[45]

Editor's Note

The authors of this chapter have nicely described the current state of the diagnosis of trauma pathology today. In the unstable, dying trauma patient, we know that hemorrhagic shock is the culprit in two-thirds of instances, so we proceed with bilateral chest tubes and laparotomy when indicated. Fortunately, these cases are much less common than hemodynamically stable injured individuals. In these folks, advances in imaging technology have led to a radical change in our method of identifying injuries. Ultrasonography and CT scanning have replaced diagnostic peritoneal lavage and plain x-rays in the delineation of injuries. This has reduced the number of unnecessary interventions. As technology improves, the diagnosis of clinically relevant abnormalities following trauma will likely become faster and more accurate.

REFERENCES

1. Teixeira PG, Inaba K, Hadjizacharia P, Brown C, Salim A, Rhee P, et al. Preventable or potentially preventable mortality at a mature trauma center. *J Trauma.* 2007;63(6):1338–46; discussion 1346-7.
2. Rozycki GS, Ballard RB, Feliciano DV, Schmidt JA, Pennington SD. Surgeon-performed ultrasound for the assessment of truncal injuries: lessons learned from 1540 patients. *Ann Surg.* 1998;228(4):557–67.
3. Yoshii H, Sato M, Yamamoto S, Motegi M, Okusawa S, Kitano M, et al. Usefulness and limitations of ultrasonography in the initial evaluation of blunt abdominal trauma. *J Trauma.* 1998;45(1):45–50; discussion 50-1.
4. Chiu WC, Cushing BM, Rodriguez A, Ho SM, Mirvis SE, Shanmuganathan K, et al. Abdominal injuries without hemoperitoneum: a potential limitation of focused abdominal sonography for trauma (FAST). *J Trauma.* 1997;42(4):617–23; discussion 623-5.
5. Miller MT, Pasquale MD, Bromberg WJ, Wasser TE, Cox J. Not so FAST. *J Trauma.* 2003;54(1):52–9; discussion 59-60.
6. Natarajan B, Gupta PK, Cemaj S, Sorensen M, Hatzoudis GI, Forse RA. FAST scan: is it worth doing in hemodynamically stable blunt trauma patients? *Surgery.* 2010;148(4):695–700; discussion 700-1.
7. Stengel D, Bauwens K, Sehouli J, Rademacher G, Mutze S, Ekkernkamp A, et al. Emergency ultrasound-based algorithms for diagnosing blunt abdominal trauma. *Cochrane Database Syst Rev.* 2005;(2): CD004446.
8. Glen J, Constanti M, Brohi K. Assessment and initial management of major trauma: summary of NICE guidance. *BMJ.* 2016;353:i3051.
9. Blackbourne LH, Soffer D, McKenney M, Amortegui J, Schulman CI, Crookes B, et al. Secondary ultrasound examination increases the sensitivity of the FAST exam in blunt trauma. *J Trauma.* 2004;57(5):934–38.
10. McKenney KL, McKenney MG, Cohn SM, Compton R, Nunez DB, Namias N. Hemoperitoneum score helps determine need for therapeutic laparotomy. *J Trauma.* 2001;50(4):560–64; discussion 654-6.
11. Lee BC, Ormsby EL, McGahan JP, Melendres GM, Richards JR. The utility of sonography for the triage of blunt abdominal trauma patients to exploratory laparotomy. *AJR Am J Roentgenol.* 2007;188(2):415–21.
12. Neal MD, Peitzman AB, Forsythe RM, Marshall GT, Rosengart MR, Alarcon LH, et al. Over reliance on computed tomography imaging in patients with severe abdominal injury: is the delay worth the risk? *J Trauma.* 2011;70(2):278–84.
13. Hoffman L, Pierce D, Puumala S. Clinical predictors of injuries not identified by focused abdominal sonogram for trauma (FAST) examinations. *J Emerg Med.* 2009;36(3):271–79.
14. Laselle BT, Byyny RL, Haukoos JS, Krzyzaniak SM, Brooks J, Dalton TR, et al. False-negative FAST examination: associations with injury characteristics and patient outcomes. *Ann Emerg Med.* 2012;60(3):326–34.e3.

15. Rowell SE, Barbosa RR, Holcomb JB, Fox EE, Barton CA, Schreiber MA. The focused assessment with sonography in trauma (FAST) in hypotensive injured patients frequently fails to identify the need for laparotomy: a multi-institutional pragmatic study. *Trauma Surg Acute Care Open.* 2019;4(1):e000207.

16. Holmes JF, Harris D, Battistella FD. Performance of abdominal ultrasonography in blunt trauma patients with out-of-hospital or emergency department hypotension. *Ann Emerg Med.* 2004;43(3):354–61.

17. Netherton S, Milenkovic V, Taylor M, Davis PJ. Diagnostic accuracy of eFAST in the trauma patient: a systematic review and meta-analysis. *CJEM.* 2019;21(6):727–38.

18. Gaarder C, Kroepelien CF, Loekke R, Hestnes M, Dormage JB, Naess PA. Ultrasound performed by radiologists-confirming the truth about FAST in trauma. *J Trauma.* 2009;67(2):323–27; discussion 328-9.

19. Rozycki GS, Feliciano DV, Schmidt JA, Cushman JG, Sisley AC, Ingram W, et al. The role of surgeon-performed ultrasound in patients with possible cardiac wounds. *Ann Surg.* 1996;223(6):737–44; discussion 744-6.

20. Rozycki GS, Feliciano DV, Ochsner MG, Knudson MM, Hoyt DB, Davis F, et al. The role of ultrasound in patients with possible penetrating cardiac wounds: a prospective multicenter study. *J Trauma.* 1999;46(4):543–51; discussion 551-2.

21. Tayal VS, Beatty MA, Marx JA, Tomaszewski CA, Thomason MH. FAST (focused assessment with sonography in trauma) is accurate for cardiac and intraperitoneal injury in penetrating anterior chest trauma. *J Ultrasound Med.* 2004;23(4):467–72.

22. Ball CG, Williams BH, Wyrzykowski AD, Nicholas JM, Rozycki GS, Feliciano DV. A caveat to the performance of pericardial ultrasound in patients with penetrating cardiac wounds. *J Trauma.* 2009;67(5):1123–24.

23. Matsushima K, Khor D, Berona K, Antoku D, Dollbaum R, Khan M, et al. Double jeopardy in penetrating trauma: Get FAST, get it right. *World J Surg.* 2018;42(1):99–106.

24. Inaba K, Demetriades D. The nonoperative management of penetrating abdominal trauma. *Adv Surg.* 2007;41:51–62.

25. Biffl WL, Kaups KL, Cothren CC, Brasel KJ, Dicker RA, Bullard MK, et al. Management of patients with anterior abdominal stab wounds: a Western Trauma Association multicenter trial. *J Trauma.* 2009;66(5):1294–301.

26. Smith IM, Naumann DN, Marsden ME, Ballard M, Bowley DM. Scanning and war: utility of FAST and CT in the assessment of battlefield abdominal trauma. *Ann Surg.* 2015;262(2):389–96.

27. Soffer D, McKenney MG, Cohn S, Garcia-Roca R, Namias N, Schulman C, et al. A prospective evaluation of ultrasonography for the diagnosis of penetrating torso injury. *J Trauma.* 2004;56(5):953–57; discussion 957-9.

28. Udobi KF, Rodriguez A, Chiu WC, Scalea TM. Role of ultrasonography in penetrating abdominal trauma: a prospective clinical study. *J Trauma.* 2001;50(3):475–79.

29. Boulanger BR, Kearney PA, Tsuei B, Ochoa JB. The routine use of sonography in penetrating torso injury is beneficial. *J Trauma.* 2001;51(2):320–25.

30. Rowan KR, Kirkpatrick AW, Liu D, Forkheim KE, Mayo JR, Nicolaou S. Traumatic pneumothorax detection with the thoracic US: correlation with chest radiography and CT–initial experience. *Radiology.* 2002;225(1):210–14.

31. Nandipati KC, Allamaneni S, Kakarla R, Wong A, Richards N, Satterfield J, et al. Extended focused assessment with sonography for trauma (EFAST) in the diagnosis of pneumothorax: experience at a community-based level I trauma center. *Injury.* 2011;42(5):511–14.

32. Soldati G, Testa A, Sher S, Pignataro G, La Sala M, Silveri NG. Occult traumatic pneumothorax: diagnostic accuracy of lung ultrasonography in the emergency department. *Chest.* 2008;133(1):204–11.

33. Zhang M, Liu ZH, Yang JX, Gan JX, Xu SW, You XD, et al. Rapid detection of pneumothorax by ultrasonography in patients with multiple trauma. *Crit Care.* 2006;10(4):R112.

34. Abdulrahman Y, Musthafa S, Hakim SY, Nabir S, Qanbar A, Mahmood I, et al. Utility of extended FAST in blunt chest trauma: is it the time to be used in the ATLS algorithm? *World J Surg.* 2015;39(1):172–78.

35. Fakhry SM, Watts DD, Luchette FA. Current diagnostic approaches lack sensitivity in the diagnosis of perforated blunt small bowel injury: analysis from 275,557 trauma admissions from the EAST multi-institutional HVI trial. *J Trauma.* 2003;54(2):295–306.

36. Joseph DK, Kunac A, Kinler RL, Staff I, Butler KL. Diagnosing blunt hollow viscus injury: is computed tomography the answer? *Am J Surg.* 2013;205(4):414–18.

37. Atri M, Hanson JM, Grinblat L, Brofman N, Chughtai T, Tomlinson G. Surgically important bowel and/or mesenteric injury in blunt trauma: accuracy of multidetector CT for evaluation. *Radiology.* 2008;249(2):524–33.

38. Marek AP, Deisler RF, Sutherland JB, Punjabi G, Portillo A, Krook J, et al. CT scan-detected pneumoperitoneum: an unreliable predictor of intra-abdominal injury in blunt trauma. *Injury.* 2014;45(1):116–21.

39. Hefny AF, Kunhivalappil FT, Matev N, Avila NA, Bashir MO, Abu-Zidan FM. The usefulness of free intraperitoneal air detected by CT scan in diagnosing bowel perforation in blunt trauma: experience from a community-based hospital. *Injury.* 2015;46(1):100–4.

40. Park MH, Shin BS, Namgung H. Diagnostic performance of 64-MDCT for blunt small bowel perforation. *Clin Imaging.* 2013;37(5):884–88.

41. Mahmood I, Tawfek Z, Abdelrahman Y, Siddiuqqi T, Abdelrahman H, El-Menyar A, et al. Significance of computed tomography finding of intra-abdominal free fluid without solid organ injury after blunt abdominal trauma: time for laparotomy on demand. *World J Surg.* 2014;38(6):1411–15.

42. Petrosoniak A, Engels PT, Hamilton P, Tien HC. Detection of significant bowel and mesenteric injuries in blunt abdominal trauma with 64-slice computed tomography. *J Trauma Acute Care Surg.* 2013;74(4):1081–6.

43. Gonser-Hafertepen LN, Davis JW, Bilello JF, Ballow SL, Sue LP, Cagle KM, et al. Isolated free fluid on abdominal computed tomography in blunt trauma: watch and wait or operate? *J Am Coll Surg.* 2014;219(4):599–605.

44. Khan I, Bew D, Elias DA, Lewis D, Meacock LM. Mechanisms of injury and CT findings in bowel and mesenteric trauma. *Clin Radiol.* 2014;69(6):639–47.

45. Brofman N, Atri M, Hanson JM, Grinblat L, Chughtai T, Brenneman F. Evaluation of bowel and mesenteric blunt trauma with multidetector CT. *Radiographics.* 2006;26(4):1119–31.

46. Kim HC, Yang DM, Kim SW, Park SJ. Gastrointestinal tract perforation: evaluation of MDCT according to perforation site and elapsed time. *Eur Radiol.* 2014;24(6):1386–93.

47. Firetto MC, Sala F, Petrini M, Lemos AA, Canini T, Magnone S, et al. Blunt bowel and mesenteric trauma: role of clinical signs along with CT findings in patients' management. *Emerg Radiol.* 2018;25(5):461–467.

48. Tan KK, Liu JZ, Go TS, Vijayan A, Chiu MT. Computed tomography has an important role in hollow viscus and mesenteric injuries after blunt abdominal trauma. *Injury.* 2010;41(5):475–8.

49. Benjamin ER, Siboni S, Haltmeier T, Lofthus A, Inaba K, Demetriades D. Negative finding from computed tomography of the abdomen after blunt trauma. *JAMA Surg.* 2015;150(12):1194–5.

50. Delaplain PT, Barrios C, Spencer D, Lekawa M, Schubl S, Dosch A, et al. The use of computed tomography imaging for abdominal seatbelt sign: a single-center, prospective evaluation. *Injury.* 2020;51(1):26–31.

51. Murray JA, Demetriades D, Asensio JA, Cornwell EE, 3rd, Velmahos GC, Belzberg H, et al. Occult injuries to the diaphragm: prospective evaluation of laparoscopy in penetrating injuries to the left lower chest. *J Am Coll Surg.* 1998;187(6):626–30.

52. Leppäniemi A, Haapiainen R. Occult diaphragmatic injuries caused by stab wounds. *J Trauma.* 2003;55(4):646–50.

53. Cremonini C, Lewis MR, Jakob D, Benjamin ER, Chiarugi M, Demetriades D. Diagnosing penetrating diaphragmatic injuries: CT scan is valuable but not reliable. *Injury.* 2022;53(1):116–21.

54. Dreizin D, Bergquist PJ, Taner AT, Bodanapally UK, Tirada N, Munera F. Evolving concepts in MDCT diagnosis of penetrating diaphragmatic injury. *Emerg Radiol.* 2015;22(2):149–56.

55. Dreizin D, Borja MJ, Danton GH, Kadakia K, Caban K, Rivas LA, et al. Penetrating diaphragmatic injury: accuracy of 64-section multidetector CT with trajectography. *Radiology.* 2013;268(3):729–37.

56. Hammer MM, Flagg E, Mellnick VM, Cummings KW, Bhalla S, Raptis CA. Computed tomography of blunt and penetrating diaphragmatic injury: sensitivity and interobserver agreement of CT Signs. *Emerg Radiol.* 2014;21(2): 143–49.

57. Bodanapally UK, Shanmuganathan K, Mirvis SE, Sliker CW, Fleiter TR, Sarada K, et al. MDCT diagnosis of penetrating diaphragm injury. *Eur Radiol.* 2009;19(8):1875–81.

9

Damage Control Laparotomy and Abdominal Compartment Syndrome

Christopher S. Thomas and Bruce A. Crookes

9.1 Introduction

Over the course of the past 20 years, the term "damage control" has become a part of the common vernacular among trauma surgeons, general surgeons, and orthopedists. Initially conceptualized as a temporizing measure to stabilize the victims of penetrating trauma, it is now a widely applied algorithm that has become a standard of care within the trauma community.

The term "damage control" has its origin within the U.S. Navy, where it was intended to describe a technique in which the damaged hull of a ship undergoes rapid assessment and stabilization, so that it may return to the controlled environment of port [1]. Although the original application of the term "damage control" to surgery is attributed to Rotondo et al. [2] in 1993, the origins of the surgical technique can be traced back to Pringle [3], who first applied hepatic packing to arrest hemorrhage. Most authors, however, attribute the formalization of the technique to Stone [4], who, in 1983, described the technique of laparotomy truncation in the setting of exsanguinating hepatic hemorrhage. Stone and his associates terminated the initial laparotomy of patients with hepatic injury once the patient became coagulopathic.

With an increase in semiautomatic weapons use in the late 1980s and faced with an average of 2.7 shots per body [5], traumatologists saw a concomitant increase in mortality. From this crucible of interpersonal violence arose the sentinel report by Rotondo et al. [2], and the term "damage control" was applied to trauma surgery for the first time.

The damage control sequence is commonly employed to avoid the "lethal triad" of hypothermia (defined as a core body temperature of <35°C), coagulopathy, and acidosis. Although there is no formal definition of the damage control technique, its steps are commonly acknowledged to include the following three-part sequence [6, 7]:

1. Operating room (OR) (Part I)
   a. Rapid control of hemorrhage
   b. Control or containment of contamination
   c. Restoration of vascular flow when required
   d. Intraabdominal packing
   e. Temporary abdominal closure

2. Intensive care unit (ICU) (Part II)
   a. Core rewarming
   b. Optimization of hemodynamics
   c. Correction of coagulopathy
   d. Ventilatory support
   e. Secondary survey and injury identification
3. OR (Part III)
   a. Pack removal
   b. Definitive repair of injuries

The purpose of this chapter is to provide an evidence-based review of the literature concerning the indications for the implementation of damage control techniques, the morbidity and mortality associated with the use of damage control, and the optimal technique for the temporary closure of the abdominal wall.

9.2 Does a "Damage Control" Approach Improve Mortality?

Reports of damage control procedures have denoted mortality rates ranging from 16% to 69% [2, 8]. In a collective review of 961 damage control patients, published in 1994, Rotondo et al. [7] delineated a cumulative mortality rate of 58% from all of the known, published damage control series. A more recent series, however, has shown a continued improvement in mortality rates. Johnson et al. [8] performed a retrospective cohort series comparing their damage control experience with that at their center from 10 years earlier. While the historical control group had a mortality rate of 58%, Johnson et al. had a mortality rate of 10% for their more recent series. The authors postulated that this was due to improved ICU care, increased experience with the open abdomen, and improved temperature control. Wang et al. [9] reported survival of 61.5% when damage control techniques were utilized to manage hemorrhagic shock in patients with blunt abdominal trauma. Most recently, the U.S. military has successfully employed the damage control paradigm, yielding a 16% mortality rate [10].

DOI: 10.1201/9781003316800-9

Asensio et al. [11] examined the mortality rate in damage control patients before and after the institution of intraoperative guidelines and found a consistent mortality rate of 24% pre- and post-implementation. Interestingly, the combination of a vascular injury and rectal injury resulted in a mortality rate of 36% and was found to be the most deadly injury complex. Nicholas et al. [12] used a retrospective cohort analysis to find that in penetrating abdominal trauma, an increasing application of damage control techniques resulted in a statistically significantly higher survival rate (73.3%). Unfortunately, it carried with it a significant morbidity load, including sepsis, intraabdominal abscess, and gastrointestinal fistula rate.

The combination of damage control resuscitation concepts with damage control laparotomy (DCL) has seemingly continued to decrease mortality rates even further. Cotton et al. [13] compared outcomes in 282 patients who underwent DCL before damage control resuscitation techniques with outcomes in 108 DCLs coupled with damage control resuscitation: The 24-hour and 30-day survival were significantly higher with the addition of damage control resuscitation (88% vs. 97% and 76% vs. 86%).

RECOMMENDATION

The application of damage control techniques appears to have decreased mortality rates, although absolute mortality reduction is difficult to quantify due to improvements in critical care and resuscitation. Practitioners of this resuscitation paradigm should consider combining the technique with a damage control resuscitation algorithm.

Grade of recommendation: C.

9.3 How Do We Preoperatively Identify the Damage Control Patient?

The decision to employ a damage control technique initiates a sequence of events that require an intense utilization and commitment of resources: The patient must now undergo at least two operations, the ICU must assume the responsibility for a complex and time-consuming resuscitation, and the surgeon and the OR staff are obligated to return to the OR within the next several days after the injury. Thus, the decision to convert to a damage control approach is crucial.

The majority of trauma patients will not require a damage control technique. Multiple authors have attempted to characterize patients who would benefit from a damage control approach, with most employing objective markers, including mechanism of injury, injury severity score (ISS), temperature, pH, coagulopathy, lactate levels, and the number of units of blood transfused.

Wyrzykowski, in the definitive text *Trauma* [14], advocates that "In trauma patients, relative pre-operative indications for DCL include systolic blood pressure (SBP) <90 mmHg with penetrating torso, blunt abdominal, or severe pelvic trauma, and the need for resuscitative thoracotomy."

Asensio et al. [15] retrospectively evaluated 548 patients for prehospital characteristics that predicted "exsanguination syndrome." Using a logistic regression model, they identified several independent risk factors for survival upon presentation to the emergency department (ED): Penetrating trauma, spontaneous ventilation, and the absence of an ED thoracotomy. As a result, the authors of this chapter recommend that patients arriving in the ED with a Revised Trauma Score (RTS) ≤5, patients requiring ≥2,000 mL of crystalloids or ≥2 units of packed red blood cells (PRBCs) for resuscitation, and those patients who have a pH of ≤7.2 are in the early stages of exsanguination syndrome and were excellent candidates for a damage control approach.

Preoperative indications for DCL in nontrauma patients have been published [16] and are similar to traumatic indications. In a review of 455 patients undergoing DCL for emergency abdominal surgery over the past 10 years, the indications for DCL have included uncontrolled bleeding during elective surgery, hemorrhage from complicated gastroduodenal ulcer disease, generalized peritonitis, acute mesenteric ischemia, and "other sources of intra-abdominal sepsis" [16]. Unfortunately, there are insufficient data to validate guidelines for emergency general surgery operations.

RECOMMENDATION

A "damage control approach" should be considered with any trauma patient who has any of the following characteristics:

- RTS ≤5
- Patients who require ≥2,000 mL of crystalloids for their resuscitation in the ED
- Patients who require ≥2 units of PRBCs for their resuscitation in the ED
- Patients who have a pH ≤7.2
- Systolic blood pressure (SBP) <90 mmHg with penetrating torso, blunt abdominal, or severe pelvic trauma and the need for resuscitative thoracotomy

Grade of recommendation: C.

9.4 How Do We Intraoperatively Identify the Damage Control Patient?

Once the patient is in the OR, how does one know when to convert to a "damage control" technique?

Rotondo et al. [2], in the original report on damage control, began to employ a damage control technique once a patient had received more than 10 units of PRBCs before the termination of the laparotomy, but did not evaluate the effectiveness of transfusion requirement as a trigger point for conversion to damage control. Cue et al. [17] noted that coagulopathy began to occur in patients who had received more than 15 units of PRBCs during their initial resuscitation and operation and recommended abdominal packing before reaching that transfusion threshold. Burch et al. [18] performed a retrospective review of 200 patients who were treated for over 7.5 years utilizing damage control techniques. This group used a logistic regression analysis to show that the two most powerful predictors of mortality were the rate of red cell transfusion (units per hour) and pH. When plotted as a scatter plot, these two variables correctly identified patient death within 48 hours of injury 77% of the time. Asensio et al. [15] identified the following values as predictive of survival once a trauma patient was in the OR: ISS ≤20, spontaneous ventilation in the ED, OR blood product replacement of <4,000 mL, no ED or OR thoracotomy, and the absence of abdominal vascular injury. His group recommended that damage control techniques be employed when transfusion volumes are >4,000 mL of PRBCs (or >5,000 mL if both PRBCs and whole blood are used), total OR volume of resuscitation is >12,000 mL (crystalloid and blood products), or when pH is ≤7.2 and temperature is 34.2°C and volume of blood product is ≥5,000 mL.

Sharp and Locicero [19], in a case series of 39 patients, identified several intraoperative risk factors for mortality, including a pH <7.18, a temperature of 31°C, a prothrombin time of 16 seconds, a partial thromboplastin time of 50 seconds, and a transfusion of 10 units or more as being predictive of outcome. Patients with four to five risk factors had a 100% mortality rate, although this represents a small subset of the overall study (three patients). Those who had two to three risk factors had an 83% mortality rate, and those with zero to one risk factor had an 18% mortality rate.

Several reviews of damage control indicate that a damage control technique should be employed in the following circumstances [6, 7, 20, 21]:

1. Inability to achieve hemostasis owing to a recalcitrant coagulopathy
2. Inaccessible major venous injury
3. Time-consuming procedure in the patient with suboptimal response to resuscitation
4. Management of extraabdominal life-threatening injury
5. Reassessment of intraabdominal contents
6. Inability to reapproximate abdominal fascia due to splanchnic reperfusion-induced visceral edema

Consensus statements, however, list the intraoperative indications for DCL in trauma patients to include "nonsurgical" bleeding, pH ≤7.18, temperature ≤33°C, transfusion of ≥10 units of blood, total fluid replacement >12 L, and estimated blood losses of ≥5 L [4, 19]. This also includes patients with evidence of visceral edema, peak inspiratory pressures >40 cm H$_2$O, or intraabdominal pressure >21 mm Hg during attempted closure [22–26]. While these indications represent the application of sound surgical judgment, evidence-based guidelines to definitively support their implementation are lacking at present.

RECOMMENDATION

In the OR, a damage control technique should be considered when, and if, the following criteria apply:

- Patients who require transfusion of ≥10 units of blood or a total fluid replacement of >12 L
- Patients who have had an ED or OR thoracotomy
- Patients who have a pH ≤7.2
- Patients who have a temperature of ≤34°C
- If the patient has an inaccessible major venous injury
- If the surgeon cannot achieve hemostasis owing to a recalcitrant coagulopathy
- If the definitive operative repair is a time-consuming procedure in the patient with suboptimal response to resuscitation
- If the patient requires the management of an extraabdominal life-threatening injury
- If the patient will require a reassessment of intraabdominal contents
- If the surgeon cannot reapproximate the abdominal fascia due to splanchnic reperfusion-induced visceral edema
- Patients with peak inspiratory pressures >40 cmH$_2$O or intraabdominal pressure >21 mmHg during attempted closure

Grade of recommendation: D.

9.5 When Should We Terminate the Initial Damage Control Operation?

In Rotondo et al.'s [2] initial description of the technique, the authors retrospectively included those patients who had a penetrating injury resulting in exsanguination from an abdominal source and who had received more than 10 units of PRBCs before completion of the laparotomy.

It would seem obvious that the need to terminate an operation would be based on the factors of coagulopathy, acidosis, or hypothermia. Ferrara et al. [27] examined a series of 45 trauma patients who required massive transfusions. They found that nonsurvivors were more likely to have had penetrating injuries (88% vs. 55%), received more transfusions (26.5 vs. 18.6), had lower pH (7.04 vs. 7.18), had lower core temperatures (31°C vs. 34°C), and had a higher incidence of clinical coagulopathy (73% vs. 23%). Severe hypothermia occurred in 80% of nonsurvivors vs. 6% of survivors.

Garrison et al. [28] examined a series of 70 consecutive patients who underwent a damage control operation to control hemorrhage, comparing survivors and nonsurvivors. Significant differences included ISS (29 vs. 38), initial pH (7.3 vs. 7.1), platelet count (229,000 vs. 179,000), prothrombin time

(14 seconds vs. 22 seconds), partial thromboplastin time (42 seconds vs. 69 seconds), and duration of hypotension (50 vs. 90 minutes).

RECOMMENDATION

Damage control operations should be rapidly terminated and the patient should be transferred to the ICU when the patient meets any of the following criteria:

- Core temperature ≤34°C
- pH ≤7.2
- Prothrombin time ≥ twice normal
- Partial thromboplastin time ≥ twice normal

Grade of recommendation: B.

9.6 What Is the Best Method to Temporarily Close the Abdomen to Prevent Long-Term Morbidity?

Historically, multiple methods have been described to temporarily close the open abdomen, ranging from simple towel clips, to the "Bogota Bag," to polytetrafluoroethylene patches, to the Wittman Patch, to vacuum closures [29]. As damage control laparotomies have become more prevalent, there has also been an evolution in the methods used to close the abdomen. Offner et al. [30] retrospectively compared methods utilized to temporarily close the open abdomen, including primary fascial closure, towel clips, and the "Bogota Bag." The group found that primary fascial closure led to a statistically higher incidence of abdominal compartment syndrome, acute respiratory distress syndrome (ARDS), and multisystem organ failure.

Barker et al. reported a case series of 717 general surgical and trauma patients who had a vacuum-type closure of their abdominal wall, in which the overall complication rate was 15.5% (14.7% in trauma patients) [29]. In this series, 68.1% of the patients underwent primary fascial closure of their abdomen. Garner et al. [31] achieved a 90% (13 out of the 14 patients) primary closure rate when the incision was managed with a vacuum closure dressing. Hougaard et al. [32] published a retrospective review of 115 patients who underwent temporary abdominal closure with a negative pressure wound dressing (either vacuum-assisted closure [VAC] or AbThera) for open abdomens secondary to abdominal compartment syndrome, damage control surgery, diffuse peritonitis, or wound dehiscence. This group achieved a 92% secondary fascial closure rate, a 17% mortality rate, and a 3.5% fistula rate.

Cothren et al. [33] used a modified closure technique, combining a vacuum dressing with persistent fascial tension (using #1 PDS suture) to accomplish a 100% fascial closure rate. Using a similar technique, Miller et al. [34] closed 88% of patients with an open abdomen, with a mean time to closure of 9.5 days. One patient who was successfully closed developed an incisional hernia.

Miller et al. [35] have published the largest series in the literature (344 patients) that examined closure techniques of the open abdomen. His group found that complications began to escalate after 8 days from the initial operative intervention to fascial closure. Patients undergoing primary closure had significantly fewer complications than those patients undergoing temporary abdominal closure (skin closure only, split-thickness skin graft, and/or absorbable mesh) or prosthetic closures, despite equivalent mean ISS scores between the groups. Pommerening et al. [36] analyzed 499 patients who underwent DCL and noted that only 327 (65.5%) achieved primary fascial closure; they found that each hour delay in return to the OR (24 hours after initial laparotomy) was associated with a 1.1% decrease in the odds of primary fascial closure. In another analysis by Pommerening et al. [37], 301 of the 501 DCLs achieved primary fascial closure. Primary skin closure was associated with an increased risk of superficial abdominal site infection, but not fascial dehiscence. Of the patients who achieved skin closure, 85.6% did not develop abdominal surgical site infections and were spared the morbidity of managing an open wound at discharge.

RECOMMENDATION

Temporary closure of the open abdomen during the index operation may be accomplished using an X-ray cassette drape, Jackson-Pratt drains, and an Ioban drape. Temporary closure of the open abdomen, after the index operation, is best accomplished with a combination of a vacuum-type device and a fascial tensioning system. Delays to the OR should be avoided to obtain primary fascial closure. Abdominal closure is best accomplished by hospital day number 8 to reduce morbidity.

Grade of recommendation: C.

9.7 What Is the Morbidity Rate from a Damage Control Approach?

Carrillo et al. report a morbidity rate of 56% in their case series of 14 patients [38]. Nicholas et al. [12] denoted that an increase in the use of damage control techniques resulted in higher rates of sepsis, intraabdominal abscesses, and gastrointestinal fistulas. Rotondo and Zonies [7] delineated a 40% morbidity rate when all damage control series were summated. Morris et al. [39] found an overall complication rate of 1.09 complications per patient, with eight positive blood cultures, six intraabdominal abscesses, and abdominal compartment syndrome in 16 patients.

Abikhaled et al. [40] compared groups of damage control patients who were packed, noting that patients who were packed for more than 72 hours had statistically significantly lower rates of abscess and mortality. The duration of packing, however, may be more indicative of ongoing physiologic instability rather than serving as a conduit for higher mortality. In a cohort of 67 octogenarians undergoing DCL,

Goussous et al. [41] examined 111 patients who underwent DCL (79 for sepsis and 32 for hemorrhage) and noted different complication rates between the two populations: Overall morbidity (81% vs. 66), mortality (19% vs. 22%), intraabdominal abscess (18% vs. 16%), deep wound infection (9% vs. 9%), enterocutaneous fistula (8% vs. 6%), and primary fascial closure (58% vs. 59%) all differed between groups.

Cheatham and Safcsak [42] prospectively examined the effects of delayed abdominal closure post-hospital. Patients who were discharged with a chronic incisional hernia were compared with patients discharged with primary fascial closure and with the general population, utilizing the SF-36 version 2 health survey at regular intervals for 2 years post-decompression. Cheatham's group looked at quality-adjusted life years and successful return to employment. At 6 months post-decompression, physical and social functioning were significantly decreased among patients with an open abdomen when compared with the general population, but not in patients whose abdomens were closed before discharge. At 18 months post-decompression and after formal abdominal closure, patients who had been discharged with an open abdomen demonstrated normal physical and mental health perception. When compared with the general population at the 18-month time point, both groups of patients exhibited decreased, but identical, quality-adjusted life years (1.20 ± 0.11 vs. 1.23; $p = 0.39$) and a similar ability to resume employment (41% vs. 55%; $p = 0.49$).

RECOMMENDATION

Expected complication rates from damage control laparotomies range from 25% to 40% of patients, with the most common complications being intraabdominal abscesses and enterocutaneous fistulae. Patients who are discharged with an open abdomen should return to a quality of life that is similar to that of patients who are discharged with a closed abdomen by 18 months post-discharge.

Grade of recommendation: C.

9.8 What Is Abdominal Compartment Syndrome and How Should Patients Be Screened and/or Monitored for the Development of Intraabdominal Hypertension?

Abdominal compartment syndrome (ACS) has evolved conceptually from a postoperative concern of trauma surgeons to a potentially preventable cause of multiple organ dysfunction for all critically ill patients. The World Society of Abdominal Compartment Syndrome (WSACS) met in 2004; established consensus definitions in 2006 to guide clinicians in the diagnosis of ACS; published evidence-based recommendations for the diagnosis, management, and prevention of ACS in 2007; and released research recommendations in 2009 [22]. An update of definitions and guidelines using the Grading of

Recommendations Assessment, Development, and Evaluation (GRADE) methodology was published by WSACS in 2013 [43].

The WSACS defined intraabdominal hypertension (IAH) as a "sustained or repeated pathological elevation in intraabdominal pressure (IAP) ≥12 mmHg." Furthermore, it defined ACS as "sustained IAP >20 mmHg that is associated with new organ dysfunction/failure." It also subclassified ACS into primary ACS (due to primary abdominal or pelvic pathology), secondary ACS (due to non-abdominopelvic pathology), and recurrent ACS (redevelopment of ACS after treatment). New definitions added in 2013 by the WSACS included polycompartment syndrome (elevated compartment pressures in two or more anatomic regions) and abdominal compliance (change in volume over the change in IAP). Also, a classification of open abdomen complexity was created [43].

Importantly, the physical examination has been shown to lack sufficient sensitivity to diagnose IAH. Thus, direct measurement of IAP is the preferred diagnostic test for IAH. The WSACS recommends intermittent IAP measurement via the urinary bladder with an instillation volume of 25 mL of sterile saline, the pressure transducer zeroed at the midaxillary line, the patient in the supine position, and at end expiration [43]. This determination was based on reliability, simplicity, and low cost, especially when performed in a standardized fashion [44].

According to surveys of surgeons and anesthesiologists in multiple countries, detection and management of IAH and ACS are inconsistent, and physicians tend to wait until there is an associated organ dysfunction before proceeding to decompressive laparotomy instead of using a critical threshold IAP [45]. Cheatham and Safcsak demonstrated in a prospective observational study that routinely monitoring IAP in ICU patients at risk for IAH/ACS every 4 hours in the ICU via the intravesicular technique to guide resuscitation and need for decompression, as per the WSACS guidelines, significantly increases patient survival and the rate of fascial closure following abdominal decompression [46].

RECOMMENDATION

Intermittent IAP measurement via the urinary bladder should be performed in patients identified to be at risk for IAH/ACS, based on an assessment of the risk factors mentioned earlier. At-risk individuals demonstrating IAH (IAP ≥12 mmHg) should have serial measurements performed during their ICU course to monitor for the development of worsening IAH or ACS requiring intervention.

Grade of recommendation: B.

9.9 Is There an IAP Threshold Level that Mandates Intervention in IAH/ACS?

As mentioned previously, IAP >20 mmHg in the presence of organ dysfunction defines ACS as a condition requiring acute intervention. Nevertheless, no threshold value for IAP exists that can be universally applied to all patients. An alternative parameter, abdominal perfusion pressure (APP), defined as the difference between mean arterial pressure and IAP, has been studied as a resuscitation endpoint. One retrospective trial identified an APP value of ≥50 mmHg as being correlated with lower mortality in surgical and trauma patients [47]. Several other studies in mixed populations of medical and surgical patients identified a critical APP value of ≥60 mmHg as imparting improved survival [48]. Unfortunately, there are no studies to date that define one threshold IAP value for intervention, but the aforementioned study by Cheatham demonstrated that surgical decompression as a prophylactic intervention for IAP of 28 ± 8 and APP of 46 ± 15 mmHg improved survival and the subsequent fascial closure [46].

RECOMMENDATION

In patients being monitored for IAP, there appears to be a benefit in keeping APP ≥50–60 mmHg.

Grade of recommendation: C.

9.10 Are There Any Effective Nonsurgical Strategies for Treating IAH/ACS?

The standard treatment for ACS remains decompressive laparotomy, and the progression of IAH, organ failure, or failed management of nonoperative strategies should not delay its utilization. Nevertheless, the use of screening IAP measurement inevitably leads to the identification of a population of patients with isolated IAH or with evolving ACS. Such patients may be candidates for nonsurgical interventions aimed at reducing IAP. These interventions may theoretically prevent the development of ACS and its associated organ dysfunction while simultaneously sparing the patient the morbidity associated with a decompressive laparotomy and an open abdomen. These interventions include sedation, analgesia, diuretics, hemofiltration/ultrafiltration, gastric/colonic decompression, prokinetic agents, neuromuscular blockade, supine positioning, limitation of fluid resuscitation, albumin resuscitation, damage control resuscitation, and catheter decompression. These nonsurgical strategies for treating IAH/ACS revolve around the principles of improving abdominal wall compliance, decreasing intra-abdominal and intra-luminal volume, decreasing capillary leak, and other measures to optimize regional perfusion. Achieving an ideal fluid balance that maintains perfusion yet does not unnecessarily increase third-space volume is also synergistic with decreasing ACS and its associated morbidity.

Although sedation and analgesia might be expected to have favorable effects on IAH by decreasing abdominal muscle tone, no clinical data exist to support such intervention. Similarly, no clinical studies of active fluid withdrawal

by either diuretic therapy or renal replacement therapies have been conducted. Similarly, neither gastrointestinal decompression nor prokinetic drug therapy has been studied as a treatment for IAH.

Both prone positioning and head-of-bed elevation have been shown to increase IAP, and both positioning maneuvers are becoming more commonplace in the ICU. Head elevation is used to reduce aspiration risk, and prone positioning is used as an adjunct to mechanical ventilation in the management of patients with ARDS. Although supine positioning may minimize IAP, no evidence exists as to whether the IAP benefit is of sufficient magnitude to offset the greater risk of aspiration or to preclude prone positioning in the ARDS patient.

Fluid administration is a critical consideration in the management of IAH/ACS. Volume resuscitation is necessary to maintain adequate intravascular volume and support organ perfusion in critically ill patients. Excessive or supranormal fluid resuscitation, however, is an independent risk factor for IAH/ACS and is a frequent cause of secondary ACS. In one retrospective study, volume resuscitation to a supranormal level of oxygen delivery was found to be associated with a significantly increased incidence of IAH and ACS, organ failure, and decreased survival [49].

The use of catheter decompression to reduce IAP may be an effective alternative to decompressive laparotomy, especially when the elevation in IAP results from intraperitoneal fluid accumulations such as hemoperitoneum, ascites, or abscess. Percutaneous decompression has been reported as a successful treatment for ACS in a retrospective case series [50]. A second small prospective study demonstrated that percutaneous catheter drainage performed in conjunction with aggressive IAP and APP monitoring resulted in the successful reduction of IAP and augmentation of APP in 8 of 12 trauma patients [50].

RECOMMENDATIONS

1. DCL remains the standard treatment of ACS. There are no systematic reviews or randomized controlled trials that compare DCL to nonsurgical strategies in patients with ACS.

2. Neuromuscular blockade and supine positioning may be used as adjunctive measures in the treatment of IAH after careful consideration of the potential adverse consequences of such therapies.

3. In patients at risk for IAH or ACS, care must be taken to provide sufficient resuscitation to support adequate organ perfusion while avoiding overly zealous volume administration.

4. Percutaneous catheter decompression may be an option in cases of IAH/ACS due to intraperitoneal fluid collections.

Grade of recommendation: 1. B; 2. C; 3. B; 4. C.

TABLE 9.1

Damage Control Laparotomy: Question Summary

No.	Question	Answer	Grade	References
1	Does a damage control approach improve mortality?	The application of damage control techniques appears to have decreased mortality rates, although absolute mortality reduction is difficult to quantify due to improvements in critical care and resuscitation. Practitioners of this resuscitation paradigm should consider combining the technique with a damage control resuscitation algorithm.	C	[2, 7–13]
2	How do we preoperatively identify the damage control patient?	A damage control approach should be taken with any trauma patient who has any of the following: RTS<5, require >2L crystalloid resuscitation, require >2 units PRBCs, have a pH <7.2, and/or have an SBP <90 mmHg with penetrating torso, blunt abdominal, or severe pelvic trauma and the need for ED thoracotomy.	C	[14–16]
3	How do we intraoperatively identify the damage control patient?	In the OR, a damage control technique should be considered when, and if, certain criteria apply (see criteria earlier).	D	[2, 4, 6, 7, 17–21]
4	When should we terminate the initial "damage control" operation?	Damage control operations should be rapidly terminated and the patient should be transferred to the ICU when the patient has a temperature <34°C, pH <7.2, PT or PTT > twice normal.	B	[2, 27, 28]
5	What is the best method to temporarily close the abdomen to prevent long-term morbidity?	Temporary closure of the open abdomen is best accomplished with a combination of a vacuum-type device and a fascial tensioning system. Delays to the OR should be avoided to obtain primary fascial closure. Abdominal closure is best accomplished by hospital day number 8 to reduce morbidity.	C	[29, 32–37]
6	What is the morbidity rate from a damage control approach?	Expected complication rates from damage control laparotomies range from 25% to 40% of patients, with the most common complications being intraabdominal abscesses and enterocutaneous fistulae. Methods to avoid these complications are unclear from the literature. Patients who are discharged with an open abdomen should return to a quality of life that is similar to that of patients who are discharged with a closed abdomen by 18 months post-discharge.	C	[7, 12, 38, 40–42]
7	How should patients be screened and/or monitored for the development of IAH/ACS?	Intermittent IAP measurement via the urinary bladder should be performed in patients identified to be at risk for IAH/ACS, based on an assessment of the risk factors mentioned earlier.	B	[43–46]
		At-risk individuals demonstrating IAH (IAP ≥12 mmHg) should have serial measurements performed during their ICU course to monitor for the development of worsening IAH or ACS requiring intervention.	B	[43–46]
8	Is there an IAP threshold level that mandates intervention in IAH/ACS?	In patients being monitored for IAP, there appears to be a benefit in keeping APP ≥50–60 mmHg.	C	[46]
9	Are there any effective nonsurgical strategies for treating IAH/ACS?	Decompressive laparotomy remains the standard treatment of ACS. There are no systematic reviews or randomized controlled trials that compare decompressive laparotomy to nonsurgical strategies in patients with ACS.	B	[49, 50]
		Neuromuscular blockade and supine positioning may be used as adjunctive measures in the treatment of IAH after careful consideration of the potential adverse consequences of such therapies.	C	[49, 50]
		In patients at risk for IAH or ACS, care must be taken to provide sufficient resuscitation to support adequate organ perfusion while avoiding overly zealous volume administration.	B	[49, 50]
		Percutaneous catheter decompression may be an option in cases of IAH/ACS due to intraperitoneal fluid collections.	C	[49, 50]

Disclaimer

There were no sources of funding or conflicts of interest in the writing of this chapter.

Editor's Note

This excellent chapter reviews two topics in surgery that are relatively new to the field: The use of abbreviated operations and the management of abdominal compartment syndrome. "Damage control" was employed in a limited manner in the past, but has become increasingly popular for the management of the unstable, critically ill patient undergoing surgery. It seems like most of the patients we operate emergently on now are "on death's door." Abbreviating an operation to permit the correction of a multitude of pathophysiologic parameters permits the surgeon to return to the operating room with a potentially survivable patient. Some surgeons have expressed concerns that the pendulum has swung too far and we are failing to close patients who could have their operation completed.

One of the reasons to avoid primary fascial closure in patients with catastrophic injury or illness is the potential for the development of abdominal compartment syndrome. This has been well studied, and abdominal pressures are now a routine part of the management of patients after major abdominal operations or significant resuscitations [51]. When an open abdomen or chest is required either initially or following compartment syndrome, it seems prudent to use the least expensive, disposable technique for temporary closure.

REFERENCES

1. Defense Do. Surface ship survivability. Naval War Publication 3– 2031. Washington DC: US Government Printing Office; 1983.
2. Rotondo MF, Schwab CW, McGonigal MD, et al. 'Damage control': an approach for improved survival in exsanguinating penetrating abdominal. Injury J Trauma 1993;35:375–82; discussion 82-3.
3. Pringle JH. V. notes on the arrest of hepatic hemorrhage due to trauma. Ann Surg 1908;48:541–9.
4. Stone HH, Strom PR, Mullins RJ. Management of the major coagulopathy with onset during laparotomy. Ann Surg 1983;197:532–5.
5. Schwab CW. Violence: America's uncivil war–presidential address, sixth scientific assembly of the Eastern Association for the Surgery of Trauma. J Trauma 1993;35:657–65.
6. Moore EE, Burch JM, Franciose RJ, Offner PJ, Biffl WL. Staged physiologic restoration and damage control surgery. World J Surg 1998;22:1184–90; discussion 90-1.
7. Rotondo MF, Zonies DH. The damage control sequence and underlying logic. Surg Clin North Am 1997;77:761–77.
8. Johnson JW, Gracias VH, Schwab CW, et al. Evolution in damage control for exsanguinating penetrating abdominal injury. J Trauma 2001;51:261–9; discussion 9-71.
9. Wang SY, Liao CH, Fu CY, et al. An outcome prediction model for exsanguinating patients with blunt abdominal trauma after damage control laparotomy: a retrospective study. BMC Surg 2014;14:24.
10. Smith IM, Beech ZK, Lundy JB, Bowley DM. A prospective observational study of abdominal injury management in contemporary military operations: Damage control laparotomy is associated with high survivability and low rates of fecal diversion. Ann Surg 2014;261 (4):765–73.
11. Asensio JA, Petrone P, Roldan G, Kuncir E, Ramicone E, Chan L. Has evolution in awareness of guidelines for institution of damage control improved outcome in the management of the posttraumatic open abdomen? Arch Surg 2004;139:209–14; discussion 15.
12. Nicholas JM, Rix EP, Easley KA, et al. Changing patterns in the management of penetrating abdominal trauma: the more things change, the more they stay the same. J Trauma 2003;55:1095–108; discussion 108-10.
13. Cotton BA, Reddy N, Hatch QM, et al. Damage control resuscitation is associated with a reduction in resuscitation volumes and improvement in survival in 390 damage control laparotomy patients. Ann Surg 2011;254:598–605.
14. Feliciano DV, Mattox KL, Moore EE. Trauma. 6th ed. New York: McGraw-Hill, Medical; 2008.
15. Asensio JA, McDuffie L, Petrone P, et al. Reliable variables in the exsanguinated patient which indicate damage control and predict outcome. Am J Surg 2001;182:743–51.
16. Weber DG, Bendinelli C, Balogh ZJ. Damage control surgery for abdominal emergencies. Br J Surg 2014;101:e109–e18.
17. Cue JI, Cryer HG, Miller FB, Richardson JD, Polk HC, Jr. Packing and planned reexploration for hepatic and retroperitoneal hemorrhage: critical refinements of a useful technique. J Trauma 1990;30:1007–11; discussion 11-3.
18. Burch JM, Ortiz VB, Richardson RJ, Martin RR, Mattox KL, Jordan GL, Jr. Abbreviated laparotomy and planned reoperation for critically injured patients. Ann Surg 1992;215:476–83; discussion 83-4.
19. Sharp KW, Locicero RJ. Abdominal packing for surgically uncontrollable hemorrhage. Ann Surg 1992;215:467–74; discussion 74-5.
20. Moore FA, Nelson T, McKinley BA, et al. Is there a role for aggressive use of fresh frozen plasma in massive transfusion of civilian trauma patients? Am J Surg 2008;196:948–58; discussion 58-60.
21. Shapiro MB, Jenkins DH, Schwab CW, Rotondo MF. Damage control: collective review. J Trauma 2000;49: 969–78.
22. Cheatham ML, Malbrain ML, Kirkpatrick A, et al. Results from the international conference of experts on intra-abdominal hypertension and abdominal compartment syndrome. II. recommendations. Intensive Care Med 2007;33:951–62.
23. Diaz JJ, Jr., Cullinane DC, Dutton WD, et al. The management of the open abdomen in trauma and emergency general surgery: part 1-damage control. J Trauma 2010;68:1425–38.
24. Oelschlager BK, Boyle EM, Jr., Johansen K, Meissner MH. Delayed abdominal closure in the management of ruptured abdominal aortic aneurysms. Am J Surg 1997;173:411–5.
25. Raeburn CD, Moore EE, Biffl WL, et al. The abdominal compartment syndrome is a morbid complication of postinjury damage control surgery. Am J Surg 2001;182:542–6.

26. Rasmussen TE, Hallett JW, Jr., Noel AA, et al. Early abdominal closure with mesh reduces multiple organ failure after ruptured abdominal aortic aneurysm repair: guidelines from a 10-year case-control study. J Vasc Surg 2002;35:246–53.

27. Ferrara A, MacArthur JD, Wright HK, Modlin IM, McMillen MA. Hypothermia and acidosis worsen coagulopathy in the patient requiring massive transfusion. Am J Surg 1990;160:515–8.

28. Garrison JR, Richardson JD, Hilakos AS, et al. Predicting the need to pack early for severe intra-abdominal hemorrhage. J Trauma 1996;40:923–7; discussion 7-9.

29. Barker DE, Green JM, Maxwell RA, et al. Experience with vacuum-pack temporary abdominal wound closure in 258 trauma and general and vascular surgical patients. J Am Coll Surg 2007;204:784–92; discussion 92-3.

30. Offner PJ, de Souza AL, Moore EE, et al. Avoidance of abdominal compartment syndrome in damage-control laparotomy after trauma. Arch Surg 2001;136:676–81.

31. Garner GB, Ware DN, Cocanour CS, et al. Vacuum-assisted wound closure provides early fascial reapproximation in trauma patients with open abdomens. Am J Surg 2001;182:630–8.

32. Hougaard HT, Ellebaek M, Holst UT, Qvist N. The open abdomen: temporary closure with a modified negative pressure therapy technique. Int Wound J 2014;11 Suppl 1:13–6.

33. Cothren CC, Moore EE, Johnson JL, Moore JB, Burch JM. One hundred percent fascial approximation with sequential abdominal closure of the open abdomen. Am J Surg 2006;192:238–42.

34. Miller PR, Meredith JW, Johnson JC, Chang MC. Prospective evaluation of vacuum-assisted fascial closure after open abdomen: planned ventral hernia rate is substantially reduced. Ann Surg 2004;239:608–14; discussion 14-6.

35. Miller RS, Morris JA, Jr., Diaz JJ, Jr., Herring MB, May AK. Complications after 344 damage-control open celiotomies. J Trauma 2005;59:1365–71; discussion 71-4.

36. Pommerening MJ, DuBose JJ, Zielinski MD, et al. Time to first take-back operation predicts successful primary fascial closure in patients undergoing damage control laparotomy. Surgery 2014;156:431–8.

37. Pommerening MJ, Kao LS, Sowards KJ, Wade CE, Holcomb JB, Cotton BA. Primary skin closure after damage control laparotomy. Br J Surg 2014;102 (1):67–75.

38. Carrillo C, Fogler RJ, Shaftan GW. Delayed gastrointestinal reconstruction following massive abdominal trauma. J Trauma 1993;34:233–5.

39. Morris JA, Jr., Eddy VA, Blinman TA, Rutherford EJ, Sharp KW. The staged celiotomy for trauma. Issues in unpacking and reconstruction. Ann Surg 1993;217:576–84; discussion 84-6.

40. Abikhaled JA, Granchi TS, Wall MJ, Hirshberg A, Mattox KL. Prolonged abdominal packing for trauma is associated with increased morbidity and mortality. Am Surg 1997;63:1109–12; discussion 12-3.

41. Goussous N, Jenkins DH, Zielinski MD. Primary fascial closure after damage control laparotomy: sepsis vs haemorrhage. Injury 2014;45:151–5.

42. Cheatham ML, Safcsak K. Longterm impact of abdominal decompression: a prospective comparative analysis. J Am Coll Surg 2008;207:573–9.

43. Kirkpatrick AW, Roberts DJ, De Waele J, et al. Intra-abdominal hypertension and the abdominal compartment syndrome: updated consensus definitions and clinical practice guidelines from the World Society of the Abdominal Compartment Syndrome. Intensive Care Med 2013;39:1190–206.

44. Malbrain ML, Cheatham ML, Kirkpatrick A, et al. Results from the international conference of experts on intra-abdominal hypertension and abdominal compartment syndrome. I. definitions. Intensive Care Med 2006;32:1722–32.

45. Kaussen T, Otto J, Steinau G, Höer J, Srinivasan PK, Schachtrupp A. Recognition and management of abdominal compartment syndrome among German anesthetists and surgeons: a national survey. Ann Intensive Care 2012;2 Suppl 1:S7.

46. Cheatham ML, Safcsak K. Is the evolving management of intra-abdominal hypertension and abdominal compartment syndrome improving survival? Crit Care Med 2010;38:402–7.

47. Cheatham ML, White MW, Sagraves SG, Johnson JL, Block EF. Abdominal perfusion pressure: a superior parameter in the assessment of intra-abdominal hypertension. J Trauma 2000;49:621–6; discussion 6-7.

48. Malbrain M. Abdominal Perfusion Pressure as a Prognostic Marker in Intra-Abdominal Hypertension. In: Vincent J-L, ed. Intensive Care Medicine: Annual Update 2002. New York, NY: Springer New York; 2002:792–814.

49. Balogh Z, McKinley BA, Cocanour CS, et al. Supranormal trauma resuscitation causes more cases of abdominal compartment syndrome. Arch Surg 2003;138:637–42; discussion 42-3.

50. Parra MW, Al-Khayat H, Smith HG, Cheatham ML. Paracentesis for resuscitation-induced abdominal compartment syndrome: an alternative to decompressive laparotomy in the burn patient. J Trauma 2006;60:1119–21.

51. Hong JJ, Cohn SM, Perez JM, Dolich O, McKenney MG. Prospective study of the incidence and outcome of intra-abdominal hypertension and the abdominal compartment syndrome. Br J Surg 2002;89:591–596.

10

Coagulopathy in the Trauma Patient

Bardiya Zangbar and Peter M. Rhee

10.1 Introduction

Trauma is the leading cause of death for individuals 46 years and younger [1], and since hemorrhagic shock is the leading cause of trauma-related deaths, the mechanism and protocols that deal with this type of shock are a crucial part of treatment. Hemorrhagic shock can be compounded by trauma-induced coagulopathy (TIC), which is a hypocoagulable state that can develop immediately after injury and deteriorates with increasing tissue hypoperfusion [2]. TIC is a disease state that includes impairments in clot formation, hemostasis, and ultimate breakdown of the clot due to disorders in both inflammatory and coagulopathic pathways.

Acute coagulopathy of trauma is described as derangements in both intrinsic and extrinsic pathways and activation of the protein C pathway, which increases with the severity of the injury and predicts significantly greater mortality. About one-quarter to one-third of trauma patients are known to have TIC at the time of admission [3], which is present even before iatrogenic crystalloid infusion can worsen the coagulation cascade by dilution. It is well known that massive crystalloid infusion frequently leads to irreversible situations by further driving the lethal triad to exhaustion. Fresh-frozen plasma (FFP) has been considered an effective alternative for volume expansion, as it provides coagulation factors along with volume support to arrest the initial triggers for the development of TIC. Animal studies have shown that FFP can resuscitate without causing an increase in the inflammatory cascade. Further studies led by the PROPPER trial suggested balanced resuscitation results in better outcomes for trauma patients [4]. Ultimately the principles of damage control resuscitation (DCR) comprising permissive hypotension, early use of ratio-based blood products, minimization of crystalloid resuscitation, and factor replacement therapy have become the pillars of our resuscitation doctrines in trauma patients. This approach has been shown to limit the development of hypothermia and acidosis, which are known factors that aggravate TIC. However, transfusion-related adult respiratory distress syndrome and transfusion-associated circulatory overload are rare complications that are attributed to the transfusion of blood components containing plasma, preventing their liberal use in less critical situations.

An alternative and historical practice which has recently gained favor is whole blood transfusion. Fresh whole blood transfusion has been used as a safe and efficacious method of resuscitation since World War I without causing adult respiratory distress syndrome, multiple organ dysfunction syndromes,

or TIC [5]. This method has been replaced with component therapy mostly due to the ability to store blood components, without compelling evidence regarding its effectiveness. Only a single randomized trial was performed during this transition period [6]. Whole blood resuscitation in civilian trauma centers remains controversial, and TIC continues to be a major problem when resuscitating with artificial crystalloids and colloids.

In this chapter, we aim to address and provide evidence to help identify the optimal method of measuring TIC, treatment strategies of blood product use and the optimal ratio, type of factor replacement, the role of permissive hypotension, and the use of adjunct therapy in preventing TIC.

10.2 Measuring Trauma-Induced Coagulopathy

The rate of trauma patients receiving massive transfusions remains low; however, patients requiring this intervention are at highest risk for TIC. The identification of TIC can be achieved by conventional lab tests, including a platelet count; fibrinogen level; and coagulation assays such as prothrombin time (PT), activated partial thromboplastin time (aPTT), and international normalized ratio (INR). The major limiting factor with these assays is the time to obtain the results.

Viscoelastic hemostatic assays (VHAs), such as thromboelastography (TEG) and rotational thromboelastometry (ROTEM), have emerged as coagulation tests that detect thrombin formation and fibrinolysis, thus providing information about the global process of coagulation (Figure 10.1) [7]. These modern assays provide several measurements in a single run and provide actionable data within half the time, as short as 5 minutes in some newer models [8, 9].

TIC has been traditionally defined as prolongation of PT and INR. However, several studies have shown that these VHAs may be abnormal after injury despite normal activity levels of coagulation factors. There is a vast array of coagulation changes in severely injured trauma patients that leads to different stages of hemostasis from hypocoagulation to hypercoagulation and fibrinolysis [10]. TIC is a complex process involving not only platelets and coagulation factors but also tissue factors, endothelium, and the immune system, which integrate in a coordinated cascade of events. Defining this process with a single test is incomplete and imprecise. Moreover, PT, aPTT, and INR are performed under optimal conditions

DOI: 10.1201/9781003316800-10

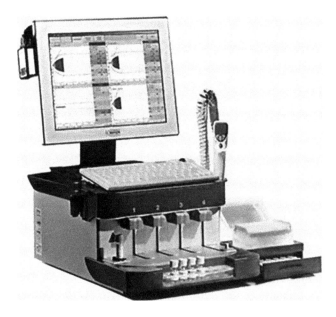

FIGURE 10.1   Thromboelastography.

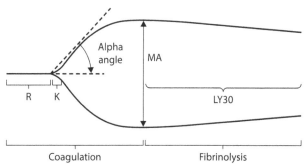

FIGURE 10.2   Thromboelastograph.

inside a blood vessel, while the transducer system connected to the pin detects changes in clot strength. Both devices are point-of-care assays and provide similar measurements to reflect the stages of clot formation, clot strength, and fibrinolysis (Figures 10.2 and 10.3).

of coagulation in a laboratory, i.e., 37°C and normal physiologic pH. These ex vivo laboratory assays fail to account for at least some of the important events such as hypothermia and acidosis on the coagulation cascade [11]. Of note, conventional coagulation assays are conducted on plasma, and therefore they do not take into account the role of platelet function in clot formation. Consequently, VHAs were considered a better alternative and had the potential to become the gold-standard test to define TIC. On the other hand, there has been valid criticism regarding the reproducibility of some older versions of VHAs. Disagreement on specific thresholds on hyperfibrinolysis and lack of adequate research evidence regarding the accuracy of TEG and ROTEM lead to recommendations that these tests should only be used for research purposes [12].

In recent years, VHAs have gained more approval with further enhancement of their detection speed and new studies suggesting a dynamic cutoff value rather than a fixed value, which combined with injury severity assessment and other physiological and clinical data, provide a better definition for TIC. This is particularly important since in the setting of abnormal values of these assays, ultimately the clinical picture of the patient drives the decision-making. Also, with normal values of these assays in a clinically deteriorating patient, terminating blood product transfusion and switching back to crystalloid transfusion would make the situation worse. There is other growing evidence, outside the field of trauma, that is reinforced by a multicenter randomized controlled trial that shows VHA-guided transfusion strategy reduces red blood cell (RBC) transfusions, platelet transfusions, and major bleeding in patients undergoing cardiac surgery [13].

TEG and ROTEM are the most widely used VHAs to assess and manage TIC [14]. Both assays are based on the same principle but slightly differ from each other in the mechanics involved. TEG involves the rotation of a cylindrical cup filled with whole blood around a suspended pin inside, while ROTEM involves the pin oscillating inside a stationary cup. The movement of the cup mimics the sluggish venous flow

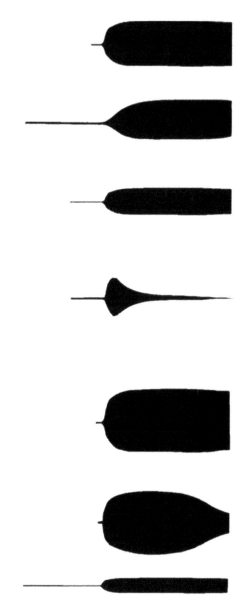

FIGURE 10.3   Interpretation of the thromboelastograph.

VHA technology has existed for the past 70 years; however, major enhancements have only been accomplished within the last decade. These legacy devices have been gradually supplanted with cartridge systems and more portable point-of-care bedside testing iterations such as Sonoclot®, Quantra®, and ClotPro®. New-generation VHA devices are user-friendly and do not require extensive laboratory expertise but only a short training period. Since the advent of the COVID-19 pandemic there has been a rapid growth in the literatures changing the acceptance of VHA-guided patient resuscitation.

Overall, VHAs have been shown to be more sensitive than conventional coagulation assays in detecting TIC and its complex coagulation abnormalities [15]. They have shown to be useful in guiding resuscitation in these patients. The ability to detect hyperfibrinolysis facilitates the initiation of antifibrinolytic therapy in these patients, which eventually reduces mortality [16, 17].

Despite these advantages, TEG and ROTEM have limitations. They come with relatively higher costs than the conventional coagulation assays. They are unable to detect specific platelet receptor abnormalities without the use of specialized testing [18]. In addition, patients treated with direct-acting oral anticoagulants (DOACs), direct thrombin inhibitors (DTIs), or warfarin also require specialized reagents and testing. Without modification and additional modules, they are unable to detect the effect of antiplatelet therapy (aspirin and clopidogrel) or factor Xa (FXa) inhibitors (apixaban, rivaroxaban, edoxaban) [19]. VHAs are not sensitive to detect von Willebrand disease (vWD) since the activation of von Willebrand factor (vWF) requires high shear rate forces. Point-of-care testing, while potentially providing useful information to guide resuscitation, is not often embraced by some centers, as it is sometimes difficult to incorporate the results into the electronic medical records. Central laboratories of hospitals are burdened with the added costs and responsibility of maintaining and calibrating the machines.

Thus, there is a lack of class I, II, or III studies to determine the best tool to diagnose TIC and determine resuscitation therapy in trauma patients. VHAs have been gaining popularity recently, especially after the COVID-19 pandemic, with some studies in nontrauma settings providing evidence in favor of their effectiveness in improving outcomes. However, their implementation nationally is still limited to major academic trauma centers.

RECOMMENDATION

aPTT and PT/INR continue to remain the standard for measuring coagulopathy.

Grade of recommendation: C.

10.3 Prehospital Resuscitation and Optimum Blood Product Type and Ratio

Management of hemorrhagic shock in a prehospital setting includes first mechanically stopping the bleeding, which essentially is direct pressure or application of a tourniquet when this fails. "Stop the Bleed" campaigns have raised awareness of hemorrhage control. However, while use of the tourniquets in the military may have saved lives, there are currently still no data to support the need or utility for tourniquet use in the civilian sector, although it has been postulated. Because improvised tourniquets are potentially more harmful, the use of standard windlass-type tourniquets is encouraged to first responders and in Stop the Bleed kits found in airports and public spaces. The issue is that in the civilian sector, the use of tourniquets is often overused by first responders and the critical step of direct pressure is often skipped. Unless the tourniquet cuts off the arterial flow, the source of bleeding is often made worse as the tourniquets become venous tourniquets. When the source of hemorrhage is truncal and not amiable to direct pressure or the use of tourniquets, restoring circulatory blood volume with the right product and re-establishing hemostasis, while remaining within the boundaries of "damage control resuscitation" principles and rapidly transporting the patient to a trauma center, is the only option [20, 21]. Boundaries of "damage control resuscitation" in the prehospital phase include permissive hypotension. There are broad variations both globally and even regionally in executing the previously mentioned management facts that makes the development of a uniform guideline difficult. Differences from the "fibrinogen replacement" emphasis in European guidelines compared to the "plasma and platelets first" approach in the United States, to the lack of blood banks in underserved areas compared to the availability of the point-of-care latest generation of VHA make the recommendations almost regionally dependent. Still, some aspects of prehospital care can be the focus of management regardless of the geographical location of the traumatic event. It is generally recommended that prehospital providers establish IV access and start the initial volume resuscitation only during transport to minimize scene time. While the ideal fluid type for resuscitation has always been a matter of debate, isotonic fluids have been, until recently, considered the "ideal fluid" for resuscitation in trauma patients. This stems historically from the work of Shires and Canizaro during the pre–Vietnam War era that proposed the use of isotonic fluids in a 3:1 ratio to replace intravascular blood and fluid losses. Large-volume isotonic fluid replacement temporarily improves blood pressure; however, it does not improve the oxygen-carrying capacity needed to correct the tissue hypoxia associated with shock. Large-volume crystalloid resuscitation has been associated with hyperfibrinolysis [22], partially through dilution of circulating antifibrinolytic proteins, and is independently associated with morbidity [23, 24]. The use of crystalloids causes a temporary expansion in the intravascular compartment, but most of this fluid redistributes into the interstitial and intracellular compartments within an hour. Current insights also show that crystalloids induce neutrophil activation and increased inflammatory responses in trauma patients [25, 26]. Studies have shown that increased use of large amounts of crystalloids increases mortality, hospital and intensive care unit length of stay, acute respiratory distress syndrome, and abdominal compartment syndrome [27, 28]. There are also concerns about metabolic acidosis associated with the supraphysiologic concentrations of chloride in normal saline. Maintaining permissive hypotension with low-volume crystalloid resuscitation in a prehospital setting was initially thought to improve outcomes in trauma patients. However, further analysis showed the improvement is limited to trauma patients with tamponade physiology. These findings have led to a paradigm shift away from an aggressive resuscitation with crystalloids to less aggressive and more hemostatic resuscitation.

The concept of "damage control" is derived from the U.S. Navy and referred to the utilization of resources in a prioritized fashion to contain the intake of water or the spread of conflagration and defer the definitive repair in order to return a ship safely to shore during an emergency. The same concept has been adopted by trauma surgeons beginning in the 1980s to both surgery and eventually also to resuscitation. Damage control resuscitation aims to minimize blood loss and coagulopathy by combining permissive hypotension, early and balanced use of blood products, and the use of additional hemostatic drugs and to minimize the use of crystalloids. The evidence is mostly based on military sources that showed improved survival with the use of fresh whole blood for resuscitation in trauma patients [29, 30]. In the civilian sector, fresh whole blood is not available due to logistical reasons, and thus stored whole blood has come into favor. However, it must be pointed out that fresh whole blood is not the same as cold-stored whole blood. Storage of whole blood even in the most optimum conditions at 4°C causes it to lose platelet and clotting factor activity and undergo morphological changes in RBCs. However, cold-stored whole blood was evaluated for use in a civilian academic Level 1 trauma center, without any adverse reaction [31]. The advent of component therapy allowed for the separation and storage of whole blood components in conditions that help maintain their functionality. Although fresh whole blood seems to be the ideal fluid for resuscitation, its availability and storage make it an unfeasible option in the civilian trauma setting, and its role remains controversial.

Between 3% and 17% of trauma patients require massive transfusion (MT), defined as the need for more than 10 units of packed red blood cells (PRBCs) in 24 hours [32, 33]. Despite the use of PRBCs, many of these trauma patients continued to become coagulopathic due to the combined effects of TIC and dilutional coagulopathy from using crystalloid or artificial colloids. Dilutional coagulopathy also occurred when large amounts of PRBCs were used to treat anemia, which can dilute the remaining coagulation factors. Because the loss of whole blood cannot be replaced by merely using crystalloids and PRBC, the idea of resuscitating early with all three blood components, i.e., PRBC, FFP, and platelets, in an attempt to reconstitute whole blood in a nearly physiologic ratio came into use. These observations called for the development of MT protocols and early use of fixed PRBC, FFP, and platelet ratios during resuscitation. These protocols provided RBCs for the delivery of oxygen and the coagulation factors that are lost through or consumed during blood loss. Additionally, fixed-ratio resuscitation is an excellent way to restore blood volume with blood products containing oncotic particles. The development of these MT protocols has shown improvement in outcomes in trauma patients [33, 34]. Also the definition for the early use of blood products has been matured to focus on shorter intervals. The greatest advantage of the use of predefined ratios exists within the first 3–4 hours, when most deaths in trauma

patients occur from exsanguinating hemorrhage [35–38]. This demonstrates the need to identify patients requiring MT at the time of arrival. Some studies have developed scoring systems to predict the need for MT. Although several scoring systems have been proposed, the positive predictive value remains low, and this represents a major challenge in identifying patients at risk for TIC.

Numerous retrospective studies from both civilian and military centers consistently reported lower 24-hour mortality with the use of PRBC:FFP ratios close to 1:1 [32, 39–42]. The independent effect of high versus low platelet:PRBC ratios as well as high versus low FFP:PRBC ratios was also studied showing improved survival with the combination of high plasma and high platelet to RBC ratios [40]. The retrospective nature of these studies brought up the argument that the observed advantage might be a survivor bias [43]. This debate was partially resolved after the large multi-institutional Pragmatic, Randomized Optimal Platelet and Plasma Ratios (PROPPR) trial that randomized patients to receive 1:1:1 versus 2:1:1 ratios of PRBC, FFP, and platelets found some survival benefit at 24 hours but no statistical difference in 30-day mortality with 1:1:1 ratio [4]. In addition, the increased ratio of plasma transfusion is associated with a heightened risk for transfusion-related acute lung injury and is the most common cause of transfusion-related deaths. Recently a single-center study has shown low titer O-type whole blood (LTOWB) transfusion improves survival with reduced transfusion volumes [44]. Further studies are needed to investigate the value of LTOWB transfusions since O-type blood has a low vWf activity level and outcome profiles in massive postinjury transfusion within different TIC phenotypes are unknown.

RECOMMENDATIONS

Accumulating data demonstrate whole blood transfusion can be a potentially lifesaving method of resuscitation in severely injured trauma patients. Evidence from the PROPPR trial shows no difference in survival at 30 days with a PRBC:FFP:platelet ratio of 1:1:1.

Grade of recommendation: B.

10.4 Adjuvant Therapies

Despite adapting the damage control resuscitation principles, including the permissive hypotension strategy, in the prehospital setting, often a limited-volume administration is needed. The fluid of choice for resuscitation is often crystalloid due to its wide availability and low cost. The challenge, however, is to identify which crystalloid should be the first line of treatment. Resuscitation with hypertonic saline (HTS) has been extensively studied and has shown a significant reduction in resuscitation volumes and improvement in the immunological response [45, 46]. However, a recent meta-analysis of clinical studies showed no survival benefits with the use of HTS with and without dextran as compared to normal saline [47].

Conversely, it has been shown that the use of HTS is safe and may be advantageous in scenarios where carrying large amounts of crystalloids or colloids is logistically disadvantageous such as in the military setting or austere environments.

HTS continues to have a major role in traumatic brain injury (TBI) resuscitation, with higher concentrations of up to 23.4% being used in both adult and pediatric TBI patients [48]. Studies show clear benefits in reducing cerebral edema and thus improving cerebral perfusion pressure in TBI patients. The theoretical risk of central pontine myelinolysis (CPM) has not been observed with the use of HTS. The real downside to the use of HTS in trauma patients is the possibility of hyperchloremic metabolic acidosis; however, human studies have shown consistently that this may not clinically matter, as all the hypertonic saline studies have shown that outcome is equivalent and not inferior. Human studies have also demonstrated safety with the use of 5% HTS for resuscitation in trauma patients, and this formulation is currently available, whereas the researched concentration of 7.5% is not available [49, 50].

Prothrombin complex concentrate (PCC) is a plasma-derived blood product with a 25 times higher concentration of coagulation factors than FFP, which reduces the volume needed to replete these lost factors in trauma patients. PCC has additional benefits, as unlike FFP, PCC is present in lyophilized form, and therefore, it does not require the thawing needed for FFP, thus expediting therapy. Three-factor PCC contains factors C, S, II, IX, and X. Four-factor PCC additionally contains factor VII, which is present in small amounts in three-factor PCC. A retrospective study suggested the use of four-factor PCC compared to three-factor PCC is associated with a rapid reversal of INR and reduction in transfusion requirement [51]. Multiple studies, as well as clinical trials comparing the combined use of PCC and FFP with FFP alone, showed accelerated correction of INR [52, 53].

Hyperfibrinolysis is seen in up to 7% of trauma patients with hemorrhagic shock and is a known factor that aggravates TIC [54]. Hyperfibrinolysis is associated with elevated levels of tissue plasminogen activator (tPA) released from Weibel–Palade vesicles in the endothelium. This hyperfibrinolysis is often followed by a fibrinolysis shutdown and is associated with higher mortality [55]. Tranexamic acid (TXA) is an antifibrinolytic agent that is used to inhibit hyperfibrinolysis and reduce blood loss by strengthening clot formation in trauma patients [56]. With the raised interest in the role of TXA in trauma resuscitation, in 2010, the CRASH-2 trial as a double-blinded, prospective, randomized, placebo-controlled trial, was performed in 274 hospitals in 40 countries. This study showed that there is a decreased risk of mortality if TXA is used within 3 hours of injury [16]. Although the CRASH-2 trial provides Level I evidence that shows a statistically significant survival advantage with the use of TXA, the main criticism is that this may lack clinical significance. Another criticism of this study is that the survival advantage was also shown in patients who did not have significant blood loss. The Military Application of Tranexamic Acid in Trauma Emergency Resuscitation (MATTERs) trial was a retrospective study on soldiers receiving at least 1 unit of PRBC, which supported the results of the CRASH-2 trial [57]. In this study when they did a subgroup analysis on a patient receiving MT (more than 10 units of PRBC), they found that there were improved measures of coagulopathy and survival

with TXA use. Based on these findings, the military Tactical Combat Casualty Care Committee has recommended its use in the military setting. The Study of Tranexamic Acid During Air and Ground Medical Prehospital Transport (STAAMP) trial was a multicenter randomized controlled trial of TXA versus placebo, given within 2 hours of injury in the prehospital setting to patients with shock. No significant difference in the primary outcome of 30-day mortality was identified. However, in a subgroup analysis, patients with severe shock (systolic blood pressure <70 mmHg) who received TXA within 1 hour of injury had a significant reduction in 30-day mortality [58]. The exact mechanism by which TXA confers a survival benefit is still uncertain and may be more related to the attenuation of host inflammatory response than improving hemostasis. Also, it remains unclear which group of patients would benefit the most from TXA administration. The following CRASH-3 study showed a survival benefit of early TXA administration in patients with mild-to-moderate but not severe TBI [59].

Recombinant activated factor VII (rFVIIa) has been suggested as an adjunct for control of traumatic hemorrhage as part of DCR [60]. rFVIIa is approved by the Food and Drug Administration (FDA) for use in hemophilia but has been extensively used for off-label purposes, including trauma. rFVIIa activates factor Xa at the site of tissue injury by creating a complex with tissue factor and also on the surface of platelets. Two parallel randomized, placebo-controlled, double-blind trials were conducted to determine the use of rFVIIa in blunt and penetrating trauma patients. rFVIIa effectively reduced the RBC transfusion requirement and the need for MT in patients with blunt trauma without any increased risk for thromboembolic complications [61]. Other studies have also reported improved 24-hour survival with the use of rFVIIa in trauma patients with hemorrhagic shock [62]. However, the routine use of rFVIIa is limited mainly by its high cost and decreased efficacy with coexisting hypothermia and acidosis [63].

RECOMMENDATIONS

PCC is the recommended therapy for warfarin reversal. Although a survival advantage has not been shown with PCC, it has been shown to effectively and quickly treat coagulopathy. While there are some data supporting the use of TXA therapy in the trauma population, much of the major study trial was conducted in developing countries or in the military setting. TXA is popular due to its low cost and high safety profile. In addition, it is difficult to discern the reason TXA is beneficial, as half of the study population was not bleeding.

Grade of recommendation: B.

10.5 Permissive Hypotension: What Do We Know about It?

During World War I, the Harvard Medical Unit concluded that aiming toward higher blood pressure by administration of crystalloids may deteriorate the situation since much-needed blood may be lost due to higher blood pressure [64]. Hypotensive resuscitations with systolic blood pressures of 80–90 mmHg were practiced during World War II and were thought to be beneficial before surgery [65]. Although this practice has long been recognized as helpful, the earliest high-quality human studies were conducted in the 1990s [66]. In this iconoclastic study Bickell et al. showed that delayed prehospital fluid resuscitation in penetrating trauma patients was associated with lower mortality and fewer postoperative complications. Carrick et al. included both penetrating and blunt trauma patients in a randomized controlled trial showing the lower mean arterial pressure (MAP) target did not increase the mortality in trauma patients [67]. Leaving a trauma patient hypotensive may seem counterintuitive to clinicians since logically, a higher blood pressure should equate to better organ perfusion. However, data have shown that achieving near-normal blood pressure may disrupt normal hemostasis and may increase uncontrolled hemorrhage, as it could "pop off" the clot of bleeding sources and worsen TIC. Although there were many critics of these studies, eventually the previously proposed use of prehospital large-volume resuscitation began to lose traction. All animal models of hemorrhage have shown a reduction in mortality with hypotensive resuscitation [68–70]. Similarly, a significant review of human studies has shown a reduction in the incidence of coagulopathy with a reduced volume of prehospital fluids [71]. Dutton et al. performed a randomized study in hemorrhagic shock patients, where one group had a target systolic blood pressure (SBP) of >100 mmHg and the other 70 mmHg. They found no difference in the duration of hemorrhage and mortality rate in the two groups and concluded that titration of fluids to a lower-than-normal SBP did not affect mortality [72]. Following these studies, Advanced Trauma Life Support (ATLS) changed their aggressive resuscitation strategy to a more balanced resuscitative strategy and accepted the possible beneficial role of permissive hypotension in exsanguinating trauma patients.

The role of permissive hypotension stems from a logical argument that the goal of prehospital resuscitation in exsanguinating trauma patients is to maintain blood pressure just enough to maintain adequate tissue perfusion to the vital organs. The goal of prehospital resuscitation should not be achieving the normal figures of blood pressure, as achieving those high pressures in trauma patients disrupts clots and potentially worsens bleeding.

The most important question in this regard has been what pressure is adequate to maintain normal tissue perfusion without increasing the risk of mortality. Animal models showed that a MAP of 45–50 mmHg may be adequate to maintain the perfusion of the brain and heart, and renal perfusion can be upheld when MAP was sustained above 50 mmHg [68, 70, 73]. Other animal studies showed that achieving a MAP of 60 mmHg or an SBP of 90 mmHg maintains adequate tissue perfusion [74]. Pressures above this have been shown to worsen the bleeding in uncontrolled hemorrhage models [75]. Also it has been shown that maintaining a MAP of around 60 mmHg for 60–90 minutes is safe and does not increase the risk of an irreversible shock state by inducing end-organ damage and mortality [76]. Whereas the optimal blood pressure target for permissive hypotension has yet to be defined, based on the currently available literature, an SBP of 90–100 mmHg is likely safe for most patients. For patients with coexisting TBI, permissive hypotension is still currently contraindicated [77, 78]. TBI patients require high blood pressure to maintain adequate cerebral perfusion pressure because of the raised intracranial pressures from ongoing cerebral edema. However, resuscitation with crystalloid solutions may increase cerebral edema. According to the latest guidelines for the management of TBI, an SBP >100 mmHg is recommended for patients aged 50–69 and an SBP >110 mmHg is recommended for patients younger than 49 or older than 70 years [77].

The role of permissive hypotension needs to be understood in its context and that permissive hypotension in uncontrolled hemorrhagic shock is not an alternative to definitive hemorrhage control. Hypotensive resuscitation with restricted use of fluids is most applicable in the scenario where rapid transport to a trauma center for definitive hemorrhage control can be carried out.

RECOMMENDATIONS

SBPs of 90–100 mmHg appear to be safe in patients who are about to get definitive control of hemorrhage. Permissive hypotension is considered to be contraindicated in patients with brain injuries.

Grade of recommendation: C.

TABLE 10.1

Clinical Questions

Question	Answer	Grade of Recommendation	References
How do we measure coagulopathy: INR versus TEG?	• aPTT and PT/INR continue to remain the standard for measuring coagulopathy.	C	[12, 15, 20]
What is the optimum blood product ratio?	• Whole blood transfusion can be a potentially lifesaving method of resuscitation in severely injured trauma patients. • A PRBC:FFP:platelet ratio of 1:1:1 shows no difference in survival at 30 days.	B	[4]
What adjuvant measures are available?	• PCC is the recommended therapy for warfarin reversal. • TXA is popular due to its low cost and high safety profile. • The data supporting its use are problematic.	B	[16, 58, 59]
What do we know about permissive hypotension?	• Maintaining relative hypotension in hemorrhaging trauma patients can reduce mortality in certain subpopulations.	A	[68–73]

TABLE 10.2

Levels of Evidence

Subject	Year	References	Level of Evidence	Strength of Recommendation	Findings
MT protocols	2008, 2010	[33, 34]	III	B	MT protocols improve outcomes.
PRBC:FFP ratio	2014	[4]	I	B	Early empiric use of PRBC and FFP at ratios of 1:1 shows no difference in mortality in 30 days. Twenty-four-hour mortality was reduced due to exsanguination.
HTS	2017	[47]	I	A	Resuscitation with HTS does *not* improve outcomes in patients requiring MT.
Factor VIIa for trauma	2005	[61]	II	B	rFVIIa reduces blood product requirement and the need for MT in patients with blunt trauma with impacting mortality.
Antifibrinolytics	2010, 2019	[16, 59]	I	B	TXA lowers mortality if used within 3 hours of injury. May be beneficial in mild to moderate TBI. Aspects of available data are problematic.

Disclaimer

There are no identifiable conflicts of interest to report. The authors have no financial or proprietary interest in the subject matter or materials discussed in the chapter.

Editor's Note

The highly controversial topic of this chapter, trauma-induced coagulopathy, is of great interest to the trauma community. The authors have nicely summarized the data and have delineated the evidence to support current protocols. Unfortunately, many aspects of our management have been adopted too eagerly, in my opinion, related to the clinical scenario, massive exsanguination after trauma. First, the monitoring of coagulopathy should probably involve complementary tests along with clinical assessment rather than a single modality. Second, the data for reversal of coagulopathy support early availability of blood products (or, even better, whole blood). The blood product ratio does not appear to be as important as providing it as rapidly as possible. No 30-day mortality advantages have been demonstrated. The same can be said about factor VIIa and hypertonic saline. TXA, because it is inexpensive and seemingly safe, has been implemented despite major issues with the large problematic clinical trial that supported its use after trauma, despite the fact that half the patients were not bleeding.

REFERENCES

1. Rhee P, Joseph B, Pandit V, Aziz H, Vercruysse G, Kulvatunyou N, Friese RS. Increasing trauma deaths in the United States. Ann Surg. 2014;260(1):13–21.
2. Cohen MJ, West M. Acute traumatic coagulopathy: from endogenous acute coagulopathy to systemic acquired coagulopathy and back. J Trauma. 2011;70(5 Suppl):S47–S49.
3. MacLeod JB, Lynn M, McKenney MG, Cohn SM, Murtha M. Early coagulopathy predicts mortality in trauma. J Trauma. 2003;55(1):39–44.
4. Holcomb JB, Tilley BC, Baraniuk S, Fox EE, Wade CE, Podbielski JM, del Junco DJ, Brasel KJ, Bulger EM, Callcut RA, et al. Transfusion of plasma, platelets, and red blood cells in a 1:1:1 vs a 1:1:2 ratio and mortality in patients with severe trauma: the PROPPR randomized clinical trial. JAMA. 2015;313(5):471–82.
5. Kornblith LZ, Howard BM, Cheung CK, Dayter Y, Pandey S, Busch MP, Pati S, Callcut RA, Vilardi RF, Redick BJ, et al. The whole is greater than the sum of its parts: hemostatic profiles of whole blood variants. J Trauma Acute Care Surg. 2014;77(6):818–27.
6. Cotton BA, Podbielski J, Camp E, Welch T, del Junco D, Bai Y, Hobbs R, Scroggins J, Hartwell B, Kozar RA, et al. A randomized controlled pilot trial of modified whole blood versus component therapy in severely injured patients requiring large volume transfusions. Ann Surg. 2013;258(4):527–32; discussion 32-3.
7. Enriquez LJ, Shore-Lesserson L. Point-of-care coagulation testing and transfusion algorithms. Br J Anaesth. 2009; 103(Suppl 1):i14–22.
8. Barrett CD, Moore HB, Vigneshwar N, Dhara S, Chandler J, Chapman MP, Sauaia A, Moore EE, Yaffe MB. Plasmin thrombelastography rapidly identifies trauma patients at risk for massive transfusion, mortality, and hyperfibrinolysis: a diagnostic tool to resolve an international debate on tranexamic acid? J Trauma Acute Care Surg. 2020;89(6): 991–8.
9. Kelly JM, Rizoli S, Veigas P, Hollands S, Min A. Using rotational thromboelastometry clot firmness at 5 minutes (ROTEM((R)) EXTEM A5) to predict massive transfusion and in-hospital mortality in trauma: a retrospective analysis of 1146 patients. Anaesthesia. 2018;73(9):1103–9.
10. Brohi K, Cohen MJ, Ganter MT, Schultz MJ, Levi M, Mackersie RC, Pittet JF. Acute coagulopathy of trauma: hypoperfusion induces systemic anticoagulation and hyperfibrinolysis. J Trauma. 2008;64(5):1211–7; discussion 7.
11. Moore HB, Gando S, Iba T, Kim PY, Yeh CH, Brohi K, Hunt BJ, Levy JH, Draxler DF, Stanworth S, et al. Defining trauma-induced coagulopathy with respect to future implications for patient management: communication from the SSC of the ISTH. J Thromb Haemost. 2020; 18(3):740–7.

12. Hunt H, Stanworth S, Curry N, Woolley T, Cooper C, Ukoumunne O, Zhelev Z, Hyde C. Thromboelastography (TEG) and rotational thromboelastometry (ROTEM) for trauma induced coagulopathy in adult trauma patients with bleeding. Cochrane Database Syst Rev. 2015 Feb 16;2015(2):CD010438.

13. Bouzat P, Guerin R, Boussat B, Nicolas J, Lambert A, Greze J, Maegele M, David JS. Diagnostic performance of thromboelastometry in trauma-induced coagulopathy: a comparison between two level I trauma centres using two different devices. Eur J Trauma Emerg Surg. 2021;47(2): 343–51.

14. Gonzalez E, Moore EE, Moore HB. Management of trauma-induced coagulopathy with thrombelastography. Crit Care Clin. 2017;33(1):119–34.

15. Martini WZ, Cortez DS, Dubick MA, Park MS, Holcomb JB. Thrombelastography is better than PT, aPTT, and activated clotting time in detecting clinically relevant clotting abnormalities after hypothermia, hemorrhagic shock and resuscitation in pigs. J Trauma. 2008;65(3):535–43.

16. Collaborators C-t, Shakur H, Roberts I, Bautista R, Caballero J, Coats T, Dewan Y, El-Sayed H, Gogichaishvili T, Gupta S, et al. Effects of tranexamic acid on death, vascular occlusive events, and blood transfusion in trauma patients with significant haemorrhage (CRASH-2): a randomised, placebo-controlled trial. Lancet. 2010;376(9734):23–32.

17. Cotton BA, Faz G, Hatch QM, Radwan ZA, Podbielski J, Wade C, Kozar RA, Holcomb JB. Rapid thrombelastography delivers real-time results that predict transfusion within 1 hour of admission. J Trauma. 2011;71(2):407–14; discussion 14-7.

18. Bochsen L, Wiinberg B, Kjelgaard-Hansen M, Steinbruchel DA, Johansson PI. Evaluation of the TEG platelet mapping assay in blood donors. Thromb J. 2007;5:3.

19. Walsh M, Thomas S, Kwaan H, Aversa J, Anderson S, Sundararajan R, Zimmer D, Bunch C, Stillson J, Draxler D, et al. Modern methods for monitoring hemorrhagic resuscitation in the United States: why the delay? J Trauma Acute Care Surg. 2020;89(6):1018–22.

20. Gonzalez E, Moore EE, Moore HB, Chapman MP, Chin TL, Ghasabyan A, Wohlauer MV, Barnett CC, Bensard DD, Biffl WL, et al. Goal-directed hemostatic resuscitation of trauma-induced coagulopathy: a pragmatic randomized clinical trial comparing a viscoelastic assay to conventional coagulation assays. Ann Surg. 2016;263(6):1051–9.

21. Holcomb JB, Jenkins D, Rhee P, Johannigman J, Mahoney P, Mehta S, Cox ED, Gehrke MJ, Beilman GJ, Schreiber M, et al. Damage control resuscitation: directly addressing the early coagulopathy of trauma. J Trauma. 2007;62(2): 307–10.

22. Cotton BA, Harvin JA, Kostousouv V, Minei KM, Radwan ZA, Schochl H, Wade CE, Holcomb JB, Matijevic N. Hyperfibrinolysis at admission is an uncommon but highly lethal event associated with shock and prehospital fluid administration. J Trauma Acute Care Surg. 2012;73(2): 365–70; discussion 70.

23. Moore HB, Moore EE, Gonzalez E, Wiener G, Chapman MP, Dzieciatkowska M, Sauaia A, Banerjee A, Hansen KC, Silliman C. Plasma is the physiologic buffer of tissue plasminogen activator-mediated fibrinolysis: rationale for plasma-first resuscitation after life-threatening hemorrhage. J Am Coll Surg. 2015 Mar;220(5):872–9.

24. Neal MD, Hoffman MK, Cuschieri J, Minei JP, Maier RV, Harbrecht BG, Billiar TR, Peitzman AB, Moore EE, Cohen MJ, et al. Crystalloid to packed red blood cell transfusion ratio in the massively transfused patient: when a little goes a long way. J Trauma Acute Care Surg. 2012;72(4):892–8.

25. Rhee P, Burris D, Kaufmann C, Pikoulis M, Austin B, Ling G, Harviel D, Waxman K. Lactated Ringer's solution resuscitation causes neutrophil activation after hemorrhagic shock. J Trauma. 1998;44(2):313–9.

26. Rhee P, Wang D, Ruff P, Austin B, DeBraux S, Wolcott K, Burris D, Ling G, Sun L. Human neutrophil activation and increased adhesion by various resuscitation fluids. Crit Care Med. 2000;28(1):74–8.

27. Joseph B, Zangbar B, Pandit V, Vercruysse G, Aziz H, Kulvatunyou N, Wynne J, O'Keeffe T, Tang A, Friese RS, et al. The conjoint effect of reduced crystalloid administration and decreased damage-control laparotomy use in the development of abdominal compartment syndrome. J Trauma Acute Care Surg. 2014;76(2):457–61.

28. Kasotakis G, Sideris A, Yang Y, de Moya M, Alam H, King DR, Tompkins R, Velmahos G. Inflammation, host response to injury I. Aggressive early crystalloid resuscitation adversely affects outcomes in adult blunt trauma patients: an analysis of the Glue Grant database. J Trauma Acute Care Surg. 2013;74(5):1215–21; discussion 21-2.

29. Spinella PC. Warm fresh whole blood transfusion for severe hemorrhage: U.S. military and potential civilian applications. Crit Care Med. 2008;36(7 Suppl):S340–S5.

30. Spinella PC, Perkins JG, Grathwohl KW, Beekley AC, Holcomb JB. Warm fresh whole blood is independently associated with improved survival for patients with combat-related traumatic injuries. J Trauma. 2009;66(4 Suppl): S69–S76.

31. Yazer MH, Jackson B, Sperry JL, Alarcon L, Triulzi DJ, Murdock AD. Initial safety and feasibility of cold-stored uncross matched whole blood transfusion in civilian trauma patients. J Trauma Acute Care Surg. 2016;81(1):21–6.

32. Borgman MA, Spinella PC, Perkins JG, Grathwohl KW, Repine T, Beekley AC, Sebesta J, Jenkins D, Wade CE, Holcomb JB. The ratio of blood products transfused affects mortality in patients receiving massive transfusions at a combat support hospital. J Trauma. 2007;63(4): 805–13.

33. Nunez TC, Young PP, Holcomb JB, Cotton BA. Creation, implementation, and maturation of a massive transfusion protocol for the exsanguinating trauma patient. J Trauma. 2010;68(6):1498–505.

34. Cotton BA, Gunter OL, Isbell J, Au BK, Robertson AM, Morris JA, Jr., St Jacques P, Young PP. Damage control hematology: the impact of a trauma exsanguination protocol on survival and blood product utilization. J Trauma. 2008;64(5):1177–82; discussion 82-3.

35. Meyer DE, Cotton BA, Fox EE, Stein D, Holcomb JB, Cohen M, Inaba K, Rahbar E, Group PS. A comparison of resuscitation intensity and critical administration threshold in predicting early mortality among bleeding patients: a multicenter validation in 680 major transfusion patients. J Trauma Acute Care Surg. 2018;85(4):691–6.

36. Savage SA, Sumislawski JJ, Zarzaur BL, Dutton WP, Croce MA, Fabian TC. The new metric to define large-volume hemorrhage: results of a prospective study of the critical administration threshold. J Trauma Acute Care Surg. 2015;78(2):224–9; discussion 9-30.

37. Nunns GR, Moore EE, Stettler GR, Moore HB, Ghasabyan A, Cohen M, Huebner BR, Silliman CC, Banerjee A, Sauaia A. Empiric transfusion strategies during life-threatening hemorrhage. Surgery. 2018;164(2):306–11.

38. Sperry JL, Guyette FX, Brown JB, Yazer MH, Triulzi DJ, Early-Young BJ, Adams PW, Daley BJ, Miller RS, Harbrecht BG, et al. Prehospital plasma during air medical transport in trauma patients at risk for hemorrhagic shock. N Engl J Med. 2018;379(4):315–26.

39. Gunter OL, Jr., Au BK, Isbell JM, Mowery NT, Young PP, Cotton BA. Optimizing outcomes in damage control resuscitation: identifying blood product ratios associated with improved survival. J Trauma. 2008;65(3):527–34.

40. Holcomb JB, Wade CE, Michalek JE, Chisholm GB, Zarzabal LA, Schreiber MA, Gonzalez EA, Pomper GJ, Perkins JG, Spinella PC, et al. Increased plasma and platelet to red blood cell ratios improves outcome in 466 massively transfused civilian trauma patients. Ann Surg. 2008;248(3):447–58.

41. Sperry JL, Ochoa JB, Gunn SR, Alarcon LH, Minei JP, Cuschieri J, Rosengart MR, Maier RV, Billiar TR, Peitzman AB, et al. An FFP:PRBC transfusion ratio >/=1:1.5 is associated with a lower risk of mortality after massive transfusion. J Trauma. 2008;65(5):986–93.

42. Teixeira PG, Inaba K, Shulman I, Salim A, Demetriades D, Brown C, Browder T, Green D, Rhee P. Impact of plasma transfusion in massively transfused trauma patients. J Trauma. 2009;66(3):693–7.

43. Snyder CW, Weinberg JA, McGwin G, Jr., Melton SM, George RL, Reiff DA, Cross JM, Hubbard-Brown J, Rue LW, 3rd, Kerby JD. The relationship of blood product ratio to mortality: survival benefit or survival bias? J Trauma. 2009;66(2):358–62; discussion 62-4.

44. Williams J, Merutka N, Meyer D, Bai Y, Prater S, Cabrera R, Holcomb JB, Wade CE, Love JD, Cotton BA. Safety profile and impact of low-titer group O whole blood for emergency use in trauma. J Trauma Acute Care Surg. 2020;88(1):87–93.

45. Rhee P, Koustova E, Alam HB. Searching for the optimal resuscitation method: recommendations for the initial fluid resuscitation of combat casualties. J Trauma. 2003; 54(5 Suppl):S52–S62.

46. Stanton K, Alam HB, Rhee P, Llorente O, Kirkpatrick J, Koustova E. Human polymorphonuclear cell death after exposure to resuscitation fluids in vitro: apoptosis versus necrosis. J Trauma. 2003;54(6):1065–74; discussion 75-6.

47. de Crescenzo C, Gorouhi F, Salcedo ES, Galante JM. Prehospital hypertonic fluid resuscitation for trauma patients: a systematic review and meta-analysis. J Trauma Acute Care Surg. 2017;82(5):956–62.

48. Wu AG, Samadani U, Slusher TM, Zhang L, Kiragu AW. 23.4% hypertonic saline and intracranial pressure in severe traumatic brain injury among children: a 10-year retrospective analysis. Pediatr Crit Care Med. 2019;20(5): 466–73.

49. Joseph B, Aziz H, Snell M, Pandit V, Hays D, Kulvatunyou N, Tang A, O'Keeffe T, Wynne J, Friese RS, et al. The physiological effects of hyperosmolar resuscitation: 5% vs 3% hypertonic saline. Am J Surg. 2014;208(5):697–702.

50. DuBose JJ, Kobayashi L, Lozornio A, Teixeira P, Inaba K, Lam L, Talving P, Branco B, Demetriades D, Rhee P. Clinical experience using 5% hypertonic saline as a safe alternative fluid for use in trauma. J Trauma. 2010;68(5):1172–7.

51. Zeeshan M, Hamidi M, Kulvatunyou N, Jehan F, O'Keeffe T, Khan M, Rashdan L, Tang A, Zakaria ER, Joseph B. 3-factor versus 4-factor PCC in coagulopathy of trauma: four is better than three. Shock. 2019;52(1):23–8.

52. Joseph B, Aziz H, Pandit V, Hays D, Kulvatunyou N, Yousuf Z, Tang A, O'Keeffe T, Green D, Friese RS, et al. Prothrombin complex concentrate versus fresh-frozen plasma for reversal of coagulopathy of trauma: is there a difference? World J Surg. 2014;38(8):1875–81.

53. Jehan F, Aziz H, O'Keeffe T, Khan M, Zakaria ER, Hamidi M, Zeeshan M, Kulvatunyou N, Joseph B. The role of four-factor prothrombin complex concentrate in coagulopathy of trauma: a propensity matched analysis. J Trauma Acute Care Surg. 2018;85(1):18–24.

54. Moore HB, Moore EE, Neal MD, Sheppard FR, Kornblith LZ, Draxler DF, Walsh M, Medcalf RL, Cohen MJ, Cotton BA, et al. Fibrinolysis shutdown in trauma: historical review and clinical implications. Anesth Analg. 2019;129(3):762–73.

55. Gall LS, Vulliamy P, Gillespie S, Jones TF, Pierre RSJ, Breukers SE, Gaarder C, Juffermans NP, Maegele M, Stensballe J, et al. The S100A10 pathway mediates an occult hyperfibrinolytic subtype in trauma patients. Ann Surg. 2019;269(6):1184–91.

56. Moore HB, Moore EE, Chapman MP, Hansen KC, Cohen MJ, Pieracci FM, Chandler J, Sauaia A. Does tranexamic acid improve clot strength in severely injured patients who have elevated fibrin degradation products and low fibrinolytic activity, measured by thrombelastography? J Am Coll Surg. 2019;229(1):92–101.

57. Morrison JJ, Dubose JJ, Rasmussen TE, Midwinter MJ. Military application of tranexamic acid in trauma emergency resuscitation (MATTERs) study. Arch Surg. 2012;147(2):113–9.

58. Guyette FX, Brown JB, Zenati MS, Early-Young BJ, Adams PW, Eastridge BJ, Nirula R, Vercruysse GA, O'Keeffe T, Joseph B, et al. Tranexamic acid during prehospital transport in patients at risk for hemorrhage after injury: a double-blind, placebo-controlled, randomized clinical trial. JAMA Surg. 2020.

59. Collaborators C-t. Effects of tranexamic acid on death, disability, vascular occlusive events and other morbidities in patients with acute traumatic brain injury (CRASH-3): a randomised, placebo-controlled trial. Lancet. 2019; 394(10210):1713–23.

60. Holcomb JB. Use of recombinant activated factor VII to treat the acquired coagulopathy of trauma. J Trauma. 2005;58(6):1298–303.

61. Boffard KD, Riou B, Warren B, Choong PI, Rizoli S, Rossaint R, Axelsen M, Kluger Y; NovoSeven Trauma Study Group. Recombinant factor VIIa as adjunctive therapy for bleeding control in severely injured trauma patients: two parallel randomized, placebo-controlled, double-blind clinical trials. J Trauma. 2005;59(1):8–15; discussion-8.

62. Rizoli SB, Nascimento B, Jr., Osman F, Netto FS, Kiss A, Callum J, Brenneman FD, Tremblay L, Tien HC. Recombinant activated coagulation factor VII and bleeding trauma patients. J Trauma. 2006;61(6):1419–25.

63. Fries D. The early use of fibrinogen, prothrombin complex concentrate, and recombinant-activated factor VIIa in massive bleeding. Transfusion. 2013;53(Suppl 1):91S–5S.

64. Cannon WB, Fraser J. The preventive treatment of wound shock. JAMA. 1918;70:618–21.

65. Beecher HK. Preparation of battle casualties for surgery. Ann Surg. 1945;121(6):769–92.

66. Bickell WH, Wall MJ, Jr., Pepe PE, Martin RR, Ginger VF, Allen MK, Mattox KL. Immediate versus delayed fluid resuscitation for hypotensive patients with penetrating torso injuries. N Engl J Med. 1994;331(17):1105–9.

67. Carrick MM, Morrison CA, Tapia NM, Leonard J, Suliburk JW, Norman MA, Welsh FJ, Scott BG, Liscum KR, Raty SR, et al. Intraoperative hypotensive resuscitation for patients undergoing laparotomy or thoracotomy for trauma: early termination of a randomized prospective clinical trial. J Trauma Acute Care Surg. 2016;80(6):886–96.

68. Mapstone J, Roberts I, Evans P. Fluid resuscitation strategies: a systematic review of animal trials. J Trauma. 2003; 55(3):571–89.

69. Burris D, Rhee P, Kaufmann C, Pikoulis E, Austin B, Eror A, DeBraux S, Guzzi L, Leppaniemi A. Controlled resuscitation for uncontrolled hemorrhagic shock. J Trauma. 1999;46(2):216–23.

70. Dunser MW, Takala J, Brunauer A, Bakker J. Re-thinking resuscitation: leaving blood pressure cosmetics behind and moving forward to permissive hypotension and a tissue perfusion-based approach. Crit Care. 2013;17(5):326.

71. Kwan I, Bunn F, Chinnock P, Roberts I. Timing and volume of fluid administration for patients with bleeding. Cochrane Database Syst Rev. 2014 Mar 5;2014(3):CD002245.

72. Dutton RP, Mackenzie CF, Scalea TM. Hypotensive resuscitation during active hemorrhage: impact on in-hospital mortality. J Trauma. 2002;52(6):1141–6.

73. Aizawa C, Honda N, Yoshitoshi Y. Depletion of the renal medullary osmotic gradient following hemorrhagic hypotension in hydropenic rabbits. Jpn Heart J. 1969;10(2): 177–84.

74. Kentner R, Safar P, Prueckner S, Behringer W, Wu X, Henchir J, Ruemelin A, Tisherman SA. Titrated hypertonic/hyperoncotic solution for hypotensive fluid resuscitation during uncontrolled hemorrhagic shock in rats. Resuscitation. 2005;65(1):87–95.

75. Sondeen JL, Coppes VG, Holcomb JB. Blood pressure at which rebleeding occurs after resuscitation in swine with aortic injury. J Trauma. 2003;54(5 Suppl):S110–S7.

76. Palmer L, Martin L. Traumatic coagulopathy—part 2: resuscitative strategies. J Vet Emerg Crit Care (San Antonio). 2014;24(1):75–92.

77. Carney N, Totten AM, O'Reilly C, Ullman JS, Hawryluk GW, Bell MJ, Bratton SL, Chesnut R, Harris OA, Kissoon N, et al. Guidelines for the management of severe traumatic brain injury, fourth edition. Neurosurgery. 2017;80(1) 6–15.

78. Nevin DG, Brohi K. Permissive hypotension for active haemorrhage in trauma. Anaesthesia. 2017;72(12):1443–8.

11

Traumatic Brain Injury

Morgan Crigger and Ara J. Feinstein

Traumatic brain injury (TBI) continues to be a major cause of death and disability. Despite the human and economic toll, there remains a paucity of high-quality clinical studies in the field. The Centers for Disease Control and Prevention noted that there were approximately 223,135 TBI-related hospitalizations in 2019 and 64,362 TBI-related deaths in 2020 [1]. Most injuries are due to motor vehicle crashes, assaults, and falls, with falls more prevalent as age increases. TBI is viewed as a dual cerebral insult composed of primary and secondary processes [2]. The primary injury occurs at the time of impact with immediate damage to brain cells. These injuries subsequently become progressively vulnerable to further damage due to secondary cerebral changes such as intracranial hypertension (ICH), decreases in cerebral perfusion pressure (CPP), and cerebral hypoxia [3]. Treatment of these patients is often complicated by concomitant injuries that affect the ability of the clinician to effectively manage TBI. To improve outcomes, questions arise regarding monitoring, intervention, and pharmacologic management of these patients.

11.1 Should Routine Repeat Head CT Scans Be Performed in Stable Patients without Neurologic Change?

Head computed tomography (CT) is an invaluable tool in the evaluation of patients with suspected TBI. Most institutions obtain a head CT for any patient with blunt trauma and a Glasgow Coma Scale (GCS) score of less than 15. Repeat head CT scans are routinely performed to evaluate the progression of intracranial bleeding or to assess the need for neurosurgical intervention. Given the increased cost and risk of moving critically ill patients, several studies have called this practice into question.

Sifri et al. prospectively evaluated 130 consecutive patients with minor head injury (GCS ≥13 and loss of consciousness or amnesia) and intracranial bleeding on an initial CT scan that did not require immediate intervention [4]. Ninety-nine of these patients (76%) had no deterioration of their exam before the second CT. Twelve patients had worsened bleeding on repeat CT (9%), but none of these required neurosurgical intervention. In contrast, of the 31 (24%) patients who had deterioration of their neurologic

exam before the second CT, 14 (11%) had worsening CT scans and 2 (1.5%) required surgical intervention. After the initial CT, a stable neurologic exam has a negative predictive value of 100% in predicting the lack of neurosurgical intervention.

Brown et al. prospectively studied 100 consecutive TBI patients with an abnormal initial head CT that did not require immediate neurosurgical intervention [5]. Sixty-eight of these patients underwent 90 repeat CT scans. Eighty-one (90%) of these scans were performed without neurologic change, and none of these patients required medical or surgical intervention for TBI, despite the apparent worsening on 19 (23%) scans. Of the nine CT scans done in the setting of a deteriorating mental status, six (67%) showed worsening bleeding requiring one medical and two surgical interventions. In a subsequent study, Brown et al. prospectively examined 274 patients with an abnormal head CT not requiring immediate intervention [6]. Patients were stratified into mild (GCS 13–15), moderate (GCS 9–12), and severe (GCS ≤8) injury groups. Only two patients (0.7%) had changes on repeat CT that required intervention in the absence of clinical deterioration; both were in the severe injury group.

Fattah et al. prospectively studied 145 consecutive patients with a GCS of 13–15 with intracranial hemorrhage [7]. These subjects were divided into two groups: 92 (63%) in the "routine" repeat CT group and 53 (37%) in the "selective" repeat CT group. Six subjects (11%) in the selective group received repeat scans due to physical exam changes, with one (1.9%) having a progression of hemorrhage that did not require intervention. Overall, the patients in the selective group had significantly fewer scans with shorter intensive care unit (ICU) and hospital lengths of stay.

The definitive study was performed by Joseph et al. who prospectively studied 1,129 trauma patients with intracranial hemorrhage on initial head CT [8]. These were divided into two groups: Routine repeat head CT within 6 hours (1,099) and repeat head CT due to deteriorating neurologic exam (30). In the routine group, 216 (20%) had worsened on a CT scan. Four of these patients required intervention. All four of these patients had a presentation GCS ≤8 and were intubated. In the selective group, 30 patients underwent repeat head CT for a decline in the neurologic exam. Sixteen (53%) of these scans showed progression, and 12 (40%) required an intervention. No patient without a change in

DOI: 10.1201/9781003316800-11

TABLE 11.1

Summary of Data Results

Trial (Ref. No.)	Year	Level of Evidence	Intervention/ Design	Randomized Groups (*n*)	Primary Endpoint	Interpretations/Comments
[4]	2006	IIb	Prospective, observational study	130 patients with minor TBI/ICH underwent serial CT scans to observe the progression of ICH.	Neurologic deterioration, neurosurgical intervention	In patients with a minimal head injury and normal neurologic exam, repeat head CT should not be performed.
[5]	2004	IIb	Prospective, observational study	100 TBI patients with abnormal CT scans were observed for use of repeat head CT and clinical outcomes.	Neurologic deterioration, number of head CTs performed, neurosurgical intervention	In patients with TBI and abnormal initial head CT, repeat head CT is not warranted unless there is an acute change in neurologic status.
[6]	2007	IIb	Prospective, observational study	274 TBI patients with abnormal initial CT scans were observed for use of repeat head CT and clinical outcomes.	Neurologic deterioration, medical and neurosurgical intervention	Repeat head CT is warranted in patients who sustain TBI and clinically decline, as it often results in the need for intervention; routine repeat head CT is not warranted in patients with GCS >8 with an out change in neurologic status.
[7]	2012	IIb	Prospective, observational study	145 patients with GCS 13–15 divided into routine repeat head CT and "selective" repeat head CT groups	Neurologic deterioration, progression of ICH, and neurosurgical intervention	The use of selective repeat head CT results in a decreased number of head CTs, ICU days, and hospital length of stay for TBI patients with GCS 13–15.
[8]	2014	IIb	Prospective, observational study	1,129 patients with ICH after TBI were divided into routine repeat head CT at 6 hours and selective head CT groups	Neurologic deterioration, progression of ICH	In the absence of a deteriorating neurologic examination, repeat head CT is not warranted in the TBI setting.

neurologic examination required any type of neurologic intervention (Table 11.1).

RECOMMENDATION

Patients with intracranial hemorrhage with a GCS of 13–15 and no change in the neurologic exam do <u>not</u> require a routine repeat CT scan.

Grade of recommendation: B.

11.2 Does the Use of Continuous Hypertonic Saline vs. Standard Care Improve Outcomes?

Patients with severe TBI and increased intracranial pressure (ICP) have been managed with mannitol and hypertonic (3–20%) saline to reduce ICP. Continuous prophylactic hyperosmolar therapy has not been recommended as resuscitation fluids in neurointensive care because data on its effects on long-term clinical outcomes are scarce [9]. To address this, a multicenter randomized clinical trial (RCT)—the Continuous Hyperosmolar Therapy for Traumatic Brain-Injured Patients (COBI)—was conducted to study if a continuous infusion of 20% hypertonic saline solution improves neurologic outcomes at 6 months in patients with moderate to severe TBI [9]. Patients aged 18–80 years with moderate to severe TBI were

enrolled. Within 24 hours after trauma, a 1-hour bolus infusion of 20% hypertonic saline solution adapted to patients' serum sodium levels to limit the risk of severe hypernatremia was injected, followed by a continuous infusion of 20% hypertonic saline solution also adapted to patients' serum sodium levels [9]. Sodium levels were monitored every 8 hours and dosages were adjusted based on the results. The intervention was continued for a minimum of 48 hours and as long as a patient was considered at risk of ICH. It was stopped when all specific therapies against ICH were suspended for 12 hours or more [9]. The primary outcome was the Glasgow Outcome Scale-Extended (GOS-E) score 6 months after the trauma. They found that continuous 20% hypertonic saline was significantly associated with increased serum sodium levels and increased blood osmolarity. They also found a reduced risk of ICH in the first 2 days of treatment, but a rebound effect to high ICPs was noted after cessation on day 4. Six months after the trauma, the distribution of GOS-E scores was not significantly different between the two groups (Table 11.2).

RECOMMENDATION

Continuous hypertonic saline infusion is safe and initially lowers ICPs; however, there is a rebound effect noted. More studies need to be performed to better assess this treatment, and we cannot recommend for or against use at this time.

Grade of recommendation: B.

TABLE 11.2

Summary of Data Results

Trial (Ref. No.)	Year	Level of Evidence	Intervention/Design	Randomized Groups (n)	Primary Endpoint	Interpretations/Comments
[9]	2021	Ib	Multicenter randomized clinical trial	370 patients were assigned to receive continuous infusions of 20% hypertonic saline solution plus standard care (n = 185) or standard care alone (controls; n = 185).	Extended Glasgow Outcome Scale score	Treatment with continuous infusion of 20% hypertonic saline compared with standard care did not result in a significantly better neurologic status at 6 months.

11.3 Do Procoagulants Decrease Intracranial Hemorrhage in Coagulopathic TBI Patients?

The use of novel hemostatic agents in the setting of trauma to reverse coagulopathy has been a growing area of interest over the past decade. The frequency of intracranial hemorrhage in the setting of TBI has been reported to be as high as 75%. Furthermore, patients who sustain a TBI while taking oral anticoagulation have a 30-day mortality approaching 60% [10]. Coagulopathy in the setting of secondary TBI due to ongoing hemorrhage, pretraumatic use of anticoagulants, and liberal administration of crystalloid result in the worsening of ICH and increased mortality [11]. Several agents have been investigated in trauma populations to reverse coagulopathy, including factor VII, prothrombin complex concentrate (PCC), and tranexamic acid (TXA). PCC is a combination of Food and Drug Administration (FDA)–approved vitamin K–associated clotting factors to reverse coagulopathy from warfarin use in patients with acute hemorrhage. There are two available versions of the drug: a four-factor formulation containing factor VII and a three-factor formulation without factor VII. Factor VII is available in recombinant form (rFVIIa) and has been studied in trauma populations. TXA is an antifibrinolytic agent that is often used in the setting of surgical bleeding, but recent studies have focused on its use in trauma.

Joseph et al. conducted a retrospective study of 85 coagulopathic TBI patients who received either PCC (n = 64) or rFVIIa (n = 21) [12]. Coagulopathy was either medication-related or acquired from trauma. The groups were not similar, with patients in the PCC group being significantly older, with a lower Injury Severity Score (ISS), more likely to be on warfarin preinjury, and receiving fewer blood products before treatment. The authors found lower mortality and cost in the PCC group, but this is difficult to interpret given the differences in the patient populations of the two groups.

Yanamadala et al. retrospectively compared PCC to fresh-frozen plasma (FFP) in 33 patients taking warfarin who sustained TBI with ICH, with 5 patients receiving PCC as their sole pharmacologic source of coagulopathy reversal [10]. Time to reversal was significantly shorter for the PCC group (65 minutes PCC vs. 265 minutes FFP). The time to anesthesia

induction was also significantly shorter in the PCC group (159 minutes PCC vs. 307 minutes FFP).

The CRASH-2 trial studied the use of TXA in trauma patients and found that the use of TXA within 3 hours of injury reduced the risk of death due to bleeding and reduced hospital costs [13]. Although this study did not use TBI specifically as its inclusion criteria, Perel et al. performed a nested study of the patients within the CRASH-2 study who sustained TBI. The study compared mortality, mean hemorrhage growth, and the presence of new ischemic lesions in the TXA and placebo groups. Although the TXA group appeared to have lower mortality, less progression of hemorrhage, and fewer new ischemic foci, none of the analyses reached statistical significance [14]. These data prompted the CRASH-3 trial to quantify the effects of TXA on head injury–related death, disability, and adverse events [15].

The CRASH-3 trial was a randomized, placebo-controlled trial of TXA that enrolled patients within 3 hours of injury with the primary endpoint of in-hospital death within 28 days of injury. They enrolled patients with TBI from 175 hospitals in 29 countries. They found that the risk of head injury–related death was decreased in the TXA group with a mild-to-moderate head injury but not in patients with severe head injury [15]. Similarly, Yutthakasemsunt et al. performed a randomized, placebo-controlled trial in 238 patients with TBI and GCS 4–12. There were no statistically significant improvements in mortality, ICH progression, or Glasgow Outcome Scale in patients receiving TXA, stressing the need for larger studies [16].

Jokar et al. performed a single-blinded RCT on 40 patients with a traumatic ICH. All patients received conservative ICH treatment, either intravenous TXA or placebo. They found that the ICH volume increased significantly less in the TXA group compared to the placebo group [17] (Table 11.3).

RECOMMENDATION

TXA, when given within 3 hours of TBI, may decrease the risk of head injury–related death in mild to moderate TBI and may aid in slowing the expansion of known ICH.

Grade of recommendation: C.

TABLE 11.3

Summary of Data Results

Trial (Ref. No.)	Year	Level of Evidence	Intervention/ Design	Randomized Groups (*n*)	Primary Endpoint	Interpretations/Comments
[10]	2014	IIb	Prospective, observational study	Prospective analysis of 33 patients undergoing correction of coagulopathy with either PCC or FFP while treated for TBI	Time to INR correction, time delay until surgical intervention	Patients who were treated with PCC had faster correction of INR and shorter delay to surgical intervention; however, the study is very small and underpowered.
[14]	2012	Ib	Nested, randomized, controlled trial derived from CRASH-2 study	Nested data from the CRASH-2 trial of TBI patients who were randomized to treatment with TXA or placebo	Death, need for surgical intervention, intracranial hemorrhage growth from admission to 24–48 hours after admission	Patients receiving TXA had less progression of ICH and lower mortality; however, the findings failed to reach statistical significance.
[15]	2019	Ib	Randomized, placebo-controlled trial	12,737 patients with TBI to receive TXA (6,406 [50.3%] or placebo [6,331 [49.7%], of whom 9,202 (72.2%) patients were treated within 3 hours of injury	Head injury–related death in hospital within 28 days of injury in patients treated within 3 hours of injury	TXA is safe in patients with TBI and that treatment within 3 hours of injury reduces head injury–related death. Patients should be treated as soon as possible after injury.
[16]	2013	Ib	Randomized, double-blinded trial	238 mild to severe TBI patients were randomized to receive TXA or a placebo	Death Progressive intracranial hemorrhage on CT scan 24 hours after initial scan	No statistically significant difference in the progression of intracranial hemorrhage or mortality between TXA and placebo groups.
[17]	2017	Ib	Single-blinded, randomized control trial	40 patients received conservative treatment for ICH, as well as either intravenous TXA or placebo	The extent of ICH growth at 48 hours after admission was measured by brain CT scan	ICH volume increased significantly less in the TXA group than in the placebo group.

11.4 When Should DVT Prophylaxis Be Initiated in TBI?

Chemical deep venous thrombosis (DVT) prophylaxis has been an intense area of research in the trauma literature. Grade B recommendations support low-molecular-weight heparin (LMWH) as the most effective method of prophylaxis to prevent DVT in trauma patients without TBI [18]. Prophylactic therapy for DVT and pulmonary embolism (PE) in patients with TBI must always be balanced against the risk of expansion of intracranial hematoma and rebleeding [19]. This necessitates balancing evidence-based guidelines with prophylactic regimens that are individualized based on the injury patterns and risks of each patient.

Phelan et al. analyzed 62 patients randomized to enoxaparin (*n* = 34) or placebo (*n* = 28) after moderate TBI and a stable CT scan 24 hours after admission [20]. Subclinical, radiographic TBI progression rates on the scans performed 48 hours after injury and 24 hours after the start of treatment were 5.9% for enoxaparin and 3.6% for placebo, a treatment effect difference of 2.3%, which was not significant. No clinical TBI progressions occurred, and one DVT occurred in the placebo arm. The study only randomized a small percentage of the total patients screened, with a large number excluded due to a TBI being too severe. Although lacking in power, it does suggest that in patients with moderate TBI, initiation of enoxaparin 24 hours after TBI with a stable repeat CT is safe.

In a prospective, nonrandomized study, Norwood et al. analyzed the use and safety of LMWH (enoxaparin) in patients with intracranial hemorrhage injuries following blunt trauma [21]. The medication was started 24 hours after injury or craniotomy except in patients with concomitant splenic injury being conservatively managed. Head CT scans were carried out on admission, 24 hours after admission, and at various times during hospitalization. Although only 4% of patients managed nonoperatively had an expansion of their hematoma while on enoxaparin, 9.1% of patients receiving surgical intervention suffered postoperative bleeding. This bleeding rate caused the study authors to change their protocol so that the drug was started later (24 hours after surgical intervention). Venous color flow duplex studies were performed within 24 hours of hospital discharge on 101 of the 150 patients and found a 2% DVT incidence in enoxaparin-treated patients (which they compare to historic controls), and no patient in the study group was documented to have suffered a PE. In a follow-up study in 2008, Norwood et al. prospectively followed 525 patients with TBI who received enoxaparin within 48 hours of admission [22]. Only 26% of eligible patients were enrolled in the study, with many being excluded for concomitant injuries or the surgeon's reluctance to initiate venous thromboembolism (VTE) prophylaxis. After starting enoxaparin, 18 (3.4%) patients had progression of their hemorrhage by serial CT. Six of these patients (1.1%) required a craniotomy. Salottolo et al. retrospectively analyzed 255 patients receiving enoxaparin or heparin for DVT prophylaxis after TBI with stable repeat head CT [23]. Therapy was initiated early (<72 hours) in 108 patients and late (≥72 hours) in 147 patients. Rates of hemorrhage progression or DVT did not differ significantly in patients who received VTE prophylaxis early or late. There were significant differences in the demographics of the two groups, and given the small sample size, it is difficult to conclude this study.

A retrospective evaluation of unfractionated heparin (UFH) use for DVT prophylaxis in patients sustaining severe closed head injuries (Abbreviated Injury Scale Score of >3) was carried out by Kim et al. [24]. They compared 47 patients who received UFH early after injury (<72 hours) versus 17 patients treated late after injury (>72 hours). They did not exclude patients with splenic and hepatic lacerations managed conservatively. They demonstrated no increase in the risk of increased intracranial bleeding in either group by CT and/or change in physical exam, but also no difference in the rate of DVT, PE, or death between the two groups. No conclusions as to the efficacy of UFH as a prophylactic agent for DVT can be drawn from this study, but it does suggest that prophylactic doses of heparin can be safely administered early to patients with TBI.

Dudley et al. retrospectively analyzed 287 patients with moderate to severe (GCS 3–12) TBI treated with dalteparin or enoxaparin initiated at 48–72 hours postinjury after a minimum of two stable head CT scans [25]. They reported only one patient with a symptomatic expansion of ICH and no difference in DVT rates between groups.

In a retrospective cohort study, Koehler et al. reviewed 669 patients with TBI who received enoxaparin after TBI [26]. Two hundred and sixty-eight patients received prophylaxis early (<72 hours), and 401 patients received prophylaxis late (>72 hours). Following prophylaxis, no patients required craniotomy, and there was no difference in the rate of hemorrhage progression between the early and late groups. No deaths were attributable to DVT prophylaxis, but one patient in the late group died of PE (Table 11.4).

TABLE 11.4
Summary of Data Results

Trial (Ref. No.)	Year	Level of Evidence	Intervention/ Design	Randomized Groups (n)	Primary Endpoint	Interpretations/Comments
[18]	2002	IIb	Prospective, nonrandomized, observational study	LMWH is given 24 hours after admission or 24 hours after surgery to patients with TBI	Expansion of IH or prevention of DVT/PE	The study group was small and nonrandomized. Variable study protocol changed during the study due to bleeding complications. There was a trend toward the safety of LMWH in TBI patients with CT scan follow-up.
[19]	2012	Ib	Randomized, double-blinded trial	62 TBI patients randomized to LMWH or placebo 24 hours after admission	Radiologic worsening of TBI	TBI progression rates 24 hours after injury in patients receiving LMWH were similar to the placebo group; only a small subset of patients was randomized, but the study suggests that VTE prophylaxis is safe to use in TBI patients.
[20]	2008	IIb	Prospective, nonrandomized, observational study	525 patients received enoxaparin 48 hours after sustaining TBI	Intracranial bleeding complications, discharge GCS, death	Use of enoxaparin 48 hours after sustaining TBI was deemed safe in the setting of stable head CT.
[21]	2011	IIb	Retrospective, observational study	255 patients with TBI and stable head CTs were analyzed for use of chemical VTE prophylaxis before or after 72 hours	VTE occurrence	There were no differences in outcomes between groups receiving chemical VTE prophylaxis before or after 72 hours from injury; however, given the small sample size and variable demographics, it is difficult to derive a conclusion from this study.
[22]	2002	IIb	Retrospective, observational study	64 patients with TBI and Abbreviated Injury Scale score of >3 divided into early (<72 hours) vs. late (>72 hours) administration of UFH	Intracranial bleeding related to UFH administration	There was no significant difference between the two groups of DVT prevention (4% early vs. 6% late) with no major increases in intracranial bleeding. Groups are too small to draw major conclusions.
[23]	2010	IIb	Retrospective, observational study	287 TBI patients treated with enoxaparin or dalteparin prophylaxis 48–72 hours after injury	Symptomatic expansion of ICH, the occurrence of VTE	There was no difference between the expansion of ICH or VTE occurrence in patients receiving either drug.
[24]	2011	IIb	Retrospective cohort study	669 TBI patients received chemical VTE prophylaxis either before or after 72 hours from injury	Progression of ICH, the occurrence of VTE/PE	There was no difference in the progression of ICH between early and late administration of chemical VTE prophylaxis; there were no deaths attributed to VTE prophylaxis; however, one patient died of PE in the late group.

RECOMMENDATION

Early initiation (72 hours after injury) of heparin or LMWH in patients with moderate TBI and without clinical or radiologic decline is supported by Level II data.

Grade of recommendation: B.

11.5 Is Standard Use of Antiepileptic Drugs for Seizure Prophylaxis Beneficial in Patients with TBI?

Posttraumatic seizure activity occurs both early and late after injury. Brain seizure activity is known to dramatically increase cerebral metabolic requirements, glucose metabolism [27], and ICP [28]. If untreated, the overall risk of seizure activity following TBI in patients with no previous history of epilepsy is 2–5%. However, this varies widely depending on the age, mechanism of injury, and severity of TBI [29]. The presence of early seizures (<7 days) after TBI has not been substantiated to correlate with increased mortality in trauma patients but is predictive of the development of late seizure activity [30]. As such, patients who suffer post-TBI seizures have been shown to have significantly worse long-term functional outcomes as compared to patients who do not suffer seizure activity [31]. Therefore, pharmacologic suppression of post-TBI seizure activity is part of an overall brain-protective strategy.

In a systematic review of Class I and Class II data, phenytoin was effective when used as prophylaxis against early post-TBI seizures given for 7 days following TBI [32]. Phenytoin demonstrated a significant benefit (3.4% early seizure rate vs. 13.3% in the placebo group) in suppressing post-TBI seizures in patients with severe brain injuries. They further evaluated adverse events and drug complications and found that there were few serious side effects from antiepileptic drug usage. From these data, the authors make practice recommendations for adult patients with severe TBI (defined as prolonged loss of consciousness, amnesia, intracranial hematoma or brain contusion on CT scan, and/

or depressed skull fracture). These include prophylactic treatment with phenytoin, beginning with an intravenous loading dose as soon as possible after an injury to decrease the risk of early (<7 days) post-TBI seizures. The same study reviewed the use of antiepileptic drugs in late (>7 days) post-TBI seizures. From their review, they concluded that data do not support the use of phenytoin for more than 7 days, as there was no difference in late post-TBI seizures in the antiepileptic drug–treated group (10.0%) vs. placebo group (8.4%). From these data, the authors made additional practice guideline recommendations that prophylactic treatment with phenytoin, carbamazepine, or valproate should not routinely be used beyond the first 7 days after injury in an attempt to decrease the risk of post-TBI seizures.

Szaflarski et al. randomized 46 TBI and 6 stroke patients to receive either phenytoin or levetiracetam after severe TBI [33]. Patients were monitored in the ICU with an electroencephalogram (EEG) for 72 hours and clinically thereafter. There was no difference in early seizures (levetiracetam 5/34 vs. phenytoin 3/18) or at 6 months (levetiracetam 1/20 vs. phenytoin 0/14). Surprisingly, patients in the levetiracetam group experienced significantly better 6-month outcomes than patients in the phenytoin arm by GOS-E and Disability Rating Scale.

Inaba et al. prospectively studied 813 consecutive blunt TBI patients admitted to two Level I trauma centers (mean admission GCS 12) [34]. Patients received either levetiracetam (407) or phenytoin (406). Although not randomized, the groups were similar in demographics. There were six seizures in each group (1.5%). This suggests that both drugs are effective in preventing seizures in the first 7 days after injury.

Younus et al. performed a prospective RCT and studied whether phenytoin or levetiracetam influenced long-term seizure risk in TBI. The patients were given either phenytoin or levetiracetam, and EEGs were obtained to monitor for seizure activity. They failed to determine a significant relationship between the antiepileptic drug used with the initial EEG and seizure activity. However, a significant correlation between the antiepileptic drug used was found with EEG and seizure activity on subsequent follow-up. Patients who took levetiracetam had decreased incidence of abnormal EEG and seizure activity on follow-up [35] (Table 11.5).

TABLE 11.5

Summary of Data Results

Trial (Ref. No.)	Year	Level of Evidence	Intervention/ Design	Randomized Groups (*n*)	Primary Endpoint	Interpretations/Comments
[32]	2007	Ia	A systematic review of the existing literature	Review of data Levels I–IV from the decade of 1996–2006	Suppression of seizure, duration of medication use	A summary of pooled data suggests benefits to antiepileptic drugs in early (<7 days) postinjury seizure prophylaxis.
[33]	2010	Ib	Randomized, controlled, single-blinded trial	52 patients randomized to receive either phenytoin or levetiracetam	Seizure occurrence, death	There were no differences between the two groups in preventing early seizures; the levetiracetam group had better functional outcomes on long-term follow-up.
[34]	2013	IIb	Prospective, observational study	813 patients with TBI received either phenytoin or levetiracetam	Seizure occurrence within 7 days	Seizure occurrence was the same for both groups, suggesting that both medications are efficacious in preventing early post-TBI seizures.
[35]	2018	Ib	Prospective randomized control trial	140 patients with TBI were given either phenytoin or levetiracetam	Compare the efficacy of phenytoin and levetiracetam for seizure prophylaxis	The decreased tendency of seizures and abnormal EEG on follow-up with the use of levetiracetam.

RECOMMENDATION

There is a significantly lower risk of early (<7 days) postinjury seizures in patients with severe head injuries who are treated with either levetiracetam or phenytoin.

Grade of recommendation: B.

11.6 Do ICP Monitoring and Therapy Directed at Lowering ICP Improve Outcome?

In the management of patients with TBI, ICP monitoring has been one of the most important measures for goal-directed therapy. It is widely accepted that ICH (ICP >20 mmHg) is strongly associated with TBI-related mortality [36]. Thus, guidelines have been developed to minimize TBI-related mortality due to ICH. The Brain Trauma Foundation (BTF) 2007 guidelines recommend that all patients with head trauma, a GCS of 3–8, and abnormal CT imaging should have some form of ICP monitoring. It also recommends ICP monitoring in patients with severe TBI and a normal CT scan if two of the following conditions are met: The patient is more than 40 years old, the presence of posturing is observed, or systolic blood pressure <90 mmHg. It also recommends that treatment for ICH be initiated when ICP reaches the threshold of greater than 20 mmHg [37]. However, these guidelines are not based on any randomized controlled data and are derived solely from Class II and Class III evidence. As the most recent guidelines were released, several studies have been published that question the efficacy of ICP-directed therapy in patients with TBI. These studies argue that improved outcomes associated with ICP monitoring may be coincidental with other improvements in TBI care.

An RCT involving ICP monitoring was published by Chestnut et al. [38]. The trial included 324 patients with severe TBI being treated in two different facilities that were randomized to a treatment protocol utilizing intraparenchymal ICP monitoring to guide therapy or treatment based on imaging and clinical examination. The primary outcome of the study was based on a composite of survival time, functional status at 3 and 6 months, and neuropsychological status at 6 months. There were no significant differences between the two groups regarding the primary outcome composite score, 6-month mortality, length of ICU stay, or adverse events. The imaging and clinical exam group did have a significantly greater time interval over which brain-specific therapy was provided (mannitol, hypertonic saline, etc.).

In a retrospective review of data from a prospective database, Farahvar et al. examined 223 patients managed without ICP monitors and 1,084 patients managed with ICP monitors during the first 48 hours after admission with TBI [39]. They demonstrated that patients in the ICP monitoring group had a significant decrease in mortality at 2 weeks, citing mortality of 19.6% in the monitored group versus 33.2% in the nonmonitored population. This is difficult to interpret, however, as the non–ICP monitoring group had significantly higher proportions of patients over the age of 60 years and with pupillary changes compared to the ICP monitoring group. Cremer et al. produced a retrospective cohort study comparing the outcomes of TBI patients from two different trauma centers [40]. One of the centers did not use ICP monitoring and relied on treating patients by maintaining mean arterial pressures of 90 mmHg and providing therapeutic interventions based on clinical observations and CT imaging (122 patients). The other center used ICP monitoring with goals of therapy directed at maintaining an ICP <20 mmHg and CPP >70 mmHg (142 patients). Outcomes for the two populations were similar for in-hospital mortality (34% without ICP monitoring vs. 33% with ICP monitoring) and functional outcomes. However, the ICP-directed group had prolonged mechanical ventilation time, as well as increased use of sedatives, vasopressors, mannitol, and barbiturates. Shafi et al. also produced a retrospective review of 1,646 patients with severe TBI from the National Trauma Data Bank comparing outcomes in patients with and without ICP monitoring [41]. This study found that only 43% of studied patients that met BTF criteria underwent placement of an ICP monitor and that among those patients there was a 45% reduction in survival when compared to the non–ICP monitored group (Table 11.6).

RECOMMENDATION

There are insufficient data to support the use of ICP monitoring in TBI.

Grade of recommendation: B.

11.7 Does the Use of a Hypothermia Protocol for TBI Treatment Improve Morbidity and Mortality?

Prophylactic hypothermia has been proposed as a potential treatment for TBI. The theoretical mechanism of action is to reduce cerebral inflammation that occurs after TBI to limit further injury. Multiple studies have been conducted with mixed and mostly negative results.

Cooper et al. performed a multinational randomized trial of early prophylactic hypothermia versus standard of care. The hypothermia group was sustained for at least 72 hours at 33–35°C followed by slow rewarming [42]. The primary outcome was the percentage of favorable outcomes using GOS-E. They found that prophylactic hypothermia compared with normothermia after severe TBI did not increase favorable neurologic outcomes, and no benefit from prophylactic hypothermia was seen in any of the secondary outcomes [42].

Andrews et al. also conducted an RCT of therapeutic hypothermia for elevated ICPs. One hundred and ninety-five patients over the age of 18 with a primary closed TBI were selected and enrolled. The primary outcome was the GOS-E score. They found that hypothermia plus standard care did not result in outcomes better than those with standard care alone, and the trial was ended early due to safety concerns. These results suggest that outcomes were worse with hypothermia than with standard care alone [43].

TABLE 11.6

Summary of Data Results

Trial (Ref. No.)	Year	Level of Evidence	Intervention/ Design	Randomized Groups (*n*)	Primary Endpoint	Interpretations/Comments
[38]	2012	Ib	Randomized, double-blinded trial	TBI patients treated with or without ICP monitoring	Survival time, impaired consciousness, functional status at 3 and 6 months, neuropsychological status at 6 months	Management of TBI using ICP monitoring to keep ICP <20 mmHg does not improve outcomes compared to treating patients based on imaging/ symptoms.
[39]	2012	IIb	A retrospective cohort of data from a prospectively maintained database	Outcomes comparison of patients with TBI who underwent ICP monitoring vs. without ICP monitoring	Mortality at 2 weeks from injury	Patients undergoing ICP monitoring had lower mortality rates at 2 weeks than nonmonitored patients.
[40]	2005	IIb	Retrospective cohort study with prospective outcome assessment	Outcomes comparison of patients with TBI who underwent ICP monitoring vs. without ICP monitoring	Mortality, GCS at 12 months	For patients surviving for more than 24 hours after injury, ICP monitoring provided no benefit to survival or functional outcomes.
[41]	2008	IIb	Retrospective cohort study, nonrandomized data	Outcomes comparison of patients with TBI who underwent ICP monitoring vs. without ICP monitoring	Survival to discharge	Patients who were treated with ICP monitoring per BTF guidelines were associated with worse survival outcomes when controlling for injury/TBI severity, comorbidities, and need for craniotomy.

Feng et al. took a different approach to hypothermia. They hypothesized that lowering the metabolic rate by 50–60% of the resting metabolic rate would represent a more appropriate target for therapeutic hypothermia compared with reaching a fixed body temperature and would result in more favorable clinical outcomes after severe TBI [44]. They also used proton nuclear magnetic resonance (1HNMR) metabolomics technology to analyze the brain and body circulation metabolism pool profiles of these different hypothermia targets [44]. Eighty-eight severe TBI patients were enrolled, 44 in the metabolic-targeted hypothermia treatment (MTHT) and 44 in the body temperature-targeted hypothermia treatment (BTHT). They found that compared with the BTHT group, mortality was reduced, length of ICU stay was reduced, and the neurologic function recovery was slightly better with the MTHT group.

Hui et al. studied the safety and efficacy of 5 days of mild hypothermia (34–35°C) in severe TBI with severe ICH. They enrolled 302 patients in 14 hospitals aged 18–65 and divided them into two groups: 156 in the hypothermia group and 146 in the normothermia group. The primary outcome was the GOS score at 6 months. There was no difference in favorable outcomes and mortality between groups, but in patients with an initial ICP >30 mm Hg, hypothermic treatment significantly increased favorable outcomes over the normothermia group [45]. They also found that long-term mild hypothermia did not increase the risk or number of complications (Table 11.7).

RECOMMENDATION

Hypothermia for TBI patients does not appear to improve outcomes and mortality.

Grade of recommendation: A.

11.8 Does a Decompressive Craniectomy for Severe TBI Improve Outcomes?

There is an ongoing debate about the efficacy of decompressive craniectomy (DHC) used to reduce ICP. Clinical trials have shown that DHC can improve the survival and prognosis of patients with TBI. However, several case series have reported that in patients with TBI, DHC can lead to similar or worse outcomes compared with the medical treatment [46]. Several meta-analyses and RCTs have attempted to better clarify the efficacy of this procedure with mixed results. To better address this question, Lu et al. performed an updated meta-analysis to assess the efficacy and safety of DHC compared with medical therapy for the treatment of TBI [46].

Lu et al. included 7 RCT studies with a total of 779 patients with TBI in their meta-analysis and found that the DHC group demonstrated significantly lower rates of mortality, postoperative ICP levels, postoperative hematoma, and significantly shorter hospital length of stay. Unfortunately, in line with the literature, the rate of unfavorable outcomes was higher in the DHC group compared with the medical therapy group [46].

Hutchinson et al. performed an international, multicenter, parallel-group, superiority RCT to compare secondary decompressive craniectomy with continued medical management for refractory ICH after TBI. Patients with an ICP above 25 mmHg for 1–12 hours despite maximum medical therapy either underwent DHC with medical therapy or continued medical therapy. In the surgical arm, a unilateral frontotemporoparietal or bifrontal craniotomy was performed. The exact type of craniectomy was left up to the surgeons. The primary outcome was the rating GOS-E scale at 6 months. They found that DHC in patients with TBI and

TABLE 11.7

Summary of Data Results

Trial (Ref. No.)	Year	Level of Evidence	Intervention/ Design	Randomized Groups (n)	Primary Endpoint	Interpretations/Comments
[42]	2018	Ib	Multinational randomized control trial	293 patients: 132 in the hypothermia group and 161 in the normothermia group, received the full trial protocol	Percentage of favorable outcomes using GOS-E	Prophylactic hypothermia compared with normothermia after severe TBI did not increase favorable neurologic outcomes, and no benefit from prophylactic hypothermia was seen in any of the secondary outcomes
[43]	2015	Ib	Randomized controlled trial	195 participants were randomly assigned to the hypothermia group and 192 to the control group	GOS-E score at 6 months after injury	Hypothermia plus standard care did not result in outcomes better than those with standard care alone, and the trial was ended early due to safety concerns.
[44]	2017	Ib	A pilot single-blind, randomized controlled trial	44 severe TBI patients in the metabolic-targeted hypothermia treatment (MTHT) and 44 cases in the body temperature-targeted hypothermia treatment (BTHT)	Mortality	Compared with the BTHT group, mortality was reduced, length of ICU stay was reduced, and the neurologic function recovery was slightly better with the MTHT group.
[45]	2021	Ib	A prospective, multicenter, randomized, controlled trial	302 patients: 156 in the hypothermia group and 146 in the normothermia group	GOS score at 6 months	No difference in favorable outcomes and mortality between groups. For patients with an initial ICP >30 mm Hg, hypothermic treatment significantly increased favorable outcomes over the normothermia group.

refractory ICH resulted in 22% lower mortality but higher rates of vegetative state and severe disability than medical management [47].

Mendelow et al. compared early (within 12 hours) hematoma evacuation with initial conservative medical treatment. They randomized 82 patients to early surgery and 85 to medical treatment. They found that 30 (37%) of the early surgical arm had an unfavorable outcome and 40 (47%) of the medical treatment arm had an unfavorable outcome, showing an absolute benefit in favorable outcomes of 10.5% with the surgical arm. There were significantly more deaths in the first 6 months in the initial conservative treatment group [48] (Table 11.8).

TABLE 11.8

Summary of Data Results

Trial (Ref. No.)	Year	Level of Evidence	Intervention/ Design	Randomized Groups (n)	Primary Endpoint	Interpretations/Comments
[46]	2020	Ia	Meta-analysis of 7 RCTs	779 patients with TBI	Mortality, a favorable outcome, unfavorable outcome, postoperative intracranial pressure (ICP), adverse events with hematoma, and hospital stay.	The DHC group demonstrated significantly lower rates of mortality, postoperative ICP levels, postoperative hematoma, and significantly shorter hospital lengths of stay
[47]	2016	Ib	International, multicenter, parallel-group, superiority, randomized controlled trial	408 patients: 206 were assigned to the surgical group and 202 to the medical group	GOS-E scale at 6 months	Decompressive craniectomy in patients with traumatic brain injury and refractory intracranial hypertension resulted in 22% lower mortality but higher rates of vegetative state, lower severe disability, and upper severe disability than medical management
[48]	2015	Ib	Randomized controlled trial	167 patients: 82 patients to early surgery and 85 to medical treatment	GOS-E scale at 6 months	The absolute benefit of 10.5% improvement in favorable outcomes with the surgical arm. There were significantly more deaths in the first 6 months in the initial conservative treatment group

<table>
<tr><td>

RECOMMENDATION

DHC appears to lower mortality but is associated with increased unfavorable outcomes.

Grade of recommendation: B.

</td></tr>
</table>

11.9 Does Amantadine after TBI Improve Cognition and Level of Consciousness?

TBI patients are known to suffer from long-term disability, including but not limited to loss of memory; concentration disorders; and increases in irritability, depression, and violence [49]. A larger portion (15%) of patients with severe TBI cannot follow simple commands for 4 weeks after the injury and may suffer from mental performance issues up to 10 years after a concussion [49]. Certain neurotransmitters are affected after a severe TBI, including dopamine, which has been shown to increase during an acute injury and drop below preinjury levels later. Dopamine is thought to be effective in stimulating the frontal lobe and plays an important role in behavior, mood, speech, motor control, hypothalamus functions (including knowledge), and environmental awareness [49]. Amantadine hydrochloride (AMH), which is a dopamine receptor agonist, has been shown to stimulate the nervous system after TBI and possibly aid in recovery.

Ghalaenovi et al. performed a double-blinded RCT of 40 patients to determine if AMH can improve the level of consciousness in patients with moderate to severe TBI. They also investigated if the use of AMH in the acute phase of the postinjury period for 6 weeks can improve arousal, responsiveness, cognition, and function 6 months later [49]. They found that the GCS score increased between the first and seventh day after drug initiation; however, amantadine did not lead to reportable effects on the patient's level of consciousness, memory, disability, cognition, mortality, and performance [49] (Tables 11.9 and 11.10).

<table>
<tr><td>

RECOMMENDATION

There is insufficient evidence to recommend the use of amantadine to aid in cognitive improvement in TBI patients.

Grade of recommendation: B.

</td></tr>
</table>

TABLE 11.9

Summary of Data Results

Trial (Ref. No.)	Year	Level of Evidence	Intervention/ Design	Randomized Groups (*n*)	Primary Endpoint	Interpretations/Comments
[49]	2018	Ib	A double-blind, randomized, controlled trial	40 patients grouped into AMH (19 patients) and placebo (21 patients)	Evaluate the effects of AMH on arousal, responsiveness, cognition, and function of the patients with moderate-severe TBI after 7 days of the study drug and after 4.5 months after completing 6 weeks of treatment	GCS score rose between the first and seventh day after drug initiation; however, amantadine did not lead to reportable effects on the patient's level of consciousness, memory, disability, cognition, mortality, and performance.

TABLE 11.10

Summary of Data Results

Summary of Recommendations				
Question	Answer	Levels of Evidence	Grade of Recommendation	References
Does repeat head CT determine the need for intervention?	Patients with intracranial hemorrhage with a GCS of 13–15 and no change in the neurologic exam do *not* require a routine repeat CT scan.	IIb	B	[4–8]
does the use of hypertonic saline vs. standard care improve outcomes?	Continuous hypertonic saline infusion is safe and initially lowers ICP; however, there is a rebound effect noted. More studies need to be performed to better assess this treatment, and we cannot recommend for or against use at this time.	Ib	B	[9]
Do procoagulants decrease intracranial hemorrhage related to TBI?	TXA, when given within 3 hours of TBI, may decrease the risk of head injury–related death in mild to moderate TBI and may aid in slowing the expansion of known ICH.	Ib–IIb	C	[10–17]
When and how should DVT prophylaxis be initiated?	Early initiation (72 hours after injury) of heparin or LMWH in patients with moderate TBI and without clinical or radiologic decline is supported by Level II data.	Ia–IIb	B	[18–24]

(Continued)

TABLE 11.10 (Continued)

Summary of Data Results

Summary of Recommendations				
Question	Answer	Levels of Evidence	Grade of Recommendation	References
Is seizure prophylaxis beneficial?	There is a significantly lower risk of early (<7 days) postinjury seizures in patients with severe head injuries who are treated with either levetiracetam or phenytoin.	Ia–IIb	B	[32–35]
Does the use of ICP monitoring improve outcomes?	Despite expert guidelines, there are insufficient data to support the use of ICP monitoring in TBI.	Ia–IIb	B	[38–41]
Does the use of a hypothermia protocol for TBI treatment improve morbidity and mortality?	Hypothermia for TBI patients does not appear to improve outcomes and mortality.	Ib	A	[42–45]
Does a decompressive craniectomy for severe TBI improve outcomes?	Decompressive craniectomy appears to lower mortality but is associated with increased unfavorable outcomes.	Ia-Ib	B	[46–48]
Is using amantadine to improve cognition and level of consciousness recommended?	There is insufficient evidence to recommend the use of amantadine to aid in cognitive improvement in TBI patients.	Ib	B	[49]

Editor's Note

The topic of the management of traumatic brain injury can be infuriating for the clinician. Unfortunately, all of the Level I data related to TBI has demonstrated that the standard of care employed for decade, was in fact harmful. Examples of this include hyperventilation, volume restriction, and steroids. There is also accumulating data that ICP monitoring is of little or no value. Large studies investigating hypothermia and progesterone have found no benefit.

While there are excellent prospective data that clearly show zero benefits from repeated head CT scans in neurologically stable patients with traumatic brain injury, this continues to be routinely performed at most trauma centers. There is high-quality evidence that hyperosmolar therapy provides no benefit (RCT using 3% saline), but we continue to employ this modality. Increasing serum sodium levels and placing unnecessary central venous catheters for this unproven treatment are associated with negative consequences.

Decompressive craniectomy is controversial because it is typically used as a last-ditch salvage intervention in moribund patients with devastating brain injuries. The benefits of the procedure seem logical: Decompress the edematous brain tissue. However, efficacy has been hard to prove. Finally, amantadine is often prescribed despite a paucity of supportive data.

Therefore, if one takes the conservative view that we should manage patients based on logical and/or proven therapy, it appears that much of our current neurocritical care for traumatic brain injury (such as hyperosmolar therapy, ICP monitoring, and amantadine) should be abandoned.

REFERENCES

1. Centers for Disease Control and Prevention. National Center for Health Statistics: Mortality Data on CDC WONDER. Accessed 2022, https://wonder.cdc.gov/mcd.html.
2. Sarrafzadeh AS, Peltonen EE, Kaisers U, et al. Secondary insults in severe head injury: Do multiply injured patients do worse? *Crit Care Med*. 2001;*29*:1116–1123.
3. Carlson A, Schermer C, Lu S. Retrospective evaluation of anemia and transfusion in traumatic brain injury. *J Trauma*. 2006;*61*:567–571.
4. Sifri ZC, Homnick AT, Vaynman A, et al. A prospective evaluation of the value of repeat cranial computed tomography in patients with a minimal head injury and an intracranial bleed. *J Trauma*. October 2006;*61(4)*:862–867.
5. Brown CV, Weng J, Oh D, et al. Does routine serial computed tomography of the head influence management of traumatic brain injury? A prospective evaluation. *J Trauma*. November 2004;*57(5)*:939–943.
6. Brown CV, Zada G, Salim A, et al. Indications for routine repeat head computed tomography (CT) stratified by severity of traumatic brain injury. *J Trauma*. June 2007;*62(6)*: 1339–1344.
7. Abdel-Fattah KR, Eastman AL, Aldy KN. A prospective evaluation of the use of routine repeat cranial CT scans in patients with intracranial hemorrhage and GCS score of 13 to 15. *J Trauma Acute Care Surg*. September 2012;*73(3)*:685–688.
8. Joseph B, Aziz H, Pandit V. A three-year prospective study of repeat head computed tomography in patients with traumatic brain injury. *J Am Coll Surg*. July 2014;*219(1)*: 45–51.
9. Roquilly A, Moyer JD, Huet O, et al. Effect of continuous infusion of hypertonic saline vs standard care on 6-month neurological outcomes in patients with traumatic brain injury: The COBI randomized clinical trial. *JAMA*. May 25, 2021; *325(20)*:2056–2066.
10. Yanamadala V, Walcott B, Fecci P, et al. Reversal of warfarin associated coagulopathy with 4-factor prothrombin complex concentrate in traumatic brain injury and intracranial hemorrhage. *J Clin Neurosci*. 2014;*21*: 1881–1884.
11. Perel P, Roberts I, Shakur H, et al. Haemostatic drugs for traumatic brain injury. *Cochrane Database Syst Rev*. 2010;*5(1)*:CD007877.
12. Joseph B, Pantelis H, Aziz H. Prothrombin complex concentrate: An effective therapy in reversing the coagulopathy of traumatic brain injury. *J Trauma Acute Care Surg*. 2012;*74(1)*:248–253.

13. Roberts I, Shakur H, Coats T, et al. The CRASH-2 trial: A randomized controlled trial and economic evaluation of tranexamic acid on death, vascular occlusive events and transfusion requirement in bleeding trauma patients. *Health Tech Assess.* 2013;*17(10)*:1–79.

14. Perel P, Al-Shahi Salman R, Morris Z. CRASH-2 (Clinical Randomization of An Antifibrinolytic in Significant Hemorrhage) intracranial bleeding study: The effect of tranexamic acid in traumatic brain injury—A nested randomized, placebo-controlled trial. *Health Tech Assess.* 2012;*17(10)*:1–11.

15. CRASH-3 Trial Collaborators. Effects of tranexamic acid on death, disability, vascular occlusive events and other morbidities in patients with acute traumatic brain injury (CRASH-3): a randomized, placebo-controlled trial. *Lancet.* November 9, 2019;*394*(10210):1713–1723.

16. Yutthakasemsunt S, Kittiwatanagul W, Piyavechvirat P, et al. Tranexamic acid for patients with traumatic brain injury: A randomized, double-blinded, placebo-controlled trial. *BMC Emerg Med.* 2013;*22(13)*:20.

17. Jokar A, Ahmadi K, Salehi T, et al. The effect of tranexamic acid in traumatic brain injury: A randomized controlled trial. *Chin J Traumatol.* February 2017;*20*(1):49–51.

18. Rogers FB, Cipolle MD, Velmahos G, et al. Practice management guidelines for the prevention of venous thromboembolism in trauma patients: The EAST practice management guidelines work for the group. *J Trauma.* 2002;*53*: 142–164.

19. Hammond F, Meighben M. Venous thromboembolism in the patient with acute traumatic brain injury: Screening, diagnosis, prophylaxis and treatment issues. *J Head Trauma Rehabil.* 1998;*13(1)*:36–50.

20. Phelan HA, Wolf SE, Norwood SH, et al. A randomized, double-blinded, placebo-controlled pilot trial of anticoagulation in low-risk traumatic brain injury: The Delayed Versus Early Enoxaparin Prophylaxis I (DEEP I) study. *J Trauma Acute Care Surg.* December 2012;*73(6)*:1434–1441.

21. Norwood SH, McAuley CE, Berne JD, et al. Prospective evaluation of the safety of enoxaparin prophylaxis for venous thromboembolism in patients with intracranial hemorrhagic injuries. *Arch Surg.* 2002;*137*:696–702.

22. Norwood SH, Berne JD, Rowe SA. Early venous thromboembolism prophylaxis with enoxaparin in patients with blunt traumatic brain injury. *J Trauma.* November 2008; *65(5)*:1021–1026.

23. Salottolo K, Offner P, Levy AS. Interrupted pharmacologic thromboprophylaxis increases venous thromboembolism in traumatic brain injury. *J Trauma.* January 2011;*70(1)*:19–24.

24. Kim J, Gearhart MM, Zurick A, et al. Preliminary report on the safety of heparin for deep venous thrombosis after severe head injury. *J Trauma.* 2002;*53*:38–43.

25. Dudley RR, Aziz I, Bonnici A. Early venous thromboembolic event prophylaxis in traumatic brain injury with low-molecular-weight heparin: Risks and benefits. *J Neurotrauma.* December 2010;*27(12)*:2165–2172.

26. Koehler DM, Shipman J, Davidson MA. Is early venous thromboembolism prophylaxis safe in trauma patients with intracranial hemorrhage? *J Trauma.* February 2011;*70(2)*: 324–329.

27. Darbina O, Rissob JJ, Carreb E. Metabolic changes in rat striatum following convulsive seizures. *Brain Res.* 2005; *1050*:124–129.

28. Shah AK, Fuerst D, Sood S. Seizures lead to elevation of intracranial pressure in children undergoing invasive EEG monitoring. *Epilepsia.* June 2007;*48(6)*: 1097–1103.

29. Wang HC, Chang WN, Chang HW. Factors predictive of outcome in posttraumatic seizures. *J Trauma.* 2008;*64(4)*: 883–888.

30. Jeremitsky E, Omert L, Dunham CM. Harbingers of poor outcome the day after severe brain injury: Hypothermia, hypoxia, and hypoperfusion. *J Trauma.* 2003;*54*:312–319.

31. Asikainen I, Kaste M, Sarna S. Early and late posttraumatic seizures in traumatic brain injury rehabilitation patients: Brain injury factors causing late seizures and influence of seizures on long-term outcome. *Epilepsia.* 1999;*40(5)*: 584–589.

32. Bratton SL, Chestnut RM, Ghajar J, et al. Antiseizure prophylaxis. *J Neurotrauma.* 2007;*24(S1)*:S83–S86.

33. Szaflarski JP, Sangha KS, Lindsell CJ. Prospective, randomized, single-blinded comparative trial of intravenous levetiracetam versus phenytoin for seizure prophylaxis. *Neurocrit Care.* April 2010;*12(2)*:165–172.

34. Inaba K, Menaker J, Branco BC. A prospective multicenter comparison of levetiracetam versus phenytoin for early posttraumatic seizure prophylaxis. *J Trauma Acute Care Surg.* March 2013;*74(3)*:766–771.

35. Younus SM, Basar S, Gauri SA, et al. Comparison of phenytoin versus levetiracetam in early seizure prophylaxis after traumatic brain injury, at a Tertiary Care Hospital in Karachi, Pakistan. *Asian J Neurosurg.* October–December 2018;*13*(4):1096–1100.

36. Marmarou A, Anderson R, Ward J, et al. Impact of ICP instability and hypotension on outcome in patients with severe head trauma. *J Neurosurg.* 1991;*75*:S59–S66.

37. Brain Trauma Foundation; American Association of Neurological Surgeons; Congress of Neurological Surgeons. Guidelines for the management of severe traumatic brain injury. *J Neurotrauma.* 2007;*24(Suppl 1)*:S1–S106.

38. Chestnut R, Temkin N, Carney N, et al. A trial of intracranial-pressure monitoring in traumatic brain injury. *N Engl J Med.* December 2012;*367(26)*:2471–2481.

39. Farahvar A, Gerber L, Chiu Y, et al. Increased mortality in patients with severe traumatic brain injury treated without intracranial pressure monitoring. *J Neurosurg.* October 2012;*117(4)*:729–734.

40. Cremer L, van Dijk G, Wensen E, et al. Effect of intracranial pressure monitoring and targeted intensive care on functional outcome after severe head injury. *Crit Care Med.* 2005;*33(10)*:2207–2213.

41. Shafi S, Diaz-Arrastia R, Madden C, et al. Intracranial pressure monitoring in brain-injured patients is associated with worsening of survival. *J Trauma.* 2008;*64*: 335–340.

42. Cooper DJ, Nichol AD, Bailey M, et al.; POLAR Trial Investigators and the ANZICS Clinical Trials Group. Effect of early sustained prophylactic hypothermia on neurologic outcomes among patients with severe traumatic brain injury: The POLAR randomized clinical trial. *JAMA.* December 4, 2018;*320*(21):2211–2220.

43. Andrews PJ, Sinclair HL, Rodriguez A, et al.; Eurotherm3235 Trial Collaborators. Hypothermia for intracranial hypertension after traumatic brain injury. *N Engl J Med.* December 17, 2015;*373*(25):2403–2412.

44. Feng JZ, Wang WY, Zeng J, et al. Optimization of brain metabolism using metabolic-targeted therapeutic hypothermia can reduce mortality from traumatic brain injury. *J Trauma Acute Care Surg.* August 2017;*83*(2):296–304.

45. Hui J, Feng J, Tu Y, Zhang W, et al. Safety and efficacy of long-term mild hypothermia for severe traumatic brain injury with refractory intracranial hypertension (LTH-1): A multicenter randomized controlled trial. *EClinicalMedicine.* January 28, 2021;*32*:100732.

46. Lu G, Zhu L, Wang X, Zhang H, Li Y. Decompressive craniectomy for patients with traumatic brain injury: A pooled analysis of randomized controlled trials. *World Neurosurg.* January 2020;*133*:e135–e148.

47. Hutchinson PJ, Kolias AG, Timofeev IS, et al. Trial of decompressive craniectomy for traumatic intracranial hypertension. *N Engl J Med.* September 22, 2016;*375*(*12*): 1119–1130.

48. Mendelow AD, Gregson BA, Rowan EN, et al. Early surgery versus initial conservative treatment in patients with traumatic intracerebral hemorrhage (STITCH[Trauma]): The first randomized trial. *J Neurotrauma.* September 1, 2015;*32*(*17*):1312–1323.

49. Ghalaenovi H, Fattahi A, Koohpayehzadeh J, et al. The effects of amantadine on traumatic brain injury outcome: A double-blind, randomized, controlled, clinical trial. *Brain Inj.* 2018;*32*(8):1050–1055.

12

Traumatic Spinal Cord Injuries

Moti Cordoba and Yoram Klein

12.1 Introduction

Spine injuries are common in the modern urban trauma setting. Although rare, spinal cord injury (SCI; 1.3% of all trauma patients) carries an extremely high rate of morbidity and mortality. The annual incidence of SCI is approximately 54 cases per 1 million people in the United States, or 17,730 new traumatic SCIs each year. Given that those who die at the scene of injury are not included, the true incidence is probably higher. The estimated number of people with SCI in the United States is estimated to be about 291,000 (range 249,000–363,000). The average yearly expenses and the estimated lifetime costs vary greatly according to the neurological impairment (1.5–3 million dollars/year); the total annual cost of treating SCI patients is billions of dollars. Although surgical techniques have dramatically improved and the ability to get spinal stability and alignment enable earlier rehabilitation of the patients, the neurological recovery and the postinjury life expectancy of this population have not changed significantly over the years [1].

The etiologies of SCI include (1) high-energy motor vehicle collisions (MVCs)—approximately 39%; most are thoracic and lumbar; (2) high fall injuries—approximately 32%; most are in the thoracolumbar zone; (3) acts of violence/penetrating trauma (primarily gunshot wounds)—approximately 13%; (4) sports injuries/recreation activities (diving being the most common sport causing SCI)—approximately 8%; most are cervical; and (5) miscellaneous causes—approximately 7%. Three other statistical points are worth mentioning. The male-to-female ratio for these injuries is 3:1, with higher occurrence in non-Hispanic black distribution of age at injury significantly shifted from unimodal (the early 2000s) to bimodal distribution (2019). Survival relates strongly to the extent of neurological impairment and the patient's age. The life expectancy for SCI patients has not improved since the 1980s and remains significantly lower than the general population.

i. *Pathophysiology*: SCI is characteristically composed of primary and secondary injuries. The primary injury is divided into four categories: Impact plus persistent compression, impact alone with transient compression, distraction, and laceration or transection. This mechanical injury compromises the neural tissue, disrupts the vasculature, and gives rise to several molecular processes. Unlike the immediate mechanical primary injury, the second injury effect is slower and mainly involves ischemic, inflammatory, and immune processes, which promote neuronal apoptosis [2].

ii. *Neurological Assessment*: The initial neurological examination of the SCI patient is essential for the assessment of the level of injury and the prognosis. The examination should include sensory, motor, and proprioception evaluation together with perianal sensation, rectal sphincter tone, and bulbocavernosus reflex [3]. Since its introduction in 1969, the Frankel classification provided a simple and acceptable, though nonspecific, scheme for the categorization of SCI. Patients are classified as follows: A. Complete—the absence of motor or sensory function below the level of the lesion; B. sensory only—sensation present but no motor function below level of the lesion; C. motor useless—sensation + motor function 2–3/5 (without practical application); D. motor useful—sensation present with motor function of 4/5 (practical); and E. normal sensory and motor function. The Frankel classification has several limitations, the main one being that the level of the injury is not incorporated into the classification. Introduced in 1992, the American Spinal Injury Association (ASIA) Impairment Scale replaced the previously utilized Frankel classification to describe the severity of SCI. The ASIA classification combines the assessments of motor, sensory, and sacral functions, thus addressing the shortcomings of previous scoring systems. The ASIA classification involves both a motor and sensory examination to determine the sensory level and motor level for each side of the body, the single neurological level of injury (NLI), and whether the injury is complete or incomplete. Since its introduction, the ASIA classification underwent several revisions, with the most recent in 2019. In this last revision, the zone of partial preservation (ZPP) definition has been refined. The ZPPs represent important pieces of information for the characterization of the extent of preserved functions below the sensory and motor levels. As such, ZPPs are among the most important predictors of neurological recovery [4].

iii. *SCI defined*:

a. *Complete SCI*: There is no motor or sensory function caudal to the level of injury, and the bulbocavernosus reflex is present.

DOI: 10.1201/9781003316800-12

b. *Spinal shock*: Defined as a complete SCI with absent bulbocavernosus reflex. It should not be confused with neurogenic shock, which is a hemodynamic condition characterized by hypotension and bradycardia. Only after the reappearance of the bulbocavernosus reflex can we reevaluate the neurologic status of the patient and classify him or her as one of the incomplete or complete SCI syndromes.

c. *Incomplete spinal cord injuries (ICSCIs)*: There is some motor or sensory function below the level of injury. There are a few formal types of ICSCI:

  i. Central cord syndrome is the most common ICSCI and presents as quadriplegia, with perianal and sacral sparing. About 75% of the patients will have partial recovery of motor function.

  ii. Brown-Sequard syndrome is a unilateral SCI (usually due to penetrating trauma resulting in cord hemisection) characterized by motor deficit and loss of proprioception ipsilateral to the injury and contralateral loss of pain and temperature sensation. Most of these patients gain partial recovery with bowel and bladder continence and usually walking ability.

  iii. Anterior cord syndrome is a relatively common ICSCI characterized by complete motor and sensory loss with residual deep sensation and proprioception of the trunk and lower extremities. The prognosis of this syndrome is poor, and only 10% of them show some motor recovery.

  iv. Posterior cord syndrome is a rare ICSCI and is characterized by loss of proprioception and deep sensation but intact motor functioning. The patient usually ambulates in a "tabes dorsalis gait."

12.1.1 Initial Management

As with every other severe trauma patient, initial management includes securing a patent airway, controlling adequate oxygenation, and managing hemodynamics and perfusion.

Head injury with a depressed level of consciousness due to MVC is the most common indication for definitive airway control in trauma patients. Unfortunately, cervical spine injury (CSI) is more common among these patients. The overall incidence of CSI is found to be around 2%, and patients with a Glasgow Coma Score (GCS) of less than 8 have an incidence of more than 10% [5]. Upper cervical spine ligamentous injuries, with or without vertebral fractures, are among the most common injuries in acceleration-deceleration MVC injuries and represent unstable injuries that mandate head–neck immobilization with airway control [6]. Although extremely rare, the worsening of cervical spinal cord damage due to airway control maneuver is a dreaded complication [7].

12.2 What Is the Impact of Airway Maneuvers on Cervical Spine Movement?

Numerous studies have tried to define spinal movement during airway management in patients with intact and injured cervical spines. Nevertheless, the evidence is limited due to the heterogeneity of the measurement techniques and the controversy about the clinical importance of the biomechanical findings. Both basic and advanced airway maneuvers were found to cause movement in different segments of the cervical spine. Even presumably safe maneuvers, such as chin lift and jaw thrust, were found to cause movements that theoretically might jeopardize the cord.

Advanced airway interventions, such as blind nasotracheal intubation and direct laryngoscopy and orotracheal intubation (DLOI) were also found to cause relative segmental cervical spine movement (to a lesser extent than the preintubation maneuver) in patients with normal and injured cervical spines. The most accentuated movements were found to be at the atlantooccipital and atlantoaxial joints, but other portions of the cervical spine were affected as well [8]. Occipital-cervical injuries warrant special attention, as these injuries are common, and accentuated pathological motion at the atlantooccipital and atlantoaxial joints has been documented during airway control, intubation, and cervical collar application.

No significant difference in the movement was found between curved or straight laryngoscope blades [9]. Although the measured movements can be considered within the physiological margins in the intact cervical spine, the injured spine might be still compromised by these maneuvers. This is the reason for the application of spine immobilization during airway intervention. The most common immobilization technique is manual inline axial stabilization (MIAS), which was found to be most effective in limiting segmental movement to 1–3 mm in various airway maneuvers [10].

In their paper, Lennarson et al. compared segmental cervical motion during DLOI in cadavers with and without a complete subaxial injury. They found that in the setting of complete C4–C5 destabilization, immobilization effectively eliminated distraction and diminished angulation but increased subluxation. Although intubation without stabilization causes less subluxation than immobilization, it has intermediate results and increased angulation compared with either intervention [11].

RECOMMENDATIONS

The accumulated experimental data suggest that airway management in the trauma patient with suspected CSI may inflict spinal movement. Manual inline axial stabilization of the neck during the airway intervention can safely be applied and significantly limit the allegedly dangerous spine motion.

Grade of recommendation: B.

12.3 What Is the Preferred Way to Achieve Tracheal Intubation in Patients with Suspected CSI?

There are several options for achieving definitive airway control in a trauma patient with suspected CSI. Traditionally, DLOI was considered unsafe for patients with unstable CSI, and blind nasotracheal intubation and surgical cricothyroidotomy were recommended as better options in that scenario. In the past decade, many series demonstrated the safety of DLOI. Although all series were retrospective, one fact is evident: Neurological deterioration after orotracheal intubation is an extremely rare event even in patients with unstable CSI. In a review article from 2006, Crosby summarized the results of 12 retrospective series examining the outcome of tracheal intubations in patients with CSI, most of them unstable. The accumulated number of DLOIs was 395; only two experienced neurological deterioration, and that was not attributed to the airway intervention [12].

Regardless of the evident safety of DLOI, awake nasotracheal intubation is an option that many anesthesiologists choose as the preferred technique for definitive airway control in patients with suspected CSI [13]. This maneuver can be done blindly or, more commonly in recent years, with a fiberoptic endoscope. Minimal spine movement, the ability to continue the neurological examination after the intubation, and maintaining airway-protective reflexes are some of the advantages of this procedure. The potential disadvantages are the slow learning curve that causes many caregivers to be uncomfortable with the procedure [14] and the potential for desaturation that might aggravate secondary cord injury [15]. Although nasotracheal intubation may be an accepted method and is suitable for certain scenarios in trauma patient management, we strongly recommend two-person endotracheal intubation with inline stabilization over it.

No significant differences in success rate or safety were found between flexible and rigid endoscopes in establishing a controlled airway in patients with a compromised cervical spine [16]. Bathory et al. showed improved laryngoscopic view with video laryngoscopy when compared with DLOI, with some studies suggesting better first-attempt success rates with video laryngoscopy. Nonetheless, cervical spine motion may not be affected any less with video laryngoscopy as compared with direct laryngoscopy [17].

RECOMMENDATIONS

DLOI is a safe and effective option for securing the airway in a trauma patient with suspected CSI. Grade of recommendation: B. No data exist to support one technique over the other. Because no special equipment or advanced expertise is needed for DLOI, it is probably preferred in emergencies.

Grade of recommendation: C.

SCIs might inflict respiratory failure and hemodynamic compromise, which can lead to hypoxemia and hypotension that might increase the chance of secondary cord injury and worsen the neurological outcome. Cervical spinal cord injury might cause respiratory muscle paresis and paralysis, causing decreased ventilatory efficiency, hypoxemia, and hypoventilation. Patients with cervical SCI are at significant risk for ventilatory failure. This risk varies based on the level and completeness of injury. Ventilatory support is needed for the majority of patients with C5 and higher injuries and virtually all patients with C3 and higher injuries in the acute phase. Adequate fluid resuscitation and hemodynamic improvement were found to correlate with better neurological outcome [18].

High SCI (usually above the level of T6) can be associated with disruption of the sympathetic chain that can cause hypotension and bradycardia. This condition, called neurogenic shock, is caused by unopposed parasympathetic vasodilation and bradycardia. The reported incidence of neurogenic shock varies greatly according to the diagnostic definition that is being applied. In their paper from 2008, Guly et al. found that the incidence of classic neurogenic shock is 19.3% [19]. Since then, several studies assessed the incidence of neurogenic shock, considering the different clinical definitions, and found that neurogenic shock incidence in cervical SCI ranges between 19% and 30% [20]. In most patients, adequate perfusion pressure can be maintained with fluid administration. Despite a lack of evidence-based literature on the subject, if the systolic blood pressure of at least 90 mmHg, mean arterial pressure of 85 mmHg, and normal perfusion status are not achieved, administration of a vasoactive drug should be considered once hypovolemia from blood loss is excluded [21].

12.4 What Criteria Should Be Used to Exclude Cervical Spine Injury in Trauma Patients?

Two major research projects have been published in an attempt to establish a set of criteria by which a significant CSI can be safely ruled out based on clinical evaluation alone. Other smaller prospective studies reached the same conclusion. The NEXUS study enrolled 34,069 patients. There were five criteria for the definition of a low probability of CSI: No midline cervical tenderness, no focal neurological deficit, normal alertness, no intoxication, and no painful, distracting injury. The decision instrument missed 8 of the 818 patients who eventually were diagnosed with CSI (sensitivity, 99.0%; 95% confidence interval [CI] 98.0–99.6%). The negative predictive value was 99.8% (95% CI, 99.6%–100%), the specificity was 12.9%, and the positive predictive value was 2.7% [22]. The Canadian study enrolled 8,924 adults with blunt trauma to the head and neck, with normal vital signs and a GCS of 15. Among the study population, there were 151 (1.7%) patients diagnosed with clinically important CSI. The decision to order cervical spine radiography was based on three questions: (1) Is there any high-risk factor present that mandates radiography (i.e., age 65 years, dangerous mechanism, or paresthesias in extremities)? (2) Is there any low-risk factor present that allows safe assessment of a range of motion (i.e., simple rear-end MVC, sitting position in emergency department, ambulatory at any time since injury, delayed onset of neck pain, or absence of midline cervical spine tenderness)? (3) Is the patient able to actively rotate the neck 45 degrees to the left and right?

The results were 100% sensitive (95% CI 98–100%) and 42.5% specific (95% CI 40–44%) for identifying clinically important cervical spine injuries [23]. In 2003, a prospective comparison of the two criteria sets was published. There were 169 important CSIs among the 8,283 study patients. The Canadian cervical spine rule was more sensitive than the NEXUS rule (99.4% versus 90.7%, $p < 0.001$), more specific (45.1% versus 36.8%, $p < 0.001$), and resulted in lower radiography rates [24].

RECOMMENDATIONS

Both the NEXUS and the Canadian cervical spine rule set of criteria can be safely used to clinically clear the cervical spine in adult asymptomatic patients with blunt trauma. Patients who meet the low-risk criteria do not need any further radiographic investigation.

Grade of recommendation: A.

National Emergency X-Radiography Utilization Study (NEXUS) Criteria

1. Normal alertness (i.e., GCS 15)
2. No focal neurological deficit
3. No intoxication
4. No painful distracting injury
5. No midline tenderness

The Canadian C-Spine Rule

For alert (GCS score = 15) and stable trauma patients when cervical spine injury is a concern.

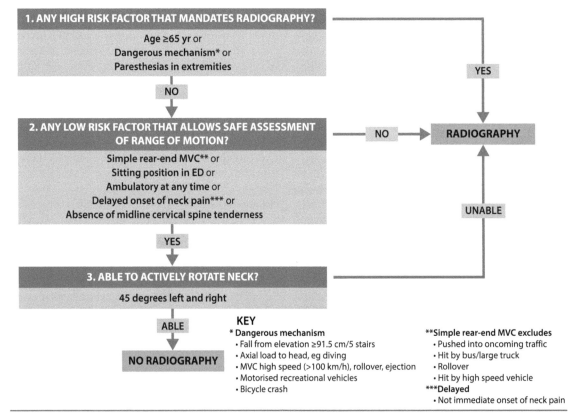

www.sira.nsw.gov.au/acutewhiplash

12.5 What Imaging Study Is Needed to Clear the Cervical Spine in the Obtunded Patient?

Another controversial issue is the clearance of the cervical spine in the comatose patient. Clearing the cervical spine in these circumstances is important mainly to allow removal of the cervical collar and thus preventing side effects (neck and scalp pressure sores and elevated intracranial pressure) and improving the nursing and physical therapy care. In the alert blunt trauma patient, the definitive clearance is done by the combination of computed tomography (CT) and clinical exam, as mentioned, before normal clinical exam practically rules out significant ligamentous injuries that can be missed in the CT. Coma or deep sedation in the intensive care unit prevents meaningful physical examination. Three options were traditionally suggested: Passive flexion–extension fluoroscopy, magnetic resonance imaging (MRI), and clearing of the cervical spine based on the CT alone. The limitations of the flexion–extension study were mentioned earlier. The passive flexion-extension study was also found to be unreliable in detecting cervical spine instability in comatose patients [25].

The difficulties and risk of taking ventilated patients with multiple trauma to the MRI have led to attempts to show the safety of clearing the cervical spine based on normal CT alone. Currently, the most comprehensive study was a meta-analysis, published by Raza et al. in 2013, which included 10 prospective studies. The authors found a cumulative negative predictive value and a specificity of cervical spine CT of 99.7% (95% CI 99.4–99.9%). The positive predictive value and sensitivity were 93.7% (95% CI 84.0–97.7%). They concluded that clearing the cervical spine based on the CT is safe and recommended [26].

SUMMARY AND RECOMMENDATIONS

In the obtunded trauma patient, the cervical spine can be safely cleared based on a normal CT. MRI should be reserved for the selected patients (e.g., those with neurological deficits, those with abnormal cervical CT findings, and those planned for spine surgery).

Grade of recommendation: B.

12.6 What Is the Imaging Modality of Choice to Evaluate the Spine?

Active flexion–extension cervical spine radiography has been suggested as adjacent to normal static radiographs in cases of continued neck tenderness or stiffness after blunt trauma. However, it rarely can add important information to the alert patient where muscle guarding typically will not allow for more than a few degrees of motion due to pain. Moreover, it has been demonstrated that the threshold cervical range of motion needed to detect even significant instability is approximately 30 degrees of flexion or extension, which is more than most pain patients can perform [27]. In addition, one must consider the fact that the cervical flexion–extension motions required in the setting of possible CSI may increase the risk of damage to the spinal cord or aggravate any existing damage.

Finally, flexion–extension radiographs became a rare choice due to their high rate of technical inadequacy and the fact that they add little information to CT or MRI, which became more available in recent years [28]. Traditionally, evaluation of the thoracic, lumbar, and sacral spine was done with plain radiographs augmented with CT in cases of evident fracture or technical inadequacy. In recent years, the availability of the high-resolution fast multislice CT scanner makes it the screening modality of choice. With most victims of high-energy blunt trauma needing torso CT, regenerating the spine images is more effective than plain radiographs with proven cost reduction [29, 30].

A known low sensitivity, together with the cumbersome task of obtaining at least three views (lateral, anteroposterior, and open-mouth odontoid), have led many trauma centers to choose cervical spine CT with coronal reconstruction as the primary screening modality for suspected CSI in patients with multiple trauma. The superiority of this approach was shown in a meta-analysis published in 2005. Despite some methodological flaws and the fact that no randomized controlled study was included, the authors presented a pooled sensitivity for plain radiography of 52% (95% CI 47–56%) versus a pooled sensitivity for CT of 98% (95% CI 96–99%) [31]. The American College of Orthopedic Surgeons now recommends routine cervical spine screening via CT scan instead of plain radiography [32]. The three-view radiographic study should be performed only when CT is not readily available and should not be considered a substitute for CT. Lateral cervical plain radiographs in the resuscitation area cannot rule out unstable CSI, so the information gained will not change the management of the patient. This is why we do not recommend this study. The assumption that CSI increases the risk for other thoracolumbar spine injuries has been proven in a large retrospective study based on the nationwide trauma database. The occurrence of thoracolumbar spine fracture was doubled from 6.9% to 13.06% if a concomitant cervical spine fracture was found [33].

MRI is the most sensitive imaging method for the evaluation of the neck structure, including soft tissue (ligaments, intervertebral discs, etc.) and neural structures. Therefore, it is an appealing modality for the diagnosis of a suspected injured spine. However, its relatively low availability and the technical problems of scanning trauma patients in the acute phase preclude its routine use during the initial evaluation. MRI is an important follow-up study in patients with CT signs that are suggestive of ligamentous or soft tissue and disc rupture injuries (noncongruent facet joins, chip avulsion fractures of end plates adjacent to disc space, and distended disc space). These may represent severely unstable cervical injuries that are reduced via muscle spasm and guarding in the alert patient, and in this scenario, MRI may add important additional information that no other modality can detect. MRI is also usually performed in patients with SCI to document the injury to the spinal cord itself and for reserved for cases of spinal-related signs and symptoms that are not explained by findings in the CT (i.e., continued neck pain or motion limitation or unexplained clinical neurological findings) [34]. As mentioned, MRI is more capable of detecting soft tissue injuries; some recent studies showed that in terms of clinical decision-making, MRI is best utilized in patients requiring spine surgery for CT-proven thoracic and lumbar spine injuries [35].

RECOMMENDATIONS

In patients where spine clearance cannot be achieved with clinical examination, CT of the cervical spine with reconstruction is the screening modality of choice. Views reconstructed from the thoracic and abdominal CT are adequate for the evaluation of the thoracic and lumbar spine. MRI should be preserved for selected cases of clinical/radiological discrepancy or inadequate CT.

Grade of recommendation: B.

12.6.1 Medical Management of Spinal Cord Damage

Inflicting direct forces such as laceration, compression, and distraction on the spinal cord create primary damage and cell death on impact. A secondary insult can occur within minutes as a result of hypoxia or hypoperfusion. The resulting inflammatory process, combined with other metabolic derangements, might further increase neural and glial cell apoptosis. These events will eventually lead to a worse neurological outcome. The relative contribution of the secondary insult to the final neurological outcome is unknown but estimated to be no higher than 10% [36], and it is still the focus of numerous research projects.

Several studies focus on the effort to promote neural tissue recovery and regeneration. Autologous incubated macrophages, oscillating field stimulation, autologous bone marrow cell transplantation with granulocyte-macrophage colony-stimulating factor, embryonic stem cell transplantation, and autologous olfactory ensheathing cell transplantation are all in various stages of clinical studies after showing promising results in animal models. However, none have yet produced any evidence to support use in any human clinical condition [37–40].

Recent innovations (e.g., stem cell secretome therapy, gene-based therapy) have been shown to promote neuronal growth, vascular remodeling, and cellular survival in animal models and in vitro models [41, 42]. Science and technology are advancing at an astonishing rate, improving the ability to successfully translate these techniques to clinical implications.

12.7 Should High-Dose Corticosteroids Be Used in Trauma Patients with SCI?

Few issues in medicine have stirred up as much controversy and dispute as the issue of corticosteroid administration in SCI. The complexity of the interpretation of evidence-based data and its influence on medicolegal considerations are demonstrated in a survey of 60 Canadian neurosurgeons and orthopedic spine surgeons about their practice. Approximately 75% of the responders routinely prescribe steroids for acute SCI, but 70% of them do so due to fear of litigation or peer criticism. Only 17% of them believe that steroids improve their patient's neurological outcomes [43]. The first study on the administration of methylprednisolone (MP) was published in 1984 [44]. In 1992, the National Spinal Cord Injury Study (NASCIS II) was published with high-profile professional and popular media coverage. It was a prospective, randomized, double-blind, controlled, multicenter trial with 487 patients randomized to high-dose MP, naloxone, or placebo. A 1-year follow-up study summarized the results. No significant neurological improvement was achieved, and an insignificant trend toward increased complication rate (mainly infectious) was demonstrated. A post hoc analysis found that patients who received high-dose MP within 8 hours of their injury showed a statistically significant, although questionable, improvement in motor and sensory scores at 6 months [45]. The next pivotal study (NASCIS III) randomized 499 patients and compared 24 and 48 hours of MP administration with no significant

outcome differences. Again, post hoc analyses showed that the 48-hour MP group had a slightly better motor outcome if the drug was given 3–8 hours after the trauma. The sensory scores were equal between the groups. As in all other similar studies, an increased infectious complications rate was evident [46]. In general, the same results were also obtained subsequently, including several prospective randomized studies.

In 2013, the American Association of Neurological Surgeons and the Congress of Neurological Surgeons stated that the use of glucocorticosteroids in acute SCI is not recommended. A 2014 survey of the Cervical Spine Research Society reported that overall, 55% of institutions continue to prescribe glucocorticosteroids in the setting of acute SCI. When comparing to earlier reports, it is clear that the use of glucocorticosteroids in the setting of acute SCI is declining [47].

SUMMARY AND RECOMMENDATIONS

Current data do not support the routine use of high-dose MP in patients with SCI.

Grade of recommendation: B.

12.8 Surgical Intervention: Timing

12.8.1 What Is the Optimal Timing to Operate on a Patient with Spinal Injury?

The effect of early surgery on neurological outcomes remains a debatable topic. Vaccaro et al. designed a prospective randomized controlled study to determine whether the functional outcome is improved in patients with traumatic cervical SCI who underwent early surgery (<72 hours after injury) compared with those who underwent late surgery (>5 days after injury). They revealed no significant neurological benefit for the early surgical intervention [48].

Fehlings et al. conducted a meta-analysis study, which provide the following recommendations: (1) Urgent decompression is recommended in case of bilateral locked facets and incomplete tetraplegia or neurological deterioration; (2) urgent decompression in any acute CSI is a reasonable practice option [49].

The dilemma of timing is much more complicated in multitrauma patients with an associated spinal injury. Though advocating urgent decompression, Fehling et al. found that in this setting, it is extremely difficult to obtain an MRI of the cervical spine and to prepare the patients for urgent surgery in the face of physiological insult that often mandates lifesaving efforts and intensive care unit stay [50]. Dai et al. retrospectively summarized their experience with 147 patients who sustained blunt high-energy multitrauma with thoracolumbar fractures. Although it is not the preferable study design in terms of evidence-based medicine, it is worthwhile to learn its results and conclusions. There was no statistically significant correlation between the timing of thoracolumbar surgery and the complication rate. Neither the severity of the injury nor the timing of surgery had any significant effect on the recovery rate [51].

One criticism of these earlier studies is that the threshold definition of early versus late surgery was randomly defined at 72 hours. Animal models and clinical data have demonstrated that if any recovery is to be expected in the face of continuous cord compression and SCI, decompression and removal of cord pressure are to be achieved within 12–24 hours and optimally even within 6 hours. Therefore, this earlier trial that defined the threshold at 72 hours compared two groups, both of which had surgery at a "late" stage. New trials that compare decompression surgery within 24 hours and after 24 hours have consistently shown a marked neurological improvement of two grades in SCI patients and represent a new trend toward very early surgery [52–54].

Published in 2012, the prospective nonrandomized STASCIS trial compared outcomes in 313 patients with acute cervical SCI in those who received surgery within 24 hours (182 patients, mean 14.2 hours) and those who received a late operation (131 patients, mean 48.3 hours). In the multivariate analysis, after adjusting for preoperative neurological status and steroid administration, the odds of at least a two-grade AIS improvement were 2.8 times higher among those who underwent early surgery as compared to those who underwent late surgery (odds ratio [OR] = 2.83, 95% CI: 1.10–7.28). Mortality and complication rates were similar in both groups [54].

In their paper from 2020, Haghnegahdar et al. evaluated the safety and efficacy of early (<24 hours) compared with late (24–72 hours) decompressive surgery after thoracic and thoracolumbar (T1–L1) SCI. Seventy-three injured patients were included in this single-center randomized controlled trial (RCT). Of these, 37 received early surgery and 36 underwent late surgery. In the early group 45.9% of patients and in the late group 33.3% of patients had a ≥1-grade improvement in ASIA Impairment Scale (AIS ([OR] 1.70, 95% [CI]: 0.66–4.39, *p* = 0.271); significantly more patients in the early (24.3%) than late (5.6%) surgery group had a ≥2-grade improvement in AIS (OR 5.46, 95% CI: 1.09–27.38, *p* = 0.025) [55].

RECOMMENDATIONS

To date, there are no defined standards regarding the timing of decompression and stabilization in acute SCI. The literature does infer urgent spinal cord decompression in the face of evolving neurological deficits or specific lesions.

Grade of recommendation: D.

Editor's Note

The treatment of spinal cord injury lacks high-quality evidence to guide management. For some time, high-dose steroids were adopted despite the fact that the clinical trial data were fatally flawed and the medical community was aware of this fact. More recently, there has been an aggressive campaign aimed at pushing mean arterial pressures to much higher-than-normal levels ("MAP greater than 85 mmHg"). This is based upon three small retrospective Level III studies. Despite the paucity of data, spine surgeons continue to demand that the trauma patient with partial or complete spinal cord injury receive massive fluid resuscitation and high-dose pressors to elevate their blood pressure. This has resulted in organ dysfunction (specifically bowel ischemia) and poor overall outcomes. This practice should be avoided until quality data are provided to support its use.

REFERENCES

1. National Spinal Cord Injury Statistical Center, Facts and Figures at a Glance. Birmingham, AL: University of Alabama at Birmingham, 2020.
2. Alizadeh A, Dyck SM, Karimi-Abdolrezaee S. Traumatic spinal cord injury: An overview of pathophysiology, models and acute injury mechanisms. *Front Neurol*. March 22, 2019;10:282. DOI: 10.3389/fneur.2019.00282. PMID: 30967837; PMCID: PMC6439316.
3. Browner BD, Jupiter JB, Levine AM, et al. *Skeletal Trauma: Fractures, Dislocations, Ligamentous Injuries.* WB Saunders: Philadelphia, PA; 1998.
4. ASIA and ISCoS International Standards Committee. The 2019 revision of the International Standards for Neurological Classification of Spinal Cord Injury (ISNCSCI)—What's new? *Spinal Cord*. 2019;57:815–817. DOI: 10.1038/s41393-019-0350-9
5. Demetriades D, Charalambides K, Chahwan S, et al. Nonskeletal cervical spine injuries: Epidemiology and diagnostic pitfalls. *J Trauma*. 2000;48:724–727.
6. Dreiangel N, Ben-Galim P, Lador R, Hipp JA. Occipito-cervical dissociative injuries: Common in blunt trauma fatalities and better detected with objective CT-based measurements. *Spine J*. August 2010;10(8):704–707.
7. Lador R, Ben-Galim P, Hipp JA. Motion within the unstable cervical spine during patient maneuvering: The neck pivot-shift phenomenon. *J Trauma*. January 2011;70(1):247–251.
8. Sawin PD, Todd MM, Traynelis VC, et al. Cervical spine motion with direct laryngoscopy and orotracheal intubation: An in vivo cinefluoroscopic study of subjects without cervical abnormality. *Anesthesiology*. 1996;85:26–36.
9. Gerling MC, Davis DP, Hamilton RS, et al. Effects of cervical spine immobilization technique and laryngoscope blade selection on an unstable cervical spine in a cadaver model of intubation. *Ann Emerg Med*. 2000;36:293–300.
10. Lennarson PJ, Smith D, Todd MM, et al. Segmental cervical spine motion during orotracheal intubation of the intact and injured spine with and without external stabilization. *J Neurosurg*. 2000;92:201–206.
11. Lennarson PJ, Smith DW, Sawin PD, Todd MM, Sato Y, Traynelis VC: Cervical spinal motion during intubation: Efficacy of stabilization maneuvers in the setting of complete segmental instability. *J Neurosurg*. 2001;94(2 suppl):265–270.
12. Crosby ET. Airway management in adults after cervical spine trauma. *Anesthesiology*. 2006;104:1293–1318.
13. Rosenblatt WH, Wagner PJ, Ovassapian A, et al. Practice patterns in managing the difficult airway by anesthesiologists in the United States. *Anesth Analg*. 1998;87:153–157.
14. Ezri T, Szmuk P, Warters RD, et al. Difficult airway management practice patterns among anesthesiologists practicing in the United States: Have we made any progress? *J Clin Anesth*. 2003;15:418–422.

15. Fuchs G, Schwarz G, Baumgartner A, et al. Fiberoptic intubation in 327 patients with lesions of the cervical spine. *J Neurosurg Anesth*. 1999;11:16–11.

16. Cohn AI, Zornow MH. Awake endotracheal intubation in 520 patients with cervical spine disease: A comparison of the Bullard laryngoscope and the fiberoptic bronchoscope. *Anesth Analg*. 1995;81:1283–1286.

17. Bathory I, Frascarolo P, Kern C, Schoettker P. Evaluation of the GlideScope for tracheal intubation in patients with cervical spine immobilization by a semi-rigid collar. *Anaesthesia*. 2009;64:1337–1341.

18. Vale FL, Burns J, Jackson AB, et al. Combined medical and surgical treatment after acute spinal cord injury: Results of a prospective pilot study to assess the merits of aggressive medical resuscitation and blood pressure management. *J Neurosurg*. 1997;87:239–246.

19. Guly HR, Bouamra O, Lecky FE; Trauma Audit and Research Network. The incidence of neurogenic shock in patients with isolated spinal cord injury in the emergency department. *Resuscitation*. 2008;76:57–62.

20. Dave S, Cho JJ. Neurogenic Shock. [Updated 2022 Feb 10]. In: *StatPearls [Internet]*. StatPearls Publishing: Treasure Island (FL); 2022. Available from: https://www.ncbi.nlm. nih.gov/books/NBK459361/

21. Hadley MN, Walters BC, Grabb PA, et al. Blood pressure management after acute spinal cord injury. *Neurosurgery*. 2002;50(Suppl):58–62.

22. Hoffman JR, Mower WR, Wolfson AB, et al. Validity of a set of clinical criteria to rule out injury to the cervical spine in patients with blunt trauma. National Emergency X-Radiography Utilisation Study Group. *N Engl J Med*. 2000;343:94–99.

23. Stiell IG, Wells GA, Vandemheen KL, et al. The Canadian C-spine rule for radiography in alert and stable trauma patients. *JAMA*. 2001;286:1841–1848.

24. Stiell IG, Clement CM, McKnight RD, et al. The Canadian C-spine rule versus the NEXUS low-risk criteria in patients with trauma. *N Engl J Med*. 2003;349:2510–2518.

25. Freedman I, van Gelderen D, Cooper DJ, Fitzgerald M, Malham G, Rosenfeld JV, Varma D, Kossmann T. Cervical spine assessment in the unconscious trauma patient: A major trauma service's experience with passive flexion-extension radiography. *J Trauma*. June 2005;58(6):1183–1188.

26. Raza M1, Elkhodair S, Zaheer A, Yousaf S. Safe cervical spine clearance in adult obtunded blunt trauma patients based on a normal multidetector CT scan—A meta-analysis and cohort study. *Injury*. November 2013;44(11): 1589–1595.

27. Hwang H, Hipp JA, Ben-Galim P, Reitman CA. Threshold cervical range of motion is necessary to detect abnormal intervertebral motion in cervical spine radiographs spine. *Spine*. April 2008;33(8):E261–E267.

28. Insko EK, Gracias VH, Gupta R, et al. Utility of flexion and extension radiographs of the cervical spine in the acute evaluation of blunt trauma. *J Trauma*. 2002;53:426–429.

29. Sheridan R, Peralta R, Rhen J, et al. Reformatted visceral protocol helical computed tomographic scanning allows conventional radiographs of the thoracic and lumbar spine to be eliminated in the evaluation of blunt trauma patients. *J Trauma*. 2003;55:655–669.

30. Brandt MM, Wahl WL, Yeom K, et al. Computed tomographic scanning reduces cost and time of complete spine evaluation. *J Trauma*. 2004;56:1022–1026.

31. Holmes JF, Akkinepalli R. Computed tomography versus plain radiography to screen for cervical spine injury: A meta-analysis. *J Trauma*. 2005;58:902–905.

32. Mulkens TH, Marchal P, Daineffe S, et al. Comparison of low-dose with standard-dose multidetector CT in cervical spine trauma. *Am J Neuroradiol*. 2007;28:1444–1450.

33. Winslow JE III, Hensberry R, Bozeman WP, et al. Risk of thoracolumbar fractures doubled in victims of motor vehicle collisions with cervical spine fractures. *J Trauma*. 2006;61:686–687.

34. Karpova A, Arun R, Cadotte DW, Davis AM, Kulkarni AV, O'Higgins M, Fehlings MG. Assessment of spinal cord compression by magnetic resonance imaging—Can it predict surgical outcomes in degenerative compressive myelopathy? A systematic review. *Spine*. 2013;38(16): 1409–1421.

35. Khoury L, Chang E, Hill D, Shams S, Sim V, Panzo M, Vijmasi T, Cohn S. Management of thoracic and lumbar spine fractures: Is MRI necessary in patients without neurological deficits? *Am Surg*. March 1, 2019;85(3):306–311. DOI: 10.1177/000313481908500338. PMID: 30947780.

36. Young W, Yen V, Blight A. Extracellular calcium ion activity in experimental spinal cord contusion. *Brain Res*. 1982;235:105–113.

37. Knoller N, Auerbach G, Fulga V, et al. Clinical experience using incubated autologous macrophages as a treatment for complete spinal cord injury: Phase I study results. *J Neurosurg Spine*. 2005;3:173–181.

38. Shapiro S, Borgens R, Pascuzzi R, et al. Oscillating field stimulation for complete spinal cord injury in humans: A phase I trial. *J Neurosurg Spine*. 2005;2:3–10.

39. Yoon SH, Shim YS, Park YH, et al. Complete spinal cord injury treatment using autologous bone marrow cell transplantation and bone marrow stimulation with granulocyte macrophage-colony stimulating factor: Faze me/II clinical trial. *Stem Cells*. 2007;25:2066–2073.

40. Féron F, Perry C, Cochrane J, et al. Autologous olfactory ensheathing cell transplantation in human spinal cord injury. *Brain*. 2005;128:2951–2960.

41. Pajer K, Bellák T, Nógrádi A. Stem cell secretome for spinal cord repair: Is it more than just a random baseline set of factors? *Cells*. November 18, 2021;10(11):3214. DOI: 10.3390/ cells10113214. PMID: 34831436; PMCID: PMC8625005.

42. Zavvarian MM, Toossi A, Khazaei M, Hong J, Fehlings M. Novel innovations in cell and gene therapies for spinal cord injury. *F1000Res*. April 22, 2020;9:F1000 Faculty Rev-279. DOI: 10.12688/f1000research.21989.1. PMID: 32399196; PMCID: PMC7194487.

43. Hurlbert RJ, Moulton R. Why do you prescribe methylprednisolone for acute spinal cord injury? *Can J Neurol Sci*. 2002;29:236–239.

44. Bracken MB, Collins WF, Freeman DF, et al. Efficacy of methylprednisolone in acute spinal cord injury. *JAMA*. 1984;251:45–52.

45. Bracken MB, Shepard MJ, Collins WF, et al. Methylprednisolone or naloxone treatment after acute spinal cord 1-year follow-up data. *J Neurosurg*. 1992;76:23–31.

46. Bracken MB, Shepard MJ, Holford TR, et al. Administration of methylprednisolone for 24 or 48 hours or tirilazad mesylate for 48 hours in the treatment of acute spinal cord injury. *JAMA*. 1997;277:1597–1604.

47. Schroeder GD, Kwon BK, Eck JC, Savage JW, Hsu WK, Patel AA. Survey of cervical spine research society members on the use of high-dose steroids for acute spinal cord injuries. *Spine (Phila Pa 1976)*. May 20, 2014;39(12):971–7. DOI: 10.1097/BRS.0000000000000297. PMID: 24583739.

48. Vaccaro AR, Daugherty RJ, Sheehan TP, et al. Neurologic outcome of early versus late surgery for cervical spinal cord injury. *Spine*. 1997;22:2609–2613.

49. Fehlings MG, Perrin RG. The role and timing of early decompression for cervical spinal cord injury: Update with a review of recent clinical evidence. *Injury*. 2005;36(Suppl 2): S13–S26.

50. Fehlings MG, Cuddy B, Dickman C, Fazl M, Green B, Hitchon P, Northrup B, Sonntag V, Wagner F, Tator CH. Surgical treatment for acute spinal cord injury studies pilot study #2: Evaluation of a protocol for decompressive surgery within 8 hours of injury. *Neurosurg Focus*. January 1999;6(1):e3.

51. Dai LY, Tao WF, Zhou O. Thoracolumbar fractures in patients with multiple injuries: Diagnosis and treatment—A review of 147 cases. *J Trauma*. 2004;56:348–355.

52. Wilson JR, Singh A, Craven C, Verrier MC, Drew B, Ahn H, Ford M, Fehlings MG. Early versus late surgery for traumatic spinal cord injury: The results of a prospective Canadian cohort study. *Spinal Cord*. November 2012; 50(11):840–843.

53. Umerani MS, Abbas A, Sharif S. Asian: Clinical outcome in patients with early versus delayed decompression in cervical spine trauma. *Spine J*. August 2014;8(4):427–434.

54. Fehlings MG, Vaccaro A, Wilson JR, Singh A, W Cadotte D, Harrop JS, Aarabi B, Shaffrey C, Dvorak M, Fisher C, Arnold P, Massicotte EM, Lewis S, Rampersaud R. Early versus delayed decompression for traumatic cervical spinal cord injury: Results of the surgical timing in acute spinal cord injury study (STASCIS). *PLoS One*. 2012;7(2):e32037. DOI: 10.1371/journal.pone.0032037. Epub 2012 Feb 23. PMID: 22384132; PMCID: PMC3285644.

55. Haghnegahdar A, Behjat R, Saadat S, Badhiwala J, Farrokhi MR, Niakan A, Eghbal K, Barzideh E, Shahlaee A, Ghaffarpasand F, Ghodsi Z, Vaccaro AR, Sadeghi-Naini M, Fehlings MG, Guest JD, Derakhshan P, Rahimi-Movaghar V. A randomized controlled trial of early versus late surgical decompression for thoracic and thoracolumbar spinal cord injury in 73 patients. *Neurotrauma Rep*. September 18, 2020;1(1):78–87. DOI: 10.1089/neur.2020.0027. PMID: 34223533; PMCID: PMC8240887.

13

Facial Injuries

Yinglun Wu, Paolo Rigor, and Joseph H. Shin

13.1 Introduction

Facial injuries are among the most common emergencies seen in an acute care setting. They range from simple soft tissue lacerations to complex facial fractures associated with significant craniomaxillofacial injuries with soft tissue loss. The management of these injuries generally follows standard surgical management priorities, but is rendered more complex by the nature of the numerous areas of overlap in management areas such as airway, neurologic, ophthalmologic, and dental. In addition, the significant psychological nature of injuries affecting the face and the resultant aftermath of scarring can have devastating and long-lasting consequences. Even though these injuries are exceedingly common, they are cared for by a large group of different specialists and, as such, have a remarkably heterogeneous presentation and diverse treatment schema. Nonetheless, guiding principles in the care of these injuries will provide the basis for the best possible outcomes. The following questions will hopefully guide general management and provide a framework for understanding the principles in the acute care of patients with facial injuries and trauma.

13.2 What Is the Proper Timing and Method of Closure? What Is the Optimal Subsequent Care for Facial Lacerations and Wounds after Closure?

There remains little standardization in the method of repair of traumatic lacerations and the subsequent care of these wounds, primarily because of the numerous different specialties involved in caring for the trauma patient. We reviewed the available literature to provide best practice guidelines to address the optimal timing of wound closure, the closure technique and material utilized, the type of dressing, and adjunctive measures for a facial laceration.

The timing of facial skin laceration closure is the same as that of any open wound. Previously, it was thought that the presence of contaminating factors in wounds would generally not allow closure after 6 hours [1]. However, there has been an evolving body of literature in recent years that seems to dispute the long-standing "golden period" hypothesis. Clinical practice is slightly more variable in the management of facial trauma because of the uniquely sensitive nature of facial scarring and the exceptionally rich blood supply of the face.

To date, there have been multiple studies comparing early vs. delayed primary laceration repair. In a prospective cohort study done in 2014 by Quinn et al., they examined 2,663 patients with traumatic lacerations to see whether the timing of closure influenced infection rates. They found no difference in infection rates in wounds closed before or after 12 hours. However, their higher infection rates were seen in patients with diabetes, lower extremity lacerations, contaminated lacerations, and lacerations greater than 5 cm [2].

In 2013, Rui-feng et al. published a prospective randomized controlled trial (RCT) addressing whether primary closure of a dirty wound is possible. The authors randomly divided 600 facial lacerations inflicted by a dog bite into two groups, those closed primarily and those left open to allow for healing by secondary intention, and measured the infection rate and time to healing. The group found that primary closure of the dirty wound did not have an increased incidence of infection over the group left to heal by secondary intention and primary closure predictably shortens the time to healing. They concluded that immediate primary closure of dirty wounds after thorough irrigation and debridement was the preferred approach [3]. In a similar study published by Paschos et al. in 2013, the authors performed an RCT comparing primary closure vs. healing by secondary intention following dog bite wounds. Of the 168 patients enrolled in the study, the authors found that wounds closed before 8 hours had an overall infection rate of 4.5% compared to 22.2% for wounds closed after 8 hours. Interestingly, head and neck dog bite wounds exhibited both improved cosmesis and lower infection rates compared to other parts of the body, which supports the practice of repairing facial lacerations when feasible [4].

Regarding the suturing technique, Gandham and Menon published a prospective RCT in 2003 in which they compared the cosmetic appearance of skin lacerations closed by either the traditional or dynamic sliding loop suture technique. Two independent observers blinded to the technique used a visual analogue cosmetic scale to assess the aesthetic result and found no statistical difference in cosmetic outcomes between the two groups [5]. Then in 2005, Singer et al. conducted a prospective RCT that compared the short-term wound infection, dehiscence rates, and cosmetic outcome after 3 months of traumatic facial lacerations closed with either a single or double layer of sutures. The study included 65 patients, all with simple, linear, nonbite, and nongaping (<10 mm in width) wounds. Wounds were evaluated at the time of closure, 5 days later, and again 3 months later. Both the patient and a researcher who was

DOI: 10.1201/9781003316800-13

blinded to the number of suture layers assessed cosmesis at the 3-month follow-up. The authors demonstrated that although skin closure with a single layer of suture was 7 minutes shorter, no statistical difference was found between groups regarding the aesthetic result. Therefore, the cosmetic outcome was not improved by the addition of a second layer of deep sutures to simple interrupted percutaneous sutures for the treatment of nongaping facial lacerations [6].

Traditional management of facial lacerations includes closure of the skin with a nonabsorbable suture, citing the low tissue reactivity that minimizes scar formation and the high tensile strength preventing dehiscence. However, several studies comparing absorbable and nonabsorbable sutures in adults reported no statistically significant difference in infection rate or wound appearance [7–11]. In 2008, Luck et al. conducted a prospective, randomized controlled trial comparing absorbable catgut sutures and nonabsorbable nylon sutures for the closure of pediatric facial lacerations. The authors showed that there was no statistically significant difference between the two groups in the rates of infection, wound dehiscence, keloid formation, parental satisfaction, and cosmetic outcome [12]. However, in 2013, the same group published again a nearly identical prospective RCT comparing absorbable and nonabsorbable sutures for skin closure of facial lacerations in the pediatric population. The results largely echoed those of the previous study with no statistical difference in the rate of infection, wound dehiscence, and keloid formation. The aesthetic results were judged using a visual analog scale (VAS) by caregivers and three blinded physicians. As in the prior study, there was no difference in caregiver VAS score; however, the 2013 results of the physician group found that nonabsorbable sutures resulted in a better cosmetic outcome. One of the reasons for this disparity could be accounted for by the difference between treatments of absorbable sutures at the first physician visit; in 2008, any remaining suture was removed, and in 2013, remaining suture was not removed, allowing it to completely resorb. Up to 50% of catgut repairs were still intact by day 9, while all nylon was removed by day 7; thus, the longer time to absorption possibly allowed for greater tissue reactivity and could account for the difference in cosmetic outcome [13]. Most recently in 2016, Xu et al. performed a meta-analysis of RCTs that compared outcomes of absorbable vs. nonabsorbable sutures for skin closure. A total of 1,748 patients were analyzed in 19 RCTs. The authors concluded that there was no significant difference in the incidence of wound infections, cosmetic outcomes, scar formation, wound dehiscence, and patients' or caregivers' satisfaction [14].

Cyanoacrylates, commonly referred to as tissue adhesives, have revolutionized wound care because of the inexpensive, painless, and relatively easy means to repair low-tension facial lacerations. They provide good tensile strength and bactericidal or bacteriostatic properties and obviate the need for suture removal. A 2009 Cochrane review included 11 studies comparing tissue adhesive with standard wound closure, with the aesthetic result being the primary outcome and the secondary outcomes being patient pain, time of the procedure, and any complications, including wound infection or dehiscence. There was no difference in the cosmetic outcomes between the suture and tissue adhesive; pain and procedure time statistically significantly favored tissue adhesive, while only a small increased rate of wound dehiscence was found with tissue adhesives [15].

Two of the studies included in the Cochrane review compared different types of tissue adhesives, one of which was published by Zempsky et al. comparing Steri-Strip® and Dermabond® for closure of pediatric facial lacerations. They conducted a prospective randomized trial that consisted of 100 children divided into two groups: One was treated with Steri-Strips and the other was given Dermabond. The pain was measured using a 100-mm pain VAS, and the cosmetic outcome was measured by two blinded cosmetic surgeons using a 100-mm VAS. There was no statistical difference in pain, cosmetic score, or wound complication rates. The authors concluded that the use of Steri-Strips for skin closure was less expensive and provided a clinically equivalent result when compared with Dermabond [16].

A more recent study by Fontana et al. published in 2021 even goes so far as to suggest that in the case of simple facial lacerations, tissue adhesives may be superior to traditional laceration repair with sutures. In this study, physicians used either traditional suturing techniques or applied Epiglu®. However, one important caveat in the study design is that the choice of treatment modality was left to the discretion of the treating physician. Thus, one significant limitation of this study is its single-blinded design, as it is conceivable that treating physicians might selectively apply tissue adhesives in more favorable, less hostile wounds [17].

Botulinum toxin has also been studied as a therapeutic option to improve the quality of wound healing after facial laceration closure. In 2013, Ziade et al. addressed this issue by conducting a prospective RCT of 30 postoperative patients with facial wounds randomized into patients who received botulinum toxin within 72 hours of repair and those who did not. The rationale behind this hypothesis is that botulinum toxin–induced immobilization of muscle activity around the healing wound reduces the muscle tension that acts on the wound edges, thereby decreasing the repeated microtrauma and the opportunity for hypertrophic and hyperpigmented scars to form. After 1-year follow-up, the cosmetic outcome was judged by the patient, an independent evaluator, and six physicians using the VAS based on photographs. No statistically significant difference was found between the two groups based on patient and independent evaluator assessment; however, the physician group found a statistically significant improvement in scarring in the group that underwent postoperative botulinum injection [18].

In a recent study by Kim et al. in 2019, the authors performed a randomized, double-blinded, controlled trial to evaluate the efficacy of botulinum toxin type A (BoNTA) on scar formation following forehead laceration repair. Twenty-four patients received 5 IU/cm BoNTA and 21 patients received saline, with follow-ups at 1, 3, and 6 months. Scars were analyzed with the patient and observer scale, Stony Brook Scar Evaluation Scale (SBSES), VAS, and biopsies. In all scar scales, favorable changes were the largest in the BoNTA groups; statistical significance was reached on the SBSES and VAS. Interestingly, skin biopsies showed less collagen deposition in the dermal layer of the BoNTA group [19].

The utility of ablative and nonablative lasers for the treatment of scars has been well described, and recently, this approach has been applied to minimize scarring from traumatic facial lacerations. A case series published in 2012 describes the use of ablative fractional resurfacing for traumatic facial scars using an Er:YAG laser after primary repair during the immediate postoperative period. All patients had treatment initiated 1 month after primary repair with laser treatment, occurring four times at monthly intervals. The results obtained 1 month after the last treatment revealed improvement as measured by the cosmetic scale used by patients, independent evaluators, and 10 physicians. The authors concluded that laser treatment is a safe and effective adjunct to postoperative care of facial lacerations; however, more studies, including RCTs, are required [20]. In a more recent study, researchers compared fractional ablative resurfacing to fully ablative lasers in the treatment of postoperative scarring. Twenty-two patients were enrolled in the split-scar study following excision from dermatologic surgery. One half of the scar was treated with fully ablative Er:YAG, whereas the other half was treated with fractionated Er:YAG. Scars were treated at monthly intervals for 3 months, with follow-up at 1 and 2 months after the final treatment. Patients were assessed via the patient observer self-assessment scale (POSAS) along with a 5-point Likert scale to assess erythema, height, texture, and overall cosmetic appearance. The results showed that patients and physicians alike overwhelmingly preferred the fractionated Er:YAG laser over the fully ablative laser [21].

RECOMMENDATIONS

There appears to be little difference noted in terms of the outcome of the treatment of lacerations and injuries, depending on the method of repair. Early expeditious repair should be undertaken within 12 hours, if feasible. Either absorbable or nonabsorbable sutures may be considered equivalent. The timing of facial suture removal is generally best done between 5 and 7 days (Grade of recommendation: B). The advent of tissue adhesives has obviated the need for sutures in cases of nongaping simple facial lacerations and is equally efficacious. Grade of recommendation: B. Botulinum toxin administered postoperatively may be effective in improving the appearance of scars (Grade of recommendation: B). The use of fractionated laser resurfacing for traumatic facial scars using an Er:YAG laser shows early promise. Grade of recommendation: C

13.3 What Is the Proper Timing of Repair of Facial Fractures, Especially in the Setting of Neurologic Trauma/Other Injuries?

Facial injuries, in particular facial fractures, have long been noted to be associated with concomitant head and cerebral injuries. A retrospective review of trauma in motorcycle riders found the odds of traumatic brain injury (TBI) were 3.5 times greater with a facial injury than without a facial injury and 6.5 times greater with a facial fracture than without a facial fracture. Additionally, while significantly increased odds of TBI were observed for fractures of all bones of the face, the highest odds of TBI were found in riders with fractures to bones of the upper face [22].

The timing of the repair of facial fractures in polytrauma patients, specifically patients with TBI, has been controversial. It is accepted that the outcome of facial fractures is improved by early repair, as demonstrated in the orthopedic literature. Delay of fracture fixation impedes the restoration of both function and aesthetic results by allowing fibroblast migration and potentially increasing scarring, leading to a poor result. The historical concern of the deleterious impact on functional neurological outcomes posed by the risks of anesthesia during operative intervention has been the basis of a delayed approach to operative repair. A study by Derdyn et al. retrospectively examined clinical and radiographic data in patients with displaced facial fractures and cerebral trauma. They found that a statistically significant worse neurological outcome was predicted by the presence of upper-level facial fracture, low presenting Glasgow Coma Scale (GCS), intracranial hemorrhage, displacement of midline cerebral structures, and multisystem trauma. More importantly, they found no significant difference in survival between individuals who underwent early, middle, or late operative intervention for facial fractures [23]. Furthermore, in 2007, another retrospective review of patients with TBI and facial fractures sought to determine if a difference in postoperative complications was changed by the timing of the repair of facial fractures. Of the 99 patients studied, they found an 11% complication rate, and on multivariate logistic regression model analysis, it was found that the odds of a postoperative complication were increased not only by a prolonged surgical procedure but also by a delay in surgical repair [24]. Similarly, Wang et al. in 2007 performed a prospective cohort study to examine whether the timing of noncranial surgery in patients with TBI had any effect on neuropsychological and functional outcomes, morbidity, or mortality. They divided patients into early (<24 hours) vs. late surgery (>24 hours) after injury and evaluated patients at 6 months postinjury. They found that early timing of orthopedic and facial fracture fixation under general anesthesia was not associated with worse neuropsychological or functional outcomes compared to late surgery [25].

Similarly, in 2008 Janus et al. retrospectively reviewed 34 charts of patients who underwent midface fracture repair at a Level 1 trauma center. The early repair was defined as postinjury days 1–5; late repairs occurred after day 6. There was no statistically significant difference between the two groups concerning operative time, the median number of screws used for repair, complication rate, and estimated operative blood loss (although there was a trend toward increased blood loss in the early treatment group). The authors also suggest that midface fractures should be repaired before 14 days, as after this period bone begins to heal and manipulation becomes more difficult [26]. In a retrospective review of 255 patients with orbital wall fractures, Yu et al. found that patients treated within 2 weeks of an orbital wall fracture had a significantly higher diplopia resolution rate than patients treated within 2–4 weeks and more than 4 weeks after sustaining a fracture (58% vs. 38.1%), which suggests that the timing of repair influences diplopia outcome [27]. With regard to mandibular fractures, Czserwinski et al. in 2008 conducted a retrospective review of 177 patient charts of patients with mandible fractures and found that delay in facial fracture treatment of more than 72 hours showed no increased rate of infection [28]. Furthermore, in a systematic review of orbital floor blowout fractures, Damgaard et al. identified five studies with 442 patients and divided patients into early (<14 days) vs. late (>14 days) treatment groups. Patients in the late group had a significantly higher odds ratio of 3.3 for persistent diplopia compared to the early group, with no significant difference in enophthalmos [29].

Hurrel et al. in 2014 performed a systematic review examining the effect of timing on the management of facial fractures. The PubMed database was searched from 1979 to 2013 and a total of 30 studies were identified. Twenty-eight of the studies were case series, with the majority being retrospective in nature. The findings were conflicted: Eighteen studies found no statistically significant relationship between treatment delay and treatment outcome. Nine found that treatment delay was associated with worse outcomes, with the remaining three with conflicting results [30]. Although no definitive conclusions could be drawn, it appears that facial fractures should be reduced as soon as it is safe and feasible to do so.

RECOMMENDATION

The current data support performing early repair of facial fractures as soon as the patient's condition stabilizes. There appears to be little to gain from significant delays in fracture management and no increase in complications from early (postinjury days 0–5) repair. The benefits of early repair in the neurologically stable patient appear to outweigh any possible issues related to delay.

Grade of recommendation: C.

13.4 Are Antibiotics Indicated in the Management of Facial Lacerations or Facial Fractures and, If So, When?

Antibiotics are used widely in surgery and the management of facial injuries. Growing awareness of the efficacy of antibiotic use in a perioperative setting must be balanced with the emerging threat of complications of prolonged use, the most serious of which is the development of antibiotic-resistant organisms. The profusion of opinion on the use of antibiotics is complicated again by the heterogeneous and varied presentations of the injuries, as well as those presenting with dental and oral injuries with their exceedingly high risk of subsequent infection.

It has generally been accepted that patients with simple lacerations do not require either pretreatment or posttreatment antibiotic use [31]. In bite wounds, however, antibiotics

are typically recommended. In 2015, Jaindl et al. reviewed 5,248 consecutive bite wound patients at a Level I trauma center and found a correlation between the timing of antibiotic administration and the rates of infection. Infection rates within 24 hours of antibiotic administration were 29.3% compared to 65% <48 hours, and 81.1% <72 hours, respectively. In the same study, the authors found a sixfold increased risk of infection following cat bites than dog bites [32]. The management of facial fractures and the use of antibiotics in these cases are more complicated. The presence of colonization and bacterial load in the paranasal sinuses and normal flora in the nasal and respiratory tract and then in the oral mucosa represent possible sources of bacterial contamination and the potential for subsequent infection. Therefore, the use of perioperative antibiotic treatment in these cases has a justifiable basis. In 1987, Chole and Yee studied 101 patients with facial fractures in a prospective RCT that investigated the role of the administration of cefazolin 1 g intravenously 1 hours before surgery and 8 hours later. They concluded that perioperative antibiotic use reduces the incidence of postoperative infection by demonstrating a reduction in facial and mandibular fracture infection rates from 42% to 9% and 44% to 13%, respectively [33].

In a prospective study that included 90 patients, Heit et al. compared the efficacy and cost of 1 g daily of ceftriaxone and 2 million units of penicillin G every 4 hours in patients with compound mandible fractures undergoing surgery. Two patients in each group developed infections. They therefore conclude that ceftriaxone is equally effective and carries a lower cost than penicillin G without any increase in systemic toxicity. They also suggest that adding metronidazole to the regimen may extend anaerobic coverage [34].

Abubaker and Rollert conducted a prospective RCT study in 2001 evaluating the use of antibiotics postoperatively following mandibular fracture treatment. Thirty patients were randomly assigned into two groups, and each group received penicillin G, 2 million U intravenously, every 4 hours through the preoperative period, intraoperative period, and for 12 hours postoperatively. In addition, the study group received penicillin VK, 500 mg every 6 hours for 5 days postoperatively, and the control group received an oral placebo using the same schedule for the same duration. Patients were evaluated for signs of infection after 1, 2, 4, and 6 weeks. The study reports that in uncomplicated mandibular fractures, the use of postoperative antibiotic prophylaxis does not seem to reduce the infection rate. However, one important limitation of this study was its relatively small sample size [35].

In 2006, Miles et al. sought to determine the benefit of postoperative antibiotic treatment of mandible fractures. They studied 291 patients who underwent open reduction and internal fixation (ORIF) of mandibular fractures in a prospective randomized trial. The study group received 2.4 mIU of intramuscular penicillin G benzathine or, if allergic, a 5- to 7-day regimen of oral clindamycin. No antibiotics were given postoperatively to the control group. The follow-up period was 5–8 weeks. The authors did not find statistically significant effectiveness in the use of postoperative antibiotics when addressing open mandibular fractures with ORIF techniques. They conclude that there is no benefit to the use of postoperative antibiotics in patients with open mandible fractures [36].

More recently in a systematic review by Mundinger, the authors divided facial fractures into facial thirds. Studies supported the use of perioperative antibiotics in all facial thirds, but only preoperative antibiotics were used in comminuted mandible fractures. Postoperative antibiotics were not supported in any facial third [37].

Finally, Andreasen et al. published a systematic review in 2006 regarding the role of prophylactic administration of antibiotics in the treatment of maxillofacial fractures. They concluded that 1-day administration of antibiotics is as effective as a 7-day course. Additionally, the authors believe that because of the very low infection incidence in maxillary, zygoma, and condylar fractures, antibiotic treatment does not seem necessary [38]. In a systematic review and meta-analysis performed in 2019, they examined the role of antibiotic prophylaxis in facial fractures. In total, 13 studies met all inclusion and exclusion criteria. They found that postoperative antibiotic prophylaxis, when added to a standard preoperative and/or perioperative antibiotic regimen, showed no significant difference in the risk of surgical site infection [39]. In 2020, Delapin et al. performed a similar systematic review that, again, did not show any difference in the rates of surgical site infection with the addition of postoperative antibiotic prophylaxis for facial fractures after ORIF [40].

RECOMMENDATION

There is little to no role for antibiotic use in a prophylactic manner for facial injuries. There may be value for a 1-day perioperative antibiotic course in patients with fractures of the maxilla or mandible.

Grade of recommendation: C.

13.5 Which Treatment Is Better for Mandible Fractures: Closed or Open Reductions?

Despite many years of experience with the management of mandible fractures with both a closed approach (maxillomandibular fixation [MMF]) and the use of ORIF, there remains significant controversy about management by proponents of each depending on the situation as well as the type of fixation. The intervention is aimed at realignment of the fractured segments and prevention of movement by immobilization of the fractured bone, thereby allowing the osseous union to occur. In closed reduction, the bone ends or fragments are realigned either manually or using traction devices, and in open reduction, the fracture site is exposed and then internal fixation is carried out. The benefit of ORIF is clear, as it has been shown that early mobilization and return to functionality are of vital importance to the patient. MMF still has a very important role in those patients who cannot tolerate a longer operation or potentially in complex fractures that require a combination of techniques or potentially in injuries affecting the condyle.

In 2010, Singh et al. conducted a prospective RCT study to compare these two options for the treatment of displaced subcondylar fractures of the mandible angulated between 10 and 35 degrees or when the ascending ramus was shortened by more than 2 mm. Clinical and radiographic data were collected 6 months following the intervention, and the authors concluded that while both treatment options for condylar fractures of the mandible yielded acceptable results, the open treatment was superior in all objective and subjective functional parameters except occlusion [41].

Eckelt et al. coordinated a prospective randomized multicenter study in 2006, which included 66 patients with mandibular condylar process displaced fractures divided into two groups according to their modality of treatment: Open or closed reductions. Patients had a follow-up at 6 weeks and 6 months. There was no statistically significant difference in either clinical complications or accuracy of fracture reduction based on radiographs. However, patients who underwent open reduction presented statistically significant improvement in mandible mobility and subjective functional index, as well as a statistically significant reduction in disturbance of function, disturbance of occlusion, subjective pain, and discomfort [42].

Collins et al. published in 2004 a prospective RCT that studied 90 patients with mandible fractures, comparing the outcomes of using 2-mm locking plates versus 2-mm nonlocking plates. The theoretical advantages of locking plates include less screw loosening, greater stability across the fracture site, less precision required, and less alteration in an osseous and occlusal relationship. The difference in overall complication rates according to the type of plate used was not statistically significant, and operative time was the same [43].

Kaplan et al. conducted a prospective randomized single-blinded study to compare outcomes of patients who underwent ORIF of displaced mandible fractures followed by either immediate mobilization or 2 weeks of MMF. Twenty-nine patients were followed and examined at 6 weeks, 3 months, and 6 months after surgery. The rates of infection, wound breakdown, and inferior alveolar nerve paresthesia, as well as the dentition quality and the quality of occlusion, did not show any statistically significant difference between either patients after immediate mobilization or patients who underwent MMF [44].

All the aforementioned studies were included in a Cochrane review published in 2013, which included 14 studies totaling 830 mandibular fractures not affecting the condyle comparing open and closed management. The review included studies with different interventions, including different plate materials, use of one or two lag screws, microplate versus miniplate, early and delayed mobilization, eyelet wires versus intraoperative intermaxillary fixation, and intramural versus transbuccal approach, which was composed of small trials with even smaller sample sizes for each comparison and outcome. As a result, the authors concluded that there was inadequate evidence to support open or closed reduction for the treatment of mandibular fractures without condylar involvement [45] (Table 13.1).

Management of mandibular condylar fractures remains an area of considerable debate. Al-Moraissi et al. conducted a systematic review and meta-analysis to examine whether ORIF or closed treatment is superior. Twenty-three studies were

TABLE 13.1

Summary of Questions and Recommendations

Question	Answer	Level of Evidence	Grade of Recommendation	References
What is the proper method and timing of closing and caring for facial lacerations and injuries after closure?	Repair should be performed within 6–12 hours with either absorbable or nonabsorbable sutures.	IIB	B	[1–14]
For nongaping, simple facial lacerations, is suture repair superior to the use of tissue adhesives?	There is no significant difference between the use of tissue adhesives vs. suture repair in simple, nongaping facial lacerations.	IIB	B	[15–17]
Does postoperative use of botulinum toxin improve scarring after primary repair for facial lacerations?	Postoperative care with botulinum toxin may improve the outcome.	IIB	B	[18–19]
Does postoperative use of fractional Er:YAG laser improve scarring for facial lacerations?	Postoperative care with fractional Er:YAG laser may improve the outcome.	IIB	C	[20–21]
What is the proper timing of repair of facial fractures, especially in the setting of neurologic trauma/other injuries?	Early repair in the neurologically stable patient appears to outweigh any possible issues related to delay.	IIIB	C	[22–30]
Are antibiotics indicated in the management of facial lacerations or facial fractures and, if so, when?	Prophylactic antibiotics in nonbite wounds are not necessary. In fractures, perioperative antibiotic use reduces the incidence of infection. The postoperative antibiotic does not seem to reduce the infection rate.	IIB	C	[31–40]
Which treatment is better for mandible fractures: Closed or open reduction?	Performance of open reduction and internal fixation with appropriate-size fixation is critical in the development of the best possible result and patient outcome.	IIB	B	[41–47]

examined, including 5 RCTs, 16 controlled trials, and 2 retrospective studies. Overwhelmingly, the studies show a statistically significant improvement of ORIF over closed treatment for maximal interincisal opening, laterotrusive movement, protrusive movement, malocclusion, pain, and chin deviation on mouth opening. Thus, the result of the meta-analysis confirmed that ORIF provided both superior clinical and functional outcomes compared to the closed treatment group for the management of mandibular condylar fractures [46].

Patel et al. performed a small, prospective RCT to evaluate bite force in patients treated for unilateral mandibular condyle fractures via open vs. closed approaches. Twenty patients were randomized to either intermaxillary fixation ($N = 10$) or ORIF ($N = 10$) and then evaluated 1 week, 1 month, and 3 months after surgery. Not only were patients treated in the ORIF group able to achieve higher maximum bite forces, but they required less time to reach their maximum bite force than those in the IMF group [47].

Technological advances in the composition of rigid fixation with titanium alloys, the development of self-drilling and self-tapping screws, and locking plates have greatly expanded the armamentarium of the surgeon caring for the patient with facial fractures. The use of MMF is well tolerated, especially in medically compromised patients. However, when possible, the performance of ORIF with appropriate-size fixation yields the best possible result and patient outcome. Early motion and rehabilitation will allow for greater functional improvement and allow for maximal patient benefit, especially regarding feeding and nutrition. Six weeks of rigid fixation and a liquid diet have a significant impact on the patient's overall weight and return to function. Therefore, optimal timing of surgery and use of optimal rigid fixation when possible are indicated.

RECOMMENDATIONS

The authors support the use of ORIF for the treatment of condylar fractures to achieve greater functional improvement.

Grade of recommendation: B.

Editor's Note

For the general and trauma surgeon, this chapter is fascinating. It provides evidence that facial lacerations can be repaired up to 12 hours following injury; that absorbable sutures are equivalent to nonabsorbable sutures for repair, with sutures removed at 5–7 days; that Steri-Strips and skin adhesives have the equivalent healing results as suturing in areas without tension; that Botox post-repair can improve cosmesis; and that laser therapy can improve scar deformity. The use of prophylactic antibiotics is not indicated for facial lacerations or beyond the immediate perioperative period in the management of complex facial fractures. Early repair of facial fractures appears beneficial in neurologically stable trauma patients.

REFERENCES

1. Edlich RF, Rogers W, Kaufman D, Kasper G, Tung MS, Wangeensteen OH. Studies in the management of the open contaminated wound: I optimal timing for closure of the contaminated open wound; II comparison of resistance to infection of the open and closed wound during healing. *Am J Surg.* 1969;*117*:323–329.

2. Quinn JV, Polevoi SK, Kohn MA. Traumatic lacerations: What are the risks for infection and has the 'golden period' of laceration care disappeared? *Emerg Med J.* 2014;*31*(2): 96–100.

3. Rui-Feng C, Li-Song H, Ji-Bo Z, et al. Emergency treatment on facial laceration of dog bite wounds with immediate primary closure: A prospective randomized trial study. *BMC Emerg Med.* 2013;*13*:1–5.

4. Paschos NK, Markis EA, Gantsos A, Georgoulis AD. Primary closure versus non-closure of dog bite wounds. A Randomized controlled trial. *Injury.* 2014;*45*(1):237–240.

5. Gandham SG, Menon D. Prospective randomized trial comparing traditional suture technique with the dynamic sliding loop suture technique in the closure of skin lacerations. *Emerg Med J.* 2003;*20*:33–36.

6. Singer AJ, Gulla J, Hein M, Marchini S, Chale S, Arora BP. Single-layer versus double-layer closure of facial lacerations: A randomized controlled trial. *Plast Reconstr Surg.* 2005; *116*:363–368.

7. Fosko SW, Heap D. Surgical pearl: An economical means of skin closure with absorbable suture. *J Am Acad Dermatol.* 1998;*39*:248–250.

8. Gabel EA, Jimenez GP, Eaglstein WH, et al. Performance comparison of nylon and an absorbable suture material (Polyglactin 910) in the closure of punch biopsy sites. *Dermatol Surg.* 2000;*26*:750–752.

9. Guyuron B, Vaughan C. A comparison of absorbable and nonabsorbable suture materials for skin repair. *Plast Reconstr Surg.* 1992;*89*(2):234–236.

10. Scaccia FJ, Hoffman JA, Stepnick DW. Upper eyelid blepharoplasty. A technical comparative analysis. *Arch Otolaryngol Head Neck Surg.* 1994;*120*:827–830.

11. Missori P, Polli FM, Fontana E, et al. Closure of skin or scalp with absorbable sutures. *Plast Reconstr Surg.* 2003;*112*:924–925.

12. Luck RP, Flood R, Eyal D, Saludades J, Hayes C, Gaughan J. Cosmetic outcomes of absorbable versus nonabsorbable sutures in pediatric facial lacerations. *Pediatr Emerg Care.* 2008;*24*(3):137–142.

13. Luck R, Tredway T, Gerard J, et al. Comparison of cosmetic outcomes of absorbable versus nonabsorbable sutures in pediatric facial lacerations. *Pediatr Emerg Care.* 2013; *29*(6):691–695.

14. Xu B, Xu B, Wang L, et al. Absorbable versus nonabsorbable sutures for skin closure: A meta-analysis of randomized controlled trials. *Ann Plast Surg.* 2016;*76*(5):598–606.

15. Farion KJ, Russell KF, Osmond MH, et al. Tissue adhesives for traumatic lacerations in children and adults. *Cochrane Database Syst Rev.* 2002;(3):CD003326. Art. Updated Issue 1, 2009.

16. Zempsky WT, Parrotti D, Grem C, Nichols J. Randomized controlled comparison of cosmetic outcomes of simple facial lacerations closed with Steri Strip Skin Closures or Dermabond tissue adhesive. *Pediatr Emerg Care.* 2004; *20*(8):519–524.

17. Fontana S, Schiestl CM, Landolt MA, et al. A prospective controlled study on long-term outcomes of facial lacerations in children. *Front Pediatr.* 2021;8:616151.

18. Ziade M, Domergue S, Batifol D, et al. Use of botulinum toxin type A to improve treatment of facial wounds: A prospective randomized study. *J Plast Reconstr Aesthet Surg.* 2013;*66*(2):209–214.

19. Kim SH, Lee SJ, Lee JW, Jeong HS, Suh IS. Clinical trial to evaluate the efficacy of botulinum toxin type A injection for reducing scars in patients with a forehead laceration. *Medicine (Baltimore).* 2019;*98*(34):e16952.

20. Kim SG, Kim EY, Kim YJ, et al. The efficacy and safety of ablative fractional resurfacing using a 2,940-Nm Er: YAG laser for traumatic scars in the early posttraumatic period. *Arch Plast Surg.* 2012;*39*(3):232–237.

21. Tidwell WJ, Owen CE, Kulp-Shorten C, Maity A, McCall M, Brown TS. Fractionated Er: YAG laser versus fully ablative Er: YAG laser for scar revision: Results of a split scar, double-blinded, prospective trial. *Lasers Surg Med.* 2016;*48*(9):837–843.

22. Kraus, JF, Rice TM, Peek-Asa C, et al. Facial trauma and the risk of intracranial injury in motorcycle riders. *Ann Emerg Med.* 2003;*41*(1):18–26.

23. Derdyn C, Persing JA, Broaddus WC, Delashaw JB, Jane J, Levine PA, Torner J. Craniofacial trauma: An assessment of risk related to the timing of surgery. *Plast Reconstr Surg.* 1990;*86*(2):238–245.

24. Shibuya TY, Karam AM, Doerr T, et al. Facial fracture repair in the traumatic brain injury patient. *J Oral Maxillofac Surg.* 2007;*65*(9):1693–1699.

25. Wang MC, Temkin NR, Deyo RA, Jurkovich GJ, Barber J, Dikmen S. Timing of surgery after multisystem injury with traumatic brain injury: Effect on neuropsychological and functional outcome. *J Trauma.* 2007;*62*(5):1250–1258.

26. Janus SC, MacLeod SP, Odland R. Analysis of results in early versus late midface fracture repair. *Otolaryngol Head Neck Surg.* 2008;*138*(4):464–467.

27. Yu DY, Chen CH, Tsay PK, Leow AM, Pan CH, Chen CT. Surgical timing and fracture type on the outcome of diplopia after orbital fracture repair. *Ann Plast Surg.* 2016;*76*(Suppl 1):S91–S95.

28. Czerwinski M, Parker WL, Correa JA, Williams HB. Effect of treatment delay on mandibular fracture infection rate. *Plast Reconstr Surg.* 2008;*122*(3):881–885.

29. Damgaard OE, Larsen CG, Felding UA, Toft PB, Von Buchwald C. Surgical timing of the orbital "blowout" fracture: A systematic review and meta-analysis. *Otolaryngol Head Neck Surg.* 2016;*155*(3):387–390.

30. Hurrell MJL, Batstone MD. The effect of treatment timing on the management of facial fractures: A systematic review. *Int J Oral Maxillofac Surg.* 2014;*43*(8):944–950.

31. Cummings P, Del Beccaro MA. Antibiotics to prevent infection of simple wounds: A meta-analysis of randomized studies. *Am J Emerg Med.* 1995;*13*(4):396–400.

32. Jaindl M, Oberleitner G, Endler G, Thallinger C, Kovar FM. Management of bite wounds in children and adults-an analysis of over 5000 cases at a level I trauma center. *Wien Klin Wochenschr.* 2016;*128*(9–10):367–375.

33. Chole RA, Yee J. Antibiotic prophylaxis for facial fractures. A prospective, randomized clinical trial. *Arch Otolaryngol Head Neck Surg.* 1987;*113*(10):1055–1057.

34. Heit JM, Stevens MR, Jeffords K. Comparison of ceftriaxone with penicillin for antibiotic prophylaxis for compound mandible fractures. *Oral Surg Oral Med Oral Pathol Oral Radiol Endod.* 1997;*83(4)*:423–426.

35. Abubaker AO, Rollert MK. Postoperative antibiotic prophylaxis in mandibular fractures: A preliminary randomized, double-blind, and placebo-controlled clinical study. *J Oral Maxillofac Surg.* 2001;*59(12)*:1415–1419.

36. Miles BA, Potter JK, Ellis E III. The efficacy of postoperative antibiotic regimens in the open treatment of mandibular fractures: A prospective randomized trial. *J Oral Maxillofac Surg.* 2006;*64(4)*:576–582.

37. Mundinger GS, Borsuk DE, Okhah Z, Christy MR, Bojovic B, Dorafshar AH, Rodriguez ED. Antibiotics and facial fractures: Evidence-based recommendations compared with experience-based practice. *Craniomaxillofac Trauma Reconstr.* 2015 Mar;*8(1)*:64–78.

38. Andreasen JO, Jensen SS, Schwartz O, Hillerup Y. A systematic review of prophylactic antibiotics in the surgical treatment of maxillofacial fractures. *J Oral Maxillofac Surg.* 2006;*64(11)*:1664–1668.

39. Habib AM, Wong AD, Schreiner GC, et al. Postoperative prophylactic antibiotics for facial fractures: A systematic review and meta-analysis. *Laryngoscope.* 2019;*129*(1):82–95.

40. Delaplain PT, Phillips JL, Lundeberg M, et al. No reduction in surgical site infection obtained with post-operative antibiotics in facial fractures, regardless of duration or anatomic location: A systematic review and meta-analysis. *Surg Infect (Larchmt).* 2020;*21*(2):112–121.

41. Singh, V, Bhagol, A Goel M, et al. Outcomes of open versus closed treatment of mandibular subcondylar fractures: A prospective randomized study. *J Oral Maxillofac Surg.* 2010;*68(6)*:1304–1309.

42. Eckelt U, Schneider M, Erasmus F, Gerlach KL, Kuhlisch E, Loukota R, Rasse M, Schubert J, Terheyden H. Open versus closed treatment of fractures of the mandibular condylar process-a prospective randomized multi-centre studying. *J Craniomaxillofac Surg.* 2006;*34(5)*:306–314.

43. Collins CP, Pirinjian-Leonard G, Tolas A, Alcalde R. A prospective randomized clinical trial comparing 2.0-mm locking plates to 2.0-mm standard plates in treatment of mandible fractures. *J Oral Maxillofac Surg.* 2004;*62(11)*: 1392–1395.

44. Kaplan BA, Hoard MA, Park SS. Immediate mobilization following fixation of mandible fractures: A prospective, randomized study. *Laryngoscope.* 2001;*111(9)*:1520–1524.

45. Nasser M, Pandis N, Fleming PS, et al. Interventions for the management of mandibular fractures. *Cochrane Database Syst Rev.* 2013;7:CD006087.

46. Al-Moraissi EA, Ellis E. Surgical treatment of adult mandibular condylar fractures provides better outcomes than closed treatment: A systematic review and meta-analysis. *J Oral Maxillofac Surg.* 2015;*73*(3):482–493.

47. Patel K NA, Girish G, Akarsh R, Nikhila G, Bhat P, Shabadi N. Comparative evaluation of bite force in patients treated for unilateral mandibular condylar fractures by open and closed methods. *Dent Traumatol.* 2022;*38*(3): 223–228.

14

Ocular Trauma

Erin Jennings and Yasha Modi

14.1 Introduction

Ocular trauma represents the leading cause of monocular blindness globally and accounts for an estimated one-third of all eye-related emergency department (ED) visits in the United States each year [1]. While ocular trauma represents a small percentage of general trauma cases, these injuries can be devastating and are often associated with permanent poor visual outcomes if not managed rapidly and appropriately in the acute care setting. Due to the niche nature of the ocular injury and the complexity of ocular imaging modalities, many acute care physicians rely on ophthalmologic consultation for trauma management in the ED. However, rapid recognition of serious eye injury and early intervention are critical to ensure the best possible visual outcome, deeming it critical for nonophthalmic physicians to be capable of recognizing and treating these conditions. Many studies have examined the incidence, injury characteristics, patient demographics, and visual outcomes of eye trauma. These studies have yielded important insights into the ocular trauma patient population and the high likelihood of visual impairment associated with these injuries. However, due to the relative rarity of these injuries within the trauma spectrum and the lack of follow-up for ocular trauma patients, there is a paucity of data that exists within the literature highlighting Level 1 evidence-based management and standard-of-care treatment, specifically in the acute care setting, for these types of injuries.

Therefore, the goal of this review is to serve as a guide for acute care physicians, written by ophthalmic surgeons, for the rapid diagnosis and initial management of the most common ocular traumatic conditions seen in the acute care setting. The recommendations arising from this review are based on the strongest available level of evidence and are intended to familiarize nonophthalmic physicians with recent advances in diagnosis and primary interventions for these ocular conditions.

14.2 Major Ocular Traumas

14.2.1 Ruptured/Open Globe Injury

Open globe injuries (Figure 14.1) are defined by full-thickness lacerations of the cornea or sclera (Figure 14.2) and represent a major cause of permanent vision loss worldwide. These injuries have the potential to result in substantial visual loss. While definitive treatment is surgical closure of the wound by a trained ophthalmic surgeon, rapid diagnosis and preliminary management in the acute care setting can prevent lifelong, vision-threatening sequelae. Open globe injuries represent perhaps the most feared ocular trauma, with an incidence of 4.49 per 100.000 population in the United States. Per analysis of the U.S. Nationwide Emergency Department Sample (NEDS), open globe injuries are most commonly caused secondary to penetrating or blunt trauma and are more rarely seen with falls, motor vehicle crashes, and injury by firearm or machinery [1].

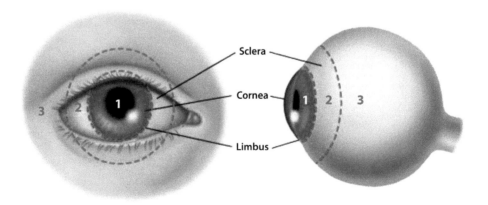

FIGURE 14.1 Zones of injury. (From image as seen on UpToDate [Andreoli CM, Gardiner MF. Open globe injuries: Emergent evaluation and initial management. In UpToDate, Post TW, Ed., UpToDate, Waltham, MA].)

DOI: 10.1201/9781003316800-14

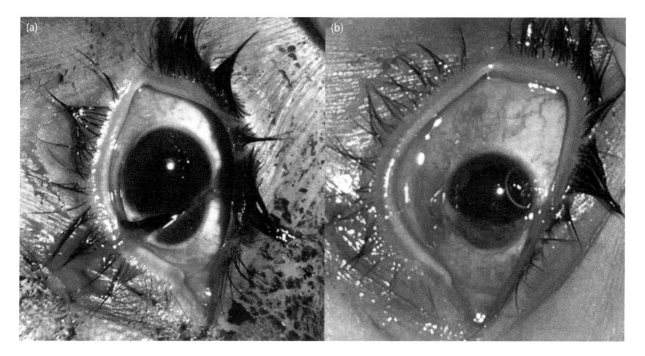

FIGURE 14.2   Ruptured globe: (a) Zone 2 trauma demonstrating full-thickness injury to the cornea, limbus, and anterior sclera. (b) Day 1 after globe repair with 10-0 nylon sutures closing the cornea and limbus and a small air bubble in the anterior chamber demonstrating a formed globe. (Images courtesy of Dr. Vikram Paranjpe.)

14.2.1.1 Assessment of Injury and Diagnostic Workup

Open globe injury is an ocular emergency and therefore requires an accurate physical examination and history assessment to appropriately and rapidly diagnose this condition. Slit lamp examination is not necessarily needed for this condition, with many of the common ocular signs visible through pen light examination or indirect ophthalmoscope, including deep or shallow anterior chamber compared to the contralateral eye; peaked or irregular pupil; positive Seidel test (Seidel test is utilized to reveal leaks from the cornea, sclera, or conjunctiva following injury or surgery—it is conducted by applying a moistened fluorescein strip to the area of suspected leak or rupture then visualizing the injured site under cobalt blue light to evaluate for green flow; if the flow is evident, this indicates a positive test); limitation of extraocular motility; intraocular contents outside the globe; and history of trauma, fall, or sharp object entering the globe.

CT scan can be used for detecting and localizing the intraocular foreign body (IOFB). This is particularly true for metallic foreign bodies. MRI, as a rule, should be avoided for initial imaging when evaluating open globe injuries, as any ferromagnetic metallic foreign body may yield a devastating outcome due to the movement of the IOFB at the time of MRI acquisition.

While many studies have been conducted in regard to predicting the visual outcome of patients after open globe ocular trauma, the most commonly accepted system within the literature (and clinically) is the Ocular Trauma Score (OTS, see later) [2]. Calculating the OTS (and recognizing the components of the scoring rubric) as an acute care physician is helpful when considering management and visual prognosis of the patient (Tables 14.1 and 14.2).

TABLE 14.1

Method for Deriving OTS Score

Initial Visual Factor	Raw Points	
A. Initial raw score (based on initial visual acuity)		
	NPL =	60
	PL or HM =	70
	1/200 to 19/200 =	80
	20/200 to 20/50 =	90
	>20/40 =	100
B. Globe rupture		−23
C. Endophthalmitis		−17
D. Perforating injury		−14
E. Retinal detachment		−11
F. Relative afferent pupillary defect (RAPD)		−10
Raw score sum = sum of raw points		

Abbreviation: NPL: No perception of light; PL: Perception of light; HM: Hand movements.

TABLE 14.2

Estimated Probability of Follow-Up Visual Acuity Category at 6 Months

Raw Score Sum	OTS Score	NPL	PL/HM	1/200 to 19/200	20/200 to 20/50	>20/40
0–44	1	73%	17%	7%	2%	1%
45–65	2	28%	26%	18%	13%	15%
66–80	3	2%	11%	15%	28%	44%
81–91	4	1%	2%	2%	21%	74%
92–100	5	0%	1%	2%	5%	92%

Abbreviation: NPL: Nil perception of light, PL: Perception of light, HM: Hand movements.

TABLE 14.3

Zones of Injury

Zones of Injury	
Zone 1	Full-thickness injury to cornea or limbus
Zone 2	Full-thickness injury to anterior 5 mm or sclera
Zone 3	Full-thickness injury more than 5 mm posterior to the limbus

Note: The posterior-most extent of rupture represents the zone. For instance, if the entirety of the cornea is lacerated but the rupture extends to the anterior sclera, this would represent a zone 2 rupture.

14.2.1.2 Primary Intervention and Management

Once open globe injury has been diagnosed and assessed (appropriate zone, Table 14.3 and Figure 14.1) and OTS scored, primary intervention in the acute care setting is critical to maximizing the visual prognosis. Primarily, a rigid shield should be placed around the eye to minimize further ocular manipulation or intraocular exposure. The patient should be admitted to the hospital for surgical exploration and repair by an ophthalmic surgeon. Furthermore, the elevation of the head of the bed to 30 degrees and medical management of pain and nausea should be addressed to avoid any additional increase in intraocular pressure (IOP) from inadvertent Valsalva maneuvers.

The recommended emergency room treatment for open globe injury is tetanus prophylaxis for those determined necessary by current Centers for Disease Control and Prevention (CDC) protocol, in addition to broad-spectrum systemic antibiotic coverage for typical pathogens commonly associated with posttraumatic endophthalmitis, including *Clostridium*, *Bacillus*, and coagulase-negative *Staphylococcus aureus*, which typically includes oral (PO) or IV cephalosporins, fluoroquinolones, and/or IV vancomycin [3].

A retrospective review by Keil et al. between 2000 and 2019 at the University of Michigan found intravitreal antibiotics (most commonly vancomycin + ceftazidime) to be particularly effective in preventing endophthalmitis in those with open globes, organic foreign bodies, delayed presentation (>24 hours), and signs and symptoms of endophthalmitis (hypopyon, increased pain with vitritis) [4]. Current recommendations for open globes with or without IOFBs include prompt injection of intravitreal antibiotics within 24 hours to reduce the risk of

endophthalmitis. These intravitreal antibiotics are frequently administered after globe repair surgery.

> Are prophylactic antibiotics (intravitreal and systemic) warranted in open globe injury?
>
> Prophylactic systemic and intravitreal antibiotics reduce the risk of endophthalmitis in open globes with or without a foreign body.
>
> Grade of recommendation: B.

14.2.2 Intraocular or Intraorbital Foreign Body

The presence of an ocular foreign body (OFB) is considered an ocular emergency, requiring urgent diagnosis and treatment to maximize the chances of visual improvement and prevent globe loss. OFB patients are typically male, with injury most often occurring in the workplace (i.e., hammering). The most common material is metal [3]. OFBs can cause vision damage by direct tissue injury and bleeding at the time of injury or secondarily through the development of intraocular infection or retinal detachment [3]. Foreign body injuries involving the globe are classified as either intraocular or extraocular (more often intraorbital) and penetrating or perforating. The definitions of penetrating/perforating injuries are dependent on anatomical points of reference. A penetrating injury, by definition, penetrates an anatomical reference point (i.e., cornea, globe) without exiting that reference point (Figure 14.3). A perforating injury, by definition, involves two full-thickness lacerations with an entrance and exit within the anatomic reference point. For example, a perforating injury of the cornea is considered a penetrating injury of the globe.

An extensive literature review conducted by Kuhn et al. (the same group that developed the OTS) reported foreign bodies typically enter through the cornea (65%), sclera (25%), or limbus (10%). Symptoms can vary widely, from foreign body sensation, light sensitivity, and pain [3]. Approximately 20% of patients may also be asymptomatic, so a high suspicion must be maintained based on the mechanism of injury [3]. Ability to confirm the presence or absence of a foreign body, and further

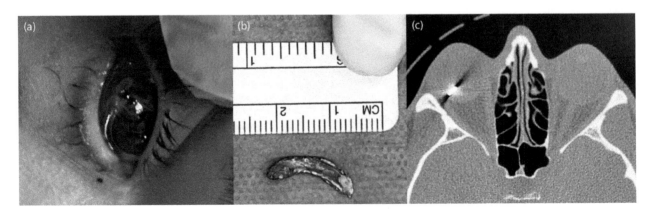

FIGURE 14.3   (a) Penetrating intraocular foreign body as seen on external examination (b) measuring 1.5 cm. (c) Visualization of IOFB on CT orbits without contrast. (Images courtesy of Dr. Vikram Paranjpe.)

determine IOFB location and material if present, is critical to establishing the choice of primary intervention in the acute care setting of a patient with this type of ocular trauma.

14.2.2.1 Assessment of Injury and Diagnostic Workup

Frequently these traumas coexist with an open globe injury, which changes overall management, as described earlier. Not all IOFBs can be visualized on examination, specifically for penetrating injuries of the globe. Therefore, timely imaging is critical. Earlier studies advocated for X-ray as the initial imaging modality of choice (specifically for metallic IOFBs) [5]. However, after conducting a systematic review, Jung et al. recommended CT scan as the primary approach to detection, as CT is easily and rapidly attained in emergency rooms and is a more sensitive modality capable of detecting the widest array of foreign body material [6]. MRI should never be the primary modality, as this is contraindicated in the scenario of metallic IOFB.

14.2.2.2 Primary Intervention and Management

Once a foreign body is detected, urgent and appropriate primary intervention is essential in maintaining the patient's best posttraumatic visual acuity. In the ED, a rigid shield (i.e., Fox Shield or another rigid device) should be placed over the affected eye to prevent further injury with accidental eyelid rubbing or touching [3].

In cases of suspected IOFB, the patient is at increased risk of infection, with studies reporting a presence of endophthalmitis ranging from 5% to 17% of cases [3]. The recommended treatment for all IOFBs follows that of open globe injury noted earlier. In regard to the timing of removal of IOFB, ocular surgery is the definitive treatment of choice, and prompt referral to ophthalmology is indicated. The decision to primarily or secondarily remove the IOFB should be based on the decision of the operating surgeon, comfort with removal, the material of the foreign body, and the risk of collateral damage. Timing of removal can vary depending on these factors, as research has demonstrated delayed removal, with appropriate management, does not adversely affect visual outcome or risk of endophthalmitis [4, 7].

What is the most sensitive imaging modality for primary detection of IOFB?

CT scan is the most sensitive imaging modality for primary detection of IOFB.

Grade of recommendation: B.

Does the timing of IOFB removal change visual outcomes?

Delayed surgical IOFB removal does not adversely affect visual outcome or risk of endophthalmitis. Prompt intravitreal antibiotics and primary globe closure, however, are essential.

Grade of recommendation: B.

14.2.3 Ocular Chemical Injury

Ocular chemical injuries vary in severity and are responsible for 11.5–22.1% of ocular traumatic injuries [8]. Two of the largest epidemiologic studies were conducted in the United States and reported an incidence of 51–56 per million, with injury being more common in men, typically due to alkali (53.6%) substances and secondary to work-related injuries (with assault being the second most common mechanism of injury) [9]. Chemical injury or ocular surface exposure to an unknown chemical is considered an ocular emergency and requires immediate recognition and treatment to minimize permanent damage. Management and overall visual prognosis are dependent on a variety of factors, the most important being establishing alkali vs. acid chemical, initial grading of ocular chemical injury, and assessment of injury timing (phases of healing).

14.2.3.1 Immediate Management: Irrigation

Unlike many other ocular pathologies, chemical burn injuries require immediate intervention before ocular assessment. The single most important factor in acute management and prognosis is a timely intervention with ocular irrigation. Rinsing solutions may include water, normal saline, Ringer's lactate, phosphate buffer, Diphoterine®, and Cederroth®. The most effective irrigation remains undetermined, as there is a dearth of studies comparing various solutions, but the current standard of care is the use of isotonic solutions including lactate Ringer's or balanced salt solution (BSS) to prevent corneal edema—swelling that may arise as a result of irrigation with hypotonic fluids (tap water). Timely delivery remains the most critical factor in overall prognosis, and therefore irrigation should never be delayed for the choice of irrigating solution.

While no evidence suggests the total length of irrigation, the consensus among ophthalmic specialists is the eye should be irrigated for at least 30 minutes, using 1–3 liters of fluid in total. pH should be checked using pH paper every 15 minutes until the pH is neutralized (target range: 6–8). Irrigation systems (i.e., the Morgan Lens), when available, may be employed to facilitate irrigation [10]. However, there should be no delay in irrigation if this apparatus is not available.

14.2.3.2 Assessment of Injury and Diagnostic Workup

After irrigation, assessment of injury using a classification system should be employed to further guide treatment and prognosis in the acute care setting. The most commonly used systems are the Roper-Hall and Dua classifications. Research has shown the Dua classification to provide superior prognostic predictive value in severe ocular burns when compared to Roper-Hall classification, secondary to its ability to subclassify chemical burns based on both conjunctival and limbal injury [11]. Furthermore, it is easier to employ without a detailed slit lamp examination, as it does not require an assessment of the depth of corneal injury. The Dua system includes assessment and severity of conjunctival (bulbar conjunctiva up to and including fornices) and limbal involvement, ranging from grades I to VI (Table 14.4). "Involvement" of these regions is defined by the

TABLE 14.4

Chemical Injury of the Eye

Grade	Prognosis	Clinical Findings	Conjunctival Involvement	Analog Scale*
I	Very good	0 clock hours of limbal involvement	0%	0/0%
II	Good	≤3 clock hours of limbal involvement	<30%	0.1–3/1–29.9%
III	Good	>3–6 clock hours of limbal involvement	>30–50%	3.1–6/31–50%
IV	Good to guarded	>6–9 clock hours of limbal involvement	>50–75%	6.1–9/51–75%
V	Guarded to poor	>9 to <12 clock hours of limbal involvement	>75 to <100%	9.1–11.9/75.1–99.9%
VI	Very poor	Total limbus (12 clock hours) involved	Total conjunctiva (100%) involved	12/100%

* The analog scale records the amount of limbal involvement in clock hours of affected limbus/percentage of conjunctival (bulbar) involvement; the analog scale allows for combining features of the different grades, which is more compatible with real clinical situations.

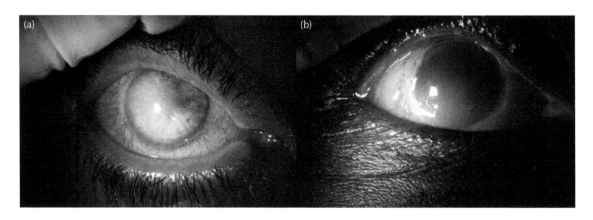

FIGURE 14.4   Chemical burn. (a) Grade I injury with demonstrated corneal epithelial staining and limbal blanching; however, there is no presence of limbal or conjunctival involvement. (b) Grade VI injury with total loss of limbal stem cells and destruction of the proximal conjunctival epithelium. The cornea is completely opaque and porcelainized, and it is extremely prone to melting in the acute or intermediate time frames after injury. (Images courtesy of Dr. Anat Galor.)

presence of fluorescein staining for the Dua system indicating loss of epithelialization from the injury (Figure 14.4). However, in practice, physicians should associate the blanching of the limbal vessels with limbal ischemia [12].

14.2.3.3 Further Management

Patients should be referred immediately to an ophthalmologist with subspecialty training in corneal trauma, when available. Appropriate management for chemical burns requires managing the ocular inflammatory response and promoting epithelialization of the cornea. Management in the acute care setting of burns classified by the Dua system is summarized next, based on an updated review of the literature by Sharma et al (Table 14.5) [10].

> What classification system can be reliably used in the acute care setting to guide initial management and predict visual outcomes?
>
> The Dua classification system provides superior diagnostic and prognostic value in severe ocular burns when compared to the Roper-Hall classification.
>
> Grade of recommendation: A.

TABLE 14.5

Treatment of Chemical Burns to the Eye

Grade I–II	**Standard Medical Therapy:** • Topical lubrication and artificial tears every 1–2 hours • Topical broad-spectrum antibiotics (erythromycin, Polytrim, Viagmox, or Bacitracin) every 4 hours • Topical steroids every 1–2 hours
Grade III–V	**Standard Medical Therapy +:** • Topical Na+ ascorbate (10%) drops every 2 hours • Topical Na+ citrate 10% drops every 2 hours • Oral vitamin C 500 mg QID • Oral doxycycline 100 mg BID • Topical umbilical cord serum (if available) 20% 10 × a day
Grade VI	**Standard Medical Therapy (as Grade III–V) + Early Surgical Intervention** (done by a trained ophthalmologist): • Surgical intervention includes amniotic membrane transplant/Prokera placement or tenonplasty to re-establish limbal vascularity

14.2.4 Orbital Compartment Syndrome and Retrobulbar Hemorrhage

Orbital compartment syndrome (OCS) is a rare, vision-threatening, time-sensitive condition characterized by rapid elevation of intraocular and intraorbital pressure within the closed compartment of the orbit leading to irreversible blindness. Recognition and management by the acute care physician are critical, as treatment is curative without requiring imaging or ophthalmic expertise.

The pathogenesis of OCS is similar to that of limb compartment syndrome: Swelling or bleeding occurs within a confined compartment (in this case the orbit, which has a volume of approximately 30 mL). The IOP rises, which exceeds the perfusion pressure of the blood supply to the optic nerve, thus causing permanent optic nerve and retinal damage.

The most common etiology of OCS is hemorrhage of the intraorbital tissue (retrobulbar hemorrhage) often seen secondary to severe facial trauma, specifically with orbital-facial fractures [13]. The most common iatrogenic cause of OCS is ocular surgical trauma (reported in orbital, eyelid, and lacrimal surgery) or following periocular or retinal injections. Less common causes of OCS include nonophthalmologic surgeries (oral-maxillofacial, sinus), facial/periocular chemical burns, and actions that lead to increased accumulation of fluid into the orbit, including prolonged proning often seen following neurosurgical/spinal surgeries.

14.2.4.1 Assessment of Injury and Diagnostic Workup

OCS is a clinical diagnosis and therefore requires an accurate physical examination and history assessment to appropriately and rapidly diagnose this condition. A comprehensive review of the literature conducted by McCallum et al. reports the most common clinical signs of OCS are the following [13]: Proptosis, ophthalmoplegia, decreased visual acuity (commonly with no light perception [NLP]), relative afferent pupillary defect (RAPD), tense globe resistant to retropulsion, tight eyelids in the partially retracted position, elevated IOP (normal IOP: 8–20 mmHg), and diplopia.

While one or more of these clinical signs are typically present on examination, there have been case reports documenting elevated IOP as the only presentation of OCS, especially if the patient is unconscious in the setting of facial/orbital trauma [13]. Therefore, an accurate historical assessment for the presence of any of the common etiologies listed is critical, and high suspicion of OCS must be maintained when examining patients with clinical histories associated with this condition.

While ancillary testing with a CT scan can help establish the diagnosis of OCS (with typical findings of retrobulbar/intraorbital hemorrhage), it is generally agreed upon within the literature that emergent management should not be delayed for radiographic imaging.

14.2.4.2 Primary Intervention and Management

If OCS is suspected based on physical examination and historical assessment, urgent orbital decompression via lateral canthotomy and inferior cantholysis (LCC) is the mainstay of treatment. This procedure entails cutting the lateral canthal tendon and its inferior crus to allow for additional anterior eye protrusion, thus lowering IOP by effectively increasing the orbital volume. This procedure is now commonly taught as part of the residency curriculum of acute care physicians and surgeons.

While there is no consensus in the literature for precise indications for LCC, general guidelines call for emergent surgical intervention if IOP is >35–40, especially if accompanied by additional common signs and symptoms of OCS, including proptosis, ophthalmoplegia, and RAPD [13–15]. In regard to timing for the intervention, decompression should occur within 2 hours of injury. The timing of intervention is based on research conducted by Hayreh et al., which reported irreversible retinal ischemia after clamping the optic nerve in rhesus monkeys after 105 minutes [16].

Medical therapy has been used as adjunctive therapy with surgical decompression to lower intraorbital pressure, including the use of corticosteroids, osmotic agents, and aqueous suppressants. However, their effectiveness has not been established within the literature [11].

Ultimately, the performance of an LCC is a temporary measure until the retrobulbar hemorrhage or alternative etiology can be evacuated, and thus ophthalmology must be consulted when this condition is first considered on the differential.

Lateral Canthotomy and Inferior Cantholysis Procedure Instructions:

1. Position patient supine with head of the bed elevated to 10–20 degrees with eyelids and head stabilized.
2. Clean and irrigate lateral canthus area with antiseptic (chlorhexidine or betadine) and drape area.
3. Inject 1–2 mL of local anesthetic with epinephrine into the planned incision site (lateral canthus to the rim of the orbit); aim the tip of the needle away from the globe.
4. Use a needle driver or hemostat to approximate the path of the incision site and lock in place for about 20 seconds to 1 minute to provide hemostasis; then remove.
5. To perform a canthotomy, cut from lateral canthus to rim of orbit using fine scissors (ideally Wescott or iris scissors); can also use suture removal scissors if only scissors readily available. Cut along the path of crushed tissue made in the previous step; the incision should be 1–2 cm in length.
6. Lift the lateral portion of the inferior eyelid with forceps to expose the lateral canthal tendon.
7. To perform cantholysis, identify and cut the inferior crus of the lateral canthal ligament (identify by using scissors to "strum" the area to feel for tension/inferior crus). Point scissors away from the globe.

8. Recheck IOP. If IOP remains high and further exposure is necessary, can perform superior cantholysis using the same technique.

9. Apply antibiotic ointment to the area of the incision.

YouTube video of procedure: https://www.youtube.com/watch?v=kcB50sVOBKs

---

Does timing of ocular decompression affect visual outcomes in cases of ocular compartment syndrome?

Patients who decompressed beyond 2 hours have reported poorer visual outcomes.

Grade of recommendation: B.

While there is no consensus in the literature for precise indications for LCC, general guidelines call for emergent surgical intervention if IOP is >35–40 mm Hg, especially if accompanied by additional common signs and symptoms of OCS, including proptosis, ophthalmoplegia, or RAPD.

Grade of recommendation: B.

14.2.5 Traumatic Hyphema

Hyphema is defined by the accumulation of blood in the anterior chamber of the eye. The most common etiology of this condition is blunt or penetrating trauma of the ocular and periocular region, causing shearing of the small vessels supplying the iris, ciliary body, and trabecular meshwork. According to an analysis of all hyphema-related ED cases in the NEDS, the incidence of traumatic hyphema is 0.52/100,000 and predominately occurs in males after an assault and athletic accidents [17]. While relatively rare, vision-threatening sequelae of traumatic hyphema may include corneal blood staining, secondary hemorrhage, increased IOP with resultant optic atrophy, and peripheral anterior synechiae. Although corneal blood staining may be transient, children can develop amblyopia and permanent loss of vision if the blood is slow to clear. Thus, it is critically important for the acute care physician to astutely recognize and properly manage this condition.

14.2.5.1 Assessment of Injury and Diagnostic Workup

Patients with hyphema typically present with signs and symptoms commonly associated with trauma to the ocular region, including blurry vision, photophobia, and pain. Hyphema is frequently assessed via slit lamp examination. However, hyphemas greater than grade 1 can often be recognized and assessed via pen lamp examination alone (Figure 14.5). Grading of hyphema severity is classified by the depth of settled red blood

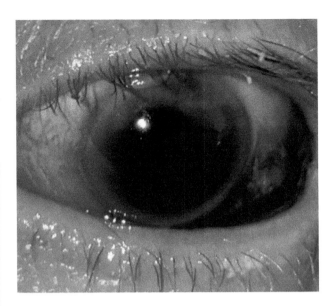

FIGURE 14.5   Grade 3 traumatic hyphema demonstrating three-fourths filling of the anterior chamber. (Image courtesy of Dr. Sheel Patel.)

TABLE 14.6

Hyphema Grading

Grade	Criteria
0	Microhyphema, circulating RBC only
1	Less than one-quarter of the anterior chamber
2	More than one-quarter to one-half of the anterior chamber
3	More than one-half to three-fourths of the anterior chamber
4	Total filling or "eight ball" hyphema

cells within the anterior chamber (Table 14.6). Accurate grading is valuable for both management and prognosis, as the risk of elevated IOP and secondary complications are greater with larger hyphemas.

14.2.5.2 Management

Primary management of a traumatic hyphema should include elevation of the head of the bed to at least 30–45 degrees, protection of the eye with a shield, and no exertional activity. The most feared complication of hyphema is secondary hemorrhage, as this is associated with elevated IOP, optic atrophy, and corneal blood staining. Visual outcomes after hyphema are worse in cases of secondary hemorrhage; preventing rebleeding remains a key goal. Those at higher risk for rebleeding include patients with bleeding diatheses or on blood thinners, patients with sickle cell disease or trait, and more darkly pigmented patients irrespective of sickle cell status [18, 19].

The literature supports the use of steroids to reduce rebleeds (both topical and systemic). It's unclear if antifibrinolytics (aminocaproic acid, tranexamic acid), applied topically as an ophthalmic gel or taken orally, reduce rebleeds. The most recent Cochrane review reports a lack of statistical significance in the use of antifibrinolytics due to the small occurrence of rebleeds [18]. A larger study is needed to prove their usefulness statistically. If used, there should be caution in patients with a history of gastrointestinal conditions or low blood pressure, as the use of these antifibrinolytics (specifically aminocaproic acid) has been linked to complications including GI upset and systemic hypotension. Antifibrinolytics should be avoided in pregnant patients [18, 19].

> What medications (systemic or topical) prevent rebleeds of traumatic hyphemas?
>
> The literature supports the use of steroids and antifibrinolytics to reduce rebleeds. There is insufficient evidence to support or refute the use of antifibrinolytics in traumatic hyphema.
>
> Grade of recommendation: B.

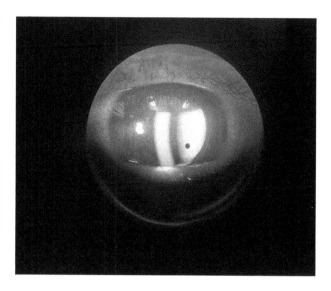

FIGURE 14.6 Metallic corneal foreign body visualized under a slit lamp. (Image courtesy of Dr. Stephanie Choi.)

14.3 Minor Ocular Traumas

14.3.1 Corneal Abrasions and Foreign Bodies

Corneal abrasions and foreign bodies are ophthalmic injuries that are commonly seen and treated in the acute care setting. While these are considered relatively benign injuries in comparison to the more invasive traumas discussed earlier, without proper acute care management, these injuries can quickly evolve into sight-threatening complications, including corneal ulceration, bacterial keratitis, corneal erosions, and traumatic iritis, all of which can dramatically impact visual potential.

14.3.1.1 Assessment of Injury and Diagnostic Workup

The most common associated symptoms of corneal abrasion and foreign body include pain, photophobia, foreign body sensation, discomfort of the eye, blurry vision, and a history of scratching the eye. The demographic for a corneal foreign body, in particular, is the same as that seen with IOFB injury (males who work with metal or in construction). These injuries often are subtle in appearance, and therefore if there is any suspicion, examination under a slit lamp is essential (Figure 14.6). Furthermore, the use of fluorescein dye will help distinguish frank corneal epithelial defects, as these drops only penetrate the corneal stroma and basement membrane. One must additionally examine closely for the presence of perforation or IOFB.

14.3.1.2 Management

For cases of superficial corneal foreign body, an attempt can be made to remove the object with a cotton swab or 27–30 G hypodermic needle under direct visualization via slit lamp. Irrigation with saline and the use of a topical anesthetic should be implemented before removal. A residual rust ring may be present after removal. The ring can often be removed with an ophthalmic burr or Alger brush. However, if the ring is deemed to be too deep for removal (dependent on the comfort and skill level of the provider), a close ophthalmic follow-up can be scheduled within the week to leave time for the rust to migrate to the corneal surface (with a second attempt at rust removal) [20].

The use of short-term topical antibiotics for both corneal abrasion and following corneal foreign body removal is widely accepted as standard practice. The antibiotics (e.g., fluoroquinolone QID) should continue until re-epithelialization occurs (within a few days) [20].

While widely accepted as standard prophylaxis given the low-risk nature of the intervention, a Cochrane review conducted by Algarni et al. failed to demonstrate the efficacy of antibiotic prophylaxis to prevent ocular infection or accelerate epithelial healing [21]. However, this practice persists given the low risk of the antibiotic drop weighed against the devastating visual consequences of infectious keratitis involving the visual axis.

> Do topical antibiotics prevent infection or alter epithelial healing in corneal abrasions?
>
> While widely accepted as standard prophylaxis given the low-risk nature of the intervention, the literature has failed to demonstrate the efficacy of antibiotic prophylaxis to prevent ocular infection or accelerate epithelial healing. This practice persists given the low risk of the antibiotic drop weighed against the devastating visual consequences of infectious keratitis involving the visual axis.
>
> Grade of recommendation: B.

TABLE 14.7

Summary of Essential Questions and Answers

Question	Answer	Levels of Evidence	Grade of Recommendation	References
Do intravitreal and systemic antibiotics prevent posttraumatic bacterial endophthalmitis? Does their use affect outcomes in eyes that are already infected?	Prophylactic systemic and intravitreal antibiotics reduce the risk of endophthalmitis in open globes with or without a foreign body.	2A, 2B	B	[3, 4]
What is the most sensitive imaging modality for primary detection of IOFB?	CT scan	2A	B	[6]
Does the timing of IOFB removal change visual outcomes?	Delayed surgical IOFB removal does not adversely affect visual outcome or risk of endophthalmitis. Prompt intravitreal antibiotics and primary globe closure, however, are essential.	2C	B	[7]
Chemical injuries: What classification system can be reliably used in the acute care setting to guide initial management and predict visual outcomes?	The Dua classification provides superior diagnostic and prognostic value in severe ocular burns when compared to the Roper-Hall classification.	1B	A	[11]
Are there specific clinical indications for lateral canthotomy and cantholysis in orbital compartment syndrome (OCS)?	While there is no consensus in the literature for precise indications for LCC, general guidelines call for emergent surgical intervention if IOP is >35–40 mm Hg, especially if accompanied by additional common signs and symptoms of OCS, including proptosis, ophthalmoplegia, or RAPD.	2A	B	[13]
Does timing of ocular decompression affect visual outcomes in cases of ocular compartment syndrome?	The literature indicates patients who decompressed beyond 2 hours have reported poorer visual outcomes.	2A	B	[13]
What medications prevent rebleeds after traumatic hyphema?	The literature supports the use of steroids and antifibrinolytics to reduce rebleeds. There is insufficient evidence to support or refute the use of antifibrinolytics in traumatic hyphema.	2A, 1A	B	[18, 19]
Do topical antibiotics prevent infection or alter epithelial healing in corneal abrasions?	While widely accepted as standard prophylaxis given the low-risk nature of the intervention, the literature has failed to demonstrate the efficacy of antibiotic prophylaxis to prevent ocular infection or accelerate epithelial healing. This practice persists given the low risk of the antibiotic drop weighed against the devastating visual consequences of infectious keratitis involving the visual axis.	2A	B	[21]

REFERENCES

1. Mir TA, Canner JK, Zafar S, Srikumaran D, Friedman DS, Woreta FA. Characteristics of Open Globe Injuries in the United States From 2006 to 2014. JAMA Ophthalmol. 2020 Mar 1;138(3):268–275. DOI: 10.1001/jamaophthalmol.2019.5823. PMID: 31971539; PMCID: PMC6990674.

2. Kuhn F, Maisiak R, Mann L, et al. The Ocular Trauma Score (OTS). Ophthalmol Clin North Am. 2002;15(2):163–165.

3. Loporchio D, Mukkamala L, Gorukanti K, Zarbin M, Langer P, Bhagat N. Intraocular foreign bodies: A review. Surv Ophthalmol. 2016 Sep-Oct;61(5):582–596. DOI: 10.1016/j.survophthal.2016.03.005. Epub 2016 Mar 17. PMID: 26994871.

4. Keil JM, Zhao PY, Durrani AF, Azzouz L, Huvard MJ, Dedania VS, Zacks DN. Endophthalmitis, visual outcomes, and management strategies in eyes with intraocular foreign bodies. Clin Ophthalmol. 2022 May 3;16:1401–1411. DOI: 10.2147/OPTH.S358064. PMID: 35535124; PMCID: PMC9078426.

5. Otto PM, Otto RA, Virapongse C, et al. Screening test for detection of metallic foreign objects in the orbit before magnetic resonance imaging. Invest Radiol. 1992;27(4):308–311. DOI: 10.1097/00004424-199204000-00010

6. Jung HC, et al. Intraocular foreign body: Diagnostic protocols and treatment strategies in ocular trauma patients. J Clin Med. 2021 April 25;10(9):1861. DOI: 10.3390/jcm10091861

7. Colyer MH, Weber ED, Weichel ED, Dick JS, Bower KS, Ward TP, Haller JA. Delayed intraocular foreign body removal without endophthalmitis during Operations Iraqi Freedom and Enduring Freedom. Ophthalmology. 2007 Aug;114(8):1439–1447. DOI: 10.1016/j.ophtha.2006.10.052. Epub 2007 Feb 28. PMID: 17331579.

8. Baradaran-Rafii A, Eslani M, Haq Z, Shirzadeh E, Huvard MJ, Djalilian AR. Current and upcoming therapies for ocular surface chemical injuries. Ocul Surf. 2017 Jan;15(1): 48–64. DOI: 10.1016/j.jtos.2016.09.002. Epub 2016 Sep 17. PMID: 27650263; PMCID: PMC5191942.

9. Bizrah M, Yusuf A, Ahmad S. An update on chemical eye burns. Eye (Lond). 2019 Sep;33(9):1362–1377. DOI: 10.1038/s41433-019-0456-5. Epub 2019 May 13. PMID: 31086244; PMCID: PMC7002428.

10. Sharma N, Kaur M, Agarwal T, Sangwan VS, Vajpayee RB. Treatment of acute ocular chemical burns. Surv Ophthalmol. 2018 Mar-Apr;63(2):214–235. DOI: 10.1016/j.survophthal.2017.09.005. Epub 2017 Sep 19. PMID: 28935121.

11. Gupta N, Kalaivani M, Tandon R. Comparison of prognostic value of roper hall and dua classification systems in acute ocular burns. Br J Ophthalmol. 2011 Feb;95(2):194–198. DOI: 10.1136/bjo.2009.173724. Epub 2010 Aug 30. PMID: 20805137.

12. Dua HS, King AJ, Joseph A. A new classification of ocular surface burns. Br J Ophthalmol. 2001 Nov;85(11): 1379–1383. DOI: 10.1136/bjo.85.11.1379. PMID: 11673310; PMCID: PMC1723789.

13. McCallum E, Keren S, Lapira M, Norris JH. Orbital compartment syndrome: An update with review of the literature. Clin Ophthalmol. 2019 Nov 7;13:2189–2194. DOI: 10.2147/OPTH.S180058. PMID: 31806931; PMCID: PMC6844234.

14. Ballard SR, Enzenauer RW, O'Donnell T, Fleming JC, Risk G, Waite AN. Emergency lateral canthotomy and cantholysis: A simple procedure to preserve vision from sight threatening orbital hemorrhage. J Spec Oper Med. 2009 Summer;9(3):26–32. DOI: 10.55460/1CLD-XJUV. PMID: 19739474.

15. Rowh AD, Ufberg JW, Chan TC, Vilke GM, Harrigan RA. Lateral canthotomy and cantholysis: Emergency management of orbital compartment syndrome. J Emerg Med. 2015 Mar;48(3):325–330. DOI: 10.1016/j.jemermed.2014.11.002. Epub 2014 Dec 16. PMID: 25524455.

16. Hayreh SS, Weingeist TA. Experimental occlusion of the central artery of the retina. IV: Retinal tolerance time to acute ischemia. Br J Ophthalmol. 1980 Nov;64(11): 818–825. DOI: 10.1136/bjo.64.11.818. PMID: 7426553; PMCID: PMC1043826.

17. Zafar S, Canner JK, Mir T, Srikumaran D, Channa R, Goldberg MF, Thorne J, Woreta FA. Epidemiology of hyphema-related emergency department visits in the United States between 2006 and 2015. Ophthalmic Epidemiol. 2019 Jun;26(3):208–215. DOI: 10.1080/09286586.2019.1579917. Epub 2019 Feb 22. PMID: 30794001

18. Walton W, Von Hagen S, Grigorian R, et al. Management of traumatic hyphema Surv Ophthalmol. 2002;47(4):297–334.

19. Gharaibeh A, Savage HI, Scherer RW, Goldberg MF, Lindsley K. Medical interventions for traumatic hyphema. Cochrane Database Syst Rev. 2013 Dec;12:CD005431.

20. Ahmed F, House RJ, Feldman BH. Corneal abrasions and corneal foreign bodies. Prim Care. 2015 Sep;42(3):363–375. DOI: 10.1016/j.pop.2015.05.004. Epub 2015 Jul 31. PMID: 26319343.

21. Algarni AM, Guyatt GH, Turner A, Alamri S. Antibiotic prophylaxis for corneal abrasion. Cochrane Database Syst Rev. 2022 May 27;5(5):CD014617. DOI: 10.1002/14651858. CD014617.pub2. PMID: 35622535; PMCID: PMC9139695.

15

Neck Trauma

Katherine R. Iverson and Marc A. de Moya

15.1 Introduction

The neck has been an area that has spawned much debate and research in trauma over the past several decades. It is a region packed with vital structures vulnerable to both blunt and penetrating mechanisms. Penetrating neck injuries, defined as penetration of the platysma, account for approximately 5–10% of all injuries [1]. Blunt neck injuries, including aerodigestive, vascular, and nerve injuries, affect approximately 0.7–4.2% of all significant blunt trauma patients. This excludes the most common neck structure injured, the cervical spine. This chapter will focus on a few of the most commonly asked questions regarding the evaluation and treatment of aerodigestive and vascular injuries in the neck.

In 1969, Cook County investigators divided the neck into three zones [2]. Roon and Christensen recapitulated this classification in 1979 [3] to standardize therapy and research efforts. Zone I refers to the area from the clavicles to the cricoid cartilage, Zone II refers to the area from the cricoid cartilage to the angle of the mandible, and Zone III refers to the area from the angle of the mandible to the base of the skull. However, since the first description of the three zones of the neck in 1969, much has changed in how we approach, image, and treat patients with neck trauma. While the three zones are still commonly used to describe and discuss these injuries, modern diagnostic and management practices are no longer limited by this classification.

Mandatory exploration of the neck was the standard of care soon after World War II but led to a negative exploration rate of approximately 56% [4]. In the 1960s, routine operative explorations were challenged in the abdomen by Nance and Cohn [5] and in the neck by Shirkey et al. [6]. This initial push for nonoperative management eventually led to a more careful selection of operative candidates. Clinicians began to use the hard signs of vascular injury—(1) active external hemorrhage, (2) expanding hematomas, (3) bruit or thrill over the wound, (4) pulse deficit, and (5) a central neurologic deficit—to select operative candidates. Hard signs of tracheobronchial injuries include (1) bubbling from the wound, (2) massive subcutaneous emphysema, (3) airway compromise, or (4) hemoptysis. Some consider crepitance, dysphagia, and hematemesis soft signs of digestive tract injuries. Hard signs of digestive tract injuries usually do not manifest themselves immediately but are more insidious, leading to neck cellulitis and sepsis.

To decrease the number of negative neck explorations, more emphasis has been placed on the physical exam, new imaging technology, and close observation. As our technology has improved, so has the incidence of occult injuries, raising questions about treatment. In a series of 146 patients with penetrating neck trauma, 25% of the external wounds did not correlate with the zone of the internal injury, which questions the value of zone-specific treatment algorithms [7]. Similar findings have been obtained in additional studies, including a review of 298 patients with vascular or aerodigestive penetrating injuries, in which at least 23% of patients had internal injuries outside of the corresponding external neck zone [8]. A "nonzonal" approach to penetrating neck injuries is currently favored, with further testing and management guided by physical exam. What follows are common clinical questions regarding neck trauma, with the discussion forming a foundation for the current assessment and treatment algorithms. The following recommendations are focused on the most recent literature.

15.2 Assessment of Neck Trauma

15.2.1 How Good Is the Physical Exam to Rule Out a Significant Aerodigestive or Vascular Injury?

The initial evaluation of a patient with a suspected neck trauma is the physical exam. Clinicians have been unsure of how reliable the physical exam is as a predictor of a significant aerodigestive or vascular injury. Atteberry et al. studied 28 patients with penetrating zone II neck injuries [9]. They compared the physical exam with angiographic, operative, and ultrasonic findings. There were no missed injuries, although the follow-up period was short. The same group performed a follow-up study with a larger series in 2000 after having instituted strict physical exam–driven protocols for neck trauma [10]. This follow-up study with 145 patients over 8 years confirmed their earlier study. Again, the false-negative rate was approximately 0.3%, which was quoted to be equivalent to false-negative rates of angiograms. The false-positive rate was 10%. In 1997, Demetriades et al. [11] reviewed their experience with 223 patients and claimed that the negative predictive value of physical exams was 100% for vascular or aerodigestive injuries requiring treatment. An additional review of 200 patients by Isaza-Restrepo et al. in 2020 similarly found a sensitivity of 97.4% and negative predictive value of 98.7% for using physical exam soft signs of injuries to predict the CT

DOI: 10.1201/9781003316800-15

need for surgical repair, with specificity and positive predictive value notably less than 50% [12]. Physical exam after penetrating neck injury is more sensitive for major vascular injury, while aerodigestive injuries remain more elusive to diagnose. Of particular concern is the lack of significant signs following stab wounds to the cervical esophagus.

In penetrating neck trauma, cervical esophageal injuries occur in 0.5–7% and carry associated high morbidity and mortality, especially with delay in treatment. Meyer et al. reported clinical exam findings indicative of an esophageal injury in approximately 68% of patients with penetrating neck injuries [13]. Weigelt et al. [14] discovered that up to 50% of esophageal injuries were missed in those stabbed. Based on clinical exams, they describe a 100% sensitivity in the physical exam for gunshot wound victims. The early clinical findings described for an esophageal injury include crepitance [15], hematemesis, anterior tracheal deviation, odynophagia, dysphagia, or hoarseness. If the diagnosis is delayed, complications as a result of contamination arise, including abscess, sepsis, mediastinitis, or neck cellulitis. Further diagnostic testing is often warranted if there is a high level of suspicion for these injuries, given the morbidity and mortality associated with delay in treatment or missed injury.

The role of physical exams in blunt neck trauma is not as clear. In those with angiographically confirmed carotid/vertebral injuries, some report that up to approximately 60% of patients lack any hard signs of injury. Therefore, the physical exam in blunt trauma is not consistently accurate in detecting vascular injuries. Esophageal injury secondary to blunt trauma has been reported but is exceedingly rare. Tracheobronchial injuries have similar findings as penetrating traumatic injuries with an equivalent sensitivity.

RECOMMENDATION

Physical exam is adequate to rule out significant airway and vascular injuries in the case of penetrating trauma. Caution is required when ruling out an esophageal injury based on physical exam and observation, and additional diagnostics may be warranted.

Grade of recommendation: B.

15.2.2 Are Both Esophagoscopy and Swallow Studies Necessary to Rule Out Esophageal Injuries?

Esophageal injuries can occur in both blunt and penetrating trauma; however, it is exceedingly rare to have a blunt cervical esophageal injury. The lack of more obvious signs, particularly in stab wounds, has led clinicians to use other diagnostic methods to rule out an esophageal injury. The early treatment of esophageal injuries significantly decreases complications and costs [16–18]. The delay in treatment may lead to stricture, dysfunction, and infectious complications.

The diagnostic modalities that one may choose from include a fluoroscopic or CT esophagogram with water-soluble contrast, flexible esophagoscopy, or rigid esophagoscopy. Some have found that esophagograms were 90% accurate, while esophagoscopy was 86–95% accurate [19, 20]. Weigelt et al. [14] reported a 100% sensitivity for the combination of esophagograms followed by rigid esophagoscopy if the esophagogram was equivocal in 118 patients with penetrating neck trauma. Srinivasan et al. [21] in a retrospective study of 55 patients discovered that flexible endoscopy yielded a sensitivity of 100% and specificity of 92.4%. However, recommendations are limited by a small number of esophageal injuries and overall a small number of patients. CT esophagography has become increasingly used where available due to reports of higher sensitivity than a fluoroscopic exam for diagnosing upper digestive tract injuries with a reported sensitivity of 95% [22].

RECOMMENDATION

Contrast esophagography, if completely negative, may effectively rule out an esophageal injury; however, esophagoscopy should be added in those cases where the esophagography is equivocal.

Grade of recommendation: C.

15.2.3 How Reliable Is CT Scan for Ruling Out a Vascular or Aerodigestive Tract Injury?

Since the advent of the modern-day CT scan, our diagnostic accuracy has significantly improved, not only achieving better patient selection but also detecting smaller injuries. Once the trauma community began to challenge the notion of mandatory explorations, the reliance on better imaging modalities evolved. Gracias et al. [23] reported that if the trajectory of the injury was distant from vital structures, no further imaging was necessary. Mazolewski et al. examined the role of CT angiography and found that when compared with operative findings, the CT was 100% sensitive and 91% specific in a group of 14 patients [24]. Eastman et al. [25] compared 146 high-risk patients with both CT angiograms (CTA) and digital subtraction (DS) angiograms. Of the 46 positive findings on digital subtraction, one false-negative CTA was discovered. This injury was a grade I vertebral artery injury. They concluded that the sensitivity, specificity, positive predictive value, negative predictive value, and accuracy were 97.7%, 100%, 100%, 99.3%, and 99.3%, respectively. One other study similar to the parallel CTA versus DS angiogram design was performed by Malhotra et al. in 2007. Malhotra et al. [26] did not agree with the Eastman trial and found the sensitivity, specificity, and positive and negative predictive values to be 74%, 86%, 65%, and 90%, respectively. However, if the initial values are eliminated from the study, the sensitivity and specificity values approach the Eastman values. In the discussion, Malhotra suggests that the early data may have been affected by the initial learning curve. Nevertheless, this study provided a warning that the initial optimism for CTA needs to be tempered and critically analyzed further. In 2014, Paulus et al. [27] published a series of patients comparing 64-channel multidetector CTs to DS angiograms and found there was a 68%

sensitivity versus the 51% sensitivity from their earlier study and the negative predictive value was 97.5%. In addition, 62% of the injuries missed were grade I injuries with no significant sequelae. They concluded that 64-channel multidetector CTs were now reliable enough to use as a screening modality for blunt cerebrovascular injury (BCVI). It bears mentioning that nearly 40% of BCVIs are missed with current techniques in CTA based on this study. However, this is of supposedly minimal consequence given the minimal grade of the majority of these injuries with anticipated equivalent long-term outcomes for these patients. A systematic review and meta-analysis of 693 patients by Morales-Uribe et al. demonstrated a 97% sensitivity and 99% specificity for CTA in diagnosing vascular injuries, naming CTA as the gold standard for the identification of these injuries in neck trauma. Sliker et al. [28] compared the use of a whole-body CT protocol with a dedicated CTA for visualization of neck injuries and found them to be equivalent. Both modalities had high sensitivities and specificities for ruling out a cerebrovascular injury.

Inaba et al. [29] report on 106 patients with penetrating neck trauma. No injuries requiring intervention were missed by the CT scan, and it appeared that this potentially reduced the number of unnecessary explorations. A systematic review of 13 studies regarding the accuracy of CTA in penetrating neck trauma by Ibraheem et al. [30] in 2020 reported a sensitivity of 89.5–100% in patients with soft signs of injury and a specificity of 61–100%. This review demonstrated improved accuracy of vascular injury identification over airway or digestive tract injuries. Specific to aerodigestive injuries in penetrating trauma, a CTA had a sensitivity of 92% and specificity of 88% on systematic review in 2021, with some esophageal injuries missed with this modality alone [31]. There has been an ongoing debate regarding the use of CT scan to rule out esophageal injuries, with CTA missing some of these injuries, but a dedicated CT esophagogram demonstrating a high rate of diagnosis.

RECOMMENDATIONS

1. A 16-slice CT scan can accurately identify vascular injuries and the trajectory of bullets.

   Grade of recommendation: B.

2. A 64-slice CT scan can have a high enough negative predictive value to be used to rule out significant cerebrovascular injury.

   Grade of recommendation: B.

3. Reformatted images help detect tracheobronchial injuries.

   Grade of recommendation: C.

4. CT scan cannot be used to rule out an esophageal injury, but CT esophagogram has a high sensitivity for identifying esophageal injuries.

   Grade of recommendation: C.

15.2.4 What Is the Role of Color Flow Doppler Imaging to Determine Vascular Injury?

Color flow Doppler imaging is noninvasive and readily available. In some series, the sensitivity when compared to DS angiography reaches 90–95% [32]. Demetriades et al. [33] and Ginzburg et al. [34] have both published duplex sensitivities and specificities approaching 100%. However, the limitations of ultrasound include the inability to detect nonocclusive injuries with preserved flow, such as intimal flaps and pseudoaneurysms. The technique also fails to detect high internal carotid injuries, which are the most common area injured in blunt trauma patients.

RECOMMENDATION

Duplex ultrasound may be used to rule out an arterial injury in zone II; however, it is limited in zone I or III.

Grade of recommendation: C.

15.2.5 What Are the Risk Factors for Blunt Carotid/Vertebral Arterial Injuries?

Although the signs and symptoms of significant neck trauma secondary to penetrating mechanisms tend to be fairly straightforward, those for blunt trauma are more obtuse. In the study by Miller et al., only approximately 34% of carotid artery injuries were diagnosed by ischemic changes confirmed by either a CTA or DS angiogram [35]. Thirty-eight percent of carotid artery injuries were diagnosed based on suspicion given injury patterns and mechanisms. In Fabian's 1996 study [36] of 87 BCVIs, his group suggested in their discussion that the higher incidence of BCVIs in their trial was a result of "aggressive neurosurgical screening." Based on this and other suggestions, the "at risk" group was more actively sought after. The Denver group screened all those patients with mechanisms compatible with severe cervical hyperextension/rotation or hyperflexion, displaced midface or complex mandibular fractures, closed head injury consistent with diffuse axonal injury, near hanging, seat belt sign across the neck, basilar skull fractures particularly involving the carotid canal, and cervical body fractures [37]. In addition to this list, some have advocated the presence of Horner's syndrome to suggest enough force to produce a BCVI, although in a recent study Malhotra et al. [26] discovered that the presence of Horner's syndrome was rarely associated (<10%) with BCVI, suggesting that it may not be necessary to add to the list of risk factors. These recent studies are based on studies almost 30 years ago that analyzed the associated injuries and found a high incidence associated with complex facial trauma, direct neck blows, cervical spine fractures, and near hanging [38–40].

In 2014, Bruns et al. [41] published a series of 256 patients with BCVI and found that 30% of the patients had no radiographic or physical findings, suggesting the need for additional imaging using the aforementioned screening criteria. Similarly, two studies out of Indiana, Jacobson et al. [42] and Harper et al. [43], found that 37% (17/46) and 16% (25/160) of their patients identified with BCVI, respectively, did not meet typical Denver screening criteria. They recommended more broad screening criteria to include a CTA on any patients undergoing CT cervical spine or chest as part of their traumatic workup based on mechanisms to better capture these injured patients.

Subsequently, the initial Denver criteria have now been expanded to include additional high-risk mechanisms for BCVI following a study by Geddes et al. in 2016 where the authors found a lower incidence of missed injuries with this approach (2.99% vs. 2.36%) [44]. The expanded criteria now include the factors listed here:

Signs/symptoms of BCVI

- Arterial hemorrhage from neck/nose/mouth
- Cervical bruit in patients <50 years
- Expanding cervical hematoma
- Focal neurological deficit
- Neurological exam incongruous with head CT findings
- Stroke on secondary CT scan

Risk factors for BVCI

High-energy transfer mechanism with:

- Le Fort II or III
- Mandible fracture
- Complex skull fracture/basilar skull fracture/occipital condyle fracture
- Severe traumatic brain injury (TBI) with Glasgow Coma Score (GCS)<6
- Cervical spine fracture, subluxation, or ligamentous injury at any level
- Near hanging with anoxic brain injury
- Seat belt abrasion with significant swelling, pain, or altered mental status
- TBI with thoracic injury
- Scalp degloving
- Thoracic vascular injury
- Blunt cardiac rupture
- Upper rib fracture

RECOMMENDATIONS

1. Cervical spine fractures, carotid canal fractures, seat belt sign, unilateral neurologic deficits, near hanging, Le Fort II or III, mandible fractures, skull base fractures, upper rib fractures, and additional significant blunt head and thoracic injuries in conjunction with high-energy mechanisms.

   Grade of recommendation: B.

2. A high mechanism of injury with concomitant signs of injury may also contribute to a high risk for BCVI.

   Grade of recommendation: B.

15.3 Treatment of Neck Trauma

15.3.1 Should Penetrating Neck Injuries Be Selectively Observed or Always Explored?

In 1956, Fogelman and Stewart demonstrated that mandatory exploration was associated with few complications and diminished mortality [45]. Since that time, several authors have challenged the concept of mandatory explorations. This challenge comes as a result of improved technologies and more careful critical analysis of the physical exam. Mandatory exploration produced a negative exploratory rate of approximately 50–60% [4, 46, 47]. Over the past decade, larger prospective observational trials have demonstrated success with a more selective approach. Biffl et al. [48] demonstrated in a series of 128 asymptomatic patients by a physical exam that only one patient had a missed injury. This injury was from an ice pick. They went on to describe that only 15% of the patients required adjuvant tests. Velmahos et al. [49] described in a large retrospective series that 3% of explorations were unnecessary, and in the monitored group, 9% had missed injuries; however, interpretation of the high missed injury rate was difficult. Additional retrospective reviews have since been performed, demonstrating the safety of the selective surgical exploration based on physical exam findings and diagnostic testing with the benefit of avoiding unnecessary operations [61, 62]. The only randomized clinical trial comparing mandatory exploration with selective observation was Golueke et al. [52], where there was no difference in hospital stay, morbidity, or mortality in 160 patients.

RECOMMENDATION

Mandatory exploration and selective exploration have equivalent outcomes. Selective exploration is the current management of choice with careful attention to a physical exam and adjunctive diagnostic imaging.

Grade of recommendation: B.

15.3.2 How Should BCVIs Be Treated?

Much has been written concerning carotid injuries, but little is known about how to best treat the spectrum of carotid and vertebral injuries. The overall incidence of BCVIs is between 0.33% and 1% of all traumas. In 1994, a Western Trauma Association multi-institutional trial described 60 carotid artery injuries [53]. The overall mortality was 43%, and moderate to bad neurologic complications were present in over 22%. In 1996, Fabian et al. [36] described the treatment and outcomes of 87 blunt carotid artery injuries over 11 years. The use of heparin with a goal of partial thromboplastin time (PTT) of 40–50 seconds seemed to independently improve outcomes. In 1999, Biffl et al. [55, 59] developed a grading system for studying and categorizing blunt carotid injuries: Grade I = <25% luminal stenosis, grade II = >25% luminal stenosis or intimal flap, grade III = pseudoaneurysm, grade IV = complete occlusion, and grade V = transection with active extravasation.

They studied 76 patients with 109 blunt carotid injuries and determined that based on their protocol they had favorable outcomes with the use of systemic anticoagulation; however, the study lacked any controls. In 2001, Miller et al. [35] described 139 BCVIs in 96 patients. Of these, 75 were carotid artery injuries and 64 were vertebral artery injuries. The overall stroke rate for carotid injuries was 31%, and the overall stroke rate for vertebral injuries was 14%. A systematic review of 19 studies by Murphy et al. [54, 57, 58, 60] in 2021 for the treatment of asymptomatic BCVI reported better outcomes (decreased cerebrovascular accidents) with antiplatelet or anticoagulation treatment, but no specific treatment modality recommendation could be concluded. In this review, the overall incidence of stroke in patients diagnosed with BCVI who did not receive treatment (usually due to concomitant injuries such as TBI) was 25% in this review compared to 3% stroke risk in patients receiving any treatment.

RECOMMENDATION

Systemic anticoagulation with either IV heparin (PTT 40–50 seconds) or antiplatelet therapy decreases stroke rate in grade II–IV injuries.

Grade of recommendation: C.

15.3.3 Does Endovascular Repair Confer an Outcome Advantage Over Medical Therapy for Grade II and III Traumatic BCVI?

There are no randomized controlled trials exploring this question. Four trials attempt to address the issue and one review with a meta-analysis. In 2005, Cothren et al. [37] reviewed their institution's experience with stenting for BCVI. Of the 46 patients with grade III (pseudoaneurysm) injuries, 50% underwent carotid stents. Of those who underwent carotid stents, 21% had a complication related to the stent and 45% occlusions, whereas 5% of those who were treated medically had a 5% occlusion rate.

In 2011, DiCocco et al. [55] described their series of selective endovascular stent repairs for grade II and III BCVI. They reported an occlusion rate of 4% when stents were used with appropriate medical therapy, suggesting some patients with severe injuries may benefit from stenting.

This was followed up in 2014 by Burlew et al. [56] who reviewed 195 patients with grade II or III injuries. After the aforementioned 2005 report they published, they only performed stents on 2% of patients and found that no patients (109) who were treated with medical therapy suffered a stroke. In addition, they found that none of those patients with grade II injuries had a rupture of the pseudoaneurysm. They concluded that stenting should only be reserved for those with large pseudoaneurysms.

Shahan et al. [57] studied the treatment modalities and outcomes for BCVI patients treated by an interventional radiology (IR) team compared to a multidisciplinary team at their institution. The multidisciplinary group had a lower rate of stenting performed in 8.9% (21/237) of patients as compared to 34% (44/128) of patients in the IR-treated group, with no significant difference in stroke between groups (4.2% vs. 3.9%, respectively). They concluded that anticoagulation with heparin was adequate for most patients with BCVI, but stenting still had a role in significant carotid injuries such as enlarging pseudoaneurysms and vessel narrowing secondary to dissection. A review in 2022 of seven retrospective studies comparing antithrombotic therapy with endovascular therapy showed no significant difference between stroke rates in these two groups in a meta-analysis [58].

RECOMMENDATION

There is no appreciable difference in outcomes when comparing endovascular stents to medical therapy, including those with grade II and III injuries. Stenting should be reserved for large pseudoaneurysms and vessel narrowing secondary to dissection.

Grade of recommendation: C.

TABLE 15.1

Summary of Clinical Recommendations

Question No.	Question	Answer	Grade	References
1	Is a physical exam adequate to rule out significant aerodigestive or vascular injury in penetrating trauma?	A physical exam is adequate to rule out significant airway and vascular injuries. Caution is required when ruling out an esophageal injury based on physical exam and observation, and additional diagnostics may be warranted.	B	[9–15]
2	Are both esophagoscopy and fluoroscopic studies required to rule out esophageal injuries?	Contrast esophagography, if completely negative, may effectively rule out an esophageal injury; however, esophagoscopy should be added in those cases where the esophagography is equivocal.	C	[14, 16–22]
3	How reliable is a CT scan for ruling out a vascular or aerodigestive tract injury?	A 16-slice CT scan can accurately identify vascular injuries and the trajectory of bullets.	B	[23–31, 59, 60]

(Continued)

TABLE 15.1 (Continued)

Summary of Clinical Recommendations

Question No.	Question	Answer	Grade	References
		A 64-slice CT scan can have a high enough negative predictive value to be used to rule out significant BCVI.	B	
		Reformatted images help detect tracheobronchial injuries.	C	
		CT scan cannot be used to rule out an esophageal injury, but a CT esophagogram has a high sensitivity for identifying esophageal injuries.	C	
4	Can color flow Doppler rule out a vascular injury?	Duplex ultrasound may be used to rule out an arterial injury in zone II; however, it is limited in zone I or III.	C	[32–34]
5	What are the risk factors for BCVI?	Cervical spine fractures, carotid canal fractures, seat belt sign, unilateral neurologic deficits, near hanging, Le Fort II or III, mandible fractures, skull base fractures, upper rib fractures, and additional significant blunt head and thoracic injuries in conjunction with high-energy mechanisms.	B	[26, 35–44]
		A high mechanism of injury with concomitant signs of injury may also contribute to a high risk for BCVI.	B	
6	Is selective exploration safe for penetrating neck trauma?	Mandatory exploration and selective explorations have equivalent outcomes. Selective exploration is the current management of choice with careful attention to a physical exam and adjunctive diagnostic imaging.	B	[45–52, 61, 62]
7	How should BCVIs be treated?	Systemic anticoagulation with either IV heparin (PTT 40–50 seconds) or antiplatelet therapy decreases stroke rate in grade II–IV injuries.	C	[35, 36, 54]
8	Does endovascular repair confer an outcome advantage over medical therapy for grade II and III traumatic BCVI?	There is no appreciable difference in outcomes when comparing endovascular stents to medical therapy, including those with grade II and III injuries. Stenting should be reserved for large pseudoaneurysms and vessel narrowing secondary to dissection.	C	[37, 55–58]

Editor's Note

Over the past four decades there have been substantial changes in our management of neck trauma, as elegantly delineated by the authors of this chapter. Recognition of the inaccuracies of our physical exam, particularly in the setting of blunt trauma, has led to the widespread use of CT scanning as an accurate, reliable way to exclude major injuries, the rare esophageal injury notwithstanding. There appears to be little value in characterizing the various anatomic zones of injury in assessing penetrating neck injuries, as this area is now assessed and managed as a continuum.

It is clear that the use of endovascular stents has replaced open, operative interventions in many vascular injuries of the neck, particularly after blunt trauma. As injuries in this area often require complex operative exposures and can be quite difficult, this advance has been adopted rapidly by clinicians.

The major area of controversy remains in the evaluation of the neck after blunt trauma to determine the presence of blunt vascular injury and subsequent therapy. While these injuries can result in neurologic injury, rarely does someone develop sequelae after arrival. There are excellent prospective data demonstrating that the most advanced CTA still misses about 40% of blunt cerebrovascular injuries (identified by angiography) and that approximately 10% of injured patients with this lesion had zero risk factors. So, clearly, many of these "injuries" are being missed, which leads to the obvious question if any occult blunt cerebrovascular injury is worth treating. One could dispel with CTA altogether and just give everyone a daily aspirin when they are discharged, as it is uncertain if our interventions significantly impact outcomes. No randomized trials exist assessing the value of aggressive evaluation and treatment of blunt cerebrovascular injuries. Also, recognize that studies showing the value of anticoagulation compare patients with blunt cerebrovascular injuries with head injury (precluding anticoagulation) with those without head injury, confounding interpretation of neurologic outcomes.

REFERENCES

1. Demetriades D, Asensio JA, Velmahos G, et al. Complex problems in penetrating neck trauma. *Surg Clin North Am.* 1996;6(4):661–683.
2. Monson DO, Saletta JD, Freeark RJ. Carotid vertebral trauma. *J Trauma.* 1969;9:987–999.
3. Roon AJ, Christensen N. Evaluation and treatment of penetrating cervical injuries. *J Trauma.* 1979;19(6):391–397.

4. Elerding SC, Manart FD, Moore EE. A reappraisal of penetrating neck injury management. *J Trauma*. 1980;*20*: 695–697.

5. Nance FC, Cohn I, Jr. Surgical judgment in the management of stab wounds of the abdomen. A retrospective and prospective analysis based on a study of 600 stabbed patients. *Ann Surg*. 1969;*170*:569–645.

6. Shirkey AL, Beall AC, Jr., Debakey ME. Surgical management of penetrating wounds of the neck. *Arch Surg*. 1963;*86*:955–963.

7. Low GM, Inaba K, Chouliaras K, et al. The use of the anatomic 'zones' of the neck in the assessment of penetrating neck injury. *Am Surg*. 2014;*80*(*10*):970–974.

8. Madsen AS, Bruce JL, Oosthuizen GV, Bekker W, Smith M, Manchev V, Laing GL, Clarke DL. Correlation between the level of the external wound and the internal injury in penetrating neck injury does not favour an initial zonal management approach. *BJS Open*. 2020 Aug;*4*(*4*):704–713. doi: 10.1002/bjs5.50282. Epub 2020 Jun 11. PMID: 32525254; PMCID: PMC7397367.

9. Atteberry LR, Dennis JW, Menawat SS, Frykberg ER. Physical examination alone is safe and accurate for the evaluation of vascular injuries in penetrating zone II neck trauma. *J Am Coll Surg*. 1994;*179*(*6*):57–62.

10. Sekharan J, Dennis JW, Veldenz HC, et al. Continued experience with physical examination alone for evaluation and management of penetrating zone 2 neck injuries: Results of 145 cases. *J Vasc Surg*. 2000;*32*(*3*):483–489.

11. Demetriades D, Theodorou D, Cornwell E III, et al. Evaluation of penetrating injuries of the neck: Prospective study of 223 patients. *World J Surg*. 1997;*21*:41–48.

12. Isaza-Restrepo A, Quintero-Contreras JA, Escobar-DiazGranados J, Ruiz-Sternberg ÁM. Value of clinical examination in the assessment of penetrating neck injuries: A retrospective study of diagnostic accuracy test. *BMC Emerg Med*. 2020 Mar 9;*20*(*1*):17. doi: 10.1186/s12873-020-00311-4. PMID: 32151240; PMCID: PMC7063736.

13. Meyer JP, Barrett JA, Schuler JJ, et al. Mandatory vs selective exploration for penetrating neck trauma. A prospective assessment. *Arch Surg*. 1987;*122*:592.

14. Weigelt JA, Thal ER, Snyder WH III, et al. Diagnosis of penetrating cervical esophageal injuries. *Am J Surg*. 1987;*154*:619–622.

15. Goudy SL, Miller FB, Bumpous JM. Neck crepitance: Evaluation and management of suspected upper aerodigestive tract injury. *Laryngoscope*. 2002;*112*:791–795.

16. Symbas PN, Hatcher CR, Jr., Vlasis SE. Esophageal gunshot injuries. *Ann Surg*. 1980;*191*:703–707.

17. Shama DM, Odell J. Penetrating neck trauma with tracheal and esophageal injuries. *Br J Surg*. 1984;*71*:534–536.

18. Asensio JA, Chahwan S, Fornao W, et al. Penetrating esophageal injuries: Multicenter study of the American Association for the Surgery of Trauma. *J Trauma*. 2001;*50*:289.

19. Noyes LD, McSwain NE, Jr., Markowitz IP. Panendoscopy with arteriography versus mandatory exploration of penetrating wounds of the neck. *Ann Surg*. 1986;*204*:21–31.

20. Arantes V, Campolina C, Valerio SH, de Sa RN, Toledo C, Ferrari TA, Coelho LG. Flexible esophagoscopy as a diagnostic tool for traumatic esophageal injuries. *J Trauma*. 2009 Jun;*66*(*6*):1677–1682. doi: 10.1097/TA.0b013e31818c1564. PMID: 19509631.

21. Srinivasan R, Haywood T, Horwitz B, et al. Role of flexible endoscopy in the evaluation of possible esophageal trauma after penetrating injuries. *Am J Gastroenterol*. 2000;*95*(*7*): 1725–1729.

22. Conradie WJ, Gebremariam FA. Can computed tomography esophagography reliably diagnose traumatic penetrating upper digestive tract injuries? *Clin Imaging*. 2015 Nov-Dec;*39*(*6*):1039–1045. doi: 10.1016/j.clinimag.2015.07.021. Epub 2015 Jul 19. PMID: 26264956.

23. Gracias VH, Reilly PM, Philpott J, et al. Computed tomography in the evaluation of penetrating neck trauma: A preliminary study. *Arch Surg*. 2001;*136*:1231–1235.

24. Mazolewski PJ, Curry JD, Browder T, et al. Computed tomographic scan can be used for surgical decision making in Zone II penetrating neck injuries. *J Trauma*. 2001; *51*:315–319.

25. Eastman AL, Chason DP, Perez CL, et al. Computed tomographic angiography for the diagnosis of blunt cervical vascular injury: Is it ready for primetime? *J Trauma*. 2006;*60*(*5*):925–929.

26. Malhotra AK, Camacho M, Ivatury RR, et al. Computed tomographic angiography for the diagnosis of blunt carotid/vertebral artery injury: A note of caution. *Ann Surg*. 2007;*246*(*4*):632–642.

27. Paulus EM, Fabian TC, Savage SA, et al. Blunt cerebrovascular injury screening with 64-channel multidetector computed tomography: More slices finally cut it. *J Trauma Acute Care Surg*. 2014;*76*(*2*):279–283.

28. Sliker CW, Shanmuganathan K, Mirvis SE. Diagnosis of blunt cerebrovascular injuries with 16-MDCT: Accuracy of whole-body MDCT compared with neck MDCT angiography. *AJR*. 2008;*190*:790–799.

29. Inaba K, Munera F, McKenney M, et al. Prospective evaluation of screening multislice helical computed tomographic angiography in the initial evaluation of penetrating neck injuries. *J Trauma*. 2006;*61*(*1*):144–149.

30. Ibraheem K, Wong S, Smith A, Guidry C, McGrew P, McGinness C, Duchesne J, Taghavi S, Harris C, Schroll R. Computed tomography angiography in the "no-zone" approach era for penetrating neck trauma: A systematic review. *J Trauma Acute Care Surg*. 2020 Dec;*89*(*6*): 1233–1238. doi: 10.1097/TA.0000000000002919. PMID: 32890346.

31. Paladino L, Baron BJ, Shan G, Sinert R. Computed tomography angiography for aerodigestive injuries in penetrating neck trauma: A systematic review. *Acad Emerg Med*. 2021 Oct;*28*(*10*):1160–1172. doi: 10.1111/acem.14298. Epub 2021 Sep 28. PMID: 34021515.

32. Kuzniec S, Kauffman P, Molnar LJ, et al. Diagnosis of limb and neck arterial trauma using duplex ultrasonography. *Cardiovasc Surg*. 1998;*6*:358–366.

33. Demetriades D, Theodorov D, Cornwell E III, et al. Penetrating injuries to the neck in patients in stable condition: Physical examination, angiography or color flow imaging. *Arch Surg*. 1995;*130*:971–975.

34. Ginzburg E, Montavo B, Leblang S, et al. The use of duplex ultrasound in penetrating neck trauma. *Arch Surg*. 1996;*131*:691–693.

35. Miller PR, Fabian TC, Bee TK, et al. Blunt cerebrovascular injuries: Diagnosis and treatment. *J Trauma*. 2001; *51*(*2*):279–286.

36. Fabian TC, Patton JH, Croce MA, et al. Blunt carotid injury: Importance of early diagnosis and anticoagulant therapy. *Ann Surg.* 1996;*223(5)*:513–525.

37. Cothren CC, Moore EE, Ray CE, et al. Carotid artery stents for blunt cerebrovascular injury: Risks exceed benefits. *Arch Surg.* 2005;*140(5)*:480–486.

38. Stringer WL, Kelly DL. Traumatic dissection of the extra-cranial internal carotid artery. *Neurosurgery.* 1980;*6*:123.

39. Perry MO, Snyder WH, Tahl ER. Carotid artery injuries are caused by blunt trauma. *Ann Surg.* 1980;*192*:74.

40. Davis JW, Holbrook TL, Hoyt DB et al. Blunt carotid artery dissection: Incidence, associated injuries, screening, and treatment. *J Trauma.* 1990;*30*:1514.

41. Bruns BR, Tesoriero R, Kufera J, et al. Blunt cerebrovas-cular injury screening guidelines: What are we willing to miss? *J Trauma Acute Care Surg.* 2014;*76(3)*:691–695.

42. Jacobson LE, Ziemba-Davis M, Herrera AJ. The limita-tions of using risk factors to screen for blunt cerebrovas-cular injuries: The harder you look, the more you find. *World J Emerg Surg.* 2015;*10*:46. doi: 10.1186/s13017-015-0040-7

43. Harper PR, Jacobson LE, Sheff Z, Williams JM, Rodgers RB. Routine CTA screening identifies blunt cerebrovascular injuries missed by clinical risk factors. *Trauma Surg Acute Care Open.* 2022 Aug 26;*7(1)*:e000924. doi: 10.1136/tsaco-2022-000924. PMID: 36101794; PMCID: PMC94228.

44. Geddes AE, Burlew CC, Wagenaar AE, Biffl WL, Johnson JL, Pieracci FM, Campion EM, Moore EE. Expanded screening criteria for blunt cerebrovascular injury: A big-ger impact than anticipated. *Am J Surg.* 2016 Dec;*212(6)*:1167–1174? doi: 10.1016/j.amjsurg.2016.09.016. Epub 2016 Sep 29. PMID: 27751528.

45. Fogelman M, Stewart R. Penetrating wounds of the neck. *Am J Surg.* 1956;*91*:581–596.

46. Saletta JD, Lowe RJ, Lim LT, et al. Penetrating trauma of the neck. *J Trauma.* 1976;*16*:579–587.

47. Bishara RA, Pasch AR, Douglas DD, et al. The necessity of mandatory exploration of penetrating zone II neck injuries. *Surgery.* 1986;*100*:655–660.

48. Biffl WL, Moore EE, Rehse DH, et al. Selective manage-ment of penetrating neck trauma based on cervical level of injury. *Am J Surg.* 1997;*174*:678–682.

49. Velmahos GC, Souter I, Degiannis E, et al. Selective surgi-cal management in penetrating neck injuries. *Can J Surg.* 1994;*37*:487–491.

50. Teixeira, F, Menegozzo, CAM, Teixeira F., Menegozzo CAM, Netto SDdC, et al. Safety in selective surgical explo-ration in penetrating neck trauma. *World J Emerg Surg.* 2016;*11*:32. doi: 10.1186/s13017-016-0091-4

51. Sperry JL, Moore EE, Coimbra R, Croce M, Davis JW, Karmy-Jones R, McIntyre RC Jr, Moore FA, Malhotra A, Shatz DV, Biffl WL. Western Trauma Association critical decisions in trauma: Penetrating neck trauma. *J Trauma Acute Care Surg.* 2013 Dec;*75(6)*:936–940. doi: 10.1097/TA.0b013e31829e20e3. PMID: 24256663.

52. Golueke PF, Goldstein AS, Sclafani SJ, et al. Routine ver-sus selective exploration of penetrating neck injuries: A ran-domized prospective study. *J Trauma.* 1984;*24*:1010–1014.

53. Cogbil TH, Moore EE, Meissner M, et al. The spectrum of blunt injury to the carotid artery: A multicenter perspective. *J Trauma.* 1994;*37(3)*:473–479.

54. Cothren CC, Biffl WL, Moore EE, Kashuk JL, Johnson JL. Treatment for blunt cerebrovascular injuries: Equivalence of anticoagulation and antiplatelet agents. *Arch Surg.* 2009;*144(7)*:685–690. doi: 10.1001/archsurg.2009.111

55. DiCocco JM, Fabian TC, Emmett KP, et al. Optimal outcomes for patients with blunt cerebrovascular injury (BCVI): Tailoring treatment to the lesion. *J Am Coll Surg.* 2011;*212(4)*:549–557.

56. Burlew CC, Biffl WL, Moore EE, et al. Endovascular stent-ing is rarely necessary for the management of blunt cerebro-vascular injuries. *J Am Coll Surg.* 2014;*218*:1012–1017.

57. Shahan CP, Sharpe JP, Stickley SM, Manley NR, Filiberto DM, Fabian TC, Croce MA, Magnotti LJ. The changing role of endovascular stenting for blunt cerebrovascular inju-ries. *J Trauma Acute Care Surg.* 2018 Feb;*84(2)*:308–311. doi: 10.1097/TA.0000000000001740. PMID: 29370049.

58. Priola SM, Ku JC, Palmisciano P, Taslimi S, Mathieu F, Pasarikovski CR, Malhotra A, Umana GE, Scalia G, Tomasi SO, Raudino G, Yang VXD, da Costa L. Endovascular and antithrombotic treatment in blunt cerebrovascular injuries: A systematic review and meta-analysis. *J Stroke Cerebrovasc Dis.* 2022 Jun;*31(6)*:106456. doi: 10.1016/j.jstrokecerebrovasdis.2022.106456. Epub 2022 Apr 4. PMID: 35390729.

59. Biffl WL, Moore EE, Offner PJ et al. Blunt carotid arte-rial injuries: Implications of a new grading scale. J Trauma. 1999;47(5):845.

60. Murphy PB, Severance S, Holler E, et al. Treatment of asymptomatic blunt cerebrovascular injury (BCVI): a sys-tematic review. Trauma Surgery & Acute Care Open 2021; 6:e000668. doi: 10.1136/tsaco-2020-000668.

61. Sriussadaporn S, Pak-Art R, Tharavej C, et al. Selective management of penetrating neck injuries based on clinical presentations is safe and practical. *Int Surg.* 2001;*86*:90–93.

62. Nason RW, Assuras GN, Gray PR, et al. Penetrating neck injuries: Analysis of experience from a Canadian trauma centre. *Can J Surg.* 2001;*44*:122–126.

16

Resuscitative Thoracotomy*

Christopher R. Reed and Suresh K. Agarwal

16.1 Introduction

Resuscitative thoracotomy (RT) is the performance of left anterolateral thoracotomy, potentially but not necessarily with extension to the right chest (i.e., "clamshell' thoracotomy), in a patient with cardiovascular collapse after traumatic injury. It is almost always performed in the emergency department with the intent to relieve immediately reversible causes of shock (cardiac tamponade, exsanguinating supradiaphragmatic injury) followed by temporarily clamping the descending thoracic aorta to maximize coronary and cerebral perfusion and facilitating open cardiac massage. The procedure exposes the already moribund patient to substantial morbidity and puts the healthcare team at risk of exposure to bloodborne pathogens [1]. It is also a resource-intensive procedure that has the potential to salvage patients with severe, irreversible anoxic encephalopathy. Over the past several decades, there has been increasing interest in defining, standardizing, and refining the criteria for RT to prevent utilizing this technique in futile situations [2]. The conditions under which RT is performed largely preclude validation in clinical trials. Research on this topic has, therefore, been limited to observational studies. Additionally, the definition of "signs of life" and specific indications and protocols for RT are inconsistent across trauma centers and in the published literature, which makes rigorous study and protocol development particularly difficult [3]. In the era of evidence-based medicine, there is little evidence on which to establish concrete practice guidelines for this resource-intensive procedure, although there is understandably considerable enthusiasm for doing so with available data. The most familiar recommendations for the performance of RT typically consider the anatomic location of the injury (if known), mechanism, and the presence of signs of life in the emergency department versus prehospital only—all of which unsurprisingly have associations with survival and long-term neurological prognosis [4].

In the absence of conclusive evidence to guide management, the decision to perform RT continues to rely on the clinical judgment of trauma physicians. Although institutional protocols have been advocated, the heterogeneity of patient and injury factors in such cases continues to demand a risk-benefit analysis on a case-by-case basis [5]. The likelihood of a favorable outcome must be balanced against the misuse of limited resources, the potential for occupational exposure to bloodborne pathogens, and the monetary cost of performing a potentially futile procedure. Appropriate patient selection, therefore, requires thorough knowledge of the available literature and appropriate application to each unique scenario with careful consideration of the injury burden and mechanism, the patient's physiologic status, and prehospital resuscitation efforts.

16.2 Is There a Length of Prehospital CPR Time Beyond Which the Performance of Resuscitative Thoracotomy for Penetrating Trauma Should Be Considered Futile?

Multiple large, retrospective studies agree that the best outcomes after RT are in patients with penetrating thoracic injuries with signs of life on arrival to the emergency department [6]. Stab wounds and those injuries causing cardiac tamponade which can be relieved during RT have the best outcomes. This is unsurprising, as blunt trauma sufficient to cause cardiac arrest is likely associated with multiple life-threatening injuries simultaneously, and prehospital arrest suggests that a patient is arriving in an unsalvageable state of uncertain chronicity. In a 26-year review of 959 patients who underwent emergency department thoracotomy (EDT), Powell et al. found that among 26 survivors requiring prehospital cardiopulmonary resuscitation (CPR), 21 (81%) were neurologically functional at discharge [7]. Patients with cardiac stab wounds and pericardial tamponade were the most likely to benefit from RT, even if they arrived in asystole. Among these five survivors, four (80%) patients requiring CPR for less than 15 minutes experienced good functional outcomes. In contrast, of those patients with a penetrating injury who required more than 15 minutes of prehospital CPR, none survived. These findings are illustrative and representative of the most recent major trauma society guideline update specifically addressing patient selection for RT (Eastern Association for the Surgery of Trauma, 2015), which conditionally recommends RT for patients with prehospital CPR and a penetrating

---

* The authors would like to acknowledge Dr. Joseph J. DuBose and Dr. Mina L. Boutrous for their previous edition of the chapter.

DOI: 10.1201/9781003316800-16

mechanism (i.e., no pulse and no signs of life prehospital) but specifically avoids making any conclusion concerning the duration of CPR. It is worthwhile to note that cardiac arrest is likely to be the most powerful indicator of outcome, beyond any injury or patient factors. In a series of 60 consecutive patients with penetrating cardiac wounds, the specific mechanism (stabbing versus gunshot wound) was less important than the occurrence of cardiac arrest in predicting outcomes [8]. The authors of the guideline agree, and it has been described that prehospital assessment of salvageability, reversibility of shock state, and even palpation of pulses is unreliable, and therefore it is not possible to assign a specific time at which RT becomes futile [9].

RECOMMENDATION

Based on available retrospective literature, the most favorable outcomes following RT are achieved in patients with penetrating thoracic injuries and who have required CPR for less than 15 minutes. Patients with tamponade following cardiac stab wounds appear to be the most likely to benefit in this scenario. Conclusive evidence of an association between a specific duration of prehospital CPR and optimal outcome, however, has not been identified, and no evidence-based recommendation can be made for a concrete threshold.

Grade of recommendation: C.

16.3 Should Resuscitative Thoracotomy Be Performed on Blunt Trauma Patients Who Lose Vitals in the Prehospital Setting?

Any discussion regarding the consequences of an aggressive intervention must compare this outcome to the standard of care in the absence of the intervention. Patients presenting after blunt traumatic injury sufficient to effect cardiac arrest with last signs of life prehospital or in-hospital have predictably poor outcomes overall without RT, with estimated in-hospital survival of 0.001% and 0.5%, respectively [2]. Although favorable outcomes are relatively poor following RT after blunt trauma, they must be interpreted in the context of what is otherwise an essentially nonsurvivable insult. The largest retrospective reviews have documented that an average of 1.4% of these patients will survive; 2% of those presenting in shock and less than 1% if no vital signs are present on arrival [6, 10, 11]. In the most pessimistic series, which was notably from the 1970s to 1990s, Powell et al. identified no survivors among those who had undergone RT for blunt trauma after more than 5 minutes of CPR [7]. Conversely, in a series of 38 patients injured by blunt mechanisms who required CPR after a witnessed arrest, Fialka et al. reported 4 RT survivors (10.5%) following CPR for a mean of 13 minutes. All four survivors were neurologically intact on discharge [12]. A more contemporary, single-center series of RT performed for all injury mechanisms specifically in the context of prehospital

CPR showed predictably poor but unexpectedly similar neurologic outcomes among both blunt and penetrating patients, with most survivors discharged with functional independence [13]. Although this series of 93 patients undergoing RT for prehospital arrest agreed with prior studies showing improved survival among penetrating trauma victims (4% survival to discharge for penetrating mechanism versus 1.3% survival to discharge for blunt mechanism), the overall survival with independence at discharge was about 2% for both groups. This study provides even further evidence that there are insufficient data to perform or withhold RT among patients with prehospital arrest based on injury mechanism alone.

RECOMMENDATION

Based on the retrospective data available, RT after blunt trauma is associated with a low overall rate of survival (1–10%). However, these results should be interpreted in the context of nearly universal lethality of cardiac arrest after blunt trauma with standard resuscitation efforts. Therefore, the decision to perform RT after blunt trauma must be made with careful consideration of the patient's overall injury burden, as well as whether signs of life are present on arrival to the emergency department. Patients presenting after blunt traumatic arrest without signs of life (electrical activity, pupillary response, or any extremity movement/spontaneous ventilation) are rarely salvageable with or without RT. Regardless, there are insufficient data to recommend always performing or always withholding RT in the setting of blunt traumatic arrest in the prehospital setting, especially given similar overall functional outcomes for both penetrating and blunt injury mechanisms [13].

Grade of recommendation: C.

16.4 Is Resuscitative Thoracotomy Effective at Reducing Mortality in Patients with Extrathoracic Injuries?

Resuscitative thoracotomy may improve survival in agonal patients with extrathoracic injuries. Several of the largest reports describing outcomes of the procedure include survivors with abdominal injuries. Mechanistically, it is not surprising that temporary control of abdominopelvic hemorrhage via descending thoracic aortic clamp while allowing for resuscitation and transport to the operating room for laparotomy improves survival in these patients. Interestingly, Seamon et al. reported a series of RT survivors in which 35% had extrathoracic injuries. The majority of these were abdominal penetrating injuries from gunshot wounds. The authors concluded that the finding appeared counterintuitive and that surgeons should revisit long-standing reluctance to perform RT for patients with extrathoracic injuries, especially when those injuries are penetrating abdominopelvic injuries in nature [14]. Sheppard et al. further described 27 patients undergoing RT for nontorso injuries [15]. They noted 100% mortality in patients with penetrating head injuries undergoing RT but had three (11%) survivors with penetrating neck or extremity injuries.

RECOMMENDATION

Small retrospective reports have suggested that the use of RT may facilitate salvage in a select group of agonal patients with exsanguinating vascular injuries in the abdomen and pelvis. Aortic occlusion likely provides temporary control of exsanguinating vascular injury and may allow sufficient stability for transfer to the operating room and definitive control. However, the salvage of patients with injuries to the neck or extremities is rarely described, and head injury sufficient to cause hemorrhagic shock and arrest is associated with poor outcomes after RT. Given that conventional RT increases blood flow to these vascular beds, this is not surprising.

Grade of recommendation: C.

16.5 Can Resuscitative Endovascular Balloon Occlusion of the Aorta Serve as a Potential Replacement for Conventional Resuscitative Thoracotomy?

Since its first description and commercial availability for use in trauma patients in the 2000s and 2010s, respectively, resuscitative endovascular balloon occlusion of the aorta (REBOA) has seen increasing enthusiasm at select centers [16]. The goal of the procedure is to provide proximal control of truncal hemorrhage using a percutaneous transfemoral endovascular balloon inflated in the aorta. In appropriately selected patients (and injuries) and when deployed by a skilled practitioner, it may provide the benefits of an aortic cross-clamp without the morbidity inherent to RT [17]. Recently, the first results from a large American Association for the Surgery of Trauma (AAST) prospective, nonrandomized comparison of REBOA versus RT were reported [18]. This ambitious multicenter study, coined Aortic Occlusion for Resuscitation in Trauma and Acute Care Surgery (AORTA), included 46 REBOA patients and compared them to 68 open aortic occlusion patients over the course of 2 years. Most open aortic occlusion patients underwent conventional RT. The initial results are exciting and suggest that REBOA may be lifesaving in appropriately selected patients with life-threatening retroperitoneal hemorrhage. Balloon deployment in zones I, II, and III was included in the study, and both hemodynamic improvement and overall survival were comparable to that seen with conventional RT. Complications were remarkably uncommon (2% access vessel pseudoaneurysm, 4% embolization), especially when considering the relative morbidity of RT. Given that the procedure is still gaining popularity and more data are needed to support its use, high-volume centers with access to and experience with REBOA should continue to define its use and the appropriate patient population for its application. It is important to reiterate

that the study was not randomized, and conventional RT patients were more likely to be hypotensive, were more hypotensive overall, and were more likely to be receiving CPR on arrival to the ED. Also of note, the vast majority of REBOAs were deployed by attending trauma or vascular surgeons, as compared to RT, which was most often performed by trainees. As national experiences accrue with this technique, it will be necessary to consider the implications of this training gradient in future studies. The endovascular and catheter-directed skills required for rapid and safe deployment of REBOA may favor high-volume centers with significant experience and resources with the technique. Several groups have introduced curricula designed to familiarize trauma providers with REBOA, including the Endovascular Skills for Trauma and Resuscitative Surgery course, to both improve the effectiveness of the intervention and improve its application across institutions. However, all of the centers included in the AORTA study were high-volume centers, where the increased acuity and experience with novel techniques may facilitate REBOA.

RECOMMENDATION

In summary, a single large, nonrandomized, multicenter, recent prospective study of REBOA compared to open aortic occlusion typically by RT has demonstrated early but exciting results with low complication rates and comparable hemodynamic improvement and survival rates. However, conventional RT was applied more frequently in patients with worse hypotension and with CPR ongoing. Future work should disseminate and standardize training and application of the device to allow the rigorous and widespread study of REBOA outside of select centers to allow a formal recommendation regarding the place of REBOA in the care of the agonal patient.

Grade of recommendation: C.

16.6 Should Bilateral Anterolateral ("Clamshell") Thoracotomy Be Routinely Performed during Resuscitative Thoracotomy?

The most common and best-described approach to RT involves a long left anterolateral thoracotomy in the fourth or fifth interspace. This incision can be made expediently without any specialized equipment beyond a rib retractor and provides good access to the left lung hilum, pericardium, heart, and descending aorta. It is possible to extend the incision across the body of the sternum to the right chest to facilitate additional exposure of the mediastinum and, ultimately, the right pleural and hilar structures. This so-called "clamshell" thoracotomy has traditionally been selectively employed after traumatic arrest when there is clinical suspicion for ongoing, uncontrolled hemorrhage in the right chest or additional exposure of the heart and thoracic great vessels is required for hemorrhage control sufficient to proceed to the operating room. There is little doubt that this dramatic extension of the conventional RT incision across the bony and soft tissue structures can improve retraction and visualization of the mediastinal and right pleural structures [19]. There has been recent interest in defining whether routinely employing this incision during RT improves exposure and therefore hemorrhage control. A study of non-surgical staff and resident physicians in emergency medicine comparing clamshells to traditional RT on fresh human cadavers aimed to define the benefits of routine clamshell thoracotomy [20]. The overall success rate of their subjects (defined by delivery of the heart and aortic clamp placement) was 53%, with most failures related to inadequate aortic clamping. There was no difference overall in the success rate of the procedure for all physicians, although there was a slight improvement in procedural success only for staff (not resident) physicians with clamshell versus traditional anterolateral RT.

It is important to consider the additional morbidity incurred by the extension of this incision across the sternal body. Short-term consequences of this incision include obligate laceration of both internal thoracic arteries with pursuant potentially problematic hemorrhage in immediate and delayed fashions, as well as the need for a more complex repair (i.e., with sternal wires, additional perichondral sutures). Perhaps more importantly, the longer-term consequences of semicontrolled, semisterile incision of the sternum should be considered: Sternal wound dehiscence, nonunion, and chronic pain and debility are unfortunately familiar foes from the lung transplant population. Finally, most surgeons are comfortable with adequate exposure of the left lung hilum, pericardium, heart, and descending aorta through a conventional RT incision.

RECOMMENDATION

Therefore, we recommend that the decision to extend a left anterolateral thoracotomy RT incision be made based on the clinical circumstances on a case-by-case basis, including the patient's physiologic response to aortic cross-clamping and resuscitation, as well as the injury pattern, including the most likely projectile trajectory.

Grade of recommendation: D.

16.7 Should Organ Procurement Be Considered a Conditionally Positive Outcome of Resuscitative Thoracotomy?

Although the primary goal of any surgeon caring for a critically injured patient in the hyperacute setting is to maximize life and limb salvage while minimizing debility, patients undergoing RT may regain physiologic stability but ultimately be neurologically devastated from either their injuries or hypoxia. It is therefore important to consider this situation in the context of a global shortage of lifesaving organs from healthy donors without any short-term solutions. Schnüriger et al. described a series of 11 trauma patients undergoing RT from 2006 to 2009 that survived to the intensive care unit

(ICU) but had subsequent brain death and ultimately resulted in the donation of six kidneys, two livers, two pancreases, and one small bowel [21]. Only three patients had poor organ function after their resuscitation as a contraindication to transplant. Another single institutional series of 340 patients arriving without signs of life after traumatic injury identified 24 organs procured from 12 donors over 13 years, with 4% of all such moribund patients ultimately eligible for and ultimately donating at least one organ [13]. It is reasonable to consider the donation of healthy organs that would otherwise be squandered after trauma as an ancillary benefit of RT and maximal resuscitation, although most surgeons understandably would never consider RT for the sole purpose of organ salvage [22]. However, the goals of maximizing salvage of patients with the best chances of meaningful recovery and maximizing the chance of successful organ donation are not conflicting interests, as nicely demonstrated in a recent cost analysis that also examined clinical variables and outcomes, including survival and organ donation after traumatic arrest [23].

RECOMMENDATION

Given the overall low survival rate, only a small number of patients with posttraumatic arrest requiring RT ultimately go on to become organ donors in the ICU. Even this relatively small number of donations, of course, has massive implications for recipients in their transplant region. The decision to proceed with RT should be made with the intent to maximize the likelihood of a favorable outcome for the injured patient, which does not conflict with the potential for organ donation.

Grade of recommendation: C.

16.8 Does Resuscitative Thoracotomy Expose Healthcare Providers to Increased Risk of Bloodborne Pathogen Exposure?

There is a high seroprevalence of the human immunodeficiency virus (HIV), hepatitis B virus (HBV), and hepatitis C virus (HCV) in the trauma patient population overall. Interestingly, both penetrating and blunt populations have high seroprevalence rates, with blunt trauma patients historically at increased risk compared to penetrating [24–26]. There is no doubt among physicians who have performed RT that there is a relatively high risk of needlestick or laceration on the part of treating clinicians owing to the rapid rate of performance and reliance on multiple sharp instruments with many participants in the resuscitation working in tandem. This risk must be considered inherent in the performance of the procedure and is probably best quantified in a 2018 multicenter prospective observational study from Nunn et al. in which the study team surveyed 1,360 ED healthcare providers of different professions and ultimately identified a 7.2% exposure rate during RT (22 events) [27]. The authors calculated a 6 in 1,000,000 HIV seroconversion rate and 1 in 10,000 HCV conversion rate per

TABLE 16.1

Questions, Answers, and Evidence Regarding Emergency Thoracotomy

Question	Answer	Grade of Recommendation	Level of Evidence	References
Is there a length of prehospital CPR time beyond which the performance of resuscitative thoracotomy for penetrating trauma should be considered futile?	According to retrospective data, RT after more than 15 minutes of prehospital CPR may be futile, but many factors are associated with futility, and each case must be considered individually.	C	IV	[6, 7]
Should resuscitative thoracotomy be performed on blunt trauma patients who lose vitals in the prehospital setting?	Limiting RT use to patients with penetrating injuries results in better survival rates.	C	IV	[6, 7, 10–12]
Is resuscitative thoracotomy effective at reducing mortality in patients with extrathoracic injuries?	RT may facilitate salvage in a select group of agonal patients with vascular injuries to the neck, extremities, or (especially) the abdomen and pelvis.	C	IV	[14, 15]
Can resuscitative endovascular balloon occlusion of the aorta serve as a potential replacement for conventional resuscitative thoracotomy?	Although early results are very exciting, REBOA deserves further study to adequately define the ideal patient population and overcome its inherent learning curve before head-to-head comparison with RT.	C	IV	[18]
Should bilateral anterolateral ("clamshell") thoracotomy be routinely performed during resuscitative thoracotomy?	There are no large, high-quality studies to suggest that surgeons should routinely extend conventional left anterolateral RT incisions across the sternum, and clinical judgment should continue to guide this decision.	D	V	[19, 20]
Should organ procurement be considered a conditionally positive outcome of resuscitative thoracotomy?	Although efforts in the emergency setting should be focused on the patient being treated, RT survivors who are neurologically devastated may donate vital organs, and the preservation of organs is not at odds with caring for the injured patient.	D	V	[21–23]
Does resuscitative thoracotomy expose healthcare providers to an increased risk of bloodborne pathogen exposure?	Occupational exposures to bloodborne pathogens during RT are uncommon but not rare, and PPE may mitigate the risk.	C	IV	[27]

RT, highlighting the extremely low but nonzero risk and noting that personal protective equipment appeared to mitigate the risks of exposure in their study further.

RECOMMENDATION

The risk of bloodborne pathogen exposure during RT should be considered a risk to the healthcare team that is (1) greater than in other procedures performed under less exigent circumstances, (2) mitigated in part by universal precautions, and (3) is not, by itself, a contraindication to performing the potentially lifesaving procedure.

Grade of recommendation: C.

Editor's Note

With the absence of clinical trials to guide us, the decision to perform an emergency department thoracotomy (EDT) has undergone considerable modifications over the past 50 years. There was a time that EDT was routine in every trauma patient presenting dead on arrival to the hospital who did not have rigor mortis. The typical question at the Morbidity and Mortality conference, "was the patient warm," if answered in the affirmative, was considered adequate justification. At the time, the procedure was often performed in patients in moderate to severe shock, which elevated the survival statistics reported from major urban centers. In patients presenting without vital signs, we now recognize a 2% rate of neurologic survivors, but another 3% or so of patients can be resuscitated but brain dead and give up a major organ for transplantation. The impact of the duration of time in cardiac arrest and the mechanism of injury reflect individual providers' clinical experience, and no patient should be denied EDT based exclusively on the number of minutes of transport. Patient selection should therefore be individualized. Of note, REBOA has not been subjected to a rigorous clinical trial, but it represents another modality for gaining aortic occlusion, like thoracotomy, and is related to the skill of the provider and frequency of institutional use. Thus, all of the recommendations in this chapter are based on limited clinician experience and none of them on rigorous prospective research.

REFERENCES

1. Seamon MJ, Ginwalla R, Kulp H, Patel J, Pathak AS, Santora TA, Gaughan JP, Goldberg AJ, Tedaldi EM. (2011). HIV and hepatitis in an urban penetrating trauma population: Unrecognized and untreated. J Trauma. 71(2):306–310; discussion 311.

2. Seamon MJ, Haut ER, Van Arendonk K, Barbosa RR, Chiu WC, Dente CJ, Fox N, Jawa RS, Khwaja K, Lee JK, et al. (2015). An evidence-based approach to patient selection for emergency department thoracotomy: A practice management guideline from the Eastern Association for the Surgery of Trauma. J Trauma Acute Care Surg. 79(1):159–173.

3. Hall BL, Buchman TG. (2005). A visual, timeline-based display of evidence for emergency thoracotomy. J Trauma. 59(3):773–777.

4. Burlew CC, Moore EE, Moore FA, Coimbra R, McIntyre RC, Jr., Davis JW, Sperry J, Biffl WL. (2012). Western Trauma Association critical decisions in trauma: Resuscitative thoracotomy. J Trauma Acute Care Surg. 73(6):1359–1363.

5. Aihara R, Millham FH, Blansfield J, Hirsch EF. (2001). Emergency room thoracotomy for penetrating chest injury: Effect of an institutional protocol. J Trauma. 50(6):1027–1030.

6. Rhee PM, Acosta J, Bridgeman A, Wang D, Jordan M, Rich N. (2000). Survival after emergency department thoracotomy: Review of published data from the past 25 years. J Am Coll Surg. 190(3):288–298.

7. Powell DW, Moore EE, Cothren CC, Ciesla DJ, Burch JM, Moore JB, Johnson JL. (2004). Is emergency department resuscitative thoracotomy futile care for the critically injured patient requiring prehospital cardiopulmonary resuscitation? J Am Coll Surg. 199(2):211–215.

8. Buckman RF, Jr., Badellino MM, Mauro LH, Asensio JA, Caputo C, Gass J, Grosh JD. (1993). Penetrating cardiac wounds: Prospective study of factors influencing initial resuscitation. J Trauma. 34(5):717–725; discussion 725-717.

9. Hunt RC, Carroll RG, Whitley TW, Bryan-Berge DM, Dufresne DA. (1994). Adverse effect of helicopter flight on the ability to palpate carotid pulses. Ann Emerg Med. 24(2):190–193.

10. Cothren CC, Moore EE. (2006). Emergency department thoracotomy for the critically injured patient: Objectives, indications, and outcomes. World J Emerg Surg. 1:4.

11. Hunt PA, Greaves I, Owens WA. (2006). Emergency thoracotomy in thoracic trauma-a review. Injury. 37(1):1–19.

12. Fialka C, Sebok C, Kemetzhofer P, Kwasny O, Sterz F, Vecsei V. (2004). Open-chest cardiopulmonary resuscitation after cardiac arrest in cases of blunt chest or abdominal trauma: A consecutive series of 38 cases. J Trauma. 57(4):809–814.

13. Alarhayem AQ, Cohn SM, Muir MT, Myers JG, Fuqua J, Eastridge BJ. (2017). Organ donation, an unexpected benefit of aggressive resuscitation of trauma patients presenting dead on arrival. J Am Coll Surg. 224(5):926–932.

14. Seamon MJ, Fisher CA, Gaughan JP, Kulp H, Dempsey DT, Goldberg AJ. (2008). Emergency department thoracotomy: Survival of the least expected. World J Surg. 32(4):604–612.

15. Sheppard FR, Cothren CC, Moore EE, Orfanakis A, Ciesla DJ, Johnson JL, Burch JM. (2006). Emergency department resuscitative thoracotomy for nontorso injuries. Surgery. 139(4):574–576.

16. Stannard A, Eliason JL, Rasmussen TE. (2011). Resuscitative endovascular balloon occlusion of the aorta (REBOA) as an adjunct for hemorrhagic shock. J Trauma. 71(6):1869–1872.

17. Brenner ML, Moore LJ, DuBose JJ, Tyson GH, McNutt MK, Albarado RP, Holcomb JB, Scalea TM, Rasmussen TE. (2013). A clinical series of resuscitative endovascular balloon occlusion of the aorta for hemorrhage control and resuscitation. J Trauma Acute Care Surg. 75(3):506–511.

18. DuBose JJ, Scalea TM, Brenner M, Skiada D, Inaba K, Cannon J, Moore L, Holcomb J, Turay D, Arbabi CN, et al. (2016). The AAST prospective Aortic Occlusion for Resuscitation in Trauma and Acute Care Surgery (AORTA) registry: Data on contemporary utilization and outcomes of aortic occlusion and resuscitative balloon occlusion of the aorta (REBOA). J Trauma Acute Care Surg. 81(3):409–419.

19. Simms ER, Flaris AN, Franchino X, Thomas MS, Caillot JL, Voiglio EJ. (2013). Bilateral anterior thoracotomy (clamshell incision) is the ideal emergency thoracotomy incision: An anatomic study. World J Surg. 37(6):1277–1285.

20. Newberry R, Brown D, Mitchell T, Maddry JK, Arana AA, Achay J, Rahm S, Long B, Becker T, Grier G, et al. (2021). Prospective randomized trial of standard left anterolateral thoracotomy versus modified bilateral clamshell thoracotomy performed by emergency physicians. Ann Emerg Med. 77(3):317–326.

21. Schnuriger B, Inaba K, Branco BC, Salim A, Russell K, Lam L, Plurad D, Demetriades D. (2010). Organ donation: An important outcome after resuscitative thoracotomy. J Am Coll Surg. 211(4):450–455.

22. Peetz AB, Kuzemchak MD, Streams JR, Patel MB, Guillamondegui OD, Dennis BM, Betzold RD, Gunter OL, Karp SJ, Beskow LM. (2021). Regional ethics of surgeon resuscitation for organ transplantation after lethal injury. Surgery. 169(6):1532–1535.

23. Love KM, Brown JB, Harbrecht BG, Muldoon SB, Miller KR, Benns MV, Smith JW, Baker CE, Franklin GA. (2016). Organ donation as an outcome of traumatic cardiopulmonary arrest: A cost evaluation. J Trauma Acute Care Surg. 80(5):792–798.

24. Kaplan AJ, Zone-Smith LK, Hannegan C, Norcross ED. (1992). The prevalence of hepatitis C in a regional level I trauma center population. J Trauma. 33(1):126–128; discussion 128-129.

25. Caplan ES, Preas MA, Kerns T, Soderstrom C, Bosse M, Bansal J, Constantine NT, Hendrix E, Caplan M. (1995). Seroprevalence of human immunodeficiency virus, hepatitis B virus, hepatitis C virus, and rapid plasma reagin in a trauma population. J Trauma. 39(3):533–537; discussion 537-538.

26. Sloan EP, McGill BA, Zalenski R, Tsui P, Chen EH, Duda J, Morris M, Sherer R, Barrett J. (1995). Human immunodeficiency virus and hepatitis B virus seroprevalence in an urban trauma population. J Trauma. 38(5):736–741.

27. Nunn A, Prakash P, Inaba K, Escalante A, Maher Z, Yamaguchi S, Kim DY, Maciel J, Chiu WC, Drumheller B, et al. (2018). Occupational exposure during emergency department thoracotomy: A prospective, multi-institution study. J Trauma Acute Care Surg. 85(1):78–84.

17

Chest Wall Trauma

John K. Bini

Trauma to the chest wall is common and may account for up to one-quarter of all traumatic deaths. Because thoracic trauma accounts for a significant portion of traumatic morbidity and mortality, proper management of these injuries has the potential to significantly and positively impact trauma outcomes. Many clinical questions surround the management of chest wall trauma, and significant clinical equipoise exists. Unfortunately, this is one area where robust data-guiding management is often lacking. Questions exist regarding the optimal management of acute open pneumothorax, optimal treatment for tension pneumothorax, autotransfusion for hemothorax, optimal chest drainage tube size, surgical stabilization of multiple rib fractures (MRFs) or flail chest, and timing of video-assisted thoracoscopic surgery (VATS) for evacuation of retained hemothorax. The lack of Level 1, Level 2, and in some cases Level 3 evidence makes answering all these questions in the setting of an evidence-based text impracticable. This chapter will answer and make recommendations in areas where sufficient evidence exists, specifically in the areas of surgical stabilization of the chest wall, autotransfusion, selection of chest tube size, and timing of VATS for evacuation of retained hemothorax.

17.1 Should Open Reduction and Internal Fixation Be Performed Routinely on Trauma Patients with Multiple Rib Fractures?

It has been reported that up to 25% of annual traumatic deaths result from chest trauma. A flail chest may be seen in as many as 6% of patients (82 of 1417) sustaining blunt chest trauma [1–3]. Mortality rates of up to 12% (84 of 711) for patients with MRFs and up to 33% (30 of 92) for patients with a flail chest have been reported [4–6]. A study of 181,331 adults in the National Trauma Data Bank showed the odds ratio for death for younger patients and patients over 64 years of age. If two patients have similar severity of injuries, the one with rib fractures will have a substantially higher expected risk of death than the one without. This effect is more pronounced for older patients [6].

Studies have demonstrated a direct correlation between the number of rib fractures and intrathoracic injury, morbidity, and mortality [3]. In particular, patients who have had a flail chest with pulmonary contusions often report long-term dyspnea and chest pain and have abnormal test results on spirometry [7]. Bulger et al. [8] found that elderly patients with rib fractures had twice the mortality and thoracic morbidity compared with younger patients with similar injuries. In their study, for each additional rib fracture in an elderly patient, mortality increased by 19%, and the risk of pneumonia increased by 27%.

Rib fractures are frequently associated with pulmonary contusions [5], and MRFs predispose patients to pulmonary insufficiency and compromised ventilation. In patients with a flail chest, paradoxical chest wall motion and pain can result in low tidal volumes, alveolar collapse, arteriovenous shunting, and hypoxemia, resulting in prolonged mechanical ventilation [9]. This may cause complications such as pneumonia and sepsis [10, 11]. Because the stability of the chest wall is intimately related to the ability to ventilate and subsequently oxygenate, it may seem almost intuitive that stabilization of the bony thorax would result in improved ventilation and ultimately improve outcomes in this patient population. Therefore, the structural integrity of the chest wall provides a theoretical advantage of improved lung functional reserve following surgical stabilization secondary to the restoration of greater lung volumes.

Nonoperative management has been associated with substantial pain and discomfort [9]. Fractured ribs managed nonoperatively are cyclically displaced during breathing while they are healing. This may lead to malunion or nonunion, which may require future surgery [12, 13]. The key to nonoperative management relies fully on various pain control methods (IV and oral narcotics, nonsteroidal antiinflammatory medications, intercostal and paravertebral blocks, patient-controlled analgesia, pleural catheters, and epidural analgesia), pulmonary toilet, and, if necessary, positive pressure mechanical ventilation. Reported long-term problems are rare, and most broken ribs heal uneventfully.

Ultimately, significant clinical equipoise exists regarding the management of rib fractures surgically, and operative intervention remains controversial [14]. Reported short-term benefits of open reduction and internal fixation (ORIF) for rib fractures and flail chest include earlier restoration of pulmonary function [9, 11, 15], fewer complications associated with mechanical ventilation [10, 11, 16, 17], and more intensive care unit (ICU)– and hospital-free days [9, 11]. Some of the potential long-term benefits of surgical fixation may be reduced long-term pain, pulmonary dysfunction, and skeletal deformity [18].

Tanaka et al. [11] randomized 37 patients 5 days after injury to be treated with surgical fixation or internal pneumatic stabilization. Ventilator management was the same for both groups, and at 1 month following injury, patients who underwent surgery required less ventilator support ($p < 0.05$) and had lower

DOI: 10.1201/9781003316800-17

rates of pneumonia ($p < 0.05$), more ICU-free days ($p < 0.05$), and lower medical costs ($p < 0.05$) than patients treated with intubation and mechanical ventilation. They also showed that patients who underwent surgical stabilization had improved early forced expiratory volume in 1 second (FEV_1) and significantly more of them were able to return to their previous employment 6 months after injury.

Granetzny et al. [19] conducted a randomized trial of 40 patients with flail chest. The operatively treated group was compared with patients treated with external adhesive plaster. Eighty-five percent of the patients in the surgical group achieved chest wall stability, while only 50% of the nonoperative group achieved stability. The operatively managed patients required an average of 2 days on the ventilator, while the nonoperative patients spent an average of 12 days on the ventilator. Pulmonary function tests at 2 months indicated that the operatively treated group had a significantly less restrictive pattern ($p < 0.001$), as indicated by the measurement of forced vital capacity and total lung capacity. The surgical group also had significantly fewer days in the ICU and as inpatients ($p < 0.001$) along with having a lower rate of pneumonia ($p = 0.014$) [19].

Pieracci et al. [20] conducted a multicenter, prospective, controlled, clinical trial (12 centers) comparing surgical stabilization of rib fracture (SSRF) in 110 patients within 72 hours to medical management of patients with three or more ipsilateral, severely displaced rib fractures without flail chest. The primary outcome was the numeric pain score (NPS) at a 2-week follow-up. Narcotic consumption, spirometry, pulmonary function tests, pleural space complications (tube thoracostomy or surgery for retained hemothorax or empyema >24 hours from admission), and both overall and respiratory disability–related quality of life (RD-QoL) were also compared. Of the 110 subjects, 51 (46.4%) underwent SSRF. NPS was significantly lower in the operative as compared with the nonoperative group (2.9 vs. 4.5, $p < 0.01$), and RD-QoL was significantly improved (disability score, 21 vs. 25, $p = 0.03$). Pleural space complications were significantly lower in the operative group. The authors concluded that SSRF performed within 72 hours improved the primary outcome of NPS at a 2-week follow-up among patients with three or more displaced fractures in the absence of a flail chest.

Marasco et al. [21] conducted a prospective multicenter randomized controlled trial (RCT) comparing rib fixation to nonoperative management of nonventilated patients with at least three consecutive rib fractures. A total of 124 patients were enrolled at four sites between 2017 and 2020. Sixty-one patients were randomized to operative management and 63 to nonoperative management. No differences were seen in the primary endpoint of Pain Rating Index at 3 months or in the QoL measures. Return-to-work rates improved between 3 and 6 months, favoring the operative group. No improvements in pain or QoL at 3 and 6 months in patients undergoing rib fixation for nonflail, non-ventilator-dependent rib fractures were seen.

Liang et al. [22] published a meta-analysis to evaluate the clinical prognosis of surgical fixation of MRFs. They looked at (1) hospital-related endpoints (including duration of mechanical ventilation, ICU length of stay [LOS], and hospital LOS), (2) complications, (3) pulmonary function, and (4) pain scores.

Authors searched PubMed, Embase, and Cochrane databases for randomized and prospective studies published before January 2018. The surgical group had a reduced duration of mechanical ventilation, ICU LOS, and hospital LOS. Complications likewise were less common in the surgical group, including pneumonia, mortality, chest wall deformity, dyspnea, chest wall tightness, and incidence of tracheostomy. There were no differences between the surgical and nonsurgical groups in terms of pulmonary function, such as forced vital capacity and pain scores. The authors concluded that their meta-analysis supported surgical fixation, rather than conservative treatment, for MRFs.

Long et al. [23] conducted a meta-analysis to determine the optimal treatment for MRFs. Six databases (PubMed, Medline, Embase, Cochrane, Cnki, Wanfang Database) were queried for RCTs published before January 2020. MRFs were treated either with ORIF or conservative treatment involving 538 MRF patients (260 were treated surgically vs. 278 conservatively) were included for analysis. Surgical treatment resulted in a shorter length of hospital stay and duration of mechanical ventilation, with a lower risk of complications, including pneumonia and chest wall deformity. After excluding one study with significant heterogeneity, the analysis showed that the rate of tracheostomy was lower in the surgical group. The authors concluded that in patients with MRFs, surgical treatment resulted in faster recovery, a lower risk of complications, and a better prognosis than nonoperative treatment.

Thus, the practice of surgical rib stabilization has generated a significant amount of interest in recent years. Some studies claim surgical stabilization can decrease mortality; shorten mechanical ventilation days, hospital LOS, and ICU LOS; and decrease the incidence of pneumonia and the need for tracheostomy. Selection bias is a significant concern, and it appears sicker patients who are likely to have worse outcomes are less likely to undergo surgical management. The literature does not fully address surgery-specific complications such as the need for reoperation, nonunion, malunion, and surgical site complications. If a study is designed to explore the potential benefits, it needs to have a very specific pain management protocol that must be complied with in both the surgical and nonsurgical arms to get truly valid data. To date, that is a glaring weakness of the study design and may be difficult to do secondary to resource limitations such as the availability of anesthesia providers to place epidural catheters and differences in regional pain management practice patterns. The current evidence has yet to delineate the patient population that may benefit from chest wall stabilization.

RECOMMENDATION

The current body of literature does not support the routine use of surgical stabilization in patients with multiple rib fractures. The standard management of chest wall injury remains excellent for aggressive multimodal pain control and early mobilization to allow adequate pulmonary toilet.

Grade of recommendation: B.

17.2 In Trauma Patients with Traumatic Hemothorax Who Require Blood Transfusion, Should Blood Collected from the Hemothorax Routinely Be Autotransfused?

Historically, autotransfusion has been described in both civilian and military literature [24, 25]. In 1957, Ferrara published an article in the *Southern Medical Journal* describing the technique at his facility for performing autotransfusion in the setting of a traumatic hemothorax [26]. The technique of autotransfusion with blood drained from a hemothorax has been described clinically for nearly 80 years [27]. Concerns regarding the safety of transfused blood have prompted reconsideration of the use of allogeneic (from an unrelated donor) red blood cell (RBC) transfusion and a range of techniques to minimize transfusion requirements [28].

Although the practice of autotransfusion is well described historically, it is not well studied in the trauma population. It has been most rigorously studied in the cardiac surgery population [18, 26, 29, 30]. In the trauma literature, the majority of clinical reports are case series and case reports that are descriptive in nature [18, 24, 25, 31]. There are prospective randomized studies in the trauma literature; however, they primarily look at the variance in laboratory indicators of coagulation and not clinical outcomes or studies of efficacy [32–34].

Body et al. [29] conducted a multicenter prospective trial to determine the efficacy and safety of autotransfusion of mediastinal blood in 617 patients undergoing elective primary coronary artery bypass grafting. They found that shed mediastinal blood was ineffective as a blood conservation method and may be associated with a greater frequency of wound infection [29]. Helm et al. [26] conducted a prospective randomized study of patients undergoing coronary artery bypass or cardiac valve surgery to determine the benefit of the acute removal and reinfusion of fresh autologous blood around the time of cardiopulmonary bypass—a technique known as intraoperative autologous donation (IAD). They concluded that autotransfusion did not affect postoperative bleeding or platelet and coagulation factor transfusion requirements [26]. Ward et al. [18] prospectively randomized 35 consecutive cardiac surgery patients into two groups and found that neither group demonstrated transfusion-related complications, and autotransfusion of shed mediastinal blood did not decrease the need for homologous blood transfusion [18]. Eng et al. [30] conducted a prospective, randomized, controlled study in two matched groups of 20 patients undergoing elective coronary artery bypass surgery. There was no statistically significant difference in the clinical outcome, overall blood loss, use of platelets, fresh-frozen plasma and colloids, hematological indices, renal and hepatic functions, or clotting mechanism [30].

Broadie et al. [32] collected from the body cavities of 31 trauma victims with indications for intraoperative transfusion. Blood was collected at thoracotomy or laparotomy before the institution of any anticoagulant measures and was assessed for clotting competence, the presence of fibrinogen, the presence of soluble fibrin monomers, and the appearance of fibrin degradation products. The prothrombin time, partial thromboplastin

time, and thrombin time of this blood were markedly elevated; fibrinogen was absent; soluble fibrin monomer was absent, and fibrin degradation products were markedly elevated. They concluded that the blood collected from body cavities is incoagulable [32].

Lassié et al. [27] conducted a prospective study that assessed an autotransfusion system in 30 patients suffering from a hemothorax. The retransfusion took place in less than 4 hours, and patients with an isolated hemothorax did not receive any homologous blood. The shed blood was analyzed and found to have decreased platelets and fibrinogen and was incoagulable. Its hematocrit was lower than the patient's, but the concentration of 2,3-diphosphoglycerate (DPG) remained normal [27].

Barriot et al. [31] reviewed 18 patients with life-threatening traumatic hemothorax who received prehospital autotransfusion. Hemorrhagic blood was not coagulable and had a hematocrit of 20% ± 4%, few platelets, and low fibrinogen levels. Five patients died from irreversible hemorrhagic shock. Thirteen patients were alive on admission to the hospital, underwent emergency surgery, and were discharged alive. During autotransfusion, hematocrit decreased from 24% ± 3% to 19% ± 3%, and systolic arterial pressure increased from 78 ± 11 to 88 ± 12 mmHg. On admission to the hospital, platelet count was 90,800 ± 21,400/mm^3, prothrombin time 48% ± 3%, partial thromboplastin time 197% ± 18%, plasma-free hemoglobin levels 21 ± 7 mg/100 mL, and serum potassium levels 3.6 ± 0.5 mmol/L. No serious complications were attributed to autotransfusion [31].

Ahmed et al. [35] reported on a large series of patients undergoing autotransfusion during the Somali Civil War between 1992 and 2001. This was a retrospective study that looked at 45,900 war-wounded patients, 13,770 of whom had chest injuries. There was no blood bank and a lack of donors; therefore, it was necessary to set up a system for immediate autotransfusion in patients with massive hemothorax from penetrating chest war wounds. A total of 137 patients had autotransfusion. There were five deaths (3.6% mortality rate), and no major complications were detected in the autotransfusion patients who survived [35].

A group of investigators at the University of Texas Health Science Center in San Antonio, Texas, conducted two prospective studies looking at blood from trauma patients who received thoracostomy tubes [33, 34]. The first study was a prospective descriptive study of adult patients from whom ≥50 mL of blood was drained within the first 4 hours after chest tube placement. Pleural and venous blood samples were analyzed for coagulation, hematology, and electrolytes. The group enrolled 22 subjects. The measured coagulation factors of hemothorax were significantly depleted compared with venous blood: International normalized ratio (>9 in contrast to 1.1, $p < 0.001$), activated partial thromboplastin time (aPTT; >180 in contrast to 28.5 seconds, $p < 0.001$), and fibrinogen (<50 in contrast to 288 mg/dL, $p < 0.001$). The mean hematocrit (26.4 in contrast to 33.9, $p = 0.003$), hemoglobin (9.3 in contrast to 11.8 g/dL, $p = 0.004$), and platelet count (53 in contrast to 174 K/µL, $p < 0.001$) of hemothorax were significantly lower than venous blood. Hemothorax blood contains significantly decreased coagulation factors and has lower hemoglobin when compared with venous blood [33].

The second study was a prospective descriptive study of 34 adult patients with traumatic chest injuries necessitating tube thoracostomy. Pleural and venous samples were analyzed for coagulation, hematology, and electrolytes at 1–4 hours after drainage. Pleural samples were also analyzed for their effect on the coagulation cascade via mixing studies. Coagulation factors were significantly depleted in hemothorax blood compared with venous blood: International normalized ratio (>9 vs. 1.1, $p < 0.001$) and aPTT (>180 vs. 24.5 seconds, $p < 0.001$). Mixing studies showed a dose-dependent increase in coagulation dilutions through 1:8 ($p < 0.05$). The authors concluded that an evacuated hemothorax does not vary in composition significantly with time and is incoagulable alone. Mixing studies with hemothorax plasma increased coagulation, raising safety concerns if the hemothorax blood were to be autotransfused [34].

Carless conducted a Cochrane review [28] in 2010 to examine the evidence for the efficacy of cell salvage in reducing allogeneic blood transfusion and the evidence for any effect on clinical outcomes. They selected RCTs with a concurrent control group in which adult patients scheduled for nonurgent surgery were randomized to cell salvage (autotransfusion) or to a control group who did not receive the intervention. Data were independently extracted, and the risk of bias was assessed. The primary outcomes were the number of patients exposed to allogeneic red cell transfusion and the amount of blood transfused. Overall, the use of cell salvage reduced the rate of exposure to allogeneic RBC transfusion by a relative 38% (risk ratio [RR] 0.62; 95% confidence interval [CI], 0.55–0.70). The absolute reduction in risk of receiving an allogeneic RBC transfusion was 21% (95% CI, 15–26%). In orthopedic procedures, the RR of exposure to RBC transfusion was 0.46 (95% CI, 0.37–0.57) compared with 0.77 (95% CI, 0.69–0.86) for cardiac procedures. The use of cell salvage resulted in an average saving of 0.68 units of allogeneic RBCs per patient (weighted mean difference [WMD] −0.68; 95% CI, −0.88 to −0.49). Cell salvage did not adversely impact clinical outcomes. The authors concluded that cell salvage is efficacious in reducing the need for allogeneic red cell transfusion in adult elective cardiac and orthopedic surgery [28]. Although this review is quite comprehensive, especially regarding the cardiac and orthopedic literature, it does not specifically address trauma patients with autotransfused hemothoraces.

Harrison et al. [36] developed a model of hemothorax autotransfusion and looked at its impact on coagulopathy. The authors included adult trauma patients from whom greater than 140 mL of hemothorax was evacuated within 1 hour of tube thoracostomy. Hemothorax was sampled 1 hour after evacuation. Ten subjects were enrolled based on inclusion criteria. In hemothorax samples analyzed alone, no thrombus was formed in any coagulation test (aPTT >180). In 1-hour specimens mixed at a clinically relevant dilution, hemothorax was mixed with normal pooled plasma (NPP) and with patients' own thawed plasma (PTP). Hemothorax + NPP had a median aPTT value of 26.0, whereas hemothorax mixed with PTP had a median aPTT value of 21.7. Thus, the mixture of hemothorax + PTP demonstrated a statistically significantly lower aPTT than the mixture of hemothorax + NPP ($P = 0.01$).

Additionally, the mixture of hemothorax and PTP shows a statistically significantly lower aPTT value than PTP alone ($P = 0.03$), indicating a hypercoagulable state. The authors concluded that hemothorax demonstrates coagulopathy when analyzed independently, but is hypercoagulable when mixed with NPP or PTP. Furthermore, mixing studies show a statistically significantly lower aPTT when hemothorax is mixed with PTP versus hemothorax mixed with NPP. Traumatic hemothorax has been demonstrated to predictably contain low fibrinogen, low hematocrit, and low platelet counts. When analyzed on its own, shed hemothorax demonstrates coagulopathy. However, when mixed with NPP at physiologically relevant dilutions, hemothorax demonstrates accelerated coagulation. They concluded autotransfusion of hemothorax would likely produce a hypercoagulable state in vivo and should not be used in place of other blood products to resuscitate a trauma patient. The autotransfusion of hemothorax may, however, be of use in a resource-limited environment where other blood products are not available [36].

Mitchell et al. [37] hypothesized that induction of coagulopathic changes by shed hemothorax blood may be due to increases in cellular microparticles (MPs) and that these may also affect recipient platelet function. Shed hemothorax blood was obtained from 17 adult trauma patients under an institutional review board–approved prospective observational protocol. Blood samples were collected every hour up to 4 hours after thoracostomy tube placement. The effects of shed hemothorax frozen plasma (HFP) and isolated hemothorax microparticles (HMPs) on coagulation and platelet function were assessed through mixing studies. HFP was also assessed for von Willebrand factor (vWF) antigen levels and multimer content and plasma-free hemoglobin. ROTEM showed that diluted HFP and isolated HMP samples decreased clotting time, clotting formation time, and increased α angle, irrespective of sample concentrations when compared with diluted control plasma. Isolated HMP inhibited platelet aggregation. MP concentrations in HFP were significantly increased. vWF multimer analysis revealed a significant loss of high molecular weight multimers in HFP samples. The authors concluded that HFP induces plasma hypercoagulability that is likely related to increased tissue factor and phosphatidylserine expression originating from cell-derived MP. In contrast, platelet dysfunction is induced by HMP, potentially aggravated by depletion of high molecular weight multimers of vWF. Thus, autologous transfusion of shed traumatic hemothorax blood may induce a range of undesirable effects in patients with acute traumatic coagulopathy [37].

RECOMMENDATION

Current evidence does not support the routine autotransfusion of traumatic hemothorax. We recommend that autotransfusion be considered when transfusion is required in a patient with a large traumatic hemothorax and resources are limited.

Grade of recommendation: C.

17.3 Should Small-Bore Chest Drainage Catheters Be Used Rather than Large-Bore Tubes for Traumatic Hemothorax?

In elective cardiac surgery, blood accumulating inside chest cavities can lead to serious complications if it is not drained properly [38]. In trauma patients, a similar argument can be made. The optimal chest tube size for the drainage of traumatic hemothoraces and pneumothoraces is unknown [39, 40]. Patients experience increasing discomfort with increasing drain size [38]. Smaller tube sizes may cause less pain and possibly result in improved respiratory effort and pulmonary toilet. The concern with smaller tubes is whether or not they will adequately drain a hemothorax. Because life-threatening conditions can result from chest tube occlusion after thoracic surgery, large-bore tubes are generally employed to optimize patency [38].

Rahman et al. [41] studied the effect of tube size on the management of empyema. They prospectively enrolled a total of 405 patients with pleural infection in a multicenter study investigating the utility of fibrinolytic therapy. The combined frequency of death and surgery and secondary outcomes (hospital stay, change in chest radiograph, and lung function at 3 months) were compared in patients receiving different size chest tubes. Tubes were stratified according to size as follows: <10 Fr, 10–14 Fr, 15–20 Fr, and >20 Fr. They did find that smaller, guidewire-inserted chest tubes cause substantially less pain than blunt dissection–inserted larger tubes, without any impairment in clinical outcome in the treatment of pleural infection. The authors concluded that smaller-size tubes may be the initial treatment of choice for pleural infection, and randomized studies are now required [41].

Rivera et al. [42] conducted a retrospective trauma registry review of tube thoracostomies at a Level 1 trauma center after the center adopted the practice of using small catheter tube thoracostomy (SCTT) as a less invasive method to manage nonemergent chest injuries. During their study period, 565 tube thoracostomies were performed on 359 patients: 252 were deemed emergent and 157 were nonemergent. Of the patients receiving nonemergent tubes, 63 received large catheter tube thoracostomy (LCTT) and 107 received SCTT. The average duration of SCTT was shorter than nonemergent LCCT (5.5 days vs. 7 days, $p < 0.05$). The rate of occurrence of fibrothorax was significantly lower for SCTT compared with nonemergent LCTT (0% vs. 4.2%, $p < 0.05$). The authors concluded that SCTT was effective in managing chest trauma, and data supported their institutional practice of adopting image-guided small catheter techniques in the management of chest trauma in stable patients [42].

Kulvatunyou et al. [40] hypothesized that 14 Fr pigtail catheters (PCs) could drain blood as well as large-bore 32–40 Fr chest tubes. They prospectively collected data on all bedside-inserted PCs in patients with traumatic hemothorax or hemopneumothorax during 30 months (July 2009 through December 2011) at a Level 1 trauma center. They compared their PC prospective data with trauma registry–derived retrospective chest tube data (January 2008 through December 2010). In the study population, they found that 36 patients received PCs and 191 received chest tubes. The primary outcome was the initial drainage output. Secondary outcomes were tube duration, insertion-related complications, and failure rate. The mean initial output was similar between the PC group and the chest tube group. Tube duration, rate of insertion-related complications, and failure rate were all similar between groups. This led Kulvatunyou et al. to conclude that 14 Fr PCs drained blood as well as large-bore chest tubes. They also stated that to make any definitive clinical recommendations, they would need a larger sample size and possibly a well-designed prospective study [40].

Inaba et al. [39] attempted to address the specific issues of adequate drainage and pain as they relate to chest tube size in trauma patients by conducting a prospective observational trial between 2007 and 2010. They collected demographic and outcome data, including the efficacy of drainage, complications, retained hemothoraces, residual pneumothoraces, need for additional tube insertion, VATS, and thoracotomy. The data were then analyzed by tube size stratified as either small (28–32 Fr) or large (36–40 Fr). A total of 353 chest tubes (small, 186; large, 167) were placed in 293 patients. Of the 275 chest tubes inserted for a hemothorax, 144 were small (52.3%) and 131 were large (47.7%). The volume of blood drained initially and the total duration of tube placement were similar for both groups (small 6.3 ± 3.9 days vs. large 6.2 ± 3.6 days; adjusted [adj.] $p = 0.427$). No statistically significant difference in tube-related complications, including pneumonia (4.9% vs. 4.6%; adj. $p = 0.282$), empyema (4.2% vs. 4.6%; adj. $p = 0.766$), or retained hemothorax (11.8% vs. 10.7%; adj. $p = 0.981$), was found. The need for tube reinsertion, image-guided drainage, VATS, and thoracotomy was the same (10.4% vs. 10.7%; adj. $p = 0.719$). For patients with a pneumothorax requiring chest tube drainage ($n = 238$), there was no difference in the number of patients with an unresolved pneumothorax (14.0% vs. 13.0%; adj. $p = 0.620$) or those needing reinsertion of a second chest tube. The mean visual analog pain score was similar for small and large tubes (6.0 ± 3.3 and 6.7 ± 3.0; $p = 0.237$). These findings led the investigators to conclude that tube size did not affect the efficacy of drainage. They also concluded that tube size did not impact tube-associated complication rates or pain [39].

Tanizaki et al. [43] conducted a retrospective review of all patients with chest trauma requiring tube thoracostomy within the first 2 hours from arrival over 7 years. Small chest tubes (20–22 Fr) were compared with a large tube (28 Fr). The primary outcome was tube-related complications. Secondary outcomes included additional invasive procedures, such as additional tube insertion and thoracotomy. The authors looked at 124 tube thoracostomies (small: 68, large: 56) performed in 116 patients. There were no significant differences between the small- and large-tube groups in age, gender, injury mechanism, systolic blood pressure, heart rate, and injury severity score. Both groups were similar in the posterior direction of tube insertion, initial drainage output, and duration of tube insertion. There was no significant difference in the primary outcomes of tube-related complications, including retained hemothorax. Secondary outcomes, including the need for additional tube placement or thoracotomy, were also similar. The study concluded that for patients with chest trauma, emergent insertion of 20–22 Fr chest tubes has no difference in the efficacy of drainage, rate of complications, and need for additional invasive procedures compared with a large tube (28 Fr) [43].

Bauman et al. [44] conducted a study to analyze cumulative experience and outcomes with PCs in patients with traumatic hemothorax/hemopneumothorax. They analyzed all trauma patients who required chest drainage for hemothorax/ hemopneumothorax from 2008 to 2014. Primary outcomes were initial drainage output in milliliters, tube insertion-related complications, and failure rate. During the 7 years, 496 trauma patients required chest drainage for traumatic hemothorax/hemopneumothorax: 307 by chest tubes and 189 by PCs. All primary outcomes were similar, except that the initial drainage output for PCs was higher (425 mL vs. 300 mL). PCs had similar outcomes to chest tubes in terms of failure rate and tube insertion–related complications, and the initial drainage output from PCs was not inferior to that of chest tubes [44].

Kulvatunyou et al. [45] performed a multi-institution prospective RCT comparing 14 Fr PCs with 28–32 Fr chest tubes in the management of patients with traumatic hemothorax from July 2015 to September 2020. The primary outcome was failure rate, defined as a retained hemothorax requiring a second intervention. Secondary outcomes included daily drainage output, tube days, ICU and hospital LOS, and insertion perception experience (IPE) score on a scale of 1–5 (1, tolerable experience; 5, worst experience). A total of 119 patients participated in the trial, 56 were randomized to PCs and 63 to chest tubes. The primary outcome, failure rate, was similar between the two groups (11% PCs vs. 13% chest tubes, $p = 0.74$). All other secondary outcomes were also similar, except PC patients reported lower IPE scores. They concluded small caliber 14 Fr PCs are equally as effective as 28–32-Fr chest tubes in their ability to drain traumatic hemothorax with no difference in complications. Patients reported better IPE scores with PCs over chest tubes, suggesting that PCs are better tolerated [45]. This study is the most impactful in that it compared not only differences in size but the technique. Not requiring blunt dissection to place the PC does impact the patient's improved pain scores that this study demonstrated.

RECOMMENDATION

Small-bore chest tubes are as effective as large-bore drains in patients with traumatic hemothoraces. Smaller tubes reduce patient discomfort during insertion and should be used in the nonemergent setting for stable trauma patients with either a hemothorax or pneumothorax.

Grade of recommendation: C.

17.4 When Should VATS Be Performed in Trauma Patients Who Have a Retained Hemothorax after Initial Tube Thoracostomy?

In patients suffering blunt chest wall trauma, hemothorax is a frequent occurrence that is initially treated with tube thoracostomy. Despite this initial treatment, a significant number of patients will manifest a retained hemothorax. Although the true incidence of retained hemothorax is not known, we do know that it is a strong predictor of empyema, fibrothorax, and subsequent poor outcomes [46, 47]. The presence of retained hemothorax on postplacement chest X-ray (CXR) is an independent predictor of the development of empyema in 33% of patients [48]. Historically the options for management of a retained hemothorax have been to place an additional chest tube, perform open thoracotomy for evacuation of the clot, installation of thrombolytics into the pleural cavity, and VATS. Because VATS is only slightly more invasive than additional tube thoracostomy, in facilities that can perform VATS, it has become the treatment of choice to ensure adequate evacuation of a retained hemothorax and avoidance of subsequent complications [46, 47, 49, 50]. Ultimately, there remains significant clinical equipoise about the timing of the performance of this procedure [46, 47].

Dubose et al. [46] conducted an American Association for the Surgery of Trauma multicenter prospective observational trial, enrolling patients with the placement of a chest tube within 24 hours of trauma admission and RH on subsequent computed tomography of the chest. Demographics, interventions, and outcomes were analyzed. Interventions were at the surgeon's discretion and included observation, additional thoracostomy tube placement or image-guided percutaneous drainage (IGPD), intrapleural thrombolysis, VATS, and thoracotomy. Logistic regression analysis was used to identify the independent predictors of successful intervention for each of the management choices chosen and complications. Retained hemothorax was identified in 328 patients from 20 centers. VATS was the most commonly used initial procedure in 33.5%. Independent predictors of successful VATS as definitive treatment were the absence of an associated diaphragm injury (odds ratio [OR], 4.7 [1.6 –13.7]; p 0.005), use of periprocedural antibiotics for thoracostomy placement (OR, 3.3 [1.2–9.0]; p 0.023), and volume of RH 900 cc (OR, 3.9 [1.4–13.2]; p 0.03). No relationship between the timing of VATS and the success rate was identified. VATS can be performed with high success rates, although the optimal timing is unknown [46].

Meyer et al. [50] conducted a prospective randomized trial comparing the efficacy of additional tube thoracostomy to the VATS procedure. Over 4 years, 39 patients were randomized to a second chest tube or VATS. Patients receiving VATS had shorter duration of tube drainage (2.53 +/– 1.36 versus 4.50 +/– 2.83 days, $p < 0.02$), spent fewer days in the hospital (5.40 +/– 2.16 versus 8.13 +/– 4.62 days; $p < 0.02$), and had reduced hospital costs by 42%. Of the patients who were randomized to receive VATS as their primary treatment for retained hemothorax, none required conversion to a thoracotomy. In the group of patients who received an additional chest tube, 10 of them (41.7%) required an additional procedure, and they were randomized to VATS or thoracotomy. The authors concluded that VATS for retained hemothoraces decreases the duration of tube drainage, the length of hospital stay, and hospital cost [50]. They showed that early intervention with VATS was more efficient and economical than the placement of an additional chest tube.

Oğuzkaya et al. [49] performed a retrospective review over 10 years in 65 patients with retained hemothorax and compared those managed with intrapleural streptokinase to those managed with VATS. VATS is associated with significantly shorter hospital LOS and decreased need for additional therapy. They found that patients undergoing the VATS procedure had more success in evacuation when they looked at conversion rates to open thoracotomy and had significantly shorter hospital stays and concluded VATS is a more effective procedure than intrapleural streptokinase for the treatment of post-traumatic retained hemothorax [49].

Ziaour et al. [51] conducted a systematic review to analyze the optimal time range to evacuate traumatic retained hemothorax. They combined data from six cohort studies for a total of 476 patients. They broke the patients down into three groups based on the timing of the performance of VATS. Group A was from 1 to 3 days, Group B was from 4 to 6 days, and Group C was 7 days and beyond. When they looked at the successful evaluation of the hemothorax, they found that group A had a significantly higher success rate when compared to Group C. When looking at hospital LOS group patients went home 7 days sooner than Group B and Group B patients went home 18.1 days sooner than Group C. They concluded that when the choice to evacuate a retained hemothorax was VATS, the procedure should be done within the first 3 days of hospitalization [51].

Lin et al. [47] retrospectively looked at 136 patients who received VATS for the management of retained hemothorax between 2003 and 2011. They stratified patients into three groups. Group 1 patients had their VATS performed between days 2 and 3, group 2 had their VATS performed between days 4 and 6, and group 3 patients had VATS performed on day 7 or beyond. There were no statistical differences in the demographics between any of the groups. Group 3 had higher rates of positive microbial cultures in pleural collections and sputum, longer duration of chest tube insertion, and ventilator use. The LOS in the hospital and the ICU was longer in group 3 compared to the other groups. The need for repeat VATS was lowest in group 1. The study showed that early VATS reduced the risk of infectious complications, and the authors concluded that should be done within 3 days of the original trauma. For cases where surgery is delayed due to other injuries or patient stability, they concluded that VATS should be performed on or before posttrauma day 6 [47].

Morales Uribe et al. [52] conducted a retrospective cohort study of all patients who received VATS for evaluation of a retained hemothorax. They had data on 139 patients over 8 years. They looked at the success of the procedure. Failure was defined as reaccumulation of the hemothorax

or the need for an additional procedure either VATS or thoracotomy. They reviewed their data at predetermined break points of 3 days, 4 days, 5 days, 6 days, and 7 days. Data showed that when VATS was performed after posttrauma day 5 the risk of needing a thoracotomy and/or additional procedures increased in a statistically significant manner. These data show that there are better outcomes and shorter hospital stays when that is performed before posttrauma day 5 [52].

Huang et al. [53] recognized that evacuation of a retained hemothorax is often delayed as a result of other injuries, particularly in patients with traumatic brain injuries concurrent with their chest trauma. To that end, they conducted a prospective trial over 7 years. Sixty-one patients enrolled with intracranial hemorrhage that did not require craniotomy received VATS due to a retained hemothorax or pneumothorax. Patients were divided into two groups according to the time from trauma to VATS. Group 1 had its procedure within the first 4 days and group 2 had its procedure sometime after 4 days. The clinical outcomes included hospital LOS, ICU LOS, infection rates, ventilator days, and the number of days requiring chest tube drainage. They found that patients in group 1 had fewer ventilator days and shorter hospital and ICU LOS (6.77 vs. 18.55, $p = 0.016$; 20.63 vs. 35.13, $p = 0.003$; 8.97 vs. 17.65, $p = 0.035$). Patients in group 2 also had a higher incidence of positive cultures from the pleural fluid that was drained when compared to group 1. This study is extremely important because it addresses one of the reasons often given for delaying or not performing the VATS procedure. The study showed that it could be performed safely in brain hemorrhage patients without indication for surgical decompression. The clinical outcomes were much better in the patients with brain injury who had their procedure done within 4 days of their original trauma [53].

Abid et al. [54] conducted a prospective cohort study in 2019 and 2020. They enrolled 160 patients prospectively who underwent VATS to attain hemothorax. They defined retained hemothorax as an estimated retained volume after an initial tube thoracostomy of 500 cc. One hundred and three patients underwent the procedure during the first 4–7 days after their trauma while the remainder underwent that between 8 and 14 days after trauma. The patients in the early cohort were statistically more likely to have complete lung expansion, reduced air leaks, earlier removal of the chest tube, and decreased LOS in the hospital. This study showed that it was effective for the management of retained hemothorax and also showed that there were better outcomes when the procedure was performed early rather than in a delayed manner [54].

Of patients who receive a tube thoracostomy for management of a hemothorax, a significant number will have a retained hemothorax. Management options have included observation, placement of additional tube thoracostomy, use of thrombolytics, open thoracotomy, and VATS. VATS has emerged as a reliable, safe, most frequently used, and preferred method for the evacuation of a retained hemothorax [46]. The ability to perform this procedure may vary from institution to institution based on available surgical expertise, credentialing requirements, and operating room availability. Although the exact timing of when to perform the procedure has yet to be fully elucidated, early versus delayed performance increases the likelihood of successful evacuation of the hemothorax and reduces the number of complications [47, 51–54]. The data indicate that early VATS decreases the length of hospital stay, length of ICU stay, days of chest drainage, ventilator days, and number of additional required procedures [47, 51–54].

RECOMMENDATION

VATS is effective, safe, and the preferred method for evacuation of retained hemothorax. The literature shows the early evacuation of retained hemothorax with VATS leads to improved outcomes. We recommend that VATS be performed within 3 days of trauma for retained hemothorax.

Grade of recommendation: B.

EBM Summary Table

Question	Answer	Grade	References
Should open reduction and internal fixation be performed routinely on trauma patients with multiple rib fractures?	The current body of literature does not support the routine use of surgical stabilization in patients with multiple rib fractures. The standard management of chest wall injury remains excellent for early aggressive multimodal pain control and early mobilization to allow adequate pulmonary toilet.	B	[11, 19–23]
In Trauma patients with traumatic hemothorax who require blood transfusion, should blood collected from the hemothorax routinely be autotransfused?	Current evidence does not support the routine autotransfusion of traumatic hemothorax. We recommend that in the clinical scenario where transfusion is required and a significant traumatic hemothorax exists in a resource-limited or austere environment, the clinician should consider the urgency of the situation and balance the risks and benefits of autotransfusion for patients on an individual basis.	C	[18, 26–37]
Should small-bore chest drainage catheters be used rather than large-bore tubes for traumatic hemothorax?	The body of literature and clinical experience show smaller tubes reduce patient discomfort during insertion and should be used in the nonemergent setting for stable trauma patients with either a hemothorax or pneumothorax.	C	[39–45]
When should VATS be performed in trauma patients who have a retained hemothorax after initial tube thoracostomy?	We recommend that VATS be performed within 3 days of trauma for retained hemothorax. In patients with absolute contraindications to early performance, all efforts should be made to complete evacuation within 6 days to optimize clinical outcomes.	B	[47, 50–54]

Editor's Note

As one of the few trauma surgeons (hopefully) who has experienced a flail chest personally, I can attest to the pain incurred. However, nonsteroidal antiinflammatory medications and a strong dose of "biting the bullet" allowed me to go home the next day and deal with the discomfort. Therefore, I am naturally skeptical when clinicians suggest the great value of operative fixation of rib fractures. It is clear that excellent results can be seen in the majority of patients when adequate pain control and pulmonary toilet are utilized. While there are likely some patients who might benefit from operative fixation of their chest wall, it is unclear who this subpopulation represents. In my experience, many trauma centers struggle to meet the basic objective of pain control in the setting of chest wall injury. Multimodality pain regimens, including NSAIDs and regional analgesic blocks are often underutilized. Instead, narcotics administered as patient-controlled analgesia are employed with limited success. Lidoderm patches, intravenous acetaminophen, and gabapentin are all proven to be of little to no value in this setting, yet are frequently used. Optimizing pain control utilizing proven modalities appears prudent.

REFERENCES

1. Bergeron E, Lavoie A, Clas D, Moore L, Ratte S, Tetreault S, Lemaire J, Martin M. Elderly trauma patients with rib fractures are at greater risk of death and pneumonia. *J Trauma.* 2003;*54*:478–485.
2. Holcomb JB, McMullin NR, Kozar RA, Lygas MH, Moore FA. Morbidity from rib fractures increases after age 45. *J Am Coll Surg.* 2003;*196*:549–555.
3. Sirmali M, Türüt H, Topcxu S, Gülhan E, Yazici U, Kaya S, Tasxtepe I. A comprehensive analysis of traumatic rib fractures: Morbidity, mortality, and management. *Eur J Cardiothorac Surg.* 2003;*24*:133–138.
4. Brasel KJ, Guse CE, Layde P, Weigelt JA. Rib fractures: Relationship with pneumonia and mortality. *Crit Care Med.* 2006;*34*:1642–1646.
5. Ciraulo DL, Elliott D, Mitchell KA, Rodriguez A. Flail chest as a marker for significant injuries. *J Am Coll Surg.* 1994;*178*:466–470.
6. Kent R, Woods W, Bostrom O. Fatality risk and the presence of rib fractures. *Annu Proc Assoc Adv Automot Med.* 2008;*52*:73–82.
7. Landercasper J, Cogbill TH, Lindesmith LA. Long-term disability after flail chest injury. *J Trauma.* 1984;*24*:410–414.

8. Bulger EM, Arneson MA, Mock CN, Jurkovich GJ. Rib fractures in the elderly. *J Trauma*. 2000;*48*:1040–1047.

9. Ahmed Z, Mohyuddin Z. Management of flail chest injury: Internal fixation versus endotracheal intubation and ventilation. *J Thorac Cardiovasc Surg*. 1995;*110*:1676–1680.

10. Lardinois D, Krueger T, Dusmet M, Ghisletta N, Gugger M, Ris HB. Pulmonary function testing after operative stabilization of the chest wall for the flail chest. *Eur J Cardiothorac Surg*. 2001;*20*:496–501.

11. Tanaka H, Yukioka T, Yamaguti Y, Shimizu S, Goto H, Matsuda H, Shimazaki S. Surgical stabilization of internal pneumatic stabilization? A prospective randomized study of management of severe flail chest patients. *J Trauma*. 2002;*52*:727–732.

12. Cacchione RN, Richardson JD, Seligson D. Painful non-union of multiple rib fractures managed by operative stabilization. *J Trauma*. 2000;*48*:319–321.

13. Slater MS, Mayberry JC, Trunkey DD. Operative stabilization of a flail chest six years after injury. *Ann Thorac Surg*. 2001;*72*:600–601.

14. Nirula R, Diaz JJ, Jr., Trunkey DD, Mayberry JC. Rib fracture repair: Indications, technical issues, and future directions. *World J Surg*. 2009;*33*:14–22.

15. Voggenreiter G, Neudeck F, Aufmkolk M, Obertacke U, Schmit-Neuerburg KP. Operative chest wall stabilization in flail chest—Outcomes of patients with or without pulmonary contusion. *J Am Coll Surg*. 1998;*187*:130–138.

16. Karev DV. Operative management of the flail chest. *Wiad Lek*. 1997;*50(Suppl 1)*:205–208.

17. Velmahos GC, Vassiliu P, Chan LS, Murray JA, Berne TV, Demetriades D. Influence of flail chest on outcome among patients with severe thoracic cage trauma. *Int Surg*. 2002;*87*:240–244.

18. Ward HE, Smith RR, Landis KP, et al. Prospective, randomized trial of autotransfusion after routine cardiac operations. *Ann Thorac Surg*. 1993;*56(1)*:137–141.

19. Granetzny A, Abd El-Aal M, Emam E, Shalaby A, Boseila A. Surgical versus conservative treatment of flail chest. Evaluation of the pulmonary status. *Interact Cardiovasc Thorac Surg*. 2005;*4*:583–587.

20. Pieracci FM, Leasia K, Bauman Z, et al. A multicenter, prospective, controlled clinical trial of surgical stabilization of rib fractures in patients with severe, nonflail fracture patterns (Chest Wall Injury Society NONFLAIL). *J Trauma Acute Care Surg*. 2020;*88(2)*:249–257.

21. Marasco SF, Balogh ZJ, Wullschleger ME, et al. Rib fixation in non-ventilator-dependent chest wall injuries: A prospective randomized trial. *J Trauma Acute Care Surg*. 2022;*92(6)*:1047–1053.

22. Liang YS, Yu KC, Wong CS, Kao Y, Tiong TY, Tam KW. Does surgery reduce the risk of complications among patients with multiple rib fractures? A meta-analysis [published correction appears in Clin Orthop Relat Res. 2019 Mar;477(3): 667]. *Clin Orthop Relat Res*. 2019;*477(1)*:193–205.

23. Long R, Tian J, Wu S, Li Y, Yang X, Fei J. Clinical efficacy of surgical versus conservative treatment for multiple rib fractures: A meta-analysis of randomized controlled trials. *Int J Surg*. 2020;*83*:79–88.

24. Symbas PN. Autotransfusion from hemothorax: Experimental and clinical studies. *J Trauma*. 1972;*12(8)*: 689–695.

25. Ferrara, BE. Autotransfusion: Its use in acute hemothorax. *South Med J*. 1957;*50*:516–519.

26. Helm RE, Klemperer JD, Rosengart TK, et al. Intraoperative autologous blood donation preserves red cell mass but does not decrease postoperative bleeding. *Ann Thorac Surg*. 1996;*62*:1431–1441.

27. Lassié P, Sztark F, Petitjean ME. Autotransfusion, with blood drained from a hemothorax, using the ConstaVac device. *Ann Fr Anesth Reanim*. 1994;*13(6)*:781–784.

28. Carless PA, Henry DA, Moxey AJ, O'Connell D, Brown T, Fergusson DA. Cell salvage for minimizing perioperative allogeneic blood transfusion. *Cochrane Database Syst Rev*. 2010;*(4)*: CD001888.

29. Body SC, Birmingham J, Parks R, et al. Safety and efficacy of shed mediastinal blood transfusion after cardiac surgery: A multicenter observational study. Multicenter Study of Perioperative Ischemia Research Group. *J Cardiothorac Vasc Anesth*. 1999;*13(4)*:410–416.

30. Eng J, Kay PH, Murday AJ, et al. Postoperative autologous transfusion in cardiac surgery. A prospective, randomized study. *Eur J Cardiothorac Surg*. 1990;*4(11)*:595–600.

31. Barriot P, Riots B, Viarst P. Prehospital autotransfusion in life-threatening hemothorax. *Chest*. 1988;*93(3)*:522–526.

32. Broadie TA, Glover JL, Bang N, et al. Clotting competence of intracavitary blood in trauma victims. *Ann Emerg Med*. 1981;*10(3)*:127–130.

33. Salhanick M (1), Corneille M, Higgins R, et al. Autotransfusion of hemothorax blood in trauma patients: Is it the same as fresh whole blood? *Am J Surg*. 2011;*202(6)*:817–821.

34. Smith WZ, Harrison HB, Salhanick MA, et al. A small amount can make a difference: A prospective human study of the paradoxical coagulation characteristics of hemothorax. *Am J Surg*. 2013;*206(6)*:904–909.

35. Ahmed AM, Riye MH, Baldan M, Autotransfusion in penetrating chest war trauma with haemothorax: The Keysaney hospital experience. *East Cent Afr J Surg*. 2003;*8(1)*:51–54.

36. Harrison HB, Smith WZ, Salhanick MA, et al. An experimental model of hemothorax autotransfusion: Impact on coagulation. *Am J Surg*. 2014;*208(6)*:1078–1082.

37. Mitchell TA, Herzig MC, Fedyk CG, et al. Traumatic hemothorax blood contains elevated levels of microparticles that are prothrombotic but inhibit platelet aggregation. *Shock*. 2017;*47(6)*:680–687.

38. Shalli S, Saeed D, Fukamachi K, et al. Chest tube selection in cardiac and thoracic surgery: A survey of chest tube related complications and their management. *J Card Surg*. 2009;*24(5)*:503–509.

39. Inaba K, Lustenberger T, Recinos G, et al. Does size matter? A prospective analysis of 28–32 versus 36–40 French chest tube size in trauma. *J Trauma*. 2012;*72*:422–427.

40. Kulvatunyou K, Joseph B, Friese RS, et al. 14 French pigtail catheters placed by surgeons to drain blood on trauma patients: Is 14-Fr too small? *J Trauma Acute Care Surg*. 2012;*6*:1423–1427.

41. Rahman NM, Maskell NA, Davies CW, et al. The relationship between chest tube size and clinical outcome in pleural infection. *Chest*. 2010;*137(3)*:536–543.

42. Rivera L, O'Reilly EB, Sise MJ, et al. Small catheter tube thoracostomy: Effective in managing chest trauma in stable patients. *J Trauma*. 2009;*66*:393–399.

43. Tanizaki S, Maeda S, Sera M, et al. Small tube thoracostomy (20–22 Fr) in emergent management of chest trauma. *Injury.* 2017;*48*(9):1884–1887.

44. Bauman ZM, Kulvatunyou N, Joseph B, et al. A prospective study of 7-year experience using percutaneous 14-French pigtail catheters for traumatic hemothorax/hemopneumothorax at a level-1 trauma center: Size still does not matter. *World J Surg.* 2018;*42*(1):107–113.

45. Kulvatunyou N, Bauman ZM, Zein Edine SB, et al. The small (14 Fr) percutaneous catheter (P-CAT) versus large (28–32 Fr) open chest tube for traumatic hemothorax: A multicenter randomized clinical trial. *J Trauma Acute Care Surg.* 2021;*91*(5):809–813.

46. DuBose J, Inaba K, Demetriades D, et al. Management of post-traumatic retained hemothorax: A prospective, observational, multicenter AAST study. *J Trauma Acute Care Surg.* 2012;*72*(1):11–316. doi:10.1097/TA.0b013e318242e368

47. Lin HL, Huang WY, Yang C, et al. How early should VATS be performed for retained haemothorax in blunt chest trauma? *Injury.* 2014;*45*(9):1359–1364. doi:10.1016/j.injury.2014.05.036

48. Mowery NT, Gunter OL, Collier BR, et al. Practice management guidelines for the management of hemothorax and occult pneumothorax. *J Trauma.* 2011;*70*(2):510–518. doi:10.1097/TA.0b013e31820b5c31

49. Oğuzkaya F, Akçali Y, Bilgin M. Videothoracoscopy versus intrapleural streptokinase for management of post traumatic retained haemothorax: A retrospective study of 65 cases. *Injury.* 2005;*36*(4):526–529. doi:10.1016/j.injury.2004.10.008

50. Meyer DM, Jessen ME, Wait MA, Estrera AS. Early evacuation of traumatic retained hemothoraces using thoracoscopy: A prospective, randomized trial. *Ann Thorac Surg.* 1997;*64*(5):1396–1401. doi:10.1016/S0003-4975(97)00899-0

51. Ziapour B, Mostafidi E, Sadeghi-Bazargani H, Kabir A, Okereke I. Timing to perform VATS for traumatic-retained hemothorax (a systematic review and meta-analysis). *Eur J Trauma Emerg Surg.* 2020;*46*(2):337–346. doi:10.1007/s00068-019-01275-2

52. Morales Uribe CH, Villegas Lanau MI, Petro Sánchez RD. Best timing for thoracoscopic evacuation of retained post-traumatic hemothorax. *Surg Endosc.* 2008;*22*(1):91–95. doi:10.1007/s00464-007-9378-6

53. Huang FD, Yeh WB, Chen SS, et al. Early management of retained hemothorax in blunt head and chest trauma. *World J Surg.* 2018;*42*(7):2061–2066. doi:10.1007/s00268-017-4420-x

54. Abid A, Ahmad T, Shaikh KA, Nasreen S, Sikander N, Mazcuri M. Video assisted thoracoscopy as a therapeutic modality in evacuating retained or clotted haemothoraces. *J Pak Med Assoc.* 2021;*71*(5):1428–1431. doi:10.47391/JPMA.288

18

Injury to the Thoracic Great Vessels

Mark Cockburn

18.1 Introduction

Chest injury from blunt trauma is a significant cause of morbidity and mortality. Most of the literature published on injury to the thoracic great vessels has focused on the aorta and on blunt thoracic aortic injury (BTAI), which is a devastating injury that requires early recognition to minimize morbidity and mortality. It has been estimated that there are about 8,000 cases of blunt aortic injury (BAI) each year in the United States [1]. Approximately 80–85% die at the scene or in transport [2]. This injury most commonly results from motor vehicle collisions [3], but we have seen an increase in fatalities from this injury among pedestrians hit by cars [4]. The remaining mechanisms for this injury include falls from heights and crushing chest injuries.

18.2 What Is the Ultimate Imaging Modality for Diagnosing Blunt Thoracic Aortic Injury?

The chest X-ray is a good screening tool and is usually one of the first studies obtained on the trauma patient. Angiography remains the standard by which most other diagnostic tests are compared. There are Level 2 data that have supported helical or spiral computed tomographic scanners as having an extremely high negative predictive value and may be used to rule out BTAI [3]. As only 20% of the 8,000 BTAIs (or 1,600 patients in the entire United States each year) survive to reach the hospital, this lesion is rarely seen at trauma centers, and it is easy for an imaging technique to have a high negative predictive value (as there are very few "true positive" studies).

TABLE 18.1

Clinical Questions

Question	Answer	Grade of Recommendation
What is the ultimate imaging modality for diagnosing BTAI?	CT angiography of the chest has become the study of choice for making the diagnosis of BTAI.	B
What modality should be used to follow MAIs from blunt trauma?	Multidetector CT angiography of the chest has become the modality for following MAIs.	B
What medications should we use in the medical management of MAI, and for how long should patients be required to take these medications?	β-Blockade and intravenous vasodilator therapy should be used for the medical management of MAIs.	B
When is nonoperative management to be considered?	MAIs can be managed nonoperatively with specific medical treatment protocols to control heart rate and blood pressure.	B
What is the target blood pressure to maintain when nonoperative management or delayed surgical therapy is considered?	Controlling the heart rate and blood pressure (systolic between 100 and 120 mmHg) using β-blockade and intravenous vasodilator is effective in preventing rupture of BTAI.	B
Which operative technique should be used for the repair of descending thoracic aortic injuries? Is any technique superior?	Some form of distal perfusion should be used because neurologic complications seem to correlate with ischemia time.	B
Are endovascular stent procedures superior to open vascular procedures?	Endovascular stent grafts are associated with less mortality, fewer postoperative neurologic complications including paraplegia, and fewer systemic complications than open procedures.	B

Abbreviations: BTAI: Blunt thoracic aortic injury, MAI: Minimal aortic injury.

DOI: 10.1201/9781003316800-18

However, accurate early detection remains crucial, as delays in the diagnosis of aortic tears lead to poor outcomes. A review of the literature comparing CT angiography of the chest with catheter-based angiography for diagnosing clinically significant BTAI resulted in six studies directly comparing the two. The sensitivities of both tests were very high, but the overall specificity is lower for CT compared to aortography. CT scanning of the chest with intravenous contrast is now readily available, less invasive, less time-consuming, and provides other secondary information, including other injuries [5].

RECOMMENDATION

CT of the chest with intravenous contrast is strongly recommended for making the diagnosis of blunt thoracic aortic injury. Helical CT scan has become the diagnostic test of choice.

Level of evidence: 2b. Grade of recommendation: B.

18.3 What Medications Should We Use in the Medical Management of Minimal Aortic Injuries?

Minimal aortic injury (MAI) has traditionally been defined as a subcentimeter intimal defect without external contour deformity. The current definition of MAI is a subcentimeter intimomedial abnormality without external contour deformity. The increased experience with the conservative management of localized intramural hematomas without external contour abnormalities has contributed to these injuries being included in the definition of MAIs [6]. As a direct result of the significant advances in multidetector CT imaging and the increased frequency of use of CT angiography, MAI is being recognized more frequently. An additional benefit of the advancement in CT technology has been the ability to grade BTAIs. The grading of BTAI adopted by the Society for Vascular Surgery consists of four grades: I, intimal tear; II, intramural hematoma; III, pseudoaneurysm; and IV, rupture [7]. The management of MAIs historically had created some anxiety among surgeons and left some questions unanswered. What modalities should be used to follow these injuries? How often should follow-up studies be obtained? What medications should be used in the medical management of these injuries, and for how long should patients be required to take these medications? What should the target blood pressure be? Within the past decade, with the increased recognition of these injuries and the comfort of managing these injuries, some of these questions have been answered.

Malhotra et al. published their paper in 2001 describing their experience with MAIs. They conducted a retrospective review of all patients suspected of BTAI seen on screening helical CT (HCT) over the study period from July 1994 to June 2000. All patients with BTAI were admitted to the trauma intensive care unit, and all received short-acting β-blockade infusion (esmolol or labetalol) to control heart rate (<90 beats/min) and blood pressure (systolic blood pressure <120 mmHg). Sodium nitroprusside was added to the regimen when β-blockade alone did not adequately control blood pressure. Patients were changed to oral antihypertensive therapy over the following 5–7 days. Eight of the nine patients with MAI were managed nonoperatively [8].

Kepros et al. reviewed their experience with MAIs [9]. All patients with MAI were managed nonoperatively based on the limited and superficial nature of their aortic injury. Their management strategy included serial transesophageal endoscopy (TEE) studies to visualize and monitor the progression or resolution of injury, hypotension (systolic blood pressure between 80 and 90 mmHg), and prevention of tachycardia (heart rate between 60 and 80 beats/min) using β-blockade, close invasive monitoring in the surgical intensive care unit, and standard intravenous fluid resuscitation using serum lactate levels and base deficit as endpoints of adequate tissue perfusion. TEE was more sensitive in diagnosing aortic intimal injuries compared with aortic arch angiography or HCT of the chest. Nonoperative management was completed in all cases. Complete resolution of all intimal tears was documented by TEE within 3–19 days (mean = 9.4 ± 6.6 days). There were no complications related to the aortic injuries in any of the patients during a mean follow-up of 16.8 months. Thus, TEE appears to be a good modality for diagnosing and following these MAIs.

Kidane et al. performed a retrospective review of their Level 1 trauma center's database to identify patients who had a BTAI between October 1998 and March 2010. CT scans of those who were initially treated nonoperatively were reviewed to determine the extent of BTAI as either MAI (intimal flap with minimal or no periaortic hematoma) or more severe injuries (pseudoaneurysm and greater periaortic hematomas). They reviewed follow-up CT scans and clinical information to determine the natural history of these lesions and the clinical outcomes related to their nonoperative management. Sixty-nine patients with BTAIs were identified during the study period; 10 were initially untreated and were included in this study. The degree of injury included intimal flaps ($n = 7$, 70%), pseudoaneurysms with minimal hematoma ($n = 2$, 20%), and circumferential intimal tear ($n = 1$, 10%). Duration of clinical follow-up ranged from 1 month to 6 years (median = 2 months) after discharge, whereas CT radiologic follow-up ranged from 1 week to 6 years (median = 6 weeks). Seven (70%) patients had complete resolution or stabilization of their MAI, one (10%) with circumferential intimal tear showed extension of the injury at 8 weeks postinjury and underwent successful repair, and two (20%) were lost to follow-up. Thus, there appears to be a subset of patients with BTAI who require no surgical intervention. This includes those with limited intimal flaps, which often resolve. Radiologic surveillance is mandatory to ensure MAI resolution and identify any progression that might prompt repair [10].

MAIs are being diagnosed more frequently by high-resolution multidetector CT scanners and imaging protocols, making contrast CT the best screening and diagnostic test for BTAI [9]. More specifically, MAIs have been detected with more frequency using CT angiography. Recent studies have used CT angiography to follow the MAIs. There remains no consensus on the timing of repeat imaging [11].

The medical management of MAIs consists of anti-impulse therapy with β-blockade to maintain systolic blood pressure below 100–120 mmHg, and a heart rate of 60–90 beats/min appeared to prevent progression and rupture of MAIs [12].

RECOMMENDATIONS

1. Multidetector CT angiography of the chest has become the modality of choice for following MAIs.

   Level of evidence: 2b. Grade of recommendation: B.

2. β-Blockade and intravenous vasodilator therapy should be used for the medical management of MAIs. Controlling the heart rate and blood pressure (systolic between 100 and 120 mmHg) using β-blockade and intravenous vasodilator is effective in treating patients with MAIs.

   Level of evidence: 2b. Grade of recommendation: B.

18.4 What Is the Target Blood Pressure to Maintain When Nonoperative Management or Delayed Surgical Therapy Is Considered?

The nonoperative management of blunt aortic injuries stemmed from studies reporting the use of medical management of these injuries in patients who were poor operative candidates due to advanced age or comorbidities that prohibit emergency thoracic surgery [13, 14]. Unstable patients who require laparotomy or patients with severe closed head injuries who require craniotomies also undergo medical management of the BTAI [15–17].

The concerns with the nonoperative management of BTAIs are risks of subsequent rupture of the aorta and the development of chronic thoracic aneurysms. Reports estimate that the risk of aortic rupture is less than 4% in patients presenting to the emergency room with stable hemodynamics during the initial workup; however, once rupture occurred, survival is rare [18, 19]. Hirose et al. showed that only 1.5% of patients died of aortic rupture if they survived the initial few hours [20]. Pate's study showed that only 7% of patients with a history of acute aortic injury developed chronic thoracic aneurysms over 7–48 years [18]. Interestingly, some patients have regression of the aortic injury with antihypertensive management.

The use of antihypertensives for BTAI was based on the successful management of type B dissection [18]. In 1995, Pate described two cases of aortic rupture during nonoperative management when blood pressure was not adequately managed [18]. Camp, in his study from 1997, and Pate in a follow-up study in 1999, published their results showing that there was no aortic rupture using a blood pressure control strategy during a waiting period for delayed surgery or among medically managed patients [11, 21]. Pate used the β-blockade when the cardiac rate was >90 beats/min and the systolic blood pressure was >100 mmHg. When the systolic blood pressure persisted at levels of >100 mmHg after β-blockade, an intravenous vasodilator (usually nitroprusside) was used to control the pressure.

Sandhu et al. looked retrospectively at the Memorial Hermann Trauma experience with patients admitted with BTAI between 1999 and 2015 [22]. Nonoperative management consisted of anti-impulse therapy with β-blockade and, when indicated, the addition of a vasodilator. The goal for nonoperative management was a systolic blood pressure between 100 and 120 mmHg accompanied by a heart rate between 60 and 90 beats/min.

Thus, it appears that MAIs can be managed nonoperatively with specific medical treatment protocols to control heart rate and blood pressure. Similarly, patients who are poor operative candidates can have their injuries managed nonoperatively with the same treatment protocols (β-blockade and intravenous vasodilator). Patients who are initially managed nonoperatively because of concerns of concomitant injuries and whose follow-up studies reveal the resolution of the aortic injury can continue to be managed nonoperatively on β-blockade and intravenous vasodilator. There are no Level 1 data that have answered this question specifically. Pate's study provides Level 2b data. There are also references to a target systolic blood pressure quote between 100 and 110 mmHg (Pate), 110 mmHg (Hirose), less than 120 mmHg (Malhotra), and between 80 and 90 mmHg (Kepros).

RECOMMENDATION

Controlling the heart rate and blood pressure (systolic between 100 and 120 mmHg) using β-blockade and intravenous vasodilator is effective in preventing rupture of BTAI.

Level of evidence: 2b. Grade of recommendation: B.

18.5 Which Operative Technique Should Be Used for Open Repair of Descending Thoracic Aortic Injuries?

The first description of thoracic endovascular repair (TEVAR) of a BTAI was in 1997 [23], and since then TEVAR for BTAI has gained significant traction and has largely replaced open repair for BTAI [24]. However, regarding the open repair of BTAIs, the optimal open technique remains controversial. Open repair of aortic injury is best accomplished with some form of distal perfusion, either bypass or shunt [3].

Cardarelli et al. looked at the University of Maryland's 30 years of experience with traumatic aortic rupture [25]. There were 219 patients with a diagnosis of traumatic aortic rupture between 1971 and 2001. Patients were divided according to surgical technique. There were 82 patients in the clamp-and-sew technique group (group A), 64 patients in the passive shunt group (group B), and 73 patients in the heparin-less partial cardiopulmonary bypass (group C). Mortality was 18 patients for group A (21.9%), 23 patients for group B (35.9%), and 13 patients for group C (17.8%) ($p = 0.03$). Paraplegia occurred in 15 of the 64 survivors in group A (23.4%), 7 of the 41 survivors in group B (17%), and 0 of the 60 survivors in group C ($p = 0.0005$). Aortic occlusion without lower body perfusion for longer than 30 minutes ($p = 0.004$) and surgical technique without lower body bypass support ($p = 0.0005$) were associated with paraplegia. They concluded that the use of heparin-less distal cardiopulmonary bypass in the authors' hands is safe and is associated with a reduced incidence of paraplegia.

Whitson et al. describe their experience with the repair of this injury [26]. They did a retrospective review (1991–2004) of patients with traumatic thoracic aortic injuries to evaluate whether or not an individualized approach to operative management provides acceptable neurologic outcomes. Ninety-one percent of the 67 patients who met the study criteria had concomitant injuries. Distal aortic perfusion was used in 81% of cases (75% left heart bypass, 6% cardiopulmonary bypass), and 19% underwent the clamp-and-sew technique without heparinization. There were no spinal cord deficits or adverse cerebral events related to repair. If the definitive repair was completed, the mortality was 16%. They concluded that judicious use of clamp-and-sew techniques can achieve excellent neurologic outcomes, equivalent to distal aortic perfusion.

RECOMMENDATION

For open repairs of BTAI, distal perfusion has been shown to decrease the incidence of paraplegia compared to the clamp-and-sew technique when the aortic cross-clamp time exceeds 30 minutes. Some form of distal perfusion should be used since neurologic complications seem to correlate with ischemia time.

Level of evidence: 2a. Grade of recommendation: B.

18.6 Are Endovascular Stent Procedures Superior to Open Vascular Procedures?

Patients with blunt aortic injuries frequently have significant associated injuries that can preclude them from immediate surgical repair. Endovascular grafts have been used since 1991 for the repair of abdominal aortic aneurysms, and this approach was first described as an alternative to open repair by Parodi et al. [27]. Since then, there has been improvement in stent graft technology, which has led to the use of stent grafts for the treatment of traumatic BTAIs. Most studies published on the use of this technology for the treatment of BAIs have been retrospective. In 2001, Fujikawa et al. published the first prospective case study on the use of endovascular stent grafting for the treatment of traumatic BTAIs [28]. They treated six patients who had sustained BTAIs confirmed by digital subtraction angiogram with stent grafts. All patients had injuries to the aortic isthmus. All patients except one had an event-free clinical course.

One patient died because of a rupture of the ascending aorta. They concluded that an endovascular stent graft is a valid therapeutic option with minimal surgical invasion for patients with acute-phase aortic injury. In 2004, Ott et al. published their review of 18 patients who underwent repair of a BTAI over 11 years, comparing the outcomes of patients treated with endovascular repair and open repair. Six of these patients had an endovascular repair and 12 had an open repair. There were no significant differences in demographics, injury, or crash statistics between the two groups. The open group had a 17% early mortality rate, a paraplegia rate of 16%, and an 8.3% incidence of recurrent laryngeal nerve injury compared to a 0% rate of mortality, paraplegia, and recurrent laryngeal nerve injury in the endovascular group. A definite trend toward decreased morbidity, mortality, intensive care unit length of stay, and the number of ventilator days was seen with endovascular repair. There was a clear trend toward improved outcomes after endovascular repair of thoracic aortic injuries compared with the standard open repair in the setting of trauma [29]. In 2004, Dunham et al. published their retrospective review of 28 patients treated with endovascular stent grafts for BTAIs. Twelve patients were excluded because injuries occurred more than 30 days before grafting or under a different protocol or the procedure was performed in a different center, leaving 16 patients for review. Technical success was achieved in all patients, no graft-related complications were detected during follow-up, and no patient developed postoperative paraplegia. There was one postoperative mortality secondary to comorbid injury. There was one patient with a preoperative traumatic carotid dissection who demonstrated a postoperative stroke and another patient who required thoracentesis for pleural effusion. They concluded that endovascular stent graft repair of BTAIs can be performed safely [30].

In 2006, Andrassy et al. published their retrospective review of all patients treated for acute and chronic traumatic injury of the thoracic aorta and compared the outcome of the endovascular approach versus surgery [31]. In the study period of 14 years, 46 patients were treated. The overall 30-day mortality was 16% in patients treated for acute or contained rupture ($n = 31$) and not significantly different after endovascular versus open repair (13.3% vs. 18.8%). There was no mortality in the patients undergoing elective stent grafting or open surgery for chronic posttraumatic aortic aneurysms ($n = 15$). Conversion and/or operative revision following stent graft implantation occurred in three patients (12.5%). Neurologic complications were absent in the stent graft group (0 of 24), whereas paraplegia ($n = 2$) or minor neurologic deficits ($n = 3$) developed following open surgery (5 of 22; 22.7%; $p = 0.013$). The length of intensive care and overall hospital stay was significantly shorter for patients after elective stent graft treatment compared to open surgery ($p = 0.045$). They concluded that minimally invasive endovascular repair for patients with acute and chronic posttraumatic aneurysms is an equally effective treatment option compared with open surgery, with advantages regarding perioperative neurologic complications and duration of hospital stay under elective circumstances.

Demetriades et al. published the results of a prospective, multicenter study assessing the early efficacy and safety of endovascular stent grafts in traumatic thoracic aortic injuries and comparing outcomes with standard operative repair [32]. The decision for open or endovascular repair was the surgeon's preference. One hundred and twenty-five patients (64.9%) were selected for stent grafts and 68 (35.2%) for operative repair. Stent grafts were selected in 71.6% of the 74 patients with major extrathoracic injuries and 60% of the 115 patients with no extrathoracic injuries. Twenty-five patients in the stent graft group (20%) developed 32 device-related complications. There were 18 endoleaks (14.4%), of which 6 needed open repairs. Procedure-related paraplegia developed in 2.9% in the open repair group and 0.8% in the stent graft group ($p = 0.28$). Multivariate analysis adjusting for severe extrathoracic injuries, hypotension, Glasgow Coma Scale (GCS), and age revealed that the stent graft group had significantly lower mortality (adjusted odds ratio, 8.42; 95% confidence interval [CI], 2.76–25.69; adjusted p-value < 0.001) and fewer blood transfusions (adjusted mean difference, 4.98; 95% CI, 0.14–9.82; adjusted p-value, 0.046) than the open repair group. Among the 115 patients without major extrathoracic injuries, higher mortality and higher transfusion requirements were also found in the open repair group (adjusted odds ratio for mortality, 13.08; 95% CI, 2.53–67.53; adjusted p-value, 0.002; and adjusted mean difference in the transfusion units, 4.45; 95% CI, 1.39–7.51; adjusted p-value, 0.004). Among the 74 patients with major extrathoracic injuries, significantly higher mortality and pneumonia rates were found in the open repair group (adjusted p-values 0.04 and 0.03, respectively). Multivariate analysis also showed that centers with a high volume of endovascular procedures had significantly fewer systemic complications (hospital length of stay [adjusted p-value = 0.005]) than low-volume centers. They concluded that most surgeons at the centers in the study select stent grafts for traumatic thoracic aortic ruptures, irrespective of associated injuries, injury severity, and age. Stent graft repair is associated with significantly lower mortality and fewer blood transfusions, but there is a considerable risk of serious device-related complications.

Estrera et al. reviewed their experience between January 1, 1997, and January 1, 2012, on the data regarding 338 patients who presented with suspected BTAI that were entered into the University of Texas Medical School at Houston Trauma Centre Registry [33]. A total of 175 patients (52%) underwent thoracic aortic repair; 29 (17%) had open repair with aortic cross-clamping, 77 (44%) had open repair with distal aortic perfusion, and 69 (39%) had a thoracic endovascular aortic repair. Outcomes were determined, including early mortality, morbidity, length of stay, and late survival. Multiple logistic regression analysis was used to compute adjusted estimates for the effects of the operative technique. The early mortality for all patients with BTAI was 41% (139/338). The early mortality rate was 17% (27/175) for operative aortic interventions, 4% (3/69) for thoracic endovascular aortic repairs, 31% (11/29) for open repairs with aortic cross-clamping, and 14% (11/77) for open repairs with distal aortic perfusion. The survival rate for thoracic endovascular aortic repair at 1 and 5 years were 92% and 87%, respectively. The survival rate for open repair at 1, 5, 10, and 15 years was 76%, 75%, 72%, and 68%, respectively. They concluded that BTAI remains associated with significant early mortality. Delayed selective management, when applied with open repair with distal aortic perfusion and the use of thoracic endovascular aortic repair, has been associated with improved early outcomes. The long-term durability of thoracic endovascular aortic repair is unknown, necessitating close radiographic follow-up [33].

A multicenter study by the Western Trauma Association, published in 2017, reported on data collected from eight verified trauma centers. This retrospective study looked at all patients with BTAI admitted between January 1, 2006, and June 30, 2016 [34]. Of the 316 patients with BTAI, 57 (18%) were in extremis and died before any treatment. Two hundred and fifty-nine patients were treated surgically of which TEVAR was performed in 176 (68%), open repair in 28 (10.8%), the hybrid technique in 4 (1.5%), and nonoperative management in 51 (19.7%). Similar Injury Severity Score (ISS), chest Abbreviated Injury Score (AIS), Trauma and Injury Severity Score (TRISS), and probability of survival were found in both the TEVAR group and the open repair group. These two groups differed, however, in median age (open: 28 with interquartile range [IQR] 19–51; TEVAR: 46 with IQR 2–4; $p < 0.001$). The overall in-hospital mortality was 6.6% (TEVAR: 5.7%, open: 10.7%, nonoperative: 3.9%; $p = 0.535$). There were two deaths among the 240 patients who survived to discharge (one at 9 months and one at 8 years). Both patients had been treated with TEVAR, and their deaths were unrelated to the procedure. Of the patients who received stent grafts, surveillance CT scans were not obtained in 37.6%. The study concluded that TEVAR should be the treatment of choice when anatomically suitable, with open repair to be used for more proximal injuries and that there needs to be process improvement in CT imaging follow-up of TEVAR.

The EAST guidelines committee's 2015 update on the evaluation and management of BTAI also looked at the question of "should an endovascular repair be performed versus open repair to minimize the risk of mortality, stroke, paraplegia, and renal failure" [5]. The committee identified 38 articles after their PubMed search that they felt were appropriate for the construction of their guidelines. Thirty-seven studies reported on mortality outcomes, 21 studies reported on the incidence of paralysis, and 12 studies reported on the incidence of stroke. One article was excluded because the methodology was significantly different from the other studies. Regarding renal failure, the available studies did not give consistent or sufficient data, specifically on the onset of renal failure whether before or after operative intervention. Forty-five comparative studies (1997–2013) were identified of which 37 were used in the final analysis. Overall mortality (reported by all 37 studies) was lower for the endovascular repair compared to open repair (8% vs. 19%, respectively; risk ratio [RR] of 0.56, 95% CI 0.44–0.73). The incidence of paraplegia (reported by all 37 studies) was also lower for the endovascular repair compared to open repair (0.5% vs. 3%, respectively; RR of 0.36, 95% CI 0.19–0.71). Twenty-one of the 37 studies reported stroke, and the endovascular group was found to have a slightly higher incidence of stroke compared to the open group (2.5% vs. 1%, respectively; RR 1.48, 95% CI 0.67–3.27) [5].

RECOMMENDATION

Endovascular stent grafts are associated with less mortality, fewer postoperative neurologic complications including paraplegia, and fewer systemic complications than open procedures.

Level of evidence: 2a. Grade of recommendation: B.

18.7 Penetrating Injuries of the Aorta

There are fewer numbers of studies published on penetrating injury to the aorta compared to BTAI. Penetrating injury to the thoracic aorta accounts for approximately 1% of traumatically injured aortas [35]. Mortality from such injuries has not changed in the past decade, and open surgical repair remains the gold standard in emergent situations. Endovascular stent grafts have been used successfully for the management of BTAIs, and there are case reports in the literature describing the use of endovascular stent grafts in penetrating injuries to the aorta [36].

Demetriades et al. conducted a retrospective analysis of all patients with penetrating aortic injuries admitted over 5 years [37]. The abdominal aorta was injured in 72% of 93 patients and the thoracic aorta in 28%. Eighty-two percent of the patients were admitted in shock and 41% with unrecordable blood pressure. Victims with thoracic aortic injuries were more likely to have unrecordable blood pressure on admission than patients with abdominal aortic injuries (73% vs. 28.4%) and more likely to require an emergency room thoracotomy (76.9% vs. 20.9%). There were no survivors among the 36 patients who required an emergency room thoracotomy. The overall mortality was 80.6% (87.5% for gunshot wounds and 64.7% for knife wounds). Patients with abdominal aortic injuries were three times more likely to survive than those with thoracic aortic injuries (23.9% vs. 7.7%) [37]. Since this study by Demetriades et al., no one has published an extensive series of their experience with penetrating injuries to the aorta.

Injury to the thoracic vena cava is extremely rare and is usually fatal. Most of the literature published on these injuries are case studies and describes the experience in the management of these injuries. Management involves surgical repair, and there are not enough papers to render any Level 1, 2, or 3 data.

RECOMMENDATIONS

Injury to the thoracic aorta, gunshot wounds, unrecordable blood pressure on admission, and the need for emergency room thoracotomy are important predictors of mortality.

Level of evidence: 2b.

Editor's Note

Because the number of patients arriving alive at trauma centers with aortic injuries is very small each year (i.e., less than 2,000 total per year in the United States), there is little prospective high-quality evidence to inform our management. There have been some huge improvements in outcomes in these patients, however, due to advances in technology. CT angiography of the chest has completely replaced the aortogram for the diagnosis of blunt thoracic aortic injury. As this imaging modality is more widely available and requires fewer resources than an aortogram, aortic lesions are now identified more readily and rapidly. Once aortic injury is suspected, medications to lower blood pressure and slow heart rate (decreasing the force of cardiac contraction) are now employed to lower the risk of aortic rupture. This management protocol employs an understanding of the pathophysiology of this disease, derived from the cardiovascular surgeon's experience with aortic aneurysms. When the diagnosis is confirmed and the patient is deemed stable to undergo an operative intervention, endovascular stenting is now routinely utilized with superior outcomes.

Diagnosis change to CTA from cxr/aortogram; immediate treatment w esmolol; the intimal tear treated nonop; definitive treatment nonop in the unstable, and endovascular.

REFERENCES

Diagnosis of BAI

1. Jackson DH. Of TRAs and ROCs. *Chest.* 1984;*85*:585–587.
2. Smith RS, Chang FC. Traumatic rupture of the aorta: Still a lethal injury. *Am J Surg.* 1986;*152*:660–663.
3. Nagy K, Fabian T, Rodman G, et al. Guidelines for the diagnosis and management of blunt aortic injury: An EAST practice management guidelines work group. *J Trauma.* 2000;*48*(6):1128–1143.
4. Burkhart HM, Gomez GA, Jacobson LE, et al. Fatal blunt aortic injuries: A review of 242 cases. *J Trauma.* 2001;*50*:113–115.
5. Fox N, Schwartz D, Salazar JH, et al. Evaluation and management of blunt traumatic aortic injury: A practice management guideline from the Eastern Association for the Surgery of Trauma. *J Trauma Acute Care Surg.* January 2015;*78*(1): 136–46.

Minimal Aortic Injuries

6. Heneghan RE, Aarabi S, Quiroga E, et al. Call for a new classification system and treatment strategy in blunt aortic injury. *J Vasc Surg.* 2016;*64*(1):171–176.
7. Lee WA, Matsumura JS, Mitchell RS, et al. Endovascular repair of traumatic thoracic aortic injury: Clinical practice guidelines of the society for vascular surgery. *J Vasc Surg.* 2011;*53*:187–192.
8. Malhotra AK, Fabian TC, Croce MA, et al. Minimal aortic injury: A lesion associated with advancing diagnostic techniques. *J Trauma.* 2001;*51*:1042–1048.
9. Kepros J, Angood P, Jaffe CC, et al. Aortic intimal injuries from blunt trauma: Resolution profile in nonoperative management. *J Trauma.* 2002;*52*:475–478.

10. Kidane B, Abramowitz D, Harris JR, DeRose G, Forbes TL. Natural history of minimal aortic injury following blunt thoracic aortic trauma. *Can J Surg.* December 2012;*55(6)*: 377–381.

Nonoperative Management of Blunt Traumatic Aortic Injuries

11. Kapoor H, Lee JT, Orr NT, et al. Minimal aortic injury: Mechanisms, imaging manifestations, natural history, and management. *Radiographics.* 2020;*40(7)*:1834–1847.
12. Harris DG, Rabin J, Starnes BW, et al. Evolution of lesion-specific management of blunt thoracic aortic injury. *J Vasc Surg.* 2016;*64*:500–555.
13. Camp PC, Shackford SR. Outcome after blunt traumatic aortic laceration: Identification of a high-risk cohort. *J Trauma.* 1997;*43*:413–422.
14. Camp PC, Rogers RB, Shackford SR, et al. Blunt traumatic thoracic aortic lacerations in the elderly: An analysis of outcome. *J Trauma.* 1994;*37*:418–423.
15. Borman KR, Aurbakken CM, Weigelt JA. Treatment priorities in combined blunt abdominal and aortic trauma. *Am J Surg.* 1982;*144*:728–732.
16. Hudson HM, Woodson J, Hirsch E. The management of traumatic aortic tear in the multiply-injured patient. *Ann Vasc Surg.* 1991;*5*:445–448.
17. Maggisano R, Nathens A, Alexandrova NA, et al. Traumatic rupture of the thoracic aorta: Should one always operate immediately? *Ann Vasc Surg.* 1995;*9*:44–52.
18. Pate JW, Fabian TC, Walker W. Traumatic rupture of the aortic isthmus: An emergency? *World J Surg.* 1995;*19*: 119–126.
19. Fabian TC, Richardson JD, Croce MA, et al. Prospective study of blunt aortic injury: Multicenter trial of the American association for the surgery of trauma. *J Trauma.* 1997;*42*:374–383.
20. Hirose H, Gill IS, Malangoni MA. Nonoperative management of traumatic aortic injury. *J Trauma.* 2006;*60*:597–601.
21. Pate JW, Gavant ML, Weiman DS, Fabian TC. Traumatic rupture of the aortic isthmus: Program of selective management. *World J Surg.* 1999;*23*:59–63.
22. Sandu HK, Leonard SD, Perlik A, et al. Determinants and outcomes of nonoperative management for blunt traumatic aortic injuries. *J Vasc Surg.* February 2018;*67(2)*:389–398.

Operative Technique for Repair of Blunt Traumatic Thoracic Aortic Injuries

23. Semba CP, Kato N, Kee ST, et al. Acute rupture of the descending thoracic aorta: Repair with use of endovascular stent-grafts. *J Vasc Interv Radiol.* 1997;*8*:337–342.
24. Scalea TM, Feliciano DV, DuBose JJ, et al. Blunt thoracic aortic injury: Endovascular repair is now the standard. *J Am Coll Surg.* April 2019;*228*(4):605–610.

25. Cardarelli MG, McLaughlin JS, Downing SW, et al. Management of traumatic aortic rupture: A 30-year experience. *Ann Surg.* 2002;*236(4)*:465–469.
26. Whitson BA, Nath DS, Knudtson JR, et al. Is Distal aortic perfusion in traumatic thoracic aortic injuries necessary to avoid paraplegic postoperative outcomes? *J Trauma.* 2008;*64*:115–120.

Endovascular Treatment of Blunt Traumatic Aortic Injuries

27. Parodi JC, Palmaz JC, Barone HD. Transfemoral intraluminal graft implantation for abdominal aortic aneurysms. *Ann Vasc Surg.* 1991;*5*:491–499.
28. Fujikawa T, Yukioka T, Ishimaru S, et al. Endovascular stent grafting for the treatment of the blunt thoracic aortic injury. *J Trauma.* February 2001;*50(2)*:223–229.
29. Ott MC, Stewart TC, Lawlor DK, et al. Management of blunt thoracic injuries: Endovascular stents versus open repair. *J Trauma.* 2004;*56*:565–570.
30. Dunham MB, Zygun D, Petrasek P, et al. Endovascular stent grafts for acute blunt aortic injury. *J Trauma.* 2004; *56*:1173–1178.
31. Andrassy J, Weidenhagen R, Meimarakas G, et al. Stent versus open surgery for acute and chronic traumatic injury of the thoracic aorta: A single-center experience. *J Trauma.* 2006;*60*:765–772.
32. Demetriades D, Velhamos GC, Scalea TM, et al. Operative repair or endovascular stent graft in blunt traumatic thoracic aortic injuries: Results of an American association for the surgery of trauma multicenter study. *J Trauma.* 2008; *64*:561–571.
33. Estrera A, Miller C, Guajardan-Salinas G, Coogan S, Charlton-Ouw K, Safi H, Azizzadeh A. Update on blunt thoracic aortic injury: Fifteen-year single-institution experience. *J Thorac Cardiovasc Surg.* March 2013;*145(3)*: S154–S158.
34. Shackford SR, Dunne CE, Karmy-Jones R, et al. The evolution of care improves outcomes in blunt thoracic aortic injury: A Western Trauma Association multicenter study. *J Trauma Acute Care Surg.* December 2017;*83(6)*: 1006–1013.

Penetrating Injuries of the Aorta

35. Cornwell EE III, Kennedy F, Berne TV, et al. Gunshot wounds to the thoracic aorta in the '90s: Only prevention will make a difference. *Am Surg.* 1995;*61*:721–723.
36. Fang TD, Peterson DA, Kirilcuk NN, et al. Endovascular management of a gunshot wound to the thoracic aorta. *J Trauma.* 2006;*60*:204–208.
37. Demetriades D, Theodorou D, Murray J, et al. Mortality and prognostic factors in penetrating injuries of the aorta. *J Trauma.* 1996;*40*:761–763.

19

Cardiac Trauma

Adam Lee Goldstein and Dror Soffer

19.1 Introduction

Cardiac injury remains a small percentage of trauma patients being received at trauma centers, despite a continual improvement in prehospital care and an unfortunate increase in penetrating trauma over the last few years [1–4]. The majority of cardiac trauma patients still die in the prehospital setting; nevertheless, when these victims do present, an accurate index of suspicion, precise diagnosis, and rapid intervention are vital to optimize survival. There are major differences between penetrating and blunt cardiac injury (BCI) in the presentation of the patient to the trauma bay, associated injuries, diagnostic methods, and therapeutic interventions. Depending on the mechanism of injury and management of these patients, low mortality is obtainable [5]. An important evolution in the care of cardiac trauma, especially in penetrating trauma, is to think "outside the (cardiac) box" and rule out cardiac injury to any thoracic and upper abdomen trauma in which the mechanism

may have led to cardiac injury [6]. This is especially true in the setting of hemothorax after penetrating injury, where the hemothorax might be the only clinical sign of cardiac injury. In these patients, imaging modalities are not sensitive for the initial diagnosis of cardiac injury; therefore, pericardial window should be considered and utilized early.

Even with the continual advances in trauma care, there remains a paucity of recommendations and guidelines in the management of traumatic cardiac injury. This chapter focuses on relevant topics of debate while reviewing the current evidence-based knowledge in the management of penetrating cardiac injury and BCI from their presentation to definitive care in the hospital setting. New sections for this edition will focus on the variable presentations and treatments of tamponade and damage control surgery in cardiac trauma. Relevant questions and answers regarding the care of these patients that are covered in this chapter are summarized in Table 19.1.

TABLE 19.1

Question Summary

No.	Question	Answer	Level of Evidence	Grade	Reference
1.	How do you rule out BCI?	The combination of repeated normal troponin levels with a normal ECG	1, 2	C	[2–21]
2.	What is the role of CCT in both penetrating and blunt cardiac trauma?	It is useful in both penetrating and blunt trauma for the diagnosis of cardiac injury along with associated chest injuries, but in penetrating trauma, it is not more sensitive or specific than in the US.	1	B	[2, 7, 22–27]
3.	When does the stable BCI patient need continuous ECG monitoring and for how long?	When there are changes in the ECG and/or elevated cardiac enzymes. Patients admitted for monitoring with neither ECG nor enzyme abnormalities may be monitored for only 24 hours.	2	C	[12, 28, 29]
4.	How do you initially manage a pericardial effusion secondary to trauma?	A quick diagnosis, followed by a pericardial window in the operating room (or thoracotomy in the ER if the patient is extremis), prepared to open the chest if necessary.	2	B	[30–36]
5.	How do you manage a foreign body in the heart?	Nonoperable and noninvasive conservative therapy is safe when the foreign object does not cause hemodynamic compromise or has a clear risk of causing embolization, infection, or fistulization.	3	C	[37–39]
6.	What are damage control techniques for unstable patients?	A finger, staples, suture, Foley catheter, and Satinsky clamp all may be used for initial hemorrhagic control.	3	C	[40–42]
7.	Must one use pledgets when suturing the heart?	There are not enough data to show that pledgets are beneficial in cardiac trauma surgery.	4	C	[43–47]

Abbreviations: BCI: Blunt cardiac injury, CCT: Chest CT, US: Ultrasound.

19.2 How Do You Rule Out Blunt Cardiac Injury?

BCI in a stable patient seems an elusive diagnosis and is easily missed because of a high incidence of associated injuries. In an autopsy-based study looking at 1,597 fatalities due to blunt trauma, 11.9% were found to have a cardiac injury. In the subset with cardiac trauma, motor vehicle crashes were the cause of 56% of the BCIs, followed by falls from significant heights (38%) and crush injuries (4%) [2]. The majority of BCI patients had associated injuries that included the thorax, abdominal cavity, and spine [7]. Another postmortem study found that sternal fractures were found in 76% of patients with BCI due to falls from a certain height, and the conclusion was made that any fall greater than 6 m (20 ft) with a sternal fracture should undergo an immediate and thorough cardiac evaluation [8]. Following studies showed that sternal fractures alone were not significantly associated with BCI [8] and only pulmonary coinjuries were found to have a significant correlation with BCI [10]. Patients with sternal fractures from any mechanism were found to have BCI in only 5% of these cases. In a large National Trauma Bank Analysis (USA), the most common associated chest injuries to BCI were first hemopneumothorax (odds ratio [OR] 9.53), followed by sternal fractures (OR 5.52), esophageal injury (OR 5.47), and thoracic aortic injury (OR 4.82) [11]. Therefore in particular, the "combo" of sternal fractures with pulmonary injury (radiographic evidence of contusion, hemothorax, pneumothorax, and especially hemopneumothorax), with a sternal fracture in blunt trauma requires BCI workup.

A laboratory test, electrocardiography, and imaging modalities are essential in the diagnosis when BCI is clinically suggested, yet there remains a lack of strong evidence (or consensus) in the literature to support evidence-based clinical practice/recommendations. Commonly used diagnostic modalities for BCI are electrocardiogram (ECG), cardiac enzymes, chest X-ray (CXR), echocardiography, and most recently, chest computed tomography (CCT).

Currently, the only Level 1 recommendation for the initial diagnosis of BCI is to perform an ECG [12]. However, ECG alone is not sufficient in ruling out significant BCI, and several patients with normal ECG will be further diagnosed as having significant BCI [12]. Again, we cannot emphasize enough that the first step for optimizing care in these patients, and a chance for survival, is a high index of suspicion based on the traumatic mechanism. In all patients with possible BCI who are admitted, a follow-up ECG is a must to evaluate for further change or normalization.

A prospective study of 333 patients presenting after blunt thoracic trauma was able to demonstrate a negative predictive value (NPV) of 100% when combining a normal ECG and the cardiac-specific serum troponin I (cTnI) at admission and after 8 hours to rule out significant BCI. This study concluded that in the absence of other reasons for hospitalization, such patients may be safely discharged from the emergency room [9, 14].

A prospective study evaluated 187 patients with blunt cardiac trauma and concluded that cTnI levels below 1.05 µg/L in asymptomatic patients at admission and within the first 6 hours after admission ruled out myocardial injury, whereas positive cTnI levels more than 1.05 µg/L mandate further cardiologic workup for the detection and management of myocardial injury. This study further described how the peak levels of pathologic cTnI correlated with the occurrence of (and severity of) ventricular arrhythmias [15, 16]. The higher/highest cTnI levels during hospitalization also correlated with overall mortality [17]. Therefore cTnI trends must be monitored closely. A new cardiac enzyme, heart-type fatty acid-binding proteins (H-FABPs), has begun to show clinical significance, yet there is currently no evidence for its utility in BCI [18].

CXR is a must for all blunt trauma (especially chest) patients. CXR has a low sensitivity for assisting in the diagnosis of BCI. Yet what is important is to notice signs of significant force to the chest that may increase the level of suspicion for BCI, such as first rib fractures [19].

A formal transthoracic echocardiogram (TTE) has not been found useful in the initial assessment and diagnosis of BCI. No correlation was found between significant BCI and pathologic findings during TTE [20]. An analysis of 213 patients with significant BCI and a positive cTnI found only 49% to have evidence of heart injury on TTE [21]. The only current utilization of TTE has been found in patients with clinically established significant BCI who have persistent dysrhythmias and/or are hemodynamically unstable (i.e., hypotension and/or unexplained depressed cardiac index).

A study from the United States found the cardiac portion of the focused assessment with sonography in trauma (FAST) exam to have limited utility in the majority of blunt trauma patients. This study evaluated 777 FAST exams and found blunt hemopericardium to be extremely rare and that the rate of incidental effusion was higher, thus leading to a significant amount of false-positive results. Hemopericardium or cardiac rupture was only present if at least one of three identified high-acuity variables were present: Major mechanism of injury, hypotension, or emergency intubation [22].

RECOMMENDATION

BCI may be ruled out with a normal ECG and two normal serum cTnI measurements at the time of admission and after 8 hours. There is no role for a TTE in the initial diagnosis of BCI in asymptomatic patients, but it is recommended in symptomatic patients with dysrhythmias or hemodynamic instability and/or pathologic changes in ECG/cardiac enzymes. The cardiac component of the FAST exam is not diagnostic for BCI. A routine CXR is highly recommended to better understand the overall trauma load to the chest.

Level of evidence: 2. Grade of recommendation: C.

19.3 What Is the Role of Chest CT Scan in Both Penetrating and Blunt Cardiac Trauma?

The diagnostic workup for the hemodynamically stable patient with penetrating chest injury has changed over the years with the continued increased use of CCT during the initial evaluation despite inconclusive evidence. The utilization of CCT in this patient population has increased up to 3.5-fold without a clear benefit when compared to delayed follow-up CXR and/or FAST exams. CXR and FAST, when combined, had an equal sensitivity and increased specificity compared to CCT in identifying penetrating cardiac injuries needing intervention [23]. In the 1990s, trauma centers began questioning the value of CCT in the management of stable thoracic trauma patients with suspected cardiac injury. A group led by Nagy at Cook County Hospital advocated the use of CCT when ultrasound (US) was not immediately available [24]. This report identified the benefits of being able to identify trajectories and retained missile locations while balancing the disadvantage of having to transport the patient. Similar sensitivities, specificities, and accuracy in identifying penetrating cardiac trauma were reported between US (90–96%, 96–97%, and 96%, respectively) and CCT (100%, 96.6%, and 96.7%, respectively). In 2012, the question of the potential use of CCT in penetrating cardiac injury was still unanswered, and another study examined the utility of CCT in stable patients and the potential diagnostic value of hemopericardium and/or pneumopericardium seen on CCT. They found CCT to have a sensitivity of 76.9%, specificity of 99.7%, positive predictive value of 90.9%, and NPV of 99.1%. They concluded that CCT is a potentially useful modality for the evaluation of cardiac injuries in stable patients and that hemopericardium and/or pneumopericardium on CCT is highly specific for significant cardiac injury [24]. In CCT, cardiac penetrating injury is found as hemopericardium, pneumopericardium, intracardiac foreign bodies, extravasation of contrast material from the cardiac chambers, or coronary artery/cardiac vein/valvular injury [25]. CCT in the setting of cardiac penetrating trauma in a stable patient still has not been proven superior to a competent FAST of the pericardium, specifically when dealing with cardiac injuries. Nevertheless, CCT has gained popularity in this setting and has been found to be beneficial and cost-efficient in identifying cardiac injury in a manner equivalent to US while being able to provide additional information regarding injuries to other thoracic organs [26].

As in penetrating trauma, CCT is being used more frequently as a diagnostic modality in stable blunt trauma patients. More specifically, CCT using ECG-gating techniques has been able to improve resolution by minimizing imaging artifacts caused by cardiac motion [12]. Despite being rarely utilized in the emergency setting, the ECG-gating scans have been shown not to slow down the diagnostic workup; have better resolution of the cardiac thoracic aorta; and have an inferior resolution of the lung parenchyma, spine, and ribs but without compromising the detection of lesions or fractures [7]. An advantage of gated CCT is the ability to visualize the coronary vessels and aid in the diagnosis of acute myocardial infarction (AMI) together with the clinical and biochemical picture [27]. This is important in ruling out an AMI in the symptomatic patient as the primary event leading to the blunt trauma (e.g., a driver having an AMI leading to an automobile accident) or secondary to the BCI (e.g., a myocardial hematoma compressing a coronary vessel). CCT is capable of identifying hemopericardium and diagnosing cardiac tamponade, rupture, septal tears, valvular injury, herniation, cardiovascular injury,

and other pathologies in the chest affecting the heart (such as extrapericardial mediastinal hematomas) after blunt trauma [28]. Despite the increased use of computed tomography in any trauma patient, there is a current trend to increase the skill and comfort level of using advanced chest US techniques in the initial assessment of chest trauma (beyond FAST), which has shown high sensitivity to both cardiac, soft tissue, and skeletal pathologies [17]. The CCT should not be depended on for the diagnosis of cardiac injury, yet it does provide useful information regarding overall chest injury. An important limitation of CCT/FAST to be aware of is the setting of hemothorax. When the mechanism/trajectory raises the possibility of cardiac injury and there is a hemothorax, CCT (or FAST) is not sensitive in ruling out cardiac injury, and an early pericardial window in the operating room is necessary [6].

RECOMMENDATION

For penetrating trauma, CCT is not more accurate or useful than FAST together with CXR in identifying cardiac injury. Nevertheless, CCT is of value, with an increased advantage over FAST/TTE and CXR in diagnosing other injuries in the chest cavity, while also being able to diagnose cardiac injury with high specificity and sensitivity. CCT in blunt trauma is more specific than the FAST exam and useful in identifying hemopericardium.

With penetrating trauma specifically, no imaging modality is sensitive enough to rule out cardiac injury in the setting of hemothorax; therefore, in these cases, an early pericardial window is recommended.

Level of evidence: 2. Grade of recommendation: B.

19.4 When Does the Stable BCI Patient Need Continuous ECG Monitoring and for How Long?

A large number of stable patients after BCI who are in no need of emergent surgery will present to the emergency room symptomatic with, or without, changes in the ECG and/or a rise in cTnI. As noted earlier, cardiac arrhythmias are considered to be one of the most common manifestations of BCI, and the question remains on how to proceed with these patients by either discharging them or admitting them for observation ± further workup.

A classic review from 1989 determined that patients who will develop life-threatening arrhythmias or relative complications are identified in the emergency room by conduction abnormalities in the initial ECG. This group recommended that stable patients be triaged (e.g., need for monitored/unmonitored bed or to be discharged) based on the initial ECG, and if there are abnormalities and no other injury requiring intensive care, patients should be monitored for at least 48 hours [29]. The reason behind a 48-hour "window" was not clear in this study. In a prospective study of 336 patients, Cachecho et al. concluded that young patients with minor blunt thoracic trauma and normal or minimally abnormal ECG did not benefit from cardiac monitoring [30]. Another prospective study from Toronto, Canada, followed 312 patients after BCI for new cardiac arrhythmias and found that all arrhythmias were present on admission and that the majority were of atrial fibrillation type. They had no recommendations regarding the need and length of continuous ECG monitoring [13].

As the world population ages, elderly patients might also have a clinical myocardial infarction that is the cause of an increasing cardiac enzyme and/or changes in the ECG. This must be understood and treated appropriately, especially if emergency surgery is needed for other traumatic injuries.

RECOMMENDATIONS

There is clear evidence for those needing continuous monitoring when arrhythmia is present in the emergency room and/or cardiac enzymes are abnormal. For patients without these findings, there is no evidence for the need for continuous ECG monitoring. However, in certain high-risk patient populations (either determined by individual risk factors, such as age, or severity of trauma kinematics) 24 hours of observation and monitoring is recommended.

Level of evidence: 2. Grade of recommendation: C.

19.5 How Do You Initially Manage a Pericardial Effusion Secondary to Trauma?

A pericardial effusion secondary to trauma is an impending catastrophic event if not acknowledged, managed, and definitively treated with the utmost urgency. The result will be physiological cardiac tamponade with a rapid hemodynamic collapse. The lack of a cardiac effusion on the initial survey does not rule out full-thickness damage to the myocardium due to the possible drainage of blood into the pleural space as a result of concurrent damage to the pericardium. Therefore, a high level of suspicion, together with continual re-evaluation, must occur in these patients. Even with a cardiac injury, a number of these patients will respond to resuscitation and resemble the response to fluids seen with hemorrhagic shock. This is especially true with patients suffering more from cardiac compressive shock (cardiac tamponade/tension pneumothorax) due to a rapid increase in the preload. Nevertheless, any response in these patients is usually transient, and it is a known pitfall and may lead the treating team to proceed to further diagnostic modalities (CT scan) rather than operative exploration. Within a short time, the patient becomes unstable [31, 32].

Despite studies showing the potential safety and efficacy of pericardiocentesis [33, 34], we practice and strongly encourage the safest approach, a pericardial window in the operating

room followed by sternotomy/thoracotomy as needed. There might be a role for pericardiocentesis at centers without the operative capacity to attempt to stabilize a patient before transferring, yet this remains controversial without evidence-based guidelines. A study by Chestovich et al. showed that even a positive result on the pericardial window does not mandate the immediate opening of the chest. If after the drainage there is no sign of active bleeding after lavage and the patient is responsive to resuscitation, then the evacuation of the effusion together with lavage and drainage is safe and effective [35]. Studies have found that up to 25% of positive pericardial windows will not need further intervention/surgery [36]. There is a significant number of traumatic pericardial effusions/tamponade from either bleeding from surrounding tissue (pericardium, mediastinum) and not because of damage to the heart wall; therefore, this group is a prime example where a pericardial window would likely be sufficient [37].

RECOMMENDATION

Even in a stable or responsive patient, a pericardial effusion must be dealt with immediately. The safest approach is in the operating room performing a pericardial window while being prepared to continue rapidly opening the chest.

Level of evidence: 2. Grade of recommendation: B.

19.6 How Do You Manage a Foreign Body in the Heart?

There are multiple approaches and techniques to treat a foreign body in the heart, depending on the characteristics of the impaled or retained object and the resources available at the hospital. Over the past decade, advances in interventional radiologic techniques or minimally invasive surgical approaches have been able to replace previously mandatory open-heart procedures and successfully retrieve retained intracardiac objects [38]. Reviews of case reports, editorials, and case-related analyses have formed current recommendations for these traumatic events that are not infrequent at major trauma centers.

One common theme in the past decades has been the observation that many cases of retained foreign bodies, especially in the myocardium, may be treated conservatively, nonoperatively, and without retrieval if they are asymptomatic and unlikely to cause problems. The main deciding factor for retrieval in asymptomatic patients is the shape and location of the foreign body [39]. For example, sharp foreign bodies that have a significant chance for perforation are recommended to be removed, in contrast to bullets that are embedded in the myocardium and will eventually form fibrous capsules, remaining asymptomatic.

Complications, or anticipated complications, that would require removal are the perceived likelihood or occurrence of embolization (due to size and location), erosion (into the bronchial system or cause of fistulas within the heart), or infection (nonmetal objects). In a 1989 study, Symbas et al. retrospectively analyzed 24 gunshot patients with bullets retained in the heart, in which 14 were managed successfully without surgical intervention. Their results suggest that the management of bullets in the heart should be "individualized according to the patient's clinical course" and that bullets left in the heart are tolerated well if they remain asymptomatic [40]. One major issue with retaining foreign bodies to the heart is their unpredictable nature, with many clinicians recommending surgery even in the stable patient to avoid future catastrophic events [39].

RECOMMENDATION

Foreign bodies in the heart may be treated conservatively in stable, asymptomatic patients if there is determined to be little risk of embolization, infection, or fistula formation.

Level of evidence: 3. Grade of recommendation: C.

19.7 What Are Damage Control Techniques for Unstable Patients?

The unstable patient with suspected cardiac trauma must be operated on immediately. The preferable location is in the operating room, but if too unstable, then a left lateral thoracotomy is performed in the emergency room. In the operating room, a pericardial window is the first procedure performed to evaluate and potentially treat cardiac injury/sequelae. The pericardial window may be subxiphoid, trans-diaphragmatic, or transpleural depending on other concurrent injuries [41]. A pericardial window should never be performed in the emergency department because of the inability to control significant hemorrhage.

For immediate repairs to holes in the heart, the options range from an available finger, surgical staples, or any suture. A Satinsky clamp is also useful for temporary hemorrhage control in atrial injury. We recommend against using a Foley catheter due to the potential of the balloon causing an increased size of the hole in the heart, making a difficult situation even worse. Important technical pearls include using a U-stitch directly under cardiac vessels when the injury is in proximity to these vessels, the use of nonabsorbable sutures, and the option of packing with an open chest and negative pressure dressing [36]. A cardiopulmonary bypass is an important potential tool when treating cardiac trauma, yet is rarely utilized. Depending on the resources of the treating center, this may be a necessary option during the initial surgery, yet might be preferable during a second surgery 24–48 hours later after successful hemorrhagic control and the patient has further stabilized [42]. Regardless of the procedure, all patients undergoing emergent surgery should have a transesophageal echocardiogram within the first 6 hours after surgery to evaluate future structural damage to the heart and major vasculature [43].

RECOMMENDATIONS

Any general surgeon treating trauma patients needs to have the basic tools for damage control cardiac surgery. A sternotomy remains the access of choice, yet depends on the stability of the patient and capabilities of the surgeon. Priority remains to stop the bleeding from holes in the heart, preserve cardiac vessels, and diagnose further structural damage.

Level of evidence: 3. Grade of recommendation: C.

19.8 Is There an Advantage of Using Pledgets When Suturing the Heart?

The role of pledgets in cardiac surgery is a widely debated yet hardly researched topic. A search over the past several decades yielded few published studies on cardiac suturing techniques. Despite other techniques, such as a prolene suture buttressed with polytetrafluoroethylene [44], no comparison studies are allowing for evidence-based recommendations. In 1981, a study was conducted between nonpledgeted sutures and pledget-supported sutures and the potential for dehiscence of sutured atrioventricular valves. Pledget-supported sutures were found to be advantageous with higher suture line strength than nonpledgeted stitches [45]. In 1984, the role of pledgets in mitral valve replacements was evaluated. A prospective cohort study found the yield force of initial disruption of pledgeted sutures to be comparable to that of nonpledgeted sutures and recommended their use for mitral valve surgery [44]. In 1996, a study on cardiac suturing was conducted on canines, comparing pledget sutures to a stapling device for the rapid closure of cardiac wounds. The authors compared gross blood loss, hemodynamic instability, and the integrity of the repair. They concluded that stapling was faster, had similar integrity, and carried less risk of accidental needlesticks than traditional repair [46]. In other somewhat-dated reports, the potentially fatal complications of pledget suturing have been described. Two deaths occurred as a result of the embolization of cotton pledgets following aortic valve replacement [46], and another case reported an embolization to the pulmonary arteries [48]. More recent reviews on cardiac trauma mention the use of pledgets only for the repair of myocardial lacerations/holes in older patients and not for the younger population, with no clear reason behind this [36].

RECOMMENDATION

There is minimal evidence available suggesting that pledget usage in elective cardiac valve surgery is beneficial, and there are few studies examining the use in the repair of traumatic cardiac injury. In contrast, there have also been several reports showing how complications directly from pledget use may be life-threatening. Despite their popularity, there is no evidence that pledget use is beneficial in the suture repair of cardiac injuries.

Level of evidence: 4. Grade of recommendation: C.

Editor's Note

Patients presenting with cardiac tamponade (or the more common cause of cardiac compressive shock, tension pneumothorax) respond to fluid resuscitation in a manner indistinguishable from the more common hemorrhagic shock trauma patient. This can make the diagnosis of cardiac tamponade extremely difficult to discern. Therefore, a high index of suspicion must be maintained in patients with proximity penetrating chest and abdominal injuries or severe blunt thoracic injury.

Cardiac injury is very rare after blunt trauma and occurs in patients after only the most severe chest injuries. Stable patients with troponin leak do not appear to be a risk for subsequent complications and do not require monitoring. Patients with malignant arrhythmias and pump failure have significant damage and need critical care support.

Penetrating injuries traveling through or into the cardiac box must be evaluated for cardiac injury, as about 25% of patients with this lesion present without any signs or symptoms. In the setting of hemothorax, all patients require a pericardial window, as both ultrasound and 2-D echocardiography notoriously miss the injuries. These comments are based purely on clinical experience, as there are no high-quality data from prospective clinical trials concerning this unusual injury.

REFERENCES

1. Campbell NC, Thomsen SR, Murkart DJ, Meumann CM, Van Middelkoop I, Botha JB. Review of 1198 cases of penetrating cardiac trauma. Br J Surg. 1997;84:1737–40.
2. Turan AA, Karayel FA, Akyildiz E, Pakis I, Uzun I, Gurpinar K, Atilmis U, Kir Z. Cardiac injuries caused by blunt trauma: an autopsy based assessment of the injury pattern. J Forensic Sci. 2010;55(1):82–84.
3. Sutherland M, McKenney M, Elkbuli A. Gun violence during COVID-19 pandemic: Paradoxical trends in New York City, Chicago, Los Angeles, and Baltimore. Am J Emerg Med. 2021 Jan 1;39:225–6.
4. Goldman S, Bodas M, Lin S, Radomislensky I, Levin L, Bahouth H, Acker A, Bahouth H, Bar A, Becker A, Braslavsky A. Gunshot casualties in Israel: A decade of violence. Injury. 2022 Aug 8;53(10):3156–62.
5. Degiannis E, Loogna P, Doll D, Bonanno F, Bowely DM, Smith MD. Penetrating cardiac injuries: Recent experiences in South Africa. World J Surg. 2006;30(7):1258–64.
6. Jhunjhunwala R, Mina MJ, Roger EI, Dente CJ, Heninger M, Carr JS, Dougherty SD, Gelbard RB, Nicholas JM, Wyrzykowski AD, Feliciano DV. Reassessing the cardiac box: A comprehensive evaluation of the relationship between thoracic gunshot wounds and cardiac injury. J Trauma Acute Care Surg. 2017 Sep 1;83(3):349–55.
7. Yousef R, Carr JA. Blunt cardiac trauma: A review of the current knowledge and management. Ann Thorac Surg. 2014;98:1134–40.
8. Mandal AK, Sanusi M. Penetrating chest wounds: 24 years experience. World J Surg. 2001;25(9):1145–49.
9. Dominguez F, Beekley AC, Huffer LJ, Gentlesk PJ, Eckart RE. High-velocity penetrating thoracic trauma with suspected cardiac involvement in a combat support hospital. Gen Thorac Cardiovasc Surg. 2011;59:547–52.
10. Fokin AA, Knight JW, Yoshinaga K, Abid AT, Grady R, Alayon AL, Puente I. Blunt cardiac injury in patients with sternal fractures. Cureus. 2022 Mar 4;14(3):1–11.
11. Grigorian A, Milliken J, Livingston JK, Spencer D, Gabriel V, Schubl SD, Kong A, Barrios C, Joe V, Nahmias J. National risk factors for blunt cardiac injury: Hemopneumothorax is the strongest predictor. Am J Surg. 2019 Apr 1;217(4):639–42.
12. Clancy K, Velopulos C, Bilaniuk JW, Collier B, Crowley W, Kurek S, Lui F, Nayduch D, Sangosanya A, Tucker B, Haut ER, Eastern Association for the Surgery of Trauma. Screening for blunt cardiac injury: An eastern association for the surgery of trauma practice management guideline. J Trauma Acute Care Surg. 2012;73(Suppl 4):S301–S306.
13. Fulda GJ, Giberson F, Hailstone D, Law A, Stillabower M. An evaluation of serum troponin T and signal-averaged electrocardiography in predicting electrocardiographic abnormalities after blunt chest trauma. J. Trauma Acute Care Surg. 1997 Aug 1;43(2):304–12.
14. Nagy K, Lohmann C, Kim DO, Barrett J. Role of echocardiography in the diagnosis of occult penetrating cardiac injury. J Trauma. 1995;38(6):859–62.
15. Kang N, Hsee L, Rizoli S, Alison P. Injury. Int J Care Injured. 2009;40:919–27.
16. Tang CC, Huang JF, Kuo LW, Cheng CT, Liao CH, Hsieh CH, Fu CY. The highest troponin I level during admission is associated with mortality in blunt cardiac injury patients. Injury. 2022 Jun 10;53(9):2960–66.
17. Abd Ella TF, Salem SA, Zytoon AA. The potential benefit of emergency ultrasound plus MDCT for the diagnosis of major chest trauma … a diagnostic test accuracy study. Egypt J Hosp Med. 2021 Apr 1;83(1):1270–8.
18. Fadel R, El-Menyar A, ElKafrawy S, Gad MG. Traumatic blunt cardiac injuries: An updated narrative review. Int J Crit Illn Inj Sci. 2019 Jul;9(3):113.
19. Shenoy KS, Jeevannavar SS, Baindoor P, Shetty S. Fatal blunt cardiac injury: Are there any subtle indicators? Case Rep. 2014 Feb 12;2014:bcr2013203149.
20. O'Connor JO, Ditillo M, Scalea T. Penetrating cardiac injury. J R Army Med Corps. 2009;155(3):185–90.
21. Kang N, Hsee L, Rizoli S, Alison P. Penetrating cardiac injury: Overcoming the limits set by nature. Injury. 2009;40:919–27.
22. Jacob S, Sebastian JC, Cherian PK, Abraham A, John Sk. Pericardial effusion impending tamponade: A look beyond Beck's triad. Am J Emerg Med. 2009;27(2):216–19.
23. Burack JH, Kandil E, Sawas A, O'Neill PA, Sclafani SJ, Lowery RC, Zenilman ME. Triage and outcomes of patients with mediastinal penetrating trauma. Ann Thorac Surg. 2007;83(2):377–82.
24. Nagy KK, Roberts RR, Smith RF, Joseph KT, An GC, Bokhari F, Barrett J. Trans-mediastinal gunshot wounds: Are "stable" patients really stable? World J. Surg. 2002;26:1247–50.
25. Teixeira PG, Georgiou C, Inaba K, Dubose J, Plurad D, Chan LS, Toms C, Noguchi TT, Demetriades D. Blunt cardiac trauma: lessons learned from the medical examiner. J Trauma. 2009;67(6):1259–64.
26. Turk EE, Tsokos M. Blunt cardiac trauma caused by fatal falls from height: an autopsy-based assessment of the injury pattern. J Trauma. 2004;57:301–4.

27. Wall MJ, Tsai P, Mattox KL. "Heart and Thoracic Vascular Injuries," in Trauma, 7th edition. ed. Mattox KL, Moore EE, Feliciano DV. McGraw-Hill. 2013.

28. Mascaro M, Trojian TH. Blunt cardiac contusions. Clin Sports Med. 2013;32(2):267–71.

29. Dubrow TJ, Mihalka J, Eisenhauer DM, de Virgilio C, Finch M, Mena IG, Nelson RJ, Wilson SE, Robertson JM. Myocardial contusion in the stable patient: what level of care is appropriate? Surgery. 1989 Aug 1;106(2):267–74.

30. Cachecho R, Grindlinger GA, Lee VW. The clinical significance of myocardial contusion. J Trauma. 1992;33(1):68–71; discussion-3.

31. Stutsrim A, Lundy M, Nunn A, Avery M, Miller P, Meredith JW, Carmichael S. Blunt cardiac trauma and pericardial effusion. J Trauma Acute Care Surg. 2021 Jul 1; 91(1):e24–e6.

32. Fitzgerald M, Spencer J, Johnson F, Marasco S, Atkin C, Kossmann T. Definitive management of acute cardiac tamponade secondary to blunt trauma. Emerg Med Australas. 2005 Oct;17(5–6):494–9.

33. Omoto K, Tanaka C, Fukuda R, Tagami T, Unemoto K. Comparison of the effectiveness of pericardiocentesis and surgical pericardiotomy in the prognosis of patients with blunt traumatic cardiac tamponade: A multicenter study using the Japan Trauma Data Bank. Acute Med Surg. 2022 Jan;9(1):e768.

34. Choo TL, Wong KY, Chen CK, Tan TH. Successful drainage of a traumatic haemopericardium with pericardiocentesis through an intercostal approach. Emerg Med Australas. 2010 Dec;22(6):565–7.

35. Chestovich PJ, McNicoll CF, Fraser DR, Patel PP, Kuhls DA, Clark E, Fildes JJ. Selective use of pericardial window and drainage as the sole treatment for hemopericardium from penetrating chest trauma. J Trauma Acute Care Surg. 2018 Aug 1;3(1):e000187.

36. González-Hadad A, Ordoñez CA, Parra MW, Caicedo Y, Padilla N, Millán M, García A, Vidal-Carpio JM, Pino LF, Herrera MA, Quintero L. Damage control in penetrating cardiac trauma. Colombia Médica. 2021 Jun;52(2): 1–12.

37. Rodgers-Fischl PM, Makdisi G, Keshavamurthy S. Extrapericardial tamponade after blunt trauma. Ann Thorac Surg. 2021 Jan 1;111(1):e49–e50.

38. Gilchrist, I. C. Foreign body in the heart: Be careful how you remove it. Catheter Cardiovasc Interv. 2012;80(3):497.

39. Chen Q, Zhang S, Jiang N. The unpredictable foreign body in heart. Indian J Surg. 2021 Aug;83(4):1041–2.

40. Symbas PN, Vlasis-Hale SE, Picone AL, Hatcher CR, Jr. Missiles in the heart. Ann Thorac Surg. 1989;48(2):192–4.

41. Selvakumar S, Newsome K, Nguyen T, McKenny M, Bilski T, Elkbuli A. The role of pericardial window techniques in the management of penetrating cardiac injuries in the hemodynamically stable patient: where does it fit in the current trauma algorithm? J Surg Res. 2022 Aug 1; 276:120–35.

42. Johnson BP, Hojman HM, Mahoney EJ, Detelich D, Karamchandani M, Ricard C, Breeze JL, Bugaev N. Nationwide utilization of cardiopulmonary bypass in cardiothoracic trauma: A retrospective analysis of the National Trauma Data Bank. J Trauma Acute Care Surg. 2021 Sep 1;91(3):501–6.

43. Osman A, Fong CP, Wahab SF, Panebianco N, Teran F. Transesophageal echocardiography at the golden hour: identification of blunt traumatic aortic injuries in the Emergency Department. J Emerg Med. 2020 Sep 1;59(3):418–23.

44. Newton JR, Jr., Glower DD, Davis JW, Rankin JS. Evaluation of suture techniques for mitral valve replacement. J Thorac Cardiovasc Surg. 1984;88(2):248–52.

45. Katz NM, Blackstone EH, Kirklin JW, Bradley EL, Lemons JE. Suture techniques for atrioventricular valves: experimental study. J Thorac Cardiovasc Surg. 1981;81(4):528–36.

46. Bowman MR, King RM. Comparison of staples and sutures for cardiorrhaphy in traumatic puncture wounds of the heart. J Emerg Med. 1996;14(5):615–8.

47. Lifschultz BD, Donoghue ER, Leestma JE, Boade WA. Embolization of cotton pledgets following insertion of porcine cardiac valve bioprostheses. J Forensic Sci. 1987; 32(6):1796–800.

48. Weingarten J, Kauffman SL. Teflon embolization to pulmonary arteries. Ann Thorac Surg. 1977;23(4):371–3.

20

Injury to the Esophagus, Trachea, and Bronchus

Deborah L. Mueller and Tabitha Threatt

Dedicated to the memory of my mentor, Dr. Deborah Mueller.

The surgeon I aspire to be.

—Tabitha Threatt

David Hume, a Scottish philosopher, remarked that a wise man proportions his belief to the evidence. In the case of traumatic injuries to the esophagus and tracheobronchial tree, the evidence consists mostly of case reports, retrospective analyses, and opinions. The rarity of these injuries has prevented the accumulation of significant prospective data. This brief synopsis will cover incidence, mechanism of injury, and current practices in diagnosing and managing these rare injuries. It may not strengthen the wise physician's beliefs, but it accurately reflects the current evidence (Table 20.1).

20.1 Trachea and Bronchus

20.1.1 What Is the Incidence of Blunt and Penetrating Tracheobronchial Injuries?

Autopsy studies of blunt trauma patients reveal an incidence of tracheobronchial injury in 2.8% of fatalities [23]. In a review spanning 9 years and nearly 13,000 patients including blunt and penetrating mechanisms of injury, the incidence of tracheobronchial injury was only 0.13% [24]. The right mainstem bronchus appears to be injured more commonly in blunt trauma, perhaps due to its lack of protection by the aorta [23]. Penetrating cervical tracheal injury is more common, occurring in up to 7.5% of patients [5]. In contrast, penetrating thoracic tracheobronchial injury is rare, occurring in less than 1% of patients even with transmediastinal trajectories [25]. The mortality rate from tracheobronchial injuries in patients who survive hospital admission is 9%, which has decreased historically from 30% [26].

20.1.2 What Is the Mechanism for Penetrating and Blunt Tracheobronchial Injuries?

While most penetrating injuries from knives and bullets require no explanation, the clothesline injury pattern is unique. An obvious penetrating or subtle closed injury to the trachea can occur when a patient strikes an unseen wire while on a moving vehicle. Blunt cervical tracheal injury can occur from hyperextension or flexion and contact of the neck with the dashboard or steering wheel in a motor vehicle crash. It has also been described after a blow to the neck from a table corner, a knee, and bicycle handlebars in children [1]. Blunt thoracic

TABLE 20.1

Clinical Question Summary

Question	Answer	Levels of Evidence	Grade of Recommendation	References
What are the most common symptoms and signs of tracheobronchial injury?	Respiratory distress and subcutaneous emphysema/crepitus	IIIb, IIIb, IIIb, Ib	B	[1–4]
What is the best initial diagnostic test for tracheobronchial injury?	CT for initial screening with confirmation bronchoscopy	IIb, IV, IV, IV, IIb, IV, Ib	B	[1–3, 5–8]
Is there a role in the nonoperative management of traumatic tracheobronchial injuries?	Yes, in patients with small tears and a benign clinical presentation	IV, IV, IV, IV	C	[1, 2, 9, 10]
What are the most common symptoms and signs of esophageal injury?	Pain (neck, chest, or on swallowing) and crepitus on physical exam	Ib, IIIa, IIb, Ib, IIb	B	[6, 11–14]
What is the best initial diagnostic test for esophageal injury?	CT for initial screening with confirmation endoscopy and/or esophagography	IIb, IV, IIb, V, IV, IV, IIb	C	[13, 15–20]
Is there a role in the nonoperative management of traumatic esophageal injury?	Not enough evidence to recommend traumatic injuries at this time	IV, IV	D	[21, 22]

DOI: 10.1201/9781003316800-20

tracheobronchial injury has been reported after forceful anterior-posterior compression of the thoracic cage, rapid deceleration with shearing forces on areas of tracheal fixation, or from a closed high-pressure system if the glottis is closed during compressive forces [26]. In an analysis of 88 cases with the site of blunt tracheobronchial injury recorded, 76% occurred within 2 cm of the carina, lending credibility to the postulated mechanisms [27]. Penetrating injuries often involve the cervical trachea, while blunt tracheal injuries tend to be near the carina [28].

20.1.3 What Are the Most Reliable Initial Symptoms and Signs of Traumatic Tracheobronchial Injury?

Series that include data on symptomatology and physical findings report the most common symptom as respiratory distress and the most common physical finding as subcutaneous emphysema [1–4]. The initial chest X-ray (CXR) findings of patients in one of these series demonstrated subcutaneous emphysema in 81%, pneumothorax in 56%, and pneumomediastinum in 37% [3]. Tracheobronchial injury may be associated with small-volume hemoptysis, but massive hemoptysis associated with tracheal injury should raise suspicion for acute tracheoinnominate fistula or bronchial artery injury [29]. In most case series in the literature, there are occasional patients with a delay in diagnosis due to minimal symptoms and findings or due to findings being attributed to other etiologies.

RECOMMENDATION

Respiratory distress and subcutaneous emphysema/crepitus.

Grade of recommendation: B.

20.1.4 What Is the Best Diagnostic Test for Traumatic Tracheobronchial Injury?

Certain patients with airway injury will have obvious findings on the physical exam such as air bubbling from a penetrating neck wound. An additional subset of patients will require operative intervention immediately for injury to adjacent vascular structures, leading to the discovery of airway injury. Patients with a blunt mechanism of injury can be more difficult to diagnose.

While an initial CXR may demonstrate an abnormality, it can be normal in 12% of patients on presentation [3]. In addition, the findings on CXR such as subcutaneous emphysema, pneumothorax, and pneumomediastinum are not specific to the tracheobronchial injury. In a review of 51 blunt thoracic trauma patients who had a CXR followed by chest computed tomography (CT) demonstrating pneumomediastinum, only 10% had tracheobronchial injury [30]. More often pneumomediastinum was ascribed to the Macklin effect originally described in 1939, when blunt alveolar rupture leads to air

dissection along bronchovascular sheaths and into the mediastinum. Injuries to the right mainstem bronchus typically present with pneumomediastinum and pneumothorax, whereas left mainstem bronchus injuries may present with isolated pneumomediastinum [28].

In this era of high-quality rapid imaging with CT, many patients will undergo CT as part of their trauma evaluation. In a prospective trial of multidetector computed tomographic angiography (MDCTA) for penetrating cervical wounds, MDCTA was 100% sensitive for aerodigestive injury [6]. Overall specificity was 97.5%, with three of the five false-positive studies demonstrating air tracking suspicious for an aerodigestive injury that was subsequently ruled out by other diagnostic modalities. In a retrospective review of 18 patients with either blunt or penetrating tracheobronchial injury who underwent both chest CT and bronchoscopy, Scaglione et al. described radiologic findings that showed the site of injury was detectable by CT in 94% of cases [7]. Findings included overdistension of the endotracheal cuff (>4 cm), endotracheal cuff herniation through a tracheal wall defect, displacement of the endotracheal tube, tracheal/bronchial wall discontinuity, enlargement of the bronchus, and the "fallen lung" sign. In a prospective study of 24 patients suspected to have a tracheobronchial injury, Faure et al. demonstrated the multiplanar reconstruction of CT images had a diagnostic sensitivity of 100% and a specificity of 82%. All injuries in this study were confirmed by surgery, bronchoscopy, or autopsy [8]. Notably, this level of diagnostic accuracy with CT may require experienced radiologists to utilize specific scanning techniques.

Bronchoscopy with direct visualization of the airway remains a good diagnostic tool for tracheobronchial injury. While most injuries are obvious, a few can be subtle to the eye. Peribronchial tissue can make the airway tree seem intact with only a slight distraction from the cartilaginous rings [31]. Kiser et al. found reports of 46 patients with repair of chronic tracheobronchial obstruction from 3 months to 34 years after injury [27]. Repeat bronchoscopy may be necessary if suspicion of the injury is high but the initial bronchoscopy appeared normal. Since bronchoscopy is more invasive, it is more commonly utilized as a confirmatory diagnostic procedure, especially since false positives can occur with CT screening.

RECOMMENDATION

CT for initial screening followed by bronchoscopy for confirmation.

Grade of recommendation: B.

20.1.5 What Are the Surgical Management Options for Tracheobronchial Injuries?

The principles of surgical repair are, for the most part, consistent throughout the literature [2, 3, 24, 29, 32]. Injuries proximal to the aortic arch (cervical trachea) are approached through a collar or anterior sternocleidomastoid incision and may require a partial sternotomy. The mediastinal trachea and right mainstem bronchus are best approached through a right posterolateral thoracotomy at the level of the fifth rib to avoid the aorta. The left mainstem bronchus is best approached through a left posterolateral thoracotomy. The high mediastinal tracheal injury with associated vascular injury may also be approached through a sternotomy [3]. Debridement of devitalized tissue is recommended with the use of absorbable sutures, with knots secured exterior to the airway to prevent granulation tissue formation in the airway. Minimal dissection of the lateral aspects of the trachea will prevent ischemia to the repair. The use of a tracheostomy, while touted by some authors, is discouraged by others, who suggest that extubation and avoidance of positive pressure ventilation in the postoperative period are best for healing the injury [2].

In the setting of larger destructive wounds, several centimeters of the trachea can be resected and primary anastomosis performed. More length can be obtained if the spine fracture has been eliminated and the neck can be flexed. There are additional maneuvers to gain length for tracheal repair that are beyond the scope of this chapter. Most authors recommend buttressing complex repairs with flaps of the pericardium or intercostal muscle in the chest or strap muscles or the sternocleidomastoid in the neck [3, 24, 29, 32]. Alternatively, the use of a silicone T-tube placed in the trachea to extend from below the vocal cords to the carina with an airway maintained by cannulating the horizontal exteriorized limb with an endotracheal tube has been described in at least 16 traumatic tracheal injuries [33]. This maneuver allows damage control in an unstable patient with the repair of the airway in a more elective manner, or the T-tube can serve as a stent while healing by secondary intention occurs. Extracorporeal membrane oxygenation (ECMO) has arisen as an adjunct and bridge to the surgical management of severe tracheal injuries [34].

20.1.6 What Is the Role of Nonoperative Management for Tracheobronchial Injuries?

Nonoperative management of small iatrogenic injuries of the trachea sustained during endotracheal intubation has been described by multiple authors [2, 9]. The largest of these types of injuries managed nonoperatively was 5 cm [10]. Duval et al. described five children with noniatrogenic traumatic tracheobronchial injuries that were successfully managed nonoperatively with intubation and antibiotics [1]. A retrospective review of adults at one institution over 10 years described a nonoperative approach for both iatrogenic and traumatic tracheobronchial injuries [2]. While 89% of iatrogenic intubation injuries in these adults were managed nonoperatively, only 27% of traumatic injuries met their criteria to be managed nonoperatively. Surgical management was performed if patients had concomitant esophageal injury, progressive subcutaneous or mediastinal emphysema, severe dyspnea

requiring intubation, difficulty with mechanical ventilation, pneumothorax with a persistent air leak, the presence of an open tracheal injury, or mediastinitis. All patients were followed up for 2 years with repeat bronchoscopy, and the incidence of scarring, granuloma formation, and stenosis did not appear significantly different between the nonoperative and operative groups.

It may be reasonable to allow some tracheobronchial injuries to heal by secondary intention if the patient has no associated injuries requiring surgical repair, no significant respiratory difficulty, no persistent air leak, and well-opposed edges at the site of injury. Antibiotic utilization to prevent mediastinitis is described in all of these nonoperative approaches. It is important to remember that the number of patients in all of these reports, whether operative or nonoperative, is incredibly small; therefore, the only evidence we have is experience.

RECOMMENDATION

Nonoperative management is acceptable in patients with small tears and a benign clinical presentation.

Grade of recommendation: C.

20.2 Esophagus

20.2.1 What Is the Incidence of Blunt and Penetrating Esophageal Injuries?

Traumatic injury of the esophagus is uncommon. A contemporary 7-year review of the National Trauma Data Bank (NTDB) demonstrated an incidence of 0.03% when including blunt and penetrating mechanisms [11]. Not surprisingly, in studies of penetrating trauma, the incidence of esophageal injury, both cervical and thoracic, is nearly identical to the incidence of penetrating tracheobronchial injury. Cervical esophageal injuries occurred in 8.5% of penetrating neck wounds, and thoracic esophageal injuries occurred in 1.2% of penetrating thoracic wounds [35, 36].

20.2.2 What Is the Mechanism for Penetrating and Blunt Esophageal Injuries?

The most common mechanism for penetrating esophageal injury is iatrogenic endoscopic perforation, with rates escalating significantly when therapeutic interventions such as dilation are undertaken [37]. While many articles in the literature lump iatrogenic and noniatrogenic injuries together to achieve a better number of esophageal injuries to analyze, the average trauma patient has significant other associated injuries that may affect the presentation, management, and outcome. The focus of this chapter will remain strictly on noniatrogenic traumatic esophageal injuries to allow a narrower focus on the true presentation, diagnosis, and management of these specific types of injuries. Gunshot wounds are responsible for the majority of noniatrogenic penetrating esophageal injuries in the United States [37].

Blunt cervical esophageal injury is thought to occur from a sudden blow to a hyperextended neck, similar to cervical tracheal injury, with the esophagus stretched against the cervical spine [38]. In the most extensive review published of 63 patients with blunt esophageal injury, Beal et al. demonstrated that 82% of the injuries occurred in the cervicothoracic esophagus, defined as the esophagus from origination to the tracheal carina [39]. Interestingly, in this same series, 56% had concomitant tracheal injuries. When both the trachea and esophagus are injured at the level of the carina, Martel et al. suggest this disruption is best described as "acute tracheoesophageal burst injury," resulting from an acute increase in tracheal intraluminal pressure after rapid compression of the thoracic cavity with a closed glottis leading to rupture of the membranous trachea and the adjacent esophagus [12]. This mechanism was delineated clearly in a case report of a 14-year-old boy struck abruptly in the chest while lying flat and sustaining a tracheoesophageal injury [13].

20.2.3 What Are the Most Reliable Initial Symptoms and Signs of Traumatic Esophageal Injury?

In a large retrospective series of 405 penetrating esophageal injuries, Asensio et al. state that most patients had no symptoms or signs on initial presentation [14]. However, if one looks closely at the hospital course of these patients, the early mortality defined as death in the emergency room or operating room was 14.6%. These patients may have had symptoms or signs of esophageal injury, but the urgency of other injuries probably superseded any detailed examination or documentation. Another 175 patients went directly to the operating room, and careful evaluation for symptoms or signs may have been appropriately abbreviated. Delving into single-center studies of penetrating cervical trauma, several authors report that symptoms or signs were present in 70–100% of patients with esophageal injury [4, 15, 40, 41]. The symptoms in these studies include dysphagia, odynophagia, dysphonia, hoarseness, and hematemesis. Beal et al. also demonstrated that 66% of patients with blunt esophageal injury had symptoms including neck pain, chest pain, dyspnea, dysphagia, and/or hoarseness [39].

The most reliable physical exam finding was subcutaneous emphysema in both blunt and penetrating esophageal injuries. This sign was found in 33% of patients with blunt injuries and 45% of patients with penetrating injuries [16, 39]. The most likely etiology for crepitus on palpation is a concomitant tracheal injury, as the incidence of this finding drops to 13% in blunt trauma patients and 28% in penetrating trauma patients when only the esophagus is injured [39, 42]. The presence of subcutaneous emphysema or pneumomediastinum was also the most common finding on CXR, occurring in 30–40% of patients with both mechanisms of injury [16, 39]. It is important to note that based on these more detailed studies regarding signs and symptoms, 25% of patients may still be completely asymptomatic with minimal physical findings and a normal CXR.

RECOMMENDATION

Pain (neck, chest, or on swallowing) and crepitus on physical exam are the most reliable initial symptoms and signs of traumatic esophageal injury.

Grade of recommendation: B.

20.2.4 What Is the Best Diagnostic Test for Traumatic Esophageal Injury?

The mortality rate for traumatic esophageal injury in an NTDB review from 2007 to 2014 was 12% [11]. In this study, the majority of early deaths were from associated injuries, and 30-day mortality was higher for thoracic esophageal injuries than cervical injuries. This may be secondary to more extensive, noncontained bacterial spillage leading to more severe infectious and inflammatory complications in the thorax. In patients stable enough to undergo diagnostic studies, it appears that infectious morbidity is increased secondary to the delay in operative repair that occurs with a lengthy diagnostic workup. In the NTDB review, Aiolfi et al. demonstrated treatment within the first 24 hours was a protective factor for mortality, supporting the need for diagnostic efficiency. Several single-center reviews of esophageal perforation have also correlated increased mortality with diagnostic delays [17, 41–43].

CT scan has emerged as a rapidly available screening test for esophageal injury in both blunt and penetrating trauma. In stable blunt trauma patients, there are often other indications for CT of the neck and chest. In stable penetrating injury patients, CT can be obtained much more rapidly than traditional studies such as esophagography and endoscopy. Castelguidone et al. have described retrospectively the CT findings in six patients with traumatic esophageal injuries [18]. The most common findings were periesophageal air and fluid in 83% and esophageal wall thickening in 66%. Other nonspecific findings included pneumothorax, pleural effusion, and subcutaneous emphysema. Fuhrmann et al. tried to further delineate in 214 cases of traumatic pneumomediastinum if mediastinal fluid could be a predictor for esophageal perforation [19]. In this study, the *presence* of mediastinal fluid had a positive likelihood ratio of 96% and a negative predictive value of 99.5%, but the low number of esophageal injuries did not allow them to conclude that the *absence* of mediastinal fluid excludes esophageal injury, as the 95% confidence interval was 65–100%. In the largest prospective study of neck CTA for detecting significant vascular or aerodigestive injuries from penetrating trauma, sensitivity was 100% and specificity was 97.5% [6]. Notably, 98% of patients screened with CTA avoided further esophageal diagnostic studies with no missed injuries. CT has emerged as a tool to quickly screen for esophageal injury. It can potentially be definitive for diagnosis, but more often may show nonspecific yet concerning findings that should be further evaluated with endoscopy and/or esophagography.

In the 1980s an elegant prospective study of 118 stable patients with penetrating neck injury evaluated the sensitivity and specificity of barium esophagography as well as flexible and rigid esophagoscopy before operative exploration in all patients [15]. Then, barium esophagography had the best sensitivity (89%) and specificity (100%) of the diagnostic adjuncts. The combination of barium esophagography and rigid esophagoscopy was recommended to avoid any missed injuries if managing a patient nonoperatively, as flexible endoscopy had the lowest sensitivity. Major technologic advancements improving resolution and magnification with flexible endoscopy have occurred since then. Arantes et al. demonstrated in a large study of 163 patients thought to have an esophageal injury from all mechanisms that modern flexible endoscopy had a 95.8% sensitivity, 100% specificity, and 99.3% accuracy [20]. There are some advantages to flexible endoscopy, one of which is the ability to perform it in any location and expeditiously. The improved accuracy of flexible esophagoscopy has led to the recommendation to use CTA as a screening test, with flexible esophagoscopy utilized if periesophageal air/ fluid is seen [21]. Fluoroscopic esophagography in this algorithm is recommended as an adjunct to equivocal endoscopy results. If esophagography is utilized, the recommended process remains to first administer a low osmolar water-soluble contrast agent but if negative for injury follow with thin barium for the best diagnostic accuracy.

An emerging technique for evaluating esophageal trauma is CT esophagography. The majority of studies evaluating this technique involve patients that have had recent surgery; however, one study on penetrating trauma patients was published in 2015 [44]. Conradie et al. evaluated 102 hemodynamically stable patients with penetrating neck or chest trauma using oral contrast before imaging in symptomatic patients or after initial CT in asymptomatic patients with a high index of suspicion of digestive tract injury. A low osmolar iodinated contrast was mixed in a 1:1 ratio with tap water for a total of 50 mL given orally or by nasogastric (NG) tube in intubated patients, with the NG tube retracted toward the pharynx before administration. The majority of patients had confirmatory traditional studies, including fluoroscopic esophagography or endoscopy, including 50% of the patients initially suspected not to have an injury by CT. The other 50% of the patients in the no suspected injury cohort had a wound trajectory, were not in proximity to the digestive tract, or had 30-day follow-up by records or telephone to ensure no injuries were missed. CT esophagography had a sensitivity of 95% and specificity of 85.4% and 91.5% when studies were read by two radiologists blinded to all other information. More studies are needed on this promising technique that can be easily and rapidly performed with no special equipment in most emergency rooms.

CTA of the neck or chest is the best initial test to screen for esophageal injury in stable patients [21]. If CT is suggestive of but not diagnostic for esophageal injury, a confirmatory diagnostic test should be undertaken. The best confirmatory test should probably be the one that can be performed most expediently at any individual institution and is most appropriate for the clinical scenario of the patient. Currently, flexible esophagoscopy is considered as accurate as esophagography. In either case, if one test is equivocal, the second study should be undertaken to try to ensure the minimization of missed injuries.

RECOMMENDATION

CT for initial screening with confirmation endoscopy and/or esophagography is the best diagnostic test for traumatic esophageal injury.

Grade of recommendation: C.

20.2.5 What Are the Surgical Management Options for Esophageal Injuries?

The surgical options described in the literature range from primary repair to multiple variations on diversion, with drainage or even resection, and several succinct reviews of management have been published in the last decade [21, 22]. Approaches to the esophagus vary based on the anatomic location of the injury. The cervical esophagus is approached through a left cervical incision along the anterior border of the sternocleidomastoid. The upper thoracic esophagus is approached through a right fourth through sixth interspace posterolateral thoracotomy depending on perforation location, while the lower esophagus is approached through a left seventh interspace posterolateral thoracotomy [22]. Primary repair has been described with both single-layer and two-layer closures of the esophagus after debridement of devitalized tissue [16, 17, 45]. Drainage as an adjunct to primary repair was used in the majority of patients in the largest studies of noniatrogenic penetrating esophageal injuries, although never scientifically studied [14, 21, 45]. Buttressing of repairs with flaps of muscle, pleura, pericardium, omentum, and stomach have all been described, and their use seems predicated on the amount of local tissue destruction, injuries to adjacent structures such as the trachea, and the location of the primary injury [12, 14, 16, 17, 35, 43, 45]. While thoracoscopic approaches for Boerhaave syndrome have been described, this approach has not yet been described in the traumatic injury of the esophagus. Bougies and flexible endoscopy are liberally used during most operative procedures to assist in or evaluate repairs. Antibiotics, nothing by mouth (NPO), and enteral feeding are often recommended with follow-up esophagography to evaluate the integrity of the repair. After primary repair, the most common procedure performed in the largest studies of both penetrating and blunt esophageal injury and the recent NTDB review was drainage alone [11, 14, 39]. More complex esophageal resection, exclusion, or diversion only occurred in 7% of penetrating esophageal injuries and 9% of blunt esophageal injuries in these studies. Additionally, the NTDB review demonstrated decreased utilization of resection and diversion in the last decade, with only 3% (28/944) of blunt and penetrating esophageal injury patients managed with these techniques [11]. Most authors favor damage control such as drainage with repair around a T-tube or diverting esophagostomy with distal feeding access in more destructive injuries with very rare use of resection in the acute trauma setting [21, 22]. Instead, the authors suggest damage control with a delay of major reconstruction for 6–12 months to fully assess what will be necessary.

Therefore, the experience would suggest that primary repair with drainage is appropriate in most patients. Primary repair without drainage for simple stab wounds with minimal tissue destruction is also reasonable. Drainage alone, if the injury is difficult to identify or the patient's condition warrants abbreviated surgery, is a reasonable choice as well. Finally, diversion and drainage seem to be preferable to resection with or without anastomosis, but these techniques overall portend a poor prognosis, similar to delays in diagnosis given the destructive esophageal injuries that would warrant the use of these techniques.

20.2.6 Is There Any Role for Nonoperative Management in Traumatic Esophageal Injury?

For the most part, nonoperative or conservative management for esophageal perforation has focused on iatrogenic, emetogenic, and foreign body ingestion etiologies. In oropharyngeal and hypopharyngeal injuries from traumatic causes, literature has emerged supporting nonoperative treatment for patients diagnosed early with well-encapsulated extravasation that does not dissect down tissue planes in patients who have no signs of sepsis and minimal symptoms without any other indication for operative intervention [22, 46]. Less clear is the role of this strategy in the traumatic injury of the esophagus below the cricoid. This nonoperative management typically includes NPO status, NG tube placement beyond the injury for enteral feeding, administration of antibiotics, and follow-up esophagography to evaluate healing. Percutaneous drainage techniques can augment this strategy as long as the patient is clinically doing well.

Endoscopic approaches for nontraumatic esophageal perforations to include clips (through the scope and over the scope), stents (fully covered or partially covered self-expanding metal), and even endoscopic suturing can be found in the literature, but very little is known about their efficacy in trauma [47]. Case reports successfully utilizing stents in esophageal trauma have been published [48]. In addition, in the large recent NTDB review, Aiolfi et al. reported that 11 stents were used in 944 blunt and penetrating esophageal injuries, but no additional details of these cases are known [11]. Stents may have a place in the management of some injuries of the esophagus, but data regarding ideal utilization of this emerging technique is as rare as the esophageal injury itself.

RECOMMENDATION

There is not enough evidence to recommend nonoperative management of traumatic injuries at this time.

Grade of recommendation: D.

Editor's Note

Fortunately, injuries to the trachea, bronchus, and esophagus are rare. Unfortunately, this means that a single institution has limited experience with the entity, and therefore, there is little high-quality evidence supporting our current management protocols. The clinician evaluating a trauma patient would typically investigate the aerodigestive tract (both tracheobronchial

injury and esophageal injury) simultaneously, so this note will address both lesions together.

The signs and symptoms of these injuries such as subcutaneous air, pneumothorax, pneumomediastinum, and chest tube air leak in the setting of significant blunt mechanism or proximity of penetrating injury are not specific and are often absent (not sensitive). As delays in the diagnosis of these injuries (particularly esophageal injury) have a significant negative impact on patient complications and death, it is imperative that diagnostic imaging (chest CT angiogram) with bronchoscopy and/or upper endoscopy be liberally employed.

Surgical management is nicely summarized here for the aerodigestive tract. Nonoperative management of tracheobronchial and esophageal injuries appears possible in selective cases where no associated injuries mandate operative intervention. For extremely severe tracheobronchial injuries, ECMO represents a new, now more widely available modality to augment management. The evidence for these statements is based on empiric observations, not clinical trials.

REFERENCES

1. Duval EL, Geraerts SD. Management of blunt tracheal trauma in children: A case series and review of the literature. *Eur J Pediatr.* 2007;166:559–563.
2. Gómez-Caro A, Ausín P, Moradiellos FJ, et al. Role of conservative medical management of tracheobronchial injuries. *J Trauma.* 2006;61:1426–1435.
3. Rossbach MM, Johnson SB, Gomez MA, et al. Management of major tracheobronchial injuries: A 28-year experience. *Ann Thorac Surg.* 1998;65:182–186.
4. Demetriades D, Theodorou D, Cornwell E, et al. Evaluation of penetrating injuries of the neck: Prospective study of 223 patients. *World J Surg.* 1997;21:41–48.
5. Inaba K, Munera F, McKenney M, et al. Prospective evaluation of screening multislice helical computed tomographic angiography in the initial evaluation of penetrating neck injuries. *J Trauma.* 2006;61:144–149.
6. Inaba K, Branco B, Menaker J, et al. Evaluation of multidetector computed tomography for penetrating neck injury: A prospective multicenter study. *J Trauma.* 2012;72(3):576–584.
7. Scagilone M, Romano S, Pinto A, et al. Acute tracheobronchial injuries: Impact of imaging on diagnosis and management implications. *Eur J Radiol.* 2006;59:336–343.
8. Faure A, Floccard B, Pilleul F, et al. Multiplanar reconstruction: A new method for the diagnosis of tracheobronchial rupture? *Int Care Med.* 2007;31:2173–2178.
9. Ross HM, Grant FJ, Wilson RS, et al. Nonoperative management of tracheal laceration during endotracheal intubation. *Ann Thorac Surg.* 1997;63:240–242.
10. Denlinger CE, Veeramachaneni N, Krupnick AS, et al. Nonoperative management of large tracheal injuries. *J Thorac Cardiovasc Surg.* 2008;136(3):782–783.
11. Aiolfi A, Inaba K, Recinos G, et al. Non-iatrogenic esophageal injury: A retrospective analysis from the National Trauma Data Bank. *World J Emerg Surg.* 2017;12:1–7.
12. Martel G, Al-Sabti H, Mulder D, et al. Acute tracheoesophageal burst injury after blunt chest trauma: Case report and review of the literature. *J Trauma.* 2007;62:236–242.

13. Martin de Nicolas JL, Gamez AP, Cruz F, et al. Long tracheobronchial and esophageal rupture after blunt chest trauma: Injury by airway bursting. *Ann Thorac Surg.* 1996; 62:269–272.

14. Asensio JA, Chahwan S, Forno W, et al. Penetrating esophageal injuries: Multicenter study of the American Association for the Surgery of Trauma. *J Trauma.* 2001;50(2):289–296.

15. Weigelt JA, Thal ER, Snyder WH, et al. Diagnosis of penetrating cervical esophageal injuries. *Am J Surg.* 1987;154: 619–622.

16. Glatterer MS, Toon RS, Ellestad C, et al. Management of blunt and penetrating external esophageal trauma. *J Trauma.* 1985;25(8):784–792.

17. Richardson JD, Martin LF, Borzotta AP, et al. Unifying concepts in the treatment of esophageal leaks. *Am J Surg.* 1985;149:157–162.

18. Castelguidone E, Merola S, Pinto A, et al. Esophageal injuries: Spectrum of multidetector row CT findings. *Eur J Radiol.* 2006;59:344–348.

19. Fuhrmann C, Weissenborn M, Salman S. Mediastinal fluid as a predictor for esophageal perforation as the cause of pneumomediastinum. *Emerg Radiol.* 2021;28:233–238.

20. Arantes V, Campolina C, Valerio SH, et al. Flexible esophagoscopy as a diagnostic tool for traumatic injuries. *J Trauma.* 2009;66(6):1677–1682.

21. Biffl WL, Moore EE, Feliciano DV, et al. Western trauma association critical decisions in trauma: Diagnosis and management of esophageal injuries. *J Trauma Acute Care Surg.* 2015;79(6):1089–1095.

22. Petrone P, Kassimi K, Jimenez-Gomez M, et al. Management of esophageal injuries secondary to trauma. *Injury.* 2017;48: 1735–1742.

23. Madden BP. Evolutional trends in the management of tracheal and bronchial injuries. *J Thorac Dis.* 2017;9(1): E67–E70.

24. Huh J, Milliken JC, Chen JC. Management of tracheobronchial injuries following blunt and penetrating trauma. *Am Surg.* 1997;63(10):896–899.

25. Okoye OT, Talving P, Teixeira PG, et al. Transmediastinal gunshot wounds in a mature trauma center: Changing perspectives. *Injury.* 2013;44(9):1198–1203.

26. Shemmeri E, Vallières E. Blunt tracheobronchial trauma. *Thorac Surg Clin.* 2018;28(3):429–434.

27. Kiser AC, O'Brien SM, Detterbeck FC. Blunt tracheobronchial injuries: Treatment and outcomes. *Ann Thorac Surg.* 2001;71:2059–2065.

28. Moser JB, Stefanidis K, Vlahos I. Imaging evaluation of tracheobronchial injuries. *Radiographics.* 2020;40(2):515–528.

29. Zhao Z, Zhang T, Yin X, Zhao J, et al. Update on the diagnosis and treatment of the tracheal and bronchial injury. *J Thorac Dis.* 2017;9(1):E50–E56.

30. Wintermark M, Schnyder P. The Macklin effect: A frequent etiology for pneumomediastinum in severe blunt chest trauma. *Chest.* 2001;120:543–547.

31. Allan PF, Kelley TC, Taylor TL, et al. Bronchial transection: Diagnosis and management. *Clin Pulm Med.* 2006;13(3):203–208.

32. Kolestis, E, Prokakis C, Baltayiannis N, et al. Surgical decision making in tracheobronchial injuries on the basis of clinical evidence and the injury's anatomical setting: A retrospective analysis. *Injury.* 2012;43(9):1437–1441.

33. Miller BS, Shafi S, Thal ER. Damage control in complex penetrating tracheal injury and silicone t-tube. *J Trauma.* 2008;64:E18–E20.

34. Clark J, Morrison JJ, O'Connor JV. Extracorporeal membrane oxygenation support during repair of a noniatrogenic tracheal injury. *Ann Thorac Surg.* 2022;113(1):e49–e51.

35. Winter RP, Weigelt JA. Cervical esophageal trauma incidence and cause of esophageal fistulas. *Arch Surg.* 1990;125:849–851.

36. Cornwell EE, Kennedy F, Ayad IA, et al. Transmediastinal gunshot wounds a reconsideration of the role of aortography. *Arch Surg.* 1996;131:949–953.

37. Plott E, Jones D, McDermott D, et al. A state-of-the-art review of esophageal trauma: Where do we stand? *Dis Esophagus.* 2007;20:279–289.

38. Stringer WL, Kelly DL Jr, Johnston FR, et al. Hyperextension injury of the cervical spine with esophageal perforation. Case report. *J Neurosurg.* 1980;53(4):541–543.

39. Beal SL, Pottmeyer EW, Spisso JM. Esophageal perforation following external blunt trauma. *J Trauma.* 1988;28(10):1425–1432.

40. Vassiliu P, Baker J, Henderson S, et al. Aerodigestive injuries of the neck. *Am Surg.* 2001;67(1):75–79.

41. White RK, Morris DM. Diagnosis and management of esophageal perforations. *Am Surg.* 1992;58:112–119.

42. Sheely CH, Mattox KL, Beall AC, et al. Penetrating wounds of the cervical esophagus. *Am J Surg.* 1975;130:707–710.

43. Goldstein LA, Thompson WR. Esophageal perforations: A 15-year experience. *Am J Surg.* 1982;143:495–503.

44. Conradie WJ, Gebremariam FA. Can computed tomography esophagography reliably diagnose traumatic penetrating upper digestive tract injuries? *Clin Imaging.* 2015;39:1039–1045.

45. Smakman N, Nicol AJ, Walther G, et al. Factors affecting outcome in penetrating oesophageal trauma. *Br J Surg.* 2004;91:1513–1519.

46. Madsen AS, Oosthuizen GV, Bruce JL, et al. Selective non-operative management of pharyngoesophageal injuries secondary to penetrating neck trauma: A single-center review of 86 cases. *J Trauma Acute Care Surg.* 2018;85(3):541–548.

47. Gurwara S, Clayton S. Esophageal perforations: An endoscopic approach to management. *Curr Gastroenterol Rep.* 2019;21(57):1–6.

48. CR Amin R, Leonard K, Garcia N, et al. A novel endoscopic approach in the management of a penetrating esophageal gunshot wound. *Semin Thorac Cardiovasc Surg.* 2019;31(3): 622–624.

21

Spleen Injury

Danby Kang and Andrew B. Peitzman

21.1 Introduction

Injury to the spleen is common, resulting in a significant number of hospital admissions, morbidity, and occasionally death. The spleen is the second most commonly injured organ in blunt abdominal trauma and the most common reason for laparotomy after blunt injury [1, 2]. A review of 117,743 adult splenic injuries in the National Trauma Data Bank (NTDB) between 2007 and 2015 revealed that 72.9% were managed nonoperatively, 18.9% with splenectomy, 3.3% with embolization, and 1.8% with a splenic repair. Splenic injuries were grade 1–2 (55%), grade 3 (23%), grade 4 (15%), and grade 5 (7%). Importantly, splenic injury grade impacted management. Grade 1–2 splenic injury was managed nonoperatively in 84%, grade 3 in 72%, grade 4 in 52%, and grade 5 in 29% [2]. Failure of nonoperative management (NOM) decreased from 4.4% to 3.4%. Overwhelming postsplenectomy infection (OPSI) was originally described in the 1950s in asplenic children. Since that time, a greater appreciation of the immunologic role of the spleen and case series reporting an incidence of OPSI of 3–7%, with a case fatality rate of 50–70%, created an impetus for splenic salvage whenever possible [3]. NOM of splenic trauma has been enabled by the widespread availability of rapid, high-resolution computed tomography (CT) and by the frequent success of angiographic embolization of the spleen. Penetrating injury also accounts for 15% of splenic injuries. This chapter will attempt to answer some of the current management controversies involving splenic injury by evaluating the relevant data and developing evidence-based recommendations (Table 21.1).

21.2 Which Patients Are at Risk of Failing Nonoperative Management?

Selective NOM of blunt splenic injuries has become standard for hemodynamically stable patients and those who respond rapidly to initial resuscitation (responders). The minimal criteria for NOM of blunt spleen injuries have been identified as hemodynamic stability and the absence of generalized peritonitis in the setting of a reliable and reproducible exam [4].

NOM of splenic injury involves observation in a monitored setting with serial examinations, at times utilizing splenic artery embolization as an adjunct. Several recent studies have assessed predictors of failure of NOM in blunt splenic injury. The factors associated with failure of NOM were American Association for the Surgery of Trauma (AAST) injury grade of 4 or greater, higher injury severity score, early blood transfusion, moderate or large hemoperitoneum (compared with small or absent hemoperitoneum), and presence of subcapsular hematoma [5]. Large hemoperitoneum is defined as abdominal free fluid extending from the splenic recess to the pelvis, whereas small and moderate hemoperitoneum is free fluid contained in the splenic recess and free fluid extending into the pericolic gutters, respectively.

Although increasing transfusion requirements within the first 24 hours are associated with increasing failure rates of NOM, the exact transfusion level that should trigger the need for intervention is not clear. Transfusion of a single unit of packed red blood cells and transfusion requirement in the emergency department (ED) is associated with increased rates of failure of NOM [6–8]. Patients who fail NOM have a significantly longer hospital stay, higher mortality, and higher complication rate. Appropriate selection of patients who are candidates for NOM is critical.

RECOMMENDATIONS

1. Selective NOM of patients with blunt splenic trauma has a high rate of success. Criteria include hemodynamic stability and absence of peritonitis. Injury, grade, degree of hemoperitoneum, transfusion requirements, and the presence of subcapsular hematoma portend higher failure rates of NOM.

   Level of evidence: 2A. Grade of recommendation: B.

2. Need for transfusion of a single unit of blood is associated with failure of NOM. The available data neither justify nor refute a specific transfusion threshold for nonoperative failure (such as the traditional 2 units of blood). Clinical judgment must be exercised.

   Level of recommendation: None.

TABLE 21.1

Clinical Questions

Questions	Answers	Level of Evidence	Grade of Recommendation	References
Which patients are candidates for NOM of blunt spleen injury?	Hemodynamically stable patients without peritonitis	2A	B	[1–7]
	Increasing age, injury grade, size of hemoperitoneum, ISS, extravasation, or vascular abnormality on CT portend higher NOM failure.	2A	B	[1–8]
	Any transfusion of PRBCs increases the chances of NOM failure. A "transfusion threshold" for the failure of NOM has not been defined.		No recommendation	[4, 6, 8]
What is the role of NOM in penetrating spleen injury?	In selected patients (hemodynamically stable, no peritonitis, reliable exam), up to two-thirds of patients are managed successfully nonoperatively.	2A	B	[9]
Which patients should undergo splenic angiography?	The role of SAE in penetrating injury is unknown.	No recommendation		
	Hemodynamically stable patients with blunt splenic injury with either:	2A	B	[7, 10–14]
	CT evidence of contrast extravasation or other vascular injuries (pseudoaneurysm or arteriovenous fistula)	2A	B	
	AAST grades 4 and 5 injury.			
	The role of routine SAE in grade 3 injury (without extravasation or vascular abnormality) is unknown.			
What radiologic studies should be obtained in patients with splenic injuries?	CT is the imaging modality of choice for splenic injury.	2A	B	[15–19]
	Repeat CT scan should be considered before discharge for grade 3–5 injuries or change in clinical status.	2B	B	[20–25]
	Outpatient imaging is of little use in asymptomatic patients.	2B	B	[20–25]
What are the steps to prevent OPSI?	OPSI is best prevented by splenic preservation, when possible.	2B	B	[3, 25–32]
	Pneumococcus, meningococcus, and Hib vaccine should be given >14 days postsplenectomy, if feasible. They may be given earlier if follow-up is a concern.	2B	B	[3, 25–32]
	Specific vaccine recommendations are available through the CDC.			
When is it safe to resume activities after splenic injuries?	Pediatric patients: Manage according to APSA 2019 guidelines.	2A	B	[33, 34]
	Adult patients: Hospital observation for 3–5 days. Activity restrictions are similar to pediatric patients.	4	C	
How are patients with special circumstances managed nonoperatively?	Pediatric patients <18 years have a high rate of successful nonoperative management.			
	Patients over the age of 55 years: Likely to have a higher failure rate of NOM. Age alone does not preclude NOM.	2A	B	[35–38]
	Cirrhotic patients: Worse prognosis, but still high success rate for NOM.	2B	B	[4, 6, 35–40]
		2B	B	[41, 42]
		2A	B	[43–47]

Abbreviations: APSA = American Pediatric Surgical Association, CDC = Centers for Disease Control and Prevention, CT = Computed tomography, Hib = Haemophilus influenza B, ISS = Injury Severity Score, OPSI = Overwhelming post-splenectomy infection, PRBCs = Packed red blood cells, SAE = Splenic artery embolization.

21.3 What Is the Role of Nonoperative Management in Penetrating Spleen Injury?

As the role of NOM in penetrating abdominal injuries has increased in general, the rate of successful NOM in penetrating splenic injuries has increased as well. In a systematic review published by Teuben et al., 608 cases of penetrating splenic injury were studied. Of these cases, 128 patients (21%) were treated nonoperatively. These patients had an 18% failure rate, which was similar to patients who were treated operatively. Criteria used as a contraindication for NOM were hemodynamic instability, peritonitis, decreased level of consciousness, spinal cord injuries, and physical findings to indicate a hollow viscus injury, such as bloody nasogastric output or blood on digital rectal exam. All patients selected for NOM of penetrating splenic injury underwent CT to exclude concomitant intraabdominal injuries. It should also be noted that studies included in this review were all performed at Level 1 and Level 2 trauma centers, which are high-volume trauma centers, equipped to provide observation in the intensive care unit. Moreover, alternative means of NOM such as splenic artery embolization were not specifically studied in any of the studies that were reviewed [9]. A strictly selected patient population in penetrating splenic injury may safely undergo NOM in a highly monitored setting, but data thus far are only applicable in high-volume trauma centers in selected patients.

RECOMMENDATION

The current evidence suggests that in appropriately selected patients, the NOM of penetrating spleen injury can be successful, but the total percentage of penetrating splenic injury patients meeting these criteria is small (about 20%). Patients with hemodynamic instability, peritonitis, unreliable exam, or CT evidence of hollow viscus injury should undergo immediate exploration. The role of angiography in penetrating splenic injury is unknown.

Level of evidence: 2A. Grade of recommendation: B.

21.4 Which Patients Should Undergo Splenic Angiography?

Splenic artery embolization (SAE) has become an important adjunct in patients at the highest risk for NOM failure. Although many institutions have instituted splenic angiogram protocols, the efficacy and appropriate patient selection remain controversial. In addition, the utilization of splenic angioembolization (AE) is variable. The Chanine review from

the NTDB reports our recent practice are summarized as follows [2]:

National Trauma Data Bank, 2007–2015, Adult Blunt Splenic Injury [4]

Grade	NOM	Splenectomy	Angioembolization
3	72%	20%	3.5%
4	51%	39%	3%
5	29%	64%	1.6%

The World Society of Emergency Surgery (WSES) guidelines by Coccolini et al. currently recommend SAE in the following cases: Hemodynamically stable patients with vascular abnormalities such as contrast blush, pseudoaneurysm, or arteriovenous fistula seen on imaging and WSES grade 3 lesions (AAST 4–5) in the hemodynamically stable patient [4].

A retrospective study by Clements et al. reported a spleen salvage rate of 97% in patients with AAST grade 3–5 blunt splenic injuries. Interestingly, splenic angiography identified a statistically significant number of occult vascular injuries in AAST grade 3 splenic injuries [10]. Another retrospective study showed that the use of SAE overall decreased the length of stay, but more importantly, patients with AAST grade 3 splenic injury treated with SAE had a significantly better outcome when compared to those managed with observation alone [11]. These findings suggest a role for SAE in intermediate-grade splenic injury in addition to the current guidelines. However, other series report no benefit of angioembolization with grade 3 splenic injury [12, 13]. A randomized controlled trial of grade 3–5 blunt splenic injury by Arvieux et al. compared the role of prophylactic SAE versus surveillance followed by intervention only when necessary. Between the two groups, the 1-month spleen salvage rate was not significantly different. Of the group that initially underwent surveillance, 32.3% ultimately required SAE, compared to a 3.1% re-embolization rate in the prophylactic SAE group. The prophylactic SAE group also had lower pseudoaneurysm formation rates [12]. The authors concluded that both approaches have high and equivalent spleen salvage rates. However, further examination of their findings reveals a 71% failure rate in grade 4 and 5 injuries. In addition, grade 5 injuries requiring immediate splenectomy (not quantified in the paper) were excluded from the study. A more appropriate conclusion would be that for grade 3 splenic injury, both approaches have high and equivalent spleen salvage rates. On the other hand, grade 4 and certainly grade 5 splenic injuries require intervention (splenectomy or SAE) depending on patient stability. This observation emphasizes the importance of including all patients with splenic injury in the determination of the appropriateness of NOM. High-grade splenic injury, in particular grade 5, often requires immediate splenectomy [4]. This empiric embolization rather than simple observation for grade 4 and 5 splenic injury is supported by a meta-analysis by Requarth et al. [13]

Finally, there is controversy concerning factors predicting the failure of embolization. A large retrospective study revealed that 40% of patients with arteriovenous fistulas failed embolization. They also found that pseudoaneurysm and high-grade injuries were not associated with a significant failure rate. The size of the pseudoaneurysm did not predict the need for primary splenectomy [6]. Others suggest that pseudoaneurysms <1–1.5 cm do not require intervention. Embolization failure rates have been reported as 43% for high-grade injuries, 56% for large hemoperitoneum, and 59% for extravasation [14]. The conflicting literature regarding the indications and efficacy of SAE may be due to the frequency and familiarity that each institution has concerning embolization. In addition, different embolization protocols may produce different outcomes.

RECOMMENDATION

1. Hemodynamically stable patients with grade 4 or 5 blunt splenic injuries or with contrast extravasation, pseudoaneurysm, or arteriovenous fistula on CT should undergo SAE. SAE in these patients decreases the failure rate of NOM. Routine angiography in grade 3 injuries without contrast extravasation is controversial but may have some benefit in identifying occult injuries.

   Level of evidence: 2A. Grade of recommendation: B.

21.5 What Imaging Studies Should Be Obtained in Patients with Splenic Injuries?

The focused abdominal sonography for trauma (FAST) exam is generally the initial imaging study performed for blunt trauma patients. It has the advantage of being rapid, noninvasive, bedside, and easy to repeat. It has 90–93% sensitivity to the presence of hemoperitoneum. FAST is limited by the inability to detect the presence of active hemorrhage and has a reported sensitivity of only 46% for the detection of solid organ injury [15]. A positive FAST in a hemodynamically stable patient should prompt a follow-up CT scan, as abdominal ultrasound has limited utility in identifying specific solid organ injuries and characterizing the extent of the injury. There is debate about the role of CT in a stable patient with a negative FAST, but the rate of additional injuries in the abdomen found exclusively on CT after a negative FAST is 15%, leading to a change in management of 6.4% [16]. This suggests that CT should be routine even with a negative FAST in significant blunt force injury to the abdomen.

CT has long been the standard for the diagnosis and characterization of spleen injuries in hemodynamically stable patients. Benefits of CT include the ability to reliably determine the severity or grade of injury; detect contrast extravasation, pseudoaneurysm, or arteriovenous fistula; quickly estimate the degree of hemoperitoneum; and identify other significant injuries [29]. Many centers have traditionally used the single-portal venous phase as the protocol for CT in splenic injury. Dual-phase CT (portal venous phase + arterial phase) increases sensitivity and accuracy in the diagnosis of

splenic vascular injury [17, 18]. A more recent retrospective study showed that using a dual-phase CT significantly changed the spleen injury grading according to the 2018 revised AAST scale for splenic injury [19]. The value of triple-phase CT scans should be studied further.

With CT already established as the standard to assess the extent of splenic injury, recent literature evaluated the need and indications for follow-up imaging. Boukar et al. performed a systematic review of patients who underwent NOM of blunt liver and/or spleen injury with a repeat CT scan. Of the 28 selected studies including 2,646 patients, 16 studies included blunt splenic injuries and 3 evaluated concomitant liver and spleen injuries. Of the CTs performed as a routine clinical practice, only 4% led to a meaningful change in clinical course, whereas 47% of CTs that were prompted by a clinical indication led to a change in clinical management. The result was comparable when the analysis was performed separately for blunt liver and spleen injuries [20].

A more recent study by Byerly reviewed 219 patients who underwent routine repeat CT at 24 hours per institutional protocol. Of the patients included in the study, 5% went for angiography but only 4% ultimately required splenic artery embolization and 1.8% underwent splenectomy. Ninety-three percent of the patients enrolled in the study did not require additional diagnostic or therapeutic intervention [21]. These results support earlier studies [22, 23]. Unfortunately, neither of the two papers stratify the risk of finding vascular abnormalities on repeat CT based on the AAST grade of splenic injury. A retrospective study reimaged nearly all high-grade injuries at 5 ± 4.4 days. Splenic pseudoaneurysms were found in 12% of grade 3 injuries, 32% of grade 4 injuries, and 40% of grade 5 injuries [24].

In pediatric patients, a retrospective study was performed on 194 children with splenic injuries over 9 years. When comparing repeat CT prompted by a clinical change versus a routine scan without clinical change, there was no significant difference in delayed complications [25].

RECOMMENDATIONS

1. FAST plays a role as a screening tool in blunt trauma patients, but CT is the diagnostic tool of choice for splenic injury in stable trauma patients.

   Level of evidence: 2A. Grade of recommendation: A.

2. CT for diagnosis of splenic injury should at least include a portal venous phase and arterial phase.

   Level of evidence: 3B. Grade of recommendation: B.

3. Although still controversial, repeat imaging with CT should be considered before hospital discharge in patients with grades 3–5 injuries or patients with a change in physical exam or clinical status. Routine repeat imaging in patients with low-grade or asymptomatic injuries will rarely change management.

   Level of evidence: 2B. Grade of recommendation: B.

21.6 What Steps Can Be Taken to Prevent Overwhelming Postsplenectomy Sepsis?

OPSI is rare (3–7%) but carries a high mortality rate (40–70%). This heightened susceptibility to infection was described by King and Schumacker in 1952 in asplenic infants, and causative organisms were later identified as encapsulated bacteria (*Staphylococcus pneumoniae* is the causative agent in 50–90%). Vaccinations against encapsulated organisms, antibiotic prophylaxis against encapsulated organisms, and attempts at splenic salvage have been used to prevent OPSI. Determining the relative effect of each of these interventions on rates of OPSI is difficult because of the lack of long follow-up and low incidence of the disease [3].

An intact spleen is the best defense against OPSI. Since even grades 4 and 5 injuries may now be managed nonoperatively, it is important to know whether a severely injured spleen retains normal immunologic function. There are scant data regarding immunologic clinical outcomes (rates of infection or OPSI) in patients with severe spleen injury and splenic preservation, but studies evaluating immunologic surrogates of splenic function show patients with injured spleens to have higher levels of immune function than asplenic patients [25, 26]. Resende found Howell-Jolly bodies in all patients who underwent splenectomy for trauma, but none in noninjured controls or patients with subtotal splenectomy [27]. Another study showed that the immunologic profile of nonoperatively managed grade 4 or 5 injuries more closely resembled patients with spleens than those without spleens [28, 29].

Much debate remains on immune function after SAE for blunt splenic injuries. A recent review by Slater et al. shows that there is preserved splenic immune function, at least in the short-term postembolization period [28]. A smaller study by Lukies et al. looked at long-term splenic immune function by measuring IgM and memory B-cell levels in patients after SAE. This study demonstrated that patients retained measurable levels of IgM and memory B cells and did not develop OPSI in the 4.7- to 12.8-year period. However, this was only studied in seven patients, and the consensus on the long-term immunologic effect of SAE remains to be defined further [29]. The Eastern Association for the Surgery of Trauma recently published a systematic review and meta-analysis assessing immune function after splenic AE [30]. Two hundred and forty embolization patients were compared to 443 control patients who did not undergo splenectomy or embolization. Splenic immune function was not statistically different between groups. In addition, 3,974 splenectomy patients were compared with 686 splenic embolization patients. Embolization patients had more preserved splenic immune function and fewer infectious complications. The authors conditionally recommended against postsplenectomy vaccinations for patients after splenic AE.

In the uncommon circumstance that a portion of the spleen can be preserved operatively, 33–50% of the spleen must survive, with good perfusion, for immunocompetence to be maintained.

Current recommendations from the Centers for Disease Control and Prevention (CDC) recommend immunization for *S. pneumoniae* (pneumococcus), *Neisseria meningitidis* (meningococcus), and *Haemophilus influenzae* type b (Hib) following splenectomy. The two previously recommended pneumococcal vaccines were the pneumococcal conjugate (PCV13) vaccine and the pneumococcal polysaccharide (PPSV23) vaccine. An updated 2022 CDC guideline recommends the first dose of PCV15 followed by PPSV23 at least a year after PCV15. A reduced interval as short as 8 weeks can be considered in asplenic patients, however. Alternatively, a single dose of PCV20 is acceptable. Two types of meningococcal vaccines are available: MenACWY and MenB. MenACWY is a two-dose series administered 8 weeks apart, followed by revaccination every 5 years. MenB-4C is a two-dose primary series administered at least 1 month apart or three-dose primary series MenB-FHbp given at 0, 1–2, and 6 months (if dose 2 was administered at least 6 months after dose 1, dose 3 is not needed), both followed by a booster shot at 1 year and revaccination every 2–3 years. Hib vaccine is administered as a single one-time dose [31]. Postsplenectomy vaccines are commonly administered 14 days after splenectomy, as the previous study had shown the best functional antibody responses at 14 days [32]. However, this study only assessed polysaccharide pneumococcal vaccines, and it is unclear if the same time frame should apply to the other postsplenectomy vaccines. If the vaccination regimen includes a pneumococcal polysaccharide vaccine, dosing at 14 days post operation is acceptable. However, with concerns for patient follow-up, vaccines may be administered at the time of discharge from the hospital.

RECOMMENDATIONS

1. Even after severe splenic trauma, injured spleens retain most of their immune function. Therefore, splenic preservation should be the most effective prevention of OPSI.

2. Immune function after splenic artery embolization is likely preserved, but the consensus on accurate immunological markers and long-term results is lacking.

3. Pneumococcus (PCV15 followed by PPSV23 8 weeks to 1 year later or single dose of PCV20), meningococcus (two doses 1 or 2 months apart, three doses at 0, 1–2, 6 months), and Hib vaccine should be given at least 14 days postsplenectomy, but patients who are at high risk for loss to follow-up should be immunized before discharge. The most up-to-date guidelines for postsplenectomy vaccinations are available through the CDC Advisory Committee for Immunization Practices.

Level of evidence: 2B (retrospective studies and small prospective studies). Grade of recommendation: B

21.7 What Techniques of Splenic Artery Embolization Should Be Used?

SAE techniques can be divided based on the location of embolization: Proximal or distal embolization. Proximal embolization is used in multifocal injuries or CT findings showing splenic injury without an identifiable vascular injury. Because the proximal embolization technique works by decreasing the perfusion pressure to the spleen but still maintains collateral flow to the spleen, there is less risk of splenic infarct or subsequent abscess formation. Distal embolization is beneficial in splenic injury where a focal vascular abnormality or injury is readily identified on CT.

Two retrospective studies showed that the two techniques have similar success rates [48, 49]. However, the distal embolization technique had a significantly longer fluoroscopy time, which may translate to higher doses of radiation and longer procedural time [48]. Longer procedural time may have an impact on the subsequent care of a trauma patient with multiple injuries. Distal embolization also had higher rates of splenic infarction, likely due to the lack of collateral flow. While the primary success rates of SAE are similar in both techniques, proximal embolization has fewer severe complications. A review of the Nationwide Readmissions Database reported that, in addition to the early vascular complications, patients undergoing SAE had a significantly higher risk of sepsis and organ space infection than patients undergoing NOM or operative management at 1 year [50].

RECOMMENDATIONS

1. Both proximal and distal splenic artery embolization techniques have similar success rates. The distal embolization technique has a higher complication rate and should be reserved for cases where a focal vascular injury is identified.

   Level of evidence: 2A. Grade of recommendation: B.

21.8 When Is It Safe to Resume Activities after Splenic Injuries?

Evidence in support of specific time frames for observation of blunt splenic injuries and duration of restriction of physical activity is limited to guidelines devised from retrospective data, although with prospective validation of guidelines in pediatric patients. For pediatric patients, the American Pediatric Surgical Association (APSA) Trauma Committee published recommendations regarding the length of hospitalization and return to activity based on the grade of splenic injury. For pediatric patients, return time to activity is the grade of injury plus 2 weeks, which is generally accepted and considered safe [33]. Some suggest an earlier return to activity may be safe, as pediatric patients who were nonadherent to the restriction guideline had similar rates of bleeding and ED

visits as those who were adherent [34]. The hospital length of stay for grade 1–2 spleen injury was 3 days and for grade 4–6 was 4 days on average. APSA does not recommend a certain length of stay based on injury grade alone; rather, it should be based on clinical presentation [33].

RECOMMENDATIONS

1. The American Pediatric Surgical Association Trauma Committee's guidelines for the management of splenic injury have been prospectively validated and provide specific recommendations for hospital stay and physical activity restriction based on the grade of injury. A shorter duration of hospital stay may be feasible, but more data are needed.

   Level of evidence: 2A. Grade of recommendation: C.

2. Adult patients with blunt splenic injury undergoing NOM should be observed for 3–5 days. Determinants of hospital stay should be clinical, as no specific data regarding length of stay relative to the grade of injury are available. Activity restrictions similar to those recommended for children are reasonable, but supporting data are lacking.

   Level of evidence: 4. Grade of recommendation: C.

21.9 Special Circumstances in Splenic Injury

Previously identified risks for splenectomy during NOM in the pediatric patient include Glasgow Coma Scale score ≤8, grades 3–5 injury, older age, and associated injuries. A recent study used the Shock Index, Pediatric Age-Adjusted (SIPA) to predict the pediatric patient population that may require blood transfusion and/or operative management [36]. Another study by Knight et al. found that blood transfusion within 4 hours of arrival and high-grade spleen injury predicted the need for splenectomy [37]. The role of angiography in pediatric splenic injury is not as well defined as it is in adult patients. Although the use of embolization in pediatric blunt splenic trauma has been increasing, specific indications for embolization in children have yet to be determined [33]. A review of the NTDM of 14,027 pediatric patients (<18 years) with splenic injury from 2010 to 2015 revealed that only 1.7% underwent angioembolization. Designated pediatric trauma centers performed only 27 splenectomies and 23 angioembolizations. This age group was four times more likely to undergo angioembolization and seven times more likely to undergo splenectomy if treated at an adult trauma center [38].

Advanced age is traditionally considered a risk factor for failing NOM of blunt splenic injury. This is likely due to the decrease in catecholamine response and comorbidities, such as hypertension and frequent use of beta-blocking agents. Recent studies indicate that the NOM failure rate in elderly patients may not be as high as previously reported. However, elderly patients who fail NOM have a higher mortality rate than their younger counterparts. The differences become more pronounced in octogenarians compared to geriatric patients ages 65–79 [39, 40].

A case-control study looked at cirrhotic patients who sustained blunt splenic injury. The authors found that cirrhosis significantly increased the risk of mortality as well as the need for splenectomy [41]. Another retrospective study showed that cirrhosis in patients who undergo splenectomy is an independent risk factor for mortality [42].

Early initiation of chemical venous thromboembolism (VTE) prophylaxis, generally defined as within 48–72 hours, does not seem to affect failure rates of NOM. This was studied in patients with blunt solid organ injury grades 3–5. VTE prophylaxis was initiated within 72 hours if patients did not receive a massive transfusion [43]. A recent meta-analysis that included 14,675 patients supported the safety of VTE prophylaxis within 48 hours [44]. A review of the Trauma Quality Improvement Program database studied the initial VTE prophylaxis within 48 hours, 48–72 hours, or later than 72 hours. They concluded that prophylaxis can be initiated ≤48 hours in patients at low risk of bleeding and recommended an intermediate delay (48–72 hours) in patients with diabetes mellitus, splenic injury, and grade 3–5 liver injury. They noted an increased risk of VTE when deep venous thrombosis (DVT) prophylaxis was held until 72 hours after injury [45]. In addition, a review of the American College of Surgeons Trauma Quality Improvement Program of 36,187 adults with blunt abdominal solid organ injury reported initiation of VTE prophylaxis within 48 hours of injury safely decreased rates of DVT and pulmonary embolism [46].

Patients who were taking aspirin before blunt splenic injury did not require a higher rate of interventions such as embolization or splenectomy. Patients on warfarin before blunt splenic injury required a higher rate of embolization, but the use of warfarin did not affect the need for splenectomy [47]. Timing regarding the safety of resuming either aspirin or warfarin after splenic trauma was not discussed in these studies.

RECOMMENDATIONS

1. Level 2A evidence supports the previously stated American Pediatric Surgical Association guidelines for NOM of blunt spleen injuries in children.

2. The data are conflicting on the impact of advanced age on the success of NOM of a blunt spleen injury, but the higher-quality evidence suggests that older age is associated with higher NOM failure rates. Age should not preclude NOM.

   Level of evidence: 2B. Grade of recommendation: B.

3. Based on limited retrospective data, patients with cirrhosis have worse outcomes than noncirrhotic patients with blunt spleen injuries.

   Level of evidence: 2B. Grade of recommendation: B.

4. Retrospective studies and a meta-analysis show no adverse effects of early anticoagulation in blunt spleen injury. Once acute bleeding has stopped, thromboembolic chemoprophylaxis should proceed as with any other trauma patient.

   Level of evidence: 2A. Grade of recommendation: B.

Editor's Note

Splenic injury is common following blunt trauma and usually resulted in an emergency laparotomy (based typically on a positive peritoneal lavage) in the 1970 and 1980s. Certainly, patients with hemodynamic instability or peritonitis should undergo immediate celiotomy. With the use of diagnostic CT scans and the adoption of nonoperative management protocols, the likelihood of operative intervention decreased from nearly 90% to about 25%. When abdominal exploration occurs today, the patient is typically critically injured, and therefore splenic removal is performed.

Management is often impacted by the assessment of the severity of splenic injury assessed on CT imaging. This is subject to interpretation and therefore of variable reliability. In one study, we found there was a high degree of both intrarater and interrater variability in evaluating the grade of splenic injury, even with very experienced trauma radiologists. Certainly, the presence of devascularization of the spleen, a massive hemoperitoneum, active extravasation, or pseudoaneurysm is predictive of failure of nonoperative management. In these patients, the ease and safety of angiographic embolization must be balanced against the availability of surgical intervention. Most trauma surgeons today have a low threshold for angiography in a hemodynamically stable patient with severe splenic trauma.

When OPSI was originally described, it had nearly universal mortality. Today, it is a rare entity (with a much lower expected fatality rate), as splenic preservation is the mantra, particularly in children under age 4 with immature immune systems. When splenectomy or angioembolization is required, aggressive use of vaccines is needed to avoid subsequent infections by encapsulated organisms. The timing of vaccine administration is controversial, as ideally the patient should be recovered enough to mount an immune response, but we do not want patients to be lost to follow-up. So most vaccines are given at the time of discharge from the hospital.

There was a time that patients with splenic injuries were managed with prolonged bed rest. This is no longer utilized. Returning to full activities, particularly contact sports, should probably wait at least 6 weeks (the time to reach baseline wound burst strength in animal studies), and a repeat CT scan may be prudent to assess splenic healing and exclude the rare postsplenic injury pathology.

REFERENCES

1. Peitzman AB, Heil B, Rivera L, Federle MB, Harbrecht BG, et al. Blunt splenic injury in adults: A multi-institutional study of the Eastern Association for the Surgery of Trauma. J Trauma Acute Care Surg. 2000;49:177–189.

2. Chanine AH, Gilyard S, Hanna TN, Fan S, Risk B, et al. Management of splenic injury in contemporary clinical practice: A National Trauma Data Bank Study. Acad Radiol. 2021;28:S138–S147.

3. di Sabatino A, Carsetti R, Corazza GR. Post-splenectomy and hyposplenic states. Lancet [Internet]. 2011 [cited 2022 Jul 14];378(9785):86–97. Available from: https://pubmed.ncbi.nlm.nih.gov/21474172/

4. Coccolini F, Montori G, Catena F, Kluger Y, Biffl W, Moore EE, et al. Splenic trauma: WSES classification and guidelines for adult and pediatric patients. World J Emerg Surg. 2017;12:1–26.

5. Bhangu A, Nepogodiev D, Lal N, Bowley DM. Meta-analysis of predictive factors and outcomes for failure of nonoperative management of blunt splenic trauma. Injury. 2012;43:1337–46.

6. Lauerman M, Brenner M, Simpson N, Shanmuganathan K, Stein D, Scalea T. Extra-parenchymal splenic abnormalities not vascular injury predict need for primary splenectomy. Eur J Trauma Emerg Surg. 2020 Oct 1;46(5):1063–9.

7. Lopez JM, McGonagill PW, Gross JL, Hoth JJ, Chang MC, Parker K, et al. Subcapsular hematoma in blunt splenic injury: A significant predictor of failure of nonoperative management. J Trauma Acute Care Surg. 2015 Dec 1;79(6):957–9.

8. Fugazzola P, Morganti L, Coccolini F, Magnone S, Montori G, Ceresoli M, et al. The need for red blood cell transfusions in the emergency department as a risk factor for failure of non-operative management of splenic trauma: A multicenter prospective study. Eur J Trauma Emerg Surg [Internet]. 2020 Apr 1 [cited 2022 Jul 14];46(2):407–12. Available from: https://pubmed.ncbi.nlm.nih.gov/30324241/

9. Teuben M, Spijkerman R, Pfeifer R, Blokhuis T, Huige J, Pape HC, et al. Selective non-operative management for penetrating splenic trauma: A systematic review. Eur J Trauma Emerg Surg. 2019;45:979–85.

10. Clements W, Joseph T, Koukounaras J, Goh GS, Moriarty HK, Mathew J, et al. Splenic salvage and complications after splenic artery embolization for blunt abdominal trauma: The SPLEEN-IN study. CVIR Endovasc. 2020 Dec 1;3(1):1–10.

11. Han J, Dudi-Venkata NN, Jolly S, Ting YY, Lu H, Thomas M, et al. Splenic artery embolization improves outcomes and decreases the length of stay in hemodynamically stable blunt splenic injuries – A level 1 Australian Trauma centre experience. Injury. 2022 May 1;53(5):1620–6.

12. Arvieux C, Frandon J, Tidadini F, Monnin-Bares V, Foote A, Dubuisson V, et al. Effect of prophylactic embolization on patients with blunt trauma at high risk of splenectomy: A randomized clinical trial. JAMA Surg. 2020;155(12):1102–11.

13. Requarth JA, D'Agostino RB, Miller PR. Nonoperative management of adult splenic injury with and without splenic artery embolotherapy: A meta-analysis. J Trauma Acute Care Surg. 2011;71:898–903.

14. Gaarder C, Dormagen JB, Eken T, Skaga NO, Klow NE, Pillgram-Larsen J, et al. Nonoperative management of splenic injuries: Improved results with angioembolization. J Trauma [Internet]. 2006 Jul [cited 2022 Jul 14];61(1):192–8. Available from: https://pubmed.ncbi.nlm.nih.gov/16832270/

15. Rozycki GS, Knudson MM, Shackford SR, Dicker R. Surgeon-performed bedside organ assessment with sonography after trauma (BOAST): A pilot study from the WTA Multicenter Group. J Trauma [Internet]. 2005 Dec [cited 2022 Jul 14];59(6):1356–64. Available from: https://pubmed.ncbi.nlm.nih.gov/16394909/

16. van der Vlies CH, van Delden OM, Punt BJ, Ponsen KJ, Reekers JA, Goslings JC. Literature review of the role of ultrasound, computed tomography, and transcatheter arterial embolization for the treatment of traumatic splenic injuries. Cardiovasc Intervent Radiol [Internet]. 2010 Dec [cited 2022 Jul 14];33(6):1079–87. Available from: https://pubmed.ncbi.nlm.nih.gov/20668852/

17. Boscak AR, Shanmuganathan K, Mirvis SE, Fleiter TR, Miller LA, Sliker CW, et al. Optimizing trauma multi-detector CT protocol for blunt splenic injury: Need for arterial and portal venous phase scans. Radiology. 2013 Jul;268(1):79–88.

18. Uyeda JW, LeBedis CA, Penn DR, Soto JA, Anderson SW. Active hemorrhage and vascular injuries in splenic trauma: Utility of the arterial phase in multidetector CT. Radiology. 2014 Jan;270(1):99–106.

19. Hemachandran N, Gamanagatti S, Sharma R, Shanmuganathan K, Kumar A, Gupta A, et al. Revised AAST scale for splenic injury (2018): Does addition of arterial phase on CT have an impact on the grade? Emerg Radiol [Internet]. 2021 Feb 1 [cited 2022 Jul 14];28(1):47–54. Available from: https://pubmed.ncbi.nlm.nih.gov/32705369/

20. Boukar K, Moore L, Tardif PA, Soltana K, Yanchar N, Kortbeek J, et al. Value of repeat CT for nonoperative management of patients with blunt liver and spleen injury: A systematic review. Eur J Trauma Emerg Surg. 2021;47:1753–61.

21. Byerly SE, Jones MD, Lenart EK, Seger CP, Filiberto DM, Lewis RH, et al. Serial CT for nonoperatively managed splenic injuries. Am Surg [Internet]. 2022 Jul 1 [cited 2022 Jul 14];88(7):1504–9. Available from: https://pubmed.ncbi.nlm.nih.gov/35341346/

22. Haan JM, Boswell S, Stein D, Scalea TM. Follow-up abdominal CT is not necessary in low-grade splenic injury. Am Surg. 2007;73(1):13–8.

23. Weinberg JA, Lockhart ME, Parmar AD, Griffin RL, Melton SM, Vandromme MJ, et al. Computed tomography identification of latent pseudoaneurysm after blunt splenic injury: Pathology or technology? J Trauma [Internet]. 2010 May [cited 2022 Jul 14];68(5):1112–6. Available from: https://pubmed.ncbi.nlm.nih.gov/20453766/

24. Wallen TE, Clark K, Baucom MR, Pabst R, Lemmink J, et al. Delayed splenic pseudoaneurysm identification with surveillance imaging. J Trauma Care Surg. 2022;93:113–7.

25. Fletcher KL, Meagher M, Spencer BL, Morgan ME, Safford SD, Armen SB, et al. Routine repeat imaging of pediatric blunt solid organ injuries is not necessary. Am Surg 2021. Available from: https://10.1177/00031348211038587

26. Falimirski M, Syed A, Prybilla D. Immunocompetence of the severely injured spleen verified by differential interference contrast microscopy: The red blood cell pit test. J Trauma [Internet]. 2007 Nov [cited 2022 Jul 14];63(5):1087–91. Available from: https://pubmed.ncbi.nlm.nih.gov/17993955/

27. Resende V, Petroianu A. Functions of the splenic remnant after subtotal splenectomy for treatment of severe splenic injuries. Am J Surg [Internet]. 2003 Apr 1 [cited 2022 Jul 14];185(4):311–5. Available from: https://pubmed.ncbi.nlm.nih.gov/12657380/

28. Slater SJ, Lukies M, Kavnoudias H, Zia A, Lee R, Bosco JJ, et al. Immune function and the role of vaccination after splenic artery embolization for blunt splenic injury. Injury. 2022;53:112–5.

29. Lukies M, Zia A, Kavnoudias H, Bosco JJ, Narita C, Lee R, et al. Immune function after splenic artery embolization for blunt trauma: Long-term assessment of CD27 + IgM B-cell levels. J Vasc Interv Radiol [Internet]. 2022 May 1 [cited 2022 Jul 14];33(5):505–9. Available from: https://pubmed.ncbi.nlm.nih.gov/35489783/

30. Freeman JJ, Yorkgitis BK, Haines K, Koganti D, Patel N, et al. Vaccination after spleen embolization: A practice guideline from the Eastern Association for the Surgery of Trauma. Injury (accessed August 25, 2022; ahead of print). Available from: https://doi.org/10.1016/j.injury.2022.08.006

31. The Centers for Disease Control and Prevention's Advisory Committee on Immunization Practices. Recommended Adult Immunization Schedule: United States 2022.

32. Shatz DV, Schinsky MF, Pais LB, Romero-Steiner S, Kirton OC, Carlone GM. Immune responses of splenectomized trauma patients to the 23-valent pneumococcal polysaccharide vaccine at 1 versus 7 versus 14 days after splenectomy. J Trauma [Internet]. 1998 May [cited 2022 Jul 14];44(5):760–6. Available from: https://pubmed.ncbi.nlm.nih.gov/9603075/

33. Gates RL, Price M, Cameron DB, Somme S, Ricca R, Oyetunji TA, et al. Non-operative management of solid organ injuries in children: An American Pediatric Surgical Association Outcomes and Evidence Based Practice Committee systematic review. J Pediatr Surg [Internet]. 2019 Aug 1 [cited 2022 Jul 14];54(8):1519–26. Available from: https://pubmed.ncbi.nlm.nih.gov/30773395/

34. Notrica DM, Sayrs LW, Krishna N, Ostlie DJ, Letton RW, Alder AC, et al. Adherence to APSA activity restriction guidelines and 60-day clinical outcomes for pediatric blunt liver and splenic injuries (BLSI). J Pediatr Surg [Internet]. 2019 Feb 1 [cited 2022 Jul 14];54(2):335–9. Available from: https://pubmed.ncbi.nlm.nih.gov/30278984/

35. Holmes IV JH, Wiebe DJ, Tataria M, Mattix KD, Mooney DP, Scaife ER, et al. The failure of nonoperative management in pediatric solid organ injury: A multi-institutional experience. J Trauma [Internet]. 2005 Dec [cited 2022 Jul 14];59(6):1309–13. Available from: https://pubmed.ncbi.nlm.nih.gov/16394902/

36. Phillips R, Meier M, Shahi N, Acker S, Reppucci M, Shirek G, et al. Elevated pediatric age-adjusted shock-index (SIPA) in blunt solid organ injuries. J Pediatr Surg [Internet]. 2021 Feb 1 [cited 2022 Jul 14];56(2):401–4. Available from: https://pubmed.ncbi.nlm.nih.gov/33358417/

37. Knight M, Kuo YH, Ahmed N. Risk factors associated with splenectomy following a blunt splenic injury in pediatric patients. Pediatr Surg Int [Internet]. 2020 Dec 1 [cited 2022 Jul 14];36(12):1459–64. Available from: https://pubmed.ncbi.nlm.nih.gov/33044611/

38. Swendiman RA, Abramov A, Fenton SJ, Russell KW, Nance ML, et al. Use of angioembolization in pediatric polytrauma patients with blunt splenic injury in pediatric blunt splenic injury. J Ped Surg. 2021;56:2045–2051.

39. Bashir R, Grigorian A, Lekawa M, Joe V, Schubl SD, Chin TL, et al. Octogenarians with blunt splenic injury: Not all geriatrics are the same. Updates Surg. 2021 Aug 1;73(4):1533–9.

40. Warnack E, Bukur M, Frangos S, DiMaggio C, Kozar R, Klein M, et al. Age is a predictor for mortality after blunt splenic injury. Am J Surg. 2020 Sep 1;220(3):778–82.

41. Cook MR, Fair KA, Burg J, Cattin L, Gee A, Arbabi S, et al. Cirrhosis increases mortality and splenectomy rates following splenic injury. Am J Surg [Internet]. 2015 May 1 [cited 2022 Jul 14];209(5):841–7. Available from: https://pubmed.ncbi.nlm.nih.gov/25769879/

42. Lee DU, Fan GH, Hastie DJ, Addonizio EA, Karagozian R. The impact of cirrhosis on the postoperative outcomes of patients undergoing splenectomy: Propensity score matched analysis of the 2011–2017 US hospital database. Scand J Surg [Internet]. 2021 [cited 2022 Jul 14]. Available from: https://pubmed.ncbi.nlm.nih.gov/34569369/

43. Moore K, Barton CA, Wang Y, Ran R, Chi A, Rowell S, et al. Early initiation of thromboembolic prophylaxis in critically ill trauma patients with high-grade blunt liver and splenic lacerations is not associated with increased rates of failure of non-operative management. Trauma (United Kingdom). 2022. Available from: https://doi.org/10.1177/14604086211046099

44. Murphy PB, de Moya M, Karam B, Menard L, Holder E, et al. Optimal timing of venous thromboembolism chemoprophylaxis initiation following blunt solid organ injury: Meta-analysis and systematic review. Eur J Trauma Emerg Surg. 2022;48:2039–2046.

45. Gaitanidis A, Breen KA, Nederpelt C, Parks J, Saillant N, et al. Timing of thromboprophylaxis in patients with blunt abdominal solid organ injures undergoing nonoperative management. J Trauma Acute Care Surg. 2021;90:148–156.

46. Skarupa D, Hanna K, Zeeshan M, Madbak F, Hamidi M, et al. Is early chemical thromboprophylaxis in patients with solid organ injury a solid decision? J Trauma Acute Care Surg. 2019;87:1104–1112.

47. Huang JF, Hsu CP, Fu CY, Huang YTA, Cheng CT, Wu YT, et al. Preinjury warfarin does not cause failure of nonoperative management in patients with blunt hepatic, splenic or renal injuries. Injury. 2022 Jan 1;53(1):92–7.

48. Brahmbhatt A, Ghobryal B, Wang P, Chughtai S, Baah N. Evaluation of splenic artery embolization technique for blunt trauma. J Emerg Trauma Shock. 2021 Jul 1;14(3):148–52.

49. Frandon J, Rodière M, Arvieux C, Michoud M, Vendrell A, Broux C, et al. Blunt splenic injury: Outcomes of proximal versus distal and combined splenic artery embolization. Diagn Interv Imaging. 2014 Sep 1;95(9):825–31.

50. Cioci AC, Parreci JP, Lindenmaier LB, Olufajo OA, Namias N, et al. Readmission for infection after blunt splenic injury: A national comparison of management techniques. J Trauma Acute Care Surg. 2020;88:390–95.

22

Injury to the Liver

Jose Lopez-Vera, Horeb Cano-Gonzalez, Connor Hogan and Daniel J Bonville

The liver is the most commonly injured organ in patients with blunt abdominal trauma and the second most common in penetrating abdominal trauma [1]. The diagnosis and treatment of liver injuries have evolved significantly over the past five decades. In the 1960s and 1970s, the main treatment was the liberal use of exploratory laparotomy with repair, resection, or liver packing to achieve hemostasis. This approach resulted in a death rate from 20% to over 50%, including all grades of injury [2]. Currently, less than 15% of blunt injury patients undergo surgery [3]. Over the past 25 years, nonoperative management (NOM) has become the mainstay of treatment for stable patients with blunt liver injuries [4]. In penetrating trauma, the liver may be severely damaged, and the operative management of hepatic injuries remains one of the greatest technical challenges in trauma surgery; however, recent trends increasing NOM for penetrating trauma have been reported as well. These are just a few factors that have contributed to improved mortality over the past 40 years. Despite these advances, many questions regarding best practices in patients with liver injuries remained unanswered.

22.1 What Are the Criteria for Selecting Blunt Trauma Patients for Nonoperative Management?

For over 25 years, there has been an increasing quantity of data validating NOM, with or without adjuncts, as the gold standard for the management of blunt hepatic injuries [3, 4]. This includes the evidence compiled by the latest iteration of the Eastern Association for the Surgery of Trauma (EAST) guide on NOM of hepatic injuries in 2012 [5]. There are no randomized controlled trials comparing the efficacy of operative versus NOM. Three prospective cohort trials on NOM of liver injuries are published to date [6, 7], but the bulk of evidence emanates from class III references. Currently available data suggest that every hemodynamically stable patient be treated initially by NOM [4–12]. The suitability for NOM should no longer be based on the amount of hemoperitoneum, the grade of injury [13], the presence of head injury [8], Injury Severity Score (ISS), the patient's age, or even contrast extravasation [14, 15]. Concomitant or combined injuries increase the failure rate of NOM but do not preclude implementation [4].

Less than 20% of patients with blunt liver injury will require emergent laparotomy because of either the liver or associated intraabdominal injuries [16]. Associated intraabdominal injuries necessitating laparotomy, peritonitis, hemodynamic instability, and lack of appropriate clinical environment and/or availability of facilities or personnel to support adjuncts to NOM should the need arise constitute the four absolute contraindications to NOM [4, 16]. Based on the aforementioned criteria, more than 80% of blunt trauma patients are candidates for NOM, with a success rate of around 90% [6, 11, 17].

> **RECOMMENDATION**
>
> Patients with blunt liver trauma who are hemodynamically stable are the best candidates for successful NOM.
>
> Level of evidence: Class IIb–III. Grade of recommendation: B.
>
> Patients with a combination of injuries are more likely to fail NOM but should be given a trial if they are hemodynamically normal and do not have any contraindications to NOM.
>
> Level of evidence: Class III. Grade of recommendation: B.

22.2 When Should NOM Patients Be Allowed Out of Bed after Sustaining a Liver Injury?

Historically, an integral part of the NOM of liver injuries is bed rest. Only retrospective studies have addressed the question of optimal duration for bed rest in the adult population. London et al. showed no failure of NOM in patients mobilized before the third hospital day postinjury and concluded that bed rest was unnecessary [12, 18]. Teichman et al. showed that early mobilization decreased cost and length of stay, without increasing the failure of NOM. The authors studied two groups: One in which they mobilized higher-grade (grade 3 and higher) injuries with stable hemoglobin as early as 24 hours postadmissions compared with a group not mobilized as early [19]. Another systematic review showed that bed rest had no

DOI: 10.1201/9781003316800-22

clinical benefit in those with low-grade to mid-grade solid organ injuries. Studies in the pediatric population, including a prospective study, have shown it to be safe to lift bed rest restrictions after 24 hours for low-grade injuries and 48 hours for greater than grade 3 injuries [20, 21]. Other pediatric literature states that in grade 1 and 2 injuries, implementation of bed rest in NOM should be according to clinical status rather than injury severity, including hemodynamic instability, minimal abdominal pain, and tolerating diet.

RECOMMENDATION

The available evidence suggests that patients with stable vitals and hematocrit can safely ambulate after 24 hours for grades 1–3 and after 48 hours for grades >3, but this literature is not sufficient to make a definitive recommendation regarding the duration of bed rest limitations for hepatic trauma.

Level of evidence: Class III–IV. Grade of recommendation: C.

22.3 Does Drainage Prevent Complications in Surgically Treated Hepatic Injuries, and Should Routine Endoscopic Retrograde Cholangiopancreatography and Stenting Be Used for Bile Leaks?

Multiple studies have evaluated the need for systemic biliary tract drainage via T-tube choledochostomy, cholecystostomy tube, or perihepatic drains in surgically treated hepatic trauma. These studies showed an increased risk of infectious complications and abscess formation in those managed with drains. Therefore, routine drains in surgically treated hepatic trauma have not been recommended [22, 23].

At the same time, the trend in the management of complex traumatic hepatic injuries is the use of damage control surgery (DCS) and perihepatic packing. With DCS, there is the potential to have severe parenchymal damage left untreated, with the risk of having a larger and more complex postoperative bile leak with rates reported in 0.5–21% of patients [24, 25]. Of particular concern are infectious complications arising from a biliary source and the significant morbidity associated with reoperation [25].

The use of endoscopic retrograde cholangiopancreatography (ERCP) for diagnosis and management of biliary complications in surgically managed hepatic trauma was developed out of the use of ERCP in iatrogenic causes of biliary leaks. ERCP with transpapillary stenting and/or sphincterotomy is used to promote the flow of bile into the duodenum, allowing for transhepatic and intrahepatic biliary injuries to heal [25]. ERCP in the management of traumatic hepatic biliary injuries has been mostly limited to small case series and case reports, with a reported success rate of 85% [24, 25]. In a narrative review, Sealock et al. showed that endoscopic management of traumatic biliary injuries has

success rates of 90% with sphincterotomy and stenting. Its use in traumatic biliary complications by Bajaj et al. identified 11 case series published between 1999 and 2007. In this study, 69 out of the 73 patients were resolved with ERCP maneuvers [26]. Furthermore, a retrospective study by Anand et al. showed a 100% success rate in the management of biliary leaks in 26 patients with traumatic associated biliary leaks. Of the 26 patients, 23 had resolution within 3 months with an average of 47 days, with the remaining leaks closing by 7 months [27].

Hommes and Nicol evaluated the role of conservative management of intrahepatic biliary leaks and questioned the need for routine ERCP and sphincterotomy/stenting for all trauma-associated biliary injuries. In their prospective study of 412 patients, 14 patients had major bile leaks (>400 mL/day or leak >14 days) and 26 had minor leaks. The major leaks underwent ERCP with stenting, and the minor leaks were treated conservatively. All bile leaks resolved, and there was no significant difference in septic complications, intensive care unit (ICU) length of stay, and mortality between the groups treated with ERCP (major leak) and those managed conservatively (minor leak) [25]. In summary, ERCP is effective in managing posttraumatic biliary leaks. However, it needs to be determined which biliary leaks benefit from ERCP management versus those that will resolve spontaneously.

RECOMMENDATIONS

The routine use of drains after surgical treatment of liver injuries is not supported.

Level of evidence: Class IIb; grade of recommendation: B.

Selective use of ERCP in the management of posttraumatic biliary complications is effective.

Level of evidence: Class IV. Grade of recommendation: C.

22.4 Can Gunshot Wounds to the Liver of Stable Patients Be Managed Nonoperatively on Clinical Exam?

Can computed tomography (CT) scans be safely used as an adjunct to determine who can be managed nonoperatively? Although the policy of selective NOM (sNOM) of stab wounds (SWs) to the liver has gained acceptance, utilization of this strategy for gunshot wounds (GSWs) remains controversial. At its conception [27], it was based on serial physical examination by skilled practitioners, but this has now been augmented by the use of contrast-enhanced CT to aid in determining which trauma patients are candidates for sNOM.

In March 2010, the EAST published practice management guidelines for sNOM of penetrating abdominal trauma, which specifically addressed the indications for laparotomy for GSWs, postinjury imaging, and specific recommendations for sNOM [28]. It is generally agreed that all hemodynamically unstable patients or those with diffuse abdominal tenderness should undergo emergent laparotomy for penetrating abdominal injuries. Furthermore, those who are hemodynamically stable but have an unreliable clinical exam because of concomitant injuries or altered mental status require further diagnostic evaluation or should undergo exploratory laparotomy [28]. In 1991, Demetriades et al. [29] prospectively evaluated 146 patients with abdominal GSW. One hundred and five patients had peritoneal signs and underwent laparotomy, but 41 who presented with minimal peritoneal signs were managed nonoperatively, with serial abdominal exams. Seven of these (17%) required delayed laparotomy, and there were surgical complications in two of these patients but no reported morbidity. The authors concluded that sNOM was safe and theoretically reduced the negative or nontherapeutic laparotomy rate for these patients from 27 to 5. Several studies reviewed by Navsaria et al. [30] evaluating sNOM of thoracoabdominal or abdominal GSWs were subsequently published, which specifically evaluated hepatic injury. The majority of these had a small sample size but reported success rates for sNOM of liver injuries of 69–100%, and sNOM included angioembolization for active bleeding in two of these patients. Demetriades et al. [31] retrospectively reported on 928 patients with abdominal GSWs, of which 152 had liver injuries. Of the 52 with isolated liver injuries, 16 underwent sNOM. Five in this group required delayed laparotomy, four for signs of peritonitis, and one for abdominal compartment syndrome. The remaining 11 patients were successfully treated nonoperatively (69%), although one patient developed a biloma requiring percutaneous drainage.

Demetriades et al. [32] subsequently published a prospective series of 152 patients with penetrating abdominal wounds: 70.4% GSW and 29.6% SW; 73% of these patients had hepatic injury. Of the 61 stable patients who underwent CT scans, 42 had a liver injury from either SW or GSW. Based on CT findings, 39 patients (67.2%) with abdominal injuries were managed nonoperatively. Overall, of all injured patients, 28.4% of those with liver injuries were successfully managed nonoperatively, although it was not clear what percentage were from GSW. DuBose et al. [33] retrospectively studied 644 patients with abdominal GSWs, of which 144 were managed nonoperatively. Ten of these had isolated liver injury, one of whom required delayed laparotomy. The remaining nine underwent sNOM for an overall success rate of 90%.

After the EAST guidelines [28], several studies have further supported sNOM of abdominal GSW, and four specifically discuss the hepatic injury. Navsaria et al. [30] published a prospective, protocol-driven study of all liver GSW injuries presented to a Level I trauma center over 4 years. All hemodynamically stable, nonperitoneal, and neurologically intact patients with right upper quadrant or right thoracoabdominal GSW injury, even if focally tender, underwent a contrast CT scan for evaluation of the extent of their injuries. Of the 63 patients (33.3%) with a liver injury that did not meet the criteria for emergent laparotomy, all but 5 were successfully managed nonoperatively (92.1%). Two of these 58 subsequently developed short-term complications; one developed a pleurobiliary fistula and two patients experienced an infected tract hematoma.

In a retrospective series of 133 injured military personnel with penetrating abdominal injury, 32 were identified as having a hepatic injury at laparotomy (24 patients) or by CT scan (8 patients). Seven of those undergoing CT scans were successfully managed nonoperatively [33]. Starling et al. [34]

published a prospective study of 115 patients over a 7-year period with right thoracoabdominal GSW who met inclusion criteria for sNOM. All but 6 of these had an injury to the liver, and 81 also had an injury to the kidney or diaphragm determined by CT scan. Four patients, all with liver and associated injuries, failed NOM (3.5%) and underwent laparotomy, two for fecal peritonitis and one for hemoperitoneum. The remaining laparotomy was nontherapeutic.

In 2014, Navsaria et al. [35] performed a prospective trial of NOM of abdominal GSW. Of the 1,106 patients admitted, 272 (24.6%) were selected for NOM. Of these, 82 (30.1%) were followed by serial abdominal examination alone and 190 (69.9%) underwent CT scans based on the trajectory as well as serial examination. Within this latter group, hepatic injuries were seen in 79 (41.6%). The success rate of sNOM was 95.2% overall, with only 13 patients requiring delayed laparotomy, of which only 10 were therapeutic.

Much of the data supporting the use of sNOM for hepatic GSWs has come from two groups, and the numbers of those specifically with hepatic injury have been small or not clearly stated. However, overall, and notably in the more recent studies [34, 35], the trend has been toward successful sNOM for those hemodynamically stable patients with hepatic GSWs. Thus, the conclusions reached by the EAST Practice Management Group [28] stand and support that sNOM of hepatic GSWs can be safely pursued. Furthermore, they concluded that serial physical examination is reliable in detecting significant injuries after penetrating trauma to the abdomen if performed by experienced clinicians and preferably by the same team.

Although the choice of patients for sNOM was initially based on clinical examination, currently this has become highly influenced by CT scans. In 1998, two retrospective studies were published that sought to evaluate the role of CT in the management of torso GSW. Grossman et al. [36] reviewed the CT scans of 50 patients with torso GSW over 6 years that had been performed in hemodynamically stable patients to assess missile trajectory. Of the 37 abdominal/pelvic and 15 thoracic CTs, 23 were positive for transabdominal, transpelvic, or proximity to vascular structures. Of the 17 positives in the former group, 9 laparotomies were performed and 8 patients were successfully managed nonoperatively. The remaining 20 patients with negative CT were also managed nonoperatively. Three of the positive abdominal CTs showed a transhepatic tract, and in these cases, they were managed nonoperatively without complications. A retrospective study by Schellenberg et al. looked at 4,031 patients who suffered GSW to the liver between 2007 and 2014, in which 1,564 (38%) were treated with sNOM. They found that the rate of sNOM increased over time from 34.5% to 41% from 2007 to 2014. On regression analysis, sNOM is independently associated with fewer complications (odds ratio [OR], 0.811; $p = 0.003$) and lower mortality (OR 0.438; $p < 0.001$). On subgroup analysis, patients with grade 4 injury were most likely to benefit from sNOM with fewer complications (OR 0.676; $p = 0.019$) and improved mortality (OR 0.238; $p = 0.002$). They concluded that in the appropriate clinical scenario, sNOM is a safe and effective method to treat hepatic GSW [37].

The EAST Practice Guidelines [28] strongly recommended the use of an abdominopelvic CT scan as a diagnostic tool. Three studies published since the release of the EAST guidelines further support this. As noted previously, Morrison et al. [38] utilized CT scanning as an aid in the initial decision to triage the hemodynamically stable patients within the study. In this study of 133 patients with battlefield penetrating trauma, which included 32 patients with hepatic injury, the mechanism of injury was predominantly by a missile. Overall, CT had a sensitivity of 92%, a specificity of 89%, a positive predictive value of 71%, and a negative predictive value of 98%. A retrospective study of all patients with penetrating liver injuries was undertaken and reported in 2011 [36]. One hundred and seventy-eight patients with penetrating liver injuries, 70.2% as a result of GSW, were admitted over the period studied. Of the 55 hemodynamically stable patients who then underwent CT at admission, 54.5% were selected for NOM. The sensitivity and specificity of the admission CT to predict a positive laparotomy were 95.7% and 90.6%, respectively. Overall, 80.6% of isolated liver injuries were successfully managed nonoperatively. However, they recommended follow-up CT because of the high percentage of liver-related complications that they saw subsequently in both the laparotomy and sNOM groups.

RECOMMENDATIONS

NOM based on clinical evaluation, complemented with early IV contrast CT, can be implemented safely for hepatic injury secondary to GSW.

Level of evidence: Class IIb. Grade of recommendation: B.

CT with IV contrast discriminates the stable GSW patients who do not need operative management.

Level of evidence: Class IIb. Grade of recommendation: B.

22.5 Is Arterial Embolization Effective in the Management of Penetrating and Blunt Hepatic Injuries?

The use of hepatic angiography (HA) and hepatic arterial embolization (HAE) in trauma centers appears quite variable. According to Richardson et al., the use of HA and HAE to treat injuries to the liver has increased from 1% to 9% over three decades [4]. This trend has continued to rise over the last decade at some centers [11, 39]. However, in a recent report of the National Trauma Data Bank, HAE was only reported in 3% of nonoperatively managed isolated liver trauma patients with American Association for the Surgery of Trauma (AAST) liver injuries grade 4 or higher [39]. Over the last decade, there have been several studies advocating HAE as an important part of NOM of liver trauma, as well as an important adjunct to achieving hemorrhage control in patients who require emergent laparotomy.

Emergent laparotomy is undertaken based on hemodynamic status and response to initial resuscitation more than the severity grade of the injury. All experts agree that unresponsive shock and the presence of findings suggestive of associated injuries (i.e., peritonitis) are absolute indications for exploratory laparotomy and possible DCS. The efficacy for hemorrhage control of HAE in severe liver trauma has been reported to be as high as 75–100% [40–43]. Thus, mortality from severe liver injuries has reportedly decreased with the use of HAE [36, 43]. The level of morbidity, however, has been reported with significant variability by several authors. In some series, it is unclear whether the morbidity experienced in patients treated with HAE is related to the HAE or to the liver trauma itself. A large series by Kozar et al. [44] of 453 liver injuries (grades 3–4) treated with NOM revealed an HAE rate of 8% but an overall high complication rate in patients with injuries grades 4 and 5 as well as in patients with requiring blood products. Complications, in this study, did not appear to correlate with the use of HAE.

Normotensive patients who have active extravasation or pooling of IV contrast within the liver parenchyma on CT scans are candidates for HAE. Gaarder et al. [41] observed a reduction in the number of laparotomies when comparing outcomes of patients with or without the use of HA and HAE for the treatment of liver injuries (Abbreviated Injury Scale score >3) after the implementation of an angiography protocol in hemodynamically stable patients. Their nonoperative rate increased from 51% to 76% ($p > 0.05$) without increasing failure rate, mortality, transfusion, or liver-related complications.

Asencio et al. [45] showed a mortality benefit with HAE alone in NOM patients, as well as an adjunct to operative management in a prospective study of patients with AAST grades 4 and 5 from both blunt and penetrating mechanisms of injury. Hagiwara et al. [42], in a case-control study, suggested that a combination of a CT scan of grade 4 and 5 lesion and fluid requirements of >2,000 mL/hour to maintain normotension are indications for laparotomy. However, this study also revealed that many stable patients with high-grade injuries had bleeding on angiography regardless of the presence of a contrast blush on a CT scan. Nearly half of grade 3 injuries and nearly all grade 4 injuries had bleeding on HA. Furthermore, Monnin et al. [43] used a multidisciplinary approach (surgeon, interventional radiologist, and anesthetist) to perform HAE in unstable patients with high-grade injuries with a hemorrhage control rate of 100% and only two HAE-related complications. They recommend this approach to avoid immediate surgery and consider embolization to be more effective to stop arterial bleeding than surgery without a concomitant increase in failure rate or mortality.

More recently, other authors have reported high success rates with HAE but with variable rates of morbidity [11, 39, 43, 44]. Mitsuda et al. [46] in Tokyo, Japan, studied 77 patients with AAST grades 3–5 liver injuries before and after changing the *target systolic blood pressure* from >90 to >80 mmHg after initial IV fluid resuscitation to trigger the decision for immediate laparotomy. They showed increased use of HAE and decreased urgent and overall laparotomy rate as well as decreased 24-hour transfusion requirements in the group with a target for laparotomy of 80 mmHg. There was no change in mortality or liver-related morbidity during this study. In a systematic review in 2016, Green et al. showed that the efficacy rate of HAE was greater than 90% and is not without morbidity. The most frequently reported complications included hepatic necrosis, abscess formation, and bile leaks [47]. However, not all studies were in support of HAE. In 2020 Samuels et al. did a retrospective review of 1,939 patients who met the criteria, from which 116 (6%) underwent HAE. HAE was associated

TABLE 22.1

Clinical Questions

Question	Answer	Grade of Recommendation	Levels of Evidence	References
What are the criteria for selecting blunt liver trauma patients for NOM?	Hemodynamic stability regardless of CT findings (including grade, amount of hemoperitoneum, age, and TBI). These findings, however, may dictate the use of adjuncts in NOM. NOM is the standard of care for hemodynamically stable patients.	B	IIb–III	[4–19]
When should selected patients undergoing NOM be allowed to ambulate?	After 48 hours for higher-grade liver injuries and after 24 hours for injuries grade 3 or less.	C	III–IV	[18, 20–23]
Does drainage prevent complications in surgically treated hepatic injuries?	The systematic or routine use of drainage of the biliary tract does not benefit hepatic trauma patients and is associated with increased infection risk and septic complications.	B	IIb	[24, 25]
Should routine ERCP and stenting be used for bile leaks?	ERCP is a useful adjunct in the management of traumatic-associated bile leaks, but its routine use is not warranted.	C	IV	[26–28]
Can GSWs to the liver of stable patients be managed nonoperatively based on the clinical exam?	NOM based on clinical evaluation, complemented with early IV contrast CT, can be implemented safely for hepatic injury secondary to GSW.	B	IIb	[30–40]
Is CT scan an adjunct to determine who can receive NOM?	CT with IV contrast discriminates the stable GSW patients who do not need to be operated on.	B	IIb	[34–40]
Is hepatic angioembolization effective in controlling hemorrhage in liver trauma?	HAE is safe and effective in the management of severe hepatic trauma as part of NOM, as well as when performed as an adjunct to the principles of damage control.	B	IIc–III	[41–50]

with increased morbidity compared to HAE, with a larger percentage of the AE group undergoing interventional radiology drainage (13.3% vs. 2.2%; $p < 0.001$), with more ICU days (4 vs. 3 days; $p = 0.005$) and longer length of stay (10 vs. 6 days; $p < 0.001$). After successfully matching on all variables, groups did not differ with respect to mortality (5.4% vs. 3.2%; $p = 0.5$, AE vs. non-AE, respectively) or transfusion at 4–24 hours (4.4% vs. 7.5%; $p = 0.4$). They suggest that the benefits of HAE do not outweigh the risks of a stable liver injury. Observing these patients may be a more prudent approach to management [48].

The use of mandatory HA after a DCS in patients with severe liver injuries is based on the concept that ongoing arterial bleeding is difficult to rule out at the end of DCS. The role of HAE following damage control laparotomy is to control hemorrhage in inaccessible hepatic deep parenchyma regions. This approach, which has been demonstrated to be a safe adjunct procedure to perihepatic packing with therapeutic success for HAE, has been studied by several groups [39, 44, 49]. More recently, Matsumoto et al. showed that although perioperative HAE was associated with lower in-hospital mortality, it resulted in increased length of stay and increased incidence of deep and organ space surgical site infections [50]. However, this may have been because some of the most injured (higher ISS) and critically ill patients survived.

Liver-related complications in patients who were treated with HAE have been reported as hepatic necrosis, bile leak, gallbladder infarction, and hepatic abscesses. These rates vary significantly in different published reports. They appear to correlate mostly with the severity of injury grade, hemodynamic status,

and transfusion requirements [11, 39, 44, 45]. In 2012, the EAST published guidelines on the NOM of blunt hepatic injury [6]. In this guideline, the authors recommend that HAE be considered as a first-line intervention for patients who are transient responders to resuscitation and as an adjunct to potential operative intervention. The authors also concluded that HAE should be considered following laparotomy in unstable patients (Table 22.1).

In summary, HAE should be the treatment of choice for managing hemodynamically stable patients in whom a CT scan shows extravasation of contrast medium when the injury is severe (AAST grade 4 or greater) (grade of recommendation: B). More recent reports suggest the first-line use of HAE in transient responders as well. HAE has a high success rate in controlling hemorrhage and provides a safe adjunct to the principles of damage control regardless of whether bleeding appears to be controlled with perihepatic packing.

RECOMMENDATION

HAE is safe and effective in the management of severe hepatic trauma as a key component of nonoperative treatment of severe liver trauma with the known limitations that it may be associated with an increase in HAE-related complications. It can also be safely performed as an adjunct to the principles of DCS.

Level of evidence: Class IIc–III. Grade of recommendation: B.

Editor's Note

Nonoperative management is now the standard of care for hemodynamically stable patients with liver injuries. Bed rest in these patients does not seem to provide any benefit. Drains should be avoided after liver injuries and used only in selective situations such as bile leakage. ERCP appears to accelerate the resolution of biliary complications occurring following liver trauma.

A relatively new development is the nonoperative management of penetrating liver wounds, specifically gunshot wounds. The use of contrast abdominal CT scans has helped guide this care, which appears highly successful in a subset of hemodynamically stable patients without evidence of peritonitis or associated injuries. Angiographic embolization has a key role in the management of liver injuries in both the hemodynamically stable patient with active extravasation on CT scan and the postoperative laparotomy patient. Essentially all of these recommendations are based exclusively on clinical experience with very little derived from high-quality prospective clinical trials.

REFERENCES

1. Stassen NA, Bhullar I, Cheng JD, et al. Nonoperative management of blunt hepatic injury: An Eastern Association for the Surgery of Trauma practice management guideline. *J Trauma Acute Care Surg.* 2012;*73*:S288–S293.
2. Trunkey DD. Hepatic trauma: Contemporary management. *Surg Clin North Am.* 2004;*84(2)*:437–450.
3. Brillantino A, Iacobellis F, Festa P, et al. Non-operative management of blunt liver trauma: Safety, efficacy and complications of a standardized treatment protocol. *Bull Emerg Trauma.* January 2019;*7(1)*:49–54. doi: 10.29252/beat-070107. PMID: 30719466; PMCID: PMC6360015.
4. Peitzman AB, Richardson JD. Surgical treatment of injuries to the solid organs: A 50-year perspective from the journal of trauma. *J Trauma.* November 2010;*69(5)*:1011–1121.
5. Richardson J, Franklin GA, Lukan JK, et al. Evolution in the management of hepatic trauma: A 25-year perspective. *Ann Surg.* 2000;*232(3)*:324–330.
6. Malhotra AK, Fabian TC, Croce MA, et al. Blunt hepatic injury: A paradigm shift from operative to nonoperative management in the 1990s. *Ann Surg.* 2000;*231*:804–813.
7. Sherman HF, Savage BA, Jones LM, et al. Nonoperative management of blunt hepatic injuries: Safe at any grade? *J Trauma.* 1994;*37*:616–621.
8. Croce MA, Fabian TC, Menke PG, et al. Nonoperative management of blunt hepatic trauma is the treatment of choice for hemodynamically stable patients. Results of a prospective trial. *Ann Surg.* 1995;*221*:744–753; discussion 753–755.
9. Archer LP, Rogers FB, Shackford SR. Selective non-operative management of liver and spleen injuries in neurologically impaired adult patients. *Arch Surg.* 1996;*131*:309–315.
10. Wallis A, Kelly MD, Jones L. Angiography and embolization for solid abdominal organ injury in adults—A current perspective. *World J Emerg Surg.* 2010;*5*:18.
11. Stein DM, Scalea TM. Nonoperative management of spleen and liver injuries. *J Intensive Care Med.* September–October 2006;*21(5)*:296–304.
12. London JA, Parry L, Galante J, et al. Safety of early mobilization of patients with blunt solid organ injuries. *Arch Surg.* October 2008;*143(10)*:972–976; discussion 977.
13. Petrowsky H, Raeder S, Zuercher L, et al. A quarter century experience in liver trauma: A plea for early computed tomography and conservative management for all hemodynamically stable patients. *World J Surg.* February 2012;*36(2)*:247–254.
14. Cohn SM, Arango JI, Myers JG. Computed tomography grading systems poorly predict the need for intervention after spleen and liver injuries. *Am Surg.* 2009;*8*:133–139.
15. Fang JF, Chen RJ, Wong YC, et al. Pooling of contrast material on computed tomography mandates aggressive management of blunt hepatic injury. *Am J Surg.* 1998;*176*: 315–319.
16. Pachter HL, Knudson MM, Esrig B, et al. Status of nonoperative management of blunt hepatic injuries in 1995: A multicenter experience with 404 patients. *J Trauma.* 1996;*40*:31–38.
17. Li M, Yu WK, Wang XB, et al. Non-operative management of isolated liver trauma. *Hepatobiliary Pancreat Dis Int.* October 2014;*13(5)*:545–550.
18. Coimbra R, Hoyt DB, Engelhart S, et al. Non-operative management reduces the overall mortality of grades 3 and 4 blunt liver injuries. *Int Surg.* 2006;*91*:251–257.
19. Teichman A, Scantling D, McCracken B, Eakins J. Early mobilization of patients with non-operative liver and spleen injuries is safe and cost-effective. *Eur J Trauma Emerg Surg.* December 2018;*44(6)*:883–887. doi: 10.1007/s00068-017-0864-9. Epub 2017 Dec 5. PMID: 29209737.
20. Parks NA, Davis JW, Forman D, et al. Observation for nonoperative management of blunt liver injuries: How long is long enough? *J Trauma.* March 2011;*70(3)*:626–629.
21. St Peter SD, Sharp SW, Snyder CL. Prospective validation of an abbreviated bedrest protocol in the management of blunt spleen and liver injury in children. *J Pediatr Surg.* January 2011;*46(1)*:173–177.
22. Dodgion CM, Gosain A, Rogers A, et al. National trends in pediatric blunt spleen and liver injury management and potential benefits of an abbreviated bed rest protocol. *J Pediatr Surg.* June 2014;*49(6)*:1004.
23. Lucas CE, Walt AJ. Analysis of randomized biliary drainage for liver trauma in 189 patients. *J Trauma.* 1972;*12(11)*:925–930.
24. Noyes LD Doyle DJ, McSwain NE, Jr. Septic complications associated with the use of peritoneal drains in liver trauma. *J Trauma.* 1988;*28(3)*:337–346.
25. Hommes M, Nicol AJ. Management of biliary complications in 412 patients with liver injuries. *J Trauma Acute Care Surg.* 2014;*77(3)*:448–451.
26. Bajaj JS, Dua, KS. The role of endoscopy in non-iatrogenic injuries of the liver. *Curr Gastroenterol Rep.* 2007;*9*: 147–150.
27. Anand RJ, Farrada PA. Endoscopic retrograde cholangiopancreatography is an effective treatment for bile leaks after severe liver trauma. *J Trauma.* 2011;*71(2)*:480–485.
28. Shaftan GW. Indications for operation in abdominal trauma. *Am J Surg.* 1960;*99*:657–664.
29. Demetriades D, Charalambides D, Lakhoo M, Pantanowitz D. Gunshot wound of the abdomen: Role of selective conservative management. *Br J Surg.* 1991;*78(2)*:220–222.

30. Navsaria PH, Nicol AJ, Krige JE, Edu S. Selective nonoperative management of liver gunshot injuries. *Ann Surg.* 2009;*249*:653–656.

31. Demetriades D, Velhamos G, Cornwell E III, et al. Selective nonoperative management of gunshot wounds of the anterior abdomen. *Arch Surg.* 1997;*132*:178–183.

32. Demetriades D, Hadjizacharia P, Constantinou C, et al. Selective nonoperative management of penetrating abdominal solid organ injuries. *Ann Surg.* 2006;*244(4)*:620–628.

33. DuBose J, Inaba K, Teixeira PG, Pepe A, Dunham MB, McKenney M. Selective non-operative management of solid organ injury following abdominal gunshot wounds. *Injury.* 2007;*38(9)*:1084–1090.

34. Starling SV, Rodrigues BDL, Martins NPR, et al. Nonoperative management of gunshot wounds on the right thoracoabdominal. *Rev Col Bras Cir.* 2012;*39(4)*:286–294.

35. Navsaria PH, Nicol AJ, Edu S, et al. Selective nonoperative management in 1106 patients with abdominal gunshot wounds: Conclusions of safety, efficacy, and role of selective CT imaging in a prospective single-center study. *Ann Surg.* 2015;*261*:760–764.

36. Grossman MD, May AK, Schwab CW, et al. Determining anatomic injury with computed tomography in selected torso gunshot wounds. *J Trauma.* 1998;*45(3)*:446–456.

37. Schellenberg M, Benjamin E, Piccinini A, Inaba K, Demetriades D. Gunshot wounds to the liver: No longer a mandatory operation. *J Trauma Acute Care Surg.* August 2019;*87(2)*:350–355. doi: 10.1097/TA.0000000000002356. PMID: 31045732.

38. Morrison JJ, Clasper JC, Gibb I, Midwinter M. Management of penetrating abdominal trauma in the conflict environment: The role of computer tomography scanning. *World J Surg.* 2011;*35*:27–33.

39. Schnuriger B, Talving P, Barbarino R, et al. Current practice and the role of the CT in the management of penetrating liver injuries at a level I trauma center. *J Emerg Trauma Shock.* 2011;*4(1)*:53–57.

40. Polanco PM, Brown JB, Puyana JC, et al. The swinging pendulum: A national perspective of nonoperative management in severe blunt liver injury. *J Trauma Acute Care Surg.* 2013;*75*:590–595.

41. Gaarder C, Naess PA, Eken T, et al. Liver injuries—Improved results with a formal protocol including angiography. *Injury.* 2007;*38(9)*:1075–1083.

42. Hagiwara A, Murata A, Matsuda T, Matsuda H, Shimazaki S. The efficacy and limitations of transarterial embolization for severe hepatic injury. *J Trauma.* 2002;*52(6)*:1091–1096.

43. Monnin V, Sengel C, Thony F, et al. Place of arterial embolization in severe blunt hepatic trauma: A multidisciplinary approach. *Cardiovasc Intervent Radiol.* 2008;*31(5)*:875–882.

44. Kozar RA, Moore FA, Cothern CC, et al. Risk factors for hepatic morbidity following nonoperative management. *Arch Surg.* 2006;*141*:451–459.

45. Asencio JA, Petrone P, Garcia-Nunez L, Kimbrell B, Kuncir E. Multidisciplinary approach for the management of complex hepatic injuries AAST-OIS grades IV–V: A prospective study. *Scand J Surg.* 2007;*96(3)*:214–220.

46. Mitsusada M, Nakajima Y, Shirakawa M, Takeda T, Honda H. Nonoperative management of blunt liver injury: A new protocol for selected hemodynamically unstable patients under hypotensive resuscitation. *J Hepatobiliary Pancreat Sci.* 2014;*21*:205–211.

47. Green CS, Bulger EM, Kwan SW. Outcomes and complications of angioembolization for hepatic trauma: A systematic review of the literature. *J Trauma Acute Care Surg.* March 2016;*80(3)*:529–537. doi: 10.1097/TA.0000000000000942. PMID: 26670113; PMCID: PMC4767638.

48. Samuels JM, Carmichael H, Kovar A, Urban S, Vega S, Velopulos C, McIntyre RC Jr. Reevaluation of hepatic angioembolization for trauma in stable patients: Weighing the risk. *J Am Coll Surg.* July 2020;*231*(1):123–131.e3. doi: 10.1016/j.jamcollsurg.2020.05.006. Epub 2020 May 15. PMID: 32422347.

49. Misselbeck TS, Teicher EJ, Cipolle MD, et al. Hepatic angioembolization in trauma patients: Indications and complications. *J Trauma.* 2009;*67*:769–773.

50. Matsumoto S, Cantrell E, Jung K, Smith A, Coimbra R. Influence of postoperative hepatic angiography on mortality after laparotomy in Grade IV/V hepatic injuries. *J Trauma Acute Care Surg.* August 2018;*85*(2):290–297. doi: 10.1097/TA.0000000000001906. PMID: 29613955.

23

Small Bowel and Colon Injuries

David H. Livingston

Injuries to the small intestine and colon are found in less than 5% of victims of blunt abdominal trauma but are the most common injuries sustained after penetrating abdominal trauma. Despite a large experience with these injuries in both military and civilian environments, certain aspects of the management of hollow viscus injuries remain controversial. Areas of ongoing debate without definitive conclusions include (1) whether an ostomy is ever necessary for the setting of colonic trauma, (2) the management of resected bowel (colon and distal ileum) following damage control surgery, (3) the inferiority or superiority of stapled versus hand-sewn anastomosis, (4) the management of the skin incision in the setting of hollow viscus injuries, (5) the duration of antibiotics, and (6) the routine use of presacral drainage for rectal injuries.

23.1 Is an Ostomy Ever Necessary Following Colon Trauma?

The issues driving this debate include the extent of the colonic injury, the location of the injury, and the physiology of the patient. What has been definitively settled is that for almost all injuries to the colon that do not require resection and anastomosis (usually <50% of the circumference), the primary repair is all that is required. While there have been many studies examining colonic injuries, the number of patients accrued with destructive colonic injuries has been generally insufficient to definitively answer the question of when, if ever, an ostomy is required [1–4]. Other unanswered questions are whether blunt and penetrating colonic injuries should be treated similarly and whether the location of the colonic injury matters. There have been several studies that evaluated a relatively large number of patients with destructive colon wounds requiring resection [5–8]. In all series, management was left to the surgeon's discretion, and it should be noted that several of these studies take place in the same institution. This latter factor likely adds selection and institutional biases to their conclusions. Lastly, many studies conflate all intraabdominal infections with those solely due to suture line failure. Given that patients treated by primary colostomy often are "sicker" with other factors not necessarily accounted for in statistical modeling and this group often has an elevated incidence of intraabdominal infection, this adds further bias to the recommendation of performing a stoma or primary anastomosis. Risk factors that have been associated with anastomotic leak

favoring possible treatment by ostomy include hypotension on presentation, transfusion requirement of four or more units of packed red blood cells, excessive crystalloid resuscitation, an Abdominal Trauma Index >25, and some underlying medical condition. It is also generally not recommended that anastomosis be performed in the case of severe bowel wall edema. The location of the injury to the colon has been examined and often found not to correlate with suture line failure. However, it is not the location of the injury per se that is the issue, but where one performs the anastomosis and the blood supply to the cut ends of the bowel [9]. Perfusion to the colon is segmental, and some locations have a less robust blood supply or have vasculature that may be compromised from injury or resection of the injured bowel and mesentery. All of these issues may decrease the perfusion to the resected colon, especially in those patients requiring aggressive resuscitation. These specific locations are the areas of the distal transverse to the proximal sigmoid colon, where the blood supply is dependent on the connections between the left branch of the middle colic and the left colic arteries. The other location is the distal ileum, where injury or the resection or injury to the mesentery might compromise the ileocolic artery. This results in the distal ileum being supplied by ileal arcades from the distal superior mesenteric artery. In both instances, resection of additional bowel, either proximally or distally, will improve the perfusion to the cut ends of the bowel. Regardless of how a colon injury is managed, the risk of abdominal septic complications exceeds 20%, with increased colonic-related morbidity and mortality in patients who develop suture line failure.

RECOMMENDATIONS

Nondestructive or partial circumference wounds that do not require resection should be closed primarily. Destructive wounds that require resection can usually be managed with anastomosis. Factors associated with suture line failure in almost all studies are hemorrhagic shock and the transfusion requirement of four or more units of packed red blood cells. In these patients and those with major underlying medical conditions, colostomy should be considered, as the risks of suture line failure can be severe.

Grade of recommendation: B.

DOI: 10.1201/9781003316800-23

23.2 Is It Safe to Do a Colon Anastomosis Following Damage Control Laparotomy?

If a patient's physiology is sufficiently deranged to require damage control laparotomy, injuries to the intestines and specifically colon almost always include resection without reconstruction. Thus, the question upon re-exploration is, "When is it safe and advisable to perform ileocolic or colocolonic anastomosis?" Several publications have attempted to address this issue, but few are prospective and none of these are randomized [8, 10–17]. In each study, low-risk patients were selected for colonic anastomosis at the time of a repeat laparotomy after an initial damage control procedure. Depending on the study, this ranged from 46% to 82% of the patients who had initial colon resection. Factors that are deemed to make a patient at "high risk" include bowel edema, persistent acidosis, ongoing need for ionotropic support, overall medical stability and comorbidities, and prolonged interval from injury to operation. The ability to close the abdomen is strongly associated with anastomotic success, and Ott et al. and Anjaria et al. identified that inability to close the abdomen at the first relaparotomy and the risk of anastomotic leak was unacceptably high, at 27% and 19%, respectively [13, 15]. Burlew et al. in a multicenter study found that inability to get the abdomen closed by day 5 was associated with a four times increase in suture line failure [16].

> **RECOMMENDATION**
>
> It appears to be safe to perform colon anastomosis at the first relaparotomy in selected patients in whom the abdominal fascia will also be closed at that time. Factors that may influence the decision to manage the patient with a colostomy include bowel edema, persistent physiological derangements, medical comorbidities, and the prolonged interval between injury and definitive operation.
>
> Grade of recommendation: C.

23.3 When Is Hand-Sewn Anastomosis Preferable to Stapled Anastomosis—If Ever?

This question has been debated since the invention of intestinal stapling devices. In the setting of elective surgical procedures, the literature can best be summarized by stating that no outcome difference between stapled and hand-sewn anastomoses has ever been identified [18]. Early studies following trauma and emergency surgery appear to indicate a possible superiority of hand-sewn anastomosis [19–23]. However, these studies occurred before balanced hemostatic resuscitation. A meta-analysis of emergency anastomosis failed to identify the superiority of one technique over the other [24]. The postulated mechanism for an increased leak rate in patients with stapled anastomoses is bowel edema, which might explain the findings in those earlier studies, as stapling devices with fixed staple heights were never tested or designed for use in severely edematous tissue. All studies in this arena suffer from surgeon preference and inclusion bias, and

thus, even with statistical manipulation, the populations are not likely as comparable. The decision to perform one technique or the other is also at times related to the location and architecture of the anastomosis the surgeon is creating.

> **RECOMMENDATION**
>
> There is no consensus on the issue of stapled versus hand-sewn anastomosis after small bowel or colon resection for trauma. The hand-sewn anastomosis may be preferable in situations where the portion of the intestine under consideration for anastomosis is edematous or is at risk of becoming edematous, such as in a patient requiring a large-volume resuscitation. Lastly, the way the anastomosis is created within the abdomen or the need to mobilize more bowel may influence the choice of anastomosis.
>
> Grade of recommendation: D.

23.4 Should the Skin Be Closed after Laparotomy for Colon Injury?

Injury to the small intestine has not been shown to result in a high rate of infectious complications, and skin closure after small bowel trauma is generally recommended [19]. However, surgical site infection (SSI) rates have been shown to range from 2.7% to over 50% after colonic trauma [25–29]. In a nationwide analysis of Trauma Quality Improvement Program (TQIP) data, the overall superficial skin infection rate was 4.3%; however, colon, duodenal, and multiple hollow viscus injuries increased this rate 2.9, 2.0, and >3.8 times, respectively [30]. Interestingly, this same pattern was observed in military injuries; however, the baseline rate of SSIs was higher at 14% [31]. Not surprisingly, the need for transfusion was also associated with an increased rate of SSI in both studies. This has led some authors to recommend closing only the abdominal fascia and leaving the skin open. In a prospective, randomized trial published by Velmahos et al. [28], the infection rate for open wounds was noted to be 36%, whereas the infection rate in closed wounds was seen to be 65%. Wound infection was predictive of risk for wound dehiscence and necrotizing soft tissue infection. Subjecting patients to this increased risk of major complications to avoid the need to care for an open wound does not seem prudent.

> **RECOMMENDATION**
>
> Skin should be left open after laparotomy for colon trauma.
>
> Grade of recommendation: B.

23.5 What Is the Appropriate Duration of Antibiotics after Colon Injury?

The debate of antibiotic duration following trauma laparotomy in general and colon injury in particular continues. There have been a few recent studies, and almost all data and recommendations occurred before modern resuscitation and may have not been executed with the same rigor as is required of more modern trials. Three double-blind, prospective, randomized trials compared 24-hour versus longer antibiotic coverage in patients with abdominal trauma. All studies found no significant difference in infectious complications between patients randomized to 1 day versus 5 days of perioperative antibiotics [32–34]. Specifically, in 1992, Fabian et al. published a double-blind, prospective, randomized trial in 515 patients. After sustaining penetrating abdominal trauma, the patients were randomized to receive either 5 days of a broad-spectrum antibiotic postoperatively or 1 day of the same antibiotic plus 4 days of saline placebo. The patients who received 5 days of antibiotics had a slightly but statistically insignificant higher rate of abdominal infections and were more likely to develop an infection from multidrug-resistant organisms. In 1999, Cornwell et al. published the results of a study in which they randomized 63 patients to 5 days versus 1 day of antibiotics after penetrating abdominal trauma. They also found a higher infection rate (38% versus 19%) in the patients who received a longer duration of antibiotics, although statistical significance was not reached, possibly due to the small sample size. In a trial of a similar design involving 317 patients, published in 2000, Kirton et al. found similar results, although the infection rate was slightly higher in the patients who received antibiotics for 1 day as opposed to 5 days. This difference was not statistically significant. A recent Cochrane meta-analysis found that most studies on this topic had significant bias and were considered to be generally of poor quality [35].

RECOMMENDATION

Despite the lack of truly definitive trials, it is advisable to limit antibiotic prophylaxis to no more than 24 hours after laparotomy for intestinal injury. With even less data, antibiotic usage should be limited to 24 hours in the setting of an open abdomen and restarted for an additional 24 hours upon re-exploration.

Grade of recommendation: B.

23.6 Should Presacral Drains Be Used in the Management of Rectal Injuries?

The placement of presacral drains as an adjunct to colonic diversion to prevent the development of pelvic sepsis in the management of rectal injuries began during the Vietnam War and rapidly spread throughout the civilian arena [36]. The recognition of the difference between military and civilian injuries resulted in several papers questioning this dogma. As with many issues, there are far too few patients to come to firm conclusions, and even groups with a long interest in this topic have come to oppose recommendations [37, 38]. Gonzalez et al. [39] reported their results from a prospective randomized trial and found that presacral drainage did not reduce the incidence of pelvic sepsis. As this is the only prospective randomized trial on this topic in the literature and as only 48 patients were included in the study, it is difficult to consider this question as having a definitive answer. Two reports have suggested that pelvic sepsis is relatively rare in patients with penetrating rectal trauma, even in the absence of presacral drains, suggesting that they are of little utility [40, 41]. Other authors, such as Weinberg et al. [38], have argued that having a pelvic infection that is decompressed by a presacral drain is preferable to having undrained pelvic sepsis. Lastly, in almost all studies, there is too little information on the trajectory of the wounds as well as the success of the drains in reaching the zone of injury.

RECOMMENDATIONS

Based on this review of the literature, it appears that presacral drainage is not routinely necessary for rectal injuries. These data are derived almost exclusively from low-velocity, penetrating trauma patients. The author's practice is to selectively place a presacral drain(s) in patients who have obvious extraperitoneal tissue destruction or true posterior wounds where presacral drainage might be effective. The trajectory of the wounds can be easily assessed by preoperative or postoperative CT scanning, and those patients can then undergo targeted drainage as needed.

Grade of recommendation: D.

TABLE 23.1

Levels of Evidence

Question	Answer	Level of Evidence	Grade of Recommendation	References
Anastomosis or ostomy after colon resection for trauma?	Anastomosis, except for selected patients	2A	B	[1–9]
Is it safe to perform colon anastomosis after damage control laparotomy?	Yes, but only in selected patients	4	C	[10–17]
Stapled or hand-sewn anastomosis after hollow viscus injury for trauma?	Either, although hand-sewn may be better in patients with edematous bowel	4	D	[18–24]
Should the skin be closed after laparotomy for colon trauma?	No	1B	B	[25–31]
How long should antibiotics be continued after the repair of a hollow viscus injury?	No more than 24 hours	2	B	[32–35]
Should presacral drains be used in the management of rectal trauma?	No, except in selected cases	3	D	[35–41]

Editor's Note

While significant controversy remains in the care of the patient with an injury to the colon, there is considerable quality data to inform the surgeon. Primary repair is performed for minor lacerations in stable patients and has a 5% failure rate. When damage is such that colonic resection is required (more than about 50% of the circumference of the bowel is injured), anastomosis is required. In my opinion, the methods of anastomosis should be hand-sewn whenever there is bowel wall edema evident or expected, as the failure rate is higher with the use of staplers in this setting. The anastomotic failure rate after resection and anastomosis of colonic injuries remains at about 10%. Ostomy is typically reserved for the patient after damage control laparotomy or those patients in whom an anastomotic leak would be catastrophic (i.e., patients with complex underlying medical conditions such as transplant recipients, dialysis patients, and the like). The other consideration is the extent of the injury after blunt trauma or high-velocity injuries, which may preclude the ability of the surgeon to determine the extent of bowel injury. In these patients, second-look operations after an abbreviated laparotomy to assess bowel viability appear prudent.

REFERENCES

1. Stone HH, Fabian TC. Management of perforating colon trauma: Randomization between primary closure and exteriorization. *Ann Surg.* 1979;*190*:430–436.
2. Chappuis CW, Frey DJ, Dietzen CD, Panetta TP, Buechter KJ, Cohn I. Management of penetrating colon injuries. A prospective randomized trial. *Ann Surg.* 1991;*213*:492–497.
3. Sasaki LS, Allaben RD, Golwala R, Mittal VK. Primary repair of colon injuries: A prospective randomized study. *J Trauma.* 1995;*39*:895–901.
4. Gonzalez RP, Falimirsky ME, Holevar MR. Further evaluation of colostomy in penetrating colon injury. *Am Surg.* 2000;*66*:342–347.
5. Murray JA, Demetriades D, Colson M, et al. Colonic resection in trauma: Colostomy versus anastomosis. *J Trauma.* 1999;*46*:250–254.
6. Stewart RM, Fabian TC, Croce MA, Pritchard FE, Minard G, Kudsk KA. I resection with primary anastomosis following a destructive colon wound always safe? *Am J Surg.* 1994;*168*:316–319.
7. Demetriades D, Murray JA, Chan L, Ordoñez C, Bowley D, Nagy K. Penetrating colon injuries requiring resection: Diversion or primary anastomosis? An AAST prospective multicenter study. *J Trauma.* 2001;*50*:765–775.
8. Mitchao DP, Lewis MR, Strickland M, Benjamin ER, Wong MD, Demetriades D. Destructive colon injuries requiring resection: Is colostomy ever indicated? *J Trauma Acute Care Surg.* 2022 Jun 1;*92*(6):1039–1046. doi: 10.1097/TA.0000000000003513. Epub 2022 Jan 25. PMID: 35081597.
9. Dente CJ, Patel A, Feliciano DV, Rozycki GS, Wyrzykowski AD, Nicholas JM, Salomone JP, Ingram WL. Suture line failure in intra-abdominal colonic trauma: Is there an effect of segmental variations in blood supply on outcomes? *J Trauma.* 2005 Aug;*59*(2):359–366; discussion 366–8. doi: 10.1097/01.ta.0000185034.64059.96. PMID: 16294076.
10. Miller PR, Chang MC, Hoth JJ, Holmes JH IV, Meredith JW. Colonic resection in the setting of damage control laparotomy: Is delayed anastomosis safe? *Am Surg.* 2007;*73*:606–609; discussion 609–610.
11. Kashuk JL, Cothren CC, Moore EE, Johnson JL, Biffl WL, Barnett CC. Primarily repair of colon injuries is safe in the damage control scenario. *Surgery.* 2009;*146*:663–668; discussion 668–670.
12. Weinberg JA, Griffin RL, Vandromme MJ, Melton SM, George RL, Reiff DA, Kerby JD, Rue LW III. Management of colon wounds in the setting of damage control laparotomy: A cautionary tale. *J Trauma.* 2009;*67*:929–935.
13. Ott MM, Norris PR, Diaz JJ, Collier BR, Jenkins JM, Gunter OL, Morris JA Jr. Colon anastomosis after damage control laparotomy: Recommendations from 174 trauma colectomies. *J Trauma.* 2011;*70*:595–602.
14. Georgoff P, Perales P, Laguna B, Holena D, Reilly P, Sims C. Colonic injuries and the damage control abdomen: Does management strategy matter? *J Surg Res.* 2013;*181*:293–299.
15. Anjaria DJ, Ullmann TM, Lavery R, Livingston DH. Management of colonic injuries in the setting of damage-control laparotomy: One shot to get it right. *J Trauma Acute Care Surg.* 2014;*76*:594–598.
16. Burlew CC, Moore EE, Cuschieri J, Jurkovich GJ, Codner P, Crowell K, Nirula R, Haan J, Rowell SE, Kato CM, MacNew H, Ochsner MG, Harrison PB, Fusco C, Sauaia A, Kaups KL; WTA Study Group. Sew it up! A Western Trauma Association multi-institutional study of enteric injury management in the postinjury open abdomen. *J Trauma.* 2011 Feb;*70*(2):273–277. doi: 10.1097/TA.0b013e3182050eb7. PMID: 21307721.
17. Oosthuizen G, Buitendag J, Variawa S, Čačala S, Kong V, Xu W, Clarke D. Penetrating colonic trauma and damage control surgery: Anastomosis or stoma? *ANZ J Surg.* 2021 Sep;*91*(9):1874–1880. doi: 10.1111/ans.16939. Epub 2021 May 31. PMID: 34056835.
18. Neutzling CB, Lustosa SA, Proenca IM, da Silva EM, Matos D. Stapled versus handsewn methods for colorectal anastomosis surgery. *Cochrane Database Syst Rev.* 2012 Feb;*2*:CD003144.
19. Brundage SI, Jurkovich GJ, Grossman DC, et al. Stapled versus sutured gastrointestinal anastomoses in the trauma patient. *J Trauma.* 1999;*47*:500–507.
20. Brundage SI, Jurkovich GJ, Hoyt DB, et al. Stapled versus sutured gastrointestinal anastomoses in the trauma patient: A multicenter trial. *J Trauma.* 2001;*6*:1054–1061.
21. Demetriades D, Murray JA, Chan LS, et al. Handsewn versus stapled anastomosis in penetrating colon injuries requiring resection: A multicenter study. *J Trauma.* 2002;*52*:117–121.
22. Farrah JP, Lauer CW, Bray MS, McCartt JM, Chang MC, Meredith JW, Miller PR, Mowery NT. Stapled versus handsewn anastomoses in emergency general surgery: A retrospective review of outcomes in a unique patient population. *J Trauma Acute Care Surg.* 2013 May;*74*(5):1187–1192; discussion 1192-4. DOI: 10.1097/TA.0b013e31828cc9c4. PMID: 23609266.

23. Behrman SW, Bertken KA, Stefanacci HA, Parks SN. Breakdown of intestinal repair after laparotomy for trauma: Incidence, risk factors, and strategies for prevention. *J Trauma.* 1998;*45*:227–231; discussion 231–233.

24. Naumann DN, Bhangu A, Kelly M, Bowley DM. Stapled versus handsewn intestinal anastomosis in emergency laparotomy: A systemic review and meta-analysis. *Surgery.* 2015 Apr;157(4):609–18. doi: 10.1016/j.surg.2014.09.030. Epub 2015 Feb 27. PMID: 25731781.

25. Voyles CR, Flint LM Jr. Wound management after trauma to the colon. *South Med J.* 1977;*70*:1067–1069.

26. Demetriades D, Charalambides D, Pantanowitz D. Gunshot wounds of the colon: Role of primary repair. *Ann R Coll Surg Engl.* 1992;*74*:381–384.

27. Velmahos GC, Souter I, Degiannis E, et al. Primary repair for colonic gunshot wounds. *Aust N Z J Surg.* 1996;*66*: 344–347.

28. Velmahos GC, Vassiliu P, Demetriades D, et al. Wound management after colon injury: Open or closed? A prospective randomized study. *Am Surg.* 2002;*68*:795–801.

29. Seamon MJ, Smith BP, Capano-Wehrle L, Fakhro A, Fox N, Goldberg M, Martin NM, Pathak AS, Ross SE. Skin closure after laparotomy in high-risk trauma patients: Opening opportunities for improvement. *J Trauma Acute Care Surg.* 2013;*74*:433–440.

30. Durbin S, DeAngelis R, Peschman J, Milia D, Carver T, Dodgion C. Superficial surgical infections in operative abdominal trauma patients: A trauma quality improvement database analysis. *J Surg Res.* 2019 Nov;*243*:496–502. doi: 10.1016/j.jss.2019.06.101. Epub 2019 Aug 1. PMID: 31377489.

31. Bozzay JD, Walker PF, Schechtman DW, Shaikh F, Stewart L, Carson ML, Tribble DR, Rodriguez CJ, Bradley MJ; Infectious Disease Clinical Research Program Trauma Infectious Disease Outcomes Study Group. Risk factors for abdominal surgical site infection after exploratory laparotomy among combat casualties. *J Trauma Acute Care Surg.* 2021 Aug 1;*91*(2S Suppl 2):S247–S255. doi: 10.1097/TA.0000000000003109. PMID: 33605707; PMCID: PMC8324514.

32. Fabian TC, Croce MA, Payne LW, et al. Duration of antibiotic therapy for penetrating abdominal trauma: A prospective trial. *Surgery.* 1992;*112*:788–794; discussion 794–795.

33. Cornwell EE III, Dougherty WR, Berne TV, et al. Duration of antibiotic prophylaxis in high-risk patients with penetrating abdominal trauma: A prospective randomized trial. *J Gastroint Surg.* 1999;*3*:648–653.

34. Kirton OC, O'Neill PA, Kestner M, Tortella BJ. Perioperative antibiotic use in high-risk penetrating hollow viscus injury: A prospective randomized, double-blind, placebo-control trial of 24 hours versus 5 days. *J Trauma.* 2000;*49*:822–832.

35. Herrod PJ, Boyd-Carson H, Doleman B, Blackwell J, Williams JP, Bhalla A, Nelson RL, Tou S, Lund JN. Prophylactic antibiotics for penetrating abdominal trauma: Duration of use and antibiotic choice. *Cochrane Database Syst Rev.* 2019 Dec 12;*12*(12):CD010808. doi: 10.1002/14651858.CD010808.pub2. PMID: 31830315; PMCID: PMC6953295.

36. Lavenson GS, Cohen A. Management of rectal injuries. *Am J Surg.* 1971;*122*:226–230.

37. Mangiante EC, Graham AD, Fabian TC. Rectal gunshot wounds. Management of civilian injuries. *Am Surg.* 1986; *52*:37–40.

38. Weinberg JA, Fabian TC, Magnotti LJ, et al. Penetrating rectal trauma: Management by anatomic distinction improves outcome. *J Trauma.* 2006;*60*:508–514.

39. Gonzalez RP, Falimirski ME, Holevar MR. The role of presacral drainage in the management of penetrating rectal injuries. *J Trauma.* 1998;*45*:656–661.

40. Navasaria P, Edu S, Nicol AJ. Civilian extraperitoneal rectal gunshot wounds: Surgical management made simpler. *World J Surg.* 2007;*31*:1345–1351.

41. Navsaria PH, Shaw JM, Zellweger R, et al. Diagnostic laparoscopy and diverting sigmoid loop colostomy in the management of civilian extraperitoneal rectal gunshot injuries. *Br J Surg.* 2004;*91*:460–464.

24

Diaphragmatic Injuries

Fahim Habib and Marc LaFonte

Traumatic diaphragmatic injuries (TDIs) are uncommon injuries but most often are a result of penetrating trauma. They carry high mortality rates largely due to the severity of the association with other injuries [1]. The optimal approach to the evaluation and management of TDI remains poorly defined and is particularly challenging due to several factors. The diaphragm is a thin musculoaponeurotic layer at the junction of the thoracic and peritoneal cavities. As a result, it may be involved in traumatic injuries involving both of these cavities, and associated injuries are frequent. These may dominate the clinical picture, making management of the diaphragm injury secondary. When isolated, these injuries usually have no pathognomonic features; hence, they require a high index of suspicion if the diagnosis is to be made in a timely fashion. This is becoming increasingly important as nonoperative strategies are being more commonly employed in select cases of thoracoabdominal trauma. Key differences exist regarding whether the mechanism of injury is blunt or penetrating and which side the diaphragmatic injury lies on. Perhaps more importantly, emerging literature has looked at diaphragmatic injuries involving the central fibrous tendon versus peripheral muscular portions and how this may determine injury severity and the surgical approach for optimal recovery based on tendon-to-muscle ratio [2]. This effectively precludes a universal algorithm for the management of all diaphragmatic injuries. While some of these missed injuries may never manifest, the potential for an adverse outcome exists and with it an increase in morbidity and mortality, which makes prompt diagnosis and management desirable.

There is a paucity of literature to guide clinical decision-making. The overwhelming majority of publications involve case reports and case series. These usually describe the unusual and often dramatic presentation of isolated cases. Few retrospective reviews are available that summarize the practices of individual institutions. Prospective studies are even fewer and are mostly observational, directed largely toward establishing the diagnosis. The relative infrequency of these injuries adds to the challenge of rapid diagnosis. At present, there is no Level I or Level II evidence on any aspect of the diagnosis or management of TDI. As the available evidence is limited, much of what is presented in this chapter represents a summary of the current body of knowledge and the opinions of the authors.

The key questions include the following: (1) What is the optimal diagnostic modality for the diagnosis of TDI in blunt trauma? (2) What is the optimal diagnostic modality for the diagnosis of TDI in penetrating trauma? (3) What is the clinically useful classification system that guides operative management? (4) What is the optimal approach to the operative management of TDI? (5) What is the ideal suture material/prosthesis for the repair of diaphragmatic injuries? (6) What are the differences in the approach to left- versus right-sided injuries? (7) What are the consequences of missed injuries?

24.1 What Is the Optimal Diagnostic Modality for the Diagnosis of Diaphragmatic Injury in Blunt Trauma?

The gold standard for establishing the diagnosis of TDI is direct visualization of the diaphragm by using either laparotomy or the minimally invasive techniques of laparoscopy or thoracoscopy. However, given the relative rarity of the injury, the highly invasive nature of techniques for direct visualization which requires general anesthesia, and the high resource use and resultant costs, the routine use of the direct visualization approach is not advocated. Instead, a high index of suspicion is required in patients whose trauma mechanism and physical findings are suggestive of TDI, as many imaging modalities are not reliably sensitive or specific. Blunt mechanisms most commonly associated with TDI are motor vehicle collisions, falls from heights, and crush injury to the thoracoabdominal region [3]. Among vehicular crashes, those with a near-lateral principal direction of force and those associated with a significant abrupt change in velocity of 40 km/hour or greater are most likely to result in TDI [4]. In cases of penetrating trauma, wounds in the thoracoabdominal region, defined as extending from the nipple lines to the costal margins, necessitate additional evaluation.

Physical examination is notoriously unreliable. Signs and symptoms depend on the stage of presentation, which may be divided into the acute, latent, and obstructive phases [5]. In the acute phase, variable degrees of respiratory compromise occur. This is accompanied by chest and/or abdominal tenderness, reduced breath sounds in the chest, and possibly bowel sounds in the chest [6, 7]. Alternatively, the presentation may be masked by the associated injuries, leading to incidental diagnosis or missed diagnosis. The latent phase is

DOI: 10.1201/9781003316800-24

usually asymptomatic, with the diagnosis being made incidentally when bowel sounds are heard in the chest or the patient undergoes imaging for unrelated reasons. In the obstructive phase, intraabdominal contents herniate into the thoracic cavity. This may result in obstruction of the gastrointestinal tract, ischemia of the herniated organ, or compression of thoracic structures with possible mediastinal shift. The patient may, therefore, present with bowel obstruction, peritonitis, or even features suggestive of a tension pneumothorax [7, 8], a condition termed gastrothorax.

A chest X-ray is usually the initial diagnostic modality. When present, the abnormal course of the nasogastric tube with the tip in the left chest, the elevation of the hemidiaphragm over 6 cm when compared to the contralateral side, gas-containing hollow viscera within the thoracic cavity, a visceral fluid level in the pleural space, and obscuring of the diaphragmatic shadow are highly suggestive [9, 10]. Nonspecific findings on the chest X-ray that should prompt additional workup include obliteration of the diaphragmatic contour; mild elevation of the injured diaphragm; the shift of the mediastinum to the contralateral side; or evidence of additional thoracic injuries, such as a pneumothorax, pleural effusions, or rib fractures [11]. An increase in the elevation of the hemidiaphragm on the right on a repeat X-ray is another reported finding. Having the film reviewed by a radiologist increases detection. In a retrospective review, the accuracy of the diagnosis of chest X-ray increased from 23% when read by the trauma team leader in the trauma bay to 44% when interpreted by a radiologist [3]. Limitations of the technique include the fact that the film is almost always obtained in the supine position; is portable, and hence often of suboptimal quality; and patient cooperation is usually limited and may be influenced by associated injuries or by the use of positive pressure ventilation [12].

Ultrasonography is most useful for right-sided injuries where the "lung sliding sign," visualization of the hepatic veins in the chest, and loss of the hepatorenal interface have been reported [13]. Other findings include movement of the free edge of the diaphragm in pleural fluid, splenic herniation into the thorax, inability to visualize the diaphragm, and the identification of bowel loops in the chest. Using "m-mode" imaging, failure to identify the rise of the diaphragm tracing with respiratory movements is considered diagnostic [14]. However, a ruptured diaphragm will move in mechanically ventilated patients, limiting the use of this technique to spontaneously breathing patients only.

Computed tomography (CT) performed using conventional techniques has low sensitivity and moderate specificity in identifying the presence of TDI. The invention of multidetector CT (MDCT) with multiplanar reformations has redefined the role of this modality in the diagnosis of TDI. Acquired images can be reformatted in the axial, coronal, and sagittal planes. Several radiographic features are suggestive of TDI. A "segmental diaphragmatic defect" may be observed with the abrupt loss of diaphragmatic continuity [15]. While this is highly specific, it is not very sensitive for TDI. It is most useful in blunt trauma where the resultant defect is large and on the left side where there is a significant difference in the appearance of the diaphragm and adjacent

structures. A false-positive reading may result in cases of congenital defects or other nontraumatic causes of diaphragmatic discontinuity. Here, the absence of other features of acute injury, such as accompanying bleeding, may be useful. The "dangling diaphragm sign" is the inward curling of the free edge of the torn diaphragm toward the center of the body and is best visualized in coronal images [16]. The "collar sign" is a waist-like constriction of herniated viscera at the site of the diaphragmatic tear. The "contiguous injury sign," initially described by Shanmuganathan et al. is positive when there is injury immediately adjacent to both sides of the diaphragm [17]. The "dependent viscera sign" represents the loss of the normal costophrenic sulcus by the diaphragmatic injury, which then allows the intraabdominal viscera to lie in direct contact with the posterior ribs [18]. Thickening of the diaphragm to more than 10 mm represents retraction of the injured diaphragm. The simultaneous presence of a hemothorax associated with hemoperitoneum is another suggestive finding [19]. Additional tomographic signs specific to injuries to the right side of the diaphragm include the "hump sign" and the "band sign." The hump sign is the rounded herniation of hepatic tissue into the thoracic cavity through the diaphragmatic defect [10]. The band sign is the linear area of hypodensity through the liver at the level of the torn diaphragm. It represents reduced perfusion at the site of compression by the torn diaphragm and is best visualized in the portal venous phase [20].

In a retrospective case-control study using a single detector helical CT with coronal and sagittal reconstruction, the sensitivity and specificity of the technique were 82% and 75%, respectively [21]. The dependent viscera sign was the most sensitive, and the collar sign and active extravasation of contrast were the most specific [22]. The presence of pleural effusions and perisplenic hematomas was the most common reason for false-negative examination [22]. In right-sided injuries, the presence of an associated hemothorax may limit the ability to make a diagnosis. In these situations, the high position of the liver may suggest the diagnosis [23]. More recent studies have validated the use of MDCT in establishing the diagnosis [24].

Nuclear medicine scan techniques have been described, where 2.1 mCi of technetium-99 m sulfur colloid in 500 mL of sterile saline are injected into the peritoneal cavity. Imaging is performed immediately and at 2-hour and 4-hour intervals. The appearance of a large amount of radioactivity in the chest confirms the presence of a diaphragmatic defect [25].

Intraoperative evaluation of the diaphragm remains the gold standard against which all other modalities have been compared. The operative approach selected is guided by two key principles: Hemodynamic stability and clinical or radiologic evidence of associated injury. In unstable patients, emergent operative intervention is undertaken. The presence of peritoneal signs and chest tube output can assist in guidance for initial cavitary triage: Laparotomy, thoracotomy, or both [26]. The diaphragm is directly evaluated during these interventions.

In the hemodynamically stable patient with no indication for immediate operative intervention, a minimally invasive approach may be adopted. This may be achieved by using either laparoscopy or thoracoscopy. Irrespective of the modality selected, the intervention is usually deferred at least 24 hours after injury to allow for declaration of the injury. In patients remaining asymptomatic after this interval, the intervention can be directed solely toward the evaluation and management of the diaphragm. Laparoscopy for the diagnosis of traumatic diaphragmatic lacerations was initially demonstrated by Adamthwaite [27] and subsequently confirmed by Ivatury et al. [28], especially for the identification of injury in asymptomatic cases. As trauma surgeons are becoming more facile with the use of laparoscopic techniques, their use in the repair of TDI is increasing [29–31]. Laparoscopy has the advantage of being both diagnostic and therapeutic. Additional advantages of laparoscopy include shorter hospital stay, faster recovery, earlier return to normal activities, fewer analgesic requirements, fewer wound complications, and lower long-term sequelae such as adhesions and development of incisional hernias when compared to open surgery. Although technically feasible, several disadvantages of the laparoscopic approach must be recognized. The most common complication following any laparoscopic surgery is the development of a trocar site hernia. Frequently underdiagnosed, its true incidence remains unknown. With careful long-term follow-up and the use of a combination of physical examination and imaging studies, such as ultrasound and CT, incidences of >30% have been reported, especially in high-risk patients. These include those with diabetes mellitus, obesity, postoperative wound infection, need for enlargement of the fascia at the trocar site, and the presence of chronic pulmonary disease [32, 33]. Additionally, the need for the creation of a pneumoperitoneum carries the potential to induce cardiopulmonary compromise as the carbon dioxide traverses across the injury into the thoracic cavity. Other disadvantages include the potential for inadvertent injury to intraabdominal structures, inadequate visualization of portions of the diaphragm, the risk for subsequent formation of adhesions, and the inability to evacuate an associated hemothorax.

For these reasons, it is the authors' preference to utilize video-assisted thoracoscopic surgery (VATS) for the diagnosis and management of diaphragmatic injuries in asymptomatic hemodynamically stable patients with thoracoabdominal injury without indication for immediate operative indication. Like laparoscopy, VATS is performed at least 24 hours after the initial injury to allow potential intraabdominal injuries to declare themselves. Advantages that favor the use of VATS over laparoscopy include excellent visualization of the entire hemidiaphragm, the ability to evacuate a retained hemothorax, the ability to evaluate the lung and other mediastinal structures for injury, and avoidance of trocar site hernias and postoperative adhesions. VATS requires the patient to be placed in the lateral decubitus position, requires the ability to tolerate single lung ventilation, and limits the evaluation to one hemidiaphragm. Several retrospective series have validated the clinical utility of VATS in the diagnosis and management of TDI [34, 35]. Ultimately, the surgeon must select the procedure that they are most adept at applying to the particular patient based on which side of the diaphragm the preponderance of injury lies.

RECOMMENDATION

In at-risk patients, begin with a chest X-ray followed by an MDCT reformatted in the axial, coronal, and sagittal planes. If the MDCT findings are suggestive of TDI, thoracoscopy is performed to confirm the diagnosis, with the possible thoracoscopic repair versus thoracotomy based on available expertise. Laparoscopy may be similarly employed if the patient cannot be placed in the lateral decubitus position or will not tolerate single lung ventilation.

Grade of recommendation: D.

24.2 What Is the Optimal Diagnostic Modality for the Diagnosis of Diaphragmatic Injury in Penetrating Trauma?

Diaphragmatic injuries due to penetrating trauma result most often from stab wounds and gunshot wounds to the thoracoabdominal region, defined as the region extending from the nipples to the costal margin. The initial approach to these patients is determined by the hemodynamic stability of the patient. In unstable patients, emergent operative intervention is indicated. Evaluation of the diaphragm is then performed intraoperatively after hemorrhage and contamination control. In the stable patient, workup progresses from noninvasive modalities to more invasive methods until the injury has been ruled out or ruled in. A thorough workup for all patients with penetrating trauma to the thoracoabdominal region is essential, since over 40% of pericostal wounds are associated with injury to the diaphragm [36]. In contrast to blunt trauma, the resultant diaphragmatic injury is often small and may easily be missed. While gunshot wounds may occur on either side, stab wounds are more likely to occur on the left, as most assailants are right-handed.

The chest X-ray is once again the initial imaging modality of choice. Radio-opaque markers must be used to mark the site of the external injury. Determination of the resultant trajectory allows estimation of the likelihood of diaphragmatic involvement. Findings may, however, be subtle or masked by associated injuries, making diagnosis difficult. As was seen in a prospective study, 21% of patients with diaphragmatic injuries had a normal chest X-ray [17]. In another retrospective series, the chest X-ray was normal in 68% and showed only a nonspecific hemopneumothorax in the remaining 32% of patients with TDI confirmed at laparoscopy.

CT, especially with multidetector row scanners and appropriate reformatting, has over 90% accuracy in detecting the presence of TDI when the wound tract is seen extending to the diaphragm. In a retrospective series of 803 patients with penetrating torso injury over 4 years, CT had a sensitivity, specificity, and accuracy of 76%, 98%, and 91%, respectively, to detect injury and 92%, 89%, and 90%, respectively, to exclude injury [20]. Equivocal findings necessitate the use of additional diagnostic techniques. In a more recent retrospective study, the accuracy of the 64-section MDCT with tractography has been described. Here images are acquired in nonstandard planes aligned with the knife or gunshot tract. Contiguous injury on CT tractography was found to be a very sensitive sign (80–93%), and its absence can be used to reliably forego further workup with laparoscopy or thoracoscopy [18].

Magnetic resonance imaging allows superior delineation of the anatomy but is challenging to employ in the acute setting. It may not always be readily available, requires transport of a stable patient to a potentially remote location, and places the patient in a situation where adequate monitoring and access to the patient for ongoing resuscitation may not be optimal. Its use is mostly restricted to cases that are identified in the latent or obstructive phases.

Digital exploration of left-sided thoracoabdominal stab wounds has been studied as a potential diagnostic tool in the aid of diaphragmatic injury [37]. While an interesting concept, digital probing of penetrating traumatic wounds is not recommended as a definitive diagnostic guide that replaces open or laparoscopic evaluation and has the potential to be harmful in certain settings. Intraoperative evaluation of the diaphragm during laparotomy or thoracotomy remains the gold standard. Laparoscopy is a useful diagnostic modality, especially in injuries involving the left side. Improved image quality and routine availability of angled scopes have allowed almost all areas of the diaphragm to be visualized. Identification of injuries of the posterior right diaphragm may, however, still prove challenging. The utility of this technique was prospectively studied for penetrating trauma involving the left thoracoabdominal region. Of 110 patients studied, diaphragmatic injuries were identified in 26 (24%). Similar incidences were detected for anterior, lateral, and posterior wounds (22%, 27%, and 22%, respectively) [38]. A similar incidence, 22 of 108 (20%), was reported in another retrospective series [39]. As with blunt diaphragmatic injuries, it is the preferred technique when a VATS is not possible or feasible.

A thoracoscopy is an alternative approach to the identification of TDI [40]. The patient must, however, be hemodynamically stable, be able to tolerate single lung ventilation, and be able to be placed in a lateral decubitus position. There must also be the absence of any indication for emergent laparotomy or thoracotomy. Additionally, it's important to first observe these hemodynamically stable patients overnight with serial abdominal exams before excluding diaphragmatic injury, as the patient may manifest an intraabdominal injury. In a prospective study of 28 patients who met the earlier criteria, TDI was found in 9 of the 28 (32%) [41]. All injuries were confirmed and repaired at laparotomy. Associated intraabdominal injuries were present in 89%. VATS is the preferred minimally invasive approach in the asymptomatic hemodynamically stable patient.

RECOMMENDATION

In unstable patients, diagnosis is established intraoperatively. In stable patients, obtain a chest X-ray and perform a CT scan (multidetector if available). If equivocal, proceed with thoracoscopy. Laparoscopy is performed if thoracoscopy is not possible or not feasible.

Grade of recommendation: D.

24.3 What Is the Clinically Useful Classification System that Guides Operative Management?

The most popular current classification system for diaphragmatic injuries is that of the American Association for the Surgery of Trauma. Here a contusion is classified as grade I, lacerations <2 cm as grade II, lacerations 2–10 cm as grade III, lacerations ≥10 cm with tissue loss <25 cm^2 as grade IV, and lacerations with tissue loss >25 cm^2 as grade V. The clinical significance of this classification system remains unclear.

In reviewing the operative techniques described in several case reports and case series [42–45], a common theme emerges. Using this, the author proposes the following classification system:

Grade I: Contusion: No acute intervention is required; maintain a high index of suspicion for progression.

Grade II: Linear tears with viable tissue on either side of the defect that can be primarily approximated without significant tension.

Grade III: Avulsion of the diaphragm off the chest wall; reattachment is, however, possible.

Grade IV: Significant tissue loss that precludes primary repair necessitating the use of a prosthesis for repair.

RECOMMENDATION

Diaphragmatic injuries are best classified as contusions requiring no intervention, lacerations that can be primarily repaired, avulsions that can be reattached, or associated with significant tissue loss where prosthetics are utilized for adequate repair.

Grade of recommendation: D.

24.4 What Is the Optimal Approach to the Operative Management of Diaphragmatic Injuries?

The need for operative intervention in all cases of TDI has been questioned by several animal studies that suggest the potential for spontaneous healing [46–48]. In all studies, the left diaphragm protected by the relatively fixed left lobe of the animal liver prevented herniation of abdominal contents and allowed healing of the defect. In humans, this implies that a nonoperative approach may be adopted for small defects on the right side, such as those caused by knife wounds and low-velocity gunshot wounds. In contrast, on the left side, the pressure gradient between the pleural and peritoneal cavities and the constant motion of the diaphragm will likely prevent spontaneous healing and preclude nonoperative management strategies.

As the diaphragm borders the thoracic and abdominal cavities, it can be adequately approached from either side. The optimal approach is determined by the timing of injury identification, the presence of associated injuries, and the side of the injury.

For injuries identified in the acute phase, the incidence of associated intraabdominal injuries most common to the liver and spleen requiring operative intervention is as high as 89% [31]. Here the injury is best approached via a laparotomy.

If the injury presents in the latent phase, a thoracic approach is preferred. Here, compromise of intraabdominal contents is much less likely and the need for formal abdominal exploration is minimal. An abdominal component may become necessary if the herniated contents cannot be adequately reduced through the chest alone.

For injuries presenting in the obstructive phase, the initial approach can be made through the chest. If the herniated organs are viable and can easily be reduced into the abdominal cavity, the repair can be completed through the chest. If, however, there is the need to resect nonviable or marginally viable intraabdominal organs or adhesions preclude effective reduction, a combined thoracic and subcostal approach may be employed.

Left-sided injuries can be visualized well from the abdominal cavity and thus can be approached surgically this way. The liver may preclude adequate visualization on the right, especially in posteriorly located injuries. A thoracic approach is preferable in this circumstance [9, 10].

In experienced hands, laparoscopy can be employed as both a diagnostic and a therapeutic modality and is increasingly being reported in the literature [49]. Modifications of the laparoscopic approach with laparoscopically assisted mini thoracotomy have been described [50].

RECOMMENDATION

In the acute phase, approach the injury abdominally. In the latent phase, use a thoracic approach. In the obstructive phase, use an abdominal approach for the left side and a combined approach for the right side is preferred.

Grade of recommendation: D.

24.5 What Is the Ideal Suture Material/Prosthesis for Repair of Diaphragmatic Injuries?

In 13 of 105 patients available for long-term follow-up [3], two recurrences were noted. In both cases, the absorbable suture was used for repair. In all other reported cases, the nonabsorbable suture was used. As the diaphragm is a thin muscle in constant motion, the potential for wound healing may be slower compared to thicker stationary tissue. The use of nonabsorbable material, therefore, appears justified. Polypropylene,

nylon, or polyester applied as simple interrupted, continuous, or figure-of-eight sutures have all been reported. It is the author's preference to use polypropylene in the presence of contamination from associated intraabdominal injuries and braided polyester when such contamination is absent. The sutures are placed in a horizontal mattress manner. For all defects requiring more than one or two sutures, the resultant ridge of approximated tissue is oversewn with a running simple continuous stitch. In cases where the edges of the diaphragm could not be brought together primarily, the use of expanded polytetrafluoroethylene has been described [9, 23]. More recently, biologic prostheses are being used increasingly for the repair of large abdominal wall defects. Their use has also been reported in the repair of paraesophageal hernia. While the use of biologics in the repair of diaphragmatic injury has not yet been reported, it may be a potential option in the setting of contamination from intraabdominal injuries.

RECOMMENDATION

Nonabsorbable material applied as simple interrupted, continuous, or horizontal mattress sutures is appropriate. Prosthetics, preferably synthetic over biologic mesh due to cost differences, should be used when the defect cannot be closed primarily. There are no prospective trials that demonstrate any benefit of biologic over synthetic mesh in elective or emergency diaphragmatic hernia repair.

Grade of recommendation: D.

24.6 What Are the Differences in the Approach to Left- versus Right-Sided Injuries?

Injuries to the left side are three times more frequent than those on the right. This is believed to be a result of the left side being congenitally weaker and the absence of the protective effect of the liver. These factors make it less resistant to pressure. The incidence of right-sided injury identification is increasing, and this is likely due to improvements in CT technology and the severity of motor vehicle collisions.

Left-sided TDI due to blunt or penetrating trauma must be sought and repaired early. Even small defects will likely progress over time, as the diaphragm is a thin muscle, in constant motion, and is subject to differential pressure gradients between the peritoneal and pleural cavities. This pressure gradient eventually causes intraabdominal contents to herniate through, placing them at risk for obstruction or strangulation.

Management of right-sided injuries is highly dependent on the mechanism of injury. In penetrating injuries, especially due to stab wounds, the defect is often small, is sealed by the liver, and allows for the prevention of bowel herniation. In blunt injuries, there is a significant transfer of force causing a larger defect with progressive herniation of the liver. This may occur years after the initial injury and would warrant repair [9, 23].

> **RECOMMENDATION**
>
> On the left side, repair all injuries irrespective of the mechanism. On the right side, small penetrating defects can likely be managed nonoperatively. This is based on animal studies in pigs, which suggest spontaneous healing may occur in these select cases. Blunt mechanisms, especially high force, can lead to large defects that warrant operative management.
>
> Grade of recommendation: D.

24.7 What Are the Consequences of Missed Injuries?

Literature is replete with cases describing the delayed presentation of TDI that was missed at the initial evaluation. Latent periods of up to 28 years have been reported. The presentation depends on the herniation organ. Right-sided injuries are associated with progressive herniation of the liver, which compresses the lung causing progressive respiratory compromise. On the left, gastrothorax, gastrointestinal bleeding from splenic vein thrombosis due to herniation of the spleen, tension fecopneumothorax from acute rupture of a herniated colon, and symptoms of bowel obstruction have all been reported. Yet the true number of patients with unidentified diaphragmatic injuries that remain asymptomatic remains unknown. It is unlikely that this number will ever be known. The consequence of missed injuries will therefore remain anecdotal.

It does seem prudent, however, to aggressively seek out these injuries with early repair (Table 24.1).

> **RECOMMENDATION**
>
> A wide spectrum of often-dramatic consequences may result. These make early diagnosis and repair desirable.
>
> Grade of recommendation: D.

Editor's Note

Unfortunately, we have made little progress in the diagnosis of injuries to the diaphragm over the past two decades. CT scanning and ultrasound continue to have a low sensitivity in identifying this unusual entity, particularly in small wounds found after penetrating injury. Laparoscopic or thoracoscopic evaluation after a period of observation to exclude associated injuries remains the gold standard in asymptomatic patients with risk for this injury (typically in the setting of pericostal stab wounds). There is no prospective work to guide operative repair of diaphragm injuries, and therefore, the use of nonabsorbable sutures seems prudent to avoid recurrence. When a large defect mandates mesh, likewise a synthetic, nonabsorbable material appears to be the most conservative management plan. With no prospective studies other than those of the observational variety, there is little to separate opinion from anecdote regarding the diagnosis and management of diaphragmatic injuries.

TABLE 24.1

Current Evidence-Based Recommendations for Evaluation and Management of Diaphragmatic Injuries

Question	Answer	Levels of Evidence	Grade of Recommendation
What is the optimal diagnostic modality for the diagnosis of diaphragmatic injury in blunt trauma?	There is no single diagnostic modality of choice. The optimal approach is to utilize the earlier studies sequentially until the diagnosis has either been suspected to a degree where operative intervention is warranted or excluded beyond a reasonable doubt. Thoracoscopy is the preferred minimally invasive approach in the asymptomatic hemodynamically stable patient when performed at least 24 hours after the initial injury.	3b	D
What is the optimal diagnostic modality for the diagnosis of diaphragmatic injury in penetrating trauma?	In unstable patients, diagnosis is established at operation. In stable patients, obtain a chest X-ray and CT scan. If equivocal, proceed with laparoscopy or thoracoscopy.	3b	D
What is a clinically useful classification system that guides operative management?	Diaphragmatic injuries are best classified as contusions requiring no intervention, lacerations than can be primarily repaired, avulsions that can be reattached, or associated with significant tissue loss where prosthetics are used for adequate repair.	5	D
What is the optimal approach to the operative management of diaphragmatic injuries?	In the acute phase, approach the injury abdominally. In the latent phase, use a thoracic approach. In the obstructive phase, use an abdominal approach for the left side and a combined approach for the right side.	2b	D
What is the ideal suture material/prosthesis for the repair of diaphragmatic injuries?	Nonabsorbable material applied as simple interrupted, continuous, or horizontal mattress sutures is appropriate. Prosthetics, possibly biologics, should be used when the defect cannot be closed primarily.	3b	D
What are the differences in the approach to left- versus right-sided injuries?	On the left side, repair all injuries irrespective of the mechanism. On the right side, repair those due to blunt trauma and penetrating trauma only if large.	3b	D
What are the consequences of missed injuries?	A wide spectrum of often-dramatic consequences may result. These make early diagnosis and repair desirable.	4	D

REFERENCES

1. Zarour AM, El-Menyar A, Al-Thani H, Scalea TM, Chiu WC. Presentations and outcomes in patients with traumatic diaphragmatic injury: A 15-year experience. *J Trauma Acute Care Surg.* 2013;*74*:1392–1398.

2. Plessis M, Ramai D, Shah S, et al. The clinical anatomy of the musculotendinous part of the diaphragm. *Surg Radiol Anat.* May 2015;*37*:1013–1020.

3. Hanna WC, Ferri LE, Fata P, Razek T, Mulder DS. The current status of traumatic diaphragmatic injury: Lessons learned from 105 patients over 13 years. *Ann Thorac Surg.* March 2008;*85(85)*:3–1044.

4. Ryb GE, Dischinger PC, Ho S. Causation and outcomes of diaphragmatic injuries in vehicular crashes. *J Trauma Acute Care Surg.* 2013;*74*:835–838.

5. Grimes OF. Traumatic injuries of the diaphragm. *Am J Surg.* February 1975;*38(2)*:OR8, OR10, OR12.

6. Howard R, Alijani A, Munshi IA. Right-side diaphragm injury resulting from blunt trauma. *J Emerg Med.* January 2008;*34(34)*:1–85.

7. Matsevych OY. Blunt diaphragmatic rupture: Four years' expedience. *Hernia.* February 2008;*12(1)*:73–78.

8. Nishijima D, Zehbtachi S, Austin RB. Acute posttraumatic tension gastrothorax mimicking acute tension pneumothorax. *Am J Emerg Med.* July 2007;*25(6)*:734.e5–e6.

9. Igai H, Yokomise H, Kumagai K, Yamashita S, Kawakita K, Kuroda Y. Delayed hemothorax due to right-sided traumatic diaphragmatic rupture. *Gen Thorac Cardiovasc Surg.* October 2007;*55(10)*:434–436.

10. Dineen S, Schumacher P, Thal E, Frankel H. CT reconstructions of a right-sided blunt diaphragm rupture. *J Trauma.* May 2008;*64(5)*:1412.

11. Patlas MN, Leung VA, Romano L, Gagliardi N, Ponticiello G, Scaglione M. Diaphragmatic injuries: Why do we struggle to detect them? *Radiol Med.* January 2015;*120(1)*:12–20.

12. Iochum S, Ludig T, Walter F, Sebbag H, Grosdidier G, Blum AG. Imaging of diaphragmatic injury: A diagnostic challenge? *Radiographics.* October 2002;*22*:S103–S116; discussion S116–S118.

13. Kirkpatrick AW, Ball CG, Nicolaou S, Ledgerwood A, Lucas CE. Ultrasound detection of right-sided diaphragmatic injury; the "liver sliding" sign. *Am J Emerg Med.* March 2006;*24(2)*:251–252.

14. Blaivas M, Brannam L, Hawkins M, Lyon M, Sriram K. Bedside emergency ultrasonographic diagnosis of diaphragmatic rupture in blunt abdominal trauma. *Am J Emerg Med.* November 2004;*22(7)*:601–604.

15. Hammer MM, Flagg E, Mellnick VM, Cummings KW, Bhalla S, Raptis CA. Acute rupture of the diaphragm due to blunt trauma: Diagnostic sensitivity and specificity of CT. *Emerg Radiol.* 2013;*1*:143–149.

16. Desser TS, Edwards B, Hunt S, Rosenberg J, Purtill MA, Jeffrey RB. The dangling diaphragm sign: Sensitivity and comparison with existing CT signs of blunt traumatic rupture. *Emerg Radiol.* January 2010;*17(1)*:37–44.

17. Shanmuganathan K, Mirvis SE, Chiu WC, Killeen KL, Hogan GJF, Scalea TM. Penetrating torso trauma: Triple-contrast helical CT in peritoneal violation and organ injury—A prospective study in 200 patients. *Radiology.* 2004;*231*:775–784.

18. Dreizin D, Borja MJ, Danton GH, Kadakia K, Caban K, Rivas LA, Munera F. Penetrating diaphragmatic injury: Accuracy of 64-section multidetector CT with tractography. *Radiology.* 2013;*268*:729–737.

19. Nchimi A, Szapiro D, Ghaye B, Willems V, Khamis J, Haquet L, Noukoua C, Dondelinger RF. Helical CT of blunt diaphragmatic rupture. *AJR.* January 2005;*184(1)*:24–30.

20. Rees O, Mirvis SE, Shanmuganathan K. Multidetector-row CT of right hemidiaphragmatic rupture caused by blunt trauma: A review of 12 cases. *Clin Radiol.* 2005;*60*:1280–1289.

21. Stein DM, York GB, Boswell S, Shanmuganathan K, Haan JM, Scalea TM. Accuracy of computed tomography (CT) scan in the detection of penetrating diaphragm injury. *J Trauma.* September 2007;*63(3)*:538–543.

22. Larici AR, Gotway MB, Litt HI, Reddy GP, Webb WR, Gotway CA, Dawn SK, Marder SR, Storto ML. Helical CT with sagittal and coronal reconstructions: Accuracy for detection of diaphragmatic injury. *AJR.* August 2002;*179(2)*:451–457.

23. Mintz Y, Easter DW, Izhar U, Edden Y, Talamini MA, Rivkind AI. Minimally invasive procedures for diagnosis of traumatic right diaphragmatic tears: A method for correct diagnosis in selected patients. *Am Surg.* April 2007;*73(4)*:388–392.

24. Magu S, Agarwal S, Singla A. Computed tomography in the evaluation of diaphragmatic hernia following blunt trauma. *Indian J Surg.* July–August 2012;*74*:288–293.

25. May AK, Moore MM. Diagnosis of blunt rupture of the right hemidiaphragm by technetium scan. *Am Surg.* August 1999;*65(8)*:761–765.

26. Asensio JA, Arroyo H, Jr., Veloz W, Forno W, Gambaro E, Murray J, Velmahos G, Demetriades D. Penetrating thoracoabdominal injuries: Ongoing dilemma-which cavity and when? *Would J Surg.* 2002;*28*:539–543.

27. Adamthwaite DN. Traumatic diaphragmatic hernia: A new indication for laparoscopy. *Br J Surg.* 1984;*71*:315.

28. Ivatury RR, Simon RJ, Weksler B, Bayard V, Stahl WM. Laparoscopy in the evaluation of the intrathoracic abdomen after penetrating injury. *J Trauma.* 1992;*33*:101–108.

29. Cooper C, Brewer J. Laparoscopic repair of acute penetrating diaphragm injury. *Am Surg.* 2012;*78*:490–492.

30. Yahya A, Shuweiref H, Thoboot A, Ekhail M, Ali AA. Laparoscopic repair of penetrating injury to the diaphragm: An experience from a district hospital. *Libyan J Med.* 2008;*3*:138–139.

31. Mjoli M, Oosthuizen G, Clarke D, Madiba T. Laparoscopy in the diagnosis and repair of diaphragmatic injuries in left-sided penetrating thoracoabdominal trauma. *Surg Endosc.* March 2015;*29(3)*:747–752.

32. Armananzas L, Ruiz-Tovar J, Arroyo A, Garcia-Peche P, Armananzas E, Diez M, Galindo I, Calpena R. Prophylactic mesh vs. suture in the closure of umbilical trocar site after laparoscopic cholecystectomy in high-risk patients for incisional hernia: A randomized clinical trial. *J Am Coll Surg.* 2014;*218*:960–968.

33. Comajuncosas J, Hermosa J, Gris P, Jimeno J, Orbeal R, Vallverdu H, Negre JLL, Urgelles J, Estalella L, Pares D. Risk factors for umbilical trocar sites incisional hernia in laparoscopic cholecystectomy: A prospective 3-year follow-up study. *Am J Surg.* 2014;*207*:1–6.

34. Martinez M, Briz JE, Carillo EH. Video thoracoscopy expedites the diagnosis and treatment of penetrating diaphragmatic injuries. *Surg Endosc.* 2001;*15*:28–32.

35. Freeman RK, Al-Dossari G, Hutcheson KA, Huber L, Jessen ME, Meyer DM, Wait MA, DiMaio JM. Indications for using video-assisted thoracoscopic surgery to diagnose diaphragmatic injuries after penetrating chest trauma. *Ann Thorac Surg.* 2001;*72*:342–347.

36. Bodanapally UK, Shanmuganathan K, Mirvis SE, Silker CW, Fleiter TR, Sarada K, Miller LA, Stein DM, Alexander M. MDCT diagnosis of penetrating diaphragm injury. *Eur Radiol.* 2009;*19*:1875–1881.

37. Morales CH, Villegas MI, Angel W, Vasquez JJ. Value of digital exploration for diagnosing injuries to the left side of the diaphragm caused by stab wounds. *Arch Surg.* 2001;*136*:1131–1135.

38. Murray JA, Demetriades D, Asensio JA, Cornwell EE III, Velmahos GC, Belzberg H, Berne TV. Occult injuries to the diaphragm: Prospective evaluation of laparoscopy in penetrating injuries to the left lower chest. *J Am Coll Surg.* December 1998;*187(6)*:626–630.

39. Powell BS, Magnotti LJ, Schroeppel TJ, Finnell CW, Savage SA, Fischer PE, Fabian TC, Croce MA. Diagnostic laparoscopy for the evaluation of occult diaphragmatic injury following penetrating thoracoabdominal trauma. *Injury.* May 2008;*39(5)*:530–534.

40. Bagheri R, Tavassoli T, Sadrizadeh A, Mashhadi MR, Shahri F, Shojaeian R. The role of thoracoscopy for the diagnosis of hidden diaphragmatic injuries in penetrating thoracoabdominal trauma. *Interact Cardiovasc Thorac Surg.* 2009;*9*:195–197.

41. Paci M, Ferrari G, Annessi V, de Franco S, Guasti G, Sgarbi G. The role of diagnostic VATS in penetrating thoracic injuries. *World J Emerg Surg.* October 2006;*1*:30.

42. Konstantinos S, Georgios I, Christos C, Vasilissa K, Nikolaos K, Fred L, John H, Frank S. Traumatic avulsion of kidney and spleen into the chest through a ruptured diaphragm in a young worker: A case report. *J Med Case Rep.* December 2007;*1*:178.

43. Haciibrahimoglu G, Solak O, Olcmen A, Bedirhan MA, Solmazer N, Gurses A. Management of traumatic diaphragmatic rupture. *Surg Today.* 2004;*34(2)*:111–114.

44. Baldassarre E, Valenti G, Gambino M, Arturi A, Torino G, Porta IP, Barone M. The role of laparoscopy in the diagnosis and the treatment of missed diaphragmatic hernia after penetrating trauma. *J Laparoendosc Adv Surg Tech A.* June 2007;*17(3)*:302–306.

45. Matz A, Landau O, Alis M, Charuzi I, Kyzer S. The role of laparoscopy in the diagnosis and treatment of missed diaphragmatic rupture. *Surg Endosc.* June 2000;*14(6)*:537–539.

46. Zierold D, Perlstein J, Weidman ER, Wiedeman JE. Penetrating trauma to the diaphragm: Natural history and ultrasonographic characteristics of untreated injury in a pig model. *Arch Surg.* 2001;*136*:32–37.

47. Rivaben AH, Junior RS, Neto VD, Botter A, Goncalves R. Natural history of extensive diaphragmatic injury of the right side: Experimental study in rats. *Rev Col Bras Cir.* 2014;*41*:267–271.

48. Gamblin TC, Wall CE, Morgan JH, Erickson DJ, Dalton ML, Ashley DW. The natural history of untreated penetrating diaphragm injury: An animal model. *J Trauma.* 2004;*57*:989–992.

49. Baldwin M, Dagens A, Sgromo B. Laparoscopic management of a delayed traumatic diaphragmatic rupture complicated by bowel strangulation. *J Surg Case Rep.* July 2014;*2014(7)*:pii.

50. Amini A, Latifi R. Laparoscopic-assisted minithoracotomy for repair of diaphragmatic penetrating trauma. *Surg Laparosc Endosc Percutan Tech.* 2013;*23*:406–409.

25

Pancreatic and Duodenal Injuries

Abigail Coots and Adrian W. Ong

25.1 History and Epidemiology

Although pancreaticoduodenal injuries are uncommon, occurring in less than 0.5% of trauma patients [1–3], they can be associated with significant morbidity and mortality. Determinants of morbidity and mortality include the severity of the pancreaticoduodenal injuries, Injury Severity Score (ISS), concomitant injuries to other organs, major vascular injury, and shock on presentation [3–5].

25.2 Injury Classification

The organ injury scaling systems of the American Association for the Surgery of Trauma (AAST) [6] are widely used in the published literature describing these injuries. Pancreatic injuries are classified as follows: grade I: minor contusion or superficial laceration without duct injury; grade II: major contusion or laceration without duct injury or tissue loss; grade III: distal transection or parenchymal injury with duct injury; grade IV: proximal transection or parenchymal injury involving ampulla; grade V: massive disruption of the pancreatic head. Duodenal injuries are classified as follows: grade I: hematoma involving a single portion of duodenum or partial thickness laceration; grade II: hematoma involving > 1 portion or disruption < 50% of circumference; grade III: disruption of 50–75% circumference of D2 or 50–100% of circumference of D1, D3, or D4; grade IV: disruption > 75% of D2 or involvement of the ampulla or distal common bile duct; grade V: massive disruption of duodenopancreatic complex or devascularization of duodenum [6]. These will be used in this chapter for discussion.

For discussion of postoperative pancreatic fistula (POPF), definitions based on the 2016 update of the International Study Group of Pancreatic Fistula (ISGPF) [7] will be used. In this classification system, grade B and C POPF are considered "clinically relevant" as they are associated with a clinically relevant development or condition related to the POPF.

25.3 Diagnosis and Management

Pubmed.gov was searched electronically for publications from 2012 to 2022. Case reports, reviews, and case series of 10 or fewer subjects were excluded. In certain circumstances, where there was a lack of evidence-based studies, the literature search was extended prior to 2012.

These search words were utilized: ["pancreatic injury"], ["pancreatic trauma"], ["duodenal injury"], ["duodenal trauma"], ["octreotide" AND "trauma"]. The Oxford Center for Evidence-Based Medicine 2011 levels of evidence documents were used to determine the level of evidence supporting each question.

The level of evidence and recommendations for the following questions are summarized in Table 25.1.

25.3.1 Does the Addition of Pyloric Exclusion to the Primary Repair of a Duodenal Injury Reduce Complications?

Duodenal leaks occur in a substantial minority (8–32%) of patients after repair [8–11] and are a significant source of morbidity and mortality. A retrospective single-center study of 91 patients with primary duodenal repair alone found that 3 of 7 (42.9%) patients with leaks died compared to 8 of 84 (9.5%) with no leak [11]. Pyloric exclusion with or without gastrojejunostomy as an adjunct has been advocated in the past to reduce the likelihood of a postoperative leak for patients with rare severe duodenal or pancreatic injuries and combined pancreaticoduodenal injuries. No randomized trials have addressed this question, due to the uncommon occurrence of duodenal injuries.

Schroeppel et al. [8] studied 125 patients with penetrating duodenal injuries after excluding early deaths. The duodenal leak rate was 8% ($n = 10$) with two deaths related to the duodenal injury. In 46 patients who underwent primary repair, 2.1% (1/46) leaked as compared to 23.1% (3/13) who underwent pyloric exclusion. Patients with leaks were more likely to have a concomitant pancreatic injury (70% vs. 31%) and a major vascular injury (60% vs. 31%). There were no differences in repair technique, but the pyloric exclusion group had more severe injuries (grade III or higher) as compared with the primary repair group (84% vs. 25%). The authors concluded that pyloric exclusion should be considered as an adjunct when a repair is "tenuous," involving the medial duodenal wall, or when there is a concomitant pancreatic injury and recommended performing the pyloric exclusion at the initial operation if deemed appropriate for treatment of the high-grade duodenal injuries.

Another multicenter retrospective review of 372 patients analyzed surgical repair techniques for duodenal injury [9]. The majority (79%) of patients in the cohort had penetrating injuries, with 68% having another associated intraabdominal injury. The mortality rate in this study was 24%, and predictors

DOI: 10.1201/9781003316800-25

of mortality were higher ISS, associated pancreatic injury, and need for transfusion before repair; type of repair was not a predictor. In addition, 7.8% had pyloric exclusion with or without gastrojejunostomy, 10% had primary repair with retrograde decompressive duodenostomy with or without a distal feeding tube, and 1.3% had resection with primary anastomosis. In this study, patients with pyloric exclusion had a similar proportion of grade III or higher injuries compared to those with primary repair alone (86% vs. 77%). For primary repair alone, the leak rate was lower compared to that for pyloric exclusion (10% vs. 45%). The authors concluded that primary repair is sufficient for the majority of cases, while pyloric exclusion and additional tube decompression should be "reserved for special cases."

Park et al. [10] retrospectively analyzed a 17-year cohort of trauma patients from a single trauma institution with grade II and III duodenal injuries. A cohort of 49 patients was identified as having surgical intervention. Most injuries (87.8%) were from blunt mechanisms; 21 underwent primary repair alone and 19 patients had primary repair with pyloric exclusion. Leaks occurred in 16 (33%). The time from injury to initial operation and operative time were significantly longer in patients with leakage than in patients without leakage (31.4 hours vs. 9.4 hours and 214 hours vs. 180 hours, respectively). Time to duodenal repair was found to be the only factor in the multivariable analysis that was associated with the leak. Compared to primary repair, pyloric exclusion had a similar leak rate (36.8% vs. 23.8%, $p = 0.58$) and mortality. The authors concluded that pyloric exclusion might not prevent postoperative leaks and that time to surgery was a more important predictor.

Available data demonstrate that primary repair of duodenal injury is safe and effective in most injuries, regardless of AAST grade or mechanism. Pyloric exclusion with or without gastrojejunostomy is still performed as an adjunctive procedure for the repair of severe duodenal injuries, but there are insufficient data to suggest that it improves outcomes or prevents complications.

RECOMMENDATION

Primary repair is adequate for most duodenal injuries. The addition of pyloric exclusion does not lower leak rates, and its routine use is not recommended.

Level 3. Grade of recommendation: C.

25.3.2 For Blunt Pancreatic Injuries, Under What Circumstances Is Initial Nonoperative Management Acceptable?

Recognizing that most of the morbidity in blunt pancreatic trauma is related to whether the major pancreatic duct is injured, nonoperative management (NOM) has been advocated and increasingly accepted as an initial management strategy for low-grade pancreatic injuries. There is some debate, however, as to the initial approach for injuries involving the

major pancreatic duct. Although current guidelines [12] recommend operative intervention, recent studies suggest that the NOM of selected patients with major pancreatic duct injuries is acceptable.

In a large study based on the Japan Trauma Data Bank, 743 (0.25%) had pancreatic injuries [1]. For grade I/II injuries, 49% were managed with celiotomy compared to >66% of high-grade injuries. The overall mortality rate was 17.5% and was found to be associated with age, grade of pancreatic injury, Revised Trauma Score on admission, and other severe intraabdominal injuries. After adjusting for confounders, initial celiotomy was not associated with improved odds of survival for both grade I/II and grade III/IV cohorts. The authors concluded that NOM may be an acceptable strategy for selected patients even with major pancreatic duct injuries, but there was no analysis of pancreatic-related complications.

In another study utilizing the National Trauma Data Bank database, patients with isolated pancreatic injuries (20.9% of all pancreatic injuries) were studied [2]. Low-grade injuries were more likely to be managed nonoperatively (grade II, 80.5%; grade III, 48.5%; grades IV/V, 40.9%). For grade II injuries, NOM had significantly lower mortality (1.6% vs. 5.8%) and shorter hospital length of stay (LOS) (median days, 5.0 vs. 11.0) than patients treated with an operation. For grade III injuries, mortality for NOM patients was equivalent to operatively managed patients (1.2% vs. 5.2%, $p = 0.202$) with a shorter median hospital LOS for NOM patients (8 vs. 16 days, $p < 0.001$). In severe (grade IV/V) injuries, the mortality rate was higher for NOM patients (6.9% vs. 5.6%, $p = 0.032$). Multivariable analysis showed that operative treatment had higher odds of mortality (odds ratio [OR] 2.145, 95% confidence interval [CI] 1.178–3.906) when controlled for the grade of injury, gender, age, and ISS. The authors concluded that NOM of high-grade injuries was associated with increased mortality, while for grade II injuries, NOM was associated with lower mortality. This conclusion, however, was derived from univariable analysis. In addition, pancreatic-related complications were not discussed.

Kong et al. [13] examined the influence of endoscopic retrograde cholangiopancreatography (ERCP) on NOM of pancreatic injuries. Of 470 patients with blunt pancreatic injury, 132 (32%) were selected for NOM. With endoscopic management ($n = 58$), 9% failed NOM while 30% failed without endoscopic intervention ($n = 74$). In the study, 62% of grade I/II injuries were selected for NOM compared to only 9% of grade III–V injuries. No grade IV/V injuries underwent NOM. Although the authors advocated for endoscopic management to decrease the NOM failure rate, it is not clear if this applies to high-grade pancreatic injuries, since none of the grade IV/V injuries underwent NOM.

In another study [14], 5 (15%) of 33 patients with blunt grade I/II injuries underwent operative exploration but noted that none had a "pancreatic-directed procedure." It was not clear if drainage was done in any of these cases, but the authors recommended the routine use of closed suction drains. For the other 34 patients with grade III/IV injuries, the majority ($n = 26$) underwent NOM with a failure rate of 62% ($n = 16$). Factors associated with failed NOM in this cohort by multivariate analysis were the presence of pancreatic necrosis and associated organ injury, while the presence of a pseudocyst was associated with decreased odds of NOM failure. The authors recommended that NOM could be safely done in selected patients with grade III/IV injuries who are hemodynamically stable and have a walled-off fluid collection. However, these patients are probably the selected few who present in a delayed fashion for treatment.

In pediatric patients, studies have shown NOM may be feasible even when the major pancreatic duct is injured. Naik-Mathuria et al. studied 20 pediatric trauma centers treating a total of 86 patients with grade III/IV injuries [15]. Initial treatment consisted of observation (64%), percutaneous drain (24%), endoscopic drainage (10%), and needle aspiration (2%). Fifty-nine percent (*n* = 42) had an organized peripancreatic fluid collection after 7 days. Most (64%) were observed, and the rest underwent early intervention with endoscopic and percutaneous techniques. Ultimately, 26% (*n* = 11) received definitive operative or endoscopic drainage procedures for persistent pseudocyst while two patients received distal pancreatectomy for pancreatic fistula.

On the other hand, in another multicenter study of 167 pediatric patients with grade II/III injuries where 57% were managed nonoperatively, NOM compared to resection had higher rates of pseudocyst formation (18% vs. 0%) and repeat endoscopic or percutaneous intervention (26% vs. 2%) [16]. In patients in whom a pseudocyst developed after NOM, 45% eventually required an operative drainage procedure for definitive treatment. The rate of a clinically significant pancreatic leak in the resection group was 7%, and all leaks were controlled by the surgical drain placed at the index procedure. Mean times to initial (4.5 vs. 8.9 days) and goal (7.8 vs. 15.1 days) feeds were shorter in the resection group. The time to complete resolution was shorter in the resection group (22.6 vs. 38.6 days). Due to the small number of grade II injuries undergoing resection, a comparison within this cohort was not performed. The authors concluded that operative management for distal main pancreatic duct (MPD) injury was preferable to NOM.

In a secondary analysis of a multicenter database, Biffl et al. [17] compared outcomes for blunt versus penetrating pancreatic injuries. NOM was initiated in 211 (33%) of 633 blunt trauma patients with a 4% pancreatic-related complication rate. In contrast, pancreatic-related complication rates were 43% and 20% in operative intervention with resection and drainage, respectively. Based on injury grade, pancreatic-related complications after resection and drainage in grade III injuries were 41% and 29%, respectively, compared to a 20% rate for NOM. For grade I/II injuries, these operative pancreatic-related complication rates were 50% and 14%, respectively, compared to 3% in NOM patients. In multivariable analysis, high-grade injury but not resection was predictive of pancreatic-related complications. For blunt low-grade injuries, NOM resulted in better outcomes than operative intervention.

In another prior secondary analysis of the same sample including only grade I/II blunt and penetrating injuries, Biffl et al. [18] found pancreatic-related complication rates for NOM of <5% compared to rates of 20–40% with resection and drainage. The authors recommended against resection and suggested NOM over drainage where feasible.

Ando et al. [19] studied 64 patients with MPD injury based on "imaging modalities combined with clinical, intraoperative and/or pathological findings" where 11 (17%) underwent NOM initially. Of these, only two (18%) patients were successful. Nine patients had clinical sequelae, with five needing surgery and the other four requiring long-term hospitalization for 90 days or more. In contrast, those who received operations had a lower rate of pancreatic pseudocyst (11% vs. 36%) but equivalent abscess and fistula rates. The authors did not state that operative management was preferable, but recommended careful selection of patients with MPD injuries for NOM.

The current literature supports the initial attempt at NOM for low-grade injuries. For high-grade injuries, given the high pancreatic-related complication rates, operative management is preferable, but there is no consensus that operative management produces superior outcomes [2, 13, 14, 17, 19]. NOM of pancreatic injuries should follow well-established principles: Patients should be hemodynamically stable, without peritonitis, sepsis, or significant transfusion requirements, and have no other intraabdominal injuries requiring an operation. Selecting which patients to undergo NOM for pancreatic injuries needs further refinement and will require future large prospective studies. Furthermore, current studies have compared patients selected for NOM versus operation rather than comparing management strategies or algorithms per se. As a result, selection bias may limit our understanding of outcomes.

RECOMMENDATION

Patients with grade I/II blunt pancreatic injuries may be managed nonoperatively. For high-grade injuries, given the increased risk of pancreatic-related complications, an initial strategy of operative management is preferable to NOM.

If NOM is to be attempted on patients with high-grade injuries (MPD injuries), endoscopic and interventional radiologic expertise should be available.

Level 3. Grade of recommendation: C.

25.3.3 For Patients with Distal Major Pancreatic Duct Injury Undergoing Operative Management, Is Resection Preferred over Drainage?

In published reviews by national societies [12, 20], distal pancreatectomy is recommended for pancreatic injuries with a high risk for or known MPD injury. The rationale for resection is to prevent major pancreatic fistula or ascites. However, clinically significant POPF remains a significant problem with distal pancreatectomy. Lin et al. [21] found a POPF rate of 35% in 51 patients with grade III and IV injuries who underwent resection. Subsequent radiological intervention and reoperation were required in 27% of this sample.

Byrge et al. [22] analyzed a multicenter cohort of 704 patients with pancreatic injury. In this cohort, 158 patients had grade III injuries, of which 133 underwent stapled and/or sutured resection. Mortality in patients with distal pancreatectomy versus those without resection was lower but the difference was not statistically significant (6% vs. 16%, $p = 0.08$). The rates of pancreatic-related complications and hospital LOS were similar. In addition, the authors noted that pancreatic fistula after injury was an independent risk factor for the development of adult respiratory distress syndrome. In their multivariable analysis of grade III injuries, stapled resection (OR 0.21, 95% CI 0.05–0.88) was protective for pancreatic fistula development but not oversewing (OR 0.51, 95% CI 0.1–2.7) or placing a duct stitch (OR 0.65, 95% CI 0.2–1.9).

Conversely, Mosheni et al. [23] reviewed 948 patients from a national trauma database with grade III and IV penetrating pancreatic injuries, of which 653 had grade III injuries. A reported 41.7% of the cohort of grade III injury underwent distal pancreatectomy, with the remainder having drainage only. Those who had resection had a significantly higher rate of unplanned return to the intensive care unit (ICU) (4.8% vs. 1.6%, $p = 0.03$) and longer hospital LOS (median, 17 vs. 11 days, $p < 0.001$). However, no statistically significant difference in mortality was noted between the two groups (15.1% vs. 18.4%). The authors concluded that drainage remains a "viable option."

In a multicenter retrospective review analyzing the management and outcomes of high-grade pancreatic injury, distal pancreatectomy was performed in 77% of grade III injuries with drainage only for 16% [24]. Pancreatic-related complications occurred in 41% of resected patients versus 33% in drainage patients ($p = 0.32$). The authors concluded that operative drainage may be a "non-inferior alternative" to resection in selected patients. The latter two studies [23 and 24] did not use multivariable methods in their analyses. The findings of Byrge et al. [22] regarding mortality rates and pancreatic-related complications appear to support resection over drainage.

RECOMMENDATION

Distal resection is preferred over drainage. Drainage-only procedures can be considered in select circumstances such as in the setting of damage control.

Level 3. Grade of recommendation: C.

25.3.4 For Patients with Proximal Major Pancreatic Duct Injury Undergoing Operative Management, Is Resection Preferred over Drainage?

Debate exists on the optimal operative treatment of proximal MPD injuries (to the right of the superior mesenteric vessels). Options are resection of the injured pancreas, wide drainage without resection, and "central" pancreatectomy with or without enteric anastomosis.

In a study of 19 patients with blunt grade IV injuries, 12 underwent resection (distal pancreatectomy, $n = 9$; central pancreatectomy with roux-Y anastomosis) and 7 peripancreatic

drainage [25]. For those undergoing drainage without resection, six of the seven had complications: Two had pancreatitis with one death in the two from splenic artery bleeding, and four had grade B/C POPF. In the resection group, 9 of 12 developed complications (one with pancreaticojejunostomy anastomotic leakage, two had abscesses, and six had grade B POPF, with one death). While the complication rates were high in either group, the authors recommended resection where possible, as patients who have simple drainage will almost always require reoperation or endoscopic management.

In the previously mentioned study of penetrating injuries [23], of 274 grade IV injuries, 38% underwent resection (consisting of distal pancreatectomy [10.6%], proximal pancreatectomy [8.7%], total pancreatectomy [6.7%], pancreaticoduodenectomy [24%], and "other pancreatectomy" [55%]). Rates of pancreatitis, sepsis, reoperation, pulmonary embolism, and unplanned return to ICU were similar between the two groups (resection vs. nonresection). Mortality was similar (24% vs. 27%), with the nonresection group having a shorter hospital LOS (mean, 19 vs. 25.6 days). The authors concluded that resectional management was not associated with better outcomes.

In the study by Byrge et al. [22], wide external drainage was mostly employed for grade IV injuries (6/9, 66.7%). The number of patients in the grade IV and V injury groups was too small to make any definitive statements about outcomes relative to the type of procedure performed. However, when resection was compared to drainage procedures for grade IV/V injuries, drainage alone had an increased risk of pancreatic fistula/pseudocyst (OR 8.3, 95% CI 2.2, 32.9).

In the study by Biffl et al. [24], for the 59 patients with grade IV injuries, the pancreatic-related complication rate was 31% in 26 who underwent resection compared to 55% in 18 who were drained ($p = 0.07$). When both grade IV and V injuries were analyzed, there were more pancreatic-related complications in the drainage group compared to the resection group (61% vs. 32%, $p = 0.0051$). The authors concluded that drainage for grade IV and V injuries may result in worse outcomes.

Findings from three of the studies [22, 24, 25] seem to favor resection over drainage where possible. However, the increased risk of pancreatic-related complications after proximal pancreatic resection must be carefully considered [26]. Drainage alone remains an acceptable option [23], especially in damage control situation and where resection could be technically challenging. In any case, endoscopic and interventional radiologic expertise is essential in the management of pancreatic-related complications regardless of which operative strategy is chosen. Further prospective studies are needed to help refine the criteria for selecting one management strategy (resection vs. drainage) over the other.

RECOMMENDATION

Resection where possible is preferred over drainage alone, but both are acceptable options.

Level 3. Grade of recommendation: C.

25.3.5 Do Somatostatin Analogues Reduce Postoperative Pancreatic-Related Complications after Trauma?

Trauma is a risk factor for POPF, but studies evaluating the use of somatostatin analogues (SAs) in traumatic pancreatic injuries are lacking. In a study of distal pancreatectomies, trauma was associated with increased odds for clinically relevant POPF compared to elective resection (44.7% vs. 15.8%, OR =4.3, 95% CI 2.10–8.89) [27].

The benefit of SA in elective pancreatic surgery is controversial. In a randomized trial of 109 patients undergoing pancreaticoduodenectomy, those who were randomized to the octreotide group were given 100 mcg of octreotide subcutaneously before transection of the neck of the pancreas, while the control group did not receive the same. A total of 100 mcg of octreotide was continued in the study group every 8 hours for 5 days. Clinically significant POPF (grades B and C) was similar in both groups (10.9% vs. 18.5%, $p = 0.26$). Mortality was similar in both groups [28].

In a meta-analysis of 12 randomized trials of pancreatic resection examining the efficacy of octreotide, the pancreatic fistula rate was 17.9% (341 out of 1902 patients) [29]. Grades B and C POPF occurred at similar rates between the octreotide group and the control group (11.24% vs. 12.08%, relative risk [RR] = 0.91, 95% CI = 0.55–1.49), with similar rate of overall complications and mortality. "Fluid collection" was the only complication that was lower in the octreotide group (RR 0.61, 95% CI 0.42–0.89). Another meta-analysis examined different SAs on pancreaticoduodenectomy and distal pancreatectomy and included somatostatin (4 trials), octreotide (12 trials), pasireotide (1 trial), and vapreotide (1 trial) [30]. In pancreaticoduodenectomies, there was no significant effect on all POPF, clinically relevant POPF, mortality, or postoperative complications. For distal pancreatectomies, there was reduced odds of all POPF (RR 0.41, 95% CI 0.18–0.91). The authors concluded that SAs may be associated with fewer POPFs after distal pancreatectomy but also cautioned that no sufficiently powered randomized trial was identified.

In a multinational study of 2,026 distal pancreatectomies for nontraumatic reasons, clinically relevant POPF developed in 15.1% [31]. Gland texture was associated with POPF (soft vs. firm, 17.3% vs. 12.0%, $p = 0.022$), while duct size, length of pancreas resected, region of the pancreas resected, closure of the stump, method (open vs. laparoscopic vs. robotic), and prophylactic octreotide were not.

When POPF is diagnosed, it is not clear whether SA has any effect on the time to fistula closure or fistula closure rate. In a meta-analysis of seven randomized trials, the authors were unable to estimate a pooled time to closure due to "inconsistent data." Most fistulae in this meta-analysis were enterocutaneous rather than pancreatic in origin. For pancreatic fistula closure rates, there was no difference (pooled odds ratio 1.52, 95% CI, 0.88–2.61) with the use of SA [32]. The largest study [33] enrolled 102 patients with gastrointestinal fistulae (66% pancreatic) and randomized them to lanreotide (prolonged release, 30 mg intramuscular × 1) vs. placebo. The primary

outcome was a response, defined as the reduction of at least 50% of the fistula volume at 72 hours. For pancreatic fistulae, 69% who received lanreotide were responders compared to 40% in the placebo group ($p = 0.014$). However, fistula closure rates were similar.

There are no recent studies evaluating the efficacy of SA in traumatic pancreatic injuries, either for the prevention of or treatment of pancreatic leaks and fistula. Nwariaku et al. [34] retrospectively analyzed patients who were treated with octreotide postoperatively ($n = 21$) versus no octreotide ($n = 96$). Fistula rates were similar when stratified by grade of pancreatic injury (grade I, II: octreotide vs. no octreotide, 46% vs. 35%; grades III–V: 50% vs. 56%). The authors concluded that the incidence of pancreatic complications was not reduced with octreotide administration.

There may be some benefits of SAs based on meta-analyses for elective pancreatic resections. However, it is not clear if the findings from studies concerning elective pancreatic resection can be extrapolated to the context of traumatic injuries. While there may be anecdotal successes with SA, there remains no clear evidence to support the use of SAs to prevent POPF or to promote fistula closure in the trauma population.

RECOMMENDATION

Somatostatin analogues should not be used routinely as prophylaxis following traumatic pancreatic injury.

Level 3. Grade of recommendation: C.

For the treatment of postoperative pancreatic fistula, SAs may decrease fistula output but do not increase the rate of fistula closure.

Level 2. Grade of recommendation: C.

25.3.6 Should Routine Drainage Be Used after Pancreatic Resections? If So, What Type of Drain Should Be Used?

The use of drains in pancreatic resections has been thought to be essential until recently. Some have maintained that drains are frequently ineffective at controlling pancreatic leaks, could introduce infection, and promote pancreatic leaks by erosion. On the other hand, drains can facilitate early detection of a pancreatic leak or hemorrhage. The type of drains can be categorized as closed or open, and each can be either passive or with applied suction.

After elective distal pancreatectomy, a randomized trial of 344 patients stratified by pancreatic texture (soft or firm) and surgical approach (laparoscopic or open) found that for drain placement compared to no drain, there was no difference in the rates of grade II or higher complications using the Common Terminology Criteria for Adverse Events classification system (44% vs. 42%), clinically significant POPF (18% vs. 12%), intraabdominal abscess (9% vs. 8%), and 90-day mortality (0% vs. 2%). There was a higher rate of abdominal fluid collections in the group with no drains (22% vs. 9%) but no difference in postoperative percutaneous drain placement (10% vs. 10%) [35]. The authors concluded that outcomes after distal pancreatectomy were similar with or without routine drain placement.

For pancreaticoduodenectomies, in a multicenter trial of 137 patients randomized to drain versus no drain, Van Buren et al. found that in the group without drains, there was a higher rate of gastroparesis (42% vs. 24%), intraabdominal abscess (26% vs. 12%), and abdominal fluid collections (12% vs. 2%). The trial was stopped early due to excess mortality without drains (12% vs. 3%) at 90 days [36]. On the other hand, in a two-center randomized trial of pancreatic head resections, Witzigmann et al. [37] found that there was no difference in the primary endpoint of reintervention (drain, 21.3% vs. no drain, 16.6%) but that there was a higher rate of clinically significant POPF with drains (11.9% vs. 5.7%) [37]. There was no difference in mortality or relaparotomy. The authors concluded that prophylactic drains could not be recommended for pancreatic resection with pancreaticojejunal anastomosis.

In a meta-analysis including four randomized trials of drain versus no drain use in pancreatic surgery, He et al. found a reduced risk of death at 90 days (RR 0.23, 95% CI 0.06–0.90) with the use of drains, but no difference in intraabdominal infection, wound infection, or drain-related complications [38].

No such trials have been performed for traumatic pancreatic injuries, and therefore extrapolation of the earlier findings to situations where operative treatment of pancreatic injuries is frequently done urgently may not be possible. Nevertheless, given the findings of He [38] and Van Buren [36], routine drainage after operative pancreatic injuries seems justified.

The type of drain (open versus closed) has also been debated. In a quasi-randomized trial of trauma patients, Fabian et al. [39] compared sump drains to closed-suction drains in 65 patients with all grades of pancreatic injuries. In the patients who received sump drains, 12 of 24 (50%) received distal resection compared to 12 of 35 (34%) of the closed suction group. There was a higher incidence of abdominal abscesses (21% vs. 3%, $p = 0.04$) in the sump drain group. In another nonrandomized study of 320 pancreaticoduodenectomies and distal pancreatectomies, open passive drains (51%) or closed-suction drains were used. There were no differences in intraabdominal collections, sepsis, or mortality. The primary endpoint of the study, bacterial contamination from drain fluid on postoperative day 5, was similar in both groups (open passive drain, 27.5% vs. closed-suction drain, 20.6%, $p = 0.1$). Of note, although not statistically significant, in distal pancreatectomies, the primary endpoint was seen in 25.6% where open passive drains were used versus 16% with closed-suction drains [40].

In a randomized trial of 223 patients where closed-suction drains were compared to closed passive drains, Cecka et al. found that there were no differences in the rates of reintervention by any means, intraabdominal infections, POPF, or 30-day mortality [41].

These findings suggest that closed drainage systems are preferred over open drains. Outcomes appear to be similar with a closed system whether suction or no suction is applied.

RECOMMENDATION

Routine drainage after operative pancreatic trauma should be used.

Level 2. Grade of recommendation: C.

Closed drainage systems are preferable over open drains.

Level 2. Grade of recommendation: C.

25.3.7 For Postoperative Pancreatic Fistula, Is Enteral Nutrition Preferred over Parenteral Nutrition? If So, What Is the Preferred Route of Enteral Nutrition?

For severe acute pancreatitis, there are benefits to enteral over parenteral nutrition. A meta-analysis found that enteral nutrition was associated with reduced risk of mortality, infection, complications, and surgical intervention [42].

In contrast, few studies have compared enteral versus parenteral nutrition in patients with POPF. Klek et al. [43] randomized 78 patients with POPF grades B/C to receive either nutrition via an endoscopically inserted nasojejunal tube using a 1 kcal/mL low-fat, peptide-based tube feed or parenteral nutrition. No SAs were used. In the study sample, the majority underwent pancreaticoduodenectomy (45%) with only two (2.5%) having trauma as an indication for surgery. At 30 days, closure rates were 60% vs. 37% (OR 2.571, 95% CI 1.031–6.411, $p = 0.043$), respectively, for the groups receiving enteral nutrition vs. parenteral nutrition. Multivariable analysis identified enteral nutrition and initial fistula output of <200 mL/day as independent predictors of fistula closure. The median time to closure was 27 days for enteral nutrition, while no median time was reached for the parenteral nutrition group. The authors concluded that enteral nutrition was associated with a higher fistula closure rate and decreased time to closure.

In a smaller randomized study, Fujii et al. [44] assigned 30 patients with POPF after distal pancreatectomy. When POPF was diagnosed after examination of drain fluid amylase on postoperative day 5, patients were randomized to receive parenteral nutrition versus oral intake (porridge, 750 kcal/day × 3 days, then "soft rice," 1,300 kcal/day for 4 days, then "a solid diet," 1,650 kcal/day thereafter). No patient received somatostatin analogs. The primary endpoint, length of drain placement, was similar for the dietary vs. nondietary groups (median, 12 vs. 12 days). POPF progressed to be clinically relevant in five versus four patients ($p = 0.786$). There were no differences in intraabdominal abscess, readmission, or mortality. In another randomized trial of POPF after pancreaticoduodenectomy, Fujii et al. [45] randomized 59 patients to dietary intake versus no dietary intake. The length of drain placement (median, 27 vs. 26 days) and progression to grade B/C POPF (20 vs. 19) were similar. There were no differences in intraabdominal abscess, readmission, or mortality. Results from the two studies support oral feeding as an acceptable means of nutritional support when POPF is diagnosed. No large studies exist for traumatic pancreatic injuries.

It is not clear if intrajejunal feeding should be used rather than more proximal enteral feeding. Kumar et al. [46] randomized 30 patients with severe acute pancreatitis to intragastric vs. intrajejunal feeding and concluded that there was no difference in the recurrence of pain, infection, or death. Eatock et al. in a randomized trial of 50 patients with severe acute pancreatitis similarly found no difference in tolerance of diet, pain, or mortality [47]. A meta-analysis of randomized trials in severe acute pancreatitis found that the route of enteral nutrition was not associated with mortality, need for surgical intervention, exacerbation of pain, and requirement for parenteral nutrition [48]. Certainty of evidence, however,

was "very low" per the authors. It is not clear if these findings can be extrapolated to patients with POPF.

These randomized trials suggest that enteral nutrition is at least equivalent to and may be preferable to parenteral nutrition in patients with POPF.

RECOMMENDATION

For postoperative pancreatic fistula, enteral nutrition is the preferred route of nutritional support.

Level 2. Grade of recommendation: C.

There is insufficient evidence to support intrajejunal access over more proximal enteral access.

TABLE 25.1

Evidentiary Table

Question	Answer	Level of Evidence	Grade of Recommendation	References
Does the addition of pyloric exclusion to the primary repair of a duodenal perforation reduce complications?	Primary repair is adequate for most duodenal injuries. The addition of pyloric exclusion does not lower leak rates, and its routine use is not recommended.	3	C	[8–11]
For blunt pancreatic injuries, under what circumstances is initial nonoperative management acceptable?	Patients with grade I/II blunt pancreatic injuries may be managed nonoperatively. For high-grade injuries, given the increased risk of pancreatic-related complications, an initial strategy of operative management is preferable to NOM. If NOM is to be attempted on patients with high-grade injuries (MPD injuries), endoscopic and interventional radiologic expertise should be available.	3	C	[1, 2, 13–19]
For patients with distal major pancreatic duct injury undergoing operative management, is resection preferred over drainage?	Distal resection is preferred over drainage. Drainage-only procedures can be considered in select circumstances, such as in the setting of damage control.	3	C	[22–24]
For patients with proximal major pancreatic duct injury undergoing operative management, is resection preferred over drainage?	Resection where possible is preferred over drainage alone, but both are acceptable options.	3	C	[22–25]
Do somatostatin analogues reduce postoperative pancreatic-related complications after trauma?	Somatostatin analogues should not be used routinely as prophylaxis following traumatic pancreatic injury.	3	C	[34]
	For treatment of postoperative pancreatic fistula, somatostatin analogues may decrease fistula output but do not increase the rate of fistula closure.	2	C	[32, 33]
Should routine drainage be used after pancreatic resections?	Routine drainage after operative pancreatic trauma should be used.	2	C	[35–38]
If so, what type of drain should be used?	Closed drainage systems are preferable over open drains.	2	C	[39–41]
For postoperative pancreatic fistula, is enteral nutrition preferred over parenteral nutrition?	For postoperative pancreatic fistula, enteral nutrition is the preferred route of nutritional support.	2	C	[43–45]
If so, what is the preferred route of enteral nutrition?	There is insufficient evidence to support intrajejunal access over more proximal enteral access.	n/a	n/a	

Editor's Note

Because pancreatic and duodenal injuries are rare, there is little in the way of high-quality evidence to support our clinical management. Nonoperative management has been demonstrated to be successful in adults with minor pancreatic or duodenal injuries. In children, there is a much higher threshold for operative intervention, and even high-grade injuries are often managed without surgery.

The use of pyloric exclusion is now typically reserved for tenuous primary repairs of severe duodenal or pancreatic injuries or the very rare combined pancreatic and duodenal injuries. The majority of the deaths from these injuries occur early in the hospital course from associated vascular injuries and not later from pancreatic complications such as fistula. Therefore, the use of more radical surgery is rarely employed outside of the most severe injuries. In many cases, the sickest patients can only be temporized, and abbreviated laparotomy is performed. The operative choice then becomes dependent on what can be accomplished in a patient with significant tissue edema.

Resection appears prudent for distal pancreatic injuries and those involving distal major pancreatic ductal disruption. Proximal major pancreatic ductal injuries may require a more radical operation, which may have to be accomplished in stages depending on the stability of the patient. Drainage of major pancreatic injuries when utilized should employ closed-suction drains (uniquely based on quality evidence). The use of somatostatin analogs is not supported by the literature. These recommendations are based on retrospective data and reflect clinical experience.

REFERENCES

1. Simbarashe K, Sugiyama K, Kuwahara Y, et al. Epidemiological state, predictive model for mortality, and optimal management strategy for pancreatic injury: A multicentre nationwide cohort study. Injury, Int J Care Injured. 2020; 51: 59–65.
2. Siboni S, Kwon E, Benjamin E, et al. Isolated blunt pancreatic trauma: A benign injury? J Trauma Acute Care Surg. 2016; 81: 855–859.
3. O'Reilly DA, Bouamra O, Kausar A, et al. The epidemiology of and outcome from pancreatoduodenal trauma in the UK, 1989–2013. Ann R Coll Surg Engl. 2014; 97: 125–130.
4. Blocksom JM, Tyburski JG, Sohn RL, et al. Prognostic determinants in duodenal injuries. Am Surg. 2004; 70: 248–255.
5. Al-Thani H, Ramzee AF, Al-Hassani A, et al. Traumatic pancreatic injury presentation, management, and outcome: An observational retrospective study from a level 1 trauma center. Front Surg. 8: 771121. doi: 10.3389/fsurg.2021.771121
6. Moore EE, Cogbill TH, Malangoni MA, et al. Organ injury scaling, II: Pancreas, duodenum, small bowel, colon, and rectum. J Trauma. 1990; 30: 1427–1429.
7. Bassi C, Marchegiani G, Dervenis C, et al. The 2016 update of the International Study Group (ISGPS) definition and grading of postoperative pancreatic fistula: 11 years after. Surgery. 2017; 161: 584–591.

8. Schroeppel T, Saleem K, Sharpe J, et al. Penetrating duodenal trauma: A 19-year experience. J Trauma Acute Care Surg. 2016; 80: 461–465.
9. Ferrada P, Wolfe L, Duchesne J, et al. Management of duodenal trauma: A retrospective review from the Panamerican Trauma Society. J Trauma Acute Care Surg. 2019; 86: 392–396.
10. Park YC, Kim HS, Kim DW, et al. Time from injury to initial operation may be the sole risk factor for postoperative leakage in AAST-OIS 2 and 3 traumatic duodenal injury: A retrospective cohort study. Medicina. 2022; 58: 801. doi: 10.3390/medicina58060801
11. Weale RD, Kong VY, Bekker W, et al. Primary repair of duodenal injuries: A retrospective cohort study from a major trauma center in South Africa. Scand J Surg. 2019; 108: 280–284.
12. Ho VP, Patel NJ, Bokhari F, et al. Management of adult pancreatic injuries: A practice management guideline from the Eastern Association for the Surgery of Trauma. J Trauma Acute Care Surg. 2017; 82: 185–199.
13. Kong Y, Zhang H, He X, et al. Endoscopic management for pancreatic injuries due to blunt abdominal trauma decreases failure of nonoperative management and incidence of pancreatic-related complications. Injury, Int J Care Injured. 2014; 45: 134–140.
14. Koganti SB, Kongara R, Boddepalli S, et al. Predictors of successful non-operative management of grade III & IV blunt pancreatic trauma. Ann Med Surg. 2016; 10: 103–109.
15. Naik-Mathuria BJ, Rosenfeld EH, Gosain A, et al. Proposed clinical pathway for nonoperative management of high-grade pediatric pancreatic injuries based on a multicenter analysis: A pediatric trauma society collaborative. J Trauma Acute Care Surg. 2017; 83: 589–596.
16. Iqbal CW, St Peter SD, Tsao K, et al. Operative vs nonoperative management for blunt pancreatic transection in children: Multi-institutional outcomes. J Am Coll Surg. 2014; 218: 157–162.
17. Biffl WL, Ball CG, Moore EE, et al. A comparison of management and outcomes following blunt versus penetrating pancreatic trauma: A secondary analysis from the WTA multicenter trials group on pancreatic injuries. J Trauma Acute Care Surg. 2022; 93: 620–636.
18. Biffl WL, Ball CG, Moore EE, et al. Don't mess with the pancreas! A multicenter analysis of the management of low-grade pancreatic injuries. J Trauma Acute Care Surg. 2021; 91: 820–828. doi: 10.1097/TA.0000000000003293
19. Ando Y, Okano K, Yasumatsu H, et al. Current status and management of pancreatic trauma with main pancreatic duct injury: A multicenter nationwide survey in Japan. J Hepatobiliary Pancreat Sci. 2021; 28: 183–191.
20. Biffl WL, Moore EE, Croce M, et al. Western Trauma Association critical decisions in trauma: Management of pancreatic injuries. J Trauma Acute Care Surg. 2013; 75: 941–946.
21. Lin B-C, Chen R-J, Hwang T-L. Spleen-preserving versus spleen-sacrificing distal pancreatectomy in adults with blunt major pancreatic injury. BJS Open. 2018; 2: 426–432.
22. Byrge N, Heilbrun M, Winkler N, et al. An AAST-MITC analysis of pancreatic trauma: Staple or sew? Resect or drain? J Trauma Acute Care Surg. 2018; 85: 435–443.

23. Mohseni S, Holzmacher J, Sjiolin G, et al. Outcomes after resection versus non-resection management of penetrating grade III and IV pancreatic injury: A trauma quality improvement (TQIP) databank analysis. Injury, Int J Care Injured. 2018; 49: 27–32.

24. Biffl WL, Zhao FZ, Morse B, et al. A multicenter trial of current trends in the diagnosis and management of high-grade pancreatic injuries. J Trauma Acute Care Surg. 2021; 90: 776–786.

25. Lin BC, Hwang TL. Resection versus drainage in the management of patients with AAST-OIS grade IV blunt pancreatic injury: A single trauma centre experience. Injury. 2022; 53: 129–136.

26. Lv A, Qian HG, Qiu H, et al. Is central pancreatectomy truly recommendable? A 9-year single-center experience. Dig Surg. 2018; 35: 532–538.

27. Rozich N, Morris KT, Garwe T, et al. Blame it on the injury: trauma is a risk factor for pancreatic fistula following distal pancreatectomy compared to elective resection. J Trauma Acute Care Surg. 2019; 87: 1289–1300.

28. Kurumboor P, Palaniswami KN, Pramil K, et al. Octreotide does not prevent pancreatic fistula following pancreato-duodenectomy in patients with soft pancreas and non-dilated duct: A prospective randomized controlled trial. J Gastrointest Surg. 2015; 19: 2038–2044.

29. Wang C, Zhao X, You S. Efficacy of the prophylactic use of octreotide for the prevention of complications after pancreatic resection. An updated systematic review and meta-analysis of randomized controlled trials. Medicine. 2017; 96(29): e7500.

30. Schorn S, Vogel T, Demir IE, et al. Do somatostatin-analogs have the same impact on postoperative morbidity and pancreatic fistula in patients after pancreaticoduodenectomy and distal pancreatectomy? A systematic review with meta-analysis of randomized controlled trials. Pancreatology. 2020; 20: 1770–1778.

31. Ecker BL, McMillan MT, Allegrini V, et al. Risk factors and mitigation strategies for pancreatic fistula after distal pancreatectomy. Ann Surg. 2019; 269: 143–149.

32. Gans SL, van Westreenen HL, Kiewet JJS, et al. Systematic review, and meta-analysis of somatostatin analogs for the treatment of pancreatic fistula. Br J Surg. 2012; 99: 754–760.

33. Gayral F, Campion J, Regimbeau J, et al. Randomized, placebo-controlled, double-blind study of the efficacy of lanreotide 30 mg PR in the treatment of pancreatic and enterocutaneous fistulae. Ann Surg. 2009; 250: 872–877.

34. Nwariaku FE, Terracina A, Mileski WJ, et al. Is octreotide beneficial following pancreatic injury? Am J Surg. 1995; 170: 582–585.

35. Van Buren G, Bloomston M, Schmidt CR, et al. A prospective randomized multicenter trial of distal pancreatectomy with and without routine intraperitoneal drainage. Ann Surg. 2017; 266: 421–431.

36. Van Buren G, Bloomston M, Hughes SJ, et al. A randomized prospective multicenter trial of pancreaticoduodenectomy with and without routine intraperitoneal drainage. Ann Surg. 2014; 259: 605–612.

37. Witzigmann H, Diener MK, Kienkötter S, et al. No need for routine drainage after pancreatic head resection: The dual-center, randomized, controlled PANDRA trial (ISRCTN04937707). Ann Surg. 2016; 264: 528–537.

38. He S, Xia J, Zhang W, et al. Prophylactic abdominal drainage for pancreatic surgery (review). Cochrane Database Syst Rev. 2021 Dec 18; 12(12): CD010583.

39. Fabian TC, Kudsk KA, Croce MA, et al. Superiority of closed suction drainage for pancreatic trauma. A randomized, prospective study. Ann Surg. 1990; 211: 724–728.

40. Marchegiani G, Perri G, Pulvirenti A, et al. Non-inferiority of open passive drains compared with closed suction drains in pancreatic surgery outcomes: A prospective observational study. Surgery. 2018; 164: 443–449.

41. Cecka F, Jon B, Skalický P, et al. Results of a randomized controlled trial comparing closed-suction drains versus passive gravity drains after pancreatic resection. Surgery. 2018; 164: 1057–1063.

42. Wu P, Li L, Sun W. Efficacy comparisons of enteral nutrition and parenteral nutrition in patients with severe acute pancreatitis: A meta-analysis from randomized controlled trials. Biosci Rep. 2018; 38(6): BSR20181515.

43. Klek S, Sierzega M, Turczynowski L, et al. Enteral and parenteral nutrition in the conservative treatment of pancreatic fistula: A randomized clinical trial. Gastroenterology. 2011; 141: 157–163.e1.

44. Fujii T, Yamada S, Murotani K, et al. Oral food intake versus fasting on postoperative pancreatic fistula after distal pancreatectomy a multi-institutional randomized controlled trial. Medicine. 2015; 94: e2398.

45. Fujii T, Nakao A, Murotani K, et al. Influence of food intake on the healing process of postoperative pancreatic fistula after pancreatoduodenectomy: A multi-institutional randomized controlled trial. Ann Surg Oncol. 2015; 22: 3905–3912.

46. Kumar A, Singh N, Prakash S, et al. Early enteral nutrition in severe acute pancreatitis: A prospective randomized controlled trial comparing nasojejunal and nasogastric routes. J Clin Gastroenterol. 2006; 40: 431–434.

47. Eatock FC, Chong P, Menezes N, et al. A randomized study of early nasogastric versus nasojejunal feeding in severe acute pancreatitis. Am J Gastroenterol. 2005; 100: 432–439.

48. Dutta AK, Goel A, Kirubakaran R, et al. Nasogastric versus nasojejunal tube feeding for severe acute pancreatitis. Cochrane Database Syst Rev. 2020; 3(3): CD010582.

26

Abdominal Vascular Trauma

Zoe Guzman, Harsimran Panesar, Gregory Simonian, and David O'Connor

26.1 Introduction

Abdominal vascular trauma is highly lethal. Many patients with major abdominal vascular injuries die at the scene. The clinical presentation will depend on the injured vessel, the size and type of injury, intraperitoneal or retroperitoneal location, polytrauma, and time since injury. Even after prompt diagnosis, abdominal trauma involving major vessels is challenging to treat. Within the first 24 hours the mortality rate of arterial injury only, venous injury, and both arterial and venous injury are 18.2%, 21.7%, and 32.7%, respectively [1]. The most commonly injured abdominal vessels are the aorta, superior mesenteric artery (SMA), iliac arteries, inferior vena cava (IVC), portal vein (PV), and iliac veins. Mortality from abdominal vascular injuries in the modern series remains high at 20–60%, with early deaths occurring due to exsanguination and late deaths occurring due to multisystem organ failure [4]. Those patients who make it to the trauma bay should receive immediate diagnosis and targeted lifesaving management. In recent years, advancements in imaging and targeted treatment have led to immense progress in managing vascular trauma. This chapter aims to delineate the latest evidence-based management, treatment, and interventions to use in handling abdominal vascular trauma.

26.2 Initial Evaluation and Diagnosis

Abdominal vascular trauma usually presents as hypotension or expanding hematoma. When blunt traumatic abdominal injury (BTAI) is present, the focused assessment with sonography in trauma (FAST), vitals, mechanism of injury, and physical exam help categorize the severity of the patient's status. If the patient is unstable, he or she is taken immediately for surgical exploration without further imaging. When possible, a radiograph should be obtained for identifying retained objects, bullets, or fractures. An obvious penetrating abdominal trauma with hypotension, peritonitis, or abdominal distention is highly suspicious for abdominal vascular injury. The armamentarium we currently have to interrogate abdominal vessels include duplex ultrasonography, computed tomography angiography (CTA), and magnetic resonance angiography (MRA). If the patient is stable, obtaining a stat CTA is the best choice, as it is recommended due to its superior sensitivity (97%) and specificity (97%) for vascular injuries [3]. CTA will provide the most accurate information about intraabdominal, thoracic, and pelvic injuries.

Prehospital patients with suspected abdominal vascular injury should be approached with a "scoop and run" technique. Permissive hypotension (80–90 mmHg) has been demonstrated to be beneficial since it allows adequate vasoconstriction and organ perfusion in these patients [3].

TABLE 26.1

Abdominal Vascular Injuries [15, 16, 21, 22–25, 28]

	Structure	Associated Injuries [Demetriades, book]	Mortality Rate (MR)	MOI: Blunt	MOI: Penetrate
Zone 1	Abdominal aorta	Cardiac arrest (32%)	20–80%	5–20% (MR 24–92%)	67–80% (MR 68%)
	Diaphragmatic aortic injuries	Rib fractures (21%)	88–100%		
	Suprarenal aortic injuries	Pneumo-/hemothorax (25%)	98.2–100%		
	Infrarenal aortic injuries	Fractures of the thoracolumbar spine (50%)	66–72.7%		
		Traumatic brain injury (21%)			
		Abdominal degloving (7%)			
		Hemoperitoneum (39%)			
	Celiac artery	Hepatic hemorrhage with hepatic artery injury Splenic laceration	38–62%	n/a	92%
	Superior mesenteric artery	Mesenteric ischemia	33–68%	10–20%	80–90%
	Zone I		76.5%		
	Zone IV		23.1%		
	Superior mesenteric vein (SMV)		44–57%		
	Inferior mesenteric artery/branches	Mesenteric ischemia	33–45%	20%	80%
	Inferior vena cava (IVC) [Kobayashi LM]	Aortic injuries	36–75%	10%	90%
	Pararenal/infrarenal IVC		43–53%		

(Continued)

TABLE 26.1 (Continued)

Abdominal Vascular Injuries [15, 16, 21, 22–25, 28]

	Structure	Associated Injuries [Demetriades, book]	Mortality Rate (MR)	MOI: Blunt	MOI: Penetrate
Zone 2	Renal artery/vein	Kidney laceration	26–44%	50%	50%
Zone 3	Iliac arteries (IA)	Pelvic or hip fractures	43–49%	5%	95%
	Common IA	Gonadal injuries	55%		
	Internal IA	Bladder injuries	62%		
	External IA		38%		
	Iliac veins (IV)		45–50%	5%	95%
	Common IV		48%		
	Internal IV		52%		
	External IV		33%		
Zone 4	Retrohepatic and suprahepatic	Hepatic hemorrhage with hepatic artery injury	91–100%	n/a	n/a
	Portal vein	Hemorrhagic shock	50–72%	10%	90%

26.3 Imaging Techniques

26.3.1 Ultrasonography

Ultrasonography (US) is a reliable screening tool in trauma [7]. Classically, it is known for its inexpensive and noninvasive method to assess the integrity and condition of abdominal vessels. US is used in the initial trauma survey as a part of the FAST exam. Although CTA is superior, the information US provides can help guide initial treatment decisions and help in surgical planning. It is important to note that the information obtained from the US examination is operator-dependent. In addition, findings can be compromised by patient body habitus. That being said, negative US findings do not rule out other intraabdominal injuries, and a CT scan or serial sonographic exam should follow [6, 19].

26.3.2 Computed Tomography Angiography

Since the previous edition of this book, great progress has been made in the efficiency, accuracy, and accessibility of quick diagnostic imaging for trauma patients. The advantages of a CTA include rapid acquisition, detailed anatomic rendering helpful in surgical planning, wide availability, and lack of an arterial puncture. Additionally, a good-quality study provides information about other tissues such as foreign objects or fractured bones, which one cannot appreciate on catheter angiography. CTA may also be used for the detection of late complications [8–10]. Retroperitoneal arteries, including the abdominal aorta, renal artery, proximal celiac axis, and SMA, are easily assessed with an abdominal CTA. As a result, CTA has climbed to the top as the test of choice for diagnosing abdominal vascular injuries. Disadvantages include lack of portability, exposure to ionizing radiation, and requirement for iodinated contrast. CTA may also require a higher dose of contrast than catheter angiography since the contrast needs to traverse the venous system and the heart to reach the arterial tree.

26.3.4 Magnetic Resonance Angiography

The less popular imaging of choice is the MRA. This is also a noninvasive imaging technique to help evaluate the

TABLE 26.2

Imaging Studies

Imaging Test	Mechanism of Action	Indication	Drawbacks
Doppler ultrasound	High-frequency soundwaves	• *Acute*: Iatrogenic arteriovenous fistulas, pseudoaneurysms, FAST, acute arterial and venous thromboembolism. • *Chronic*: Aortoiliac and peripheral arterial disease.	Limited anatomic rendering and interoperator variability.
CTA	CT + iodinated contrast	• Evaluation of vascular tree in a stable patient. • Visualize extravasation, blockage, aneurysms, and dissections.	Lack of portability, exposure to ionizing radiation, avoided in pregnant women or children, and requirement of iodinated contrast.
MRA	MR + gadolinium	• When CTA with contrast is contraindicated OR to monitor progression of disease.	Cannot be used in patients with implanted metal or pacemakers. Cannot use gadolinium in pregnant women or those with reduced renal function. Have a longer setup time and are more technically complex.

abdominal arteries. Many times a contrast agent (gadolinium) is used for better visualization. Gadolinium can be used in individuals who have a history of allergy to iodine contrast or are at high risk of kidney failure. MRAs are time-consuming, and therefore have limited use in the acute trauma setting. Moreover, there are no data to justify its role in acute abdominal vascular trauma. It is commonly used in follow-up evaluation of arterial injury following therapy.

RECOMMENDATION

CTA is the imaging modality of choice in stable trauma patients. Duplex sonography may have roles in specific situations (intraoperative applications and patients who are difficult to move). MRA is not well described for these indications.

Grade of recommendation: B.

26.4 Abdominal Vascular Trauma: Management

26.4.1 Is There a Role for Resuscitative Thoracotomy in the Control of Exsanguination during Abdominal Vascular Injuries?

For patients arriving at the emergency department in cardiac arrest, a left anterolateral thoracotomy should be performed with aortic cross-clamping and cardiac massage. If a return of spontaneous circulation (ROSC) is obtained, the patient is taken to the operating room (OR) for completion of exploration. The survival rate of an emergency thoracotomy is about 2% [3]. The purpose of cross-clamping the thoracic aorta is to obtain proximal control of exsanguinating abdominal hemorrhage and to redistribute intravascular volume to the heart and brain. This maneuver is also used when the infradiaphragmatic aorta is in a hostile environment or is injured.

A preventive left thoracotomy to avoid cardiopulmonary collapse in the OR has been used. In a retrospective review of 470 patients with abdominal vascular injury, the mortality rate was 45%, and in patients where the aorta was injured proximal to the renal arteries, the mortality rate was 91%. Twenty-nine patients in their series had a good response to a prelaparotomy thoracotomy with aortic cross-clamping, and this resulted in systolic blood pressure (SBP) >90 mmHg within 5 minutes and 38% of patients (11/29) survived. In another retrospective review of 237 patients who underwent emergency department thoracotomy, 50 patients underwent this procedure before a laparotomy for abdominal exsanguination [11]. Resuscitative thoracotomy (RT) should remain part of the arsenal for the approach to abdominal vascular trauma.

RECOMMENDATION

Prelaparotomy thoracotomy for select patients who are in critical status from abdominal vascular trauma may have value.

Grade of recommendation: C.

26.4.2 Is There a Role for Resuscitative Endovascular Balloon Occlusion of the Aorta?

Endovascular methods to control hemorrhage and repair vascular injury are of great interest. Resuscitative endovascular balloon occlusion of the aorta (REBOA) and endovascular stenting have been utilized for this purpose. REBOA was developed to help manage noncompressible torso hemorrhaging injuries and serve as a bridge to definitive management. This is an alternative to thoracotomy in a select population. Like any intervention, REBOA comes with its risks, and appropriate patient selection is necessary to balance the potential adverse effects. Occlusion of the aorta results in tissue ischemia and reperfusion injury, resulting in organ dysfunction and cardiovascular collapse. Some have suggested there is a role for REBOA in patients with massive hemorrhage from solid organ injuries and utilization in the prehospital setting, especially in rural areas.

A recent literature review demonstrated a positive effect of REBOA when compared to RT but no differences compared to no-REBOA [13]. Trauma registry data were used to compare all patients undergoing RT or REBOA during 18 months from two Level 1 trauma centers. Of 72 RT patients, 45 (62.5%) died in the emergency department, 6 (8.3%) died in the operating room, and 14 (19.4%) died in the intensive care unit. Of the 24 REBOA patients, 4 (16.6%) died in the emergency department, 3 (12.5%) died in the operating room, and 8 (33.3%) died in the intensive care unit. In comparing the location of death between the RT and REBOA groups, there was a significantly higher number of deaths in the emergency department among the RT patients as compared with the REBOA patients (62.5% vs. 16.7%, $p < 0.001$). REBOA had fewer early deaths and improved overall survival as compared with RT (37.5% vs. 9.7%, $p = 0.003$) [5]. But it should be noted that comparing REBOA to RT introduces survival bias and bias by indication, since patients selected for RT are likely in cardiac arrest, giving them a poor prognosis. In the absence of randomized trials, REBOA has not demonstrated improved survival compared to standard treatment of severe traumatic hemorrhage. REBOA may be used for traumatic life-threatening hemorrhage below the diaphragm in patients with hemorrhagic shock who are refractory to resuscitation. REBOA is contraindicated in patients with major thoracic hemorrhage or pericardial tamponade. Finally there are insufficient data for utilization of REBOA in pediatric or geriatric patient populations [12]. Additional studies are required to create standardized guidelines for REBOA.

Despite potential advantages over thoracotomy with aortic clamping, REBOA for trauma has not been widely adopted. Training bedside clinicians and developing easier deployment devices for rapid and blind aortic occlusion have decreased the reliance on trained endovascular specialists. As more trauma centers adopt REBOA for rapid hemorrhage control, the increase in experience will allow for protocolized options in select patients.

RECOMMENDATION

REBOA can be safely performed as a temporary non-compressible torso hemorrhage control device by an acute care team with focused training for proximal aortic control. REBOA should be employed as part of a larger system of damage control resuscitation with expedient access to definitive hemorrhage control since this intervention carries a significant risk of life-threatening and limb-threatening complications.

Grade of recommendation: Not sufficient evidence.

26.4.3 Under What Circumstances Are Interventional Endovascular Techniques Superior to Open Vascular Repair?

Whether one technique is superior to the other has not been specifically studied in abdominal vascular trauma. However, the use of endovascular techniques to treat vascular injury in the trauma setting is well-established. In an analysis of the National Trauma Data Bank, the use of endovascular procedures to treat traumatic vascular injuries increased significantly from 0.3% in 2002 to 9.0% in 2010 ($P < 0.001$), with injuries to the thoracic aorta and iliac arteries accounting for the majority of the increase. Notably, patients who underwent endovascular procedures had significantly lower in-hospital mortality (12.9% vs. 22.4%; OR, 0.5; 95% confidence interval [CI], 0.4–0.6; $P < 0.001$) [18]. In a subsequent analysis of patients sustaining inferior vena cava, abdominal aortic, or thoracic aortic injuries, the incidence remained constant from 2002 to 2014, but with decreasing mortality for blunt trauma (48.8% in 2002 to 28.7% in 2014; $P < 0.001$) and concomitant increasing use of endovascular procedures (1.0% in 2002 to 30.4% in 2014; $P < 0.001$) [18]. Furthermore, in the setting of solid organ and pelvic injury, an endovascular approach utilizing embolization is well-established, saving both the patient and the organ. Another meta-analysis demonstrated that overall mortality was lower for endovascular as compared with open repair (8% vs. 19%). Rates of paraplegia were available in 12 of the 37 studies, and the incidence of paraplegia was also lower for endovascular versus open repair (0.5% vs. 3%). Rates of stroke were available in 21 of 37 studies, and the incidence of stroke was slightly higher in the endovascular group as compared with open (2.5% vs. 1%) [18]. Endovascular repair is now performed more commonly than open repair in patients with BTAI [3]. The increasing availability and advances in angiography and embolization allowed a change in the management of trauma patients over the past three decades [14]. Endovascular management has a definitive role in selected cases of infrarenal aortic injury. Patients with limited infrarenal aortic dissection, large intimal flaps, false aneurysms, or aortocaval fistulae have been treated successfully with angiographically placed stents. Delayed vascular complications due to endovascular techniques include aneurysms, arteriovenous fistulae, and arterial occlusions. Long-term follow-up of patients who have endovascular stent grafts placed is required to monitor the longevity and status of the graft.

RECOMMENDATION

Open repair of abdominal vascular injury is still considered the standard of care, although it is associated with higher mortality. Endovascular repair in trauma patients is a feasible intervention with increased survivorship in appropriately selected patients with lower postoperative complication rates.

Grade of recommendation: C.

26.4.4 Should Abdominal Vascular Injuries Be Ligated or Repaired?

As a general rule, all major named arteries should be repaired or reconstructed if at all possible. A majority of venous injuries should be ligated in the setting of damage control, whereas in stable patients formal repair of simple injuries is advisable. Endoluminal temporary shunts should be used in damage control situations that involve injuries to moderate-sized arteries (i.e., popliteal and visceral) but can be effectively used in a variety of venous and arterial vessels of varying sizes. Before any utilization of prosthetic grafts for repair, all enteric spillage should be controlled and the peritoneum should be washed out. Many patients with small intimal tears can be managed effectively nonoperatively. However, those with free rupture of the aorta or large intimal flaps require an open or endovascular approach [15]. Operative findings may include various degrees of hemoperitoneum and hematoma around the injured vascular and/or ischemic bowel. Surgical exploration should occur after temporary control of bleeding with direct pressure or cross-clamping of the aorta.

Currently, there are no standardized clinical practice guidelines for the treatment of blunt abdominal aortic trauma. Whether the vessel is ligated or repaired depends on the availability of collateral blood flow, bowel status, and the ability to deploy endoluminal shunts. Ultimately, the patient's stability, the severity of the injury, and the anatomical limitations will determine the most effective intervention. Temporary intravascular shunts (TIVSs) are utilized when an end-organ vessel is injured, such that ligation of that vessel will require removal of the extremity or organ. A retrospective study demonstrated TIVSs is an effective method to achieve a damage control procedure in vascular trauma with an overall mortality of 22.7%, with about 63% (22/35) of the patients utilizing the TIVSs as definitive repair [26].

Abdominal Aorta. Repair of the abdominal aorta is limited due to its immobility, preventing primary end-to-end anastomosis, and inability to ligate the vessel. As a result, surgeons have found success with primary suture with a polytetrafluoroethylene (PTFE) patch, end-to-end anastomosis with a Dacron graft, or omental covering of the anastomosis.

Celiac Axis. Given extensive collateral circulation, ligation of the celiac axis is well tolerated.

That being said, ligation should be used in destructive injuries and smaller injuries should undergo a primary repair. Utilization of graft or complex repairs with an end-to-end anastomosis is not required since there is an increase in mortality and ligation is well tolerated [27]. Gallbladder ischemia may occur as a consequence of celiac axis ligation requiring cholecystectomy.

Portal Venous System. First-line treatment for portal venous injuries in stable patients is lateral repair. In unstable patients, if the hepatic artery is intact, early ligation is important to gaining hemostasis. This has been associated with favorable outcomes, especially if ligation is done early [33]. Following portal vein ligation, there may be a need for massive resuscitation, and the abdomen should be left open to avoid abdominal compartment syndrome.

Superior Mesenteric Artery and Vein. The SMA is divided into zones I–IV; the more proximal the zone of injury, the higher the mortality. SMA injuries need to be primarily repaired, transposed to the aorta, or an interposition graft used. Superior mesenteric vein (SMV) injuries are concurrent with SMA injuries. SMV injuries can be repaired via primary suture, vein graft, or shunting. For unstable patients, ligation of the SMA is a tolerable intervention [31]. TVISs are most commonly used in SMA/SMV injuries. Given the high grade of bowel edema, physicians should have a low threshold for diagnosing abdominal compartment syndrome.

Inferior Mesenteric Artery and Vein. The inferior mesenteric artery (IMA) and inferior mesenteric vein (IMV) can be ligated without major consequence [31].

Inferior Vena Cava. First-line treatment for IVC injuries are lateral repairs followed by a PTFE patch. In unstable patients, ligation of the infrarenal IVC is acceptable, but ligation of suprarenal IVC injuries is associated with renal failure and has very few long-term survivors [29]. The overall mortality of patients who underwent infrarenal IVC ligation was 59% compared to those who had primary repair, at 21%. Of those who received infrarenal IVC ligation, 77% required a below-knee fasciotomy [29]. Another study, however, showed no difference in the rate of mortality between infrarenal IVC ligation versus primary repair, and none of the patients required fasciotomies [30].

Renal Artery and Vein. In stable patients, renal arterial injuries are managed with a lateral arteriorrhaphy or with primary end-to-end anastomosis. In trauma settings, the utilization of grafts is rare. In an unstable patient with unilateral renal arterial, nephrectomy is recommended if the contralateral kidney is functional. On the other hand, with renal venous injury, the vessel can be safely ligated [31]. Endovascular treatment plays a vital role in blunt renovascular trauma and is considered the first-line treatment in stable patients.

Iliac Arteries and Veins. TVISs are used in iliac arterial and venous injuries for damage control. The common and external iliac artery (IA) injuries are repaired with a lateral repair or with a PTFE interposition graft [31]. Of those who received external IA ligation, 47% required an amputation [32]. On the other hand, internal IAs can be safely ligated and iliac veins can be managed by lateral venorrhaphy or ligation. Endovascular treatment plays a vital role in blunt trauma and is considered the first-line treatment in stable patients.

RECOMMENDATION

The decision to ligate or repair abdominal vascular injuries is dependent on collateral supply, bowel status, and patient criticality. There are some situations where ligation is preferred and others where repair is required. The use of endoluminal shunts can allow for a delay in repair.

Grade of recommendation: C.

26.4.5 In Difficult Vascular Repairs, Should Anticoagulation Be Used Postoperatively? And If So, for How Long?

There is much debate regarding the use of anticoagulation following vascular trauma. Use of anticoagulation was associated with a better prognosis for overall vascular trauma outcomes (weighted OR 0.46; 95% CI 0.34–0.64; $P < 0.00001$), as well as reduced risk of amputation for both lower and upper limb vascular trauma (weighted OR 0.42; 95% CI 0.22–0.78; $P = 0.007$) and reduced occurrence of reoperation events and amputations in isolated lower limb vascular trauma (weighted OR 0.27; 95% CI 0.14–0.52; $P < 0.0001$) [21]. A major limitation with many of the studies includes a lack of prospective analysis, and therefore we recommend prospective studies to properly elucidate prognostic outcomes following the use of these anticoagulants. In a retrospective cohort study, systemic intraoperative anticoagulation (SIAC) use was associated with greater arterial patency rates (93% vs. 85%, $p = 0.02$) without increasing return to the OR for bleeding (4% vs. 6%, $p = 0.29$). After controlling for gender, admission hemodynamics, ISS, injury location, and postoperative anticoagulation, multivariable regression determined that SIAC patients were 2.6 times more likely (OR 2.6, 95% CI 1.1–6.2, $p = 0.03$) to maintain patency. Patients who maintained arterial patency were then less likely to return to the OR (9% vs. 78%, $p < 0.001$), with shorter intensive care unit (median 3 vs. 9 days, $p < 0.01$) and hospital length of stay (median 13 vs. 21 days, $p < 0.01$) [20]. The authors suggest that SIAC may improve arterial patency rates after repair, and the attributable bleeding risk of SIAC may be overstated. In a recent review, it was noted that managing vascular trauma patients remains a delicate balance, and no consensus has yet been achieved regarding the use of anticoagulation medication in the surgical repair of traumatic extremity arterial and venous injuries [21].

TABLE 26.3

Summary

Question	Answer	Levels of Evidence	Grade of Recommendation
When comparing duplex ultrasonography, computed tomographic angiography (CTA) and magnetic resonance angiography (MRA), what is the optimal modality for the evaluation of abdominal vascular trauma?	CTA is the imaging modality of choice in stable trauma patients. Duplex sonography may have roles in specific situations (intraoperative applications and patients who are difficult to move). MRA is not well described for these indications.	4–5	B
Is there a role for thoracotomy to control the aorta in abdominal vascular exsanguinations?	"Yes" for prelaparotomy thoracotomy for patients who are in critical status from abdominal vascular trauma.	4–5	C
Regarding optimal control of the aorta, is there a role for intraoperative placement of an endovascular aortic occlusion balloon?	Further studies are needed to elucidate the utility of this technology. Areas to address include developing and refining the techniques for use by trauma and endovascular personnel in these settings and establishing standard, rapid algorithms for their use. The technique needs to be adequately compared to open aortic control and ultimately evaluated for incorporation into trauma algorithms and trauma training. It is a promising area but needs more experience before its use can become standard.	4–5	Not sufficient evidence
Under what circumstances are interventional endovascular techniques superior to open vascular repair?	Whether one technique is superior to the other has not been specifically studied in abdominal vascular trauma. Angioembolization is a good method to arrest bleeding in hemodynamically stable patients with an active bleed. The indications for stent placement can be extrapolated from the vascular surgery literature, especially in studies that examine the treatment of complications like pseudoaneurysms, fistulas, and dissections.	4–5	C
Should abdominal vascular injuries be ligated or repaired?	The decision to ligate or repair is dependent on collateral supply, bowel status, and patient criticality. There are some situations where ligation is preferred and others where repair is required. The use of endoluminal shunts can allow a delay in repair. In addition, endovascular approaches for smaller injuries and complications seen later are very useful.	4–5	C
In difficult vascular repairs, should anticoagulation be used postoperatively? And if so, for how long?	There is insufficient direct evidence for a recommendation. In the authors' opinion, the best available options are to extrapolate from the available data regarding difficult vascular repairs, even if nontraumatic. Examples provided in this chapter include abdominal aortic aneurysm repairs, spontaneous dissections, iatrogenic injuries, and highlights of concurrent injuries and comorbidities that must be considered.	4–5	Not sufficient evidence

---

RECOMMENDATION

Optimal antithrombotic strategies during and after vascular surgery are still under debate, and current practice often differs from the available evidence.

Grade of recommendation: Not sufficient evidence.

26.5 Conclusion

Technological advances have contributed to the improvement in advanced imaging and endovascular approaches for treatment. However, due to the rarity of abdominal vascular injuries, there is a paucity of high-quality research to guide diagnosis or management. Most patients presenting with abdominal vascular trauma are unstable, and diagnosis is made during exploratory laparotomy. Proximal aortic control through a thoracotomy, abdominal compression, or now REBOA is a clinical decision made by the surgeon. Given the resources available and the surgeon's experience, the mode of intervention will remain the surgeon's preference. Further advancements in endovascular techniques will continue to evolve. Given the preliminary reports of endovascular surgery outcomes, one can say that the future of endovascular surgery for trauma is optimistic. But speed is of the essence, and the expertise of the surgeon and the anesthesiologist is essential to achieve optimal outcomes.

Editor's Note

Due to the fortunate rarity of abdominal vascular injuries, there is little quality research data to guide our diagnosis and management. As nicely delineated in this chapter, most of these patients are unstable from hemorrhage, and the diagnosis is made at exploratory laparotomy. Proximal aortic control used to be a clinical decision by the surgeon (via thoracotomy or abdominal compression) and now REBOA is another option. It is likely that it will remain the surgeon's preference based on the availability of resources and clinical experience that will direct management. But speed is of the essence, and prompt availability of blood products and the expertise of the surgeon and the anesthesiology team are essential in achieving optimal outcomes.

REFERENCES

1. Barbati ME, Hildebrand F, Andruszkow H, et al. Prevalence and outcome of abdominal vascular injury in severe trauma patients based on a Trauma Register DGU international registry analysis. Sci Rep. 2021;11(1):20247. Published 2021 Oct 12.
2. Brenner M, Teeter W, Hoehn M, et al. Use of resuscitative endovascular balloon occlusion of the aorta for proximal aortic control in patients with severe hemorrhage and arrest. JAMA Surg. 2018 Feb 1;153(2):130–135.
3. Fox N, Schwartz D, Salazar JH, et al. Evaluation and management of blunt traumatic aortic injury: A practice management guideline from the Eastern Association for the Surgery of Trauma. J Trauma Acute Care Surg. 2015 Jan;78(1):136–146.
4. Kobayashi L, Costantini T, Coimbra R. Mesenteric vascular trauma. In: Dua A, Desai S, Holcomb J, et al., eds. Clinical review of vascular trauma. Springer Medical Publishing, 2014:213–24.
5. Moore LJ, Brenner M, Kozar RA, Pasley J, Wade CE, Baraniuk MS, Scalea T, Holcomb JB. Implementation of resuscitative endovascular balloon occlusion of the aorta as an alternative to resuscitative thoracotomy for noncompressible truncal hemorrhage. J Trauma Acute Care Surg. 2015 Oct;79(4):523–530; discussion 530-2.
6. Stengel D, Leisterer J, Ferrada P, et al. Point-of-care ultrasonography for diagnosing thoracoabdominal injuries in patients with blunt trauma. Cochrane Database Syst Rev. 2018 Dec 12;12(12):
7. Poletti PA, Becker CD, Arditi D, et al. Blunt splenic trauma: Can contrast-enhanced sonography be used for the screening of delayed pseudoaneurysms? Eur J Radiol. 2013 Nov;82(11):1846–1852.
8. Maturen KE, Adusumilli S, Blane CE, et al. Contrast-enhanced CT accurately detects hemorrhage in torso trauma: Direct comparison with angiography. J Trauma. 2007;62(3):740–745.
9. Loupatatzis C, Schindera S, Gralla J, et al. Whole-body computed tomography for multiple traumas using a triphasic injection protocol. Eur Radiol. 2008;18(6):1206–1214.
10. Patterson BO, Holt PJ, Cleanthis M, et al. Imaging vascular trauma. Br J Surg. 2012;99(99):4–494.
11. Seamon MJ, Haut ER, Van Arendonk K, Barbosa RR, Chiu WC, Dente CJ, Fox N, Jaw RS, et al. An evidence-based approach to patient selection for emergency department thoracotomy: A practice management guideline from the Eastern Association for the Surgery of Trauma. J Trauma Acute Care Surg. 2015 July;79(1):159–173.
12. Bulger EM, Perina DG, Qasim Z, et al. Clinical use of resuscitative endovascular balloon occlusion of the aorta (REBOA) in civilian trauma systems in the USA, 2019: A joint statement from the American College of Surgeons Committee on Trauma, the American College of Emergency Physicians, the National Association of Emergency Medical Services Physicians and the National Association of Emergency Medical Technicians. Trauma Surg Acute Care Open. 2019;4(1):e000376.
13. Castellini G, Gianola S, Biffi A, et al. Resuscitative endovascular balloon occlusion of the aorta (REBOA) in patients with major trauma and uncontrolled haemorrhagic shock: A systematic review with meta-analysis. World J Emerg Surg. 2021;16(1):41. Published 2021 Aug 12.
14. Avery LE, Stahlfeld KR, Corcos AC, et al. The evolving role of endovascular techniques for traumatic vascular injury: A changing landscape. J Trauma Acute Care Surg. 2012 Jan;72(1):41–47.
15. Shalhub S, et al. Blunt abdominal aortic injury. J Vasc Surg. 2012;55:1277–1285.
16. Demetriades D, et al. Mortality and prognostic factors in penetrating injuries of the aorta. J Trauma. 1996;40:761–763.
17. He NX, Yu JH, Zhao WY, et al. Clinical value of bedside abdominal sonography performed by a certified sonographer in the emergency evaluation of blunt abdominal trauma. Chin J Traumatol. 2020 Oct;23(5):280–283. doi: 10.1016/j.cjtee.2020.07.001. Epub 2020 Jul 7.
18. Smith BK, Sheahan, MG. III, Sgroi M, et al. Addressing contemporary management of vascular trauma: Optimization of patient care through collaboration. Ann Surg. 2021 May;273(5):e171–e172.
19. Blackbourne LH, Soffer D, McKenney M, et al. Secondary ultrasound examination increases the sensitivity of the FAST exam in blunt trauma. J Trauma. 2004 Nov;57(5):934–938.
20. Maher Z, Frank B, Saillant N, et al. Systemic intraoperative anticoagulation during arterial injury repair: Implications for patency and bleeding. J Trauma Acute Care Surg. 2017 Apr;82(4):680–686.
21. Khan S, Elghazaly H, Mian A, Khan M. A meta-analysis on anticoagulation after vascular trauma. Eur J Trauma Emerg Surg. 2020 Dec;46(6):1291–1299.
22. Deree J, Shenvi E, Fortlage D, et al. Patient factors and operating room resuscitation predict mortality in traumatic abdominal aortic injury: a 20-year analysis. J Vasc Surg. 2007;45:493–497.
23. De Mestral C, et al. Associated injuries, management, and outcomes of blunt abdominal aortic injury. J Vasc Surg. 2012;56:656–660.
24. Tyburski JG, Wilson RF, Dente C, Steffes C, Carlin AM. Factors affecting mortality rates in patients with abdominal vascular injuries. J Trauma: Injury, Infection, Critical Care. 2001;50(6):1020–1026.
25. Asensio JA, Petrone P, Roldan G, et al. Analysis of 185 iliac vessel injuries: risk factors and predictors of outcome. Arch Surg 2003;138:1187–1193; discussion 1193–4.
26. Oliver JC, Gill H, Nicol AJ, Edu S, Navsaria PH. Temporary vascular shunting in vascular trauma: A 10-year review from a civilian trauma centre. S Afr J Surg. 2013 Feb 14;51(1):6–10.
27. Asensio JA, Petrone P, Kimbrell B, Kuncir E. Lessons learned in the management of thirteen celiac axis injuries. South Med J. 2005;98(4):462–466.

28. Asensio JA, Chahwan S, Hanpeter D, Demetriades D, Forno W, Gambaro E, et al. Operative management and outcome of 302 abdominal vascular injuries. Am J Surg. 2000;180(6):528–534.

29. Sullivan PS, Dente CJ, Patel S, Carmichael M, Srinivasan JK, Wyrzykowski AD, et al. Outcome of ligation of the inferior vena cava in the modern era. Am J Surg. 2010; 199(4):500–566.

30. Navsaria PH, De Bruyn P, Nicol AJ. Penetrating abdominal vena cava injuries. Eur J Vasc Endovasc Surg. 2005;30(5): 499–503.

31. Talving, P., Saar, S. & Lam, L. Management of penetrating trauma to the major abdominal vessels. Curr Trauma Rep. 2016;2:21–28.

32. Ball CG, Feliciano DV. Damage control techniques for common and external iliac artery injuries: Have temporary intravascular shunts replaced the need for ligation? J Trauma. 2010;68(5):1117–1120.

33. Talving P, Inaba K. Major abdominal veins. In: Velmahos GC, Degiannis E, Doll D, eds. Penetrating trauma. Springer, 2012.

27

Pregnant Trauma Patients

Tara DiNitto

27.1 Introduction

Trauma is a leading cause of nonobstetric morbidity and mortality in pregnancy and complicates 6–7% of all pregnancies [1]. Only 4 out of 1,000 pregnant trauma patients lead to admission; however, the delivery rate after admission is 24–38% [A]. Significant trauma occurs in 1 of 12 pregnant women. About two-thirds of these injuries are the result of a motor vehicle crash, while falls and physical abuse account for 10–31% of injuries [2]. Maternal death from trauma ranges from 10% to 20% [3, 4]. Fetal mortality of 9% has been reported [5] and increases to about two-thirds when maternal shock is present [6].

27.2 Anatomic and Physiologic Changes Unique to Pregnancy

The specific anatomic and physiologic changes that occur during pregnancy may alter the response to injury and hence necessitate a modified approach to management.

27.2.1 Cardiovascular System

Plasma volume begins to expand at 10 weeks of gestation and increases to 45% of pregravid levels by the full term. Tubular resorption of sodium and water is significantly increased [7]. This hypervolemic state is protective for the mother because fewer red blood cells are lost during hemorrhage, and hence, the oxygen-carrying capacity of the blood is less affected [8]. Thus, volume expansion may cause a false sense of security for the resuscitating physician because as much as 35% of maternal blood may be lost before the first signs of hemodynamic instability appear. Increases in plasma volume by 30–40% are accompanied by a 15% increase in red blood cell mass, resulting in the physiological anemia of pregnancy. A hypercoagulable state is common during pregnancy. Factors VII, VIII, IX, X, and XII and fibrinogen are increased, and fibrinolytic activity is reduced, putting the patient at increased risk for thromboembolic events.

Maternal heart rate increases by about 10–15 beats/minute. As the diaphragm becomes progressively more elevated secondary to the enlarging uterus, the heart is displaced to the left and upward, resulting in a lateral displacement of the cardiac apex. Each pregnant woman has some degree of benign pericardial effusion, which can be evident on the focused assessment with sonography in trauma (FAST) exam but is physiologic. Both of these changes result in an enlarged cardiac silhouette and increased pulmonary vasculature on the chest radiograph [9]. Cardiac output increases to 25% above normal. In the healthy gravida, this increased workload on the heart is well-tolerated [7]. However, in the supine position, the gravid uterus can partially obstruct the inferior vena cava, which decreases preload to the heart. This can result in diminished cardiac output, causing supine hypotensive syndrome. This syndrome is marked by dizziness, pallor, tachycardia, sweating, nausea, and hypotension. Turning the mother onto her left side restores the cardiac output.

27.2.2 Respiratory System

Secondary to uterus enlargement, the diaphragm rises about 4 cm and the diameter of the chest enlarges by 2 cm, increasing the substernal angle by 50% [7]. Care should be taken to consider these anatomical changes when thoracic procedures such as tube thoracostomies or thoracenteses are being performed. The most prominent changes in respiratory physiology include a progressive increase in tidal volume and minute ventilation. Functional residual capacity decreases because of a decline in expiratory reserve and residual volumes. Relative to these changes, the injured pregnant patient poorly tolerates hypoxia; hence, supplemental oxygen should always be placed regardless of saturation.

Progesterone stimulates the medullary respiratory center, resulting in hyperventilation and respiratory alkalosis. PCO_2 decreases to a level of 27–32 mmHg in a pregnant woman. Therefore, pregnancy is a state of partially compensated respiratory alkalosis.

27.2.3 Gastrointestinal System

Increased levels of progesterone and estrogen inhibit gastrointestinal motility, intestinal secretion, and nutrient absorption. Additionally, the angle of the gastroesophageal junction is altered such that the lower esophageal sphincter is displaced into the thorax. This alteration decreases the competency of the lower gastroesophageal sphincter, which increases the potential for aspiration as early as 8–12 weeks [10]. Care should be taken to reduce the risk of aspiration with conscious sedation or general anesthesia. It is therefore

DOI: 10.1201/9781003316800-27

prudent to insert a nasogastric tube to decompress the stomach and prevent aspiration. Furthermore, as the uterus enlarges, it displaces the intestines upward and laterally, making physical examination unreliable. The placement of laparoscopic ports or laparotomy incisions will need to be adjusted accordingly for the displacement of the intraabdominal contents.

27.2.4 Renal System

Renal blood flow increases by 30% during pregnancy. As pregnancy progresses, the ureters and bladder are compressed by the uterus, resulting in hydronephrosis and hydroureter; consequently, a dilated collecting system visualized in imaging studies is normal. Increases in blood volume and cardiac output cause a rise in glomerular filtration rate and renal plasma flow. Therefore, more plasma is filtered, reducing the serum protein concentration and, hence, the plasma oncotic pressure [11]. This change also increases the renal clearance of many substances during pregnancy, and a review of the metabolism of pharmaceutical agents before their administration to pregnant patients is recommended [12].

27.2.5 Endocrine System

The placenta produces human chorionic gonadotropin and human placental lactogen (HPL), as well as progesterone, estrogen, thyroid-stimulating hormone, and adrenocorticotropic hormone [13].

Maternal utilization of glucose is decreased, whereas maternal lipolysis is enhanced, making nutrients available to the fetus. HPL is the physiologic antagonist of insulin and contributes to the diabetogenic effect of pregnancy by causing increased peripheral resistance to insulin. The pituitary gland enlarges by approximately 135% during pregnancy and demands increased blood flow [13]. Shock may cause necrosis of the anterior pituitary gland, resulting in pituitary insufficiency or Sheehan's syndrome.

27.2.6 Reproductive System

By the end of full-term gestation, the weight of the uterus increases to 20 times its pre-pregnancy weight. Intrapelvic location protects the uterine from injury, but after the 12th week of pregnancy, it extends out of the pelvis and ascends into the abdominal cavity to displace the intestines laterally and superiorly. This makes the uterus more vulnerable to injury but protects the intraabdominal organs. With progressive uterine enlargement, uterine blood flow increases, constituting up to 20% of the cardiac output at term. Uterine veins may dilate up to 60 times, increasing the risk of massive blood loss with a pelvic injury.

27.2.7 Musculoskeletal System

The softening and relaxation of the interosseus ligaments during pregnancy cause increased mobility of the sacroiliac and sacrococcygeal joints and widening of the symphysis pubis. These changes, coupled with an enlarged uterus, disrupt the maternal center of gravity and gait stability, putting the gravida at increased risk for trauma, especially from falls.

27.3 Assessment of Pregnant Trauma Patients

The most common cause of fetal death is maternal death. A key management principle is to treat the mother first because most medical measures that aid in the resuscitation of the mother will be helpful to the fetus. The patient and fetus are best cared for using a multidisciplinary approach. While fetal evaluation is secondary to the primary resuscitation of the pregnant woman, the fetus's well-being is a valuable measurement of maternal well-being. Fetal distress appears early and represents maternal hemorrhage even if the patient is hemodynamically stable. Waiting for maternal signs of instability will further compromise the fetus. At greater than 12 weeks gestation fetal heart tones should be >120 bpm. Fetal hypoxia presents as tachycardia and as the fetal arterial oxygen concentration decreases, it causes bradycardia [42].

Assessment and establishment of the maternal airway are critical, and all pregnant patients should receive supplemental oxygen at a minimum. Late in gestation, the oropharynx is swollen from tissue edema, and endotracheal intubation of the gravid patient can be difficult; therefore, the use of a smaller-than-normal-diameter endotracheal tube, such as a 6.5 mm or less, may be necessary [14]. During pregnancy, the risk of aspiration increases, and monitoring of oxygenation is necessary. Precaution must be taken when chest tube thoracostomy is required as the gravid uterus and fetus cranially displace intraabdominal contents.

Transfer to a facility with labor and delivery (L&D) capability should be considered in a fetus >20 weeks with fetal heart tones. Providing the mother does not have life- or limb-threatening injuries, these patients should be transported as soon as possible to either the emergency room (ER) or L&D unit based on the facility's capabilities [41]. Pelvic fractures are the most common maternal injury that results in fetal death. It is imperative to get imaging on patients with suspected pelvic fractures, as the rate of fetal mortality is 35% with up to 9% mortality in the mother.

In contrast to blunt trauma, maternal mortality is increased in penetrating trauma as the gravid uterus protects the maternal internal organs, with fetal mortality being as high as 73% in these instances [6].

27.3.1 Should a β-Human Chorionic Gonadotropin Test Be Performed in Every Female Patient of Childbearing Age?

After the primary survey and stabilization of the patient, diagnostic modalities are used to determine the extent of injuries to the mother and fetus. Laboratories pertinent to the trauma setting are obtained, and all female patients of childbearing age should have a β-human chorionic gonadotropin test performed [15]. Emergent imaging should not be delayed until the results of the test are confirmed, as fetal health is determined by maternal well-being.

RECOMMENDATION

A rapid secondary survey must include an evaluation of pregnancy. This consists of the determination of fetal heart rate and movement, assessment of the uterine size and tonus, and examination of vaginal bleeding or leakage of amniotic fluid. Fetal heart tones are discernible by Doppler by the 10th week of gestation, allowing a simple and noninvasive method of monitoring. After the 20th week of pregnancy, standard continuous fetal heart rate monitoring should be employed under the obstetrician guidance [2].

Grade of recommendation: B.

All females of childbearing years should have a β-human chorionic gonadotropin test performed—emergent imaging threatening the life of the mother or fetus should not be delayed for the results.

27.3.2 Should Fetal Resuscitation Be Initiated in the Absence of Fetal Heart Tones?

If fetal heart tones are absent, resuscitation of the fetus should not be attempted. There were no fetal survivors in a series of 441 pregnant trauma patients with initially absent fetal heart tones [16].

RECOMMENDATION

If fetal heart tones are absent, resuscitation of the fetus should not be attempted.

Grade of recommendation: B.

27.3.3 What Is an Appropriate Time for Fetal Monitoring after Trauma?

Controversies exist concerning the duration of fetal monitoring following trauma. Early studies indicate that placenta abruption can occur up to 48 hours posttrauma and recommend continuous fetal monitoring during this period [17].

A widely used protocol is based on a prospective study of 60 patients at more than 20 weeks of gestation [18]. This protocol has a sensitivity of 100% for predicting adverse outcomes within 4 hours. In the prospective study, 70% of patients required more than 4 hours of fetal monitoring because of continued contractions (four or more per hour), abnormal laboratory values, or vaginal bleeding, but all of the patients discharged at the end of 4 or 24 hours had similar outcomes compared with noninjured control patients.

If fetal tachycardia is present or a nonstress test is nonreactive, monitoring usually is continued for 24 hours, but no studies exist to support this practice. Some experts recommend prolonged electronic fetal monitoring in patients with high-risk mechanisms of injury. These mechanisms include automobile versus pedestrian and high-speed motor vehicle crashes [19]. No evidence supports the use of routine electronic fetal monitoring for more than 24 hours after non-catastrophic trauma [20].

RECOMMENDATION

All pregnant trauma patients >20 weeks of gestation should have fetal monitoring for at least 6 hours.

Grade of recommendation: B.

27.3.4 May the Approach to Evaluation of Minor Trauma in Pregnancy Be Different?

Minor trauma during pregnancy requires only limited evaluation. In a prospective study of 317 patients with minor trauma, placental abruption appeared in only one case and was not predicted by conventional tests, including tocodynamometry, ultrasonography, and the Kleihauer–Betke (KB) test. This led the authors to conclude that minor trauma can be appropriately evaluated with limited radiologic, laboratory, and fetal assessment [21].

RECOMMENDATION

Minor trauma during pregnancy requires only limited evaluation.

Grade of recommendation: B.

Five conditions are associated with signaling an acute status of the pregnancy. These include vaginal bleeding, rupture of the amniotic sac, presence of contractions, bulging perineum, and abnormal fetal heart rate and rhythm.

Vaginal bleeding before the onset of full-term labor is abnormal. It is potentially indicative of preterm labor, placental abruption, or placenta previa. Rupture of the amniotic sac can allow prolapse of the umbilical cord, resulting in compression of the cord and potential compromise of fetal circulation. Suspected amniotic fluid can be tested using nitrazine paper, which will turn deep blue if the test is positive. Rupture of the amniotic sac is an obstetrical emergency because of the risk of infection and umbilical cord prolapse. Bulging of the perineum represents pressure from a presenting part of the fetus, and delivery or spontaneous abortion may be in progress. The presence of strong contractions is associated with true labor.

27.3.5 Should the KB Test Be Performed in Pregnant Trauma Patients?

Traumatic injury to the uterus can result in transplacental or fetomaternal hemorrhage. The KB test is used to detect the presence of fetal cells in maternal circulation. Because of its high sensitivity, the KB test by itself does not necessarily indicate pathologic fetal-maternal hemorrhage [22]. The KB test is recommended for injured Rh-negative patients in the second or third trimester to detect impending fetal hemorrhage and determine the risk of Rh isosensitization.

As little as 0.001 mL of fetal blood can cause sensitization in an Rh-negative mother. Therefore, all Rh-negative pregnant trauma patients should receive immunoglobulin to suppress potential immune response [16]. Recent evidence suggests that the KB test accurately predicts the risk of preterm labor, and in a patient with a negative KB test, fetal monitoring duration can be terminated [23]. When used as a predictor of preterm labor, the KB test is beneficial to all maternal trauma patients, regardless of their Rh status.

RECOMMENDATION

The KB test should be performed in all pregnant patients >12 weeks of gestation.

Grade of recommendation: B.

27.4 Diagnostic Considerations

After the maternal assessment, there is a need for rapid and accurate imaging. A pregnant patient with blunt abdominal injury or unconsciousness poses the greatest dilemma for imaging. Evaluation of the abdomen for hemoperitoneum can be performed by ultrasonography, diagnostic peritoneal lavage (DPL), computed tomography (CT) scan, or magnetic resonance imaging (MRI).

DPL can be performed safely in the pregnant patient and carries the same sensitivity as in the nonpregnant state of 96–100% detection of traumatic intraabdominal injuries [17, 41]. In these cases, DPL is performed using an open technique in a supraumbilical location. DPL is rarely used with the advent of FAST. It may be indicated when FAST is either unavailable or equivocal, particularly when the patient is hemodynamically unstable. The disadvantages of DPL include the relative invasiveness of the procedure and that, while hemoperitoneum is easily detected, the source of bleeding is not, which could lead to more operative interventions that could have been avoided with a CT scan [41]. CT evaluation should be safely used in the setting of maternal instability.

27.4.1 Should FAST Be Performed in Every Pregnant Patient with Suspected Abdominal Trauma?

FAST is an important tool performed for the diagnosis of free intraabdominal fluid. It has a sensitivity of approximately 80% [B]. FAST is less sensitive in pregnant patients than in nonpregnant trauma patients, but this examination remains highly specific and reported at up to 100% [24, 40]. There is a small amount of physiologic-free fluid in the abdomen during pregnancy; however, that amount is too small to be recognized by FAST. A study showed that in patients with negative FAST results, 96% did not need additional testing that used ionizing radiation, and therefore, ultrasound was recommended as an accurate screening tool [27]. In that study, the patients who had false-negative findings were diagnosed within 24 hours of the injury.

RECOMMENDATION

FAST should be performed in every pregnant trauma patient with suspected intraabdominal injury.

Grade of recommendation: C.

27.4.2 Should Diagnostic Radiologic Studies Be Withheld in Pregnant Trauma Patients?

During the period of major organogenesis (2–15 weeks), ionizing radiation has the highest potential for teratogenesis and neonatal neoplastic effect [2, 28, 29]. In the remainder of the pregnancy, radiation may produce growth retardation, microcephaly, and mental retardation [30]. Exposure to a cumulative dose of less than 0.05 Gy (5 rad), equivalent to the radiation dose from approximately 500 chest radiographs or 100 abdominal CT scans, has not been shown to affect pregnancy outcomes compared with control populations exposed to background radiation [31]. The American College of Obstetricians and Gynecologists stated that a 5-rad exposure to the fetus is not associated with an increased risk of fetal loss or birth defects [32]. Radiation dosage by study commonly used in trauma imaging is listed in Table 27.1. If multiple diagnostic studies are performed, particularly when radiation exposure approaches 5–10 rad, then consultation

TABLE 27.1

Fetal Radiation Exposure to Commonly Used Radiographic Studies

Imaging Study	Fetal Radiation Exposure (rad)
Plain film	
Cervical spine	0
Chest AP	0.0001
Pelvis AP	0.103
Thoracic spine	0.0001
Lumbar spine	0.090
CT	
Head	<0.05
Chest + abdomen	1.6
Abdomen + pelvis	1.6
Chest/abdomen/pelvis (angio)[1]	4.5

with a radiologist or radiation specialist should consider an alternative imaging method, such as ultrasound or MRI, when appropriate [32].

MRI is considered safe during pregnancy, as magnetic energy is not harmful to the fetus [33, 34]. The most obvious advantage of it over CT is the lack of ionizing radiation. On the other hand, most radiology providers recommend the use of gadolinium-based contrast agents, the safety of which for the fetus has never been proven (it crosses the placental barrier). Although teratogenic effects have not been observed in a small number of human studies where gadolinium has been given in pregnancy, it is clear that gadolinium should not be administered during pregnancy unless there is an essential clinical indication, particularly during the period of organogenesis [34, 35]. Moreover, MRI is a time-consuming examination, and gaining access to MRI scanners in an emergent fashion is generally impractical. Thus, MRI has no role in the evaluation of acute trauma patients, and it is more useful in the diagnosis of neurologic and musculoskeletal trauma when most life-threatening injuries were managed.

RECOMMENDATION

Radiologic studies requested for maternal evaluation should not be withheld based on their potential danger to the fetus. Common trauma imaging with a CT head, neck, chest, abdomen, and pelvis are cumulatively all under the safe dose of 5 rad [B]. Duplication of studies should be avoided, and appropriate mandatory shielding should be used whenever possible.

Grade of recommendation: C.

Prevention: Unfortunately, some pregnant women do not wear their seatbelts or wear them incorrectly due to discomfort, inconvenience, or fear of harm to the fetus. Education on the proper usage of seatbelts during pregnancy is essential. Proper use of seatbelts can lead to an 84% reduction in adverse fetal outcomes. The proper way to wear a seatbelt regardless of the trimester is a shoulder strap lying between the breasts and down alongside the abdomen with the lap belt low across the upper thighs and hip bones (below the fetus) [39].

27.5 Emergent Cesarean Section for Trauma

Emergency caesarean section (CS) is advocated for a viable fetus at >25 weeks gestation once a code is called. Perimortem cesarean delivery should be performed within 4 minutes of maternal cardiac arrest. Due to the physiologic changes during pregnancy, cardiopulmonary resuscitation only provides 30% of the needed cardiac output with the patient in a supine position. Laying the patient on their side to reduce the aortocaval compression from the gravid uterus leads to even more ineffective chest compressions [A]. This delivery must be done in the trauma bay and requires excellent multidisciplinary

communication without any deviation from the standard Advanced Cardiovascular Life Support (ACLS) protocols. The quick delivery of the fetus allows for a reported 70% fetal survival rate if the perimortem cesarean is performed within 5 minutes of maternal cardiopulmonary arrest [40].

27.5.1 What Is the Role of Perimortem Cesarean Section, and When Should It Be Performed?

Performance of an emergency CS at more than 25 weeks gestation in patients with fetal heart tones has been reported as high as 70–75% [41]. The absence of fetal heart tones ordinarily predicts fetal mortality at 100%, and an emergency CS should not be performed.

Perimortem CS should be performed in the traumatic maternal arrest with potential fetal viability when resuscitative measures have failed. The best outcomes occur if the infant is delivered within 5 minutes of maternal cardiac arrest. This means that surgery should begin 4 minutes into the arrest [16, 36]. The latest reported survival was of an infant delivered 22 minutes after documented maternal cardiac arrest [37]. Several factors must be considered when deciding whether to undertake perimortem CS [36, 38]. These include the fetus's estimated gestational age and the hospital's resources. Before 23 weeks of gestational age, delivery of the fetus may not improve maternal venous return. Therefore, aggressive maternal resuscitation is the only indicated intervention [1].

RECOMMENDATION

Perimortem CS should be considered in a moribund pregnant patient after 24 weeks of gestation with the presence of fetal heart tones. Delivery must occur within 20 minutes of maternal death, but for the best fetal viability, it should be started within 4 minutes of maternal arrest and completed in 5 minutes.

Grade of recommendation: C.

27.6 Summary

Trauma is a leading cause of nonobstetrical maternal mortality. Knowledge of anatomic and physiologic alterations in pregnancy, correct evaluation of both mother and fetus, and careful considerations of conditions specific to pregnancy are essential to ensure the best outcome. Although the literature on trauma in pregnancy is quite extensive, it is characterized by several limitations. The majority of studies are retrospective, and even prospective works do not have a matching control group. Many studies relying on hospitalized patients raise a concern of ascertainment bias, as only severe trauma cases were identified (Table 27.2). Multi-institutional retrospective data collection following prospective phone follow-up may shed more light on the existing controversies.

TABLE 27.2

Current Evidence and Recommendations

Question	Answer	Level of Evidence	Grade of Recommendation	References
Should a β-human chorionic gonadotropin test be performed on every female patient of childbearing age?	All female patients of childbearing age should have a β-human chorionic gonadotropin test performed.	II	B	[15]
Should resuscitation be initiated in the case when fetal heart tones are absent?	If fetal heart tones are absent, resuscitation of the fetus should not be attempted.	II	B	[16]
What is an appropriate time for fetal monitoring after trauma?	All pregnant trauma patients >20 weeks of gestation should have fetal monitoring for at least 6 hours.	II	B	[17, 18]
Should the approach to the evaluation of minor trauma in pregnancy be different?	Minor trauma during pregnancy requires only limited evaluation.	II	B	[21]
Should the KB test be performed in pregnant trauma patients?	The KB test should be performed in all pregnant patients >12 weeks of gestation.	II	B	[18, 23]
Should FAST be performed on every pregnant patient with suspected abdominal trauma?	FAST should be performed in every pregnant trauma patient with suspected intraabdominal injury.	III	C	[27]
Should diagnostic radiologic studies be withheld in pregnant trauma patients?	Radiologic studies necessary for maternal evaluation should not be withheld based on their potential danger to the fetus.	III	C	[29–32]
What is the role of perimortem CS, and when it should be performed?	Perimortem CS should be considered in a moribund pregnant patient after 24 weeks of gestation. Delivery must occur within 20 minutes of maternal death, but should ideally begin within 4 minutes of the maternal arrest.	III	C	[16, 36, 38]

REFERENCES

1. Muench MV, Canterio JC. Trauma in pregnancy. *Obstet Gynecol Clin N Am.* 2007;*34*:555–583.
2. Tsuei BJ. Assessment of pregnant trauma patient. *Injury.* 2006;*37*:367–373.
3. Warner MW, Salfinger SG, Rao S, et al. Management of trauma during pregnancy. *ANZ J Surg.* 2004;*74*:125–128.
4. Hyde LK, Cook LJ, Olson LM, et al. Effect of motor vehicle crashes on adverse fetal outcomes. *Obstet Gynecol.* 2003;*102*:279–286.
5. Rogers F, Rozycki G, Tuner O, et al. A Multi-institutional study of factors associated with fetal death in injured pregnant patients. *Arch Surg.* 1999;*134*:1274–1277.
6. Scorpio RJ, Esposito TJ, Smith LG. Blunt trauma during pregnancy: Factors affecting the fetal outcome. *J Trauma.* 1992;*32*(2):213–216.
7. Knudson MM, Rozycki GS, Paquin MM. 2004. Reproductive system trauma. In: Feliciano DV, Mattox KL, Moor EE (eds.), *Trauma*, 5th ed. McGraw-Hill: New York, NY, pp. 609–643.
8. Smith CV, Phalen JP. 1991. Trauma in pregnancy. In: Clark SL, Cotton DB, Hankins GDV, Phelen JP (eds.), *Critical Care Obstetrics*, 2nd ed. Blackwell: Boston, MA, p. 498.
9. Lee W, Cotton DB. 1991. Cardiorespiratory changes during pregnancy. In: Clark SL, Cotton DB, Hankins GDV, Phelen JP (eds.), *Critical Care Obstetrics*, 2nd ed. Blackwell: Boston, MA, p. 2.
10. Bynum TE. Hepatic and gastrointestinal disorders in pregnancy. *Med Clin North Am.* 1977;*61*:129.
11. Dunlop W. Serial changes in renal hemodynamics during normal human pregnancy. *Br J Obstet Gynaecol.* 1981;*88*:1.
12. Briggs GC, Freeman RK, Yaffe SJ. 1990. *A Reference Guide to Fetal and Neonatal Risk: Drugs in Pregnancy and Lactation*, 3rd ed. Williams & Wilkins: Baltimore, MD.
13. Gonzalez JG, Elizondo G, Saldiver D, et al. Pituitary gland growth during normal pregnancy: An in vivo study using magnetic resonance imaging. *Am J Med.* 1988;*85*:217.
14. Munnur U, de Boisblanc B, Suresh MS. Airway problems in pregnancy. *Crit Care Med.* 2005;*33*:S259–S268.
15. Bochicchio GV, Napolitano LM, Haan J, et al. Incidental pregnancy in trauma patients. *J Am Coll Surg.* 2001;*192*:566–569.
16. Morris JA, Jr., Rosenbower TJ, Jurkovich GJ, et al. Infant survival after cesarean section for trauma. *Ann Surg.* 1996;*223*:481–491.
17. Esposito TJ. Evaluation of blunt abdominal trauma occurring during pregnancy. *J Trauma.* 1989;*29*:1621632.
18. Pearlman MD, Tintinalli JE, Lorenz RP. A prospective controlled study of outcome after trauma during pregnancy. *Am J Obstet Gynecol.* 1990;*162*:1502–1510.
19. Curet MJ, Schermer CR, Demarest GB, Bieneik EJ III, Curet LB. Predictors of outcome in trauma during pregnancy: Identification of patients who can be monitored for less than 6 hours. *J Trauma.* 2000;*49*:18–25.
20. Grossman NB. Blunt trauma in pregnancy. *Am Fam Physician.* 2004;*70*:1303–1313.
21. Cahill A, Bastek J, Stamilio D, et al. Minor trauma in pregnancy—Is the evaluation unwarranted? *Am J Obstet Gynecol.* 2008;*198*:208.
22. Dhanraj D, Lambers D. The incidences of positive Kleihauer-Betke test in low-risk pregnancies and maternal trauma patients. *Am J Obstet Gynecol.* 2004;*190*:1461–1463.

23. Muench MV, Baschat AA, Reddy UM, et al. Kleihauer-Betke testing is important in all cases of maternal trauma. *J Trauma.* 2004;*57*:1094–1098.

24. Goodwin H, Holmes JF, Wisner DH. Abdominal ultrasound examination in pregnant blunt trauma patients. *J Trauma.* 2001;*50(4)*:689–693.

25. Richards JR, Ormsby EL, Romo MV, et al. Blunt abdominal injury in the pregnant patient: Detection with US. *Radiology.* 2004;*233*:463–470.

26. Brown MA, Sirlin SB, Farahmand N, et al. Screening sonography in pregnant patients with blunt abdominal trauma. *J Ultrasound Med.* 2005;*24*:175–181.

27. Goldman SM, Wagner LK. Radiologic ABCs of maternal and fetal survival after trauma: When minutes may count. *RadioGraphics.* 1999;*19*:1349–1357.

28. Stalberg K, Haglund B, Axelsson O, et al. Prenatal X-ray exposure and childhood brain tumours: A population-based case-control study on tumour subtypes. *Br J Canc.* 2007 3;*97(11)*:1583–1587.

29. Harvey EB, Boice JD, Jr., Honeyman M, et al. Prenatal X-ray exposure and childhood cancer in twins. *N Engl J Med.* 1985;*312(9)*:541–545.

30. Otake M, Schull WJ. Radiation-related brain damage and growth retardation among the prenatally exposed atomic bomb survivors. *Int J Radiat Biol.* 1998;*74(2)*:159–171.

31. Brent RL. Saving lives and changing family histories: Appropriate counseling of pregnant women and men and women of reproductive age, concerning the risk of diagnostic radiation exposures during and before pregnancy. *Am J Obstet Gynecol.* 2009;*200(1)*:4–24.

32. American College of Obstetricians and Gynecologists Committee Opinion #299. 2004. Guidelines for diagnostic imaging during pregnancy. Washington, DC.

33. De Wilde JP, Rivers AW, Price DL. A review of the current use of magnetic resonance imaging in pregnancy and safety implications for the fetus. *Prog Biophys Mol Biol.* 2005; *87*:335–353.

34. Nagayama M, Watanabe Y, Okumura A, et al. MR imaging in obstetrics. *Radiographics.* 2002;*22*:563–582.

35. Shellock FG, Kanal E. Safety of magnetic resonance imaging contrast agents *J Magn Reson Imaging.* 1999;*10*:477–484.

36. Katz VL, Dotters DJ, Droegemueller W. Perimortem cesarean delivery. *Obstet Gynecol.* 1986;*68(4)*:571–576.

37. Lopez-Zeno JA, Carlo WA, O'Grady JP, et al. Infant survival following delayed postmortem cesarean delivery. *Obstet Gynecol.* 1990;*76(5)*:991–992.

38. Katz V, Balderston K, DeFreest M. Perimortem cesarean delivery: Were our assumptions correct? *Am J Obstet Gynecol.* 2005;*192(6)*:1916–1920.

39. Pearce C, Martin SR. Trauma and considerations unique to pregnancy. *Obstet Gynecol Clin North Am.* 2016 Dec;*43(4)*:791–808. doi: 10.1016/j.ogc.2016.07.008. PMID: 27816161.

40. Lucia A, Dantoni SE. Trauma management of the pregnant patient. *Crit Care Clin.* 2016 Jan;*32(1)*:109–117. doi: 10.1016/j.ccc.2015.08.008. Epub 2015 Oct 19. PMID: 26600448.

41. Jain V, Chari R, Maslovitz S, Farine D; Maternal Fetal Medicine Committee, Bujold E, Gagnon R, Basso M, Bos H, Brown R, Cooper S, Gouin K, McLeod NL, Menticoglou S, Mundle W, Pylypjuk C, Roggensack A, Sanderson F. Guidelines for the management of a pregnant trauma patient. *J Obstet Gynaecol Can.* 2015 Jun;*37(6)*:553–574. English, French. doi: 10.1016/s1701-2163(15)30232-2. PMID: 26334607.

42. Krywko DM, Toy FK, Mahan ME, Kiel J. 2022. Pregnancy trauma. In: *StatPearls [Internet].* Treasure Island (FL): StatPearls Publishing. Jan–. PMID: 28613676.

43. Mehraban SS, Lagodka S, Kydd J, Mehraban S, Cabbad M, Chendrasekhar A, Lakhi NA. Predictive risk factors of adverse perinatal outcomes following blunt abdominal trauma in pregnancy. *J Matern Fetal Neonatal Med.* 2022 Dec;*35(25)*:8929–8935. doi: 10.1080/14767058.2021.2007876. Epub 2021 Dec 1. PMID: 34852716.

44. Fabricant SP, Greiner KS, Caughey AB. Trauma in pregnancy and severe adverse perinatal outcomes. *J Matern Fetal Neonatal Med.* 2021 Sep;*34(18)*:3070–3074. doi: 10.1080/14767058.2019.1678129. Epub 2019 Oct 17. PMID: 31619114.

28

Pelvic Fractures

Matthew O. Dolich and Panna A. Codner

28.1 Introduction

Pelvic fractures are reported to account for 1–3% of all skeletal injuries and are present in approximately 5% of trauma patients requiring hospitalization [1]. These fractures typically occur through a variety of blunt mechanisms, including motor vehicle collisions, pedestrian accidents, falls, and crush injuries, with penetrating mechanisms being much less common. The severity of injury varies, ranging from relatively minor (albeit painful) pubic ramus fractures to significant open-book or vertical shear injuries with substantial hemorrhage or large soft tissue wounds. Associated extrapelvic injuries are common [2], and the clinician is frequently faced with a complex decision process in a multiply injured, hemodynamically unstable patient. Patients presenting with high-energy mechanisms and unstable pelvic fracture patterns have a significant risk of in-hospital mortality [3]. Management is frequently multidisciplinary in nature, involving both trauma/acute care surgeons, orthopedic surgeons, and interventional radiologists for optimal treatment. Basic tenets of management of patients with high-energy severe fracture patterns include reduction of pelvic volume with the application of external binders or sheets, prompt initiation of damage control resuscitation, and minimizing blood loss as detailed in the sections that follow. A summary of available evidence and recommendations is contained in Table 28.1.

28.2 What Is the Role of Pelvic Fracture Stabilization with External Compression Devices, Binders, or Sheets?

As pelvic fracture hemorrhage appears to be largely venous in origin and frequently contained within the extraperitoneal spaces of the pelvis, theoretically reduction of pelvic volume may reduce the extent of bleeding via enhancing tamponade and reducing bony fracture bleeding. Early pelvic stabilization may be attempted by wrapping the pelvis in a sheet secured with clamps or application of commercially available devices such as the Trauma Pelvic Orthotic Device (T-POD). These maneuvers may be performed in the prehospital setting or in the emergency department during the initial evaluation of patients with suspected unstable pelvic fractures. Stabilization and reduction of pelvic volume appear to be best achieved when the compressive device is placed at the level of the greater trochanters. However, the misapplication is not uncommon [4, 5] with the binder resting too high or too low or used in fracture patterns not conducive to external compression (e.g., vertical shear injuries). Pelvic binders also may impede examination or vascular access for central venous or arterial line insertion in the groin. Additionally, pelvic binders may be associated with skin necrosis and deep tissue injury when left in place for prolonged periods of time.

In a recent retrospective review, Schweigkofler et al. [6] analyzed their experience with 37 patients who had pelvic binders applied in the prehospital setting. When compared with a similar group of patients not receiving a binder, they found no differences in blood transfusion requirements or mortality. Similarly, Agri et al. [7] performed a single-center retrospective study of 228 pelvic fracture patients over a 7-year period and found no mortality benefit associated with the prehospital application of pelvic binders.

Despite disappointing results in the prehospital setting, other researchers have looked at the utility of pelvic binder application after the patient's arrival in the emergency department (ED). Hsu et al. [8] retrospectively evaluated their experience with 56 pelvic fracture patients undergoing pelvic binder placement at a Level 1 trauma center. When compared with historical controls, the group that received pelvic binders in the ED had lower blood transfusion requirements and lower mortality, prompting the authors to recommend the early use of pelvic binders even before imaging is available.

In a cadaver study, Prasarn [9] compared the circumferential application of a sheet to T-POD with attention to differences in motion of the injured hemipelvis. Using electromagnetic sensors, they found no difference in sagittal, axial, or coronal motion during the application, log rolling, bed transfers, and head of bed elevation between the two groups. Based on the ready availability and low cost of bed sheets, the authors recommended circumferential pelvic sheeting for unstable pelvic fractures.

> **RECOMMENDATION**
>
> There is insufficient evidence to recommend the routine use of circumferential binders or pelvic sheet application.
>
> Grade of recommendation: D.

DOI: 10.1201/9781003316800-28

28.3 What Is the Role of Resuscitative Endovascular Balloon Occlusion of the Aorta in Patients with Hemorrhagic Shock Due to Pelvic Fracture?

During the last decade, resuscitative endovascular balloon occlusion of the aorta (REBOA) has gained increased attention as an adjunctive measure for circulatory support and temporary vascular control in patients with noncompressible torso hemorrhage, including pelvic fracture bleeding. REBOA deployment is typically described in two anatomic locations: Zone 1, or the supra celiac aorta, and zone 3, or the infrarenal aorta. The former is typically utilized in patients with intraperitoneal bleeding and shock due to injuries of the solid organs, mesentery, or abdominal blood vessels. Zone 3 control may be used for isolated pelvic fracture bleeding when concern for intraperitoneal hemorrhage is low. Newer, prepackaged kits from several commercial manufacturers have simplified insertion, minimized the need to search for multiple items during emergencies, and most importantly, enabled lower-profile access at the level of the common femoral artery. The procedure is typically performed in the ED, may be done with or without radiographic guidance, and is commonly performed in conjunction with other measures including balanced resuscitation, pelvic binder application, external fixation, preperitoneal pelvic packing, and subsequent angioembolization. Although the procedure may be lifesaving, the risk of complications remains high, and the exact indications continue to be defined.

Asmar et al. [10] conducted a retrospective review of the American College of Surgeons Trauma Quality Improvement Program (ACS-TQIP) database comparing three groups of pelvic fracture patients—those undergoing REBOA alone, those undergoing preperitoneal pelvic packing alone, and those undergoing both procedures. Overall mortality was 42%. When compared to patients undergoing pelvic packing alone, REBOA patients had lower mortality rates at 24 hours and for the entire hospitalization, lower transfusion requirements at 4 hours, and faster times to laparotomy and angioembolization, leading the authors to conclude that REBOA is less invasive than pelvic packing and is associated with improved outcomes. In a large, multicenter descriptive database study of patients with severe pelvic fractures, Harfouche [11] noted wide variability among trauma centers in the utilization of zone 3 REBOA in conjunction with other hemostatic techniques such as external fixation, angioembolization, and pelvic packing. Overall mortality in the study was 37.7%, and increasing numbers of interventions were associated with higher transfusion and complication rates. In another retrospective study of the same database, Laverty [12] found that common femoral arterial access–related complications including limb ischemia, distal embolization, and pseudoaneurysm were not uncommon, with an overall incidence of almost 10%. Tranexamic acid (TXA) use in conjunction with REBOA, as well as device caliber, appeared to be associated with an increased risk of these complications, which were associated with a greater overall length of hospital stay. Four patients (approximately 1% of the study population) underwent extremity amputation because of arterial access–related

complications. The authors suggested caution and vigilance when utilizing REBOA in patients receiving TXA, but were hopeful that newer, lower-profile devices emerging in the current market might help reduce access-related complications. Lastly, the complications and mortality associated with the utilization of REBOA should not be taken lightly. The procedure requires training, skill, and resources and can be technically challenging to perform correctly. In a recent case-control retrospective analysis of 420 patients undergoing REBOA, Joseph et al. [13] found higher rates of acute kidney injury, lower extremity amputation, and death when compared to a similar cohort of patients treated without REBOA.

RECOMMENDATION

REBOA may be considered for patients with severe pelvic fracture and hemorrhagic shock and may be utilized in conjunction with other modalities for hemorrhage control, including angioembolization, pelvic packing, and external fixation.

Grade of recommendation: C.

28.4 What Is the Role of Tranexamic Acid in Patients with Hemorrhage Due to Pelvic Fractures?

Fibrinolysis and the coagulopathy that ensues after major trauma play a major role in the balance of hemostasis and ongoing blood loss after pelvic fracture. While transfusion of fractionated or whole blood products is lifesaving in the event of major hemorrhage, massive transfusion may be associated with several deleterious effects including volume overload, acute lung injury, disease transmission, and negative immunomodulatory effects. Additionally, there is a significant cost associated with blood transfusion; thus, interventions to minimize blood loss appear to be worthwhile endeavors. One component of disordered coagulation following major trauma is hyperfibrinolysis, hence the recent interest in the therapeutic use of antifibrinolytic agents in this setting. TXA is a synthetic derivative of the naturally occurring amino acid lysine, which inhibits fibrinolysis by blocking the lysine binding sites on plasminogen, which in turn helps ameliorate fibrin degradation and improves the formation of a stable clot.

The collaborators of the CRASH-2 trial [14] investigated the effects of TXA in trauma patients with significant hemorrhage during a randomized controlled trial involving 274 hospitals in 40 countries. The study enrolled 20,211 adult trauma patients who had or were at risk for significant bleeding. The patients were assigned to receive TXA (loading dose of 1 g over 10 minutes, followed by an infusion of 1 g over 8 hours) or a matching placebo. TXA was associated with a 1.5% reduction in 28-day all-cause mortality in adult trauma patients with signs of bleeding (systolic blood pressure [SBP] <90 mmHg, heart rate >100 beats/min, or both, within

8 hours of injury). TXA had the greatest impact on reducing death caused by bleeding in the severe shock group (SBP ≤75 mmHg) (14.9% vs. 18.4%; risk ratio [RR], 0.81; 95% confidence interval [CI], 0.69–0.95). Early TXA (≤1 hour from injury) was associated with the greatest reduction (32%) in deaths caused by bleeding (5.3% vs. 7.7%; RR, 0.68; 95% CI, 0.57–0.82; $p < 0.0001$). However, TXA given between 1 and 3 hours also reduced the risk of death (4.8% vs. 6.1%; RR, 0.79; 95% CI, 0.64–0.97; $p = 0.03$). In addition, TXA treatment was not associated with an increased risk of vascular occlusive events.

Despite a subtle but significant outcome benefit, the clinical application of the CRASH-2 study results was challenged by several factors, including the inclusion criteria that diluted outpatients who were bleeding and the increase in the risk of death due to bleeding if TXA was administered beyond 3 hours. The MATTERS study [15] specifically addressed a cohort of patients who were actively bleeding. This retrospective observational study compared TXA with no TXA in patients receiving at least 1 unit of packed red blood cells (PRBCs). A subgroup of patients receiving massive transfusion (≥10 units of PRBCS) was also examined. Overall, the TXA group had lower mortality than the non-TXA group (17.4% vs. 23.9%, $p = 0.03$). This benefit was greatest in the massive transfusion group (14.4% vs. 28.1%, $p = 0.004$). The MATTERS study further supports the CRASH-2 trial in demonstrating an early mortality benefit and neutral risk profile. While neither CRASH-2 nor MATTERS specifically addressed pelvic fracture hemorrhage, their conclusions seem applicable to this population of patients, as these patients often require massive transfusions.

More recently, Spitler et al. [16] conducted a randomized prospective study of TXA in patients at a Level 1 trauma center with fractures of the pelvic ring, acetabulum, and proximal femur and examined them for differences in the amount of total blood loss, transfusion rate, and incidence of thromboembolic events. Total blood loss was significantly higher in the group that did not receive TXA (TXA =952 mL, no TXA = 1325 mL, $P = 0.02$), though transfusion rates were similar in TXA and control groups. The incidence of venous thromboembolism was not increased in the group that received TXA, and the authors concluded that TXA was both safe and appeared to decrease blood loss. Regarding the question of risk of venous thromboembolism, in a recent retrospective study, Gümüştaş [17] found no cases of symptomatic deep venous thrombosis of pulmonary embolism in a cohort of 73 consecutive patients with pelvic fractures requiring operative fixation, all of whom received TXA preoperatively.

In a recent systematic review, Shu et al. [18] sought to analyze the available data regarding TXA use in patients undergoing surgery for fractures of the pelvis and/or acetabulum. Four studies met the criteria for the review, though there was significant heterogeneity, and the overall quality of the evidence was relatively low. In their review, the authors found that TXA use was associated with a significantly lower transfusion rate (44% vs. 57%, $p = 0.02$) when compared with pelvic fracture patients not receiving TXA. There was no association between TXA use and venous thromboembolism or intraoperative blood loss.

RECOMMENDATION

TXA use may be considered as a therapeutic adjunct to potentially limit blood loss and reduce transfusion requirements in trauma patients with hemorrhage associated with severe pelvic fractures requiring surgical intervention. TXA should be administered less than 3 hours from the time of injury, according to the following regimen: 1 g bolus dose administered intravenously over 10 minutes followed by an infusion of 1 g administered intravenously over 8 hours.

Grade of recommendation: B.

28.5 What Is the Role of Preperitoneal Pelvic Packing in Hemodynamically Unstable Patients with Pelvic Fractures?

Current management of patients with hemodynamic instability related to hemorrhage from pelvic fracture has generally focused on mechanical stabilization of the pelvis, angiographic embolization of arterial hemorrhage, and prompt initiation of a balanced resuscitation. However, the belief that most pelvic hemorrhage is venous in origin coupled with the success of damage control packing techniques has generated renewed interest in pelvic packing as an adjunctive maneuver for the control of pelvic hemorrhage. Preperitoneal packing (also called extraperitoneal pelvic packing) is accomplished via a lower midline or transverse incision with the division of the skin, subcutaneous tissue, and the anterior rectus sheath, taking care to avoid entering the peritoneal cavity. The preperitoneal space is entered, and blunt dissection is used to fully develop an extraperitoneal "pocket" that extends from the symphysis pubis to the sacroiliac joint. Three or four laparotomy pads are placed on each side with the goal of tamponading venous and bony bleeding, and the midline incision is closed. The procedure may be followed by mechanical stabilization of the pelvis, laparotomy, or angiography as needed. Packs are generally removed after 24–48 hours when hemodynamic stability has been achieved. This technique did not generate much interest in North America until 2005 when a preliminary report by Smith et al. [19] described two blunt trauma patients with pelvic fracture–associated hemorrhage who underwent extraperitoneal packing and survived hospital discharge. Since that time, increasing numbers of trauma centers have adopted pelvic packing due to the relative ease of performance of the procedure as well as perceived utility as a bridge to pelvic angioembolization for control of arterial hemorrhage. Although the procedure is taught in a standardized fashion as part of the Advanced Surgical Skills for Exposure in Trauma (ASSET) course developed by the American College of Surgeons, significant local and regional practice variability still exists.

Jang [20], in a recent study at a Korean trauma center, performed a retrospective analysis of 14 patients treated with preperitoneal packing from a prospectively collected pelvic trauma database. The authors compared these patients to a matched group of patients who did not undergo pelvic packing. Mortality was significantly lower in the group that underwent pelvic packing, and the authors also found that SBP significantly increased after pelvic packing was completed. Moskowitz et al. [21], in a 10-year retrospective analysis of 14 patients with open pelvic fracture treated at a single Level 1 trauma center, found preperitoneal packing effectively controlled pelvic hemorrhage in all patients. One mortality was not associated with pelvic fracture.

In a recent retrospective single-center study, Werner et al. [22] reviewed their experience with a cohort of patients with unstable pelvic fractures and hemodynamic instability requiring 2 or more units of PRBC transfusion. The study group included patients who underwent REBOA, preperitoneal pelvic packing, or both, followed by angioembolization. Overall mortality was 14%, but there were no mortalities due to exsanguination from ongoing pelvic fracture hemorrhage. The combination of pelvic packing and REBOA was utilized in more severely injured patients and was associated with higher transfusion requirements than in patients not requiring REBOA. However, the absence of mortality due to acute pelvic fracture hemorrhage led the authors to conclude that the combination of pelvic packing and REBOA may be lifesaving in this severely injured group of patients. In 2020, the Eastern Association for the Surgery of Trauma (EAST) published a systematic review, meta-analysis, and practice management guideline [23] which included a conditional recommendation for pelvic packing while waiting for pelvic angiography.

RECOMMENDATION

There are insufficient data to support the routine use of preperitoneal pelvic packing in unstable pelvic fractures. However, it remains an option and part of the surgeon's armamentarium in hemodynamically unstable patients with suspected active ongoing hemorrhage.

Grade of recommendation: C.

28.6 Which Patients with Pelvic Fracture Warrant Early Angiography and Angioembolization?

Hemorrhage associated with pelvic fracture may come from several different sources, including branches of the internal iliac arteries, the pelvic venous plexus, and the fractured bones themselves. Multiple sources of hemorrhage may be present in a single patient, and different sources may be manifest at varying times during initial resuscitation. The challenge to the treating physician is early identification of those patients not likely to achieve early hemostasis and initiating more aggressive measures, including angioembolization, when arterial hemorrhage is suspected. One of the most widely utilized classification systems for pelvic fractures was developed by Young and Burgess more than 35 years ago [24]. This classification associates certain fracture patterns with applied force vectors such as lateral compression (LC), anteroposterior compression (APC), and vertical shear (VS). Since that time, many have

utilized the Young–Burgess classification to help guide the management of pelvic fracture patients. Recently Costantini et al. [25] conducted a prospective, multicenter observational study of patients with pelvic fracture and shock to elucidate which fracture patterns were most likely to require intervention for hemorrhage control. Of 163 patients meeting study criteria, 83% with APC type III (i.e., open book pelvic fracture with disruption of anterior and posterior sacroiliac ligaments and pubic symphysis) required intervention for hemorrhage control. Additional risk factors for requiring hemorrhage control maneuvers included VS fracture pattern, open pelvic fracture, and blood transfusion.

Over the last two decades, most trauma centers have adopted imaging protocols where the majority of patients with blunt torso trauma undergo contrast-enhanced computed tomography (CT) of the abdomen and pelvis to assess for a wide variety of injuries, including pelvic fractures. Traditionally, the presence of extravasation of intravenous contrast material, or "blush," from branches of the internal iliac artery in a patient with pelvic fractures and surrounding hematoma has been considered an indication for early pelvic angiography and embolization. While the absence of contrast extravasation has a high negative predictive value, the overall positive predictive value of a contrast blush on pelvic CT has been a bit more variable. For example, Juern et al. [26] performed a retrospective study of almost 500 pelvic fracture patients undergoing CT. Of 75 patients with a blush on CT, only 17 (23%) required therapeutic angioembolization of a bleeding arterial vessel. Of note, the negative predictive value of the absence of contrast blush was 100%. In another retrospective study, Kuo et al. [27] also found a relatively high false-positive rate when contrast extravasation was used in isolation. One plausible explanation for this is that as the resolution of multislice CT has increased over time, so has our ability to pick up transient small arterial bleeds that may be of limited clinical significance. However, when Kuo included relative or transient hypotension in the analysis, the positive predictive value of a contrast blush improved. In another large retrospective study of almost 400 pelvic fracture patients, Hammerschlag [28] found 12 who underwent diagnostic pelvic angiography, and only 4 of those benefitted from therapeutic embolization.

RECOMMENDATION

Patients with hypotension, transfusion requirements, and evidence of extravasation on contrast-enhanced CT of the pelvis should undergo urgent pelvic angiography and embolization.

Grade of recommendation: C.

28.7 What Is the Role of Fecal Diversion in Patients with Open Pelvic Fractures?

Open pelvic fracture is an uncommon clinical entity typically associated with high-energy blunt trauma mechanisms as well as crush injuries. Historically, clinicians have voiced concern about the communication of open perineal, groin, and buttock wounds with pelvic fractures generating an unacceptably high rate of osteomyelitis and pelvic sepsis. The practice of routine performance of a diverting colostomy in patients with open pelvic fractures arose largely based on these concerns. However, few studies exist that provide scientific support for this practice, and the available data are further compromised by a lack of clearly accepted criteria for defining the anatomy and severity of open pelvic fractures. For example, most studies are of a heterogeneous patient population that includes full-thickness rectal injuries, vaginal tears, perineal wounds, buttock lacerations, and groin wounds.

In the mid-1990s, Faringer et al. [29], retrospectively reviewed their experience with 33 open pelvic fracture patients. Although their overall mortality rate was relatively low (15%), wound infections occurred more commonly in the colostomy group than in those without fecal diversion (31% vs. 19%). This finding prompted the authors to suggest a more selective policy of fecal diversion in the setting of open pelvic fracture. They proposed utilizing a classification scheme based on the location of the open wound, with zone I encompassing the perineum, pubis, medial buttock, and sacrum; zone II encompassing the groin and medial thigh; and zone III including the posterolateral buttocks and iliac crest. Based on their experience, the authors advocated for fecal diversion in patients with zone I injuries.

A retrospective study published in 2018 by Hermans [30] evaluated their single-center experience at a Level 1 trauma center over 10 years with 24 patients presenting with open pelvic fractures. In this study, overall mortality was relatively low (4%) in the group with open fractures and not significantly different when compared to patients with closed pelvic fractures over the same time frame. In this study, 4 out of 11 (36%) patients with zone I injuries were managed without fecal diversion. Patients with injuries in Faringer zones II and III were managed without colostomy. Only one patient with a zone I injury developed pelvic sepsis; this patient had undergone the creation of a colostomy early during the course of hospitalization.

A systematic review of fecal diversion in preventing infection in the setting of open pelvic fracture was performed by Lunsjo and Abu-Zidan [31]. When the available data were pooled, no significant reduction in the rate of infectious complications was noted when a colostomy was performed (38% infection rate in the colostomy group vs. 35% in the noncolostomy group, $p = 0.86$). Similarly, no significant benefit for sepsis-related mortality was noted in patients undergoing fecal diversion (15% for the colostomy group vs. 9% for the noncolostomy group, $p = 0.35$).

28.8 What Is the Optimal Timing for Definitive Operative Stabilization of Pelvic Ring Fractures?

Over the last decade, there has been a trend toward decreasing the time interval from patient arrival to definitive operative stabilization of pelvic ring fractures [32, 33]. This trend has been fueled by improvements in resuscitative techniques, including damage control resuscitation, as well as initiatives to reduce hospital length of stay and medical costs. Additionally, definitive fixation of many pelvic ring fractures is now accomplished using smaller incisions, with less blood loss, using percutaneous screw fixation and plates rather than the bigger, bloodier operations of earlier decades. Additionally, early definitive fixation allows patients to regain mobility earlier in their hospitalization, hopefully ameliorating the risk of complications associated with prolonged immobility or bed rest.

In a retrospective cohort study, Tan [34] reviewed their institution's experience with 103 patients with pelvic and long bone fractures who responded to resuscitation but underwent surgery with "borderline" physiologic status. This subgroup of patients—essentially those with mild metabolic derangements including acidosis—frequently underwent delayed orthopedic repair out of concern for incurring perioperative complications. In this study, higher rates of prolonged ventilation were associated with time >4 days to definitive surgery as well as the number of units of blood transfused. Time to definitive surgery >4 days, as well as patient age and head Abbreviated Injury Scale (AIS) ≥3, were associated with an increased risk of postoperative complications.

In a retrospective analysis, Sharpe [35] examined functional outcomes in 145 patients with severe pelvic ring fractures over 18 years. Despite overall high injury severity in the study population, in multivariate analysis, time to pelvic fracture fixation was the only predictor of decreased mobility and activity following a severe pelvic fracture.

In a recent retrospective study, Taylor [36] evaluated outcomes in 287 patients with pelvic fractures requiring surgery, comparing results in those receiving surgery early (≤3 days) versus those undergoing surgery later in their hospitalization. Although there were no significant differences between the two groups in terms of ventilator-associated pneumonia, venous thromboembolism, acute kidney injury, acute respiratory distress syndrome (ARDS), or pressure ulceration, the late group experienced significantly more surgical site infections and increased hospital length of stay (11.9 +/− 0.7 days for the "early" group compared to 18.0 +/− 1.2 days for the "late" group, $P < 0.001$).

RECOMMENDATION

A diverting colostomy is not mandatory in all patients with open pelvic fractures. Selective application of fecal diversion in patients with rectal injuries, extensive perineal wounds, and disruption of the anal sphincter mechanism is reasonable.

Grade of recommendation: C.

RECOMMENDATION

Pelvic fractures should be repaired as soon as the patient is fully resuscitated and physiologically appropriate for surgery, ideally within the first 24–72 hours of injury.

Grade of recommendation: B.

28.9 What Are the Respective Roles of Early Chemical Venous Thromboembolism Prophylaxis and Prophylactic Inferior Vena Cava Filtration in Patients with Pelvic Fractures?

Since life-threatening hemorrhage is one of the most feared complications of pelvic fracture, it is certainly understandable that there might be reticence about the initiation of chemical venous thromboembolism (VTE) prophylaxis. That said, patients with pelvic fractures are often multiply injured and carry a high risk of VTE. Trauma surgeons are therefore forced to seek the appropriate balance between the risk of ongoing or recurrent hemorrhage and VTE.

To better answer this question, Benjamin et al. [37] conducted a retrospective analysis of patients with severe pelvic fractures using the ACS-TQIP database who received chemical VTE prophylaxis with either low molecular weight heparin (LMWH) or unfractionated heparin. Early VTE prophylaxis was defined as administration ≤48 hours from admission. The authors found that early VTE prophylaxis was associated with a lower incidence of VTE and improved survival. Utilization of LMWH was also an independent factor protective for both VTE and mortality, leading them to recommend LMWH for this indication.

In a 3-year, single-center retrospective review at a Level 1 trauma center, Jehan [38] analyzed data from two groups of patients with nonoperative pelvic fractures receiving chemoprophylaxis with LMWH. Patients receiving LMWH after 24 hours had a higher incidence of symptomatic deep venous thrombosis and longer hospital stay when compared to the group of patients receiving LMWH within the first hospital day.

Newer blood thinners such as direct oral anticoagulants (DOACs) have also been utilized for VTE prophylaxis in this patient population. Hamidi [39] utilized the ACS-TQIP database to perform a retrospective comparison of 852 patients with nonoperative pelvic fractures receiving either LMWH or DOAC. DOACs and LMWH were associated with similar rates of pulmonary embolism (PE), in-hospital mortality, and bleeding complications. However, DOAC use was associated with lower rates of deep venous thrombosis (DVT) (1.8% vs. 6.9%, $p < 0.01$) when compared to LMWH.

In a recent systematic review, Shu et al. [40] found that LMWH was associated with a lower risk of VTE and death and that early chemoprophylaxis within 24–48 hours of admission was associated with lower rates of both VTE and mortality.

In terms of prophylactic inferior vena cava (IVC) filter placement, the most recent evidence weighs against this practice. In a large retrospective database study, Stein et al. [41] analyzed the records of more than 1.4 million patients with orthopedic injuries including pelvic, femur, and tibia/fibular fractures using the National Inpatient Sample (NIS) database. The authors found that the majority of patients (68%) who received prophylactic IVC filters did not develop VTE and that in-hospital mortality was lower in patients who did not receive an IVC filter. Although the study was not designed to determine a causal relationship, the authors concluded that patients with these types of injuries should not have prophylactic IVC filters placed as a routine.

RECOMMENDATION

Early (within 24–48 hours of admission) chemical VTE prophylaxis with LMWH is preferred. Routine use of prophylactic IVC filtration is not recommended.

Grade of recommendation: B.

TABLE 28.1

Summary of Evidence and Recommendations

Question	Answer	Level of Evidence	Grade of Recommendation	References
What is the role of circumferential binders or sheets?	Insufficient evidence to recommend routine use	4	D	[4–9]
What is the role of REBOA?	Temporizing measures in conjunction with other maneuvers for hemorrhage control	4	C	[10–13]
What is the role of TXA?	Should be administered early to reduce blood loss in patients with shock or requiring transfusion	2	B	[14–18]
What is the role of preperitoneal pelvic packing?	Adjunctive maneuver in selected cases with shock and suspected ongoing hemorrhage.	4	C	[19–23]
Which patients should undergo pelvic angioembolization?	Patients with shock, ongoing transfusion requirements, and contrast extravasation	3	C	[26–28]
Is fecal diversion mandatory in all patients with open pelvic fractures?	No; fecal diversion should be considered in patients with rectal or perineal wounds	4	C	[29–31]
What is the optimal timing for operative pelvic fixation?	Earlier is generally better, once hemodynamic status allows; ideally 1–3 days postinjury	3	C	[32–36]
What are the respective role of early VTE prophylaxis and IVC filter placement?	Early (within 24–48 hours) prophylaxis with LMWH is preferred; IVC filter placement is not recommended	3	B	[37–41]

Editor's Note

Fortunately, only a tiny subset of the pelvic fracture population arrives hemodynamically unstable. But this subgroup has been demonstrated to routinely require more than 20 units of blood. Because these patients are exsanguinating, extreme measures have been employed as life preservers, often with little evidence of benefit. After we stopped using medical anti-shock trouser (MAST) suits, the "T-POD" became popular. It, like the MAST suit, ostensibly reduces bleeding by providing some compression of the pelvis. And also, like the MAST suit, it obscures our ability to examine the patient fully. The T-POD can also cause displacement of pelvic fractures, potentially worsening bleeding. Certainly, patients with this device in place (once they are receiving transfusions) can have the T-POD removed to determine its benefit in conjunction with the input of orthopedic surgeons. The value of REBOA in this setting is also questionable, as most patients stabilize quickly with adequate blood products. TXA is purported to be beneficial in the trauma population, but there is controversy over the large clinical trial, and there are no data on the pelvic fracture subgroup. Most of the remaining key questions reflect exclusively clinical experience and represent areas for future investigation.

REFERENCES

1. Mucha P, Farnell MB. Analysis of pelvic fracture management. J Trauma. 1984;24(5):379–386.
2. Demetriades D, Karaiskakis M, Toutouzas K, et al. Pelvic fractures: Epidemiology and predictors of associated abdominal injuries and outcomes. J Am Coll Surg. 2002;195(1):1–10.
3. Yoshihara H, Yoneoka D. Demographic epidemiology of unstable pelvic fracture in the United States from 2000 to 2009: trends and in-hospital mortality. J Trauma Acute Care Surg. 2014;76(2):380–385.
4. Naseem H, Nesbitt PD, Sprott DC, et al. An assessment of pelvic binder placement at a UK major trauma centre. Ann R Coll Surg Engl. 2018 Feb;100(2):101–105.
5. Parker WJ, Despain RW, Delgado A, et al. Pelvic binder utilization in combat casualties: Does it matter? Am Surg. 2020 Jul;86(7):873–877.
6. Schweigkofler U, Wohlrath B, Trentzsch H, et al. Is there any benefit in the pre-hospital application of pelvic binders in patients with suspected pelvic injuries? Eur J Trauma Emerg Surg. 2021 Apr;47(2):493–498.
7. Agri F, Bourgeat M, Becce F, et al. Association of pelvic fracture patterns, pelvic binder use and arterial angio-embolization with transfusion requirements and mortality rates; a 7-year retrospective cohort study. BMC Surg. 2017 Nov 9;17(1):104.
8. Hsu SD, Chen CJ, Chou YC, et al. Effect of early pelvic binder use in the emergency management of suspected pelvic trauma: A retrospective cohort study. Int J Environ Res Public Health. 2017 Oct 12;14(10):1217.
9. Prasarn ML, Conrad B, Small J, et al. Comparison of circumferential pelvic sheeting versus the T-POD on unstable pelvic injuries: A cadaveric study of stability. Injury. 2013 Dec;44(12):1756–1759.
10. Asmar S, Bible L, Chehab M, et al. Resuscitative endovascular balloon occlusion of the aorta vs pre-peritoneal packing in patients with pelvic fracture. J Am Coll Surg. 2021 Jan;232(1):17–26.
11. Harfouche M, Inaba K, Cannon J, et al. Patterns and outcomes of zone 3 REBOA use in the management of severe pelvic fractures: Results from the AAST aortic occlusion for resuscitation in trauma and acute care surgery database. J Trauma Acute Care Surg. 2021 Apr 1;90(4):659–665.
12. Laverty RB, Treffalls RN, McEntire SE, et al.; Aortic Occlusion for Resuscitation in Trauma and Acute Care Surgery (AORTA) Investigators. Life over limb: Arterial access-related limb ischemic complications in 48-hour REBOA survivors. J Trauma Acute Care Surg. 2022 Apr 1;92(4):723–728.
13. Joseph B, Zeeshan M, Sakran JV, Hamidi M, Kulvatunyou N, Khan M, O'Keeffe T, Rhee P. Nationwide analysis of resuscitative endovascular balloon occlusion of the aorta in civilian trauma. JAMA Surg. 2019 Jun 1;154(6):500–508.
14. CRASH-2 Trial Collaborators. Effects of tranexamic acid on death, vascular occlusive events, and blood transfusion in trauma patients with significant haemorrhage (CRASH-2): A randomized, placebo-controlled trial. Lancet. 2010;376: 23–32.
15. Morrison JJ, Dubose KK, Rasmussen TE, et al. Military application of Tranexamic Acid in trauma emergency resuscitation (MATTERs) study. Arch Surg. 2012;147(2):113–119.
16. Spitler CA, Row ER, Gardner WE, et al. Tranexamic acid use in open reduction and internal fixation of fractures of the pelvis, acetabulum, and proximal femur: A randomized controlled trial. J Orthopaedic Trauma. 2019;33(8):371–376.
17. Gümüştaş SA, Çelen ZE, Onay T, et al. The efficiency and safety of intravenous tranexamic acid administration in open reduction and internal fixation of pelvic and acetabular fractures. Eur J Trauma Emerg Surg. 2022 Feb;48(1):351–356.
18. Shu HT, Mikula JD, Yu AT, Shafiq B. Tranexamic acid use in pelvic and/or acetabular fracture surgery: A systematic review and meta-analysis. J Orthop. 2021 Dec 2;28:112–116.
19. Smith WR, Moore EE, Osborn P, et al. Retroperitoneal packing as a resuscitation technique for hemodynamically unstable patients with pelvic fractures: Report of two representative cases and a description of the technique. J Trauma. 2005;59(6):1510–1514.
20. Jang JY, Shim H, Jung PY, et al. Preperitoneal pelvic packing in patients with hemodynamic instability due to severe pelvic fracture: Early experience in a Korean trauma center. Scand J Trauma Resusc Emerg Med. 2016 Jan 13;24:3.
21. Moskowitz EE, Burlew CC, Moore EE, et al. Preperitoneal pelvic packing is effective for hemorrhage control in open pelvic fractures. Am J Surg. 2018 Apr;215(4)675–677.
22. Werner NL, Moore EE, Hoehn M, et al. Inflate and pack! Pelvic packing combined with REBOA deployment prevents hemorrhage-related deaths in unstable pelvic fractures. Injury. 2022 Oct;53(10):3365–3370.
23. Bugaev N, Rattan R, Goodman M, et al. Preperitoneal packing for pelvic fracture-associated hemorrhage: A systematic review, meta-analysis, and practice management guideline from the Eastern Association for the Surgery of Trauma. Am J Surg. 2020 Oct;220(4):873–888.
24. Young JW, Burgess AR, et al. Pelvic fractures: The value of plain radiography in early assessment and management. Radiology. 1986 Aug;160(2):445–451.

25. Costantini TW, Coimbra R, Holcomb JB, et al. AAST Pelvic Fracture Study Group. Pelvic fracture pattern predicts the need for hemorrhage control intervention-Results of an AAST multi-institutional study. J Trauma Acute Care Surg. 2017 Jun;82(6):1030–1038.

26. Juern JS, Milia D, Codner P, et al. Clinical significance of computed tomography contrast extravasation in blunt trauma patients with a pelvic fracture. J Trauma Acute Care Surg. 2017 Jan;82(1):138–140.

27. Kuo LW, Yang SJ, Fu CY, et al. Relative hypotension increases the probability of the need for angioembolisation in pelvic fracture patients without contrast extravasation on computed tomography scan. Injury. 2016 Jan;47(1):37–42.

28. Hammerschlag J, Hershkovitz Y, Ashkenazi I, et al. Angiography in patients with pelvic fractures and contrast extravasation on CT following high-energy trauma. Eur J Trauma Emerg Surg. 2022 Jun;48(3):1939–1944.

29. Faringer PD, Mullins RJ, Feliciano PD, et al. Selective fecal diversion in complex open pelvic fractures from blunt trauma. Arch Surg. 1994;129(9):958–963.

30. Hermans E, Edwards MJR, Goslings JC, et al. Open pelvic fracture: The killing fracture? J Orthop Surg Res. 2018 Apr 13;13(1):83.

31. Lunsjo K, Abu-Zidan FM. Does colostomy prevent infection in open blunt pelvic fractures? A systematic review. J Trauma. 2006;60(5):1145–1148.

32. Devaney GL, Bulman J, King KL, et al. Time to definitive fixation of pelvic and acetabular fractures. J Trauma Acute Care Surg. 2020 Oct;89(4):730–735.

33. Tiziani S, Halvachizadeh S, Knöpfel A, et al. Early fixation strategies for high energy pelvic ring injuries - the Zurich algorithm. Injury. 2021 Oct;52(10):2712–2718.

34. Tan JH, Wu TY, Tan JYH, et al. Definitive surgery is safe in borderline patients who respond to resuscitation. J Orthop Trauma. 2021 Jul 1;35(7):e234–e240.

35. Sharpe JP, Magnotti LJ, Gobbell WC, et al. Impact of early operative pelvic fixation on long-term self-reported outcome following a severe pelvic fracture. J Trauma Acute Care Surg. 2017 Mar;82(3):444–450.

36. Taylor NA, Smith AA, Marr A, et al. Does time to pelvic fixation influence outcomes in trauma patients? Am Surg. 2022 May;88(5):840–845.

37. Benjamin E, Aiolfi A, Recinos G, et al. Timing of venous thromboprophylaxis in isolated severe pelvic fracture: Effect on mortality and outcomes. Injury. 2019 Mar;50(3):697–702.

38. Jehan F, O'Keeffe T, Khan M, et al. Early thromboprophylaxis with low-molecular-weight heparin is safe in patients with pelvic fracture managed nonoperatively. J Surg Res. 2017 Nov;219:360–365.

39. Hamidi M, Zeeshan M, Sakran JV, et al. Direct oral anticoagulants vs low-molecular-weight heparin for thromboprophylaxis in nonoperative pelvic fractures. J Am Coll Surg. 2019 Jan;228(1):89–97.

40. Shu HT, Yu AT, Lim PK, et al. Chemoprophylaxis for venous thromboembolism in pelvic and/or acetabular fractures: A systematic review. Injury. 2022 Apr;53(4):1449–1454.

41. Stein PD, Matta F, Hughes MJ. Prophylactic inferior vena cava filters in patients with fractures of the pelvis or long bones. J Clin Orthop Trauma. 2018 Apr-Jun;9(2):175–180.

29

Extremity Vascular Injury

Eliza Fox, Andrew Lawson, and Terence O'Keeffe

29.1 Introduction

Extremity vascular injury caused by trauma remains a significant cause of mortality and morbidity in the injured patient. With technological advances, vascular surgery has changed dramatically over the past decade. Trauma surgeons are faced with these injuries daily and need to have the expertise to take care of these patients acutely. There is a growing body of evidence on which to base both diagnostic and therapeutic decisions in the acutely injured trauma patient with extremity vascular injury. This chapter will review the recent literature related to the diagnosis and management of acute vascular extremity trauma, divided into relevant clinical questions, with recommendations based on the most recent evidence.

29.2 Can a Diagnosis of Extremity Vascular Injury Be Adequately Made by Physical Exam Supplemented with Arterial Pressure Index?

Patients with "hard signs" of extremity vascular injury, including pulsatile bleeding, expanding hematoma, and pulselessness, have traditionally undergone emergent surgical exploration. This recommendation has not changed. In the absence of hard signs of vascular injury, the trauma surgeon is tasked with assessing the likelihood of occult vascular injury. The term "soft signs" has been used to describe concerning findings that may associate with vascular injury, including nonexpanding hematoma, neurological deficit, and proximity of injury trajectory to a major vascular structure.

A recent prospective multicenter study attempted to shift the distinction from hard versus soft signs of vascular injury to the identification of hemorrhagic and ischemic signs [1]. They propose that this can better inform the selection of therapeutic interventions, including the use of endovascular approaches and systemic anticoagulation in select cases. Given that the database was unable to provide sufficient clarity on the nature of these findings, it is reasonable to continue to use traditional hard signs as indicative of traumatic vascular injury.

Extremity arterial pressure indices (APIs), such as the ankle-brachial index (ABI), have long been used to augment the assessment of a patient's risk of vascular injury when an immediate operation is not indicated. A normal API is defined as ≥0.9. Both the Eastern Association for the Surgery of Trauma (EAST) and Western Trauma Associaton (WTA) algorithms for extremity vascular injury state that a patient with no concerning physical exam findings and a normal API may be discharged from the trauma bay [2, 3]. Indeed, a more recent meta-analysis determined the pooled posttest probability of arterial injury in the setting of normal physical exam and API ≥0.9 was 0% [4].

Several recent retrospective studies by Hemingway et al. have evaluated the possibility of lowering the API threshold at which computed tomographic angiography (CTA) is obtained, specifically in the setting of lower extremity injuries. In both blunt and penetrating lower extremity injuries, they found that CTA identified injuries in up to nearly 50% of patients; however, only 12% (blunt) and 35% (penetrating) required operative intervention [5, 6]. They proposed that an ABI threshold of 0.6 for blunt and 0.7 for penetrating injuries would have identified all patients requiring intervention. The follow-up of patients with radiographic abnormalities who did not undergo an operation is not well described. Although intriguing, there is insufficient evidence to support lowering the ABI threshold to 0.7.

> **RECOMMENDATION**
>
> Physical exam can adequately identify findings concerning extremity vascular injury. The API can help identify patients who require further workup for vascular injury, but in the absence of further studies, the threshold for this workup should remain at 0.9. Using API for diagnosis:
>
> Level of evidence: 2. Strength of recommendation: B.

29.3 What Role Do Tourniquets Play in the Management of Peripheral Vascular Injuries?

There has been a significant change in the use of prehospital tourniquets over the last decade, with the recognition that their use in civilian trauma has the potential to save lives, especially in mass casualty events. The Stop the Bleed campaign

DOI: 10.1201/9781003316800-29

(which came out of the Hartford consensus) focuses on tourniquet application and wound packing by bystanders and has now been taught to over 2 million people worldwide [7].

In the last edition of this book, we were forced primarily to rely on evidence from military studies, but we now have good data from the civilian arena. A single-center study published in 2019 compared a matched group of 204 patients who had prehospital tourniquets placed and showed a decrease in blood transfusions, as well as a decrease in limb complications, including amputation, in these patients [8]. Of note, the average time that the patients had the tourniquet in place was only 22.5 minutes; therefore, the results from this urban trauma center may not be applicable in rural areas.

In a multicenter study from 29 level I and II trauma centers in the United States, 1,130 tourniquets were applied on 1,392 injured limbs and these patients were compared to control patients who did not get tourniquets placed in the field [9]. They reported effective hemorrhage control by tourniquets in 87.7% of cases. The patients with tourniquets in place were also less likely to arrive in shock (13.0% vs. 17.4%). There was no difference in limb complications between groups. Of note, in this study, at least 77% of the patients had the tourniquet placed by emergency medical services (EMS), police or fire department, or a physician/nurse. This may have contributed to the effectiveness of the bleeding control.

In a separate study from 2022, the authors sounded a note of caution, as they found that a significant number of patients who had prehospital tourniquets placed did not have a major vascular injury and, by extension, did not have an indication for the tourniquet [10]. Although amputation rates were higher in the group that underwent prehospital tourniquet placement, this was not statistically significant. This suggests that we still have work to do in education and training on the appropriate placement of these devices.

RECOMMENDATION

The use of tourniquets for the management of prehospital control of peripheral vascular trauma has the potential to save lives with minimal morbidity. Tourniquet use for exsanguinating hemorrhage:

Level of evidence: 4. Strength of recommendation: C.

29.4 When Is a Computed Tomography Angiography Indicated for Extremity Vascular Trauma?

With the advent of CTA, there has been a major change in the workup of patients with suspected vascular injury, as these studies can be ordered 24/7 and have a much better safety profile than traditional angiography. Due to this convenience, there has been a significant decrease in the number of patients undergoing conventional angiography.

The clearest indication for patients to undergo a screening CTA is in the presence of abnormal ABIs. Traditionally, an ABI of less than 0.9 has been the cutoff for the need for further investigation, usually by CTA. A recent meta-analysis suggested that the performance of this test compared to a reference standard (CTA or Doppler ultrasound) was not accurate when used alone (pooled sensitivity of 49.5%; 39.3–60.1%), but the incidence of injury was low in these patients—just 14.3% across all patients [4]. Performance was improved with the addition of a physical examination (pooled sensitivity of 100%).

In a recent paper from Warwick et al., 135 CTA studies were performed with a 100% negative predictive value (when combined with a normal physical exam) [11]. A similar study by Brian et al. had similar results with a zero false-negative rate, and only one patient demonstrated a positive CTA that was not associated with an abnormal physician exam [12]. These authors concluded that the addition of CTA screening did not increase the diagnostic yield in these trauma patients without physical exam abnormalities, even those with proximity injuries and orthopedic trauma.

In a study from the PROspective Observational Vascular Injury Treatment (PROOVIT) registry in 2020, the authors compared patients with hard and soft signs and noted in patients with hard signs that 16.2% of patients still went on to get a CTA [1]. However, they also noted that those patients who were diagnosed with an injury on CTA were more likely to undergo an endovascular or hybrid repair (10.7% vs. 1.5%, $P < 0.05$). They did not comment specifically on the performance of CTA in this study, but they noted that patients who underwent CTA in the ischemic signs group received less blood and attributed this to the improved preoperative planning afforded by having this extra information available.

Similarly, a study by Bhalla et al. attempted to develop a scoring system to predict vessel transection compared to other injury types e.g. thrombosis, pseudoaneurysm, etc. [13]. While they were able to develop a score with a reasonable prediction for transection vs. thrombosis, this was not sufficiently predictive for other injury types despite the use of 64- and 128-slice scanners.

The remaining area of controversy that currently exists is whether the added information gained from obtaining a CTA in a nonhemorrhaging patient with hard signs, e.g. lack of pulse, justifies the extra ischemic time that is sacrificed to obtain this information. We remain in a data-free zone regarding this practice, and we continue to recommend immediate operative intervention in these patients rather than delaying care by obtaining a CTA study.

RECOMMENDATION

The use of CTA can help elucidate vascular injury in the presence of abnormal ABIs and no hard signs of vascular injury. Use of CTA for the diagnosis of extremity vascular injuries:

Level of evidence: 3. Strength of recommendation: B.

29.5 Which Extremity Vascular Injuries Are Appropriate for Endovascular Management?

Unlike the recommendations in favor of endovascular management of blunt thoracic aortic injury, there are no major society recommendations in favor of endovascular approaches to specific extremity vascular injuries [14]. This is likely because the use of endovascular interventions for trauma has expanded significantly over the past decade and large-scale studies and long-term follow-ups are limited. Common to all studies is the observation that the success of endovascular management is dependent on appropriate patient selection and institutional resources.

Endovascular options are particularly appealing for injuries at junctional locations (i.e. axillary-subclavian injuries) for which exposure and control may be difficult. Traditionally reserved for hemodynamically stable patients, endovascular approaches are now being recommended for some unstable patients due to the ability to achieve endoluminal hemorrhage control [15]. Boggs et al. demonstrated equivalent outcomes for axillary injuries managed by open and endovascular approaches, without a significant difference in procedural time [16]. This and other studies have shown short- and mid-term patency rates of >95%, suggesting noninferiority of endovascular management for these injuries [16, 17].

Multiple single-institution studies have evaluated the efficacy of endovascular therapy for other extremity vascular injuries, including those involving the femoral and popliteal vessels [18–20]. These studies note no difference in early limb salvage rates. A limitation common to many studies of extremity vascular trauma is the limited long-term follow-up to evaluate for complications of endovascular therapy, including stent kinking, migration, and intimal hyperplasia.

RECOMMENDATION

Endovascular management should be considered for axillary-subclavian injuries when its use will not delay hemorrhage control. Larger studies with adequate long-term follow-up are needed to support the routine use of endovascular therapy for other extremity vascular injuries.

Level of evidence: 4. Strength of recommendation: C.

29.6 Should Intravascular Shunting Be Used in the Management of Civilian Extremity Vascular Injuries?

The role of temporary intravascular shunting (TIVS) has come to the forefront in the last two decades due to the extensive experience from multiple conflicts that have involved many military organizations. The translation of this technique to civilian centers has been more haphazard, and the data have been difficult to evaluate. A recent military study looking at almost 600 patients demonstrated that only 14% of patients underwent temporary vascular shunting, with a 10% thrombosis rate of these shunts. They did not compare shunted versus nonshunted patients in this study [21].

Two multicenter civilian studies have been published in the last decade looking at these patients. The 2015 paper from the EAST organization prospectively evaluated 66 patients, and their endpoint was complications from shunt placement, defined as thrombosis, migration, and distal ischemia [22]. They had a comparable 9% risk of complications; two patients had dislodgement, three shunts thrombosed, and one patient had distal ischemia. The amputation rate was an impressively low 1.5%. They concluded that shunt complication rates were low and did not appear to be associated with dwell time in this study.

The larger American Association for the Study of Trauma (AAST)–sponsored study in 2016 was retrospective and included 213 injuries, with again low shunt thrombosis rates of 5.6% and dislodgement occurring in 1.4%. Limb salvage was again high at 96.3%. They found that the use of a noncommercial shunt (e.g. chest tube) was associated with subsequent graft failure, but no comparisons were made with patients who did not undergo shunting [23].

A cohort study performed in 2021 was notable in looking at whether TIVS placement was associated with improved outcomes, in which these patients were matched via propensity scores against nonshunted control patients [24]. They demonstrated a threefold higher likelihood of amputation in the control group compared to the TIVS patients. Other independently associated risk factors were nerve injuries, fractures, and pedestrians versus automobiles. TIVS patients were more likely to have thrombosis of the definitive repair, requiring operative intervention. Of note, follow-up was limited to only 12 days.

A systematic review of both civilian and military studies in 2022 attempted to synthesize the most recent data regarding the use of TIVS in trauma, identifying a total of 641 shunts in 564 patients [25]. As expected, there was significant heterogeneity across studies, but shunt thrombosis appeared to be lower in civilian trauma, with low rates of compartment syndrome in both groups. This review was unable to find significant advantages to the placement of TIVS other than those described in the Polcz study earlier.

There does appear to be a philosophical difference between trauma and vascular surgeons regarding the use of TIVS in vascular trauma. In a paper by Parihar et al., they showed no difference in outcomes between patients operating on either group, although the use of TIVS was less in the vascular surgery group [26]. This was a single-center study, and therefore cannot be generalized.

RECOMMENDATION

TIVS likely has a role to play in damage control situations and to allow for the repair of combined vascular/orthopedic injuries. Data showing improved outcomes in patients remain lacking, however. Use of TIVS in vascular extremity trauma:

Level of evidence: 4. Strength of recommendation: C.

29.7 What Are the Considerations in Choosing the Most Appropriate Conduit for Revascularization of an Acute Extremity Vascular Injury?

While most trauma surgeons prefer to primarily repair traumatically injured vessels, it is a frequent occurrence that the length or tension will not allow a primary repair. In such times, the surgeon performing the revascularization has to choose a conduit. The long-standing gold standard has been the saphenous vein. Recent long-term data out of the military, and published by Haney et al., demonstrate superior long-term patency when a saphenous vein was used for upper extremity vascular injuries [27]. However, there are times in which saphenous veins cannot be readily obtained such as major tissue loss, previous harvest, or a diminutive vessel.

A study by Vertrees in 2009 looked at outcomes given such a situation in combat victims in which the surgeon was forced to use a prosthetic graft due to substantial tissue loss or venous blowout. Eighty percent of the grafts remained patent in the short term [28]. This suggests that polytetrafluoroethylene (PTFE) may be readily used in the absence of a saphenous vein, either as a definitive treatment or, in the face of major contamination, as a bridge to definitive elective revascularization. A similar study was performed out of Buffalo demonstrating the virtue of a bovine carotid artery graft (BCAG) [29]. While they recommend autologous veins still be considered the standard of care, their study revealed BCAG to be a viable alternative for urgent revascularization.

RECOMMENDATION

The saphenous vein should be used as the standard of care for emergent revascularization. PTFE and BCAG can be considered if an autologous vein cannot be used.

Level of evidence: 2. Strength of recommendation: B.

29.8 Following Repair of an Acute Vascular Injury, Should Fasciotomies Be Performed Prophylactically?

Compartment syndrome following vascular injury repair is known to be due to a combination of ischemic insult and reperfusion injury. However, the indication for performing fasciotomies is not always clear. There are no large multi-institutional trials comparing patients receiving immediate fasciotomy at the time of revascularization to careful clinical observation. Practice patterns are further confounded by different definitions of compartment syndrome and a lack of uniformity in how to measure compartment syndrome.

A review of the National Trauma Data Bank (NTDB) by Farber allowed for a retrospective cohort of 543 patients undergoing early (<8 hours) fasciotomy versus 69 patients undergoing late fasciotomy following open repair of extremity vascular injury [30]. The early group had a lower amputation rate (8.5% vs. 24.6%) and shorter hospital stays (18.5% vs. 24.2%).

A great deal of our knowledge regarding the efficacy of fasciotomies in preventing the morbidity of compartment syndrome comes from the military, which has adopted a liberal policy of fasciotomy since combat data in 2008 revealed incomplete or delayed fasciotomy could be associated with additional morbidity and mortality [31]. A subsequent study in 2012 by Kragh et al. revealed that just the development of short educational programs targeted to active surgeons treating vascular injuries improved survival [32]. However, this continues to be an evolving discussion. Recent retrospective data from the military published by Kauvar et al. demonstrate the drawback to a liberal fasciotomy policy [33]. In this study, 84% of patients with vascular injury were given fasciotomy within 30 minutes of revascularization. The use of fasciotomy was associated with limb infection, motor dysfunction, and contracture.

A final area of controversy has been the timing of fasciotomies, with the standard being only patients with 6 hours of ischemia undergoing fasciotomies prophylactically. In a study looking at NTDB patients from 2019 with over 4,000 patients, the authors showed significant improvements in mortality rates with patients revascularized early (which was less than 1 hour in this study) [34]. Only early intervention was associated with improved outcomes, and fasciotomies did not influence amputation rates.

RECOMMENDATION

A liberal prophylactic fasciotomy rate following revascularization for acute traumatic vascular injury will prevent morbidity and mortality. However, the fasciotomy itself can be a source of morbidity, albeit limited.

Level of evidence: 2. Strength of recommendation: B.

29.9 What Is the Role of Anticoagulation during Revascularization of an Acute Traumatic Extremity Vascular Injury?

While the use of perioperative anticoagulation is a widely accepted practice for elective vascular surgeries, its use is still questioned by many in the setting of acute vascular trauma repair. There are no randomized trials to date, though many smaller studies show that using anticoagulation may lead to improved patency rates [35, 36]. Maher et al. published a retrospective cohort study in 2017 demonstrating improved arterial patency following repair in 393 patients without increasing the risk of bleeding [37]. However, the long-standing fear, that systemic anticoagulation in the setting of trauma, especially blunt trauma, might lead to further morbidity, remains.

In 2015, the AAST put together the PROOVIT registry, which collects ongoing multicenter data on modern vascular injuries. Loja et al. published a multicenter prospective cohort study in 2017 using PROOVIT data in which intraoperative systemic anticoagulation was not associated with a difference in the rate of repair thrombosis or limb loss, but was associated with an increase in blood product requirements and prolonged hospital stay [38].

RECOMMENDATION

While large multicenter prospective data are lacking, it does seem that there may be a benefit in utilizing anticoagulation intraoperatively for the acute repair of traumatic vascular injury, especially in isolated penetrating injury. We caution against its use in major blunt trauma, specifically when a head or visceral injury is known or suspected.

Level of evidence: 4. Strength of recommendation: C.

29.10 Conclusions

In this chapter, we have presented the best and most recent data regarding pertinent clinical questions in extremity vascular trauma. The emergent nature of this topic does not lend itself to randomized controlled trials, but with the advent of the PROOVIT registry in 2015, we are finally starting to get higher-quality data on some of the areas that remain controversial such as tourniquets and the shunting of vessels. Clinical questions do remain, however, such as whether the API threshold should be lowered, the role of postoperative anticoagulation, and the necessity of postoperative imaging. Trauma surgeons need to remain engaged in the field of vascular surgery so that these questions can be investigated and answered in the future.

	Question	Answer	Grade	Refs.
1	Can a diagnosis of extremity vascular injury be adequately made by physical exam supplemented with arterial pressure index (API)?	Physical exam with ABI is more than 90% sensitive for the presence of vascular injury.	B	[1–6]
2	What role do tourniquets play in the management of peripheral vascular injuries?	The use of tourniquets for the management of prehospital control of peripheral vascular trauma has the potential to save lives with minimal morbidity.	C	[7–10]
3	When is a computed tomography angiography (CTA) indicated for extremity vascular trauma?	The use of CTA can be helpful in elucidating vascular injury in the presence of abnormal ABIs and no hard signs of vascular injury.	B	[1, 4, 11–13]
4	Which extremity vascular injuries are appropriate for endovascular management?	Endovascular management should be considered for axillary-subclavian injuries when its use will not delay hemorrhage control.	C	[14–20]
5	Should intravascular shunting be used in the management of civilian extremity vascular injuries?	Temporary intravascular shunting can be considered in damage control situations and to allow for the repair of combined vascular/orthopedic injuries.	C	[21–26]
6	What are the considerations in choosing the most appropriate conduit for revascularization of an acute extremity vascular injury?	The saphenous vein should be used as the standard of care for emergent revascularization. PTFE and BCAG can be considered if an autologous vein cannot be used.	B	[27–29]
7	Following repair of an acute vascular injury, should fasciotomies be performed prophylactically?	A liberal prophylactic fasciotomy rate following revascularization for acute traumatic vascular injury will prevent morbidity and mortality.	B	[30–34]
8	What is the role of anticoagulation during revascularization of an acute traumatic extremity vascular injury?	There is likely benefit from intraoperative use of anticoagulation in peripheral vascular trauma, although there is insufficient evidence to use this as standard of care.	C	[35–38]

Editor's Note

The care of extremity vascular injury is informed by the data on the revascularization of patients with peripheral vascular disease. The primary difference is the typical delay in revascularization that is inherent in the transport of patients from the scene of the blunt or penetrating injury. This delay creates a fertile environment of ischemia and the need for rapid interventions (such as vascular shunts) and fasciotomy to minimize the impact of delays in reperfusion. In addition, associated bony injury, often associated with blunt force trauma and high-velocity injury, may represent additional obstacles to the success of revascularization. Recent analysis suggests that the "6-hour rule" for developing irreversible ischemia is inaccurate and that each hour of extremity ischemia increases the likelihood of limb loss and death [34]. Finally, the recognition that morbidity increases continuously with time to reperfusion suggests that reducing time to the operating room and subsequent restoration of blood flow are critical.

REFERENCES

1. Romagnoli, A.N., et al., *Hard signs gone soft: A critical evaluation of presenting signs of extremity vascular injury.* J Trauma Acute Care Surg, 2021. **90**(1): p. 1–10.
2. Feliciano, D.V., et al., *Evaluation and management of peripheral vascular injury. Part 1. Western Trauma Association/critical decisions in trauma.* J Trauma, 2011. **70**(6): p. 1551–1556.
3. Fox, N., et al., *Evaluation and management of penetrating lower extremity arterial trauma: An Eastern Association for the Surgery of Trauma practice management guideline.* J Trauma Acute Care Surg, 2012. **73**(5 Suppl 4): p. S315–S320.

4. deSouza, I.S., et al., *Accuracy of physical examination, ankle-brachial index, and ultrasonography in the diagnosis of arterial injury in patients with penetrating extremity trauma: A systematic review and meta-analysis.* Acad Emerg Med, 2017. **24**(8): p. 994–1017.

5. Hemingway, J., et al., *Lowering the ankle-brachial index threshold in blunt lower extremity trauma may prevent unnecessary imaging.* Ann Vasc Surg, 2020. **62**: p. 106–113.

6. Hemingway, J., et al., *Re-evaluating the safety and effectiveness of the 0.9 ankle-brachial index threshold in penetrating lower extremity trauma.* J Vasc Surg, 2020. **72**(4): p. 1305–1311 e1.

7. Jacobs, L.M., et al., *Improving survival from active shooter events: The Hartford consensus.* J Trauma Acute Care Surg, 2013. **74**(6): p. 1399–1400.

8. Smith, A.A., et al., *Prehospital tourniquet use in penetrating extremity trauma: Decreased blood transfusions and limb complications.* J Trauma Acute Care Surg, 2019. **86**(1): p. 43–51.

9. Schroll, R., et al., *AAST multicenter prospective analysis of prehospital tourniquet use for extremity trauma.* J Trauma Acute Care Surg, 2022. **92**(6): p. 997–1004.

10. Legare, T., et al., *Prehospital tourniquets placed on limbs without major vascular injuries, has the pendulum swung too far?* Am Surg, 2022. **88**(9): p. 2103–2107.

11. Warwick, H., et al., *Comparison of computed tomography angiography and physical exam in the evaluation of arterial injury in extremity trauma.* Injury, 2021. **52**(7): p. 1727–1731.

12. Brian, R., et al., *Computed tomography angiography is associated with low added utility for detecting clinically relevant vascular injuries among patients with extremity trauma.* Trauma Surg Acute Care Open, 2021. **6**(1): p. e000828.

13. Bhalla, D., et al., *Imaging in extremity vascular trauma: Can MDCT angiography predict the nature of injury?* Emerg Radiol, 2022. **29**(4): p. 683–690.

14. Kobayashi, L., et al., *American association for the surgery of trauma-world society of emergency surgery guidelines on diagnosis and management of peripheral vascular injuries.* J Trauma Acute Care Surg, 2020. **89**(6): p. 1183–1196.

15. Jinadasa, S.P., et al., *Endovascular management of axillo-subclavian artery injuries.* J Trauma Acute Care Surg, 2022. **92**(2): p. e28–e34.

16. Boggs, H.K., et al., *Analysis of traumatic axillo-subclavian vessel injuries: Endovascular management is a viable option to open surgical reconstruction.* Ann Vasc Surg, 2022. **79**: p. 25–30.

17. Waller, C.J., et al., *Contemporary management of subclavian and axillary artery injuries-A Western Trauma Association multicenter review.* J Trauma Acute Care Surg, 2017. **83**(6): p. 1023–1031.

18. Ganapathy, A., et al., *Endovascular management for peripheral arterial trauma: The new norm?* Injury, 2017. **48**(5): p. 1025–1030.

19. Degmetich, S., et al., *Endovascular repair is a feasible option for superficial femoral artery injuries: A comparative effectiveness analysis.* Eur J Trauma Emerg Surg, 2022. **48**(1): p. 321–328.

20. Potter, H.A., et al., *Endovascular versus open repair of isolated superficial femoral and popliteal artery injuries.* J Vasc Surg, 2021. **74**(3): p. 814–822 e1.

21. Sharrock, A.E., et al., *Management and outcome of 597 wartime penetrating lower extremity arterial injuries from an international military cohort.* J Vasc Surg, 2019. **70**(1): p. 224–232.

22. Tung, L., et al., *Temporary intravascular shunts after civilian arterial injury: A prospective multicenter Eastern Association for the Surgery of Trauma study.* Injury, 2021. **52**(5): p. 1204–1209.

23. Inaba, K., et al., *Multicenter evaluation of temporary intravascular shunt use in vascular trauma.* J Trauma Acute Care Surg, 2016. **80**(3): p. 359–364; discussion 364–365.

24. Polcz, J.E., et al., *Temporary intravascular shunt use improves early limb salvage after extremity vascular injury.* J Vasc Surg, 2021. **73**(4): p. 1304–1313.

25. Laverty, R.B., Treffalls, R.N., Kauvar, D.S. *Systematic review of temporary intravascular shunt use in military and civilian extremity trauma.* J Trauma Acute Care Surg, 2022. **92**(1): p. 232–238.

26. Parihar, S., et al., *Vascular surgeons carry an increasing responsibility in the management of lower extremity vascular trauma.* Ann Vasc Surg, 2021. **70**: p. 87–94.

27. Haney, L.J., et al., *Patency of arterial repairs from wartime extremity vascular injuries.* Trauma Surg Acute Care Open, 2020. **5**(1): p. e000616.

28. Vertrees, A., et al., *The use of prosthetic grafts in complex military vascular trauma: A limb salvage strategy for patients with severely limited autologous conduit.* J Trauma, 2009. **66**(4): p. 980–983.

29. Reilly, B., et al., *Comparison of autologous vein and bovine carotid artery graft as a bypass conduit in arterial trauma.* Ann Vasc Surg, 2019. **61**: p. 246–253.

30. Farber, A., et al., *Early fasciotomy in patients with extremity vascular injury is associated with decreased risk of adverse limb outcomes: A review of the National Trauma Data Bank.* Injury, 2012. **43**(9): p. 1486–1491.

31. Ritenour, A.E., et al., *Complications after fasciotomy revision and delayed compartment release in combat patients.* J Trauma, 2008. **64**(2 Suppl): p. S153–S161; discussion S161–S162.

32. Kragh, J.F., Jr., et al., *Compartment syndrome performance improvement project is associated with increased combat casualty survival.* J Trauma Acute Care Surg, 2013. **74**(1): p. 259–263.

33. Kauvar, D.S., et al., *Early fasciotomy and limb salvage and complications in military lower extremity vascular injury.* J Surg Res, 2021. **260**: p. 409–418.

34. Alarhayem, A.Q., et al., *Impact of time to repair on outcomes in patients with lower extremity arterial injuries.* J Vasc Surg, 2019. **69**(5): p. 1519–1523.

35. Masood, A., et al., *The utility of therapeutic anticoagulation in the perioperative period in patients presenting in emergency surgical department with extremity vascular injuries.* Cureus, 2020. **12**(6): p. e8473.

36. Khan, S., et al., *A meta-analysis on anticoagulation after vascular trauma.* Eur J Trauma Emerg Surg, 2020. **46**(6): p. 1291–1299.

37. Maher, Z., et al., *Systemic intraoperative anticoagulation during arterial injury repair: Implications for patency and bleeding.* J Trauma Acute Care Surg, 2017. **82**(4): p. 680–686.

38. Loja, M.N., et al., *Systemic anticoagulation in the setting of vascular extremity trauma.* Injury, 2017. **48**(9): p. 1911–1916.

30

Management of Extremity Trauma and Mangled Extremities

Stephanie Lumpkin and Suresh K. Agarwal

30.1 Introduction

Surgical decision-making in the setting of limb-threatening trauma is complex and time-sensitive. Although the multifaceted and emergent nature of this injury pattern has precluded the highest levels of a clinical study, evidence-based guidelines can be discerned from available clinical reviews, case series, and general clinical consensus. From the multitude of published literature on this topic, several strategies have been advocated to simplify the process and minimize morbidity and mortality from extremity trauma. The objective of this chapter is to identify and expand on evidence-based strategies that influence treatment decisions aimed at maximizing functional recovery following traumatic upper or lower extremity injury, including when to consider limb salvage versus amputation. The most recent advances in the literature have translated military combat experience to knowledge gaps in the civilian literature.

Upper and lower extremity trauma have various treatment paradigms, which reflect their unique subspecialty preferences, though this chapter focuses on the treatment of various injury patterns and complications to the extremities, such as bites, skin, and soft tissue infections. While these injuries are less severe than the subsequent mangled extremity, they are frequently seen in practice, and mismanagement can have devastating consequences.

Across the spectrum of extremity injury, the mangled lower extremity requires the greatest attention. The term *mangled extremity* describes a limb in which at least three of the four components (soft tissue, nerve, bone, vessel) are severely injured [1]. *Limb salvage* is defined as an attempt to restore structure and neurovascular function to a mangled extremity. While substantial advances have been made in reconstructive techniques, heroic measures for limb salvage do not necessarily provide superior quality of life and limb outcomes even if reconstructive efforts produce a viable limb [2–5].

Primary amputation is defined as an extremity amputation that is performed at the original operation for injury (i.e., in which limb salvage efforts were not pursued). In some cases, primary amputation may offer the patient an expedited and superior functional outcome [6, 7]. A *secondary amputation* is defined as an extremity amputation that takes place following any attempt for limb salvage (i.e., following intent to treat or intent to salvage). Secondary amputation is further divided into *early* (an amputation within 30 days following

the initial intent to salvage) and *late* (an amputation performed greater than 30 days following the initial intent to salvage). Whether early or late, a secondary amputation is performed at a subsequent operation when the measures to salvage a limb are deemed unsuccessful, futile, or detrimental to the patient.

An overarching factor that guides early decision-making is selecting the course that will optimize functional recovery. An intricate limb repair that does not enable the patient to perform activities at a level comparable to a similar patient with a primary or secondary amputation does a disservice to the patient and poses an economic burden on healthcare resources [3, 8, 9]. While there is a paucity of high-level data that guide strategies in the treatment of extremity trauma, this chapter poses relevant questions and recommendations to highlight the strongest clinical evidence on this challenging topic.

30.2 How Are Common Soft Tissue Infections Such as Human or Animal Bites, Flexor Tenosynovitis, and Hand Abscess Treated, and Are the Current Empiric Antibiotics Used Based on Clinical Evidence?

Infections of the hand can occur because of bites from humans or animals. A "fight bite" is when a closed fist punch results in the breaking of the skin by a tooth. This violates the extensor tendon and joint capsule and may injure the metacarpal head, inoculating the metacarpophalangeal (MCP) joint [10]. Because of the limited soft tissue envelope that covers the deeper structures and numerous tight compartments, bite wounds to the hand have a higher infection rate [11]. While dog bites are the most prevalent, they have the lowest infection rates (14.3%) compared to cats (37.1%) and up to 25% in human bites [12, 13].

Although most bites are polymicrobial, antibiotic selection initially is empiric and based on the most common organisms found in the mouth. This includes *Staphylococcus* species and *Eikenella corrodens* for humans and *Pasteurella* species for animals. Unusual microbial contamination can often complicate human and animal bites, as these are often associated with plants, water, and soil exposure [14]. A broad-spectrum antibiotic such as Unasyn or Augmentin is usually the first line of therapy. Tetanus prophylaxis and rabies prevention

DOI: 10.1201/9781003316800-30

should also be considered. Transmission of viruses is less common, especially after human bites, but hepatitis B and C, human immunodeficiency virus (HIV), syphilis, herpes simplex virus, and human T-lymphotropic virus–1 have been documented [15–20]. If the wound is relatively superficial, generous cleansing of the wound may be all that is needed. Deeper and more complex bites may require operative intervention and debridement of necrotic tissue. Patients should be placed on antibiotics and the hand splinted and elevated for comfort.

Hand infections can be more severe in those who are immunocompromised, including diabetics and smokers [21, 23]. Flexor tenosynovitis can occur when the infection affects the flexor tendon sheath. Purulent fluid in the synovial space surrounding the tendon denies the tendon vital nutrition, and increased pressure in the infected sheath can inhibit blood flow to the tendon, causing necrosis [23].

The classic sign of flexor tenosynovitis is Kanavel's sign: Pain on extension of a digit, the semi-flexed position of the digit, fusiform swelling of a digit, and tenderness along the flexor sheath with frequent extension into the palm [24]. Early infection, less than 24 hours after onset, can be successfully managed medically with antibiotics, elevation, and splinting. For infections with subcutaneous purulence or necrotic tendon, open exposure of the sheath and irrigation through windows sparing the A2 and A4 pulleys is necessary. In all but the most severe infections, drainage can be accomplished through the placement of an irrigation catheter at the A1 pulley (distal palmar crease) with a counter incision and drain left at the A5 pulley (volar distal interphalangeal [DIP] joint). Irrigation of the sheath is then accomplished using normal saline. The catheter may be left and irrigation attempted on the floor for the next 24–48 hours without the need to return to the operating room (OR) [25]. Other forms of hand infections like an abscess or felon need to be drained as any other abscess in the body. A longitudinal incision from the distal flexion crease to the pulp apex avoids the neurovascular bundles and permits disruption of the septal compartments [10].

Antibiotic prophylaxis (AP) is not recommended for all bites, but there is mixed evidence for bites occurring in the hand, foot, or over cartilaginous zones. A 2009 systematic review and meta-analysis were completed to assess infection rates in mammalian bites among those receiving AP vs. no AP. Overall, they did not find any benefit of AP, except in high-risk anatomical locations (hands, feet, cartilaginous zones) and human bites. Injuries located at the hand showed a higher rate of complications if not treated with AP (2% in the antibiotic group vs. 28% in the control, odds ratio [OR] 0.1 95% confidence interval [CI] 0.01–0.86) [13]. This was consistent in Cicuttin et al.'s 2022 systematic review of AP in various traumatic lesions [14].

Current guidelines show that penicillin-based antibiotics are useful in soft tissue infections. Augmentin is suitable for its broad-spectrum therapy and is commonly used in the management of open fractures [14]. The ineffectiveness of flucloxacillin, erythromycin, and cephalosporins in *Pasteurella* infections suggests that Augmentin should be used routinely in animal bites and scratches [14]. Clindamycin is a good alternative in penicillin-allergic patients unless *Pasteurella* species are

identified [15]. Oral antibiotic therapy should continue between 10 and 14 days for cellulitis and at least 3 weeks if deeper tissue is involved.

RECOMMENDATION

Augmentin is the antibiotic of choice for animal bites due to frequent Pasteurella. Thorough cleansing of the wound for shallow wounds and excisional debridements for deeper wounds may be necessary.

Level of evidence: 1. Grade of recommendation: A.

30.3 When Is It Appropriate to Operate on Scaphoid Fractures, and What Are the Diagnostic Techniques Employed?

Scaphoid fractures of the wrist are one of the most common fractures clinicians will manage. Unfortunately, it is also relatively difficult to manage, as imaging studies can often miss the fracture. Failure to immobilize scaphoid fractures risks nonunion, functional morbidity, and eventual arthritic degeneration [16]. Therefore, this injury must always be considered after significant falls on an outstretched hand.

The presenting symptom of these fractures is "snuff box" tenderness along the radial side of the wrist. Alternatively, pain with digital pressure over the scaphoid tubercle may indicate a scaphoid fracture [16]. History and physical examination alone are inadequate to rule out scaphoid fractures [17]. Imaging studies generally start with plain wrist views.

Computed tomography (CT), magnetic resonance imaging (MRI), and bone scanning are other modalities of imaging. Advanced imaging in patients with signs of a scaphoid injury within days of the injury reduces unnecessary immobilization that limits activity in patients who ultimately do not have a scaphoid fracture [17]. MRI is diagnostically superior to CT, bone scan, ultrasound, or physical examination [17]. The SMaRT (Scaphoid Magnetic Resonance Imaging in Trauma) trial found that immediate MRI in suspected scaphoid fractures was less expensive and had higher diagnostic accuracy than usual care (plain radiographs and immobilization) [18].

The traditional treatment for nondisplaced scaphoid fractures is nonoperative. The blood supply of the scaphoid bone travels from a distal to proximal direction; thus, fractures at the waist are much more likely to develop a nonunion. Displaced fractures of the scaphoid have a four times higher risk of nonunion than nondisplaced fractures when treated with a cast only [6]. Instead, aggressive conservative management should remain the mainstay for scaphoid fractures. Fracture healing can be assessed with plain radiographs or CT after 6–8 weeks of cast immobilization. In minimally displaced scaphoid fractures (<2 mm) without neurovascular compromise or suspected nonunion, nonoperative immobilization is preferred, and patient-reported outcomes at 1-year postinjury were similar between surgical and nonoperatively managed groups regarding wrist function in a SWIFFT trial [19]. Similar findings were confirmed in a meta-analysis of seven randomized controlled trials (RCTs), which found no difference in wrist function, pain, range of motion, grip strength, and union, but the operative group had higher rates of complications [20].

RECOMMENDATION

MRI is useful to diagnose scaphoid fractures. Fracture healing can be assessed with plain radiographs or CT after 6–8 weeks of cast immobilization. Surgical fixation with or without bone grafting can be performed if a gap is identified at the fracture site.

Level of evidence: 1. Grade of recommendation: A.

30.4 What Are the Indications for Replantation of Digits and Extremities?

30.4.1 Indications for Reimplantation

- Thumb
- Multiple digits
- Single-digit distal to flexor digitorum profundus (FDP) insertion
- Upper extremity and palm/Wrist/Forearm
- Proximal to elbow if a sharp amputation
- Almost any amputation in a child

30.4.2 Contraindications

- Crushed/Mangled parts
- Multilevel amputation
- Prolonged ischemia time
- Medical comorbidities
- Life-threatening injuries

30.4.3 Relative Contraindications

- Single digit in an adult
- Heavy contamination
- Self-mutilation
- Avulsion

The goals of replantation are to restore circulation and regain sufficient function and sensation of the amputated part, as well as to allow patients to return to their previous employment [22]. Not all amputees will benefit from replantation. Strict selection criteria should be defined to optimize the result.

Amputations are characterized into two main categories: Complete and incomplete [23]. Incomplete segments are connected to the proximal stump with a bridge of tissue. Incomplete amputations are further subdivided based on the viability of the remaining stump, whether the distal tissue segment maintains sufficient blood circulation and if it needs major additional microvascular reconstruction.

The injury type is the most important factor in determining the survival rate and overall functional outcome [22]. Clean-cut amputations are a good indication for replanting, whereas crush injuries and avulsion amputations have poorer outcomes [23].

The level of functional disability should be determined. For instance, the thumb should be given priority for replantation, as it is responsible for about 40% of hand function [24]. Patients with multiple-digit amputations should be given priority for replanting to preserve the hand's function [22].

In the Finger Replantation and Amputation Challenges in Assessing Impairment, Satisfaction, and Effectiveness (FRANCHISE) multicenter international cohort study, 338 adult patients with traumatic digit amputations reported less pain, less disability, higher quality of life, and improved hand function after replantation than secondary amputation [25].

Amputation at the mid-palm is also an absolute indication for replanting and is seen to have a high functional outcome when at the level of the superficial or deep palmar arch [22]. Replantation following amputation at the wrist has excellent potential for functional recovery and should be attempted.

The goal of treatment for fingertip amputations too distal for microvascular replantation is to restore a painless, minimally shortened digit and durable sensate skin on the tip [26]. Therapeutic options range from allowing the wound to heal by secondary intention, to primary closure with or without bone shortening, skin grafts, composite grafts, and local, regional, or distant flaps [26]. Composite grafts may allow the patient to maintain digital length and function while retaining a cosmetically pleasing finger. If it does not survive, finger shortening and closure can then be performed [27].

The amount of ischemia time tolerated is directly proportional to the amount of muscle present in the amputated segment. Until recently, viability times to reimplantation were based on anecdotal data and dogmatically showed that 6 hours of warm ischemia time and 12 hours of cold ischemia time were the limits. More recently, a review found that there was little consistency in the storage of the digit. The proper way to store a digit is wrapped loosely in saline-soaked gauze and placed in an airtight container. With this consistency, they suggest that delayed reimplantation can be successful, which is critical for overnight injuries and transfers from rural locations. Cooling an amputated digit allows for extended ischemia time of up to 30 hours. One must be cognizant that life-threatening complications may follow major replantation because of free radical production at the time of vascular reperfusion [28].

In addition to time, the mechanism of injury is also directly proportional to the success of reimplantation. With crush or avulsion injuries with extensive tissue disruption or contamination, such as lawnmower injuries or machinery injuries, reimplantation may not be feasible. In a systematic review of the case series, ectopic temporary reimplantation of amputated parts to a clean and viable recipient base may be considered, but there is limited evidence regarding the true indications [29].

The presence of life-threatening injuries or general conditions that prohibit a long surgical procedure is a contraindication to replantation attempts. Patients who smoke should be advised to quit smoking, as the vasoconstrictive properties of nicotine correlate with a decreased survival rate as compared to nonsmokers [30]. Diseases that deteriorate peripheral circulation, like atherosclerosis, autoimmune disease, and diabetes mellitus, can reduce survival rate and functional outcome, thus constituting a relative contraindication for replantation [24].

RECOMMENDATIONS

Indications for replantation include the thumb, multiple digits, upper extremity amputated at the wrist, mid-palm, forearm, and almost any amputation in a child.

Level of evidence: 5. Grade of recommendation: B.

Proper storage of amputated limbs and digits in saline-soaked gauze in an airtight container improves outcomes. Major limbs should be reimplanted within 6 hours and digits within 12 hours, though this time can be extended for pragmatic reasons with reasonable success. Cooling an amputated digit allows for extended ischemia time of up to 30 hours.

Level of evidence: 3. Grade of recommendation: B.

30.5 What Are the Indications for the Release of Forearm Compartment Syndrome, Hand Compartment Syndrome, and Acute Carpal Tunnel Syndrome?

Compartment syndrome is a surgical emergency. Compartment syndrome exists when fascial compartment pressures exceed perfusion pressure, leading to tissue ischemia [31]. Delaying the diagnosis can lead to functional, cosmetic, and legal ramifications. The diagnosis of compartment syndrome is often clinical with the main symptom being pain out of proportion to the injury. Paresthesias may occur early; this represents a potentially reversible state because peripheral nerves are more sensitive to ischemia than muscle [31]. Irreversible ischemia begins about 8 hours after the onset of ischemia [31]. By the time pallor, pulselessness, and poikilothermia are observed, ischemic changes may be irreversible. When the physical diagnosis is inconclusive, compartmental pressures can be measured. A value below 30 mmHg is the cutoff for inadequate perfusion to the extremity [31].

The forearm contains four interconnected compartments with a significant amount of musculature. The hand contains 10 compartments that have much less muscle mass. Even though the digits lack muscle, they can undergo increased pressures because of restriction. The median nerve is the most frequently damaged nerve in the forearm because of its course deep in the volar forearm. Some authors advocate routine decompression of the carpal tunnel in conjunction with forearm fasciotomies [32].

Although compartment syndrome has the potential for devastating consequences, if intervention is provided on a prompt basis, patients can recover fully with minimal residual dysfunction of the forearm or hand [32].

RECOMMENDATION

Compartment syndrome is a surgical emergency. When the physical exam is inconclusive, compartment pressures should be measured; a delta pressure of less than 30 mmHg signifies inadequate perfusion and should prompt emergent decompression.

Level of evidence: 1. Grade of recommendation: A.

30.6 Which Management Strategies Reduce the Impact of Ischemia and Reperfusion Injury on Limb Salvage Following Trauma?

In the setting of extremity vascular injury, the ability to save an injured limb is based on the ability to restore adequate perfusion. Over 50% of patients with severe extremity injuries will have additional injuries, many of which are life-threatening [33, 34]. Treatment of a life-threatening torso, head, or neck injury takes priority over the definitive repair of an extremity vascular injury, leaving the limb at high risk of amputation as the negative impact of ischemic time is increased [28].

While the placement of an autologous vein interposition graft is the most common and often ideal form of repair, it is a time-consuming endeavor that is not feasible in the setting of progressive coagulopathy, acidosis, and hypothermia. In the setting of life-threatening polytrauma, the successful application of damage control techniques is based on early recognition of pending patient demise with adjustment of the operative plan. Damage control strategies for extremity arterial and venous injuries include abbreviated lateral vessel repair, placement of a temporary vascular shunt (TVS), and vessel ligation with or without the performance of a primary amputation.

Many consider vessel ligation a technique of last resort, but as demonstrated over 50 years ago by DeBakey and Simeone in a series of 2,471 vascular injuries treated during World War II, ligation of a major extremity vessel does not uniformly lead to amputation [36]. The introduction of *selective vessel ligation* in the setting of extremity vessel injuries reduced the amputation rate from nearly 100% to 49%. Another example of the concept of selective vessel ligation rests in an analysis of patients with brachial artery injury, which demonstrated a twofold difference in amputation rates depending on whether the artery was ligated above (55%) or below (26%) the profunda brachii artery. A similar relationship in the rates of lower extremity amputation has been reported for femoral artery injuries: 81% lower extremity amputation rate if the ligation is above the profunda femoris artery versus 55% if ligation occurs below the profunda femoris artery.

Venous ligation is generally better tolerated than arterial ligation. While the direct impact of venous ligation on amputation rates has been reported to be low, ligation of large lower extremity veins has been found to result in thrombosis, significant venous hypertension, and postphlebitic syndrome [37, 38]. Injuries resulting from high-energy mechanisms, particularly those resulting from explosive devices or high-velocity gun-shot wounds, strip collateral venous drainage from the extremity—potentiating lifestyle-limiting venous hypertension [39]. In the largest post-Vietnam review of venous injuries, Quan et al. from Walter Reed reported a retrospective analysis of 82 patients with 103 extremity venous injuries due to combat injuries [38]. In this 2008 study, 63% of extremity venous injuries were treated by ligation, while the remaining 37% were repaired. Importantly, this study reported an 84% midterm patency of venous repair and showed that patients with extremity vein repair did not experience a higher incidence of pulmonary embolus than patients treated with venous ligation. All patients in this landmark report developed postinjury edema of the extremity, and there was a trend toward an increased deep venous thrombosis (DVT) rate (14% vs. 7%) and phlegmasia (2% vs. 0%) in the group treated by venous ligation [38].

Another tool that can be used in the setting of vascular injury is the TVS. These devices are used routinely during the performance of carotid endarterectomy but have also been utilized as a damage control adjunct as a means of quickly restoring perfusion to an extremity in the setting of vascular injury. Gifford et al. have recently reported the impact of TVS on long-term limb salvage in a case-control study of 125 patients with severe extremity injuries [40]. In this sentinel report, there were more early amputations performed in the control than in the TVS group (13% vs. 3%; $p = 0.04$); however, after nearly 2 years of follow-up, there was no significant difference in the amputation rate (17% vs. 23%; $p = 0.42$). After adjusting for a Mangled Extremity Severity Score (MESS) greater than 8, the TVS group had a significantly lower risk of amputation (hazard ratio [HR] = 0.43; $p = 0.04$). In a matched cohort analysis, patients treated initially without TVS were three times more likely to require a secondary amputation than those treated with TVS (OR 3.6, 95% CI 1.2–11.1) [41]. In a systematic review of TVS in civilian and military populations, those with shunts consistently had high injury severity scores but similar limb salvage rates as those who did not receive shunts [42]. Additionally, the Eastern Association for the Surgery of Trauma conducted a prospective, multicenter study of adults undergoing TVS for arterial injury and found that even damage control indications for surgery did not increase the amount of TVS complications (11% damage control compared to 8% non–damage control indications, $p = 0.658$) [43]. Outcomes data such as these suggest that TVS does not cause harm in the setting of extremity vascular injury and likely extends the window of opportunity for limb salvage.

RECOMMENDATIONS

Arterial ligation may be used as a damage control maneuver, understanding that there is an increased incidence of extremity amputation. Large vessel venous injuries should be repaired when feasible to avoid thromboses and phlegmasia. TVS are an effective damage control adjunct.

Level of evidence: 2. Grade of recommendation: B.

30.7 Is There a Difference in Limb Salvage Strategies in the Setting of Upper versus Lower Extremity Injury?

While severe extremity injuries are less common in the upper extremity, the complex and important function of the hand presents unique considerations that require modification in management strategies. Because of the relatively smaller size and increased collateralization, ligation of upper extremity vascular injuries is better tolerated than those of the lower extremity [35, 36]. Specifically, the radial or ulnar, but not both, can be ligated without sequela in most patients. Conversely, interwoven tendons and nerves of the upper extremity play an integral role in arm, hand, and digit function and require more meticulous debridement and repair. Finally, the relative paucity of soft tissue in the upper compared to the lower extremity makes coverage of nerve and vascular repairs more challenging in many cases.

Civilian literature, consisting of smaller case series describing blunt and penetrating injuries, reports a very high rate of upper limb salvage (95%) [44, 45]. In a systematic review of replantation versus prosthetic fitting in traumatic arm amputations, those with replantation had higher satisfaction and good function regardless of their objective functional outcomes. Notably, patients with more proximal amputations and replantations had lower functional scores but similar satisfaction scores as those with more distal replantations, whereas only 48% of above-elbow amputations obtained full use of the prosthesis [44].

In contrast, wartime injuries to the upper extremity are high-energy wounds often with penetrating, blast, and burn components. In this setting, upper extremity injuries are associated with more extensive soft tissue, nerve, and bone destruction. Data in two separate reports from the Global War on Terrorism demonstrated that upper extremity amputation rates in wartime may be as high as 10%, perhaps reflecting attempts to salvage more severely injured upper extremities than those in the civilian setting [45, 46]. Functional outcomes are greatly impacted by proximal upper extremity injuries that frequently involve the axillary structures including the brachial plexus.

RECOMMENDATIONS

Limb salvage rates are higher for upper extremities than lower extremities in the setting of civilian trauma. The rate of upper extremity amputation is higher in the setting of complex wartime injuries.

Level of evidence: 4. Grade of recommendation: D.

Three-quarters of patients with upper extremity injury report significant functional disability in the long term. Those treated with replantation report higher satisfaction.

Level of evidence: 3. Grade of recommendation: C.

30.8 What Prehospital Adjuncts Are Available That Impact Limb Salvage Following Traumatic Extremity Injury?

Tourniquets have been utilized as an adjunct for extremity hemorrhage control for over 100 years and have been reintroduced during military conflicts as a lifesaving measure while preparing for transport from the battlefield [47]. Uncontrolled hemorrhage remains a leading cause of preventable battlefield death and the second most common cause of death for civilian trauma [33]. During each recent major conflict, attention has been directed to the proper design, application, and utility of tourniquets [48].

A prospective review of tourniquet usage at a combat support hospital in Baghdad was conducted to evaluate potential adverse events associated with tourniquet usage [49]. Of 232 patients with 428 tourniquets in place, none of the 309 limbs were lost as a result of tourniquet use. There were many secondary outcomes investigated, including fasciotomy, DVT, pain, and nerve palsy. However, the only complications reported were transient nerve palsies in <2%. Nonetheless, improperly applied tourniquets may cause increased hemorrhage when placed above a venous injury, and properly placed tourniquets may cause significant pain if left in place for extended periods [50]. In 2009, Kragh et al. also prospectively reported an observed survival benefit with emergency tourniquet use to stop bleeding in major limb trauma. The authors concluded that both prehospital tourniquet use and tourniquet use when shock was absent were strongly associated with survival (90% vs. 10%; $p < 0.001$) [51].

Eighty percent of all tourniquets placed in the field for civilian extremity hemorrhage are commercial devices [52]. However, in a study of the general public with varying degrees of experience with first aid and hemorrhage control, only one-third of participants could correctly apply a commercial tourniquet [52]. In a retrospective analysis of 168 community-applied tourniquets for extremity hemorrhage, including blunt and penetrating trauma, emergency medical services (EMS) relied on the original tourniquet in 45% of cases, and 21% of these patients required vascular surgery, confirming the importance of at least trying to place a tourniquet and having them available [52]. It is a current consensus that the efficacy of tourniquet use on the battlefield is inversely related to the time in which it takes for the tourniquet to be evaluated, loosened, or removed by a surgical team.

An additional prehospital adjunct that has gained attention is the topical hemostatic agent designed to stop bleeding from large proximal arterial and venous injuries. In addition to standard pressure dressings, hemostatic agents are classified on their mechanism of action into three categories [53]:

1. Factor concentrators – quickly absorb the water content in the blood.
2. Mucoadhesive agents – adhere to the wound and physically block bleeding
3. Procoagulant supplements – deliver procoagulant materials directly to the wound.

Studies supporting the safety and efficacy of these agents have been based on large animal work that suggests that zeolite (QuikClot—factor concentrator; Z-Medica LLC, Newington, CT, USA) dressings significantly reduce blood loss after large vessel laceration and uncontrolled hemorrhagic shock. Alam et al. compared the mortality and blood loss after the application of five hemostatic agents to an iliac injury in a swine model of uncontrolled hemorrhage [53]. Animals in the zeolite group demonstrate a statistically significant mortality benefit; no animals died in the zeolite group, while mortality rates in the remaining treatment groups ranged from 28% in the chitosan (Celox—mucoadhesive, Medtrade Products Ltd. Crewe, UK) group to 100% in the untreated group. While the hemostatic properties of the zeolite dressing appear promising, the associated exothermic reaction causes tissue damage that may complicate wound healing or cause thrombosis. Despite concern and anecdotal reports that topical hemostatic agents may compromise the ability to perform vascular reconstruction and limb salvage, there are no studies that support this line of thinking.

RECOMMENDATIONS

Tourniquets should be placed early and proximal to arterial extremity injuries and remain in place until further resuscitation and evaluation by qualified teams.

Level of evidence: 2. Grade of recommendation: B.

30.9 What Strategies in Skeletal Reconstruction Impact Limb Salvage Following Traumatic Injury?

Like vascular injuries, patients with skeletal injuries will benefit most from primary definitive stabilization. Similarly, definitive stabilization is often time-consuming and represents an additional physiologic burden for the patient. Principles of damage control for orthopedic injuries include external fixation (EF) with delayed intramedullary nailing (IMN) of long bone fractures [54]. Initial small, randomized multicenter trials conducted by the European Polytrauma Study on the Management of Femur Fractures demonstrated that patients with severe polytrauma (Injury Severity Score [ISS] 22) and femur fractures exhibited a significantly greater cytokine response following early IMN versus EF followed by delayed IMN [54]. These findings were not corroborated when the same group randomized 165 patients across 10 European centers to receive either early IMN or EF followed by delayed IMN [55]. Regression analysis of the most severely injured patients (ISS 32 vs. 24) with thorax injuries (Abbreviated Injury Scale [AIS] 2.8) suggests a lower risk of pulmonary complications and sepsis if treated with early EF rather than early IMN. Conversely, stable patients did not benefit from a two-staged repair (e.g., EF followed by delayed IMN). In fact, in this less severely injured group, EF followed by delayed IMN was associated with nearly double the intensive care unit (ICU) hours (212 vs. 133) and ventilator hours nearly tripled (142 vs. 66), although neither was statistically significant.

In a Cochrane review of randomized and quasi-randomized controlled trials, antibiotic prophylaxis in open fractures reduced early infections (risk ratio [RR] 0.41 (95% CI 0.27–0.63) [56].

RECOMMENDATIONS

Severely injured patients with long bone fractures benefit from early EF followed by IMN. Less severely injured patients are best served with definitive stabilization in the form of IMN within the first 24 hours of injury. Due to the increased incidence of wound-related sepsis after open fractures, gram-negative coverage should be provided in addition to a first-generation cephalosporin for 3 days from the time of initial evaluation.

Level of evidence: 2. Grade of recommendation: B.

30.10 How Do Advances in Soft Tissue Wound Management Strategies Impact Limb Salvage?

Severe lower extremity trauma is often associated with extensive soft tissue loss. Large soft tissue wounds create an independent physiologic burden on the patient in the form of insensible fluid loss, infection, and metabolic demands during healing. Among the most commonly employed tools used to manage extremity soft tissue wounds are the negative pressure vacuum-assisted closure device (V.A.C. KCI, San Antonio, TX), tissue flaps, free tissue transfers, and skin grafts.

V.A.C. therapy (using reticulated open cell foam) acts to remove interstitial fluids that contain inflammatory cytokines that suppress the proliferative phase of wound healing and bacteria. Negative pressure wound therapy also reduces capillary afterload that increases local circulation, and a properly sealed system decreases the burden of external contamination [57–59]. The applications of V.A.C. therapy are extensive, and the techniques are especially effective when placed over properly debrided, well-vascularized tissues such as muscle and subcutaneous fat. Several case series have demonstrated that the use of the V.A.C. device decreases the time to wound closure or coverage with a skin graft without the aid of tissue flaps [58–60]. In a 2019 systematic review of V.A.C therapy, 90% of wounds were managed with V.A.C for definitive therapy and did not require additional surgeries, even minor revision [61].

There are times when immediate reconstruction can be attempted, but it is critical to note the importance of surgical expertise in the setting of decreasing free tissue transfer used in complex extremity injuries [62]. For those extremity wounds with extensive devitalized tissues, a rotational flap or free tissue transfer may be delivered into a clean wound bed to aid in definitive wound closure. This multicenter retrospective series included 532 patients receiving early (within 72 hours of injury),

delayed (between 72 hours and 3 months of injury), or late (between 3 months and 12 years of injury) free-flap transfer. Those patients undergoing delayed free tissue transfer had a significantly higher rate of wound infections (delayed 18% vs. early 2%), and the average hospitalization was over four times as long (130 days vs. 27 days). The author also highlights the steep learning curve associated with the microsurgical reconstruction of free tissue transfers, as failures occurred in 26% of the first 100 flaps and only 4% of the last 100.

RECOMMENDATIONS

Frequent and adequate surgical debridement of soft tissue wounds is paramount in the preparation of extremity soft tissue wounds. Negative pressure wound therapy (V.A.C.) as a standard surgical adjunct that aids in the management of extremity injury is associated with low infection rates and decreased time to closure or coverage with a skin graft.

Level of evidence: 2. Grade of recommendation: B.

When necessary, reconstruction of wounds using free tissue transfers should occur early and be performed by experienced subspecialists.

Level of evidence: 3. Grade of recommendation: C.

30.11 How Do Patient and Injury Characteristics Impact Decision-Making Regarding Extremity Salvage?

Six factors that influence the initial decision to amputate or attempt limb salvage are as follows:

1. Physiologic reserve of the patient
2. Extent and severity of associated injuries
3. Nature of the extremity injury
4. Preinjury functional status
5. The presence of significant comorbidities
6. Access to adequate resources during rehabilitation

Authors of the Lower Extremity Assessment Project (LEAP) assessed the relationships among these factors and the functional outcome after extremity reconstruction and limb salvage or amputation [2, 63–69]. LEAP is a multicenter prospective study of 600 patients with severe lower extremity injury who underwent either amputation or reconstruction. Results from this important study have shown that factors associated with the injury itself are the most significant in influencing the decision to amputate [68]. Specifically, muscle injury, arterial and/or deep venous injury, and absence of plantar sensation are three factors shown to be associated with a fivefold risk of amputation [2, 66, 68]. In a subsequent subset analysis of the LEAP cohort, looking at the mangled foot and ankle injuries, these patients had a significantly worse 2-year impact of disability outcomes than their below-the-knee amputation (BKA) counterparts. This was especially true if ankle arthrodesis or free flaps were required for salvage [68].

To address the absence of plantar sensation as an indication for extremity amputation, three groups of patients were selected based on the absence of plantar sensation on initial evaluation and successful limb salvage (group 1), the absence of plantar sensation and amputation (group 2), and the presence of plantar sensation and limb salvage (group 3) [65]. There was no difference in functional outcomes between the groups, and approximately half (55%) of the entire cohort had normal plantar sensation after 2 years.

These studies found no difference in functional outcome from either group based on injury characteristics or the presence of a limb. Subset analysis suggests that the factors most likely to influence the functional outcome are related to preinjury social characteristics such as level of education, income level, and access to healthcare [66].

Similar findings are reported by Sohn et al. for a cohort of 153 patients wounded during Operation Iraqi Freedom [33]. In contrast to participants in the LEAP, who were 16- to 69-year-old civilians, the injured troops in Sohn et al.'s study were young (mean 23 years), otherwise healthy, and had sustained greater percentages of high-energy complex wounds. Upon initial presentation, one-quarter was hypotensive and 80% had a base deficit ≥6. The median military ISS of the cohort was 13, all of which suggest a significant physiologic derangement as a result of their injuries. Despite the extent of their injuries, the authors report an 80% early limb salvage rate, which is comparable to that observed in the LEAP (83%) [2, 33].

In a review of patients treated with a multidisciplinary team approach, "Limb salvage was successfully achieved in 91% (29/32) of the cases. Failed limb salvages were due to flap failure (33%; 1/3), recurring periprosthetic joint infections (66%; 2/3), and concomitant reconstructive failure" [70].

RECOMMENDATIONS

Patient factors most highly correlated with extremity amputation are severe soft tissue injury, nerve injury, and vascular injury in descending order.

Level of evidence: 1. Grade of recommendation: A.

Limb salvage should be used cautiously in those with open severely injured hindfoot or ankle injuries due to worse long-term functional outcomes, especially when free flaps or arthrodesis is required.

Level of evidence: 3. Grade of recommendation: C.

30.12 What is the Role of Mangled Extremity Scores and Indices on Decision-Making in Limb Salvage?

Based on data from the previously mentioned studies and others, factors have been identified that influence functional outcomes after limb salvage. To guide the decision-making process during the initial and early management of patients with severe extremity trauma, scoring systems have been developed that incorporate several of these factors. An ideal mangled extremity scoring system needs to be simple to implement during the initial evaluation, based on readily available information, and able to predict limb salvage and functional outcome. Unfortunately, no single scoring system has been designated as ideal, and as a result, several options are now available. Among the most common are the MESS; the Predictive Salvage Index (PSI); the Limb Salvage Index (LSI); the Nerve Injury, Ischemia, Soft Tissue Injury, Skeletal Injury, Shock, and Age of Patient (NISSSA) Score; and the Hannover Fracture Scale-98 (HFA-98).

The most commonly reported scoring system, the MESS, was derived by Johansen et al. from the initial retrospective and subsequent prospective outcomes of 52 patients, 21 of whom underwent an amputation [67]. Factors considered in the calculation of a score include the following:

1. Presence or absence of skeletal/soft tissue injury (graded 1–4)
2. Presence or absence of limb ischemia (graded 1–3)
3. Presence or absence of shock (graded 0–2)
4. Patient age (graded 0–2)

Each variable is graded, and the individual scores are added to provide a score from 2 to 11. The authors of the MESS recognize limb ischemia as time-dependent and suggest limb ischemia scores be doubled if perfusion has not been restored within 6 hours of injury. The authors of the MESS found that a score ≥7 predicted amputation with 100% accuracy and scores <6 also predicted limb salvage in all cases [67]. Interestingly, patients with significant peripheral nerve deficits were excluded from the study because they were assumed to require amputation. Larger prospective trials with long-term follow-up have not successfully duplicated the results of the MESS report [10, 71, 72]. The MESS and scoring systems like it tend to have high specificities with low scores accurately able to predict limb salvage. However, the sensitivity of these metrics lacks, as their ability to predict amputation in the setting of high scores is variable (i.e., low positive predictive values).

Less commonly utilized scoring systems are available, each more complex than the MESS. Examples include the PSI developed by Howe et al. which includes the level of arterial injury, the degree of bone injury, the degree of muscle injury, and the time to surgery [73]. A score greater than or equal to 8 should be predictive of the need for amputation. The LSI designed by Russell et al. measures seven components including artery, deep vein, nerve, bone, skin, muscle, and warm ischemia time [74]. Again, variables are graded and an additive score ≥6 predicts the need for amputation. The NISSSA, developed by McNamara et al. in 1994, contains six variables including nerve injury, ischemia, soft tissue injury, skeletal injury, shock, and patient age [75]. Amputations are recommended with scores ≥11. The HFS-98 proposed in revised form by Krettek et al. is the most complex and involves the determination of fracture type, the degree of bone loss, periosteal stripping, skin injury, muscle injury, wound contamination, local circulation, systemic circulation, and neurologic function [76]. The scoring system is designed to be employed during the initial operation by the operating surgeon and ranges from 0 to 22 with a score ≥11 being predictive of amputation.

In the most comprehensive evaluation of extremity injury scoring metrics to date, the designers of the LEAP applied the criteria for each of the previously listed scoring systems to the 407 patients in their study group with the intent to evaluate long-term *functional outcomes* after attempted limb salvage [67]. In this important part of the LEAP report, there was no correlation between any ISS and reported *functional outcomes* at either 6 or 24 months.

RECOMMENDATIONS

Mangled extremity severity scoring systems have limited predictive value in terms of the need for amputation. No scoring system can reliably predict functional outcomes in a clinical setting.

Level of evidence: 1. Grade of recommendation: A.

30.13 What Is the Financial Cost of Extremity Reconstruction versus Early Amputation and the Impact on Quality of Life?

Extremity injury presents a significant physical and emotional burden for the patient as well as an economic challenge for the healthcare system, both acutely and long-term. Several groups have evaluated the costs associated with the pursuit of limb salvage as opposed to early amputation and placed these on functional outcomes [8, 65, 77]. There are significant differences in the length of hospital stay, need for rehospitalization, number of operations, and length of time to return to work in patients

receiving primary amputation versus those with limb salvage. As an example, Bondurant reported that patients who required a secondary amputation remained in the hospital for more than twice as long as those who underwent primary amputation (53 vs. 22 days) [8]. Patients in limb salvage groups also require a significantly greater number of operations than patients receiving primary amputation (19% vs. 5%) [8]. Nearly half of patients in both groups (limb salvage and primary amputation) failed to return to work within 24 months following injury, illustrating the persistent morbidity associated with severe extremity injury [8]. Finally, Bondurant documented the fiscal cost of secondary versus early primary amputation by showing a fivefold increase in the number of operations (2 vs. 7) and a doubling of hospital costs ($28,964 vs. $53,462—1988 dollars) in the secondary amputation group [8].

In a notable finding, the LEAP demonstrated no difference in the quality of life between patients with primary amputation and those with successful limb salvage at 2 years [67]. Using the validated, self-reporting questionnaire called the Sickness Impact Profile that assesses 12 categories of function including ambulation, mobility, body care, social interaction, and ability to work, the LEAP failed to show improved quality of life in those with successful limb salvage following severe extremity injury at 24 months [71]. These findings may be attributable to the increasing quality of prosthetics as well as the social and financial support required for optimal care and rehabilitation following limb salvage attempts.

RECOMMENDATION

There is no significant difference in functional outcome after limb salvage versus amputation following severe extremity injury. There is, however, a significant increase in economic, healthcare, and rehabilitation costs associated with limb salvage.

Level of evidence: 3. Grade of recommendation: C.

Levels of Evidence

No.	Subject	Year	References	Level	Strength	Findings
1	Bites	2022	Cicuttin; Medeiros	1	A	Augmentin is the antibiotic of choice for animal bites due to frequent Pasteurella. Thorough cleansing of the wound for shallow wounds and excisional debridements for deeper wounds may be necessary.
2	Scaphoid fractures	2012, 2020	Singh; Dias	1	A	MRI is useful to diagnose scaphoid fractures. Fracture healing can be assessed with plain radiographs or CT after 6–8 weeks of cast immobilization. Surgical fixation with or without bone grafting can be performed if a gap is identified at the fracture site.
3	Replantation	2001	Soucacos	5	C	Indications for replantation include the thumb, multiple digits, upper extremity amputated at the wrist, mid-palm, forearm, and almost any amputation in a child.

(Continued)

Levels of Evidence   (Continued)

No.	Subject	Year	References	Level	Strength	Findings
4	Replantation	2021	Harbour	3	B	Proper storage of amputated limbs and digits in saline-soaked gauze in an airtight container improves outcomes. Major limbs should be reimplanted within 6 hours and digits within 12 hours, though this time can be extended for pragmatic reasons with reasonable success. Cooling an amputated digit allows for extended ischemia time of up to 30 hours.
5	Compartment syndrome	2014; 2018	Garner; Kistler	1	A	Compartment syndrome is a surgical emergency. When the physical exam is inconclusive, compartment pressures should be measured; a delta pressure of less than 30 mmHg signifies inadequate perfusion and should prompt emergent decompression.
6	Limb salvage	2008	Tung	2	B	Arterial ligation may be used as a damage control maneuver, understanding that there is an increased incidence of extremity amputation. Large vessel venous injuries should be repaired when feasible to avoid thromboses and phlegmasia. Temporary venous shunts (TVS) are an effective damage control adjunct.
7	Limb salvage	2006	Clouse	4	D	Limb salvage rates are higher for upper extremities than lower extremities in the setting of civilian trauma. The rate of upper extremity amputation is higher in the setting of complex wartime injuries.
8	Limb salvage	2014	Otto	3	C	Three-quarters of patients with upper extremity injury report significant functional disability in the long term. Those treated with replantation report higher satisfaction.
9	Prehospital adjuncts	2008	Welling	2	B	Tourniquets should be placed early and above arterial extremity injuries and remain in place until further resuscitation and evaluation by qualified teams.
10	Skeletal injuries	2007	Pape	2	B	Severely injured patients with long bone fractures benefit from early EF followed by IMN. Less severely injured patients are best served with definitive stabilization in the form of IMN within the first 24 hours of injury. Due to the increased incidence of wound-related sepsis after open fractures, gram-negative coverage should be provided in addition to a first-generation cephalosporin for 3 days from the time of initial evaluation.
11	Negative pressure therapy	2019	Shine	2	B	Frequent and adequate surgical debridement of soft tissue wounds is paramount in the preparation of extremity soft tissue wounds. Negative pressure wound therapy (V.A.C.) as a standard surgical adjunct that aids in the management of extremity injury is associated with low infection rates and decreased time to closure or coverage with a skin graft.
12	Early flap reconstruction	2006	Parrett	3	C	When necessary, reconstruction of wounds using free tissue transfers should occur early and be performed by experienced subspecialists.
13	Extremity salvage decision-making	2013	Ellington	1	A	Patient factors most highly correlated with extremity amputation are severe soft tissue injury, nerve injury, and vascular injury in descending order.
14	Extremity salvage decision-making	2021	Kotsougiani	3	C	Limb salvage should be used cautiously in those with open severely injured hindfoot or ankle injuries due to worse long-term functional outcomes, especially when free flaps or arthrodesis is required.
15	Mangled extremities	2008	Ly	1	A	Mangled extremity severity scoring systems have limited predictive value in terms of the need for amputation. No scoring system can reliably predict functional outcomes in a clinical setting.
16	Quality-of-life outcomes	1995	Jurkovich	3	C	There is no significant difference in functional outcome after limb salvage versus amputation following severe extremity injury. There is, however, a significant increase in economic, healthcare, and rehabilitation costs associated with limb salvage.

Editor's Note

One of the most difficult decisions that we make as clinicians managing trauma victims is whether to perform early amputation or complex reconstructive surgery when faced with a mangled extremity. Components of that decision tree are closely examined in this chapter along with other important management questions that we face when dealing with extremity injuries. One of the issues regarding reconstruction that is naturally unclear to the uninformed injured individual and their family is what the process will entail. They have no concept of the pain and misery that will be suffered as the patient undergoes multiple operations to preserve an arm or leg. After long hospitalizations often associated with narcotic dependency, the patient often has a deformed extremity which is often less functional and more disfigured than an amputated limb. Perhaps revealing photos of a reconstructed extremity, showing something resembling Shrek's foot, would be helpful at the beginning of the process before embarking on a long, painful journey of restoration. The alternative, a quick amputation followed by fitting with one of the new, advanced prosthetic legs (or arms) would be the typical desire of most informed individuals.

REFERENCES

1. Gregory RT, Gould RJ, Peclet M, Wagner JS, Gilbert DA, Wheeler JR, Snyder SO, Gayle RG, Schwab CW. The mangled extremity syndrome (M.E.S.): A severity grading system for multisystem injury of the extremity. *J Trauma*. 1985;*25(12)*:1147–1150.
2. Bosse MJ, MacKenzie EJ, Kellam JF, et al. An analysis of outcomes of reconstruction or amputation after leg-threatening injuries. *N Engl J Med*. 2002;*347(24)*:1924–1931.
3. Fern KT, Smith JT, Zee B, et al. Trauma patients with multiple extremity injuries: Resource utilization and long-term outcome in relation to injury severity scores. *J Trauma*. 1998;*45(3)*:489–494.
4. Holbrook TL, Anderson JP, Sieber WJ, et al. Outcome after major trauma: 12-month and 18-month follow up results from the Trauma Recovery Project. *J Trauma*. 1999;*46(5)*: 765–771.
5. Katzman SS, Dickson K. Determining the prognosis for limb salvage in major vascular injuries with associated open tibial fractures. *Orthop Rev*. 1992;*21(2)*:195–199.
6. Purry NA, Hannon MA. How successful is below-knee amputation for injury? *Injury*. 1989;*20(1)*:32–36.
7. Quirke TE, Sharma PK, Boss WK, Jr., Oppenheim WC, Rauscher GE. Are type IIIC lower extremity injuries an indication for primary amputation. *J Trauma*. 1996;*40(6)*:992–996.
8. Bondurant FJ. Cotler HB, Buckle R, et al. The medical and economic impact of severely injured lower extremities. *J Trauma*. 1988;*28(8)*:1270–1273.
9. Dischinger PC, Read KM, Kufera JA, et al. Consequences and costs of lower extremity injuries. *Annu Proc Assoc Adv Automot Med*. 2004;*48*:339–353.
10. Osterman M, Draeger R, Stern P. Acute hand infections. *J Hand Surg*. 2014;*39(8)*:1628–1635.
11. Jaindl M, Grünauer J, Platzer P, Endler G, Thallinger C, Leitgeb J, Kovar FM. The management of bite wounds in children–a retrospective analysis at a level I trauma centre. *Injury*. 2012 Dec;*43(12)*:2117–21. DOI: 10.1016/j.injury.2012.04.016. Epub 2012 May 16. PMID: 22607996.
12. Bula-Rudas FJ, Olcott JL. Human and animal bites. *Pediatr Rev*. 2018 Oct;*39(10)*:490–500. DOI: 10.1542/pir.2017-0212. PMID: 30275032.
13. Medeiros I, Saconato H. Antibiotic prophylaxis for mammalian bites. *Cochrane Database Syst. Rev*. 2001:CD001738.
14. Cicuttin E, Sartelli M, Scozzafava E, Tartaglia D, Cremonini C, Brevi B, Ramacciotti N, Musetti S, Strambi S, Podda M, Catena F, Chiarugi M, Coccolini F. Antibiotic prophylaxis in torso, maxillofacial, and skin traumatic lesions: A systematic review of recent evidence. *Antibiotics (Basel)*. 2022 Jan 21;*11(2)*:139. DOI: 10.3390/antibiotics11020139. PMID: 35203743; PMCID: PMC8868174.
15. Malahias M, Jordan D, Hughes O et al. Bite injuries to the hand: Microbiology, virology and management. *Open Orthop J*. 2014;*8*:157–161.
16. Barton NJ. Twenty questions about scaphoid fractures. *J Bone Joint Surg Br*. 1992;*17*:289–310.
17. Freeland P. Scaphoid tubercle tenderness: A better indicator of scaphoid fractures? *Arch Emerg Med*. 1989;*6*:46–50.
18. Rua T, Malhotra B, Vijayanathan S, Hunter L, Peacock J, Shearer J, Goh V, McCrone P, Gidwani S. Clinical and cost implications of using immediate MRI in the management of patients with a suspected scaphoid fracture and negative radiographs results from the smart trial. *Bone Joint J*. 2019 Aug;*101-B(8)*:984–994. DOI: 10.1302/0301-620X.101B8.BJJ-2018-1590.R1. PMID: 31362557; PMCID: PMC6681676.
19. Vinnars B, Pietreanu M, Bodestedt A, et al. Nonoperative compared with operative treatment of acute scaphoid fractures. A randomized clinical trial. *J Bone Joint Surg Am*. 2008;*90(6)*:1176–1185.
20. Dias JJ, Brealey SD, Fairhurst C, Amirfeyz R, Bhowal B, Blewitt N, Brewster M, Brown D, Choudhary S, Coapes C, Cook L, Costa M, Davis T, Di Mascio L, Giddins G, Hedley H, Hewitt C, Hinde S, Hobby J, Hodgson S, Jefferson L, Jeyapalan K, Johnston P, Jones J, Keding A, Leighton P, Logan A, Mason W, McAndrew A, McNab I, Muir L, Nicholl J, Northgraves M, Palmer J, Poulter R, Rahimtoola Z, Rangan A, Richards S, Richardson G, Stuart P, Taub N, Tavakkolizadeh A, Tew G, Thompson J, Torgerson D, Warwick D. Surgery versus cast immobilisation for adults with a bicortical fracture of the scaphoid waist (SWIFFT): A pragmatic, multicentre, open-label, randomised superiority trial. *Lancet*. 2020 Aug 8;*396(10248)*:390–401. DOI: 10.1016/S0140-6736(20)30931-4. PMID: 32771106.
21. Singh HP, Taub N, Dias JJ. Management of displaced fractures of the waist of the scaphoid: Meta analyses of comparative studies. *Injury*. 2012;*43(6)*:933–939.
22. Beris AE, Lykissas MG, Korompilias AV, et al. Digit and hand replantation. *Trauma Surg*. September 2010;*130(9)*: 1141–1147.
23. Soucacos PN. Indications and selection for digital amputation and replantation. *J Hand Surg*. 2001;*26*:572–581.
24. Dec W. A meta-analysis of success rates for digit replantation. *Tech Hand Up Extrem Surg*. 2006;*10(3)*:124–129.

25. Chung KC, Yoon AP, Malay S, Shauver MJ, Wang L, Kaur S; FRANCHISE Group. Patient-reported and functional outcomes after revision amputation and replantation of digit amputations: The FRANCHISE multicenter international retrospective cohort study. *JAMA Surg.* 2019 Jul 1;*154(7)*:637–646. doi: 10.1001/jamasurg.2019.0418. PMID: 30994871; PMCID: PMC6583841.

26. Martin C, Gonzalez del Pino J. Controversies in the treatment of fingertip amputations. Conservative versus surgical reconstruction. *Clin Orthop Relat Res.* 1998;*353*:63–73.

27. Heistein J, Cook P. Factors affecting composite graft survival in digital tip amputation. *Ann Plas Surg.* 2003; *50(3)*:299–303.

28. Harbour PW, Malphrus E, Zimmerman RM, Giladi AM. Delayed digit replantation: What is the evidence? *J Hand Surg Am.* 2021 Oct;*46(10)*:908–916. DOI: 10.1016/j.jhsa.2021.07.007. Epub 2021 Aug 8. PMID: 34376294.

29. Tu, Y., Lineaweaver, W., Culnan, D., Bitz, G., Jones, K. & Zhang, F. Temporary ectopic implantation for salvaging amputated parts: A systematic review. *J Trauma Acute Care Surg.* 2018. *84*(6):985–993. DOI: 10.1097/TA.0000000000001817.

30. Wei DH, Strauch RJ. Smoking and hand surgery. *J Hand Surg.* 2013;*38(1)*:176–179.

31. Garner MR, Taylor SA, Gausden E, Lyden JP. Compartment syndrome: Diagnosis, management, unique concerns in the twenty-first century. *HSS J.* 2014;*10(2)*:143–152.

32. Kistler JM, Ilyas AM, Thoder JJ. Forearm compartment syndrome: Evaluation and management. *Hand Clin.* 2018 Feb;*34*(1):53–60. DOI: 10.1016/j.hcl.2017.09.006. PMID: 29169597.

33. Sohn VY, Arthurs ZM, Herbert GS, Beekley AC, Sebesta JA. Demographics, treatment, and early outcomes in penetrating vascular combat trauma. *Arch Surg.* 2008;*143(8)*:783–787.

34. Starnes BW, Beekley AC, Sebesta JA, et al. Extremity vascular injuries on the battlefield: Tips for surgeons deploying to war. *J Trauma.* 2006;*60(2)*:432–442.

35. Clarke P, Mollan RA. The criteria for amputation in severe lower limb injury. *Injury.* 1994;*25(3)*:139–143.

36. Debakey ME, Simeone FA. Battle injuries of the arteries in World War II: An analysis of 2471 cases. *Ann Surg.* 1946;*123(4)*:534–537.

37. Timberlake GA, Kerstein MD. Venous injury: To repair or ligate, the dilemma revisited. *Am Surg.* 1995;*61*:139.

38. Quan RW, Gillespie DL, Stuart RP, et al. The effect of vein repair on the risk of venous thromboembolic events: A review of more than 100 traumatic military venous injuries. *J Vasc Surg.* 2008;*47(3)*:571–577.

39. Rich NM, Mattox KL, Hirschberg A. 2004. *Vascular Trauma,* 2nd ed. Elsevier Saunders: Philadelphia, PA, pp. 3–73, 353–392.

40. Gifford SM, Aidinian G, Clouse WD, Fox CJ, Porras CA, Jones WT, Zarzabal LA, Michalek JE, Propper BW, Burkhardt GE, Rasmussen TE. Effect of temporary shunting on extremity vascular injury: an outcome analysis from the Global War on Terror vascular injury initiative. *J Vasc Surg.* Sep 2009;*50(3)*:549–555; discussion 555-556. doi: 10.1016/j.jvs.2009.03.051. PMID: 19595542.

41. Polcz JE, White JM, Ronaldi AE, Dubose JJ, Grey S, Bell D, White PW, Rasmussen TE. Temporary intravascular shunt use improves early limb salvage after extremity

vascular injury. *J Vasc Surg.* 2021 Apr;*73(4)*:1304–1313. doi: 10.1016/j.jvs.2020.08.137. Epub 2020 Sep 25. PMID: 32987146.

42. Laverty RB, Treffalls RN, Kauvar DS. Systematic review of temporary intravascular shunt use in military and civilian extremity trauma. *J Trauma Acute Care Surg.* 2022 Jan 1;*92(1)*:232–238. doi: 10.1097/TA.0000000000003399. PMID: 34538830.

43. Tung L, Leonard J, Lawless RA, Cralley A, Betzold R, Pasley JD, Inaba K, Kim JS, Kim DY, Kim K, Dennis BM, Smith MC, Moore M, Tran C, Hazelton JP, Melillo A, Brahmbhatt TS, Talutis S, Saillant NN, Lee JM, Seamon MJ. Temporary intravascular shunts after civilian arterial injury: A prospective multicenter Eastern Association for the Surgery of Trauma study. *Injury.* 2021 May;*52(5)*:1204–1209. DOI: 10.1016/j.injury.2020.12.035. Epub 2021 Jan 3. PMID: 33455811.

44. Joshi V, Harding GE, Bottoni DA, Lovell MB, Forbes TL. Determination of functional outcome following upper extremity arterial trauma. *Vasc Endovascular Surg.* 2007;*41(2)*:111–114.

45. Manford JD, Garard CL, Kline DG, Sternberg WC, Money SR. Management of severe vascular and neural injury of the upper extremity. *J Vasc Surg.* 1998;*27(1)*:43–49.

46. Otto IA, Kon M, Schuurman AH, van Minnen LP. Replantation versus prosthetic fitting in traumatic arm amputations: A systematic review. *PLoS One.* 2015 Sep 4;*10(9)*:e0137729. DOI: 10.1371/journal.pone.0137729. PMID: 26340003; PMCID: PMC4560425.

47. Clouse WD, Rasmussen TE, Perlstein J, et al. Upper extremity vascular injury: A current in-theater wartime report from Operation Iraqi Freedom. *Ann Vasc Surg.* 2006;*20(4)*:431–434.

48. Weber MA, Fox CJ, Adams E, et al. Upper extremity arterial combat injury management. *Perspect Vasc Surg Endovasc Ther.* 2006;*18(2)*:141–145.

49. Fox CJ, Starnes BW. Vascular surgery on the modern battlefield. *Surg Clin North Am.* 2007;*87*:1193–1211.

50. Welling DR, Burris DG, Hutton JE et al. A balanced approach to tourniquet use: Lessons learned and relearned. *J Am Coll Surg.* 2006;*203(1)*:106–115.

51. Kragh JF, Walters TJ, Baer DG, Fox CJ, Wade CE, Salinas J, Holcomb JB. Practical use of emergency tourniquets to stop bleeding in major limb trauma. *J Trauma.* 2008;*64(2)*:S38–S50.

52. Barnard LM, Guan S, Zarmer L, Mills B, Blackwood J, Bulger E, Yang BY, Johnston P, Vavilala MS, Sayre MR, Rea TD, Murphy DL. Prehospital tourniquet use: An evaluation of community application and outcome. *J Trauma Acute Care Surg.* 2021 Jun 1;*90(6)*:1040–1047. DOI: 10.1097/TA.0000000000003145. PMID: 34016927.

53. Pusateri AE, Holcomb JB, Kheirabadi BS, Alam HB, Wade CE, Ryan KL. Making sense of the preclinical literature on advanced hemostatic products. *J Trauma.* 2006;*60*:674–682.

54. Pape HC, Grimme K, Van Griensven M, et al. Impact of intramedullary instrumentation versus damage control for femoral fractures on immunoinflammatory parameters: Prospective randomized analysis by the EPOFF Study Group. *J Trauma.* 2003;*55*:7–13.

55. Pape HC, Rixen D, Morley J, et al. Impact of the method of initial stabilization for femoral shaft fractures in patients with multiple injuries at risk for complications (borderline patients). *Ann Surg*. 2007;*246(3)*:149–157.

56. Gosselin RA, Roberts I, Gillespie WJ. Antibiotics for preventing infection in open limb fractures. *Cochrane Database Syst Rev*. 2004;*2004(1)*:CD003764. DOI: 10.1002/14651858.CD003764.pub2. PMID: 14974035; PMCID: PMC8728739.

57. Pirela-Cruz MA, Machen MS, Esquivel D. Management of large soft-tissue wounds with negative pressure therapy-lessons learned from the war zone. *J Hand Ther*. 2008;*21(2)*:196–202.

58. DeFranzo AJ, Argenta LC, Marks MW, Molnar JA, David LR, Webb LX, Ward WG, Teasdall RG. The use of vacuum-assisted closure therapy for the treatment of lower-extremity wounds with exposed bone. *Plastic Reconstr Surg*. 2001; *108(5)*:1184–1191.

59. Herscovici D, Sanders RW, Scaduto JM, et al. Vacuum-assisted wound closure (VAC therapy) for the management of patients with high-energy soft tissue injuries. *J Orthop Trauma*. 2003;*17(10)*:683–688.

60. Geiger S, McCormick F, Chou R, Wandel AG. War wounds: Lessons learned from Operation Iraqi Freedom. *Plast Reconstr Surg*. 2008;*122(1)*:146–153.

61. Shine J, Efanov JI, Paek L, Coeugniet É, Danino MA, Izadpanah A. Negative pressure wound therapy as a definitive treatment for upper extremity wound defects: A systematic review. *Int Wound J*. 2019 Aug;*16(4)*:960–967. DOI: 10.1111/iwj.13128. Epub 2019 Apr 4. PMID: 30950218; PMCID: PMC7948791.

62. Parrett BM, Matros E, Pribaz JJ, Orgill DP. Lower extremity trauma: Trends in the management of soft-tissue reconstruction of open tibia-fibula fractures. *Plast Reconstr Surg*. 2006;*117(4)*:1315–1322.

63. Bosse MJ, MacKenzie EJ, Kellam JF et al. A prospective evaluation of the clinical utility of the lower-extremity injury-severity scores. *J Bone Joint Surg Am*. 2001;*83-A(1)*: 3–14.

64. Bosse MJ, McCarthy ML, Jones AL, Webb LX, Sims SH, Sanders RW, MacKenzie EJ. The insensate foot following severe lower extremity trauma: An indication for amputation? *J Bone Joint Surg Am*. 2005;*87(12)*:2601–2608.

65. MacKenzie EJ, Bosse MJ, Kellam JF, et al. Factors influencing the decision to amputate or reconstruct after high-energy lower extremity trauma. *J Trauma*. 2002;*52(4)*:641–649.

66. Treiman RL, Doty D, Gaspar MR. Acute vascular trauma: A fifteen year study. *J Surg*. 1966;*111*:469–473.

67. Johansen K, Daines M, Howey T, Helfet D, Hansen ST Jr. Objective criteria accurately predict amputation following lower extremity trauma. *J Trauma*. 1990;*30(5)*:568–572; discussion 572–573.

68. Ellington JK, Bosse MJ, Castillo RC, MacKenzie EJ; LEAP Study Group. The mangled foot and ankle: results from a 2-year prospective study. *J Orthop Trauma*. 2013 Jan;*27(1)*:43–48. DOI: 10.1097/BOT.0b013e31825121b6. PMID: 22561743.

69. MacKenzie EJ, Bosse MJ, Pollak AN, et al. Long-term persistence of disability following severe lower-limb trauma. Results of a seven-year follow-up. *J Bone Joint Surg Am*. 2005;*87(8)*:1801–1809.

70. Kotsougiani-Fischer D, Fischer S, Warszawski J, Gruetzner PA, Reiter G, Hirche C, Kneser U. Multidisciplinary team meetings for patients with complex extremity defects: A retrospective analysis of treatment recommendations and prognostic factors for non-implementation. *BMC Surg*. 2021 Mar 29;*21(1)*:168. DOI: 10.1186/s12893-021-01169-4. PMID: 33781250; PMCID: PMC8006355.

71. Jurkovich G, Mock C, MacKenzie E, Burgess A, Cushing B, deLateur B, McAndrew M, Morris J, Swiontkowski M. The sickness impact profile is a tool to evaluate functional outcomes in trauma patients. *J Trauma*. 1995;*39(4)*:625–631.

72. Ly TV, Travison TG, Castillo RC, Bosse MJ, MacKenzie EJ; LEAP Study Group. Ability of lower-extremity injury severity scores to predict functional outcome after limb salvage. *J Bone Joint Surg Am*. 2008;*90*:1738–1743.

73. Howe HR, Jr., Poole GV, Jr., Hansen KJ, Clark T, Plonk GW, Koman LA, Pennell TC. Salvage of lower extremities following combined orthopedic and vascular trauma. A predictive salvage index. *Am Surg*. 1987;*53(4)*:205–208.

74. Russell WL, Sailors DM, Whittle TB, Fisher DF, Jr., Burns RP. Limb salvage versus traumatic amputation. A decision based on a seven-part predictive index. *Ann Surg*. 1991;*213(5)*:473–480; discussion 480–481.

75. McNamara MG, Heckman JD, Corley FG. Severe open fractures of the lower extremity: A retrospective evaluation of the Mangled Extremity Severity Score (MESS). *J Orthop Trauma*. 1994;*8(2)*:81–87.

76. Krettek C, Seekamp A, Kontopp H, Tscherne H. Hannover Fracture Scale '98-re-evaluation and new perspectives of an established extremity salvage score. *Injury Int J Care Injured*. 2001;*32*:317–328.

77. Hierner R, Betz AM, Comtet JJ, Berger AC. Decision making and results in subtotal and total lower leg amputations: Reconstruction versus amputation. *Microsurgery*. 1995;*16(12)*:830–839.

31

Support of the Burned Patient

Jared S. Folwell, Garrett W. Britton, and Valerie G. Sams

31.1 Introduction

Significant advances in burn care over the past several decades have led to improved survival, particularly in young healthy patients. Through both observational and prospective basic science and clinical research, burn management no longer involves conservative wound management and deliberate observation. Instead, the science has resulted in goal-directed fluid management, early excision and grafting of burn wounds for wound closure, aggressive organ support, and directed rehabilitation strategies as the foundation for the successful management of burn patients. Primarily, these advancements involve resuscitation, wound care, prevention of infection, and critical care while work is ongoing in rehabilitation outcomes and scar management.

Burns of greater than 20% of the total body surface area (TBSA), or 10% TBSA in children and elderly adults, are severe and associated with a higher risk of mortality and other poor outcomes. In this chapter, we will consider the following relevant questions in the severely burned which will be summarized in Table 31.3.

- What are the optimal resuscitation methods and goals of resuscitation following a severe burn?
- How do we determine burn depth?
- What is the optimal approach to burn wound management according to the depth of injury?
- What is the optimal transfusion strategy in major burns, and how is blood loss best minimized during burn excision procedures?
- How are burn wounds and multidrug-resistant infections effectively minimized?
- What diagnostic procedures should be performed in patients with suspected inhalation injuries?
- What are the indications for endotracheal intubation and for tracheostomy in patients with inhalation injury?
- What mode of mechanical ventilation is most effective for patients with inhalation injury?
- What medications and fluid management strategies improve outcomes?
- What immediate treatments are safe and effective for metabolic asphyxiation by carbon monoxide or hydrogen cyanide toxicity?
- Should patients with inhalation injury be transferred to a regional burn center?

31.2 What Are the Optimal Resuscitation Methods and Goals of Resuscitation Following Severe Burn?

The primary goal of burn shock management is the restoration or maintenance of vital organ perfusion and function at the least physiologic cost. This is achieved through calculated, early replacement of circulating blood volume with IV fluids, close monitoring of the physiologic response, adjusting treatment strategies and fluid rates as needed based on patient physiology, and anticipating and mitigating edema formation. Burn shock results in significant intravascular volume depletion from interstitial and environmental fluid losses, cardiac dysfunction, and inadequate end-organ perfusion [1–5]. Fluid resuscitation is mandatory for circulatory restoration but requires judicious, calculated titration to avoid complications of over- or under-resuscitation. Delayed resuscitation leads to organ failure and death, while over-resuscitation worsens edema and associated complications, with resultant increased morbidity and mortality [6].

Consensus recommendations from the American Burn Association call for 2–4 cc/kg/%TBSA of crystalloid in the first 24 hours based on Pruitt's Modified Brooke formula and Baxter's and Shires' Parkland formula, respectively, but these guidelines are rooted in over 50-year-old data. More recent clinical experience has shown the detrimental impact of the edema of burn shock with the evolving concept of "fluid creep," the phenomenon of patients with major burns requiring resuscitation volumes that significantly exceed Parkland formula predictions (>4 mL/kg/%TBSA) [7]. Ivy et al. have previously described more than 250 cc/kg of IV fluids in the first 24 hours post burn are associated with the development of intraabdominal hypertension (IAH) and abdominal compartment syndrome (ACS). This volume of fluid (250 cc/kg) has become known as the Ivy index and has been extrapolated in many burn centers as a ceiling of resuscitation not to be exceeded due to a marked association with IAH, ACS, pulmonary, infectious, and other complications of severe burns and over-resuscitation [8].

Born out of a need for simplified fluid resuscitation management in mass casualty and combat casualty environments, Chung et al. at the U.S. Army Burn Center developed the Rule of 10s for estimating initial fluid needs. The rule of 10s calls for 10 mL LR/%TBSA (rounded to the nearest 10)/hour for patients ranging from 40 to 80 kg. Patients weighing >80 kg should receive 100 mL/hour of additional lactated Ringer's (LR) for every 10 kg of body weight over 80 kg [9]. Silico analysis comparing the Rule of 10s to the Modified Brooke and Parkland formulas demonstrated approximately 88% of 100,000 simulations of calculated initial fluid rates fell between Modified Brooke and Parkland formula estimates. In 2021, the World Health Organization's Technical Working Group on Burns (TWGB) sought to validate a simplified formula for estimating initial fluid requirements in global mass casualty scenarios in resource-limited environments. TWGB demonstrated that their formula of 100 mL/kg/24 hours effectively estimated fluid volumes within the range of current fluid guidelines for severe burns between 25–50% TBSA and 20–60% TBSA in adults and children, respectively [10]. The Department of Defense Joint Trauma System clinical practice guidelines recommend initiation of albumin at hour 8 post-burn for patients who are on a trajectory to exceed the Ivy index (250 mL/kg/%TBSA) or who are actively on >1500 mL/hour of crystalloid. The guideline further calls for cessation of colloid at 48 hours post-burn, by which time burn shock should be resolving [11].

Recently there has been a renewed interest in plasma-based resuscitation as the most appropriate colloid in burn resuscitation. Concerns over the use of plasma include the potential risk of bloodborne disease transmission, transfusion-related acute lung injury (TRALI), transfusion reactions, inconsistencies in plasma protocols, and cost. Benefits of plasma include potential reduction in overall resuscitative fluid requirements and restoration of the endothelial glycocalyx layer (EGL) [12, 13].

RECOMMENDATION

Targeted early restoration of volume and sodium losses with appropriately estimated physiologic crystalloid solutions in a simplified fashion, taking care to closely monitor and adjust the response to therapy, is key. We recommend initiation of albumin at hour 8 post-burn for patients who are on a trajectory to exceed the Ivy index (250 cc/kg) or who are receiving greater than 1500 mL/hour of crystalloid. Colloids should be stopped 48 hours post-burn, by which time burn shock should be resolving.

Grade of recommendation: B.

31.3 How Do We Determine Burn Depth?

Wound depth determination is critical to the decision to operate on burned patients. Deep partial- and full-thickness burns will not heal in a timely fashion and therefore are best treated with prompt excision and grafting. Superficial partial-thickness burns typically heal within 2–3 weeks with minimal scarring or impairment. Deep partial- and full-thickness burns take more than 3 weeks to heal, often much longer, and may result in significant hypertrophic scarring and functional impairment [6]. Partial-thickness burns that will heal

with conservative therapies are not subjected to skin grafting. Determination is typically done through clinical assessment by an expert examiner; however, this method has only 60–80% accuracy in well-done descriptive studies using histologic analysis from a biopsy of the wound as the standard [14]. While the time-honored method of expert clinical evaluation by a trained burn surgeon remains the accepted standard for assessment of burn depth outside of the more invasive gold standard of serial wound biopsies, new technologies and techniques, including laser Doppler imaging (LDI), are emerging that have the potential to improve the accuracy and consistency of burn depth assessment [15].

Superficial dermal burns (superficial partial-thickness burns) extend to the level of the papillary dermis and form characteristic blisters. Following blister debridement, the wound bed is moist, tender, and blanchable as a result of enhanced hyperemia and blood flow compared to normal skin [6]. Deep dermal burns (deep partial-thickness burns) extend into the reticular dermis and typically portend longer healing times. Deep dermal burns may blister but the wounds are less tender. Due to diminished blood flow the wound beds appear mottled pink and white with minimal blanching and delayed capillary refill [6]. Doppler technology images blood flow using laser Doppler assessment of moving red blood cells to detect vascularity and thus viability. Images are collected of normal and burned skin; normal skin has a moderate level of blood flow, while superficial burns have significantly increased blood flow associated with increased local inflammation. Deep partial- and full-thickness burns have significantly decreased blood flow. Images can be obtained at any time after injury with reasonable accuracy (>90% sensitivity and specificity with wound biopsies and requirements for surgery) [16]. However, limitations of LDI include disagreement regarding cutoff points of perfusion values, commercial cost, limited availability, topographical artifacts from scanning contoured areas (e.g., abdomen and flanks), skewing of results from tattoos, vascular disease, and anemia.

RECOMMENDATION

Burn depth may best be determined by LDI to the exclusion of clinical assessment, and for wounds in doubt, we recommend consideration of this technology.

Grade of recommendation: B.

LDI should not entirely replace expert clinical assessment, but rather should be utilized as a tool for assessing indeterminate burn depth or corroboration with physical exam findings.

31.4 What Is the Optimal Approach to Burn Wound Management According to the Depth of Injury?

All efforts should be made to avoid unnecessary excision and grafting. Superficial partial-thickness burns extend into the papillary dermis and will typically heal in 2–3 weeks with appropriate wound care. Unless there is an active infection, superficial dermal burns should be managed nonoperatively. Preventing the conversion of wounds to greater depths hinges on sound wound care and mitigation of impaired microvascular perfusion and infection. While burn wounds that have not healed within 3 weeks need excision and grafting, burns of indeterminate depth represent a diagnostic and management dilemma for burn surgeons [6, 17].

Hydrosurgery with a high-powered parallel water jet (e.g., Versajet, Smith-Nephew, Hull, UK) has shown benefit as a useful tool to debride burn wounds of variable depth. Hydrosurgical techniques may offer better wound bed preparation than standard bedside dressing changes and promote the healing of indeterminate wounds, potentially without the need for grafting. It is the opinion of these authors that the utilization of hydrosurgery for indeterminate burn wounds with ongoing meticulous postoperative wound care is a useful tool for attempting to minimize the need for skin grafting. If an indeterminate burn wound bleeds with hydrosurgical debridement at low to moderate pressure settings, we feel that reasonable healing potential exists with ongoing bedside wound care, and skin grafting may be avoided.

The goals of local wound care in partial-thickness and indeterminate-depth burns include minimizing wound complications, creating an environment for rapid healing, maximizing patient comfort, and minimizing provider effort [18]. Common topical wound care agents include petroleum-based antimicrobials and iodine-impregnated petroleum-based gauze, honey-impregnated formulations, silver-based dressings, and antipseudomonal-based therapies (e.g., mafenide acetate). No wound care option is without drawbacks, and there are no definitive data regarding which dressing or dermal agent is best for treating burn wounds while preventing infections and improving wound recovery [19].

Additional wound management options for indeterminate-depth burns include cadaveric allograft, xenograft, dermal substitutes, and synthetic skin substitutes. Cadaveric allografts and xenografts are useful as temporary biologic dressings until skin grafting in large, full-thickness burns where inadequate donor sites exist or as a biologic dressing for indeterminate-depth burns to optimize wound healing. Both require debridement of necrotic tissue and wound preparation [17]. Dermal substitutes frequently require full-thickness dermal excision prior to placement and are typically reserved for indeterminate-depth burns that have failed nonoperative management or full-thickness burns [17]. Synthetic skin substitutes are a more contemporary class of burn dressing and have been shown to promote epithelialization [20]. Biobrane is a transparent, biologic composite of nylon mesh covered with porcine type I collagen and facilitates the ingrowth of fibrin. Biobrane's transparency allows for regular wound assessment without dressing disruption. Lesher et al. demonstrated more expedient healing and shorter hospitalizations with Biobrane compared to historical controls treated with beta glucan collagen (BGC) [20]. The major disadvantage of synthetic skin substitutes is the potential for bacterial colonization and wound infection [21].

Accurate determination of burn wound depth remains paramount to appropriate management. All efforts should be made to tailor the management plan to the individual patient and utilize the principles of minimizing excision and grafting where feasible. This is best accomplished by allowing superficial partial-thickness burns to heal through sound local wound care and by providing adequate physiologic management, wound bed preparation, and meticulous wound care to indeterminate-depth burns to prevent infection, ischemia, and progression to full-thickness wounds, which mandate excision and grafting. Full-thickness wounds should be excised and grafted early.

RECOMMENDATIONS

The optimal time for burn wound excision is within 48 hours of injury to minimize infectious wound complications and expedite the length of hospital stay.

Grade of recommendation: B.

The best treatment is one that controls antimicrobial growth and allows for frequent wound assessment while minimizing dressing changes. All potential treatments have at least one drawback in this regard, but treatment with a skin substitute or a long-term silver cloth dressing appears to be the best alternative with the current technology.

Grade of recommendation: B.

31.5 What Is the Optimal Transfusion Strategy in Major Burns, and How Is Blood Loss Best Minimized During Burn Excision Procedures?

Severe burn injury is associated with the need for blood and blood product transfusions across the spectrum of resuscitation, operative, and critical care management. It is estimated that patients with major burns may have transfusion requirements exceeding an entire blood volume. Anemia in burns results from increased red blood cell destruction, decreased reticulocyte production, bone marrow suppression, hemodilution from resuscitation, iatrogenic blood draws, surgical blood loss, frequent dressing changes, and nutritional deficits [22, 23].

Estimating 0.5 mL blood loss per 1 cm^2 excised, a normal-sized man with a 50% TBSA burn excision will be predicted to lose 5000 mL of blood, or 10 units [18]. Multifactorial coagulation abnormalities are known to accompany the severely burned patient; thus balanced, judicious hemostatic resuscitation is vital to appropriate perioperative management [24] in addition to meticulous surgical technique and adjuncts to hemostasis. Adjuncts include the utilization of tourniquets during extremity burn excision, topical hemostatic agents for eschar and donor site wounds, and subcutaneous clysis or tumescence of donor sites with vasoconstrictive agents.

Tourniquet use can contribute to inadequate excision and skin graft failure due to impaired or absent punctate small vessel bleeding as a guide [25]. In a randomized controlled study of extremity wound excisions comparing tourniquets to no tourniquets in unexsanguinated extremities, O'Mara demonstrated significantly less blood loss with the use of tourniquets and no difference in graft healing [26]. Aballay et al. demonstrated significantly less blood loss and no differences in graft take with extremity exsanguination with Esmarch tourniquets in conjunction with standard pneumatic extremity tourniquets [25].

In a systematic review of topical hemostatic agents in cutaneous wounds, Groenewold et al. concluded that topical and subcutaneous vasoconstrictive therapies (namely epinephrine-based) and fibrin sealants are superior to thrombin and other hemostatic products or placebo with regard to the volume of hemorrhage and speed of hemostasis. They further noted a superiority of thrombin to K-Y jelly, mineral oil, or saline [27].

Subcutaneous clysis and tumescence of donor sites and burn eschar have been posited to reduce bleeding and possibly pain associated with burn excision and skin harvesting. Widespread adoption of this technique has been hindered by trepidation regarding potential cardiac complications from absorbed epinephrine in the setting of inhaled anesthetic use and the potential for impaired wound healing from local vasoconstriction. The data for tumescence and/or subcutaneous clysis are limited by small sample sizes, historical controls, inconsistencies in technique, solution concentrations and formulations, presence or absence of tumescent anesthetic, and site application. However, there are reasonable data to support the claim that clysis and/or tumescence may reduce blood loss without negatively impacting wound healing or significantly prolonging operative times, and without increased risk of adverse effects [28, 29].

RECOMMENDATIONS

We recommend a balanced, judicious hemostatic transfusion strategy in the burn population.

Grade of recommendation: B.

In order to mitigate perioperative hemorrhage and transfusion requirements, we recommend a multifaceted approach to include the use of pneumatic tourniquets coupled with Esmarch exsanguination for extremity burn excision, subcutaneous clysis and/or tumescence at donor sites with consideration for use at burn excision sites for small-size TBSA so as to mitigate potential systemic toxicity of epinephrine and local anesthetics, and use of topical epinephrine-impregnated solutions and/or fibrin sealant to facilitate post excision and grafting hemostasis.

Grade of recommendation: B.

31.6 How Are Burn Wound and Multidrug-Resistant Infections Effectively Minimized?

Burn wound infection is common in the severely burned due to loss of innate defense associated with the skin, the rich pabulum of the denatured protein comprising eschar, and relative burn-induced immune suppression making burn patients particularly susceptible to sepsis. These three conditions combine to result in the invasion of microorganisms into remaining viable tissue. Organisms typically causing burn wound infection are of a wide spectrum, from gram-positives and gram-negatives to opportunistic fungi and viruses.

Burn wound infection can be minimized in two ways. The first is early excision and grafting for wound closure to re-establish the skin barrier and remove the culture medium of the eschar. We have already seen that early excision of the wound in deep partial- and full-thickness burns is associated with decreased incidence of wound infection, and another study showed that wounds excised greater than 6 days from injury had increased bacterial counts and increased rate of graft loss [30]. The second is to provide topical antimicrobial therapy directly to the wound, which was shown to be beneficial in burn wounds between 40% and 80% TBSA [31]. Systemic antibiotics have almost no supportive evidence in the literature, yet are a common practice. Antimicrobial selection should be for a broad-spectrum agent effective against gram-positive and gram-negative bacteria and fungi. This is typically achieved topically with the use of silver-containing agents such as silver sulfadiazine and silver ion-containing dressings or through alternating use of 5% sulfamylon and/or Dakins' and Domboro's solutions.

RECOMMENDATION

Burn wound infection is minimized through early excision and grafting for wound closure and the use of topical antimicrobials.

Grade of recommendation: B.

31.7 Approach to the Patient with Inhalation Injury: Introduction

Smoke inhalation injury occurs as a result of the inspiration of super-heated gases and the combusted materials contained therein. Direct thermal injury of the upper airway, including the mouth, oropharynx, and larynx, may occur because of inspiring super-heated air. Injury to the lower airways, including the trachea, bronchi, and alveoli, occurs predominantly because of inspiring chemical and particulate constituents of combusted gases beyond the glottis, causing direct tissue injury. Patterns of lower airway injury are highly variable largely based on the water solubility and physical characteristics of the inhaled constituents. Lastly, systemic toxicity, or metabolic asphyxiation, may occur because of pulmonary absorption of systemic toxins, namely carbon monoxide (CO) and hydrogen cyanide (HCN) [6].

Inhalation injury (II) is common, occurring in up to 20% of fire-related injuries [32]. Death from asphyxiation is thought to be the leading cause of death in patients who die on scene, and II is thought to be a contributing factor in 60–80% of the nearly 4,000 fire-related deaths that occur annually [33]. In patients who survive to receive inpatient care, II is a known independent predictor of morbidity and mortality, with average mortality in patients with combined cutaneous burns and II approximating 25% [32]. Patients admitted with concomitant cutaneous thermal injuries will generally require more IV fluid resuscitation than controls without II. II is known to be associated with increased rates of bacterial pneumonia, pulmonary edema, and acute respiratory distress syndrome (ARDS) [34]. It is also important to recognize that II may occur in the absence of concomitant cutaneous thermal injuries [32].

31.8 What Diagnostic Procedures Should Be Performed in Patients with Suspected Inhalation Injury?

A definitive diagnosis of II need not be performed prior to referral to a regional burn center. The pretest probability of II may be estimated by history and physical examination positive for signs and symptoms to include facial burns, singed nasal or facial hair, carbonaceous deposits in the oropharynx or within expectorate, hoarseness, subjective change in voice, tachypnea, hypoxia, and dyspnea. The mechanism of injury may also predict the likelihood of II such as flame burns that occur within an enclosed space or prolonged extrication from the scene with exposure to flame or smoke. In a retrospective study of 1,058 burn-injured patients with 35% having been diagnosed with II by bronchoscopy and/or xenon-133 lung scans, Shirani et al. generated the following predictive model [35]:

$$P\,(\text{Inhalation Injury}) = ek/(1 - ek)$$

where k = −4.4165 + 1.61 (closed space) + 1.77 (facial burn) + 0.0237 (TBSA; %) + 0.0268 (age; years). P ranges from 0 to 1; values for closed space and facial burn are 0 (absent) or 1 (present).

While this model incorporates closed space, facial burns, percent TBSA, and age, most clinicians should have a high suspicion of the first two factors. The most described signs of II such as stridor, voice change, and dyspnea are frequently absent and so are not reliable.

Several radiographic techniques have been described in attempts to diagnose II, though none have demonstrated significant clinical utility. Most patients with II at the time of admission have normal chest X-rays. Thus, a normal chest radiograph cannot be used to rule out II. Chest computed tomography (CT) has also been described as a potentially more sensitive and specific measure for detecting inhalation injury than plain chest radiography. Bronchial wall thickening, perivascular fuzziness or cuffing, alveolar or interstitial pulmonary edema, consolidation, and atelectasis have been reported as common findings on chest CT [36–38]. Work is currently underway to develop methods to detect the presence and perhaps the severity of II utilizing point-of-care ultrasonography. Ultrasonographic findings that may be consistent with II include tracheal wall thickening, B-line artifact, and parenchymal consolidation [39, 40].

A flexible fiberoptic bronchoscopic survey of the airways is currently the gold standard for definitively diagnosing II.

TABLE 31.1

Abbreviated Injury Score System for Inhalation Injury Grading for Bronchoscopy

Grade	Class	Findings
0	No injury	Absence of carbonaceous deposits, erythema, edema, bronchorrhea, or obstruction
1	Mild injury	Minor or patchy areas of erythema, carbonaceous deposits in proximal or distal bronchi
2	Moderate injury	A moderate degree of erythema, carbonaceous deposits, bronchorrhea, or bronchial obstruction
3	Severe injury	Severe inflammation with friability, copious carbonaceous deposits, bronchorrhea, or obstruction
4	Massive injury	Evidence of mucosal sloughing, necrosis, or endoluminal obliteration

In addition to making the diagnosis, bronchoscopy will facilitate grading, which serves a prognostic role, as the escalating grade of II is directly related to mortality. A commonly adopted model for grading employs the Abbreviated Injury Score (AIS) for inhalation injury (Table 31.1) [41, 42]. Bronchoscopy should be performed serially, as sequelae of inhalation injury may not be apparent immediately following injury, with mucosal findings becoming more apparent 24–48 hours after injury.

RECOMMENDATION

A presumptive diagnosis of inhalation injury and a decision to transfer to a burn center can be made on clinical grounds. Definitive diagnosis requires fiberoptic bronchoscopy and/or advanced imaging techniques.

Grade of recommendation: B.

31.9 What Are the Indications for Endotracheal Intubation and for Tracheostomy in Patients with Inhalation Injury?

Respiratory failure following severe burn injury with or without II may not manifest until 24–48 hours postinjury. Due to a lack of accurate prediction models for the need for mechanical ventilation, as well as the life-threatening complications that may be associated with delayed endotracheal intubation such as airway obstruction due to edema formation, current recommendations are to have a low threshold for early endotracheal intubation in patients with suspected or confirmed II [43, 44]. Though data would suggest many patients do not require endotracheal intubation, with approximately 30% of patients extubated within 24 hours after admission, patients with burns to the face and upper airway or with clinically significant II should be considered for early endotracheal intubation (Table 31.2) [45–47].

TABLE 31.2

American Burn Association (ABA)
2011 Intubation Criteria

Full-thickness facial burn
Stridor
Respiratory distress
Airway swelling on laryngoscopy
Airway trauma
Altered mentation
Hypoxia/hypercapnia
Hemodynamic instability

RECOMMENDATIONS

Early endotracheal intubation is indicated for most symptomatic patients with inhalation injury and for patients with extensive burns during initial resuscitation.

Grade of recommendation: C.

Tracheostomy is an option for long-term airway management and may facilitate treatment to reduce pulmonary complications.

Grade of recommendation: C.

Direct thermal injury to the upper airway (including the larynx, oropharynx, mouth, and tongue) causes edema, which may progress within minutes or hours to complete airway obstruction. Orotracheal intubation of such patients after the onset of obstruction is often impossible, and immediate cricothyroidotomy should then be considered. To avoid that scenario, early endotracheal intubation is appropriate. Cotton ties (1/2-inch umbilical "tape"), rather than adhesive tape, are used to secure the endotracheal tube circumferentially around the patient's neck. The tube may become obstructed in patients with copious mucus production. This may be prevented by frequent (hourly or more) suctioning and saline flushes instilled into the endotracheal tube.

Concomitant skin burns compound airway swelling and increase the risk of airway obstruction. While II directly damages the airway, cutaneous thermal injury causes generalized edema throughout the body, including the airway. In adults, we recommend early endotracheal intubation for symptomatic patients with indicators of II, facial and/or oropharyngeal burns, and for patients with greater than 40% TBSA burns until the resuscitation period is complete (first 48 hours) even when II is absent.

Induction for endotracheal intubation must consider the risk for hypotension, as many burn patients are preload sensitive (hypovolemic) at the time of intubation. The selection of agents for induction must be well thought out and with contingencies planned such as vasopressors and IV fluids readily available to respond to induction and peri-intubation hypotension. More hemodynamically neutral agents such as ketamine should be preferred to vasodilating agents such as propofol [48]. The same considerations should be applied to premedication for direct laryngoscopy.

There is currently no consensus on the appropriate timing of tracheostomy in burn-injured patients with or without II. In patients who have an anticipated need or have demonstrated the need for prolonged mechanical ventilation, a tracheostomy is thought to allow for more frequent and efficacious airway clearance, may be more comfortable for patients and thus decrease the need for sedatives and analgesics, and promote engagement in rehabilitation, all while allowing weaning from mechanical ventilation [49, 50]. Caution should be employed when considering the percutaneous route for patients with copious purulent or bloody secretions, as may be the case in severe II. For these patients, open tracheostomy may be safer.

31.10 What Mode of Mechanical Ventilation Is Most Effective for Patients with Inhalation Injury?

The ARMA trial conducted by the ARDSNet excluded patients with burns in excess of 30% TBSA [51]; thus the results may not be fully applicable to patients with II. The principal cause of hypoxemia in ARDS induced by pulmonary contusion, systemic injury, or sepsis is alveolar flooding and an increase in a true shunt. As small airway obstruction progresses, atelectasis followed by consolidation and pneumonia ensues. Thus, ventilation of II patients, in contrast to other forms of ARDS, should focus not only on avoiding ventilator-induced lung injury but also on actively providing pulmonary toilet and recruiting and stabilizing collapsed alveoli.

The VDR-4 provides high-frequency, flow-interrupted breaths that effect the dislodgement of debris and cause its retrograde expulsion out of the airways. For this reason, we partially deflate the endotracheal tube cuff (to a minimal leak level) and frequently suction the oropharynx, as plugs and secretions in II patients can be copious. Finally, VDR-4, like airway-pressure release ventilation (APRV, also known as bilevel ventilation) enables spontaneous ventilation throughout the inspiratory and expiratory phases. This may improve patient–ventilator synchrony and, as in APRV, may have other beneficial effects on gas distribution and respiratory muscle strength. The main disadvantage of the VDR-4 is the extra training required of nurses and respiratory therapists in its operation.

RECOMMENDATION

In comparison to conventional mechanical ventilation, high-frequency percussive ventilation improves ventilation and oxygenation in patients with II and may reduce pneumonia and mortality.

Grade of recommendation: B.

Low-tidal-volume mechanical ventilation is most appropriate in the hands of those untrained in VDR or without access to VDR, along with increased pulmonary toilet adjuncts when no percussive ventilation is available.

31.11 What Medications and Fluid Management Strategies Improve Outcomes?

Patients with isolated II rarely have excessive fluid resuscitation requirements; however, in conjunction with cutaneous burns, fluid resuscitation requirements greatly increase during the first 48 hours post-burn. Resuscitation of patients with combined cutaneous burns and II should be conducted with close attention to endpoints such as the urine output to avoid too much and too little fluid.

II causes a hypercoagulable state in the lungs [52], one manifestation of which is the formation of obstructing clots and casts. Inhaled heparin is one way in which we routinely address this pathology. Because obstructing clots and casts are a common life-threatening problem after II, and because this therapy is inexpensive and does not cause systemic anticoagulation [53], we routinely provide nebulized heparin to all II patients, beginning on admission and continuing while intubated and airways remain friable.

Inhaled nitric oxide (NO), by improving blood flow to well-ventilated lung segments, modestly improves oxygenation following II [54]. Corticosteroids are to be avoided because of their immunosuppressive effects, except in those patients who are adrenally insufficient or who (rarely) have refractory bronchospasm. Bronchodilators such as albuterol, with or without N-acetylcysteine, are routinely given to intubated II patients to improve ventilation.

Patients with II are more than two times as likely to develop pneumonia than those without II [55]. In multiple studies, prophylactic antibiotics have not been shown to prevent infection in II or burn patients. When hospitalized for weeks to months, these patients are at risk of colonization and infection with multidrug-resistant organisms; this risk increases with indiscriminate antibiotic exposure. Early institution of broad-spectrum antibiotics, an aggressive diagnostic approach to include bronchoalveolar lavage, and rapid tailoring of the regimen to match organism sensitivities are crucial.

RECOMMENDATIONS

Fluid resuscitation of patients with II should be carefully titrated to physiologic endpoints such as adequacy of urine output (range 30–50 mL/hour in adults), avoiding both fluid excess and fluid restriction.

Grade of recommendation: C.

Inhaled heparin may prevent obstructing clots and casts in patients with II at low risk and cost.

Grade of recommendation: C.

While adjuncts such as proning, NO, vitamin C, and antithrombin III may be more widely available, there is not strong literature to support their use.

31.12 What Immediate Treatments Are Safe and Effective for Metabolic Asphyxiation by Carbon Monoxide or Hydrogen Cyanide Toxicity?

Along with smoke, patients may inhale compounds that impair oxygen delivery to or utilization by the tissues. CO is a product of incompletely combusted carbon-containing compounds such as cellulosics (e.g., wood, paper, coal, charcoal), natural gases (methane, butane, propane), and petroleum products. The organs most vulnerable to CO poisoning are the cardiovascular system and the brain, which are those most affected by oxygen deprivation. The diagnosis requires measurement of arterial carboxyhemoglobin (COHb) levels using a CO oximeter; the PaO_2 in these patients is frequently normal or high. A standard two-wavelength pulse oximeter will provide a falsely high SpO_2 reading even with COHb levels in the lethal range ($\geq 50\%$) because it cannot discriminate between COHb and oxygenated hemoglobin [56]. The half-life of COHb is not a function of the FiO_2, but of the PaO_2, which in II patients may be quite variable even at an FiO_2 of 100%.

The mainstay of treatment is 100% oxygen by nonrebreather mask or endotracheal tube until the COHb level is less than 5% [57] or for 6 hours [58]. Hyperbaric oxygen therapy (HBOT) has been used to treat these patients. Although HBOT accelerates the clearance of CO beyond that achieved by 100% oxygen at one atmosphere, the main rationale is the prevention of delayed neurocognitive syndrome. This features memory loss and other cognitive defects with onset 2–28 days after exposure and is thought to be caused by the binding of CO to brain mitochondrial cytochromes and by other mechanisms [58]. The American College of Emergency Physicians published a clinical policy in 2008 stating that while data support HBOT as an option for CO poisoning, its use is not mandated [59].

HCN is produced by the combustion of nitrogen-containing materials such as plastics, foam, paints, wool, and silk. It impairs cellular utilization of oxygen by binding to the terminal cytochrome (cytochrome a, a3) of the electron transport chain, causing lactic acidosis and potentially elevated mixed venous oxygen saturation. The half-life in the human body is about 1 hour. The role of HCN in fire deaths and the prevalence of HCN poisoning in patients with II is less clear than that of CO.

Diagnosis of HCN poisoning is difficult because a rapid assay is not available; HCN and CO poisoning share many features, including signs and symptoms related to the central nervous and cardiovascular systems [60]. Hydroxocobalamin (a form of vitamin B_{12}) is now available in the United States as the Cyanokit for IV injection. This drug is well-tolerated and rapidly chelates HCN [61]. The Cyanide Antidote Kit in the United States contains amyl nitrite for inhalation and sodium nitrite and sodium thiosulfate for IV injection. The nitrites oxidize hemoglobin to methemoglobin (MetHb), which chelates HCN. Sodium thiosulfate combines with HCN to form thiocyanate, which is excreted in the urine. We do not recommend the use of nitrites in patients with II and suspected HCN poisoning, as they can cause severe hypotension, and the MetHb does not transport oxygen [62]. This is problematic, particularly in patients with burn shock and impaired oxygen transport and utilization from CO and HCN.

Methemoglobinemia is another life-threatening syndrome of metabolic asphyxiation which is rarely seen in II patients. Certain smoke constituents such as NO and nitrogen dioxide oxidize hemoglobin to MetHb, a species that is incapable of carrying oxygen. This problem may also be caused by several drugs, including nitrites or topical anesthetics such as benzocaine. As with COHb, a two-wavelength pulse oximeter cannot distinguish MetHb and gives false SpO_2 readings in the 80s. Patients with high levels of MetHb may have chocolate brown-colored blood and, if light-skinned, central cyanosis. Diagnosis is by CO oximetry, and treatment consists of IV methylene blue, preferably in consultation with a poison control center [63].

RECOMMENDATIONS

CO oximetry (measurement of COHb and MetHb levels) should be performed in patients with II.

Grade of recommendation: D.

One hundred percent oxygen should be given to all patients with known or suspected COHb poisoning until the COHb is normal (less than 5%).

Grade of recommendation: D.

HBOT is an option for patients with COHb poisoning for prevention of delayed neurocognitive syndrome.

Grade of recommendation: C.

Hydroxocobalamin treatment should be given to patients with known or suspected cyanide poisoning.

Grade of recommendation: C.

31.13 Should Patients with Inhalation Injury Be Transferred to a Regional Burn Center?

II is one of the ABA criteria for burn center referral [64]. Although we are not aware of prospective data comparing the outcomes of II patients treated in burn centers versus those treated elsewhere, many of the modalities mentioned in this chapter are not routinely available outside of burn centers to include the expertise of respiratory therapists and other health-care professionals to provide optimal care to patients with this highly lethal injury. Smoke-exposed patients with an unremarkable physical examination, alert mental status, and normal blood gases and COHb levels may safely be discharged home [65]. For all II patients requiring admission, we recommend at a minimum prompt consultation with the regional burn center.

RECOMMENDATION

Consultation with the regional burn center should be performed upon admission of a patient with inhalation injury.

Grade of recommendation: D.

TABLE 31.3

Summary

Clinical Question	Answer	Recommendation Grade
What are the optimal resuscitation methods and goals of resuscitation following severe burn?	• Parkland or modified Brooke formula with isotonic crystalloid. • Initiation of albumin at post-burn hour 8 if exceeding >250 mL/kg/%TBSA or >1500 cc/hour crystalloid.	B
How do we determine burn depth?	• LDI should not entirely replace expert clinical assessment, but rather should be utilized as a tool for assessing indeterminate burn depth or corroboration with physical exam findings.	B
What is the optimal approach to burn wound management according to depth of injury?	• Excise burn wounds within 48 hours of injury to minimize infectious wound complications and expedite length of hospital stay. • Best treatment is with a skin substitute or a long-term silver cloth dressing.	B
What is the optimal transfusion strategy in major burns, and how is blood loss best minimized during burn excision procedures?	• Use a balanced, judicious hemostatic transfusion strategy in the burn population. In order to mitigate perioperative hemorrhage and transfusion requirements, we recommend a multifaceted approach to include use of tourniquets, subcutaneous clysis and/or tumescence, and use of topical epinephrine-impregnated solutions and/or fibrin sealant to facilitate post-excision and grafting hemostasis.	B
How are burn wound and multidrug-resistant infections effectively minimized?	• Burn wound infection is minimized through early excision and grafting for wound closure and use of topical antimicrobials.	B

(Continued)

TABLE 31.3 (Continued)

Summary

Clinical Question	Answer	Recommendation Grade
What diagnostic procedures should be performed in patients with suspected inhalation injury?	• A presumptive diagnosis may be made based on clinical impression alone (supporting history, mechanism, and physical exam findings). • Laryngoscopy and chest radiography or ultrasonography may support the diagnosis; however, bronchoscopy is required for definitive diagnosis.	B
What are the indications for endotracheal intubation and for tracheostomy in patients with inhalation injury?	• Early prophylactic airway control is indicated for most symptomatic patients with II and for patients with extensive burns during initial resuscitation. • Tracheostomy is an option for long-term airway management and may facilitate pulmonary clearance.	C
What mode of mechanical ventilation is most effective for these patients?	• High-frequency percussive ventilation improves ventilation and oxygenation and may reduce pneumonia and mortality.	B
What medications and fluid management strategies improve outcomes?	• Inhaled heparin may prevent obstructing clots and casts. • Avoid under- or over-resuscitation. II patients frequently require larger volumes for burn shock resuscitation, but no evidence supports initiation of resuscitation at higher infusion rates.	C
What immediate treatments are safe and effective for metabolic asphyxiation by carbon monoxide or hydrogen cyanide toxicity?	• One hundred percent oxygen should be given to all patients with CO poisoning until the COHb is normal (<5%). • Hydroxocobalamin should be considered for patients with known or suspected cyanide poisoning.	D
Should patients with inhalation injury be transferred to a regional burn center?	• Consultation with the regional burn center should be performed upon admission.	D

Note: The reader is cautioned that recommendations concerning airway management, 100% oxygen for treatment of CO poisoning, and burn center referral are considered standard of care in the United States despite the cited levels of evidence.

31.14 Conclusions

Data exist in the literature to support the use of many therapies to improve outcomes of the severely burned; however, most of these methods have not been rigorously tested. The highest grade of recommendation for these central questions for burn care is only at the class II level for the quality of evidence, and thus, only grade B recommendations can be made. Well-defined and well-conducted trials are required to provide further answers to these questions, in particular the method of resuscitation and the timing of burn excision and grafting. The advances described in this review have resulted in a significant reduction in mortality following II over the past 70 years [66]. Still, II remains a significant independent predictor of postburn death [67]. A recent ABA State of the Science symposium identified four priorities for II research: Diagnosis and grading of severity of the injury, therapeutics (mechanical ventilation, extracorporeal life support, drugs, role of tracheostomy), long-term outcomes, and basic science mechanisms [68]. Randomized controlled multicenter trials are needed to address these unsolved issues.

REFERENCES

1. Woodcock TE, Woodcock TM. Revised Starling equation and the glycocalyx model of transvascular fluid exchange: an improved paradigm for prescribing intravenous fluid therapy. British Journal of Anesthesia. 2012;108(3):384–394
2. Fleck A, Raines G, Hawker F, Trotter J, Wallace PI, Ledingham IM, Calman KC. Increased vascular permeability: a major cause of hypoalbuminaemia in disease and injury. The Lancet. 1985;325(8432):781–784
3. Soussi S, Dépret F, Benyamina M, Legrand M. Early hemodynamic management of critically Ill burn patients. Anesthesiology. 2018;129:583–589
4. Asch MJ, Feldman RJ, Walker HL, Foley FD, Popp RL, Mason AD Jr, Pruitt BA Jr. Systemic and pulmonary hemodynamic changes accompanying thermal injury. Annals of Surgery. 1973;178(2):218–221
5. Soussi S, Deniau B, Ferry A, Levé C, Benyamina M, Maurel V, Chaussard M, Le Cam B, Blet A, Mimoun M, Lambert J, Chaouat M, Mebazaa A, Legrand M; PRONOBURN group. Low cardiac index and stroke volume on admission are associated with poor outcome in critically ill burn patients: a retrospective cohort study. Annals Intensive Care. 2016;6:87
6. Herndon DN, Woodson LC, Branski LK, Enkbaatar P, Talon M. Diagnosis and treatment of inhalation injury. In: Total burn care. Available from: Elsevier eBooks+, 5th ed. Elsevier - OHCE, 2017.
7. Atiyeh BS, Dibo SA, Ibrahim AE, Zgheib ER. Acute burn resuscitation and fluid creep: it is time for colloid rehabilitation. Annals of Burns and Fire Disasters. 2012;XXV(2):59–65
8. Ivy ME, Atweh NA, Palmer J, Possenti PP, Pineau M, D'Aiuto M. Intra-abdominal hypertension and abdominal compartment syndrome in burn patients. Journal of Trauma. 2000;49(3):387–391
9. Chung KK, Salinas J, Renz EM, Alvarado RA, King BT, Barillo DJ, Cancio LC, Wolf SE, Blackbourne LH. Simple derivation of the initial fluid rate for the resuscitation of severely burned adult combat casualties: in silico validation of the rule of 10. Journal of Trauma. 2010;69(1):S49–S54

10. Leclerc T, Potokar T, Hughes A, Norton I, Alexandru C, Haik J, Moiemen N, Almeland SK. A simplified fluid resuscitation formula for burns in mass casualty scenarios: analysis of the consensus recommendation from WHO emergency medical teams technical working group on burns. Burns. 2021;47:1730–1738

11. Driscoll IR, Mann-Salinas EA, Boyer NL, Pamplin JC, Serio-Melvin ML, Salinas J, Borgman MA, Sheridan RL, Melvin JJ, Peterson WC, Graybill JC, Rizzo JA, King BT, Chung KK, Cancio LC, Renz EM, Stockinger ZT, Gurney J. Burn Care (CPG ID:12). Joint Trauma System Clinical Practice Guideline. 2016; https://jts.amedd.army.mil/assets/docs/cpgs/Burn_Care_11_May_2016_ID12.pdf

12. Du GB, Slater H, Goldfarb IW. Influences of different resuscitation regimens on acute early weight gain in extensively burned patients. Burns. 1991;17(2):17147–17150

13. Vigiola Cruz M, Carney BC, Luker JN, Monger KW, Vazquez JS, Moffatt LT, Johnson LS, Shupp JW. Plasma ameliorates endothelial dysfunction in burn injury. Journal of Surgical Research. 2019;233:459–466

14. Hemington-Gorse SJ. A comparison of laser Doppler imaging with other measurement techniques to assess burn depth. J Wound Care. 2005;14(4):151–153

15. Pape SA, Skouras CA, Byrne PO. An audit of the use of laser Doppler imaging (LDI) in the assessment of burns of intermediate depth. Burns. 2001;27(3):233–239

16. Jeng JC, Bridgeman A, Shivnan L, Thornton PM, Alam H, Clarke TJ, Jablonski KA, Jordan MH. Laser Doppler imaging determines need for excision and grafting in advance of clinical judgment: A prospective blinded trial. Burns. 2003;29(7):665–670

17. Karim AS, Shaum K, Gibson ALF. Indeterminate depth burn injury-exploring the uncertainty. Journal of Surgical Research. 2020;245:183–197

18. Bernal EB, Wolf SE. Acute care surgery and trauma: evidence-based practice. 2nd ed. 2016: Chapter 33. CRC Press.

19. Lagziel T, Asif M, Born L, Quiroga LH, Duraes E, Slavin B, Shetty P, Caffrey J, Hultman CS. Evaluating the efficacy, safety, and tolerance of silver sulfadiazine dressings once daily versus twice daily in the treatment of burn wounds. Journal of Burn Care & Research. 2021;42(6):1136–1139

20. Lesher AP, Curry RH, Evans J, Smith VA, Fitzgerald MT, Cina RA, Streck CJ, Hebra AV. Effectiveness of biobrane for treatment of partial-thickness burns in children. Journal of Pediatric Surgery. 2011;46(9):1759–1763

21. Guang Ho CW, See JL, Yang SH, Tan BK. Early experience with biobrane™ for definitive coverage of tangentially-excised partial-thickness thermal burns. World Journal of Plastic Surgery. 2021;10(1):119–124

22. Palmieri TL, Holmes JH 4th, Arnoldo B, Peck M, Potenza B, Cochran A, King BT, Dominic W, Cartotto R, Bhavsar D, Kemalyan N, Tredget E, Stapelberg F, Mozingo D, Friedman B, Greenhalgh DG, Taylor SL, Pollock BH. Transfusion requirement in burn care evaluation (TRIBE): a multicenter randomized prospective trial of blood transfusion in major burn injury. Annals of Surgery. 2017;266(4):595–602

23. Koljonen V, Tuimala J, Haglund C, Tukiainen E, Vuola J, Juvonen E, Lauronen J, Krusius T. The use of blood products in adult patients with burns. Scandinavian Journal of Surgery. 2016;105(3):178–185

24. Pidcoke HF, Isbell CL, Herzig MC, Fedyk CG, Schaffer BS, Chung KK, White CE, Wolf SE, Wade CE, Cap AP. Acute blood loss during burn and soft tissue excisions: an observational study of blood product resuscitation practices and focused review. The Journal of Trauma and Acute Care Surgery. 2015;78(601000006):S39–S47

25. Aballay AM, Recio P, Slater H, Goldfarb IW, Tolchin E, Papasavas P, Caushaj PF. The use of Esmarch exsanguination for the treatment of extremity wound burns. Annals of Burns and Fire Disasters. 2007;XX(1):22–24

26. O'Mara MS, Goel A, Recio P, Slater H, Goldfarb IW, Tolchin E, Caushaj PF. The use of tourniquets in the excision of unexsanguinated extremity burn wounds. Burns. 2002;28(7):684–687

27. Groenewold MD, Gribnau AJ, Ubbink DT. Topical haemostatic agents for skin wounds: a systematic review. BMC Surgery. 2011;11:15

28. Blome-Eberwein S, Abboud M, Lozano DD, Sharma R, Eid S, Gogal C. Effect of subcutaneous epinephrine/saline/local anesthetic versus saline-only injection on split-thickness skin graft donor site perfusion, healing, and pain. Journal of Burn Care & Research. 2013;34(2):e80–e86.

29. Fukuoka K, Yagi S, Suyama Y, Kaida W, Morita M, Hisatome I. Effect of subcutaneous adrenaline/saline/lidocaine injection on split-thickness skin graft donor site wound healing. Yonago Acta Medica. 2021;64(1):107–112

30. Barret JP, Herndon DN. Effects of burn wound excision on bacterial colonization and invasion. Plastic and Reconstructive Surgery. 2003;111(2):744–750; discussion 51–52.

31. Brown TP, Cancio LC, McManus AT, Mason AD. Survival benefit conferred by topical antimicrobial preparations in burn patients: an historical perspective. Journal of Trauma. 2004;56(4):863–866

32. 2021 burn injury summary report [Internet]. American Burn Association. American Burn Association; 2021 [cited 2022Sep23].

33. Fire-related deaths & injuries [Internet]. Injury Facts. 2022 [cited 2022Sep23]. Available from: https://injuryfacts.nsc.org/home-and-community/safety-topics/fire-related-fatalities-and-injuries/

34. Deutsch CJ, Tan A, Smailes S, Dziewulski P. The diagnosis and management of inhalation injury: an evidence based approach. Burns. 2018;44(5):1040–1051

35. Shirani KZ, Pruitt BA, Jr., Mason AD Jr. The influence of inhalation injury and pneumonia on burn mortality. Annals of Surgery. 1987;205:82–87

36. Park MS, Cancio LC, Batchinsky AI, McCarthy MJ, Jordan BS, Brinkley WW, Dubick MA, Goodwin CW. Assessment of severity of ovine smoke inhalation injury by analysis of computed tomographic scans. Journal of Trauma. 2003;55:417–427

37. Oh JS, Chung KK, Allen A, Batchinsky AI, Huzar T, King BT, Wolf SE, Sjulin T, Cancio LC. Admission chest CT complements fiberoptic bronchoscopy in prediction of adverse outcomes in thermally injured patients. Journal of Burn Care & Research. 2012;33:532–538

38. Kwon HP, Zanders TB, Regn DD, Burkett SE, Ward JA, Nguyen R, Necsoiu C, Jordan BS, York GE, Jimenez S, Chung KK, Cancio LC, Morris MJ, Batchinsky AI. Comparison of virtual bronchoscopy to fiber-optic bronchoscopy for assessment of inhalation injury severity. Burns. 2014;40:1308–1315

39. Dietrich CF, Mathis G, Blaivas M, Volpicelli G, Seibel A, Wastl D, Atkinson NS, Cui XW, Fan M, Yi D. Lung B-line artifacts and their use. Journal of Thoracic Disease. 2016 Jun;8(6):1356–1365. DOI: 10.21037/jtd.2016.04.55. PMID: 27293860; PMCID: PMC4885976.

40. Kameda T, Fujita M. Point-of-care ultrasound detection of tracheal wall thickening caused by smoke inhalation. Critical Ultrasound Journal. 2014;6(1):3.

41. Endorf FW, Gamelli RL. Inhalation injury, pulmonary perturbations, and fluid resuscitation. Journal of Burn Care & Research. 2007;28:80–83.

42. Mosier MJ, Pham TN, Park DR, Simmons J, Klein MB, Gibran NS. Predictive value of bronchoscopy in assessing the severity of inhalation injury. Journal of Burn Care & Research. 2012 Jan-Feb;33(1):65–73. DOI: 10.1097/BCR.0b013e318234d92f. PMID: 21941194.

43. Badulak JH, Schurr M, Sauaia A, Ivashchenko A, Peltz E. Defining the criteria for intubation of the patient with Thermal Burns. Burns. 2018;44(3):531–538.

44. Greenhalgh DG. Management of burns. The New England Journal of Medicine. 2019;380(24):234959.

45. Eastman AL, Arnoldo BA, Hunt JL, Purdue GF. Pre-burn center management of the burned airway: do we know enough? Journal of Burn Care & Research. 2010;31:701–705.

46. Romanowski KS, Palmieri TL, Sen S, Greenhalgh DG. More than one third of intubations in patients transferred to burn centers are unnecessary: proposed guidelines for appropriate intubation of the burn patient. Journal of Burn Care & Research. 2016;37(5):409–414.

47. American Burn Association. Advanced Burn Life Support. http://www.ameriburn.org Updated 2018. [Accessed 20 September 2022].

48. Griggs C, Goverman J, Bittner EA, Levi B. Sedation and pain management in burn patients. Clinics in Plastic Surgery. 2017;44(3):535–540

49. Delaney A, Bagshaw SM, Nalos M. Percutaneous dilatational tracheostomy versus surgical tracheostomy in critically ill patients: a systematic review and meta-analysis. Critical Care 2006;10(2):R55

50. Hosokawa K, Nishimura M, Egi M, Vincent J-L. Timing of tracheotomy in ICU patients: a systematic review of randomized controlled trials. Critical Care 2015;19:424

51. Anonymous. Ventilation with lower tidal volumes as compared with traditional tidal volumes for acute lung injury and the acute respiratory distress syndrome. The Acute Respiratory Distress Syndrome Network. The New England Journal of Medicine. 2000;342:1301–1308

52. Hofstra JJ, Vlaar AP, Knape P, Mackie DP, Determann RM, ChoiG, van der Poll T, Levi M, Schultz MJ. Pulmonary activation of coagulation and inhibition of fibrinolysis after burn injuries and inhalation trauma. Journal of Trauma. 2011;70:1389–1397

53. Yip LY, Lim YF, Chan HN. Safety and potential anticoagulant effects of nebulised heparin in burns patients with inhalational injury at Singapore General Hospital Burns Centre. Burns. 2011;37:1154–1160

54. Ogura H, Saitoh D, Johnson AA, Mason AD, Jr., Pruitt BA, Jr., Cioffi WG, Jr. The effect of inhaled nitric oxide on pulmonary ventilation-perfusion matching following smoke inhalation injury. Journal of Trauma. 1994;37:893–898

55. Liodaki E, Kalousis K, Schopp BE, Mailander P, Stang F. Prophylactic antibiotic therapy after inhalation injury. Burns. 2014 Dec;40(8):1476–1480

56. Hampson NB. Pulse oximetry in severe carbon monoxide poisoning. Chest. 1998;114:1036–1041

57. Ilano AL, Raffin TA. Management of carbon monoxide poisoning. Chest. 1990;97:165–169

58. Piantadosi CA. Carbon monoxide poisoning. The New England Journal of Medicine. 2002;347:1054–1055

59. Wolf SJ, Lavonas EJ, Sloan EP, Jagoda AS; American College of Emergency Physicians. Clinical policy: critical issues in the management of adult patients presenting to the emergency department with acute carbon monoxide poisoning. Annals of Emergency Medicine. 2008;51: 138–152

60. Baud FJ, Barriot P, Toffis V, Riou B, Vicaut E, Lecarpentier Y, Bourdon R, Astier A, Bismuth C. Elevated blood cyanide concentrations in victims of smoke inhalation. The New England Journal of Medicine. 1991;325:1761–1766

61. Borron SW, Baud FJ, Barriot P, Imbert M, Bismuth C. Prospective study of hydroxocobalamin for acute cyanide poisoning in smoke inhalation. Annals of Emergency Medicine. 2007;49:794–801.

62. Hall AH, Kulig KW, Rumack BH. Suspected cyanide poisoning in smoke inhalation: complications of sodium nitrite therapy. Journal of Toxicology Clinical Experimental. 1989;9:3–9

63. Hoffman RS, Sauter D. Methemoglobinemia resulting from smoke inhalation. Veterinary and Human Toxicology. 1989;31:168–170

64. Anonymous. Guidelines for the operation of burn centers. Resources for optimal care of the injured patient. Committee on Trauma, American College of Surgeons: Chicago, IL, pp. 79–86, 2006

65. Mushtaq F, Graham CA. Discharge from the accident and emergency department after smoke inhalation: influence of clinical factors and emergency investigations. European Journal of Emergency Medicine. 2004;11:141–144

66. Rue LW, 3d, Cioffi WG, Mason AD, McManus WF, Pruitt BA, Jr. Improved survival of burned patients with inhalation injury. The Archives of Surgery. 1993;128:772–780

67. Cancio LC, Galvez E, Jr., Turner CE, Kypreos NG, Parker A, Holcomb JB. Base deficit and alveolar-arterial gradient during resuscitation contribute independently but modestly to the prediction of mortality after burn injury. Journal of Burn Care & Research. 2006;27:289–296

68. Palmieri TL. Inhalation injury: Research progress and needs. Journal of Burn Care & Research. 2007;28:549–554

32

Electrical, Cold, and Chemical Injuries

Steven Blau and Stephanie A. Savage

32.1 Introduction

Traumatic injury to tissues is a common occurrence, and sequelae may range from relatively benign to major functional alterations or even death. The most common mechanisms include interpersonal violence and motor vehicular crashes. The less common causes of injury may often be more difficult to treat due to the lack of familiarity with the disease process, potential complications, and long-term derangements. Injuries resulting from electrical, cold, and chemical exposures fall into this latter category. In cases such as these, evidence-based medicine is a sound foundation upon which to base practice decisions (Table 32.1).

32.2 Electrical Injuries

Electrical injuries account for 3–5% of burn unit admissions annually, with a mortality rate approaching 40% (approximately 1,000 deaths annually) [1–3]. Age distribution tends to be bimodal, with the majority of injuries occurring in young children, from accidental contact with power sources, and in

adults [3]. In adult patients, electrocutions occur preferentially as a work-related injury, with electricians, linemen, and construction workers displaying the most frequent occurrence. Due to gender distribution in these trades, occurrence favors males in their fourth and fifth decade of life [4, 5].

An appropriate history aids in the diagnosis and management of these injuries, as there are multiple types of injuries. Flash injuries are caused by an arcing and are usually associated with fairly superficial burns, as there is no electrical current contact with the skin. Flame injuries are a consequence of the arc flash causing the victim's clothing to ignite. Lightning and true electrical burns produce injuries consequent to current rather than heat directly [47].

Lightning strikes are an uncommon source of electrical injury as well, with approximately 400 lightning injuries occurring annually in the United States. Though the current in a lightning bolt is between 30,000 and 110,000 A, the time of contact ranges only from 10 to 100 milliseconds, which limits the transference of energy [6]. Therefore, overall mortality is only 10–30% [7]. Simultaneous cardiac and respiratory arrests are most likely to lead to mortality and are managed with standard Adult Cardiac Life Support measures. Long-term cardiac

TABLE 32.1

Management Questions and Evidence-Based Recommendations for Electrical, Cold, and Caustic Injuries

Question	Answer	Grade of Recommendation	References
Which patients suffering electrical injury require more comprehensive monitoring, including urine myoglobin levels?	Low-voltage injuries without signs of injury do not require further monitoring. Patients with sequelae of electrical injury should be monitored closely.	C	[1, 9–14]
Is there any role for advanced imaging to evaluate muscle damage after an electrical injury?	There is little role for MRI or nuclear imaging in the management of electrical injury.	C	[11, 14–18]
What is the most appropriate method of rewarming the severely hypothermic patient?	Rewarming should wait until there is no further risk of freezing. Active rewarming is favored in patients suffering severe hypothermia.	C	[21, 22, 24–31]
What is the role of amputation in the management of significant frostbite?	Surgical debridement should be conservative, as it may take weeks to months to determine tissue viability. Early use of thrombolytic therapy may assist with tissue perfusion and preservation.	C	[22, 24, 26, 28]
What is the optimal role of endoscopy in evaluating and treating patients with caustic ingestions?	Endoscopy should be reserved for symptomatic patients or ingestions secondary to suicidal intent.	C	[32, 33, 36, 37]
Is there any role for exogenous agents to limit damage after chemical ingestion or aspiration pneumonitis?	Supportive care with antibiotics and antireflux medications is the mainstay of therapy. Steroids may have some benefits. Evidence supporting other agents is very limited.	B	[32, 38–43]

DOI: 10.1201/9781003316800-32

sequelae following lightning strikes are uncommon. Long-term neurologic sequelae may occur secondary to hypoxic injury or intracranial hemorrhage due to primary strike or secondary falls. Keraunoparalysis is a transient neurologic effect specific to lightning strikes. This transient paralysis more commonly affects the lower limbs over the upper and is attributed to parasympathetic overstimulation with secondary vascular spasms [6].

Burns related to lightning strikes tend to be linear, from the evaporation of sweat from the skin ("flashover") or punctate from current egress. Lichtenburg's figures are fern-like patterns seen under the skin, which are pathognomonic for a lightning strike but do not represent a true burn. They typically resolve within 24 hours [6, 7]. Finally, cataracts and tympanic membrane rupture are also common following these injuries. Care for victims of lightning strikes is supportive.

Electrical injuries may be especially challenging for the trauma or burn surgeon to treat, as external evidence of injury (entrance and exit wounds) frequently grossly underrepresent the true extent of tissue damage. The severity of the injury is determined by the magnitude of energy delivered, the resistance to current flow, the type of current (AC or DC), the duration of contact with the electric source, and the pathway through which the current travels [8, 9]. Mechanisms of tissue injury are varied and contribute to the difficulty of caring for these patients. The direct effect of the electric current on the tissue, especially cardiac, may result in asystole, ventricular fibrillation, or apnea in cases of respiratory muscle spasms. Electrical current may be converted to thermal energy, resulting in burns. Arcing, the transition of current across a charged space, may throw a patient, resulting in blunt injuries from falls. Tetanic contractions of muscles may also lead to fractures and the blunt disruption of soft tissues [1, 10]. Tetanic contractions are more commonly seen in low-frequency AC than in high-frequency AC. DC results in a single convulsion or contraction usually and is associated with the victim being thrown from the current source [47].

At a cellular level, three major mechanisms can result in cellular death. Joule heating results in the "frying" of tissues and disrupts the lipid bilayer. Electroporation, a process used in laboratories to introduce DNA into cells, causes the formation of temporary pores in the lipid bilayer. The influx of charged particles, especially calcium, can alter membrane gradients and lead to cellular apoptosis. Electroconformational denaturation results in a change in the orientation of proteins that results in denaturation [3]. All of these processes occur with electrical injury, contributing to tissue injury and death at the macroscopic and microscopic levels.

32.2.1 Which Patients Suffering Electrical Injury Require More Comprehensive Monitoring, Including Urine Myoglobin Levels?

With the potential injury to such varied systems as cardiac, respiratory, nervous, renal, ocular, and skeletal systems, many management conundrums arise. The pool of evidence-based data in the case of electrical injuries is primarily at Levels II and III. Owing to the uneven distribution of cardiac injury from current, with necrotic cells next to viable ones, cardiac

manifestations of electrical injury may include arrhythmias and conduction abnormalities [1, 11, 12]. Low-voltage injuries have a lesser rate of serious injury. If patients exposed to a low-voltage electric source have no evidence of injury, discharge from the emergency room is a reasonable option [13]. Purdue and Hunt proposed a series of criteria to determine whether patients require admission following electrical injury. These criteria include loss of consciousness at the scene or cardiac arrest in the field, a documented cardiac arrhythmia in the field, an abnormal electrocardiogram (ECG) (with broad criteria extending as far as bradycardia or tachycardia), or a separate indication for admission [13]. Creatine phosphokinase (CPK), CPK-MB, and serum troponin do not add to the assessment of cardiac injury [49]. Blackwell and Hayllar looked at 212 consecutive patients presenting to an Australian hospital with low-voltage electrical injury. They detected no late rhythm abnormalities in patients who originally had normal ECGs. Much like other studies, this group recommended continuous cardiac monitoring of patients with a history of loss of consciousness, documented arrhythmia, or abnormal ECG at presentation [14].

Creatine kinase (CK) levels are frequently elevated in electrical injury due to diffuse muscle damage. The average CK level following an electrical burn is 18,900 IU. Associated with this is the release of myoglobin from damaged muscle. Myoglobin may lead to renal constriction with associated ischemia and cast formation in the distal convoluted tubule. Grossly pigmented urine is highly suspicious for significant muscle damage, and urine myoglobin levels should be evaluated [15]. Some authors have even advocated using myoglobin levels as a marker for the severity of the injury, as there is an association between myoglobinuria and morbidity [16]. The presence of myoglobin in the urine following electrical injury should prompt continued close monitoring. Urine output should be maintained at a higher level, often greater than 100 cc/hour until myoglobinuria clears. There is no Level 1 evidence to support the use of urine alkalization in this process or of osmotic diuresis with mannitol [15]. Persistent myoglobinuria or elevations in CK levels should prompt evaluation for necrotic tissue requiring debridement. The theoretical advantage of sodium bicarbonate is not supported by most of the clinical literature, and mannitol has similarly not been demonstrated as a useful therapeutic intervention. The physicochemical effect of keeping the myoglobin in solution doesn't seem to be associated with a clinical advantage [48].

One of the more common electrical injuries in small children is associated with sucking or biting through the line cord of an electric appliance and producing a commissure burn. Covered with eschar, these are at risk of bleeding with labial artery injury and may come to the surgery for the management of the commissure contraction. These patients deserve appropriate close monitoring and follow-up [47].

Based on the current evidence, with the majority comprising Level III data, recommendations for the management of electrical injuries include the following points. Low-voltage (<1000 V) electrical injuries with no history of arrhythmia and a normal ECG at presentation may be discharged without further evaluation. High-voltage injuries and/or those with abnormal ECG, a history of arrhythmia, or other indications for admission should be monitored with telemetry. Patients with myoglobinuria should be monitored closely as well, with the maintenance of elevated urine output. Persistent myoglobin abnormalities are suspicious for necrotic tissue. Management is similar to that of other causes of elevated CPK.

RECOMMENDATION

Low-voltage injuries without signs of injury do not require further monitoring. Patients with sequelae of electrical injury, including recent history of cardiac arrest, arrhythmias, and myoglobinuria, should be monitored closely.

Grade of recommendation: C.

32.2.2 Is There Any Role for Advanced Imaging to Evaluate Muscle Damage?

Electrical injuries may be misleading, as the external evidence of injury may be a poor reflection of actual tissue damage. Identification of necrotic tissue is important to allow proper debridement. Although monitoring serum CK levels and urine myoglobin may provide important information, they are not very specific. Conversely, the aggressive use of early fasciotomy has been associated with increased rates of amputation, as high as 35–40% [13]. Therefore, some researchers have focused on the use of magnetic resonance imaging (MRI) or nuclear scanning to pinpoint damaged muscle.

Overall, MRI has demonstrated poor sensitivity in detecting damaged tissue in nonperfused regions, as there is a lack of local edema [17]. Xenon-133 and technetium-99 pyrophosphate radionuclide imaging are accurate predictors of tissue damage [17–20]. However, the use of these imaging modalities neither shortened the duration of hospital stay nor contributed to clinical decision-making in multiple studies [15, 19]. Therefore, there is little practical application for these diagnostic adjuncts in managing patients with electrical injuries.

Patients with significant electrical injury should be admitted to a monitored setting with telemetry and serial evaluation of laboratory values, including urine myoglobin. There is little practical utility in the use of MRI or radionuclide imaging in identifying damaged muscle or influencing clinical care.

RECOMMENDATION

There is little role for MRI or nuclear imaging in the management of electrical injury.

Grade of recommendation: C.

32.3 Cold Injuries

Frostbite remains a significant problem. While often associated with eras in which adequate heating and protection from the elements were not the norm, in modern times at-risk groups include the homeless, outdoor enthusiasts, and patients with altered mental status. Vretenar et al. identified risk factors for cold injury to include alcohol use, a history of psychiatric illness, vehicular trauma or failure, and drug abuse [21, 22]. Additionally, patient factors that may exacerbate injury include atherosclerotic disease, smoking, diabetes mellitus, and a history of prior cold-related tissue injury [23]. Cold-related injuries are more common in males, with an incidence approaching 10:1 and with a mean age of 30–49 years. Injuries preferentially affect regions distant from the core, isolated by heat conservation reflexes. Areas of frequent injury include the digits and hands, feet, nose, and ears [23].

Frostbite represents the most severe degree of tissue injury that may lead to necrosis and the potential for tissue loss. As freezing of the tissues occurs, ice crystals form in extracellular fluids. These crystals damage cell membranes, resulting in altered concentration gradients with abnormal cellular electrolyte concentrations. Further temperature decreases result in intracellular ice crystal formation and cell death. Direct tissue freezing is not the only source of cell death, however. Endothelial injury and local tissue edema from the release of inflammatory mediators lead to the occlusion of small vessels and sludging within vessels. Interruption of oxygen delivery also clearly results in tissue ischemia [23].

The degree of tissue loss is often hard to delineate at the time of the injury. Traditionally, frostbite has been described on a scale of first through fourth degree, similar to descriptive methods used to describe burn injuries. However, it is not possible to classify the degree of injury before rewarming occurs, and complete delineation of necrotic tissue is not apparent until days to weeks later. A less specific but more accurate grading system is simply classifying frostbite wounds as superficial (encompassing first and second degree) or deep (third and fourth degree). Murphy et al. note this system to be more accurate at predicting clinical outcomes than the degree system [23].

Hypothermia is the most life-threatening of the cold injury disorders, despite the lack of obvious external injury as seen in frostbite. As patients progress from mild hypothermia (32°C–35°C) to severe hypothermia (<28°C), systemic sequelae increase. Hypothermia causes decreased cardiac contractility. Combined with relative volume depletion due to fluid sequestration and cellular crystallization, patients with hypothermia experience decreased cardiac output and shock, which easily transitions to cardiac arrest. Additionally, hypothermia contributes to cardiac irritability, often resulting in intractable arrhythmias during attempts to resuscitate patients. Hypothermia leads to vasoconstriction and endothelial injury with sludging and vessel thrombosis. Cold diuresis results from the inhibition of antidiuretic hormone and cold-induced glycosuria, further contributing to volume depletion [24].

Hypothermia is a component of the "deadly triad," which includes acidosis and coagulopathy and frequently results in mortality in trauma patients. Reports of the impact of hypothermia on trauma patients from Operation Iraqi Freedom also emerged from military hospitals. In the report by Arthurs et al., they noted that no patient presenting to the 31st Combat Support Hospital with a temperature <32°C survived [25].

32.3.1 What Is the Most Appropriate Method of Rewarming the Severely Hypothermic Patient?

Rewarming the hypothermic patient may be lifesaving. However, there are conflicting descriptions of the most appropriate methods to restore normothermia. The majority of evidence regarding rewarming following cold injury is Level III or IV. The most important aspect of rewarming, as noted in multiple citations, however, is that rewarming should not occur until there is no further potential for refreezing [26]. Refreezing may convert damaged but viable tissue to frankly ischemic tissue [23, 24, 27–30]. Rapid and repeated freeze–thaw cycles promote the inflammatory response, resulting in increased production of arachidonic acid and thromboxane [31]. Limiting freeze–thaw cycles will limit the production of these inflammatory mediators.

Severe hypothermia, with temperatures less than 28°C, mandates rapid rewarming as the primary modality of therapy. As inappropriate rewarming can lead to reperfusion injury, it is important to minimize this risk while avoiding the pitfalls that accompany a hypothermic state—namely, cardiac irritability, respiratory depression, acidosis, and coagulopathy. Class 2b data using a swine model investigated the optimal rate of rewarming to improve outcomes. In this uncontrolled hemorrhage model, optimal rewarming (defined as survival without significant neurologic deficit) was achieved at 0.5°C/minute [27].

Multiple consensus statements confirm that extracorporeal rewarming with cardiopulmonary bypass is the gold standard for rewarming, especially in instances of hypothermic cardiac arrest [32]. Cardiopulmonary bypass has demonstrated fewer instances of ventricular fibrillation, better overall survival, and higher Glasgow Outcome Scores in affected patients. A further benefit of active rewarming is decreased time required for cardiopulmonary resuscitation, in which the patient risks the sequelae of possibly inadequate resuscitation (i.e., chest compressions) or thoracic trauma [33]. Active rewarming should continue until the patient's core temperature reaches 33°C–35°C. Some evidence has demonstrated that rapidly warming patients above this threshold may contribute to cerebral edema [32].

Rewarming should not occur until there is no further risk of refreezing. For hypothermic patients, active rewarming to achieve a rate of 0.5°C/minute is ideal. The cardiopulmonary bypass should be reserved for the profoundly hypothermic or in patients with cardiac irritability/instability. When used promptly, however, patients may achieve good neurologic outcomes.

RECOMMENDATION

Rewarming should wait until there is no further risk of freezing. Active rewarming is favored in patients suffering severe hypothermia.

Grade of recommendation: C.

32.3.2 What Is the Role of Amputation in the Management of Significant Frostbite?

Blood-thinning agents and thrombolytics are the areas of most vigorous research in cold injury. Hypothermia contributes to intravascular sludging, which impairs the delivery of oxygen and nutrients. During thaw cycles, endothelial damage may also contribute to thrombosis of small vessels, resulting in tissue ischemia and necrosis [24]. Delineation of nonviable tissue may take weeks to months; however, surgical debridement should be left for as late as possible [26].

Multiple studies have demonstrated the utility of technetium-99 scans in delineating areas of significant tissue injury from frostbite. In studies by Twomey et al. and Bruen et al., at-risk areas were identified and directed infusion of tissue plasminogen activator (tPA) was administered intravascularly. Both studies demonstrated the preservation of at-risk tissue. The latter study demonstrated significantly lower amputation rates when compared to patients not receiving tPA [28, 30]. The early institution of this therapy seemed to be a key component of its success.

RECOMMENDATION

Surgical debridement should be conservative, as it may take weeks to months to determine the viability of tissues. Early use of thrombolytic therapy may assist with tissue perfusion and preservation.

Grade of recommendation: C.

Rewarming is the mainstay of therapy for frostbite. In those with a poor response to rewarming who have evidence of diminished perfusion, the use of thrombolytics (in the form of tPA) with heparin should be considered if there is no known bleeding risk. Surgical debridement should be conservative.

32.4 Chemical Injuries

Injuries from chemical exposures are not common in the United States. The group at the most routine risk for a caustic burn includes laborers. In examining work-related burn injuries from 1995 to 2004, only 5.8% of burns were found to be chemical in nature as opposed to 45.8% of electrical burns and 39.6% of thermal burns [24]. Despite the very serious nature of work-related chemical burns, with morbidity and loss of productivity, caustic ingestions are a far more common source of chemical burns seen by the emergency room and surgeons. Included in the category of accidental caustic burns seen routinely would be burns to the pulmonary system due to aspiration pneumonitis. Caustic ingestion occurs in a bimodal age distribution, and the severity of the injury is often linked to the reason behind the ingestion. Caustic ingestions in young children are accidental and attributed to mistaking household cleaning items for beverages. Conversely, in adults, the most common cause of caustic ingestion is purposeful during a suicide attempt.

Overall, caustic ingestions in adults tend to be more severe due to their purposeful nature [34]. These patients may typically ingest larger volumes and not seek evaluation for prolonged periods. The extent of tissue damage depends on multiple factors including the type of agent (alkali or acid), the physical properties of the agent, agent concentration, duration of the contact, and the volume of substance ingested [35–38]. Solutions with a pH <2 or >12 tend to be highly corrosive, and solid or powdered forms may be more damaging due to the tendency to adhere to the mucosal surface [34]. Alkali ingestion results in liquefaction necrosis, with thrombosis of small vessels and local heat production compounding the injury. Similarly, acids cause liquefaction necrosis with eschar formation. By 4–7 days following the injury, mucosal sloughing begins. This allows the potential for bacterial invasion with a robust inflammatory response and deposition of granulation tissue. The tensile strength of tissue is low for the first 3 weeks, and the inflammatory response and tissue sloughing render tissues weakened starting at 48 hours. This increases the likelihood of perforation. Scar formation, which may begin as early as the second week following surgery, may result in esophageal shortening and stricture formation. A shortened esophagus has altered pressures at the lower esophageal sphincter, allowing increased acid reflux to exacerbate injuries [34].

Caustic ingestions in children are quite variable in their degree of severity. Accidental ingestions are seen more commonly in developing countries, where household cleaners and other chemicals may be stored in reused containers, thereby leading children to think the contents are potable. Twenty-six percent of children with accidental ingestions are ultimately found to have severe lesions, and 1–5% of children with accidental ingestions ultimately develop stenosis [38].

While topical chemical burns are not common, white phosphorus has been a source of significant morbidity and mortality in the military, industrial, and rural settings. White phosphorus is highly toxic in this regard and has been used in munitions, fertilizers, and the production of semiconductors. White phosphorus spontaneously ignites at 30°C and may cause severe burns when in contact with the skin. Further, if the burn allows deep invasion, white phosphorus is very lipophilic and may spread rapidly beneath the dermis. This chemical is easily absorbed via the skin, lungs, and gut and may ignite at body temperature if it dries. Further, it may cause profound electrolyte imbalances (hyperphosphatemia and hypocalcemia), which may result in fatal arrhythmias. Treatment is thorough decontamination with cold water lavage and monitoring of electrolytes if absorption is suspected [39].

Hydrofluoric acid burns are fairly unique in the burn injury produced. At high concentrations, the injury resembles that of other concentrated acids, but at low concentrations (commonly seen in emergency rooms) the complexing of calcium by fluoride ion leads to both systemic hypocalcemia and local wound injury. Management therefore includes both topical and, in some instances, systemic calcium therapy [50].

32.4.1 What Is the Optimal Role of Endoscopy in Evaluating and Treating Patients with Caustic Ingestions?

The degree of esophageal injury is assessed with endoscopy and graded on a scale of 0–IIIb [35, 38]. The primary concern during endoscopy is not in detecting perforation, which may be diagnosed with other modalities, but in differentiating minimal injury from severe injury, which then influences management. In a retrospective cohort study of 50 patients with caustic ingestions from 1988 to 2003 in Israel, the overall rate of stricture formation was 10%. However, patients with third-degree esophageal injuries had a 71% rate of stricture formation [35]. In a series of 48 pediatric patients reported in Level IIb evidence from France, 26% of the patients with accidental ingestions had severe lesions. However, this study found that all patients at risk of stenosis with severe lesions presented with symptoms, such as hematemesis and respiratory distress [38]. No particular symptom is predictive of increased severity of the esophageal lesion and thus risk of stenosis.

In light of these findings, children with accidental caustic ingestions who are asymptomatic at presentation do not require endoscopy. Owing to intent to harm, all suicidal ingestions, and patients presenting with symptoms should receive endoscopy. Endoscopy should occur within the first 48 hours, as after this time point, tensile strength is decreased and the risk of iatrogenic perforation increases [34]. Additionally, endoscopy should not proceed past circumferential burns due to the increased risk of perforation at these points. Further evaluation of the gastrointestinal tract may occur with a barium study, if necessary.

Subsequent management of patients with injury will depend on the patient's condition, injury severity, and physician practice. Although the use of nasogastric tubes to stent the esophagus and injury sites has been promulgated, some evidence indicates that this may promote stricture formation. Zargar et al., in a prospective endoscopic evaluation of 81 patients with corrosive esophageal burns, determined that all patients with grade 0–IIa burns recovered without sequelae. Further, approximately three-quarters of patients with IIb burns and all those with grades IIIa and IIIb injuries ultimately developed esophageal stricture. These authors postulated that early resection of the most severe injuries (grade IIIb) may improve outcomes as defined by morbidity and mortality [40].

The majority of the evidence in caustic injuries falls somewhere within the realm of grade C data. Endoscopy has a role in the management of patients with caustic ingestions and should be used routinely for symptomatic patients or patients with ingestion due to suicide attempts. Results of endoscopy can then be used to determine prognosis and formulate a management plan.

RECOMMENDATION

Endoscopy should be reserved for symptomatic patients or ingestions secondary to suicidal intent.

Grade of recommendation: C.

32.4.2 Is There Any Role for Exogenous Agents to Limit Damage after Chemical Ingestion or Aspiration Pneumonitis?

In light of the potentially serious effects of caustic damage to the esophagus, research has focused on interventions that may mitigate or prevent negative long-term outcomes. The most commonly used modality to prevent stricture formation is steroids [41]. While some animal models have indicated a potential benefit, evidence in human subjects is mixed. A meta-analysis retrospective review of 361 patients with corrosive esophageal injury found a stricture rate of 19% in patients treated with steroids (40–60 mg/day intravenous) and antibiotics versus a 40% stricture rate in those not receiving steroids [42]. However, a randomized controlled trial of 60 children suffering caustic ingestions and treated with steroids (2 mg/kg/day intravenous) versus no steroids found no decrease in stricture rate [43]. The only firm recommendation regarding the use of steroids in caustic ingestion patients is that antibiotics and antireflux medications should be given concurrently with steroids to mitigate the immunosuppressive effect [34, 41].

Considerable research effort continues to look at unusual adjuncts to decrease stricture formation, although most of these efforts are small studies. Halofuginone, an alkaloid plant derivative, suppresses collagen synthesis and has been shown to improve esophageal patency in rats following caustic ingestion [44]. The topical application of dilute hyaluronic acid has suppressed local inflammation and decreased stricture formation in another rat study [41]. A human study has looked at the use of biodegradable esophageal stents for patients with existing esophageal strictures. This study demonstrated temporary improvement in symptoms but little long-term benefit [45].

Finally, caustic injury secondary to aspiration pneumonitis is an intensive care unit (ICU) challenge that continues to plague clinicians. Following aspiration, one-third of patients will develop severe pulmonary symptoms, and up to 22% are at risk of acute respiratory distress syndrome (ARDS) with the associated morbidity and mortality. Aspiration may result in a profound inflammatory response, with activation of cytokines including tumor necrosis factor alpha (TNFa), interleukin (IL)-1, and IL-8. Attempts to modulate the development of ARDS increasingly focus on antiinflammatory agents and immunomodulators. Pawlik et al. examined the role of pentoxifylline, which inhibits the release of TNFa, in limiting the development of ARDS following aspiration. In this animal model ($n = 24$),

animals receiving pentoxifylline had significantly improved oxygenation, less atelectasis, and less evidence of inflammation on CT than animals in the untreated group. Mortality was also significantly less in the treated group. These results are directly opposite to findings in the ARDSNet trial using lisofylline, a pentoxifylline derivative. However, the method of drug administration and ventilatory methods were quite different between the studies, making a direct comparison between the two studies difficult [46].

Adjuncts minimizing the formation of esophageal stricture are poorly defined. The strongest evidence involves the use of steroids, though significant morbidities may occur. Nevertheless, if steroids are incorporated, they should be used in conjunction with antibiotics and antireflux agents. Additional agents are promising in animal studies but require more analysis in human trials.

RECOMMENDATION

Supportive care with the use of antibiotics and antireflux medications is the mainstay of therapy. Steroids may have some benefits as well. Evidence supporting other agents is very limited.

Grade of recommendation: C.

Editor's Note

As in many areas of surgery, the evidence guiding our management of relatively rare entities like electrical and chemical burns is not based on high-quality clinical trials, but rather on clinical experience. Therefore, the current recommendations for management are inconclusive. The authors have nicely summarized the current standard of care.

REFERENCES

1. Sples C, Trohman RG. Narrative review: Electrocution and life-threatening electrical injuries. *Ann Intern Med.* 2006;*145*:531–537.
2. Maghsoudi H, Adyani Y, Ahmadian N. Electrical and lightning injuries. *J Burn Care Res.* 2007;*28(2)*:255–261.
3. Tuttnauer A, Mordzynski SC, Weiss YG. Electrical and lightning injuries. *Contemp Crit Care.* 2006;*4(7)*:1–10.
4. Laupland KB, Kortbeek JB, Findlay C, et al. Population-based study of severe trauma due to electrocution in the Calgary Health Region, 1996–2002. *Can J Surg.* 2005; *48(4)*:289–292.
5. Fordyce TA, Kelsh M, Lu ET, et al. Thermal burns and electrical injuries among electric utility workers, 1995–2004. *Burns.* 2007;*33*:209–220.
6. Davis C, Engeln A, Johnson E, et al. Wilderness medical society practice guidelines for the prevention and treatment of lightning injuries. *Wilderness Environ Med.* 2012;*23*: 260–269.

7. Forster SA, Silva IM, Ramos MLC, et al. Lightning burn—Review and case report. *Burns*. 2013;*29*:e8–e12.

8. Bailey B, Gaudreault P, Thivierge R. Cardiac monitoring of high-risk patients after an electrical injury: A prospective multicentre study. *Emerg Med J*. 2007;*24(5)*:348–352.

9. 2005 American Heart Association Guidelines for Cardiopulmonary Resuscitation and Emergency Cardiovascular Care. Part 10.9: Electric shock and lightning strikes. *Circulation*. 2005;*112(Suppl IV)*:154–155.

10. Li M, Hamilton W. Review of autopsy findings in judicial electrocutions. *Am J Forensic Med Pathol*. 2005;*26(3)*: 261–267.

11. Pham TN, Gibran NS. Thermal and electrical injuries. *Surg Clin North Am*. 2007;*87*:185–206.

12. Purdue GF, Hunt JL. Electrocardiographic monitoring after electrical injury: Necessity of luxury. *J Trauma*. 1986;*26*:166.

13. Arnoldo B, Klein M, Gibran NS. Practice guidelines for the management of electrical injuries. *J Burn Care Res*. 2006;*27(4)*:439–447.

14. Blackwell N, Hayllar J. A three year prospective audit of 212 presentations to the emergency department after electrical injury with a management protocol. *Postgrad Med J*. 2002;*78*:283–285.

15. Arnoldo BD, Purdue GF. The diagnosis and management of electrical injuries. *Hand Clinics*. 2009;*25*:469–479.

16. Rosen CL, Adler JN, Rabban JT, et al. Early predictors of myoglobinuria and acute renal failure following electrical injury. *J Emerg Med*. 1999;*17*:783–789.

17. Fleckenstein JL, Chasson DP, Bonte FJ, et al. High-voltage electric injury: Assessment of muscle viability with MR imaging and Tc-99m pyrophosphate scintigraphy. *Radiology*. 1993;*195*:205–210.

18. Hunt JL, Lewis S, Parkey R, et al. The use of technetium 99 stannous pyrophosphate scintigraphy to identify muscle damage in acute electric burns. *J Trauma*. 1979;*19*: 409–413.

19. Hammond J, Ward CG. The use of technetium-99 pyrophosphate scanning in management of high voltage electrical injuries. *Am Surg*. 1994;*68*:886–888.

20. Clayton JM, Hayes AC, Hammond J, et al. Xenon-133 determination of muscle blood flow in electric injury. *J Trauma*. 1977;*17*:293–298.

21. Koljonen V, Andersson K, Mikkonen K, et al. Frostbite injuries treated in the Helsinki area from 1995 to 2002. *J Trauma*. 2004;*57(6)*:1315–1320.

22. Vretenar DF, Urschel JD, Parott JC, et al. Cardiopulmonary bypass resuscitation for accidental hypothermia [review]. *Ann Thorac Surg*. 1994;*58*:895–898.

23. Murphy JV, Banwell PE, Roberts AHN, et al. Frostbite: Pathogenesis and treatment. *J Trauma*. 2000;*48(1)*:171–178.

24. Biem J, Koehncke N, Classen D, et al. Out of the cold: Management of hypothermia and frostbite. *CMAJ*. 2003; *168(3)*:305–311.

25. Arthurs Z, Cuadrado D, Beekley A, et al. The impact of hypothermia on trauma care at the 31st combat support hospital. *Am J Surg*. 2006;*191*:610–614.

26. Roche-Nagle G, Murphy G, Collins A, et al. Frostbite: Management options. *Eur J Emerg Med*. 2008;*15(3)*: 173–175.

27. Alam HB, Rhee P, Honma K, et al. Does the rate of rewarming from profound hypothermic arrest influence the outcome in a swine model of lethal hemorrhage? *J Trauma*. 2006;*60(1)*:134–146.

28. Bruen KJ, Ballard JR, Morris SE, et al. Reduction of the incidence of amputation in frostbite injury with thrombolytic therapy. *Arch Surg*. 2007;*142*:546–553.

29. McGillion R. Frostbite: Case report, practical summary of ED treatment. *J Emerg Nurs*. 2005;*31(5)*:500–502.

30. Twomey JA, Peltier GL, Zera RT. An open-label study to evaluate the safety and efficacy of tissue plasminogen activator in the treatment of severe frostbite. *J Trauma*. 2005;*59(6)*:1350–1355.

31. Robson MC, Heggers JR Evaluation of hand frostbite blister fluid as a clue to pathogenesis. *J Hand Surg [Am]*. 1981;*6*:43–47.

32. Monika BM, Martin D, Balthasar E, et al. The Bernese Hypothermia Algorithm: A consensus paper on in hospital decision-making and treatment of patients in hypothermic cardiac arrest at an alpine level 1 trauma centre. *Injury*. 2011;*42*:539–543.

33. Morita S, Inokuchi S, Yamagiwa T, et al. Efficacy of portable and percutaneous cardiopulmonary bypass rewarming versus that of conventional internal rewarming for patients with accidental deep hypothermia. *Crit Care Med*. 2011;*39(5)*:1064–1068.

34. Ramasamy K, Gumaste VV. Corrosive ingestion in adults. *J Clin Gastroenterol*. 2003;*37(2)*:119–124.

35. Arevalo-Silva C, Eliashar R, Wohlgelernter J, et al. Ingestion of caustic substances: A 15 year experience. *Laryngoscope*. 2006;*116*:1422–1426.

36. Wedler V, Guggenheim M, Moron M, et al. Extensive hydrofluoric acid injuries: A serious problem. *J Trauma*. 2005;*58(4)*:852–857.

37. Mattos GM, Lopes DD, Mamede RCM, et al. Effect of time of contact and concentration of caustic agent on generation of injuries. *Laryngoscope*. 2006;*116*:456–460.

38. Lamireau T, Rebouissoux L, Denis D, et al. Accidental caustic ingestion in children: Is endoscopy always mandatory? *J Pediatr Gastroenterol Nutr*. 2001;*33*:81–84.

39. Berndtson AE, Fagin A, Sen S, et al. White phosphorus burns and arsenic inhalation: A toxic combination. *J Burn Care Res*. 2013;*35(2)*:e128–e131.

40. Zargar SA, Kuchhar R, Mehta S, et al. The role of fiberoptic endoscopy in the management of corrosive ingestion and modified endoscopic classification of burns. *Gastroint Endos*. 1991;*37*:165–169.

41. Cevik M, Demir T, Karadag CA, et al. Preliminary study of efficacy of hyaluronic acid on caustic esophageal burns in an experimental rat model. *J Pediatr Surg*. 2013;*48*:716–723.

42. Howell JM, Dalsey WC, Hartsell FW, et al. Steroids for the treatment of corrosive esophageal injury: A statistical analysis of past studies. *Am J Emerg Med*. 1992;*10*:421–425.

43. Anderson KD, Rouse TM, Randolph JG. A controlled trial of corticosteroids in children with corrosive injury of the esophagus. *N Engl J Med*. 1990;*323*:637–640.

44. Arbell D, Udassin R, Koplewitz BZ, et al. Prevention of esophageal strictures in a caustic burn model using halofuginone, an inhibitor of collagen type I synthesis. *Laryngoscope*. 2005;*115*:1632–1635.

45. Karakan T, Utku OG, Dorukoz O, et al. Biodegradable stents for caustic esophageal strictures: A new therapeutic approach. *Dis Esophagus.* 2013;*26*:319–322.

46. Pawlik MT, Schreyer AG, Ittner KP, et al. Early treatment with pentoxifylline reduces lung injury induced by acid aspiration in rats. *Chest.* 2005;*127*(2):613–621.

47. Zemaitis MR, Foris LA, Lopez RA Huecker MR. Electrical Injuries. *StatPearls*, 2023 Jul 17.

48. Somagutta A, Pagad S, Sridharan S, et al. Role of bicarbonates and mannitol in rhabdomyolysis: A comprehensive review. *Cureus.* 2020;*12*(8):e9742.

49. Arnoldo B, Klein M, Gibran NS. Practical guidelines for the management of electrical injuries. *J Burn Care Res.* 2006 Jul-Aug 27(4):439–447.

50. McKee D, Thomas A, Bailey K, Fish J. A review of hydrofluoric acid burn management. *Plast Surg.* 2014;*22*(2):95–98.

33

Wound Care Management

Aashish Rajesh, Mustafa Tamim Alam Khan, and Howard T. Wang

33.1 Introduction

The estimated prevalence of chronic nonhealing wounds in developed countries ranges from 1% to 2% within the general population. The morbidity and the associated cost of treating chronic wounds can have significant implications on the cost of healthcare. Recent studies have shown that nearly 15% of Medicare beneficiaries had at least one type of wound infection, with surgical infections forming the largest category, followed by diabetic infections.

In 2014, the total Medicare spending estimates when considering all wound types was estimated to range from $28.1 to $96.8 billion. Surgical wounds, followed by diabetic foot ulcers, accounted for the largest proportion of the cost. The majority of the wound care cost stemmed from the outpatient setting, with an estimated cost ranging from $9.9 to $35.8 billion. These numbers reiterate the enormous healthcare costs that chronic wounds impose and serve as a strong impetus for advances in wound care for optimal patient management.

33.1.1 The Principles and Phases of Wound Healing

The management of chronic wounds continues to be a significant yet understudied component of perioperative patient care. Wound healing is a dynamic process that can be influenced by both the wound microenvironment and the health and nutritional status of the individual [1].

Through the initial part of this chapter, we discuss the physiology of wound healing to set a framework for identifying the different points at which the healing process can be altered. Many factors interact with different aspects of the wound healing process and change the body's physiologic course for the healing of specific wounds. While human intervention can impact these points positively, some complex chronic wounds remain difficult to treat despite the best attempts at optimizing systemic factors and the wound microenvironment.

The wound healing process has been traditionally broken down into three integrated and often overlapping phases: Inflammation, proliferation, and maturation. In acute wounds, these processes occur in an orderly fashion and achieve the desired structural and functional restoration. However, in a chronic nonhealing wound, this repair process is often stalled at the inflammatory phase and fails to progress [2].

33.1.1.1 Inflammatory Phase

Exposure of collagen during wound formation leads to the activation of both the intrinsic and extrinsic clotting cascade. The inflammatory phase (which starts immediately upon injury and lasts 4–6 days) consists of both hemostasis and inflammation [2].

Immediately after the injury, there is the release of potent vasoconstrictors thromboxane A2 and prostaglandin 2-alpha. Additionally, a platelet plug, made from collagen, platelets, thrombin, fibronectin, and various cytokines, forms in this area. This platelet plug serves as a scaffold for other inflammatory cells, which produce cytokines and growth factors at the location of the injury [3].

As the inflammatory mediators aggregate in the wound area, the nearby blood vessels transition from vasoconstriction to vasodilation and allow for the cells of inflammation to be drawn to the injured area. The sequential arrival of neutrophils followed by macrophages (at 48–96 hours) drives the inflammatory phase of wound healing [4].

33.1.1.2 Proliferative Phase

The proliferative phase proceeds from days 4–14 from injury. This phase is highlighted by wound epithelialization, angiogenesis, granulation tissue formation, and collagen deposition [5].

Epithelialization in wounds where the basement membrane remains intact involves the epithelial progenitor cells, which remain viable and restore the normal layer of the epidermis within 2–3 days [6]. When the basement membrane has been disrupted, the epithelialization process relies on the epithelial cells located at the skin edges to proliferate in toward the wound and re-establish the protective barrier. Epithelialization is stimulated by epidermal growth factor (EGF) and transforming growth factor alpha. Angiogenesis is stimulated by tumor necrosis factor (TNF)-alpha and consists of endothelial cell migration and capillary formation [7]. The process allows for the transport of nutrients that are essential for tissue deposition needed by granulation tissue. The failure of adequate angiogenesis is often associated with a chronic nonhealing wound. The formation of the granulation tissue is the final part of the proliferative phase. The primary activating signal for granulation tissue formation comes from platelet-derived growth factors (PDGFs) and EGF, both of which are essential for activating fibroblasts. This promotes fibroblast migration and collagen synthesis [6].

DOI: 10.1201/9781003316800-33

33.1.1.3 Remodeling Phase

The remodeling phase goes on from week 2 for about a year and involves collagen deposition and organization. The initial collagen fibers that are laid down during the early parts of wound healing are thinner than the collagen of the uninjured skin. Furthermore, they tend to be oriented in a parallel fashion to the skin. However, during the remodeling phase, the initial collagen gets reabsorbed and new thicker collagen fibers are deposited. The thicker collagen fibers are also organized along stress lines. These modifications allow for increased tensile strength [6]. It should be noted that the derangement of this process can be responsible for compromised wound strength or excessive collagen deposition leading to hypertrophic scars or keloids [8].

33.1.2 The Local and Systemic Factors Affecting Wound Healing

The complex nature of wound healing leaves the process vulnerable to a myriad of both intrinsic and extrinsic stressors. The following section discusses the various local and systemic factors that affect the wound healing process.

33.1.3 Local Factors

33.1.3.1 Ischemia

Wound healing is an energy-intensive process that requires an adequate supply of oxygen and nutrients to progress satisfactorily. The proliferative phase, which is characterized by increased metabolism and protein synthesis, requires the use of a large quantity of adenosine triphosphate (ATP). This process relies on a robust blood supply, and therefore, ischemia and hypoxia around the wound can impede healing [9].

33.1.3.2 Infection

Infection and the presence of a high bacterial bioburden in the wound can lead to a prolonged inflammatory phase. It has been shown that the bacterial burden of 10^5 organisms per gram of tissue and greater is associated with the failure of wounds to close. Previous studies have shown that the presence of bacteria has the potential to suppress macrophage function and dysregulate the wound healing process [10]. The processes inhibited by infection include epithelialization, wound contraction, and collagen deposition. Bacterial endotoxins also trigger the release of collagenase, which is responsible for collagen degradation and destruction.

33.1.3.3 Foreign Bodies

The presence of foreign bodies in the wound has been shown to prolong the inflammatory phase. Previous literature has suggested that the presence of a foreign body hinders the ability to repopulate the wound bed with capillaries, epithelialize, and contract [11]. Nonviable and necrotic tissue in the wound behaves similarly to foreign bodies, and this highlights the need for thorough debridement [12].

33.1.4 Systemic Factors

33.1.4.1 Diabetes

Increased serum glucose has been shown to affect wound healing in a multifactorial manner. Hyperglycemia and associated microvascular occlusive disease can lead to increased dermal vascular permeability and leakage of albumin into the wound. The leaked albumin can severely hinder the transport of oxygen and nutrients that are required for wound healing [13]. Furthermore, sorbitol, which is a toxic by-product of glucose metabolism, can accumulate in the tissue and disrupt the phagocytic function required to degrade and remove cellular debris [14]. Additionally, hyperglycemia is associated with decreased granulation tissue formation, decreased collagen in granulation tissue, and delayed collagen maturation.

33.1.4.2 Advanced Age

Aging has been associated with higher rates of wound complications and mortality. While older patients generally have more comorbidities, studies have shown that the inflammatory and proliferative phases of wound healing become less efficient with age [15]. Animal studies have corroborated advanced age with slower epithelialization, even in cases when the dermal collagen deposition was similar to that in a younger individual [16]. Finally, wound healing in the elderly can be hindered by insufficient levels of growth factors [17].

33.1.4.3 Nutrition Status

The nutritional status of patients is paramount for the body to appropriately repair a wound. Macronutrients such as amino acids, carbohydrates, and fatty acids are the building blocks of human cells and are essential for wound healing. Hypoalbuminemia has been known to be associated with delayed healing and wound dehiscence, and the surgical literature documents wound complications in patients who are not preoperatively optimized [18]. Wound healing is a catabolic process requiring the consumption of stored fat and protein. The utilization of both micronutrient immune nutrients from a prolonged healing process can leave the patient's immune system and the regenerative capacity vulnerable. Additionally, deficiencies in vitamins and minerals that are required as cofactors in collagen production can impede collagen synthesis and cross-linking.

33.1.4.4 Smoking

Smoking is a well-known risk factor for delayed wound healing. Patients who smoke at least one pack per day are at three times higher risk of skin graft necrosis than nonsmokers. The negative impact of smoking on wound healing is multifactorial. Nicotine causes vasoconstriction, which can lead to tissue hypoxia and decreased proliferation of macrophages and fibroblasts. Increased levels of carbon monoxide in smokers have also been associated with the decreased oxygen-carrying capacity of hemoglobin through competitive inhibition. Finally, smoking also increases platelet aggregation and blood viscosity while decreasing collagen deposition [19].

33.1.4.5 Steroids

While they are often used therapeutically to decrease inflammation; the use of steroids has been shown to inhibit the ability of immunologic cells to appropriately migrate to wounds and regulate the healing process. Studies have shown that the use of corticosteroids blunts the macrophage response to chemotactic factors. The phagocytotic function of neutrophils and macrophages is less effective in the presence of corticosteroids due to their stabilizing effect on lysosomes. Furthermore, since the initial inflammatory response is hindered by steroids, studies have noted that injured cells within the wound do not produce the typical growth factor profile that facilitates wound healing. Steroids also inhibit the fibroblast genome, leading to low-secretory states with resultant decreased collagen deposition and maturation [20].

33.1.4.6 Obesity

Obesity itself is an independent risk factor for wound complications. Previous studies have shown that hypoxia may be driven by a discrepancy in the ratio of tissue to the capillary vessels in obese individuals, leading to hypoperfusion of subcutaneous adipocytes. This low oxygen tension has the potential to cause ischemia and disrupt the function of neutrophils, macrophages, and fibroblasts [21].

33.2 What Is the Optimal Way to Avoid Pressure Ulcers?

Pressure ulcers occur in areas of bony prominences, most commonly over the sacrum, heels, ischial tuberosities, greater trochanters, and lateral malleoli. The pathophysiology of pressure ulcers is related to the unrelieved pressure that can disrupt the blood supply to the subcutaneous tissues, culminating in tissue breakdown.

33.2.1 Clinical Assessment

The assessment of pressure ulcers should include a comprehensive medical evaluation including the history of the ulcer, previous wound care, risk factors, and medical comorbidities. The number, location, dimensions of the ulcer, presence of exudate, presence of sinus tracts, and necrotic tissues should all be noted. The most important aspect of evaluating a pressure ulcer involves determining the stage [22]. Pressure ulcer stages are as follows: Stage I: Intact skin with nonblanching redness; stage II: Shallow, open ulcers with a pink-red wound base; stage III: Full-thickness tissue loss with subcutaneous fat exposed; stage IV: Full-thickness tissue loss but with either muscle or bone exposed; unstageable: Full-thickness tissue loss, but the base is covered by an eschar. Synthetic dressings that maintain a moist wound environment can facilitate the healing of pressure ulcers by providing autolytic debridement. Table 33.1 describes the various synthetic dressings that can be used.

Preventive measures to avoid the development of pressure ulcers should be instituted for all at-risk patients to ensure that the subcutaneous microcirculation remains unimpeded. The Braden scale was developed in 1988 as a tool for predicting a patient's risk for developing pressure ulcers. It is a scale that consists of seven subscales (sensory perception, moisture, activity, mobility, nutrition, friction, and shear), and can provide a score between 6 and 23, with scores lower than 18 indicating a higher risk for pressure ulcer development [23]. The Agency for Health Care Policy and Research currently recommends that bedridden patients be repositioned every 2 hours. To reduce the level of shear strain on the skin, the head of the

TABLE 33.1

Synthetic Dressings for the Treatment of Pressure Ulcers

Type of Dressing	Description	Function	Indication
Transparent film	Adhesive, semipermeable polyurethane membrane that helps retain moisture	Clear polyurethane membrane with acrylic adhesive on one side	Used to manage stage I and II ulcers with little to no exudate
Hydrogel	Water- or glycerin-based amorphous gels that can be impregnated into dressings	Gels, sheets, and impregnated gauze provide an occlusive environment	Used to manage stage II, III, and IV ulcers
Alginate	Cellulose-like polysaccharide fibers that have been derived from a calcium salt of alginate (seaweed); can be found as ropes, ribbons, or pads	Calcium alginate converts to sodium salt when in contact with wound exudate, forming a hydrophilic gel that provides an occlusive environment	Can be used as primary dressing for stage III and IV ulcers, wounds with moderate to heavy exudate or tunneling, or infection
Foam (hydrophobic polyurethane sheets)	Hydrophobic polyurethane sheets are available in pads and sheets	Provide protection, absorption of exudate	For stage II to IV ulcers; can be used as a primary absorptive dressing
Hydrocolloid	Dressings are made from gelatin, pectin, and carboxymethylcellulose; available as adhesive wafers, paste, and powders	This will absorb water from wound exudates, swell, and liquefy to form a moist gel that can provide insulation, moisture retention, and protective barrier against bacteria	Can be used as a primary or secondary dressing for stage II to IV ulcers; also good for wounds with necrosis or exudate

bed should not be elevated more than 30 degrees and should be maintained at the lowest degree of elevation possible [24]. Both static and dynamic pressure-reducing devices can also be used to prevent pressure ulcers. Static devices include foam, water, gel, and air mattress or mattress overlays. Dynamic devices use power sources to redistribute localized pressure. The utilization of pressure-reducing surfaces has been shown to reduce the incidence of ulceration by 60% when compared to the standard hospital mattress. Static devices are more suitable for patients who can independently change positions, while dynamic devices may be more suitable for more debilitated patients [25].

The management of pressure ulcers requires interdisciplinary care. The initial aspect of treatment involves reducing the pressure on the skin, debriding necrotic tissue until granulation tissue is present, cleansing the wound, managing bacterial load, and selecting appropriate wound dressings. Urinary catheters, rectal tubes, and diverting ostomies may be necessary depending on size and location [26].

RECOMMENDATION

Both static and dynamic pressure-reducing devices can be used to prevent pressure ulcers in high-risk patients with moderate success.

Grade of recommendation: B.

33.3 Does Negative Pressure Wound Therapy Improve Wound Healing?

Vacuum-assisted closure (VAC) therapy is a modality of wound care that has rapidly gained popularity over the past two decades. The concept was introduced in 1997, and its proposed mechanism involves a reduction of edema in the wound bed, reduction of bacterial load, and promotion of local blood flow to augment wound healing [27]. Tissue compression by the sponge under negative pressure induces a state of hypoxia and stimulates neo-angiogenesis with local vasodilation. Additionally, the micro-deformation/micro-strain that occurs due to the VAC promotes tissue expansion with growth factor release, resulting in granulation and progressive wound closure [28].

Two types of sterile sponges are used for negative pressure wound therapy (NPWT): The black sponge (GranuFoam) made of polyurethane ether, which is hydrophobic and has a large pore size (400–600 mm), and the white sponge (Versfoam) made of polyvinyl alcohol (hydrophilic with a small pore size of 250 mm). While the former is used for large thoracic and abdominal cavity wounds, the latter is preferred for use over more superficial wounds, undermined areas, blind areas, tunnels, and sensitive structures [27]. White foam does not adhere to the underlying wound bed and does not stimulate as much granulation as black foam.

The negative pressure of 125 mmHg has been considered the optimal balance between the pressure required to stimulate granulation and that which causes tissue deformation [29]. Two modes of applying this negative pressure exist: Continuous and intermittent. While continuous NPWT is more commonly used, studies have shown that intermittent NPWT, which comprises a 5-minute on with a 2-minute off phase that is cycled, stimulates more granulation tissue growth and more pronounced wound contraction than continuous NPWT. These effects of intermittent and variable NPWT (which involves an "off" phase that goes to a subatmospheric but nonzero pressure) have been substantiated in in vivo studies [30]. Considering that pain is a major limitation of applying intermittent negative pressure at the point where the VAC sponge suctions back to –125 mmHg, recent evidence seems to favor variable and cyclic NPWT as a good trade-off that balances increased patient comfort and compliance with better granulation when compared to continuous NPWT [31].

Much of the evidence favoring NPWT has come under scrutiny since studies have been underpowered or have been funded by interested parties [32]. Multiple articles have discussed NPWT for a variety of indications, including traumatic wounds, diabetic foot ulcers, and surgical wounds, among others. A meta-analysis of 10 randomized controlled trials (RCTs) in 2011 by Suissa et al. found that NPWT afforded a significantly decreased time to healing and decreased wound size when compared to standard dressings for the management of chronic wounds [33]. However, among the 10 trials included in the meta-analysis, 9 were sponsored by Kinetic Concepts, Inc., the creator of the VAC device. Likewise, while a recent meta-analysis by Zens et al. in 2020 evaluating 48 RCTs seemed to indicate a potential benefit in favor of NPWT for wound healing and length of hospital stay, the trials included were marred by publication bias and low-quality data [34]. Such results deserve careful prospective evaluation in an unbiased clinical setting to determine the true efficacy and cost-effectiveness of NPWT. The most recent update of the Cochrane review on NPWT for surgical wounds healing by primary closure found moderate-certainty evidence for decreased surgical site infections with NPWT compared to standard closure, moderate-certainty evidence for little/no difference in dehiscence rates between NPWT and standard dressings, and imprecise results regarding seroma/hematoma and reoperation rates. Based on the included economic studies in this review, the authors also noted low-/very low-quality evidence indicating the cost-effectiveness of NPWT for a multitude of surgical indications [35].

As an alternative to the standard VAC NPWT, Dorafshar et al. from the University of Chicago conducted a randomized prospective trial of VAC versus a sealed gauze dressing to wall suction for wound management [36]. The authors found that the reduction of wound surface area and volume were similar between the two groups, while the mean cost per day and time required for dressing change were significantly higher for the VAC therapy ($4.22 versus $96.51, $p < 0.01$; 19 minutes versus 31 minutes, $p < 0.01$, respectively). Another novel technique using the NPWT concept aimed to reduce costs associated with the KCI VAC therapy includes the use of the sterile sponge of the single-use surgical hand scrub brush (E-Z Scrub 205; Becton Dickinson, Franklin Lakes, NJ) with the application of an occlusive dressing to suction, as described by Perez et al. from Switzerland [37]. Such techniques enable optimizing the cost–benefit ratio while sustaining the benefits of the NPWT concept as a means of providing higher-quality wound care, particularly in resource-limited settings.

NPWT with instillation and dwelling of a topical solution (NPWTi-d) is a modification of the traditional NPWT that has received significant attention over the past few years. The concept of NPWTi-d involves irrigating wounds between periods of negative pressure that results in wound cleansing and lowers wound fluid viscosity, thereby reducing bacterial bioburden levels, the number of debridements required, and the time to final reconstruction for the wound bed [38–40]. A recent meta-analysis by Gabriel et al. in 2021 found that wounds treated with NPWTi-d had a faster time to achieve readiness for closure and had 4.4 times higher odds of reducing bacterial counts in the wound compared to control wounds. The authors also noted a shorter overall length of therapy for the NPWTi-d group but did not find a significant difference in terms of length of hospital stay [41]. The solution used for NPWTi-d varies and ranges from saline to antiseptic solutions, including Dakin's, at various strengths. Overall, this therapy is gaining popularity for the treatment of a multitude of wounds and has been shown to have enhanced granulation tissue production, fewer operating room visits, shorter time to final surgical procedure, and easier and less painful dressing changes compared to traditional NPWT [42].

RECOMMENDATION

There is currently weak evidence for decreased healing time with NPWT wounds compared to wet-to-dry dressing. Few studies currently address the cost-effectiveness of the modality.

Grade of recommendation: B.

33.4 Do Skin Grafting and Acellular Dermal Replacement Improve Wound Outcomes after Burn and Reconstructive Surgery?

Early excision and grafting are of paramount importance in burn surgery and have been shown to positively impact survival and outcomes in burn patients [43]. Among techniques of surgical burn excision, tangential excision is preferred to preserve viable tissue identified by healthy bleeding upon serial debridement of thin burn-affected layers [44]. Alternative means include enzymatic, mechanical, biological, and hydrosurgical debridement.

Skin autografts have traditionally been used, and skin substitutes have been engineered for coverage of defects resulting from burns. The use of these techniques has spanned the entire field of reconstructive surgery [45]. Autologous split-thickness skin grafts (STSGs) comprise the epidermis and a varying amount of papillary dermis depending on the thickness specified while using the dermatome blade. These comprise the current standard of care for coverage following deep partial-thickness and full-thickness burns [45]. Autologous STSGs are also used for coverage over well-granulated wound beds and can result in epidermal coverage by neo-epithelialization from the hair follicles. While meshing an STSG can provide an increased surface for coverage of large wounds, this can also result in significant secondary contracture, limiting utilization in cosmetically sensitive areas and over mobile joints [46].

The limitations of donor site availability for STSG harvest have been addressed by a host of acellular dermal replacement matrix products. The first report of acellular dermal replacement was by Burke et al. in 1981 on a series of 10 burn patients [47]. Allografts (from cadavers and occasionally from living donors) and xenografts (from animals) have been used after multiple rounds of processing to destroy pathogens and donor cells that could elicit an immune response [48].

A multicenter prospective randomized trial found the median take of the acellular dermis to be 80% compared with 95% for controls (autograft, allograft, xenograft, or a synthetic dressing depending on the investigator's usual control). After the study, there was less hypertrophic scarring of the artificial dermis, and more patients preferred the final result of the artificial dermis to the control graft. Another multicenter trial across 13 burn centers found the acellular dermal replacement to be effective and safe in the hands of properly trained clinicians [48].

The utility of acellular dermal replacement for burn-related scarring and contracture release has been studied; however, these reports are mostly case series accruing low evidence yield. The use of an acellular dermal matrix seems to offer a better range of motion when grafted over joints in an underlay technique compared with STSG [49]. The dermal regeneration template has been advocated as a substitute for a full-thickness skin graft for large defects due to the limited availability of the same in reconstructive surgery.

The combination of NPWT with acellular dermal matrix to improve take and reduce the time for the taking of the acellular dermis has been well described in multiple studies. This is related to the expeditious tissue infiltration into the dermal template, optimized contact with the wound bed, and elimination of sheer forces [50]. A clinical trial comparing NPWT over acellular dermal matrix and STSG with the classic tie-over dressing over paraffin gauze and splint found 97.8% graft take at day 5 in the former group compared to 84% graft take in the latter. The authors noted a statistically significant improvement in time to complete healing with NPWT (5.8 days versus 8.9 days) [51]. As a further improvement of technique, Jeschke et al. found improved artificial dermis take (98% versus 78%, $p = 0.003$) when fibrin glue was added before the application of the dermal matrix and NPWT [52]. Current evidence thus seems to favor a combination of NPWT with an acellular dermal replacement for shorter healing times and simplified wound care.

RECOMMENDATION

Acellular dermal replacement offers a viable alternative to skin grafts when used in burn and reconstructive surgery. Its utility expands to contracture release, allows improved mobility when used over joints, and mitigates the risk of donor-site morbidity that is inherent to skin graft harvest. The combination of NPWT with acellular dermal matrix utilization improves wound healing times and graft take.

Grade of recommendation: B.

33.5 Does Hyperbaric Oxygen Therapy Accelerate Wound Healing?

The role of hyperbaric oxygen therapy (HBO_2) therapy for a variety of indications, including wound management, has been well documented. The Undersea and Hyperbaric Medical Society developed a list of indications for HBO_2 therapy in 1976, and this list undergoes biannual updates [53]. Dauwe et al., in a systematic review in 2014, analyzed the role of HBO_2 therapy in facilitating acute wound healing [54]. However, the heterogeneity of included data from the individual studies made it difficult to draw concrete conclusions. From the studies included in the systematic review, the authors found that HBO_2 therapy resulted in higher complete healing rates for patients with extremity crush injuries, decreased wound length and hyperemia in ultraviolet radiation–induced dermal burns, and increased partial oxygen pressures in parascapular free flaps used for lower extremity reconstruction [54, 55].

Another systematic review of RCTs from 2011 found that HBO_2 therapy identified five trials from different countries, three of which supported wound healing with HBO_2 therapy. These trials included the following outcomes in favor of HBO_2 therapy [56]:

1. Healing of crush wounds with fewer additional surgical procedures (risk ratio [RR] 1.6, 95% confidence interval [CI] 1.03–2.50) and less tissue necrosis (RR 1.70, 95% CI 1.11–2.61)
2. Quicker healing of burn wounds when compared with routine burn care
3. Higher percentage of healthy graft area when STSGs were subject to HBO_2 therapy (RR 3.50, 95% CI 1.35–9.11)

A Cochrane review updated in 2015 analyzed HBO_2 applications for chronic wounds [57]. Ten of the twelve trials included studied diabetic foot ulcers and noted a significantly increased rate of healing at 6 weeks in favor of HBO_2 therapy, a benefit that was not evident over a longer follow-up period [57]. The two other trials that reported the outcomes for venous ulcers and mixed (diabetic + venous) ulcers reported significant benefits at 6 weeks and 30 days, respectively, in terms of wound size and reduction of the wound area.

RECOMMENDATION

There is limited evidence to recommend HBO_2 therapy for wound management.

Grade of recommendation: C.

33.6 How Should We Treat Hypertrophic Scars and Keloids?

Both keloids and hypertrophic scars are characterized by the deposition of excess scar tissue resulting from increased fibroblastic activity during the wound healing process. While hypertrophic scars are contained within the boundaries of the original wound, keloids extend beyond the wound edges. The histological composition of these two entities differs: Keloids are composed of haphazardly branched and disorganized type I and type III collagen, while hypertrophic scars contain mainly type III collagen arranged parallel to the epidermal surface [58]. There is a greater genetic predisposition for keloid (compared to hypertrophic scar) formation, and a wide range of medical and surgical therapies have been developed for their management.

Among the medical treatment options, steroid injection remains the most commonly employed management modality. Steroids decrease collagen production, reduce fibroblast activity, and augment collagen degradation [59]. Following triamcinolone injection, recurrence rates of up to 50% at 5 years have been documented, and repeat injections are often required [58, 60]. A recent meta-analysis by Ren et al. found that the combination of administration of intralesional triamcinolone with 5-fluorouracil demonstrated improved scar height and erythema scores compared to triamcinolone alone [61]. Other antineoplastic drugs, including mitomycin C, bleomycin, and immune modulators including imiquimod, have been studied for keloid and hypertrophic scar management with varying efficacy [58].

Laser devices have also been evaluated for the treatment of keloids and hypertrophic scars. Lasers are classified as ablative that destroy the epidermal layer, as with erbium-doped yttrium aluminum garnet and carbon-dioxide lasers, and nonablative lasers that target the dermis, including potassium titanyl phosphate (KTP), pulsed dye (PDL), and neodymium-doped yttrium aluminum garnet (Nd-YAG). Data are limited on the role of lasers in keloid and hypertrophic scar management at this time, as these have not been adequately evaluated in RCTs [62].

Surgical excision of keloids alone results in an unacceptably high recurrence of more than 50%. However, greater success has been reported when combined with medical modalities. Ear keloids respond well to surgical excision combined with steroid injection, with a recurrence rate of approximately 15%. However, this response was not seen in keloids in other areas

TABLE 33.2

Summary of the Levels of Evidence

Question	Answer	Level of Evidence	Grade of Recommendation
What is the optimal management of pressure ulcers?	Static and dynamic pressure-reducing devices have moderate success.	IB	B
Is NPWT better than standard dressing, and is it cost-effective?	Doubtful efficacy of NPWT over standard dressings with extensive publication bias. Numerous cost-effective alternatives with comparable outcomes.	IIB	B
What is the role of skin graft/ADM after burn/reconstructive surgery?	ADM is a viable alternative to a skin graft; utility includes contracture release, allows improved mobility when used over joints, and mitigates the risk of donor-site morbidity.	IIB	B
Is there any benefit of hyperbaric oxygen therapy in wound healing?	Limited evidence to support HBO$_2$ therapy for wound management.	IIIB	C
What are the effective treatment options for keloids and hypertrophic scars?	Excision, intralesional triamcinolone injection, and radiation for selected patients.	IIA	B

of the body [63]. One of the most aggressive approaches to keloid management is a combination of surgical excision with radiation therapy. Radiation disrupts the wound healing process, and this is thought to decrease recurrence rates. A meta-analysis of 72 studies by Mankowski et al. in 2017 found a recurrence rate of 15% for brachytherapy following surgical excision of keloids [64]. However, changes in skin pigmentation and a very small risk of inducing malignancy exist with the use of radiation therapy. In the literature review from 1901 to 2009 by Ogawa et al., only five cases of carcinogenesis were reported about radiation therapy for keloids, and the authors concluded that the risk is very low, particularly if the radiosensitive organs such as the breasts and thyroid are appropriately shielded [65].

Pressure therapy and topical silicone have been studied for preventing keloid recurrence. In the recent review of 10 trials by Hsu et al. in 2017, topical silicone was not found to be significantly effective in preventing keloid recurrence [66]. A Cochrane review of 20 trials from 2013 similarly found weak benefits of silicone gel sheeting as a means of keloid treatment or prevention in high-risk individuals [67].

RECOMMENDATION

Triamcinolone injection with surgical excision lowers the recurrence risk for keloid scars. Silicone sheeting is not effective in these settings. Surgical excision followed by radiation has low recurrence rates but is usually reserved for selected patients who have lesions refractory to conventional treatment due to the risk of adverse effects from the radiation therapy.

Grade of recommendation: B.

33.6.1 Recent Advances in Wound Management

The growing interest in novel modalities for treating complex wounds has resulted in pioneering advancements based on the utilization of epidermal stem cells to facilitate wound healing. In their initial experience from a tertiary care institution in the United States, Berg et al. discussed the outcomes in eight patients from whom full-thickness skin grafts were excised, processed at a bioengineering laboratory, and returned as an autologous paste for grafting over a granulated wound bed. A silicone sheet and fibrin glue were used to seal this material over the wound, and NPWT at −75 mmHg was applied. Dressings were changed every 5–7 days for 3 weeks. The authors noted a nearly 100% survival rate for these epidermal stem cell grafts despite their application to complicated wounds resulting from multiple etiologies and found the final cosmetic appearance and functionality to be similar to that of adjacent native skin [68]. Large-scale studies in prospective settings can shed further light on these preliminary results, and harnessing epidermal stem cells for wound healing seems to hold promise for the future of advanced wound care management.

Table 33.2 provides a sumarry of the various wound care techniques and modality disucssed in prior sections.

Editor's Note

Wound healing is a well-studied field of medicine, as the authors have nicely summarized. Some of the current interventions have been adopted with little supportive data (i.e., hyperbaric oxygen) at various "wound centers" in an attempt to derive financial income from chronic wounds. The use of negative pressure wound therapy, in particular, has grabbed a major foothold in the United States with little quality data to support its use outside of skin graft sites and the diabetic foot. In fact, multiple large Cochrane reviews have failed to find a benefit of negative pressure wound therapy in the setting of acute or chronic wounds when compared to conventional dressing changes. This very expensive modality does simplify outpatient wound management, making dressing changes less frequent. In-hospital use of negative pressure wound therapy does not appear to reduce resource utilization while generating huge costs to the healthcare environment. It is the editor's experience that because of the great cost of these devices, the ability for investigators to conduct large prospective randomized trials has been severely hampered, as the manufacturers avoid rigorous examination of this widely used product.

REFERENCES

1. Schilling JA: Wound healing. Surg Clin North Am. 1976, 56:859–74. 10.1016/s0039-6109(16)40983-7
2. Velnar T, Bailey T, Smrkolj V: The wound healing process: an overview of the cellular and molecular mechanisms. J Int Med Res. 2009, 37:1528–42. 10.1177/147323000903700531
3. Lawrence WT, Diegelmann RF: Growth factors in wound healing. Clin Dermatol. 1994, 12:157–69. 10.1016/0738-081x(94)90266-6
4. Lucas T, Waisman A, Ranjan R, et al.: Differential roles of macrophages in diverse phases of skin repair. J Immunol Baltim Md. 2010, 184:3964–77. 10.4049/jimmunol.0903356
5. Wang P-H, Huang B-S, Horng H-C, Yeh C-C, Chen Y-J: Wound healing. J Chin Med Assoc JCMA. 2018, 81:94–101. 10.1016/j.jcma.2017.11.002
6. Witte MB, Barbul A: General principles of wound healing. Surg Clin North Am. 1997, 77:509–28. 10.1016/s0039-6109(05)70566-1
7. Grotendorst GR, Soma Y, Takehara K, Charette M: EGF and TGF-alpha are potent chemoattractants for endothelial cells and EGF-like peptides are present at sites of tissue regeneration. J Cell Physiol. 1989, 139:617–23. 10.1002/jcp.1041390323
8. Gauglitz GG, Korting HC, Pavicic T, Ruzicka T, Jeschke MG: Hypertrophic scarring and keloids: pathomechanisms and current and emerging treatment strategies. Mol Med Camb Mass. 2011, 17:113–25. 10.2119/molmed.2009.00153
9. Karim AS, Liu A, Lin C, Uselmann AJ, Eliceiri KW, Brown ME, Gibson ALF: Evolution of ischemia and neovascularization in a murine model of full thickness human wound healing. Wound Repair Regen Off Publ Wound Heal Soc Eur Tissue Repair Soc. 2020, 28:812–22. 10.1111/wrr.12847
10. Rico RM, Ripamonti R, Burns AL, Gamelli RL, DiPietro LA: The effect of sepsis on wound healing. J Surg Res. 2002, 102:193–7. 10.1006/jsre.2001.6316
11. Adusei KM, Ngo TB, Sadtler K: T lymphocytes as critical mediators in tissue regeneration, fibrosis, and the foreign body response. Acta Biomater. 2021, 133:17–33. 10.1016/j.actbio.2021.04.023
12. Steed DL: Debridement. Am J Surg. 2004, 187:71S–74S. 10.1016/S0002-9610(03)00307-6
13. Baltzis D, Eleftheriadou I, Veves A: Pathogenesis and treatment of impaired wound healing in diabetes mellitus: new insights. Adv Ther. 2014, 31:817–36. 10.1007/s12325-014-0140-x
14. Wilson RM, Tomlinson DR, Reeves WG: Neutrophil sorbitol production impairs oxidative killing in diabetes. Diabet Med J Br Diabet Assoc. 1987, 4:37–40. 10.1111/j.1464-5491.1987.tb00825.x
15. Van de Kerkhof PC, Van Bergen B, Spruijt K, Kuiper JP: Age-related changes in wound healing. Clin Exp Dermatol. 1994, 19:369–74. 10.1111/j.1365-2230.1994.tb02684.x
16. Freedland M, Karmiol S, Rodriguez J, Normolle D, Smith D, Garner W: Fibroblast responses to cytokines are maintained during aging. Ann Plast Surg. 1995, 35:290–6. 10.1097/00000637-199509000-00012
17. Sgonc R, Gruber J: Age-related aspects of cutaneous wound healing: a mini-review. Gerontology. 2013, 59:159–64. 10.1159/000342344
18. Dryden SV, Shoemaker WG, Kim JH: Wound management and nutrition for optimal wound healing. Atlas Oral Maxillofac Surg Clin North Am. 2013, 21:37–47. 10.1016/j.cxom.2012.12.008
19. Sørensen LT: Wound healing and infection in surgery: the pathophysiological impact of smoking, smoking cessation, and nicotine replacement therapy: a systematic review. Ann Surg. 2012, 255:1069–79. 10.1097/SLA.0b013e31824f632d
20. Wang AS, Armstrong EJ, Armstrong AW: Corticosteroids and wound healing: clinical considerations in the perioperative period. Am J Surg. 2013, 206:410–7. 10.1016/j.amjsurg.2012.11.018
21. Khan MTA, Patnaik R, Hausman-Cohen L, Panchal O, Ewart M, Lovely RS, Rajesh A: Obesity stratification predicts short-term complications after parastomal hernia repair. J Surg Res. 2022, 280:27–34. 10.1016/j.jss.2022.07.002
22. Mervis JS, Phillips TJ: Pressure ulcers: pathophysiology, epidemiology, risk factors, and presentation. J Am Acad Dermatol. 2019, 81:881–90. 10.1016/j.jaad.2018.12.069
23. Bergstrom N, Braden BJ, Laguzza A, Holman V: The Braden Scale for predicting pressure sore risk. Nurs Res. 1987, 36:205–10.
24. Rich SE, Margolis D, Shardell M, Hawkes WG, Miller RR, Amr S, Baumgarten M: Frequent manual repositioning and incidence of pressure ulcers among bedbound elderly hip fracture patients. Wound Repair Regen Off Publ Wound Heal Soc Eur Tissue Repair Soc. 2011, 19:10–8. 10.1111/j.1524-475X.2010.00644.x
25. Serraes B, van Leen M, Schols J, Van Hecke A, Verhaeghe S, Beeckman D: Prevention of pressure ulcers with a static air support surface: a systematic review. Int Wound J. 2018, 15:333–43. 10.1111/iwj.12870
26. Bluestein D, Javaheri A: Pressure ulcers: prevention, evaluation, and management. Am Fam Physician. 2008, 78:1186–94.
27. Agarwal P, Kukrele R, Sharma D: Vacuum assisted closure (VAC)/negative pressure wound therapy (NPWT) for difficult wounds: a review. J Clin Orthop Trauma. 2019, 10:845–8. 10.1016/j.jcot.2019.06.015
28. Wilkes RP, McNulty AK, Feeley TD, Schmidt MA, Kieswetter K: Bioreactor for application of subatmospheric pressure to three-dimensional cell culture. Tissue Eng. 2007, 13:3003–10. 10.1089/ten.2007.0036
29. Timmers MS, Le Cessie S, Banwell P, Jukema GN: The effects of varying degrees of pressure delivered by negative-pressure wound therapy on skin perfusion. Ann Plast Surg. 2005, 55:665–71. 10.1097/01.sap.0000187182.90907.3d
30. Malmsjö M, Gustafsson L, Lindstedt S, Gesslein B, Ingemansson R: The effects of variable, intermittent, and continuous negative pressure wound therapy, using foam or gauze, on wound contraction, granulation tissue formation, and ingrowth into the wound filler. Eplasty. 2012, 12:e5.
31. Lee KN, Ben-Nakhi M, Park EJ, Hong JP: Cyclic negative pressure wound therapy: an alternative mode to intermittent system. Int Wound J. 2015, 12:686–92. 10.1111/iwj.12201
32. Armstrong DG, Lavery LA, Diabetic Foot Study Consortium: Negative pressure wound therapy after partial diabetic foot amputation: a multicentre, randomised controlled trial. Lancet Lond Engl. 2005, 366:1704–10. 10.1016/S0140-6736(05)67695-7

33. Suissa D, Danino A, Nikolis A: Negative-pressure therapy versus standard wound care: a meta-analysis of randomized trials. Plast Reconstr Surg. 2011, 128:498e–503e. 10.1097/PRS.0b013e31822b675c

34. Zens Y, Barth M, Bucher HC, et al.: Negative pressure wound therapy in patients with wounds healing by secondary intention: a systematic review and meta-analysis of randomised controlled trials. Syst Rev. 2020, 9:238. 10.1186/s13643-020-01476-6

35. Norman G, Shi C, Goh EL, et al.: Negative pressure wound therapy for surgical wounds healing by primary closure. Cochrane Database Syst Rev. 2022, 4:CD009261. 10.1002/14651858.CD009261.pub7

36. Dorafshar AH, Franczyk M, Gottlieb LJ, Wroblewski KE, Lohman RF: A prospective randomized trial comparing subatmospheric wound therapy with a sealed gauze dressing and the standard vacuum-assisted closure device. Ann Plast Surg. 2012, 69:79–84. 10.1097/SAP.0b013e318221286c

37. Perez D, Bramkamp M, Exe C, von Ruden C, Ziegler A: Modern wound care for the poor: a randomized clinical trial comparing the vacuum system with conventional saline-soaked gauze dressings. Am J Surg. 2010, 199:14–20. 10.1016/j.amjsurg.2008.12.029

38. Horch RE, Braumann C, Dissemond J, et al.: Use of negative pressure wound therapy with instillation and dwell time for wound treatment - results of an expert consensus conference. Zentralbl Chir. 2018, 143:609–16. 10.1055/a-0713-0517

39. Yang C, Goss SG, Alcantara S, Schultz G, Lantis Ii JC: Effect of negative pressure wound therapy with instillation on bioburden in chronically infected wounds. Wounds Compend Clin Res Pract. 2017, 29:240–6.

40. Kim PJ, Lavery LA, Galiano RD, et al.: The impact of negative-pressure wound therapy with instillation on wounds requiring operative debridement: pilot randomised, controlled trial. Int Wound J. 2020, 17:1194–208. 10.1111/iwj.13424

41. Gabriel A, Kahn K, Karmy-Jones R: Use of negative pressure wound therapy with automated, volumetric instillation for the treatment of extremity and trunk wounds: clinical outcomes and potential cost-effectiveness. Eplasty. 2014, 14:e41.

42. Kim PJ, Attinger CE, Steinberg JS, et al.: The impact of negative-pressure wound therapy with instillation compared with standard negative-pressure wound therapy: a retrospective, historical, cohort, controlled study. Plast Reconstr Surg. 2014, 133:709–16. 10.1097/01.prs.0000438060.46290.7a

43. Browning JA, Cindass R: Burn Debridement, Grafting, and Reconstruction. StatPearls Publishing; 2022.

44. Edmondson S-J, Ali Jumabhoy I, Murray A: Time to start putting down the knife: a systematic review of burns excision tools of randomised and non-randomised trials. Burns J Int Soc Burn Inj. 2018, 44:1721–37. 10.1016/j.burns.2018.01.012

45. Stone Ii R, Natesan S, Kowalczewski CJ, et al.: Advancements in regenerative strategies through the continuum of burn care. Front Pharmacol. 2018, 9:672. 10.3389/fphar.2018.00672

46. Gabriel A, Shores J, Heinrich C, Baqai W, Kalina S, Sogioka N, Gupta S: Negative pressure wound therapy with instillation: a pilot study describing a new method for treating infected wounds. Int Wound J. 2008, 5:399–413. 10.1111/j.1742-481X.2007.00423.x

47. Burke JF, Yannas IV, Quinby WC, Bondoc CC, Jung WK: Successful use of a physiologically acceptable artificial skin in the treatment of extensive burn injury. Ann Surg. 1981, 194:413–28. 10.1097/00000658-198110000-00005

48. Heimbach DM, Warden GD, Luterman A, et al.: Multicenter post approval clinical trial of Integra dermal regeneration template for burn treatment. J Burn Care Rehabil. 2003, 24:42–8. 10.1097/00004630-200301000-00009

49. Motykie GD, Washington W, Sanford AP, McCauley RL, Herndon DN, Wolf SE: Outcomes of alloderm grafting in reconstructive procedures following severe thermal injuries. J Burn Care Rehabil. 2001, 22:S128. 10.1097/00004630-200103002-00162

50. Eo S, Kim Y, Cho S: Vacuum-assisted closure improves the incorporation of artificial dermis in soft tissue defects: Terudermis(®) and Pelnac(®). Int Wound J. 2011, 8:261–7. 10.1111/j.1742-481X.2011.00780.x

51. Kim EK, Hong JP: Efficacy of negative pressure therapy to enhance take of 1-stage allodermis and a split-thickness graft. Ann Plast Surg. 2007, 58:536–40. 10.1097/01.sap.0000245121.32831.47

52. Faglia E, Favales F, Aldeghi A, et al.: Adjunctive systemic hyperbaric oxygen therapy in treatment of severe prevalently ischemic diabetic foot ulcer. A randomized study. Diabetes Care. 1996, 19:1338–43. 10.2337/diacare.19.12.1338

53. Weaver LK: Hyperbaric Oxygen Therapy Indications. 172.

54. Dauwe PB, Pulikkottil BJ, Lavery L, Stuzin JM, Rohrich RJ: Does hyperbaric oxygen therapy work in facilitating acute wound healing: a systematic review. Plast Reconstr Surg. 2014, 133:208e–15e. 10.1097/01.prs.0000436849.79161.a4

55. Gehmert S, Geis S, Lamby P, et al.: Evaluation of hyperbaric oxygen therapy for free flaps using planar optical oxygen sensors. Preliminary results. Clin Hemorheol Microcirc. 2011, 48:75–9. 10.3233/CH-2011-1389

56. Eskes AM, Ubbink DT, Lubbers MJ, Lucas C, Vermeulen H: Hyperbaric oxygen therapy: solution for difficult to heal acute wounds? Systematic review. World J Surg. 2011, 35:535–42. 10.1007/s00268-010-0923-4

57. Kranke P, Bennett MH, Martyn-St James M, Schnabel A, Debus SE, Weibel S: Hyperbaric oxygen therapy for chronic wounds. Cochrane Database Syst Rev. 2015, CD004123. 10.1002/14651858.CD004123.pub4

58. Ekstein SF, Wyles SP, Moran SL, Meves A: Keloids: a review of therapeutic management. Int J Dermatol. 2021, 60:661–71. 10.1111/ijd.15159

59. Andrews JP, Marttala J, Macarak E, Rosenbloom J, Uitto J: Keloids: the paradigm of skin fibrosis - Pathomechanisms and treatment. Matrix Biol J Int Soc Matrix Biol. 2016, 51:37–46. 10.1016/j.matbio.2016.01.013

60. Morelli Coppola M, Salzillo R, Segreto F, Persichetti P: Triamcinolone acetonide intralesional injection for the treatment of keloid scars: patient selection and perspectives. Clin Cosmet Investig Dermatol. 2018, 11:387–96. 10.2147/CCID.S133672

61. Ren Y, Zhou X, Wei Z, Lin W, Fan B, Feng S: Efficacy and safety of triamcinolone acetonide alone and in combination with 5-fluorouracil for treating hypertrophic scars and keloids: a systematic review and meta-analysis. Int Wound J. 2017, 14:480–7. 10.1111/iwj.12629

62. Cho SB, Lee JH, Lee SH, Lee SJ, Bang D, Oh SH: Efficacy and safety of 1064-nm Q-switched Nd:YAG laser with low fluence for keloids and hypertrophic scars. J Eur Acad Dermatol Venereol JEADV. 2010, 24:1070–4. 10.1111/j.1468-3083.2010.03593.x

63. Forbat E, Ali FR, Al-Niaimi F: Treatment of keloid scars using light-, laser- and energy-based devices: a contemporary review of the literature. Lasers Med Sci. 2017, 32:2145–54. 10.1007/s10103-017-2332-5

64. Mankowski P, Kanevsky J, Tomlinson J, Dyachenko A, Luc M: Optimizing radiotherapy for keloids: a meta-analysis systematic review comparing recurrence rates between different radiation modalities. Ann Plast Surg. 2017, 78: 403–11. 10.1097/SAP.0000000000000989

65. Ogawa R, Yoshitatsu S, Yoshida K, Miyashita T: Is radiation therapy for keloids acceptable? The risk of radiation-induced carcinogenesis. Plast Reconstr Surg. 2009, 124: 1196–201. 10.1097/PRS.0b013e3181b5a3ae

66. Hsu K-C, Luan C-W, Tsai Y-W: Review of silicone gel sheeting and silicone gel for the prevention of hypertrophic scars and keloids. Wounds Compend Clin Res Pract. 2017, 29:154–8.

67. O'Brien L, Jones DJ: Silicone gel sheeting for preventing and treating hypertrophic and keloid scars. Cochrane Database Syst Rev. 2013, 2013:CD003826. 10.1002/14651858. CD003826.pub3

68. Berg A, Kaul S, Rauscher GE, Blatt M, Cohn S: Successful full-thickness skin regeneration using epidermal stem cells in traumatic and complex wounds: initial experience. Cureus. 2020, 12:e10558. 10.7759/cureus.10558

34

Pediatric Trauma

Benjamin Keller and Gerald Gollin

34.1 Introduction

Injuries in children are frequently managed similarly to adults. However, the unique anatomy, physiology, and psychology of children mandate care in the application of evidence obtained from studies of adults to the pediatric population. The following chapter focuses on five questions in pediatric trauma that are relevant to the daily practice of those who care for injured children.

34.2 When Is a CT Scan of the Head Indicated in Pediatric Head Trauma?

There are over 600,000 emergency department visits a year in the United States for head injuries in children 18 years old and younger [1, 2]. Among these, 60,000 were hospitalized with 2,500 deaths in 2014 [3]. The incidence of traumatic brain injury (TBI) has increased substantially, particularly among children under 4 years of age, in which the rate of TBI is twice that of older teens [4]. Computed tomography (CT) scanning is an indispensable tool in the identification of significant intracranial injuries in children.

A study of 400 children with a Glasgow Coma Score (GCS) of greater than 12 and a negative CT scan of the head found that only 4 patients were readmitted with a neurological diagnosis and only 1, who was on Coumadin, required craniotomy [5]. Based on this and similar findings in adults, most pediatric physicians have confidently discharged head-injured children with unremarkable CT scan findings. However, a protocol of CT scanning for all pediatric head injuries is neither cost-effective nor safe, considering that 1 in a 1,000 CT scans in children may result in malignancy [6]. Efforts over the last 20 years have focused on identifying all children with TBI who require admission or intervention while sparing as many of those who can be safely discharged from the emergency department from the risks of radiation from CT scanning.

Some had believed that a patient with normal mental status and no history of a loss of consciousness is at such a low risk for intracranial injury that a CT scan need not be performed. Simon et al. cast significant doubt on this in a retrospective review of 429 children with head trauma and GCS of 14 or 15 [7]. Among 219 with a GCS of 15 and a reliable history of no loss of consciousness, there were 35 intracranial injuries (16%), of which 4 required operative intervention and 1 needed intubation. Based on these findings, the authors recommended a policy of "liberal" CT scanning.

Subsequent studies have aimed to more precisely define the population at risk for intracranial injury by expanding the criteria examined beyond mental status and loss of consciousness. Haydel et al. reviewed 175 children between 5 and 17 years of age who had a loss of consciousness but a GCS of 15 and a normal neurological exam [7]. If CT scans had been obtained only in children with at least one of these six conditions: Headache, vomiting, intoxication, short-term memory loss, seizure, or physical evidence of trauma above the clavicles, intracranial injuries would have been identified with a sensitivity of 100% (95% confidence interval [CI] 73–100%) and the use of CT scanning would have been reduced by 23%. Generalizations of these criteria are limited by a very low confidence limit and the exclusion of children under 5 years of age.

In 2003, a prospective evaluation of 2,043 children with nontrivial head trauma, including 327 under 2 years of age, was published [8]. Head CT scans were done in 1,271. Of the 98 who had evidence of brain injury on CT, 96 had at least one of the following: Abnormal mental status (GCS <15), clinical signs of skull fracture, scalp hematoma (when <2 years old), or a history of vomiting. The sensitivity of an algorithm using these variables to identify patients who require CT scanning was 98% (95% CI 92.8–99.8%). To derive a decision tool to identify those at risk for the more worrisome occurrence of a head injury that requires an intervention, another set of variables (GCS <15, signs of skull fracture, vomiting, and headache) was identified for which the presence of at least one identified these more serious injuries with a sensitivity of 100% (95% CI 97.2–100%). Finally, the finding of a focal neurological deficit, GCS <15, and/or vomiting predicted all 29 cases in which a neurosurgical procedure was required, yielding a sensitivity of 100% (95% CI 90.2–100%).

The National Emergency X-Radiography Utilization Study II (NEXUS II) was a prospective, multicenter study of adults and children with blunt head trauma that sought to derive a decision tool that could be used to identify patients at risk for intracranial injury who should undergo CT scanning [9]. An algorithm was developed that identified intracranial injuries with a sensitivity of 98.3% (95% CI 97.2–99%). Oman et al. evaluated this decision instrument in the subset of 1,666 children in the original study [10]. The NEXUS II decision tool for children included seven variables: Clinical evidence of skull fracture, altered alertness, neurological deficit, persistent vomiting, scalp hematoma, abnormal behavior, and coagulopathy. The occurrence of one or more of these variables identified 136 of 138 significant injuries for a sensitivity

DOI: 10.1201/9781003316800-34

of 98.6% (95% CI 94.9–99.8%). All of the 25 clinically important injuries in children under 3 years old were identified, although the CI for this subset was largely due to the small population.

The importance of using precision in applying the two decision tools described earlier was highlighted by Sun et al. [11], who assessed a subtle modification of the criteria described by Palchak et al. [8] with the pediatric subset of the NEXUS II database. By substituting the criteria "severe headache" for "headache" and "high-risk vomiting" for "vomiting," 13 (9%) of the patients with clinically important intracranial injuries would not be identified as needing head CT scanning.

Recognition of the limitations of applying NEXUS criteria to the pediatric population, particularly the youngest patients, led to the development of pediatric-specific prediction tools for the identification of significant injuries among children with mild TBI. The Children's Head Injury Algorithm for the Prediction of Important Clinical Events (CHALICE) tool was proposed after a prospective evaluation of 766 children who underwent head CT, which found that if at least 1 of 13 conditions were present (including loss of consciousness, seizure, and evidence of basilar skull fracture), patients with an intracranial injury could be identified with a sensitivity of 98% (95% CI 96–100%) [12]. The four missed injuries included two depressed skull fractures and one case that required a craniotomy.

The Canadian Assessment of Tomography for Childhood Head Injury (CATCH) rule [13] proposed that a head CT be obtained with any of the following findings: GCS <15 at 2 hours after injury; suspected open or depressed skull fracture; history of worsening headache; irritability on examination; any sign of a basilar skull fracture; a large, boggy scalp hematoma; or a dangerous mechanism of injury. In a study of 4,060 children, in which 23 (0.6%) required neurosurgical intervention and 197 (4.9%) had some CT evidence for brain injury, the CATCH rule had a 91.3% sensitivity for predicting a neurosurgical intervention and a 97.5% sensitivity for brain injury overall. A subsequent revision [14] of the rule that added the finding of "greater than four episodes of vomiting" yielded a sensitivity of 100% for neurosurgical interventions.

In 2009, the Pediatric Emergency Care Applied Research Network (PECARN) published a multiinstitutional prospective cohort study of over 40,000 children enrolled with GCS 14–15 [2]. The authors identified prediction rules for children with a low risk of clinically significant TBIs in which CT scans could be avoided. For children less than 2 years of age, a head CT was not indicated if they have normal mental status, no temporal or parietal scalp hematoma, no loss of consciousness or loss of consciousness for less than 5 seconds, nonsevere injury mechanism, no palpable skull fracture, and acting normally per parents. These criteria had 100% sensitivity, and no child with a clinically significant head injury was missed. For children aged 2 years and older, a head CT was not needed if they had normal mental status, no loss of consciousness, no vomiting, nonsevere injury mechanism, no signs of basilar skull fracture, and no severe headache. These criteria had a 96.8% sensitivity in predicting clinically significant head injuries. Two children in this group were classified as low risk but did have a clinically significant head injury (subdural hematoma and occipital lobe contusion); neither child required neurosurgical intervention.

A study that compared the accuracy of these three pediatric algorithms [15] found that the PECARN rule resulted in the lowest incidence of missed injuries, while CATCH and CHALICE had higher sensitivities. The authors concluded that this increased specificity was not justified in light of missed injuries that required neurosurgical intervention.

RECOMMENDATION

Neurologically intact (GCS = 15) children over 2 years of age with no loss of consciousness, vomiting, severe injury mechanism, signs of basilar skull fracture, or severe headache may be safely observed in the emergency department (ED) and discharged without a head CT. In younger children with GCS = 15 and a loss of consciousness over 5 seconds, a palpable skull fracture, a temporal/parietal cephalohematoma, or progressive headache or vomiting, a head CT should be obtained.

Grade of recommendation: B.

34.3 Is There a Role for Hypertonic Saline in Pediatric Head Injuries?

Head injuries result in direct and indirect costs of 56 billion dollars [16]. Aside from prevention, the devastating impact of childhood head injuries can only be reduced by advancements in treatment. Intracranial hypertension accompanies serious brain injury and is contributed to by multiple factors. The initial injury may result in hemorrhage in the subdural, epidural, and/or subarachnoid space, thereby increasing the pressure within the rigid cranial vault in keeping with the Monro-Kellie doctrine. The secondary response to injury is characterized by the development of edema due to alterations in cerebral blood flow, ischemia, and ultimately cellular necrosis. The resultant inflammatory response, while beneficial for healing, leads to further edema and a continuing cycle of ischemia, necrosis, and inflammation. If this scenario is not controlled, herniation and global cerebral ischemia ensue.

The cornerstone of the management of brain injury in children and adults is the prevention of intracranial hypertension and the maintenance of cerebral perfusion pressure (CPP) through medical and operative interventions. Depending on the neurological examination and the intracranial pressure (ICP) and CPP, interventions such as elevation of the head of the bed, prevention of hyperthermia, and sedation may progress to mechanical ventilation with mild hyperventilation, chemical paralysis, administration of a hyperosmolar solution, barbiturate coma, and decompressive craniotomy.

The role of hyperosmolar agents in reducing experimental cerebral edema has been known for almost a century [17]. Mannitol has rheological and cerebral vasoconstrictive properties that make it a theoretically valuable agent for reducing ICP. In the early 1960s, mannitol began to be used in patients with head injury [18], but its efficacy in adults and children remains unclear [19], and the side effects in a polytrauma patient can prohibit its use. In that context, this discussion focuses on the question of whether the administration of hypertonic saline, which exerts an osmotic effect on the brain, is a safe and effective adjunct to other, more traditional, means of controlling ICP dynamics in children.

The studies that have been performed assessing hypertonic saline in pediatric head trauma have limited numbers of subjects and unique protocols. Few studies have directly compared hypertonic saline to mannitol. In 1992, Fisher et al. performed a double-blind, crossover study in 18 children with a TBI that assessed the short-term efficacy of 3% saline in reducing ICP as compared to normal (0.9%) saline (NS) [20]. Each child received a bolus of each fluid after which ICP was followed for 2 hours. On average, after administration of NS, ICP changed minimally from 19.3 mmHg to 20.0 mmHg. In contrast, after a bolus of 3% saline, ICP decreased from 19.9 to 15.8 mmHg ($p = 0.003$). After hypertonic saline infusion, there was also a reduced requirement for additional interventions to control ICP. A randomized controlled trial that compared the efficacy of hypertonic saline to lactated Ringer's solution (LR) was carried out in 35 children with a GCS <8 [21]. Subjects received either 1.75% saline, to increase serum sodium to 145–150 mEq/L, or LR for 72 hours. The group treated with hypertonic saline required fewer interventions to maintain an ICP less than 15 mmHg ($p < 0.02$), had shorter intensive care unit (ICU) stays ($p = 0.04$), and had a lower incidence of acute respiratory distress syndrome (ARDS) ($p = 0.01$) and other complications than the group that received LR.

Khanna et al. reported a prospective trial of 3% saline in 10 children with TBI in 2000 [22]. In this study hypertonic saline was continuously infused and titrated to maintain an ICP of less than 20 mmHg when other measures failed. More patients were not enrolled because standard measures, including mannitol, sedation, and hyperventilation, were usually successful in lowering ICP. The elevation in serum sodium concentration was limited to 15 mEq/L/day. At the start of therapy, the mean ICP of the subjects was 26 mmHg. A statistically significant inverse correlation between serum sodium and ICP was demonstrated. Beyond 72 hours, the frequency of ICP spikes decreased ($p < 0.01$) and CPP increased ($p < 0.01$). Reversible renal failure developed in two of the subjects. One patient, who presented 2 days after nonaccidental trauma, died.

A retrospective study of 68 children with intracranial hypertension treated with hypertonic saline was published in 2000 [23]. In this series, 3% saline was similarly used as a rescue therapy in Khanna's study when mannitol, hyperventilation, and other measures failed to maintain an ICP of less than 20 mmHg. The mean serum sodium in these cases was 160 mEq/L. Mortality was 15% and was less than what would be expected by injury severity. Two deaths were due to cerebral edema, five were as a consequence of sepsis and multisystem organ failure, and one was from ARDS. Seventy-four percent of patients had complete recovery or only moderate neurological deficits and 11% had severe deficits. When serum sodium exceeded 180 mEq/L, only one of four patients survived and that subject had severe neurological deficits. Two theoretical complications of hypertonic saline administration, central pontine myelinolysis and subarachnoid hemorrhage due to rapid brain shrinkage, did not occur in any subjects.

A 2016 study that compared the efficacy of bolus administration of hypertonic saline (2–5 mL/kg over 10–20 minutes) to other agents found that hypertonic saline led to resolution of intracranial hypertension twice as quickly as fentanyl or pentobarbital and that, while mannitol decreased ICP, only hypertonic saline increased CPP [24]. The most recent large-scale assessment of hyperosmolar therapy for TBI found substantial practice variation in the use of mannitol and hypertonic saline among hospitals and patients, although the use of mannitol was limited [19]. Hypertonic saline was associated with both decreased ICP and increased CPP, while mannitol was associated with only a lesser degree of elevation of CPP. When confounders were eliminated, however, the impact of either agent on ICP or CPP was only "modest."

The use of hypertonic saline has expanded to patients with mild TBI. In 2014, Lumba-Brown et al. reported a randomized controlled trial that compared the use of a 3% saline bolus to an NS bolus for concussive pain [25]. This study enrolled 44 pediatric patients and used a self-reported pain score at pretreatment outpatient treatment and after 2–3 days with a follow-up phone call. Subjects given 3% saline had a greater degree of improvement in their pain scale scores at 1 hour post treatment (mean improvement of 3.5 with 3% saline vs. 1.1 in the NS group, $p < 0.001$). This improvement in pain scores was also seen after 2–3 days with the 3% saline group having a mean improvement of 4.61 in their pain scores and the NS group only having a mean improvement of 3 ($p = 0.01$).

RECOMMENDATION

Although a grade C recommendation can be made for the use of hypertonic saline to reduce ICP in children, there is no evidence for associated improvements in long-term outcomes.

34.4 When Is Clinical Clearance of the Cervical Spine Appropriate in Children?

Cervical spine injuries are diagnosed in 1–2% of cases of pediatric trauma [26, 27]. As compared to adult trauma patients, the incidence of cervical spine injury in the pediatric trauma population is much lower. In children with pain and tenderness of the cervical spine or neurological deficits, it is imperative that imaging studies be obtained and interpreted carefully by a radiologist with pediatric expertise. The unique bony anatomy of the developing spine can lead to overdiagnosis of injuries, and ligamentous laxity can result in a spinal cord injury without radiological abnormality (SCIWORA), in which plain films and even CT scans may show no evidence of dangerous spinal instability. In pediatric trauma victims with no obvious signs or symptoms of injury to the cervical spine, clinicians must balance the risk of a potentially disastrous missed injury against the cost and radiation exposure of universal imaging.

The concept of "clinical clearance" of the cervical spine has evolved over the last 30 years. To reduce the time and expense of cervical spine imaging in trauma patients, investigators have worked to define the circumstances under which imaging may be omitted without resultant missed injuries. Early studies in adults [28] suggested that as many as 20% of cervical spine injuries would be missed with protocols of selective imaging based on a lack of neck pain and the mechanism of injury. Velmahos et al. [29] refined the selection criteria used to determine eligibility for a clinical clearance protocol in a prospective study of trauma victims without neck pain by eliminating cases in which patients were intoxicated and had an otherwise altered level of consciousness, a subset that accounted for most of the missed injuries in previous reports. They identified 549 cases in which there was no neck tenderness with palpation or active motion. Patients with distracting injuries and head/facial injuries were included in the subgroup analysis. Of these 549 cases, there were no cervical spine injuries identified by imaging studies. However, this cohort included only 18 patients less than 10 years of age.

A large, prospective, multicenter study evaluated the efficacy of the NEXUS decision instrument for cervical spine imaging in 31,000 trauma victims without neck pain or neurological deficit [30]. A substudy by Vicello et al. [31] focused on 3,065 patients younger than 18 years of age. There were 2,160 patients between 9 and 17, 817 between 2 and 8, and 88 less than 2 years of age. About 20% of the 3,065 cases evaluated were deemed "low risk," based on a lack of pain or midline tenderness, alertness, no neurological deficit, and no "painful distracting injury." In none of these cases was there a cervical spine injury. Thirty patients (0.98%) who did not satisfy low-risk criteria had cervical spine injuries. However, even this large study is not definitive evidence for the safety of clinical cervical spine clearance in children. This study found no cases of SCIWORA, only four injuries in children under 9 years of age, and none in those under 2, making interpretation particularly difficult in the younger child. While the sensitivity of the NEXUS instrument for the identification of cervical spine injury in children was 100%, due to the low incidence of injury in this population, the lower limit of the 95% CI for sensitivity was only 88%. To achieve a CI for a sensitivity of only 0.5%, a study of 80,000 children would be required.

The Canadian C-Spine Rule [32], described in 2001, defined high-risk factors for a cervical spine injury, including mechanism and paresthesia, and low-risk factors such as ambulation since the injury, absence of midline tenderness, and ability to actively rotate 45 degrees laterally that had 100% sensitivity and 42.5% specificity for clinically significant injury. However, this rule was based on a study population composed entirely of adults. Garton et al. [33] retrospectively reviewed the 20-year experience with cervical spine injury in children at a single institution. This study included 190 children with cervical spine injuries, many more than in the study of Vicello. The sensitivity of the NEXUS criteria for injury was 100% in those 8 and older, but 2 of the 33 patients under 8 (6 and 18 months old) were found to have cervical spine injuries despite fulfilling "low-risk" NEXUS criteria.

Pieretti-Vanmarcke et al. [34] assessed 12,537 patients younger than 3 years of age at 22 trauma centers. The incidence of cervical spine injury was 0.66%. They identified four simple clinical predictors of cervical spine injury, giving a weighted score to each: GCS <14 (3 points), $GCS_{EYE} = 1$ (2 points),

MVC (2 points), and age ≥2 years (1 point). This was labeled PEDSPINE, and a score of 0–1 had a negative predictive value of 99.9% for cervical spine injury with a sensitivity of 92.9% and specificity of 69.9%. They identified 8,707 patients who had scores of 0–1 and suggested that cervical spine clearance could be achieved without further imaging based on clinical exam. Five patients were reported as outliers, with scores <2 and with a clinically important cervical spine injury. These patients all presented with physical findings of head and neck injury and underwent CT scanning with timely identification of cervical spine injury.

Based on a comparison of 540 children with cervical spine injuries to a group of controls, the PECARN identified eight factors that were predictive of cervical spine injuries in children. [35] These included "altered mental status, focal neurological findings, neck pain, torticollis, substantial torso injury, conditions prea disposing to a cervical spine injury, diving and high-risk motor vehicle crash." In this population, the presence of one factor predicted cervical spine injury with a sensitivity of 98% and a specificity of 26%.

A Cochrane review [36] applied the NEXUS and Canadian decision rules to patient cohorts from three studies [31, 37, 38] of pediatric cervical spine injury. It concluded that there was insufficient evidence to support the use of the Canadian rule in children. While the NEXUS criteria have been better studied in children, there is still significant variability in the sensitivity (0.57–1.0) and associated low limit of the CI (0.18–0.91) for this tool in the detection of clinically relevant injuries in children.

If a child is unable to be cleared clinically, plain radiographs should still be the initial assessment tool of choice for evaluation of the cervical spine [39]. If there is a high suspicion for a cervical spine injury of a severe mechanism, a CT scan should be used. In most patients, CT should be enough to assist in ruling in or ruling out a cervical spine injury. A study published in 2013 by Gargas et al. reviewed 450 trauma patients who underwent CT imaging of the cervical spine. One hundred and seventy-three of those patients had a normal CT of the cervical spine and underwent a subsequent MRI. Five patients (2.9%) in this subset were found to have an injury that required operative intervention. Based on this, authors felt that high-resolution CT scans with sagittal and coronal reconstructions were nearly comparable to MRI for the detection of unstable cervical spine injuries. If a patient is obtunded, has an abnormal neurologic exam, there is concern for SCIWORA, or if patients require special evaluation of the soft tissue, then an MRI of the cervical spine is warranted and should be completed to help in cervical spine clearance [39].

RECOMMENDATION

A grade B recommendation may be made for clinical clearance of the cervical spine in teens and preteens who are alert and without a painful distracting injury, neurological deficit, or midline cervical tenderness (NEXUS criteria). In children under 8 who fulfill the NEXUS criteria, due to the infrequency of injury, the relative paucity of data, and the variability in patients' ability to focus during a neck examination, more clinical judgment is necessary.

34.5 How Should Blunt Pancreatic Transections Be Managed in Children?

Pancreatic injuries are rare in children, occurring in only 0.3–0.7% of trauma admissions [40–42]; however, they are present in 3–12% of children sustaining blunt abdominal trauma [40, 43]. As with other solid organs, the severity of pancreatic trauma is based on the extent and location of injury [44]. Grade I and II injuries are minor and major contusions, respectively. Distal transections and duct injuries are classified as grade III, proximal transections are grade IV, and massive disruptions of the pancreatic head are grade V. It is generally accepted that most grade I and II injuries are initially best managed nonoperatively [40, 42, 45]. Grade V injuries are often devastating due to duodenal and biliary involvement and frequently necessitate laparotomy.

The diagnosis of pancreatic injuries requires a high index of suspicion in patients sustaining blunt abdominal trauma. Serum amylase and lipase elevations are seen in pancreatic injuries; however, the values do not correlate with the grade of injury, length of stay (LOS), or mortality [41, 46]. The values can be used as a screening tool and confirm pancreatic injury on CT, magnetic resonance cholangiopancreatography (MRCP), and/or endoscopic resonance cholangiopancreatography (ERCP). There is limited value in repeated amylase and lipase levels. For children with pancreatic transections that do not involve the duodenum or bile duct (grades II and III injuries), there are several initial management strategies that have been advocated and used with success, including (1) expectant management, (2) early ERCP and ductal stenting, and (3) distal pancreatectomy [47, 48]. Due to the infrequent occurrence of pancreatic duct transection, there are no Level 1 and limited Level 2 data on which to base management. Determinations of what constitutes best practice for pediatric pancreatic transection must be made from consecutive case series and multi-institutional reviews.

In 1998, the Hospital for Sick Children in Toronto reported the outcome of nonoperative management of 35 children who sustained pancreatic injuries, including 11 cases of transection [43]. Only 5 of these 11 patients with transections developed pseudocysts. No operative intervention was required in any of the patients, although percutaneous drainage was performed in four. The average LOS was 25 days and less for those who did not develop a pseudocyst. A subsequent study from the same institution focused on nine cases managed nonoperatively [49]. Long-term follow-up (47 months) revealed complete healing of the gland in 25% of patients and body/tail atrophy in 75% of patients. None of the patients suffered endocrine or exocrine dysfunction.

Initial experiences with ductal stenting in children were in the form of case reports [47, 50] in which three cases with good outcomes were presented. In the largest series of ductal stenting, 12 children with presumed pancreatic transection underwent ERCP [42]. In 11 cases, a ductal injury was identified and an attempt was made to place a stent. Stents were technically feasible in nine cases. Three of these stents were advanced beyond the site of injury, and six were placed via the pancreatic duct into a pseudocyst. In two cases an endoscopic

cyst-gastrostomy was subsequently performed and in another, percutaneous cyst drainage was required. The remaining stented patients required no further interventions. The average LOS for the children who received stents was 27 days (3–51 days). If the cases in which a percutaneous or cyst-enteric drainage was not required, LOS was 18 days.

Multiple studies support the use of early operative intervention (less than 48–72 hours) for higher-grade pancreatic injuries when operative intervention is chosen [40, 51]. In 1999, the Children's Hospital of Pittsburg documented early operative management of pancreatic injury, usually a distal pancreatectomy, resulted in a median LOS of 11.5 days [52]. LOS was substantially longer after delayed diagnosis or failed nonoperative management.

In 2009, Wood et al. compared nonoperative vs. operative management of pancreatic injuries in children admitted to a single institution [53]. Although median LOS increased with worsening pancreatic injury grade, there was no significant difference in LOS or readmission rates in patients with grade II–IV injuries. Nonoperative management, however, was associated with an increased incidence of pancreatic complications (pancreatic pseudocyst, leak, or fistula). These complications were identified in 73% of patients treated nonoperatively as opposed to 21% of patients treated with pancreatic resection.

Recently, multi-institutional collaborations have led to better evaluation of treatment choice. In 2011, Paul et al. collected data on 131 children with grade II or III injuries from nine different Level I pediatric trauma centers [54]. Nonoperative management was associated with a higher rate of pseudocyst formation and an increased use of total parenteral nutrition (TPN), although LOS was similar. In 2013, Beres et al. reviewed 39 patients with grade III or IV pancreatic injuries from two Level I pediatric trauma centers [55]. Nonoperative management was associated with increased LOS (mean 27.5 vs. 15 days), increased days on TPN (21.8 vs. 7.9), and more complications—most commonly pseudocyst formation.

The largest multi-institutional collaboration to date is on behalf of the Pancreatic Trauma in Children (PATCH) Study Group and included 14 pediatric trauma centers with evaluation of 167 patients with grade II and III blunt pancreatic injuries [56]. Patients treated nonoperatively had a higher rate of pseudocyst formation (18% vs. 0%) and increased requirement for endoscopic or interventional radiologic procedures to manage them. Patients treated with operative resection had shorter times to initial (4.5 vs. 8.9 days) and goal (7.8 vs. 15.1 days) feedings with a corresponding decreased use of parenteral nutrition. Subset analysis was performed in patients with evidence of main pancreatic duct injury (grade III), and the results were even more compelling. For patients with grade III injuries, 44% developed a pseudocyst with an even longer delay of initial (12.7 days) and goal (26.1 days) enteral feedings. These patients also had significantly increased LOS when compared to those undergoing operative resection (17.5 vs. 12.6 days).

Endoscopic pancreatic ductal stenting is well-established for adults with ductal transections [57], but its use is limited in children, likely due to size limitations and lack of technical expertise in children's hospitals. In one of the largest pediatric series, 9 of 12 children who underwent ERCP had successful placement of a transductal stent [58] and in 3 of these, the stent extended beyond the injury into the distal duct. The median hospital stay for drained patients was 28 days but might have been lower had enteral feedings been advanced more aggressively. When endoscopic management in cases of suspected ductal disruption is employed, it should be done soon after the injury. If a ductal disruption is identified, a stent should be placed across the injury, if possible. A series that described endoscopic retrograde pancreatography (ERP) and stent placement, if indicated, in six children [59] found that pancreatectomy or endoscopic cyst-gastrostomy, with associated long LOSs, were avoided only in cases when the ERCP was done within 2 days of injury, and/or a stent traversed the site of ductal disruption. Stents were placed in children as young as 4 years of age, although the youngest patient in which a stent could be placed across the injury was 10.

RECOMMENDATION

Blunt transection of the body of the pancreas in children is best managed with a distal pancreatectomy done within 2–3 days of the injury. If a nonoperative approach is elected initially or indicated due to a delayed presentation, some patients will have a prolonged LOS. Endoscopic ductal stenting is effective but is not readily available in many pediatric trauma centers.

Grade of recommendation: B.

34.6 Damage Control Resuscitation: When Should Blood Be Used in Hypotensive Pediatric Trauma Patients and What Transfusion Ratio to Plasma?

Critically injured pediatric patients with ongoing hemorrhage and hypotension require prompt care and appropriate volume resuscitation in addition to hemorrhage control. These principles are paramount to preventing morbidity and improving survival [60]. Historically it was recommended that hypotensive pediatric trauma patients receive three isotonic saline boluses of 20 mL/kg before considering volume expansion with blood products. Up until 2018, the Advanced Trauma Life Support (ATLS) Manual (9th edition), recommended three weight-based crystalloid boluses (20 mL/kg per bolus) with consideration of blood products only after the second crystalloid bolus in the most severely injured patients [61]. This high-volume crystalloid resuscitation strategy is associated with longer periods of mechanical ventilation, prolonged ICU LOS, hospital LOS, and even mortality [62–64]. Taking cues from adult and military trauma literature, resuscitation recommendations for pediatric patients has changed significantly, with the earlier introduction of blood product resuscitation and more balanced massive transfusion protocols [65–67]. This transition to earlier and more balanced transfusions is known as damage control resuscitation.

A landmark study that began to push early balanced transfusions in civilian adults was the PROMMTT study published in 2013 [65]. This multicenter prospective cohort study analyzed the timing of transfusions and the ratio in which transfusions were administered. The study group looked at patients over 16 years of age who received at least one unit of red blood cells (RBCs) within 6 hours of admission and a smaller cohort that received more than three units of RBCs during their hospitalization. The primary outcome was hospital mortality. Those patients with higher plasma and platelet ratios to RBCs early in their resuscitation had a decreased mortality rate. Patients who had plasma to platelet transfusion ratios lower than 1:2 were three to four times more likely to die than patients with a 1:1 ratio within the first 6 hours of their hospitalization. This trend also held true at 24 hours. This study helped push balanced transfusions in adults and spurred pediatric trauma specialists to investigate the use of early and balanced transfusion in pediatric patients.

A multicenter study done by Polites et al. looked at patients 15 years or younger presenting with a shock index (heart rate/systolic blood pressure) of greater than 0.9 [68]. The goal of the study was to determine when resuscitation efforts should be switched from crystalloid to blood products in pediatric trauma patients with an elevated shock index. Two hundred and eight patients were included in the study, of which 116 (56%) required a fluid bolus and 69 patients require blood transfusions. The likelihood of transfusion increased logarithmically from 11% to 43% for those requiring more than two weight-based crystalloid boluses. This suggests that the inflection point for transitioning from crystalloid to blood product resuscitation in critically ill pediatric trauma patients is after one 20 mg/kg crystalloid bolus. Furthermore, investigators found that those who received three or more crystalloid boluses were 5.8 times more likely to require an extended hospital LOS compared to those who only received one crystalloid bolus. Based on this, authors concluded the crystalloid-sparing resuscitation is beneficial and that blood volume replacement should be considered following the first weight-based crystalloid bolus.

With more interest in early blood product utilization, interest in massive transfusion protocols (MTPs) became popular in the first and second decade of the twenty-first century. Hendrickson et al. was one of the first groups to publish their experience in implementing an MTP at the children's hospital at Emory University [69]. They formed a multidisciplinary MTP committee to create protocols and standard operating procedures for massive transfusion efforts. Their goal was for a 1:1 fresh-frozen plasma (FFP) to RBC ratio, with every other transfusion package also including either weight-adjusted platelets or cryoprecipitate. Critically ill trauma patients were studied before and after establishing their MTP. Prior to the institution of the MTP, the plasma to RBC ratio was 1:3.6, and post implementation it was 1:1.8 ($p = 0.002$). In addition, the median time to FFP administration dropped from 200 minutes to 50 minutes. From an outcomes standpoint they found a significant reduction in the median number of ventilator days (6 days pre-MTP, 2 days post-MTP) and a decrease in the median number of ICU days (9 days pre-MTP, 7 days post-MTP). There was no overall mortality benefit.

This early description and implementation of an MTP at a pediatric trauma center demonstrated feasibility, improvement in FFP:RBC transfusion ratios, improved time to FFP transfusion, and a decrease in ventilator days in patients after implementation of an MTP. Similar findings were reported by Hwu et al., who performed a retrospective study comparing injured children under 18 years of age before and after implementation of an MTP program [70]. They found that post-implementation children received more balanced transfusions in terms of both plasma and platelets to RBCs. While balanced transfusions improved, investigators were not able to demonstrate a benefit to all-cause mortality, as has been seen in larger adult data. A large limitation to these studies was the small numbers of patients who were undergoing massive transfusion.

A study done in 2019 by Cunningham et al. tried to address the problem of low sample sizes by using the Pediatric Trauma Quality Improvement Program dataset to evaluate the efficacy of high-ratio plasma to RBC transfusion protocols [71]. A retrospective review evaluated 465 children aged 18 or less who were massively transfused (>40 mL/kg blood products) within 24 hours of admission. Patients were classified into transfusion ratio categories for both plasma and platelets to RBCs (low <1:2, medium >1:2 to <1:1, and high >1:1). Children in the high-ratio plasma to RBC group had improved survival at 4 and 24 hours, which also held true when extended out to 30-day mortality compared to those who had low-ratio plasma to RBC transfusions ($p = 0.0248$). There was no mortality benefit among groups for platelets to RBCs. Similar findings of improved survival in critically ill pediatric trauma patients receiving balanced plasma to RBCs compared to those receiving 2:1 or ≥3:1 was also demonstrated by the ATOMAC Pediatric Trauma Research Network [72].

In addition to earlier use of blood products and improving transfusion balance, additional strategies that are routinely used in damage control resuscitation in adults are beginning to filter down to pediatric trauma patients as well. Two of these are the use of whole blood and the use of tranexamic acid (TXA) [73]. Initial use of whole blood in pediatric patients was reported by Leeper et al. [74]. Between June 2016 and June 2017, 18 injured children were resuscitated with whole blood without any transfusion reactions, demonstrating preliminary safety. Additional studies will be needed to help establish differences in pediatric patients resuscitated with whole blood compared to components. Another MTP adjunct is the administration of TXA. TXA is a lysine analog that prevents fibrinolysis leading to clot disruption that was popularized in adult trauma resuscitation by the CRASH-2 trial, which showed early administration of TXA in bleeding trauma patients reduced the risk of death [75]. Two studies looking at TXA use in pediatric populations have demonstrated a mortality benefit [76] or a trend toward a mortality benefit [77] without negative effects. A recent laboratory study done in a porcine hemorrhage model also demonstrated that TXA administration is safe via an intraosseous infusion and is as effective as when administered via an intravenous line [78].

RECOMMENDATION

A grade B recommendation can be made for the early use of blood products in a critically ill hypotensive pediatric trauma patient. A grade B recommendation can be made for balanced transfusions during pediatric massive transfusion events. A grade C recommendation is given to the use of whole blood and TXA in damage control resuscitation in children.

TABLE 34.1

Pediatric Trauma – Case Series

Author	References	Year	Level of Evidence	Groups	Design	Median Follow-up	Endpoint
Palchak	[8]	2003	2b	Brain injury on CT scan No brain injury on CT scan	PCS	NR	Prediction of brain injury by CT decision tool
Oman	[10]	2006	2b	Brain injury on CT scan No brain injury on CT scan	PCS	NR	Prediction of brain injury by CT decision tool
Dunning	[12]	2006	2b	Brain injury on CT scan, No brain injury on CT scan	PCS	NR	Prediction of brain injury by CT decision tool
Fisher	[20]	1992	2b	3% saline, normal saline	RCT	2 hours	ICP change
Simma	[21]	1998	2b	Lactated Ringer's, normal saline	RCT	NR	ICP, CPP, hospital and ICU stay, survival
Khanna	[22]	2000	4	3% saline	CS	72 hours	ICP spike frequency, serum sodium, renal failure
Peterson	[23]	2000	4	3% saline	CS	NR	ICP, renal failure
Vicello	[31]	2001	2b	Low risk for cervical spine injury, high risk for injury	PCS	NR	Cervical spine injury
Garton	[33]	2008	2b	Low risk for cervical spine injury, high risk for injury	RCS	NR	Cervical spine injury

(Continued)

TABLE 34.1 (Continued)

Pediatric Trauma – Case Series

Author	References	Year	Level of Evidence	Groups	Design	Median Follow-up	Endpoint
Meier	[40]	2001	4	Distal pancreatectomy, observation	CS	NR	Hospital stay, pseudocyst development
Keller	[42]	1997	4	Early diagnosis and operation, late diagnosis	RCS	12 months to 12 years	Hospital stay, pseudocyst development
Shilyansky	[43]	1998	4	Nonoperative management	CS	10 months	Time to enteral feeding, hospital stay, pseudocyst development
Wales	[49]	2001	4	Nonoperative management	CS	47 months	Time to enteral feeding, hospital stay, pseudocyst development, endocrine/exocrine dysfunction
Nadler	[52]	1999	4	Early diagnosis and operation, late diagnosis	RCS	NR	Hospital stay, morbidity
Houben	[49]	2007	4	Pancreatic ductal stenting	CS	2 years	Time to enteral feeding, hospital stay, requirement for cyst-enterostomy
Holcomb	[63]	2013	2	Transfusion ratios: Low <1:2, moderate ≥1:2 to <1:1, high ≥ 1:1	PCS	30 days	In-hospital mortality
Polites	[66]	2018	4	<1 fluid bolus, 1 fluid bolus, 2 fluid boluses, ≥3 fluid boluses	CS	NR	Requirement of transfusion, length of stay, ICU days, in-hospital death, discharge disposition
Cunningham	[69]	2019	4	*Plasma*: RBC cohorts (low, medium, high) *Platelet*: RBC cohorts (low, medium, high)	CS	NR	Mortality, ventilator days, ICU/hospital length of stay, complications
Noland	[70]	2018	4	Transfusion ratio groups (1:1, 2:1, 3:1 and greater)	CS	NR	In-hospital mortality, ICU/ hospital length of stay

Abbreviations: CPP: Cerebral perfusion pressure, CS: Case series, ICP: Intracranial pressure, ICU: Intensive care unit, NR: Not reported, PCS: Prospective cohort study, RBC: Red blood cell, RCS: Retrospective cohort study, RCT: Randomized controlled trial.

TABLE 34.2

Pediatric Trauma – Question Summary

	Question	Answer	Grade	References
1	When is a CT scan of the head indicated in pediatric head trauma?	If one of the referenced decision tools are utilized. In general, if one of the following are present: GCS <15, evidence of skull fracture, headache, vomiting, coagulopathy, or seizure.	B	[6, 8, 10]
2	Is there a role for hypertonic saline in pediatric head injury?	There is no evidence to support a reduction in mortality or even severe morbidity with hypertonic saline. There is limited evidence for its role in lowering refractory intracranial hypertension with limited side effects.	C	[17–20]
3	When is clinical clearance of the cervical spine appropriate in children?	If there is no neck pain, midline tenderness, neurological deficit, or painful distracting injury in a child older than 7. Not enough evidence in younger patients to support application of clinical clearance except in unusually mature children.	B	[25, 26]
4	How should femur fractures be managed in children?	Excluding patients under 5 and those with very proximal or distal fractures, significant contamination, or gross comminution, intramedullary rod placement results in shorter recovery time at a cost comparable to other methods.	B	[29, 32, 34]
5	How should blunt pancreatic transection be managed in children?	There is insufficient evidence to support the superiority of early pancreatectomy or nonoperative management of pancreatic transection. The incidence of this injury is likely too low to permit a large, randomized controlled trial.	C	[35, 41, 43–46, 49]

Editor's Note

The authors of this chapter have elegantly discussed major areas of controversy in the pediatric trauma population. Pediatric surgeons led the charge back in the 1980s for the use of nonoperative management of abdominal injuries. They continue to generate high-quality investigations to improve our understanding of which children are likely to have traumatic brain injuries and who can avoid the radiation risk of head CT scanning. Unfortunately, like the adult population with TBI, hyperosmolar therapy continues to have a major role despite numerous major studies revealing zero benefit. One of the major areas of style differences between pediatric and adult trauma surgeons is generated by opposing philosophies behind management of the fortunately rare complex pancreatic injury. While pediatric surgeons often judge success in these patients if operation can be avoided, despite an often long hospitalization, adult surgeons typically are more aggressive in their management style, preferring to intervene in an effort to eradicate the injury and expedite discharge. This is an area where the pediatric surgeon may well turn out to be forward-looking and, similar to their previous novel care of spleen and liver injuries, may turn out in the future to be proven correct in their conservative management scheme.

REFERENCES

CT Scan for Head Trauma

1. Langlois JA, Rutland-Brown W, Wald MM. The epidemiology and impact of traumatic brain injury: A brief overview. Journal of Head Trauma Rehabilitation 2006;21:375–8. https://doi.org/10.1097/00001199-200609000-00001.
2. Kuppermann N, Holmes JF, Dayan PS, Hoyle JD, Atabaki SM, Holubkov R, et al. Identification of children at very low risk of clinically-important brain injuries after head trauma: A prospective cohort study. The Lancet 2009;374:1160–70. https://doi.org/10.1016/S0140-6736(09)61558-0.
3. Surveillance report of traumatic brain injury-related emergency department visits, hospitalizations and deaths – United States, 2014. Centers for Disease Control and Prevention, US Department of Health and Human Services.
4. Rates of TBI-Related Emergency Department Visits by Age Group—United States, 2001–2010. CDC website 2018. https://www.cdc.gov/traumaticbraininjury/data/rates_ed_byage.html.
5. Davis RL, Hughes M, Gubler KD, Waller PL, Rivara FP. The use of cranial CT scans in the triage of pediatric patients with mild head injury. Pediatrics 1995;95:345–9. https://doi.org/10.1542/peds.95.3.345.
6. Sheppard JP, Nguyen T, Alkhalid Y, Beckett JS, Salamon N, Yang I. Risk of brain tumor induction from pediatric head CT procedures: A systematic literature review. Brain Tumor Research and Treatment 2018;6:1. https://doi.org/10.14791/btrt.2018.6.e4.
7. Haydel MJ, Shembekar AD. Prediction of intracranial injury in children aged five years and older with loss of consciousness after minor head injury due to nontrivial mechanisms. Annals of Emergency Medicine 2003;42:507–14. https://doi.org/10.1067/S0196-0644(03)00512-2.
8. Palchak MJ, Holmes JF, Vance CW, Gelber RE, Schauer BA, Harrison MJ, et al. A decision rule for identifying children at low risk for brain injuries after blunt head trauma. Annals of Emergency Medicine 2003;42:492–506. https://doi.org/10.1067/S0196-0644(03)00425-6.
9. Mower WR, Hoffman JR, Herbert M, Wolfson AB, Pollack CV, Zucker MI. Developing a clinical decision instrument to rule out intracranial injuries in patients with minor head trauma: Methodology of the NEXUS II investigation. Annals of Emergency Medicine 2002;40:505–15. https://doi.org/10.1067/mem.2002.129245.
10. Oman JA, Cooper RJ, Holmes JF, Viccellio P, Nyce A, Ross SE, et al. Performance of a decision rule to predict need for computed tomography among children with blunt head trauma. Pediatrics 2006;117:e238–e46. https://doi.org/10.1542/peds.2005-1063.
11. Sun BC, Hoffman JR, Mower WR. Evaluation of a modified prediction instrument to identify significant pediatric intracranial injury after blunt head trauma. Annals of Emergency Medicine 2007;49:325–32. https://doi.org/10.1016/j.annemergmed.2006.08.032.
12. Dunning J, Daly JP, Lomas J-P, Lecky F, Batchelor J, Mackway-Jones K, et al. Derivation of the children's head injury algorithm for the prediction of important clinical events decision rule for head injury in children. Archives of Disease in Childhood 2006;91:885–91. https://doi.org/10.1136/adc.2005.083980.
13. Osmond MH, Klassen TP, Wells GA, Correll R, Jarvis A, Joubert G, et al. CATCH: A clinical decision rule for the use of computed tomography in children with minor head injury. Canadian Medical Association Journal 2010;182:341–8. https://doi.org/10.1503/cmaj.091421.
14. Osmond MH, Klassen TP, Wells GA, Davidson J, Correll R, Boutis K, et al. Validation and refinement of a clinical decision rule for the use of computed tomography in children with minor head injury in the emergency department. CMAJ 2018;190:E816–E22. https://doi.org/10.1503/cmaj.170406.
15. Babl FE, Borland ML, Phillips N, Kochar A, Dalton S, McCaskill M, et al. Accuracy of PECARN, CATCH, and CHALICE head injury decision rules in children: A prospective cohort study. The Lancet 2017;389:2393–402. https://doi.org/10.1016/S0140-6736(17)30555-X.

Hypertonic Saline for Pediatric Head Injury

16. Thurman D. The epidemiology and economics of head trauma. In: Miller L, Hayes R, editors. Head Trauma Basic, Preclinical and Clinical Directions, New York: 2001.
17. Weed L, McKibben P. Pressure changes in the cerebrospinal fluid following intravenous injection of solutions of various concentrations. American Journal of Physiology 1919;48:512–30.
18. Wise B, Chater N. Pressure changes in the cerebrospinal fluid following intravenous injection of solutions of various concentrations. Surgical Forum 1961;12:398–9.
19. Kochanek PM, Adelson PD, Rosario BL, Hutchison J, Miller Ferguson N, Ferrazzano P, et al. Comparison of intracranial pressure measurements before and after hypertonic saline or mannitol treatment in children with severe traumatic brain injury. JAMA Network Open 2022;5:e220891. https://doi.org/10.1001/jamanetworkopen.2022.0891.

20. Fisher B, Thomas D, Peterson B. Hypertonic saline lowers raised intracranial pressure in children after head trauma. Journal of Neurosurgical Anesthesia 1992;4:4–10. https://doi.org/10.1097/00008506-199201000-00002.

21. Simma B, Burger R, Falk M, Sacher P, Fanconi S. A prospective, randomized, and controlled study of fluid management in children with severe head injury: Lactated Ringer's solution versus hypertonic saline. Critical Care Medicine 1998;26:1265–70. https://doi.org/10.1097/00003246-199807000-00032.

22. Khanna S, Davis D, Peterson B, Fisher B, Tung H, O'Quigley J, et al. Use of hypertonic saline in the treatment of severe refractory posttraumatic intracranial hypertension in pediatric traumatic brain injury. Critical Care Medicine 2000;28:1144–51. https://doi.org/10.1097/00003246-200004000-00038.

23. Peterson B, Khanna S, Fisher B, Marshall L. Prolonged hypernatremia controls elevated intracranial pressure in head-injured pediatric patients. Critical Care Medicine. 2000; 28:1136–43. https://doi.org/10.1097/00003246-200004000-00037.

24. Shein SL, Ferguson NM, Kochanek PM, Bayir H, Clark RSB, Fink EL, et al. Effectiveness of pharmacological therapies for intracranial hypertension in children with severe traumatic brain injury—Results from an automated data collection system time-synched to drug administration. Pediatric Critical Care Medicine 2016;17:236–45. https://doi.org/10.1097/PCC.0000000000000610.

25. Lumba-Brown A, Harley J, Lucio S, Vaida F, Hilfiker M. Hypertonic saline as a therapy for pediatric concussive pain: A randomized controlled trial of symptom treatment in the emergency department. Pediatric Emergency Care 2014;30:139–45. https://doi.org/10.1097/PEC.0000000000000084.

Clinical Clearance of the Cervical Spine

26. Brown RL, Brunn MA, Garcia VF. Cervical spine injuries in children: A review of 103 patients treated consecutively at a level 1 pediatric trauma center. Journal of Pediatric Surgery 2001;36:1107–14. https://doi.org/10.1053/jpsu.2001.25665.

27. Leonard JR, Jaffe DM, Kuppermann N, Olsen CS, Leonard JC. Cervical spine injury patterns in children. Pediatrics 2014;133:e1179–e88. https://doi.org/10.1542/peds.2013-3505.

28. Jacobs LM, Schwartz R. Prospective analysis of acute cervical spine injury: A methodology to predict injury. Annals of Emergency Medicine 1986;15:44–9. https://doi.org/10.1016/S0196-0644(86)80485-1.

29. Velmahos GC, Theodorou D, Tatevossian R, Belzberg H, Cornwell EE, Berne TV, et al. Radiographic cervical spine evaluation in the alert asymptomatic blunt trauma victim: Much ado about nothing? The Journal of Trauma: Injury, Infection, and Critical Care 1996;40:768–74. https://doi.org/10.1097/00005373-199605000-00015.

30. Hoffman JR, Zucker MI. Validity of a set of clinical criteria to rule out injury to the cervical spine in patients with blunt trauma. The New England Journal of Medicine 2000; 343:94–9. https://doi.org/10.1056/NEJM200007133430203.

31. Viccellio P, Simon H, Pressman BD, Shah MN, Mower WR, Hoffman JR, et al. A prospective multicenter study of cervical spine injury in children. Pediatrics 2001;108: e20–e20. https://doi.org/10.1542/peds.108.2.e20.

32. Stiell IG, Wells GA, Vandemheen KL, Clement CM, Lesiuk H, Maio VJD, et al. The Canadian C-spine rule for radiography in alert and stable trauma patients. JAMA 2001;286:1841–8. https://doi.org/10.1001/jama.286.15.1841.

33. Garton HJL, Hammer MR. Detection of pediatric cervical spine injury. Neurosurgery 2008;62:700–8. https://doi.org/10.1227/01.NEU.0000311348.43207.B7.

34. Pieretti-Vanmarcke R, Velmahos GC, Nance ML, Islam S, Falcone RA, Wales PW, et al. Clinical clearance of the cervical spine in blunt trauma patients younger than 3 years: A multi-center study of the American Association for the Surgery of Trauma. Journal of Trauma: Injury, Infection & Critical Care 2009;67:543–50. https://doi.org/10.1097/TA.0b013e3181b57aa1.

35. Leonard JC, Kuppermann N, Olsen C, Babcock-Cimpello L, Brown K, Mahajan P, et al. Factors associated with cervical spine injury in children after blunt trauma. Annals of Emergency Medicine 2011;58:145–55. https://doi.org/10.1016/j.annemergmed.2010.08.038.

36. Slaar A, Fockens MM, Wang J, Maas M, Wilson DJ, Goslings JC, et al. Triage tools for detecting cervical spine injury in pediatric trauma patients. Cochrane Database of Systematic Reviews 2017;12:CD011686 https://doi.org/10.1002/14651858.CD011686.pub2.

37. Ehrlich PF, Wee C, Drongowski R, Rana AR. Canadian C-spine rule and the national emergency X-radiography utilization low-risk criteria for C-spine radiography in young trauma patients. Journal of Pediatric Surgery 2009;44:987–91. https://doi.org/10.1016/j.jpedsurg.2009.01.044.

38. Jaffe DM, Binns H, Radkowski MA, Barthel MJ, Engelhard HH. Developing a clinical algorithm for the early management of cervical spine injury in child trauma victims. Annals of Emergency Medicine 1987;16:270–6. https://doi.org/10.1016/s0196-0644(87)80171-3.

39. Chung S, Mikrogianakis A, Wales PW, Dirks P, Shroff M, Singhal A, et al. Trauma association of Canada pediatric subcommittee national pediatric cervical spine evaluation pathway: Consensus guidelines. The Journal of Trauma 2011; 70:873–84. https://doi.org/10.1097/TA.0b013e3182108823.

Management of Pancreatic Transections

40. Meier DE, Coln CD, Hicks BA, Guzzetta PC. Early operation in children with pancreas transection. Journal of Pediatric Surgery 2001;36:341–4. https://doi.org/10.1053/jpsu.2001.20711.

41. Jobst MA, Canty TG, Lynch FP. Management of pancreatic injury in pediatric blunt abdominal trauma. Journal of Pediatric Surgery 1999;34:818–24. https://doi.org/10.1016/S0022-3468(99)90379-2.

42. Keller MS, Stafford PW, Vane DW. Conservative management of pancreatic trauma in children: The Journal of Trauma: Injury, Infection, and Critical Care 1997;42:1097–100. https://doi.org/10.1097/00005373-199706000-00019.

43. Shilyansky J, Sena LM, Kreller M, Chait P, Babyn PS, Filler RM, et al. Nonoperative management of pancreatic injuries in children. Journal of Pediatric Surgery 1998;33:343–9. https://doi.org/10.1016/S0022-3468(98)90459-6.

44. Moore EE, Cogbill TH, Malangoni MA, Jurkovich GJ, Shackford SR, Champion HR, et al. Organ injury scaling. Surgical Clinics of North America 1995;75:293–303. https://doi.org/10.1016/S0039-6109(16)46589-8.

45. Graham CA, O'Toole SJ, Watson AJ, Munro FD, Haddock G. Pancreatic trauma in Scottish children. Journal of the Royal College of Surgeons of Edinburgh 2000;45:223–6.

46. Herman R, Guire KE, Burd RS, Mooney DP, Ehlrich PF. Utility of amylase and lipase as predictors of grade of injury or outcomes in pediatric patients with pancreatic trauma. Journal of Pediatric Surgery 2011;46:923–6. https://doi.org/10.1016/j.jpedsurg.2011.02.033.

47. Canty TG, Weinman D. Management of major pancreatic duct injuries in children. The Journal of Trauma: Injury, Infection, and Critical Care 2001;50:1001–7. https://doi.org/10.1097/00005373-200106000-00005.

48. Rescorla FJ, Plumley DA, Sherman S, Scherer LR, West KW, Grosfeld JL. The efficacy of early ERCP in pediatric pancreatic trauma. Journal of Pediatric Surgery 1995;30:336–40. https://doi.org/10.1016/0022-3468(95)90585-5.

49. Wales PW, Shuckett B, Kim PCW. Long-term outcome after nonoperative management of complete traumatic pancreatic transection in children. Journal of Pediatric Surgery 2001;36:823–7. https://doi.org/10.1053/jpsu.2001.22970.

50. Çay A, İmamoglu M, Bektas Ö, Özdemir O, Arslan M, Sarihan H. Nonoperative treatment of traumatic pancreatic duct disruption in children with an endoscopically placed stent. Journal of Pediatric Surgery 2005;40:e9–e12. https://doi.org/10.1016/j.jpedsurg.2005.08.033.

51. Šnajdauf J, Rygl M, Kalousová J, Kučera A, Petrů O, Pýcha K, et al. Surgical management of major pancreatic injury in children. European Journal of Pediatric Surgery 2007;17:317–21. https://doi.org/10.1055/s-2007-965463.

52. Nadler EP, Gardner M, Schall LC, Lynch JM, Ford HR. Management of blunt pancreatic injury in children. The Journal of Trauma: Injury, Infection, and Critical Care 1999; 47:1098. https://doi.org/10.1097/00005373-199912000-00020.

53. Wood JH, Partrick DA, Bruny JL, Sauaia A, Moulton SL. Operative vs nonoperative management of blunt pancreatic trauma in children. Journal of Pediatric Surgery 2010;45:401–6. https://doi.org/10.1016/j.jpedsurg.2009.10.095.

54. Paul MD, Mooney DP. The management of pancreatic injuries in children: Operate or observe. Journal of Pediatric Surgery 2011;46:1140–3. https://doi.org/10.1016/j.jpedsurg.2011.03.041.

55. Beres AL, Wales PW, Christison-Lagay ER, McClure ME, Fallat ME, Brindle ME. Non-operative management of high-grade pancreatic trauma: Is it worth the wait? Journal of Pediatric Surgery 2013;48:1060–4. https://doi.org/10.1016/j.jpedsurg.2013.02.027.

56. Iqbal CW, St Peter SD, Tsao K, Cullinane DC, Gourlay DM, Ponsky TA, et al. Operative vs nonoperative management for blunt pancreatic transection in children: Multi-institutional outcomes. Journal of the American College of Surgeons 2014;218:157–62. https://doi.org/10.1016/j.jamcollsurg.2013.10.012.

57. Thomson DA, Krige JEJ, Thomson SR, Bornman PC. The role of endoscopic retrograde pancreatography in pancreatic trauma: A critical appraisal of 48 patients treated at a tertiary institution. Journal of Trauma and Acute Care Surgery 2014;76:1362–6. https://doi.org/10.1097/TA.0000000000000227.

58. Houben CH, Ade-Ajayi N, Patel S, Kane P, Karani J, Devlin J, et al. Traumatic pancreatic duct injury in children:

Minimally invasive approach to management. Journal of Pediatric Surgery 2007;42:629–35. https://doi.org/10.1016/j.jpedsurg.2006.12.025.

59. Ishikawa M, Shimojima N, Koyama T, Miyaguni K, Tsukizaki A, Mizuno Y, et al. Efficacy of early endoscopic intervention in pediatric pancreatic duct injury management. Pediatric Surgery International 2021;37:1711–8. https://doi.org/10.1007/s00383-021-05003-z.

Damage Control Resuscitation

60. Leeper CM, McKenna C, Gaines BA. Too little too late: Hypotension and blood transfusion in the trauma bay are independent predictors of death in injured children. Journal of Trauma and Acute Care Surgery 2018;85:674–8. https://doi.org/10.1097/TA.0000000000001823.

61. ATLS Subcommittee, American College of Surgeons Committee on Trauma, International ATLS working group. Advanced trauma life support (ATLS®): The ninth edition. The Journal of Trauma and Acute Care Surgery 2013;74:1363–6. https://doi.org/10.1097/TA.0b013e31828b82f5.

62. Acker SN, Ross JT, Partrick DA, DeWitt P, Bensard DD. Injured children are resistant to the adverse effects of early high volume crystalloid resuscitation. Journal of Pediatric Surgery 2014;49:1852–5. https://doi.org/10.1016/j.jpedsurg.2014.09.034.

63. Edwards MJ, Lustik MB, Clark ME, Creamer KM, Tuggle D. The effects of balanced blood component resuscitation and crystalloid administration in pediatric trauma patients requiring transfusion in Afghanistan and Iraq 2002 to 2012. Journal of Trauma and Acute Care Surgery 2015;78:330–5. https://doi.org/10.1097/TA.0000000000000469.

64. Mbadiwe N, Georgette N, Slidell MB, McQueen A. Higher crystalloid volume during initial pediatric trauma resuscitation is associated with mortality. Journal of Surgical Research 2021;262:93–100. https://doi.org/10.1016/j.jss.2020.12.063.

65. Holcomb JB, del Junco DJ, Fox EE, Wade CE, Cohen MJ, Schreiber MA, et al. The Prospective, Observational, Multicenter, Major Trauma Transfusion (PROMMTT) Study: Comparative effectiveness of a time-varying treatment with competing risks. JAMA Surgery 2013;148:127–36. https://doi.org/10.1001/2013.jamasurg.387.

66. Butler FK, Holcomb JB, Schreiber MA, Kotwal RS, Jenkins DA, Champion HR, et al. Fluid resuscitation for hemorrhagic shock in tactical combat casualty care: TCCC guidelines change 14-01-2 June 2014. Journal of Special Operations Medicine 2014;14:13–38. https://doi.org/10.55460/DPOC-JWIY.

67. Borgman MA, Spinella PC, Perkins JG, Grathwohl KW, Repine T, Beekley AC, et al. The ratio of blood products transfused affects mortality in patients receiving massive transfusions at a combat support hospital. Journal of Trauma 2007;63:805–13. https://doi.org/10.1097/TA.0b013e3181271ba3.

68. Polites SF, Nygaard RM, Reddy PN, Zielinski MD, Richardson CJ, Elsbernd TA, et al. Multicenter study of crystalloid boluses and transfusion in pediatric trauma— When to go to blood? Journal of Trauma and Acute Care Surgery 2018;85:108–12. https://doi.org/10.1097/TA.0000000000001897.

69. Hendrickson JE, Shaz BH, Pereira G, Parker PM, Jessup P, Atwell F, et al. Implementation of a pediatric trauma massive transfusion protocol: One institution's experience. Transfusion 2012;52:1228–36. https://doi.org/10.1111/j.1537-2995.2011.03458.x.

70. Hwu RS, Spinella PC, Keller MS, Baker D, Wallendorf M, Leonard JC. The effect of massive transfusion protocol implementation on pediatric trauma care. Transfusion 2016;56:2712–9. https://doi.org/10.1111/trf.13781.

71. Cunningham ME, Rosenfeld EH, Zhu H, Naik-Mathuria BJ, Russell RT, Vogel AM. A high ratio of plasma: RBC improves survival in massively transfused injured children. Journal of Surgical Research 2019;233:213–20. https://doi.org/10.1016/j.jss.2018.08.007.

72. Noland DK, Apelt N, Greenwell C, Tweed J, Notrica DM, Garcia NM, et al. Massive transfusion in pediatric trauma: An ATOMAC perspective. Journal of Pediatric Surgery 2019;54:345–9. https://doi.org/10.1016/j.jpedsurg.2018.10.040.

73. Evangelista ME, Gaffley M, Neff LP. Massive transfusion protocols for pediatric patients: Current perspectives. Journal of Blood Medicine 2020;11:163–72. https://doi.org/10.2147/JBM.S205132.

74. Leeper CM, Yazer MH, Cladis FP, Saladino R, Triulzi DJ, Gaines BA. Use of uncross matched cold-stored whole blood in injured children with hemorrhagic shock. JAMA Pediatrics 2018;172:491–2. https://doi.org/10.1001/jamapediatrics.2017.5238.

75. Roberts I, Shakur H, Coats T, Hunt B, Balogun E, Barnetson L, et al. The CRASH-2 trial: A randomised controlled trial and economic evaluation of the effects of tranexamic acid on death, vascular occlusive events and transfusion requirement in bleeding trauma patients. Health Technol Assess 2013;17:1–79. https://doi.org/10.3310/hta17100.

76. Eckert MJ, Wertin TM, Tyner SD, Nelson DW, Izenberg S, Martin MJ. Tranexamic acid administration to pediatric trauma patients in a combat setting: The pediatric trauma and tranexamic acid study (PED-TRAX). The Journal of Trauma and Acute Care Surgery 2014;77:852–8; discussion 858. https://doi.org/10.1097/TA.0000000000000443.

77. Hamele M, Aden JK, Borgman MA. Tranexamic acid in pediatric combat trauma requires massive transfusions and mortality. The Journal of Trauma and Acute Care Surgery 2020;89:S242–S5. https://doi.org/10.1097/TA.0000000000002701.

78. Lallemand MS, Moe DM, McClellan JM, Loughren M, Marko S, Eckert MJ, et al. No intravenous access, no problem: Intraosseous administration of tranexamic acid is as effective as intravenous in a porcine hemorrhage model. The Journal of Trauma and Acute Care Surgery 2018;84:379–85. https://doi.org/10.1097/TA.0000000000001741.

35

The Advanced-Age Trauma Patient

Juliet J. Ray, Carl I. Schulman, and Samuel Hawkins

35.1 Introduction

The projected U.S. population in 2050 of those aged 65 years and over is 83.7 million, which will be double that of 2012 [1]. As of 2010, trauma is the fifth leading cause of death in all age groups and the ninth leading cause for those 65 years and older (2.3% of deaths in this cohort) [2]. As the population ages, older patients make up an increasing portion of hospital trauma activations. One New York hospital group saw the portion of trauma activations for those 65 and older nearly double over 10 years, from 18% in 2005 to 31% in 2016 [3].

The advanced-age trauma patient can pose particular clinical challenges that, while not unique to older age groups, tend to concentrate on older patients and negatively impact their posttrauma outcomes (see Table 35.1). People of advanced age are more likely to have comorbid diseases, such as heart disease, hypertension, stroke, cancer, and diabetes. The increasingly recognized age-associated syndrome of frailty is far more prevalent in the advanced-age patient population (ranging from 15% to 80% based on study and assessment tools [4]). Older patients are more likely to be taking a beta-blocker or oral anticoagulation or antiplatelet agent. These vulnerabilities, combined with greater diversity in the patient's or family's goals of care in the setting of acute illness, make the study of the advanced-age trauma patient worthwhile for the traumatologist.

It should be acknowledged that the definition of "advanced age" and the synonym "geriatric" is not based on clear, evidence-based physiologic thresholds. The absolute age of a patient by itself is rarely meaningful in decisions regarding triage, evaluation, resuscitation, monitoring, and other aspects of management. Rather, care of the advanced-age patient involves familiarity with a combination of clinically important factors that are not unique to, but rather concentrated in patient groups of advancing age. By convention, the age threshold of 65 is used to designate advanced age. There are, however, data to suggest that those even as young as 45 years old may have poorer outcomes than their younger counterparts and that those greater than 75 years old may be at especially high risk [5, 6]. One should therefore consider the skill sets utilized in the care of advanced-age patients to be potentially applicable to any adult patient presenting to their trauma bay.

35.2 Are Advanced-Age Patients at Higher Risk for Poor Outcomes in Trauma?

There is a preponderance of evidence to suggest that elderly trauma patients have a higher level of injury-related mortality than their younger counterparts. A review of a state trauma database with over 30,000 records over 13 years showed overall mortality of 7.6% with an increase of 6.8% for each year over age 65 [7]. Age alone, however, is a poor independent risk factor for long-term trauma outcomes [6, 8, 9]. Rather, advancing age tracks with multiple other factors that increase risk, and models of risk in advanced age are attempts to account for these factors; to identify a patient's "physiologic age." A classic surrogate for the risk associated with advanced age is the presence of comorbidities, or "preexisting conditions," which are associated with an increased risk of death [6, 9, 10]. This increased risk of death varies according to the type and number of preexisting conditions and is independent of age [5, 8].

A more recent risk model applied to advanced age is that of frailty, a condition that seeks to incorporate multiple physical and physiologic vulnerabilities associated with advancing age, including functional status, mental health, and comorbid disease. A systematic review of 13 retrospective and prospective cohort studies found frail patients to have a fourfold increase in hospital and 30-day mortality, and double the rates of perioperative complications, adverse discharge, and readmission [4]. A trauma-specific frailty index has been devised and validated [11]. However, multiple frailty scoring systems are in use in trauma research and clinical practice, and multiple theories of frailty underlie those scoring systems [12, 13]. No standard currently exists for a frailty assessment that is optimal for use with trauma patients, and there is no evidence-based standard for how frailty assessments should be incorporated into the trauma care workflow. Certainly, both preexisting conditions and frailty concentrate in advanced-age patient groups and are associated with worse trauma outcomes. Unfortunately, there is no standard for how to incorporate frailty into the trauma care workflow.

RECOMMENDATIONS

Preexisting conditions and frailty affect outcomes in advanced-age trauma patients.

Level of evidence: 3. Grade of recommendation: C.

DOI: 10.1201/9781003316800-35

35.3 How Should the Decision Be Made to Continue or Remove Life-Sustaining Supportive Care after Trauma? What Clinical Factors Inform the Likelihood of Survival and Recovery after Trauma?

The combination of age, injury severity, and underlying disease makes even the most advanced modern medical care futile for certain patients. Short of diagnosing cardiac or brain death, however, there is no standard clinical threshold that permits a care team to establish futility in any specific case. Decisions to continue with or remove life-sustaining supportive care thus remain collaborative between the care team and the patient or family and require individualized consideration of a patient's values and subjective experience. For this reason, the American College of Surgeons (ACS) Committee on Trauma recommends that care teams assist patients in the early establishment of advance directives that can guide goals of care regarding the institution or continuation of lifesaving measures [14]. The number of advanced-age patients who possess an advance directive pretrauma is less than 20% in most studies [15, 16]. The process of establishing an advance directive and making these crucial decisions in the setting of acute illness is challenging, which has been one impetus for integrating palliative care processes into routine intensive care unit (ICU) care. Palliative care programs in the surgical and trauma ICU may improve rates of the adoption of advance directives and patient satisfaction, but no standard exists for the adoption of these programs [17]. Even when an advance directive is established early, the hospital course may not be significantly altered [16].

Regardless of whether absolute thresholds for futility exist, their clinical measures indicate a very high risk of death in the acute trauma setting, and that can inform goals-of-care discussions with patients and families. In one study of trauma patients over 55 years of age, those with a base deficit of 10 or worse had an 80% mortality, compared to those with mild (3–5) to moderate (6–9) base deficits, which had mortalities of 23% and 60%, respectively [18]. A review of the National Trauma Data Bank attempted to identify predictors of a 95% probability of death in advanced-age trauma patients. In the 65- to 74-year-old age group, hypotensive patients admitted with a severe thoracic and/or abdominal injury who also had severe injuries to the brain (Abbreviated Injury Scale [AIS] ≥4) or profound shock (base deficit, BD ≤–12) had a less than 5% chance of survival. For those aged 75–84, even moderate injury to the brain (AIS ≤3) and moderate shock (BD ≤–6) were associated with a less than 5% chance of survival. Finally, for those aged 85 or older, profound shock or the combination of moderate shock and moderate injury to the head was associated with a less than 5% chance of survival [19]. The Trauma Score (TS) is a composite score that incorporates blood pressure, respiratory rate, respiratory effort, Glasgow Coma Scale (GCS), and capillary refill and varies from 0 to 16. A case-matched review of 100 elderly patients showed that no patient hospitalized with severe injuries survived with a TS <9 and no advanced-age patient with a TS <7 survived to reach the hospital [20].

> **RECOMMENDATION**
>
> There is no accepted threshold for futility. Integrating palliative care processes into ICU care may increase the rate of establishment of advance directives. Clinical measures such as the elevated base deficit, elevated TS, and extensive polytrauma in advanced-age patients predict very high mortality and can be used to aid in goals-of-care discussions.
>
> Level of evidence: 3. Grade of recommendation: C.

35.4 What Is the Optimal Triage Strategy for the Advanced-Age Trauma Patient?

The ACS Committee on Trauma recommends patients older than 55 years be considered for transport to a trauma center based on the desire to maximize patient benefit based on available resources [14]. The use of "geriatric-specific" trauma criteria that included "consideration of systolic blood pressure less than 100 mmHg, any abnormality in GCS, fracture of any long bone in a motor vehicle crash, injury to two or more body regions, pedestrian struck by motor vehicle, and any fall with evidence of traumatic brain injury" significantly improved sensitivity in identifying Injury Severity Score (ISS) and other surrogate markers of the need for trauma center care [21]. It has traditionally been the finding that undertriage is common in patients over the age of 55 and even worse for those over 65 [22]. Notably, a recent statewide study of advanced-age trauma in PA found no difference in trauma outcomes based on the trauma center level [23], suggesting that even with undertriage, the triage pattern for advanced-age patients may not have a significant impact.

> **RECOMMENDATION**
>
> There is insufficient evidence to make any conclusions on the optimal triage strategy for the advanced-age trauma patient.
>
> Level of evidence: 3. Grade of recommendation: C.

35.5 What Is the Impact on Treatment and Outcome for Patients with Medication-Induced Coagulopathy?

The use of anticoagulation in the elderly is increasing and is an important consideration in the trauma population, especially in the setting of traumatic brain injury. It is generally accepted that preinjury use of anticoagulation and antiplatelet agents is associated with worse trauma outcomes [24, 25]; however, the historical data are mixed [26], and the extent to which this is true for extracranial bleeding remains controversial. A prospective study of 159 patients with a mean age of 75 ± 13 years compared to age-matched historical controls demonstrated no increased risk of fatal hemorrhagic complications in the absence of head trauma. When the intracranial injury was present, those taking warfarin had a statistically higher mortality rate [27]. No controlled studies of warfarin reversal vs. no reversal exist, and reversal strategies are based on expert consensus. An international normalized ratio (INR) threshold of >2 is associated with worse outcomes [28] and is often used as a threshold for treatment. The introduction of reversal agents such as prothrombin complex concentrate (PCC) has not been shown to change mortality [29], though PCC does cause a more rapid decrease in INR compared to fresh-frozen plasma (FFP).

Most studies show worse trauma outcomes when patients are taking antiplatelet agents. A review of 350 patients on anticoagulants and prescription antiplatelets (ACAPs) showed that anticoagulant users were more likely to have progression of intracranial hemorrhage (risk ratio [RR] = 3.23; 95% confidence interval [CI], 1.21–8.62; $p = 0.02$) and that antiplatelet users were more likely to die in the hospital (hazard ratio [HR] = 3.09; 95% CI, 1.03–9.23; $p = 0.04$) compared with non-ACAP patients [30]. In contrast, a more recent single-institution study shows no impact of antiplatelet use on mortality or length of stay [24]. More controversial than the impact of antiplatelet use on trauma outcomes is whether platelet transfusion is beneficial in these patients, especially those with intracranial bleeding. The best data on platelet transfusion and intracranial bleeding come from a randomized trial of platelet transfusion in nontrauma spontaneous intracranial hemorrhage and shows a survival detriment in the transfusion group (odds ratio [OR] 0.62 favoring no transfusion) [31]. A systematic review of the trauma literature—mostly retrospective and some prospective studies, all observational—found that the impact of platelet transfusion in traumatic intracranial hemorrhage ranged from showing benefit to showing detriment, with no clear trend [32].

Since the introduction of direct oral anticoagulation agents (DOACs), an increasing number of advanced-age trauma patients now present on these medications. These agents are as safe as vitamin K antagonists and antiplatelet medication in the setting of both intracranial and extracranial traumatic bleeding [33, 34]. While there were initially no drug-specific reversal agents for these agents, two reversal agents are now available: Idarucizumab for dabigatran and andexanet alfa for rivaroxaban and apixaban. Since the introduction of these reversal agents, no decrease in mortality has thus far been detected associated with reversal agent availability [35], though the number of patients in the literature who received drug-specific reversal for these agents is currently low.

RECOMMENDATIONS

Advanced-age patients with warfarin use, elevated INR, and intracranial hemorrhage have worse outcomes.

Level of evidence: 3. Grade of recommendation: C.

Patients on warfarin with elevated INR can receive either FFP or PCC for reversal.

Level of evidence: 3. Grade of recommendation: C.

No recommendations can be made for the use of platelet transfusion in the setting of the use of a preinjury antiplatelet agent.

Level of evidence: 3. Grade of recommendation: C.

No recommendations can be made for the use of DOAC reversal agents in the setting of the use of preinjury DOAC.

Level of evidence: 3. Grade of recommendation: C.

35.6 What Is the Impact on Treatment and Outcome for Patients on Beta-Blockers, and When Should They Be Used?

This issue is certainly not limited to the advanced-age trauma patient, but surprisingly there are few studies on beta-blocker use in trauma patients. A retrospective review of adult trauma victims found that the OR for fatal outcome was 0.3 ($p < 0.001$) for the cohort using beta-blockers compared to controls and was more pronounced in patients with a significant head injury. They concluded that beta-blocker therapy is safe and may be beneficial in selected trauma patients with or without head injury [36]. However, a study of advanced-age patients in particular found that preinjury beta-blockade had a significant association with mortality (OR 2.1, 95% CI 1.1–4.3) [37].

Bone marrow dysfunction is a known phenomenon after severe trauma that can lead to persistent anemia. Beta-blockers have been considered as an adjunctive treatment modality during the resuscitation stage of management to help mediate this response. A prospective randomized pilot trial of 45 patients was performed to evaluate the effect of propranolol treatment to decrease heart rate by 10–20% postinjury. They found that treatment safely mediated surrogate measures of bone marrow function by reducing hematopoietic progenitor cell mobilization and resulted in a faster return to baseline of the peak in granulocyte colony-stimulating factor [38]. Larger clinical trials regarding the role of beta-blockers for therapeutic hematologic benefit are needed.

35.7 Can a Physical Exam Be Used to Select Advanced-Age Trauma Patients Who Do Not Require CT Imaging?

The process of selecting which patients need advanced radiologic studies (i.e., computed tomography scans) as part of their initial trauma assessment may differ between advanced-age and younger trauma patients, and in light of the increasing volume of advanced-age trauma, there is an incentive to reduce the number of CT scans that are performed for the initial assessment of these patients. The issue is whether physical exams can be used to selectively image advanced-age patients after blunt trauma. Taking first the question of cervical spine imaging, it should be noted that the decision tools for cervical spine imaging in most frequent use (NEXUS and Canadian C-spine Rule) were derived from studies that excluded advanced-age patients, ostensibly due to the decreased sensitivity of the physical exam for clinically significant cervical spine injuries in these patients. Later studies validating these tools in advanced-age patients repeatedly found the tools to be insensitive for clinically significant cervical spine injury. Recent attempts to identify rules-based tools for cervical spine imaging in the advanced-age population are promising [39], but there are no large or prospective validation studies of these tools for advanced-age patients.

There is a similar interest in determining whether imaging of the torso (the remainder, along with the head and cervical spine CT, of the so-called "pan-scan") can be selectively used based on physical exam. The data here are mixed. One retrospective study found no difference in hospital outcomes between advanced-age patients who receive or do not receive a "pan-scan" during initial trauma assessment [40], while another retrospective study found the physical exam to be insensitive to torso injuries for which identification changes management [41]. Regardless, there exists no validated decision tool with sufficient sensitivity for clinically significant torso injury that would suggest a standard to supersede local clinical practice and consensus.

35.8 What Are the Optimal Strategies for Resuscitation and Monitoring of the Geriatric Trauma Patient?

Geriatric trauma patients are more likely to present in shock than younger patients matched for trauma and ISS [42]. In one study, the occult shock was found in 13 of 30 advanced-age patients, despite being hemodynamically stable upon initial presentation. Mortality was high in these patients (54%) [43]. A prospective cohort study of a geriatric resuscitation protocol using lactate-guided therapy found lower mortality with early recognition of occult hypoperfusion. All individuals 65 and older with admission venous lactate >2.5 had Advanced Trauma Life Support (ATLS) resuscitation initiated. Occult hypoperfusion was seen in 20.5% of the participants based on lactate level, and a significant decrease in mortality was observed over time in this group [44]. The precise cohort of patients in need of aggressive resuscitation and monitoring has yet to be determined. A trauma score <15, a base deficit of –6 or worse, or the presence of shock (systolic blood pressure [SBP] <90) have all been associated with worse outcomes and are recommended in consensus guidelines as parameters that identify patients who benefit from ICU admission [28]. Advanced-age trauma patients exhibit subtle or no signs of shock, so a heightened level of suspicion is required at all times while assessing and treating these patients.

35.9 What Are the Risk Factors for Elder Abuse and the Common Patterns of Injury to Be Recognized by the Trauma Provider?

Elder abuse can be divided into five subtypes, of which physical abuse is one. A review evaluating 838 injuries showed the most common anatomic distribution of injuries as follows: Upper extremity, 43.98%; maxillofacial, dental, and neck, 22.88%; skull and brain, 12.28%; lower extremity, 10.61%; and torso, 10.25% [45]. One case-control study showed that victims of elder abuse that resulted in traumatic injury were more likely to have more severe injuries than controls with higher mean ISS and case fatality [46]. They also were more likely to require ICU admission and mechanical ventilation. In this study, the perpetrator was most often the spouse/partner or child, and the most common types of injuries were open wounds.

To our knowledge, no studies have evaluated screening techniques for abuse in the advanced-age trauma population.

RECOMMENDATION

Over 60% of victims of elder abuse present with injury to the upper extremities, neck, and maxillofacial regions.

Level of evidence: 3. Grade of recommendation: C.

35.10 Are There Any Injury-Prevention Programs that Have Been Shown to Work for Advanced-Age Patients?

The ultimate ability to influence outcomes lies in the reduction of injuries. Injury prevention has proven to be successful for a wide variety of traumatic mechanisms. Since the majority of traumatic injuries in the advanced-age population result from falls, this has been a primary focus for injury prevention. The data are mature, supporting a variety of programs, including multimodality programs, in the reduction of falls. A recent network meta-analysis of over 150 randomized studies confirms the reduction of fall frequency after participation in multimodality programs that include components of exercise, assistive technology, environmental assessment and modifications, quality improvement strategies, and basic fall risk assessment [47].

In contrast to the robust literature on fall reduction, few studies have identified effective interventions to decrease fractures. As with fall reduction, exercise programs appear to have the greatest effect to reduce fracture risk. A prospective study with a 10-year follow-up showed that a program of back-strengthening exercises for 2 years reduced the risk of spine fractures by more than 60% [48]. A larger randomized trial showed that impact exercise in 72- to 74-year-old women reduced fracture risk by over 60% [49]. Hip protectors, which are tight-fitting garments with padding over the hip, reduce hip fractures after a fall. Multiple randomized studies exist, with hip fractures up to half as prevalent in institutionalized patients wearing hip protectors who fall [50].

RECOMMENDATION

Programs that include balance and strength training, including multimodality fall-reduction programs, are the most effective at reducing injury.

Level of evidence: 1. Grade of recommendation: A.

Targeted exercise programs and the use of hip protectors reduce injury risk in high-risk patient groups.

Level of evidence: 1. Grade of recommendation: A.

TABLE 35.1

Clinical Questions

Question	Answer	Grade of Recommendation	References
Are advanced-age patients at higher risk for poor outcomes in trauma?	Preexisting conditions and frailty worsen outcomes in advanced-age trauma patients.	C	[4–13]
How should the decision be made to continue or remove life-sustaining supportive care after trauma?	There is no accepted threshold for futility. End-of-life decisions should come out of goals-of-care discussions informed by evidence-based clinical indicators of morbidity and mortality risk.	C	[14–20, 34]
What is the optimal triage strategy for the advanced-age trauma patient?	There is insufficient evidence to make any conclusions on the optimal triage guidelines for the advanced-age trauma patient.	C	[14, 22, 23]
What is the impact on treatment and outcome for patients with medication-induced coagulopathy?	Advanced-age patients with warfarin use, elevated INR, and intracranial hemorrhage have worse outcomes.	C	[24–31]
	Patients can receive either FFP or PCC for warfarin reversal.	C	
	No recommendations can be made in support of platelet transfusion.	C	
	No recommendations can be made for DOAC reversal agent use.	C	
What is the impact on trauma outcomes for patients on beta-blockers?	It is unclear what the impact is of preinjury beta-blockade on trauma outcomes.	C	[36–37]
Can a physical exam be used to select advanced-age trauma patients who do not require CT imaging?	The physical exams do not select advanced-age trauma patients who can forgo a CT scan of the cervical spine or torso for the initial trauma assessment, even in the setting of a low-energy blunt mechanism.	C	[39–41]
What are the optimal strategies for resuscitation and monitoring of the geriatric trauma patient?	Lactate should be used to guide resuscitation in advanced-age patients, as its use frequently identifies occult shock.	B	[42–44]
What are the common patterns of injury found with elder abuse?	Over 60% of victims of elder abuse present with injury to the upper extremities, neck, and maxillofacial regions.	C	[45–46]
What injury-prevention interventions or programs work for advanced-age patients?	Multimodality programs that include balance and strength training are the most effective at reducing falls.	A	[47]
	Targeted exercise programs and the use of hip protectors reduce fall-related injuries in high-risk groups.	A	[48–50]

Editor's Note

There is very little to inform us in the literature on the subject of geriatric trauma, as the authors have nicely delineated. While this part of the population continues to grow, and most trauma centers are now inundated with elderly patients falling on their heads, chests, and hips, we have little to no information to guide our management. Most clinicians feel that the older population requires a different level of care and has inferior outcomes to the younger trauma patients. Despite the urgency of this situation, little high-quality work is available to direct our management.

REFERENCES

1. Ortman JM, Velkoff VA. May 2014. An Aging Nation: The Older Population in the United States. U.S. Department of Commerce, Economics and Statistics Administration: Washington, DC.
2. CDC. National Vital Statistics Report; Death: Leading causes for 2010, Vol. 62, No. 6, 2013
3. Konda SR, Lott A, Mandel J, Lyon TR, Robitsek J, Ganta A, Egol KA. Who is the geriatric trauma patient? An analysis of patient characteristics, hospital quality measures, and inpatient cost. Geriatr Orthop Surg Rehabil. 2020 Sep 15;11:2151459320955087. doi: 10.1177/2151459320955087. PMID: 32974077; PMCID: PMC7495933.
4. Zhao F, Tang B, Hu C, Wang B, Wang Y, Zhang L. The impact of frailty on posttraumatic outcomes in older trauma patients: A systematic review and meta-analysis. J Trauma Acute Care Surg. 2020 Apr;88(4):546–554. doi: 10.1097/TA.0000000000002583. PMID: 32205823.
5. Champion HR, Copes WS, Buyer D, Flanagan ME, Bain L, Sacco WJ. Major trauma in geriatric patients. Am J Public Health. 1989 September;79(9):1278–1282.
6. Morris JA Jr., MacKenzie EJ, Damiano AM, Bass SM. Mortality in trauma patients: The interaction between host factors and severity. J Trauma. 1990 December;30(12):1476–1482.
7. Grossman MD, Miller D, Scaff DW, Arcona S. When is an elder old? Effect of preexisting conditions on mortality in geriatric trauma. J Trauma. 2002 February;52(2):242–246.
8. Haider AH, Herrera-Escobar JP, Al Rafai SS, Harlow AF, Apoj M, Nehra D, Kasotakis G, Brasel K, Kaafarani HMA, Velmahos G, Salim A. Factors associated with long-term outcomes after injury: Results of the Functional Outcomes and Recovery after Trauma Emergencies (FORTE) multi-center cohort study. Ann Surg. 2020 Jun;271(6):1165–1173. doi: 10.1097/SLA.0000000000003101. PMID: 30550382.
9. Milzman DP, Boulanger BR, Rodriguez A, Soderstrom CA, Mitchell KA, Magnant CM. Pre-existing disease in trauma patients: A predictor of fate independent of age and injury severity score. J Trauma. 1992 February;32(2):236–243; discussion 243–244.
10. McGwin G, Jr., MacLennan PA, Fife JB, Davis GG, Rue LW III. Preexisting conditions and mortality in older trauma patients. J Trauma. 2004 June;56(6): 1291–1296.
11. Joseph, B, Pandit V, Zangbar B, Kulvatunyou N, Tang A, O'Keeffe T, Green DJ, Vercruysse G, Fain MJ, Friese RS, Rhee P. J Am Coll Surg. 2014;219(1):10–17e1. doi: 10.1016/j.jamcollsurg.2014.03.020.
12. Hamidi M, Haddadin Z, Zeeshan M, Saljuqi AT, Hanna K, Tang A, Northcutt A, Kulvatunyou N, Gries L, Joseph B. Prospective evaluation and comparison of the predictive ability of different frailty scores to predict outcomes in geriatric trauma patients. J Trauma Acute Care Surg. 2019 Nov;87(5):1172–1180. doi: 10.1097/TA.0000000000002458. PMID: 31389924.
13. Cords CI, Spronk I, Mattace-Raso FUS, Verhofstad MHJ, van der Vlies CH, van Baar ME. The feasibility and reliability of frailty assessment tools applicable in acute in-hospital trauma patients: A systematic review. J Trauma Acute Care Surg. 2022 Mar 1;92(3):615–626. doi: 10.1097/TA.0000000000003472. PMID: 34789703.
14. Committee on Trauma ACoS. 2014. Resources for the Optimal Care of the Injured Patient, 6th edn. American College of Surgeons: Chicago, IL.
15. Graw JA, Burchard R. Completion rates of advance directives in a trauma emergency room: Association with age. Emerg Med Int. 2021 Apr 20;2021:5537599. doi: 10.1155/2021/5537599. PMID: 33968449; PMCID: PMC8081623.
16. Hill LA, Waller CJ, Borgert AJ, Kallies KJ, Cogbill TH. Impact of advance directives on outcomes and charges in elderly trauma patients. J Palliat Med. 2020 Jul;23(7):944–949. doi: 10.1089/jpm.2019.0478. Epub 2020 Jan 3. PMID: 31904311
17. Mosenthal AC, Weissman DE, Curtis JR, Hays RM, Lustbader DR, Mulkerin C, Puntillo KA, Ray DE, Bassett R, Boss RD, Brasel KJ, Campbell M, Nelson JE. Integrating palliative care in the surgical and trauma intensive care unit: A report from the Improving Palliative Care in the Intensive Care Unit (IPAL-ICU) project advisory board and the center to advance palliative care. Crit Care Med. 2012 Apr;40(4):1199–1206. doi: 10.1097/CCM.0b013e31823bc8e7. PMID: 22080644; PMCID: PMC3307874.
18. Davis JW, Kaups KL. Base deficit in the elderly: A marker of severe injury and death. J Trauma. 1998 November;45(5):873–877.
19. Nirula R, Gentilello LM. Futility of resuscitation criteria for the "young" old and the "old" old trauma patient: A national trauma data bank analysis. J Trauma. 2004 July;57(1):37–41.
20. Osler T, Hales K, Baack B, et al. Trauma in the elderly. Am J Surg. 1988 December;156(6):537–543.
21. Ichwan B, Darbha S, Shah MN et al. Geriatric-specific triage criteria are more sensitive than standard adult criteria in identifying need for trauma center care in injured older adults. Ann Emerg Med. 2015 January;65(1):92–100.
22. Ma MH, MacKenzie EJ, Alcorta R, Kelen GD. Compliance with prehospital triage protocols for major trauma patients. J Trauma. 1999 January;46(1):168–175.
23. Rogers FB, Morgan ME, Brown CT, Vernon TM, Bresz KE, Cook AD, Malat J, Sohail N, Bradburn EH. Geriatric trauma mortality: Does trauma center level matter? Am Surg. 2021 Dec;87(12):1965–1971. doi: 10.1177/0003134820983190. Epub 2020 Dec 31. PMID: 33382347.

24. Narula N, Tsikis S, Jinadasa SP, Parsons CS, Cook CH, Butt B, Odom SR. The effect of anticoagulation and antiplatelet use in trauma patients on mortality and length of stay. Am Surg. 2022 Jun;88(6):1137–1145. doi: 10.1177/0003134821989043. Epub 2021 Feb 1. PMID: 33522831.

25. Nguyen RK, Rizor JH, Damiani MP, Powers AJ, Fagnani JT, Monie DL, Cooper SS, Griffiths AD, Hellenthal NJ. The impact of anticoagulation on trauma outcomes: An National Trauma Data Bank Study. Am Surg. 2020 Jul; 86(7): 773–781. doi: 10.1177/0003134820934419. Epub 2020 Jul 30. PMID: 32730098.

26. Kennedy DM, Cipolle MD, Pasquale MD, Wasser T. Impact of preinjury warfarin use in elderly trauma patients. J Trauma. 2000 March;48(3):451–453.

27. Mina AA, Bair HA, Howells GA, Bendick PJ. Complications of preinjury warfarin use in the trauma patient. J Trauma. 2003 May;54(5):842–847.

28. Calland JF, Ingraham AM, Martin N, et al. Evaluation and management of geriatric trauma: An Eastern Association for the Surgery of Trauma practice management guideline. J Trauma Acute Care Surg. 2012 November;73(5 Suppl 4): S345–S350.

29. Lumas SG, Hsiang W, Becher RD, Maung AA, Davis KA, Schuster KM. Choosing the best approach to warfarin reversal after traumatic intracranial hemorrhage. J Surg Res. 2021 Apr;260:369–376. doi: 10.1016/j.jss.2020.12.004. Epub 2020 Dec 31. PMID: 33388533.

30. Peck KA, Calvo RY, Schechter MS et al. The impact of preinjury anticoagulants and prescription antiplatelet agents on outcomes in older patients with traumatic brain injury. J Trauma Acute Care Surg. 2014 February;76(2): 431–436.

31. Baharoglu MI, Cordonnier C, Al-Shahi Salman R, de Gans K, Koopman MM, Brand A, Majoie CB, Beenen LF, Marquering HA, Vermeulen M, Nederkoorn PJ, de Haan RJ, Roos YB; PATCH Investigators. Platelet transfusion versus standard care after acute stroke due to spontaneous cerebral haemorrhage associated with antiplatelet therapy (PATCH): A randomised, open-label, phase 3 trial. Lancet. 2016 Jun 25;387(10038):2605–2613. doi: 10.1016/S0140-6736(16)30392-0. Epub 2016 May 10. PMID: 27178479.

32. Thorn S, Güting H, Mathes T, Schäfer N, Maegele M. The effect of platelet transfusion in patients with traumatic brain injury and concomitant antiplatelet use: A systematic review and meta-analysis. Transfusion. 2019 Nov;59(11):3536–3544. doi: 10.1111/trf.15526. Epub 2019 Sep 18. PMID: 31532000.

33. Puzio TJ, Murphy PB, Kregel HR, Ellis RC, Holder T, Wandling MW, Wade CE, Kao LS, McNutt MK, Harvin JA. Delayed intracranial hemorrhage after blunt head trauma while on direct oral anticoagulant: Systematic review and meta-analysis. J Am Coll Surg. 2021 Jun;232(6):1007–1016.e5. doi: 10.1016/j.jamcollsurg. 2021.02.016. Epub 2021 Mar 22. PMID: 33766725; PMCID: PMC8722268.

34. van Erp IA, Mokhtari AK, Moheb ME, Bankhead-Kendall BK, Fawley J, Parks J, Fagenholz PJ, King DR, Mendoza AE, Velmahos GC, Kaafarani HM, Krijnen P, Schipper IB, Saillant NN. Comparison of outcomes in non-head injured trauma patients using pre-injury warfarin or direct oral anticoagulant therapy. Injury. 2020 Nov;51(11):2546–2552. doi: 10.1016/j.injury.2020.07.063. Epub 2020 Aug 1. PMID: 32814636.

35. Emigh B, Kobayashi L, Kopp M, Daley M, Teal L, Haan J, Burlew CC, Nirula R, Moore F, Burruss S, Kaminski S, Dunn J, Carrick M, Schroeppel T, Thurston B, Quick J, Bosarge P, Brown CV. The AAST prospective observational multicenter study of the initial experience with reversal of direct oral anticoagulants in trauma patients. Am J Surg. 2021 Aug;222(2):264–269. doi: 10.1016/j.amjsurg.2020.12.034. Epub 2021 Jan 6. PMID: 33612255.

36. Arbabi S, Campion EM, Hemmila MR, et al. Beta-blocker use is associated with improved outcomes in adult trauma patients. J Trauma. 2007 January;62(1):56–61; discussion 61–62.

37. Neideen T, Lam M, Brasel KJ. Preinjury beta blockers are associated with increased mortality in geriatric trauma patients. J Trauma. 2008 November;65(5):1016–1020.

38. Bible LE, Pasupuleti LV, Alzate WD, et al. Early propranolol administration to severely injured patients can improve bone marrow dysfunction. J Trauma Acute Care Surg. 2014 July;77(1):54–60; discussion 59–60

39. Engelbart J, Zhou P, Johnson J, Lilienthal M, Zhou Y, Ten-Eyck P, Galet C, Skeete D. Geriatric clinical screening tool for cervical spine injury after ground-level falls. Emerg Med J. 2022 Apr;39(4):301–307. doi: 10.1136/ emermed-2020-210693. Epub 2021 Jun 9. PMID: 34108196; PMCID: PMC8655022.

40. Kim C, Sartin R, Dissanaike S. Is a "Pan-Scan" indicated in the older patient with a ground level fall? Am Surg. 2018 Sep 1;84(9):1480–1483. doi: 10.1177/000313481808400954. PMID: 30268180.

41. Kania T, Pandya S, Demissie S, Abdelhalim D, Governo C, Hawkins S, Younan D, Atanassov K, Gave A. Physical exam is not an accurate predictor of injury in geriatric patients with low-energy blunt trauma – A retrospective cohort study. Ann Med Surg (Lond). 2022 Aug 27;81:104503. doi: 10.1016/j.amsu.2022.104503. PMID: 36147051; PMCID: PMC9486729.

42. Clancy TV, Ramshaw DG, Maxwell JG, et al. Management outcomes in splenic injury: A statewide trauma center review. Ann Surg. 1997 July;226(1):17–24.

43. Scalea TM, Simon HM, Duncan AO et al. Geriatric blunt multiple trauma: Improved survival with early invasive monitoring. J Trauma. 1990 February;30(2):129–134; discussion 134–136.

44. Bar-Or D, Salottolo KM, Orlando A, Mains CW, Bourg P, Offner PJ. Association between a geriatric trauma resuscitation protocol using venous lactate measurements and early trauma surgeon involvement and mortality risk. J Am Geriatr Soc. 2013 August;61(8):1358–1364.

45. Murphy K, Waa S, Jaffer H, Sauter A, Chan A. A literature review of findings in physical elder abuse. Can Assoc Radiol J. 2013 February;64(1):10–14.

46. Friedman LS, Avila S, Tanouye K, Joseph K. A case-control study of severe physical abuse of older adults. J Am Geriatr Soc. 2011 March;59(3):417–422.

47. Dautzenberg L, Beglinger S, Tsokani S, Zevgiti S, Raijmann RCMA, Rodondi N, Scholten RJPM, Rutjes AWS, Di Nisio M, Emmelot-Vonk M, Tricco AC, Straus SE, Thomas S, Bretagne L, Knol W, Mavridis D, Koek HL. Interventions for preventing falls and fall-related fractures in community-dwelling older adults: A systematic review and network meta-analysis. J Am Geriatr Soc. 2021 Oct;69(10):2973–2984. doi: 10.1111/jgs.17375. Epub 2021 Jul 28. PMID: 34318929; PMCID: PMC8518387.

48. Sinaki M, Itoi E, Wahner HW, et al. Stronger back muscles reduce the incidence of vertebral fractures: A prospective 10 year follow-up of postmenopausal women. Bone. 2002 June;30(6):836–841.

49. Korpelainen R, Keinanen-Kiukaanniemi S, Heikkinen J, Vaananen K, Korpelainen J. Effect of impact exercise on bone mineral density in elderly women with low BMD: A population-based randomized controlled 30-month intervention. Osteoporos Int. 2006 January;17(1):109–118.

50. Parker MJ, Gillespie LD, Gillespie WJ. Hip protectors for preventing hip fractures in the elderly. Cochrane Database Syst Rev. 2004;1(3):CD001255.

36

Genitourinary Trauma

Megan Gilchrist and Joseph Love

36.1 Evidence-Based Management of Genitourinary Trauma

Management of genitourinary (GU) trauma has changed over the past few decades. Because of utilization of advanced radiographic imaging, minimally invasive interventional techniques, and improvements in resuscitation, management has become less surgically aggressive. Injury remains the leading cause of death between the ages of 4 and 45 in the United States according to the U.S. Centers for Disease Control and Prevention [1]. It is estimated that 10% of abdominal traumas involve the GU tract and frequently occur concomitantly with injuries to other abdominal organs. Urogenital trauma has an incidence of 10–20% in both adult and pediatric populations [2]. Hematuria, a hallmark of injury to the urinary tract, is not specific to the location or severity of the injury and may be absent or present during the initial evaluation. The clinician should consider the mechanism of injury, the patient's hemodynamic stability, and the resuscitative efforts required to stabilize the patient to decide the best management route. This chapter provides an evidence-based approach to the management of patient populations with traumatic injuries to the GU tract. The studies cited are mostly retrospective due to the logistics and ethics of executing prospective, randomized studies in the trauma setting.

36.1.2 Diagnostic Approach

In the absence of hemodynamic instability, computed tomography (CT) with intravenous (IV) contrast in patients with blunt trauma with evidence of gross hematuria or microscopic hematuria is recommended. A CT with IV contrast should be considered in patients presenting with clinical findings consistent with urotrauma. Obtaining both immediate and delayed imaging is recommended. Clinical findings for urotrauma include rapid deceleration, significant impact to the flank, rib fractures, flank ecchymosis, and penetrating injury. Focused assessment with sonography in trauma has low sensitivity and specificity in renal trauma and therefore is not recommended as a diagnostic tool for urotrauma but may still be beneficial in the evaluation of multisystem injured patients [2]. Suspected bladder injury should be evaluated by retrograde cystography (fluoroscopic or CT); delayed-phase CT is less sensitive and less specific due to inadequate antegrade bladder filling from renal excretion. The suspected urethral injury should be evaluated with a retrograde urethrogram.

36.2 Renal Trauma

36.2.1 When Does Renal Trauma Require Immediate Surgical Exploration?

The most commonly injured organ in the GU system is the kidney. A population-based observational study has shown that 1.2% of all trauma patients suffered renal injuries, with blunt trauma being the major cause [3]. In urogenital trauma, the kidney is involved 65–90% of the time [2]. The Injury Severity Score (assessment of the patient's global status), penetrating injury, and renal injury severity were independent predictors of the need for nephrectomy. Additional studies, utilizing both retrospective and prospective data, assessed the usefulness of the American Association for the Surgery of Trauma (AAST) injury scale, suggesting that the scale correlates with clinical outcome and the need for nephrectomy [4]. The grade of injury is determined with an IV contrast CT of the abdomen and pelvis in stable patients who have suffered blunt trauma with gross or microscopic hematuria and systolic blood pressure >90 mmHg. The scan should be obtained with IV contrast when the mechanism of injury or findings on physical examination are concerning for renal injury. The degree of hematuria does not necessarily correlate with the grade of injury and should not preclude imaging studies. Immediate and delayed imaging should be obtained to show the location of renal lacerations and the presence of extravasation from the urinary collecting system.

Depending on the severity of the injury and the patient's stability, most blunt renal injuries can be managed conservatively. The management of blunt traumatic renal injuries has shifted to nonoperative management (NOM) for the majority of cases. A 2005 systematic review of renal trauma concluded that NOM may be warranted in those patients not demonstrating exsanguination and physiologic instability from the kidney injury. NOM demonstrates decreased rates of renal exploration and nephrectomy without any increase in complications in patients with grade I–IV blunt renal injuries. These patients can be managed with close hemodynamic monitoring, bed rest, and blood transfusion if necessary. Physicians treating grade IV injuries with close observation must understand that delayed complications such as bleeding or renovascular hypertension may necessitate nephrectomy. Patients with blunt grade IV renal injury treated conservatively required delayed surgical intervention 0–40% of the time, and up to 20% required nephrectomy [5]. McGuire et al. demonstrated

DOI: 10.1201/9781003316800-36

a 9.3% complication rate with high-grade blunt injuries that were treated conservatively [6]. Retrospective data from a multicenter research consortium of 206 patients in which 154 were managed nonoperatively demonstrated hemodynamically stable patients with severe grade IV and V blunt renal trauma can be managed nonoperatively with a failure rate of 6.5% [7]. Increased failure rates of NOM in this study included patients older than 55 years and blunt injuries associated with a motor vehicle crash. Another study has shown that even grade V injuries may be amenable to NOM given the correct clinical context [8]. Patients managed conservatively were younger, had less comorbidity, and did not have imaging findings suspicious of renal pedicle injury. Although this study was limited by its small population size, NOM resulted in fewer intensive care unit (ICU) days, significantly lower transfusion rates ($p = 0.124$), and fewer complications. The clinician must consider many factors in deciding which patients can be managed conservatively.

NOM of penetrating injuries remains unclear. The majority of patients sustaining penetrating renal trauma will undergo operative intervention to address concurrent injuries based on trajectory and physiology. As a consequence, most renal injuries will be discovered during exploration in this setting. In the rare circumstance of hemodynamic stability at presentation and a truly retroperitoneal trajectory involving only the kidney, NOM could be considered. A recent observational study using the National Trauma Data Bank suggests angioembolization had increased success rates compared to surgical repair in a 481-patient cohort with high-grade renal trauma in which 44.1% had penetrating injuries [9]. NOM in penetrating renal injuries has also been associated with low complication rates in a very select group of patients. Bjurlin et al. [10] found that the selective NOM of penetrating renal injuries resulted in lower transfusion rates, shorter ICU and hospital length of stay, and decreased mortality when compared with nephrectomy, but the results were similar when compared to renorrhaphy. Patients undergoing NOM were hemodynamically stable and had an absence of the following CT findings: Gross urinary extravasation, contrast blush indicative of arterial hemorrhage, and hilar disruption. The absence of these radiographic findings was indicative of a potentially viable, salvageable kidney in a select group of patients not needing exploration of the abdomen for other concurrent additional injuries or hemodynamic instability

There is grade B evidence to support immediate intervention with surgery or angioembolization in hemodynamically unstable patients with no or minimal response to resuscitation. Again, the need for emergent intervention is not only based on the grade of the injury but also the patient's clinical status. A retrospective study of high-grade blunt renal injuries revealed that the ongoing need for fluid, blood, and blood products predicted the need for emergent intervention [6]. A higher proportion of grade V injuries required immediate intervention; however, 5.3% of patients with grade V injuries were managed nonoperatively. Others have advised that grade V vascular injuries should be treated with immediate surgical intervention, usually requiring nephrectomy.

Renal angioembolization (RAE) is important to NOM for severe blunt renal injuries in hemodynamically stable patients and has led to improved outcomes. However, the role of RAE in hemodynamically unstable patients is unclear. In a retrospective series of 26 patients, angioembolization was found to be an effective option for patients with grade IV renal trauma who have failed conservative management [11]. However, patients with grade V injuries did not respond well to embolization, and either immediate nephrectomy or death occurred. In another study, nine hemodynamically unstable patients with grade V renal injuries secondary to blunt trauma were all successfully treated with angioembolization, and none required any further intervention [12]. In a systematic review including 412 patients, a success rate of 90% in 346 stable patients and 63% in 66 unstable patients was observed [13], with success being defined as the absence of repeat RAE, nephrectomy, or death. The utilization of RAE in unstable patients should be approached with caution in blunt traumatic injury to the kidney. High-grade injuries tend to respond poorly, and increased operative intervention was demonstrated even in hemodynamically stable patients.

Urinary extravasation and renal parenchymal injuries can be managed nonoperatively in hemodynamically stable patients (grade IB) [2]. Patients with isolated urinary extravasation from parenchymal injury who were treated nonoperatively had a >90% rate of resolution of urinary leakage [14], and those taken to the operating room had a 19% nephrectomy rate. None of the patients initially treated nonoperatively required nephrectomies, but 9% required endoscopic ureteral stent placement due to persistent leakage followed by complete resolution of urinary extravasation. Follow-up CT imaging for grade III, IV, and V renal lacerations is recommended (grade C) after 36–72 hours due to association with complications, including urinoma or hemorrhage [15].

RECOMMENDATION

Hemodynamically stable patients with blunt renal injury may initially be treated nonoperatively, while hemodynamically unstable patients who do not respond to resuscitation must undergo immediate intervention, with either surgery or angioembolization.

Grade of recommendation: B.

Penetrating renal injuries require surgical intervention. Truly isolated penetrating renal injuries without hemodynamic instability may undergo angiography in rare circumstances with evidence of decreased transfusion, ICU length of stay, and mortality.

Grade of recommendation: C.

36.3 Ureteral Injury

36.3.1 How Should Traumatic Ureteral Injuries Be Repaired?

Ureteral injuries secondary to external trauma are rare—approximately 1% of all GU trauma. Most ureteral injuries are iatrogenic and usually occur in either the operating room during gynecologic, urologic, or colorectal surgery. Iatrogenic ureteral injuries usually occur in the distal third and pelvic ureter, while ureteral injuries from external trauma usually occur in the upper third of the ureter [16, 17]. Diagnosis may be missed or delayed since ureteral injuries may not manifest with obvious signs and symptoms. A high index of suspicion is necessary for prompt diagnosis and management. Ureteral injuries are associated with complex abdominopelvic trauma, complex pelvic/vertebral fractures, rapid deceleration injury, or penetrating trauma with suspected injury based on trajectory.

As with renal injuries, the management of ureteral injuries depends on the hemodynamic stability of the patient, timing, location, and extent of the injury. The AAST classifies ureteral injury as follows: Grade 1 periureteral hematoma, grade II laceration <50% transection, grade III laceration >50% transection, grade IV complete transection <2 cm length, and grade V transection with >2 cm devascularization. Stable patients with suspected ureteral injuries should be evaluated with a CT of the abdomen and pelvis with 10-minute delayed images. Ureteral injuries are suggested by contrast extravasation, delayed pyelogram, hydronephrosis, or lack of contrast in the ureter distal to the injury [18, 19]. Many ureteral injuries occur in the operating room, and visual inspection of the ureters at the time of laparotomy without imaging is recommended. Adjuncts to inspection within the operating room include IV or intraureteral injectable dyes (methylene blue or indigo carmine) as well as retrograde pyelography. The efficacy of this approach is demonstrated in a study that revealed no missed ureteral injuries during surgical exploration for patients who had a penetrating mechanism of injury [20]. A meta-analysis of ureteral injuries showed that delayed diagnosis of ureteral injuries is associated with a prolonged length of stay and increased rate of nephrectomy [21]. Primary repair is the treatment of choice unless the patient is hemodynamically unstable and complex repair is not technically feasible within a reasonable amount of time. A retrospective review showed favorable results when ureteral injuries were repaired primarily [22]. The majority of patients underwent complex repairs with nearly a 100% renal salvage rate. Deferred management with a percutaneous nephrostomy tube with or without ureteral ligation almost always resulted in significant strictures and eventual loss of ureteral length. Primary repair is the main goal, if diagnosed early and if technically feasible.

If the patient is unstable, the primary repair is not recommended. These patients should undergo temporary diversion with a nephrostomy tube, ureteral ligation, and planned delayed repair, which prevents urinary extravasation and urinoma formation; however, this is mostly based on anecdotal accounts. Placing a ureteral stent will ensure patency of the ureter in incomplete ureteral injuries if the injury was initially missed or presented in a delayed manner. Ku et al. showed that patients who underwent urinary diversion alone without a stent had a higher rate of ureteral stenosis [23]. However, if stent placement is not possible, the patient should be treated in the same manner as unstable patients.

The method of choice for ureteric repair depends on the location, extent, and mechanism of injury. In general, ureteral anastomoses should be created with absorbable sutures and spatulated ends (to minimize stricture), be tension-free, and be performed over a double J stent. A Foley should be placed to protect the anastomosis from increased pressures and a drain at the site of the repair. To allow for tension-free anastomosis, mobilization of the ureters should be performed carefully, sparing the adventitia and avoiding devascularization. If mobilization does not permit tension-free anastomosis, then ureteral reimplantation can be attempted with other maneuvers such as a psoas hitch and/or Boari flap to bring the ureter closer to the bladder. Ureteral injuries distal to the iliac vessels should be repaired either primarily if healthy enough with ureteroureterostomy over stent or with ureteral reimplant (ureteroneocystostomy) [16, 17]. Long defects >2 cm will likely require a psoas hitch or Boari flap to provide a tension-free anastomosis [17]. Injuries above the iliac vessels should be repaired primarily with ureteroureterostomy over a ureteral stent after all nonviable tissue has been debrided [16]. If unable to perform a ureteroureterostomy for injuries above iliac vessels, mobilization or psoas hitch/Boari flap can also be performed. During the acute setting, complex reconstruction such as autotransplant and bowel interposition should not be attempted [16, 17]. Autotransplant can be used with large-length ureteral loss and involves placing the affected kidney into the iliac fossa with vascular anastomoses of the renal to iliac vessels and a ureterovesicostomy. Bowel interposition, usually performed with the ileum, requires a standard mechanical and antibiotic bowel preparation. Success rates can be as high as 81%, but there are associated complications such as mucus formation, stones, recurrent infections, and metabolic acidosis [24]. These procedures are too complex and time-consuming to be appropriately performed in the trauma setting.

RECOMMENDATION

Hemodynamically stable patients with ureteral injuries should undergo primary repair or ureteral reimplant if time permits. Delayed management almost always results in significant stricture.

Grade of recommendation: C.

36.4 Bladder Trauma

36.4.1 What Types of Bladder Injuries Need to Be Surgically Repaired?

The bladder is usually protected from external trauma since it is located deep in the pelvis. Bladder injuries only occur in 1.6% of blunt abdominal trauma cases since such high forces are required to disrupt the integrity of the bony pelvis [25]. Other causes include a direct blow to a distended bladder, penetrating injuries, and other various iatrogenic causes.

Bladder injuries (60–90%) are associated with pelvic fractures, while only 2–11% of patients with pelvic fractures have bladder injuries [25]; thus, not all patients with pelvic fractures require imaging to rule out bladder injury. Gross hematuria with pelvic fracture is highly indicative of a bladder injury. A retrospective review of 53 patients with bladder rupture secondary to blunt trauma revealed that 85% with gross hematuria also sustained a pelvic fracture [26]. Stable patients with gross hematuria and pelvic fracture must have retrograde cystography (RC) to rule out bladder perforation or rupture. RC may be performed with either plain radiographs or CT; both have high specificity and sensitivity for bladder injury.

RC is also recommended in stable patients with (1) gross hematuria without pelvic fracture but with mechanisms concerning for bladder injury or (2) pelvic ring fractures and clinical suspicion for bladder rupture, although the evidence is not as strong as with gross hematuria in the setting of a pelvic fracture. Some patients with pelvic fractures with bladder injuries will present with microscopic hematuria. Patients who suffered pelvic fractures with hematuria >30 RBC/HPF (red blood cells/high power field) had an increased risk for bladder injury, while none of the patients with <30 RBC/HPF had bladder injuries [27]. Additionally, patients with wide diastasis of the symphysis pubis or sacroiliac joints and displaced fractures of the obturator ring were at increased risk for bladder injury.

The standard of care for intraperitoneal (IP) bladder rupture in the setting of blunt or penetrating external trauma is immediate surgical repair [26]. These injuries are located at the dome of the bladder and rarely heal with catheter drainage alone. Failure to repair or recognize IP bladder injuries can lead to urinary ascites, ileus, abdominal distention, peritonitis, localized abscesses, or sepsis [25]. Patients who require complex repairs, those involving the trigone or ureteral reimplantation, should undergo a postoperative cystogram to ensure complete healing of the bladder, while patients who undergo simple repairs may not necessarily need any follow-up imaging at all. All simple IP injuries had negative postoperative cystograms, while one of three of the complex IP injuries had a cystogram positive for a leak [28], with the postoperative cystogram being performed between 1 and 4 weeks. There are no prospective data to determine the optimal timing of the postoperative cystogram and catheter removal in these patients, but current practice involves obtaining the cystogram at 2 weeks.

Extraperitoneal (EP) bladder ruptures account for about 55% of all bladder injuries and are seen almost exclusively with pelvic fractures [25]. As opposed to patients with IP bladder injuries, patients with uncomplicated EP bladder injuries can be managed conservatively with Foley catheter drainage [20]. No statistical differences in outcomes were identified between patients whose EP bladder injuries were explored surgically or treated with Foley drainage [25, 29].

Patients with complicated EP bladder injuries, such as those with exposed bone spicules in the bladder lumen, potentially large EP ruptures with significant extravasation, concurrent rectal or vaginal lacerations, or bladder neck injuries, should undergo surgical repair, as patients in these circumstances will likely develop long-term sequelae if the injuries are not primarily repaired [19]. Patients undergoing open reduction and internal fixation or repair of abdominal injuries may benefit from concurrent repair of EP bladder injuries, as the typical bladder repair can be executed with little morbidity [25]. As with

IP bladder injuries, cystography should be performed for EP injuries with a high risk of leak after 2 weeks to ensure complete healing of the bladder injury [28].

Patients who undergo IP or EP bladder repair should have urethral catheter drainage without the need for a suprapubic cystotomy. Several studies have shown that the use of suprapubic tubes with urethral catheterization vs. catheterization alone does not offer any advantage in terms of altering catheter-related complications [30, 31]. Alli et al. showed that the use of urethral catheters alone is associated with shorter hospital stays and lower morbidity, including a decreased incidence of urinary tract infections (UTIs), fistula formation, and the development of urinary retention than drainage with both suprapubic and urethral catheters [31].

RECOMMENDATIONS

IP bladder ruptures in the setting of blunt or penetrating external trauma should undergo prompt surgery and be primarily repaired (grade B). Uncomplicated EP bladder injuries can be treated conservatively with Foley catheter drainage, while complicated EP bladder injuries should be primarily repaired.

Grade of recommendation: C.

36.5 Urethral Trauma

36.5.1 How Should Urethral Trauma Be Managed in the Acute Setting?

Male urethral injury can occur to the anterior urethra (penile or bulbar) or posterior urethra (proximal to the membranous urethra). The mechanism of injury tends to differ with straddle injuries (crushing of the immobile portion of the urethra between the undersurface of the pubis) and penetrating trauma affecting the anterior urethra. Posterior urethral injuries tend to be associated with pelvic fractures. Successful management of urethral trauma is dependent on prompt diagnosis. Any blood at the urethral meatus in the setting of pelvic trauma needs to be considered a significant finding and be evaluated with retrograde urethrography (RUG), which will help establish the diagnosis of urethral injury [27]; however, establishing the full extent of injury may be prevented by an external sphincter, pelvic floor, and periurethral spasm. Female urethral trauma is a result of pelvic fracture, and suspicion should be raised with labial edema and/or blood within the vaginal vault.

RECOMMENDATION

Acute management of suspected urethral injury must include RUG.

Grade of recommendation: C.

36.5.2 Should Straddle (Anterior-Crush) Injuries Be Treated Acutely or Should Management Be Delayed?

The timing of anterior crush injury repairs has been debated, and several series have provided conflicting evidence-based outcomes. RUG is required to determine a complete or incomplete injury. The most common complication related to these injuries is the subsequent development of urethral stricture, with a statistically greater likelihood of stricture formation in those who had a complete bulbar urethral rupture [32].

A retrospective study including 304 males, 197 partial and 107 complete anterior urethral injuries, suggests that endoscopic realignment is associated with a lower stricture rate than cystostomy as immediate management for partial disruption. For complete disruption, emergency anastomosis had better clinical outcomes, including a success rate of 90.4% (47 of 52 patients) with stricture in 5 patients, while a 100% stricture rate in the cystostomy subgroup necessitated urethroplasty [33].

Previous studies suggest the incidence of stricture formation is greater in those who underwent primary urethral realignment (82% vs. 35%; $p < 0.001$) [32], supporting the use of an initial suprapubic cystotomy (SP). In patients with partial urethral disruption, stricture formation occurred in 11% of patients with SP and 87% of patients who underwent realignment. Patients with complete disruption who underwent realignment demonstrated a 100% incidence of stricture formation compared to 75% treated with SP. The San Francisco General experience included only 19% of patients having primary realignment, and patients who underwent primary realignment required complex flaps or graft urethroplasty at a greater rate compared to men who underwent SP [34]. In patients with the complete bulbar disruption that occurred as a result of blunt trauma, statistically higher rates of urethral stricture formation were noted in patients who underwent delayed repair than in those who underwent immediate urethral realignment (69% vs. 31%; $p = 0.014$) [35]. Gong et al. assessed additional endpoints in another study comparing immediate and primary repair after initial SP insertion and did not find any statistical difference in stricture formation related to the time of the repair; however, a significantly shorter return to spontaneous voiding and the length of time needed for suprapubic diversion with the immediate repair was noted [36]. No differences were noted in erectile dysfunction or continence rates between the two groups, and without any outcome advantages, it does not appear that immediate primary repair is indicated in a trauma patient who likely has more serious concomitant injuries.

> **RECOMMENDATION**
>
> In bulbar urethral injuries, urinary drainage should be established with an SP tube. Primary realignment requires consideration of associated injuries, the severity of injury, bladder distention, and availability of urologic expertise and endoscopic techniques.
>
> Grade of recommendation: C.

36.5.3 What Is the Ideal Management of Posterior Urethral Injuries Associated with Pelvic Fractures?

Posterior urethral disruption has been reported in 5–25% of patients sustaining pelvic fractures. Immediate urinary drainage must be established with the placement of a suprapubic tube, and controversy exists regarding the subsequent management of urinary drainage. Traditionally, delayed repairs have been advocated, especially in those patients who may be hemodynamically unstable. The early endoscopic realignment of posterior urethral disruptions has been advocated, with long-term follow-up revealing no increased incidence of impotence, stricture formation, or incontinence compared to delayed repair, providing that the realignment is done in a fairly expeditious manner [37].

The most common complication seen in these patients is the subsequent development of urethral stricture, and long-term surveillance needs to be pursued for at least 1 year following urethral injury. Stricture formation in this group of severely ill patients who have sustained significant concomitant injuries resulting in a 51% mortality rate, is extremely high regardless of early versus delayed reconstruction but favors the early realignment group (49% vs. 100%) [37]. The delayed repair was also associated with a greater degree of complexity of the resultant stricture, further supporting early realignment.

Urethral trauma that requires a suprapubic tube raises concerns among orthopedic surgeons who worry about the proximity of a foreign body to a site of hardware insertion. On occasion, this has led on occasion to the conservative management of orthopedic injuries and possible suboptimal outcomes. However, there has not been any proven increased incidence of hardware infection despite these concerns, and orthopedic repair should occur irrespective of the need for an SP. To allay some of these fears, the urologist can place the tube as high as possible in the bladder, use a subcutaneous tunnel, and include the orthopedic surgeon in the management decision.

> **RECOMMENDATION**
>
> Placement of a suprapubic tube for immediate urinary drainage is recommended. Primary realignment in hemodynamically stable patients may be performed as long as prolonged attempts are not made.
>
> Grade of recommendation: C.

36.6 Penile and Scrotal Trauma

36.6.1 Does Penetrating Penile or Scrotal Trauma Need to Be Explored?

Penetrating penile or scrotal trauma in the civilian population usually occurs as a result of low-velocity projectiles. They are rather rare occurrences, and there is a paucity of studies in the literature, most of which come from the larger urban trauma centers in the country. Exploration of penetrating scrotal trauma occurring from either gunshot wounds (GSWs) or stab wounds (SWs) has been shown to result in testicular salvage, and exploration is indicated. Salvage rates of GSWs have been reported between 52% and 75%, with GSWs showing statistically significant higher salvage rates than SWs ($p < 0.001$) [38]. Studies such as these are consistent with the European Association of Urology (EAU) 2005 guidelines, which recommend scrotal exploration for all penetrating scrotal injuries. Only injuries that were superficial, nonpenetrating, and had low clinical suspicion of injury deep to the dartos layer were managed without surgery.

Given the high rate of testicular loss despite exploration, these outcomes may help influence preoperative counseling about patient expectations. This center advocates surgical exploration instead of ultrasound evaluation in all injuries that have penetrated or are suspected to have penetrated the dartos fascia and to perform conservative debridement. The vascularity of the scrotal contents helps to contribute to the low rate of infectious complications seen postoperatively.

GSWs to the external genitalia result in a lower incidence of urethral injury compared to SWs (6% vs. 17%) [38]. GSWs may be associated with urethral injury (15–29%), and blood at the urethral meatus is an indication to perform an RUG, which has been shown to have a sensitivity of 92%, a specificity of 100%, a positive predictive value of 100%, and a negative predictive value of 97% [39]. Spatulated primary repair of the injury should be undertaken when an injury in the anterior urethra is identified. Conservative treatment can be undertaken for superficial injuries; however, an injury to the cavernosal bodies should be repaired.

of injury and managed only the highly suspicious group with the surgical intervention [40]. None of the low-suspicion nonoperative group experienced complications related to subsequent erectile dysfunction (ED), and similarly, in the 88% of patients in the surgical group who followed up, ED did not occur. Penile curvature was noted in 5.6%. The history, physical findings, and mechanism of injury help determine treatment.

Satisfactory and painless erectile function was reported in 95% of surgical patients who underwent immediate repair, with a few long-term complications (4.7%), and ED rates were similar to a control population [41]. Urethral injury may also occur in these patients, and blood at the meatus must be evaluated either with urethrography or cystoscopy at the time of intervention. Up to 50% of patients treated conservatively have been shown to have complications of ED and penile curvature [42].

In a series of 300 patients, all undergoing repair within 48 hours of injury, reported complications included ED (0.6%), penile pain with erection or intercourse (3.3%), and mild penile curvature in 14 patients (4.6%) that did not hinder intercourse in 10 of them [43]. Older series had advocated conservative management of this problem using ice, pressure dressings, and antiinflammatories; however, complication rates in these earlier series are reported up to 53% [44].

Whether the repair of the defect in the corpora cavernosum must be treated emergently has been debated. There are no studies that show any adverse effects related to the immediate repair of the injury, and clearly, an emergent repair can be undertaken. A retrospective study of 180 patients with long-term follow-up (mean 8 years) demonstrated that regardless of early repair (within 24 hours) or delayed repair (within 7 days), no statistically significant differences in outcomes were noted (Table 36.1) [45].

> **RECOMMENDATION**
>
> Penile, urethral, or testicular injury should be explored and repaired in the hemodynamically stable patient.
>
> Grade of recommendation: C.

> **RECOMMENDATION**
>
> Penile fracture should be surgically corrected either immediately or delayed (within 7 days) to maximize outcomes such as erectile function and lack of penile deviation.
>
> Grade of recommendation: B.

36.6.2 Does Penile Fracture Need to Be Treated Emergently?

A penile fracture refers to a tear of the corpus cavernosum in an erect penis. Patients commonly complain of a snapping or popping sensation that occurs during sexual activity followed by pain, detumescence, discoloration, and penile swelling. Prompt surgical exploration and repair are recommended in patients with high suspicion of penile fracture. If equivocal signs and symptoms of penile fracture exist, ultrasound can be utilized as an adjunct. However, Koifman et al. categorized patients into either low or high suspicion

36.6.3 Testicular Rupture Management

Findings of testicular rupture include scrotal ecchymosis and swelling or inability to palpate the testicle on the exam. Ultrasound should be utilized for blunt scrotal trauma with findings concerning testicular rupture. Rupture can occur after both blunt and penetrating scrotal injuries. Surgical exploration, debridement, and repair should be performed for both blunt and penetrating trauma. If nonsalvageable, then an orchiectomy should be performed.

TABLE 36.1

Evidence-Based Management of Urotrauma

Question	Answer	Grade of Recommendation	Level of Evidence	References
When does renal trauma require immediate surgical exploration?	Hemodynamically stable patients with renal injury may initially be treated nonoperatively, while hemodynamically unstable patients who do not respond to resuscitation must undergo immediate intervention, whether via surgery or angioembolization.	B	III, IV	[1–15]
How should traumatic ureteral injuries be repaired?	Hemodynamically stable patients with ureteral injuries should undergo primary repair or ureteral reimplant if time permits. Delayed management almost always results in significant stricture.	C	III, IV	[1, 16–24]
What types of bladder injuries need to be surgically repaired?	IP bladder ruptures in the setting of blunt or penetrating external trauma should be primarily repaired.	B	III	[25–28]
	Uncomplicated EP bladder injuries should be treated conservatively with Foley catheter drainage, while complicated EP bladder injuries should be primarily repaired.	C	III	[19, 20, 25, 28–29]
How should urethral trauma be managed in the acute setting?	Acute management of suspected urethral injury must include RUG.	C	III	[27]
Should straddle injuries be treated acutely or should management be delayed?	In bulbar urethral injuries, urinary drainage should occur with a suprapubic tube. Primary realignment can be considered.	C	III	[32–36]
What is the ideal management of posterior urethral injuries associated with pelvic fractures?	Endoscopic early realignment should be attempted if possible.	C	III, IV	[1, 37]
Does penetrating penile or scrotal trauma need to be explored?	Penile, urethral, or testicular injury should be explored and repaired in the hemodynamically stable patient.	C	IV	[38, 39]
Does penile fracture need to be treated emergently?	The penile fracture should be corrected either immediately or delayed to maximize outcomes such as erectile function and lack of penile deviation.	B	III	[40–45]

Editor's Note

There is relatively little high-grade evidence to guide our management of injuries of the genitourinary tract. Essentially all of our treatment protocols are based on clinical experience and retrospective reviews. In blunt renal trauma, nonoperative management is now routine, and only hemodynamically unstable patients typically undergo operative exploration. Angiography with embolization after significant injuries to the kidneys has led to improved outcomes. It is important to recognize that there is a high complication rate with nonoperative management of major extraperitoneal bladder injuries, and some of them must be operatively repaired. Ureteral injuries are rare and can be repaired if recognized early, while urethral trauma often requires a suprapubic tube and deferred repair. Penetrating injuries to the genitourinary tract typically need operative intervention.

REFERENCES

1. Centers for Disease Control and Prevention. Leading Causes of Death Reports, 1981–2020 (February 20, 2020) Atlanta, GA: U.S. Department of Health and Human Services, Centers for Disease Control and Prevention. https://www.cdc.gov/injury/wisqars/LeadingCauses.html

2. Coccolini F, Moore EE, Kluger Y, Biffl W, Leppaniemi A, Matsumura Y, Kim F, Peitzman AB, Fraga GP, Sartelli M, Ansaloni L, Augustin G, Kirkpatrick A, Abu-Zidan F, Wani I, Weber D, Pikoulis E, Larrea M, Arvieux C, Manchev V, Reva V, Coimbra R, Khokha V, Mefire AC, Ordonez C, Chiarugi M, Machado F, Sakakushev B, Matsumoto J, Maier R, di Carlo I, Catena F; WSES-AAST Expert Panel. Kidney and uro-trauma: WSES-AAST guidelines. World J Emerg Surg. 2019 Dec 2;14:54. doi: 10.1186/s13017-019-0274-x. PMID: 31827593; PMCID: PMC6886230.

3. Wessells H, Suh D, Porter JR et al. Renal injury and operative management in the United States: Results of a population-based study. J Trauma. 2003;54:423–430.

4. Shariat SF, Roehrborn CG, Karakiewicz PI et al. Evidence-based validation of the predictive value of the American Association for the Surgery of Trauma kidney injury scale. J Trauma. 2007;62:933–939.

5. Santucci RA, Fisher MB. The literature increasingly supports expectant (conservative) management of renal trauma—A systematic review. J Trauma. 2005;59:493–501.

6. McGuire J, Bultitude MF, Davis P, et al. Predictors of outcome for blunt high-grade renal injury treated with conservative intent. J Urol. 2011;185:187–191.

7. van der Wilden GM, Velmahos GC, Joseph DK, Jacobs L, Debusk MG, Adams CA, Gross R, Burkott B, Agarwal S, Maung AA, Johnson DC, Gates J, Kelly E,

Michaud Y, Charash WE, Winchell RJ, Desjardins SE, Rosenblatt MS, Gupta S, Gaeta M, Chang Y, de Moya MA. Successful nonoperative management of the most severe blunt renal injuries: a multicenter study of the research consortium of New England Centers for Trauma. JAMA Surg. 2013 Oct;148(10):924–31. doi: 10.1001/jamasurg.2013.2747. PMID: 23945834.

8. Altman AL, Haas C, Dinchman KH, Spirnak JP. Selective non-operative management of blunt grade 5 renal injury. J Urol. 2000;164:27–30.

9. Hakam N, Amend GM, Nabavizadeh B, Allen IE, Shaw NM, Cuschieri J, Wilson MW, Stein DM, Breyer BN. Utility and Outcome of Angioembolization for High-Grade Renal Trauma Management in a Large Hospital-Based Trauma Registry. J Urol. 2022 May;207(5):1077–1085. doi: 10.1097/JU.0000000000002424. Epub 2022 Jan 4. PMID: 34981946.

10. Bjurlin MA, Jeng EI, Goble SM, et al. Comparison of non-operative management with renorrhaphy and nephrectomy in penetrating renal injuries. J Trauma. 2011;71: 554–558.

11. Breyer BN, McAninch JW, Elliott SP, et al. Minimally invasive endovascular techniques to treat acute renal hemorrhage. J Urol. 2008;179:2248–2253.

12. Brewer ME, Strnad BT, Daley BJ, et al. Percutaneous embolization for the management of grade 5 renal trauma in hemodynamically unstable patients: Initial experience. J Urol. 2009;181:1737–1741.

13. Liguori G, Rebez G, Larcher A, Rizzo M, Cai T, Trombetta C, Salonia A. The role of angioembolization in the management of blunt renal injuries: a systematic review. BMC Urol. 2021 Aug 6;21(1):104. DOI: 10.1186/s12894-021-00873-w. PMID: 34362352; PMCID: PMC8344199.

14. Alsikafi NF, McAninch JW, Elliott SP, Garcia M. Nonoperative management outcomes of isolated urinary extravasation following renal lacerations due to external trauma. J Urol. December 2006;176(6 Pt 1):2494–2497.

15. Shoobridge JJ, Corcoran NM, Martin KA, Koukounaras J, Royce PL, Bultitude MF. Contemporary management of renal trauma. Rev Urol. 2011;13(2):65–72.

16. Elliott SP, McAninch JW. Ureteral injuries from external violence: The 25-year experience at San Francisco General Hospital. J Urol. 2003;170:1213–1216.

17. Brandes S, Coburn M, Armenakas N, et al. Diagnosis and management of ureteric injury: An evidence-based analysis. BJU Int. 2004;94:277–289.

18. Carver BS, Bozeman CB, Venable DD. Ureteral injury due to penetrating trauma. South Med J. 2004;97:462–464.

19. Ortega SJ, Netto FS, Hamilton P, et al. CT scanning for diagnosing blunt ureteral and ureteropelvic junction injuries. BMC Urol. 2008;8:1–5.

20. Digiacomo JC, Frankel H, Rotondo MF, et al. Preoperative radiographic staging for ureteral injuries is not warranted in patients undergoing celiotomy for trauma. Am Surg. 2001;67:969–973.

21. Kunkle DA, Kansas BT, Pathak A, et al. Delayed diagnosis of traumatic ureteral injuries. J Urol. 2006;176(Pt 1): 2503–2507.

22. Best CD, Petrone P, Buscarini M, et al. Traumatic ureteral injuries: A single institution experience validating the American Association for the Surgery of TraumaOrgan Injury Scale grading scale. J Urol. 2005;173: 1202–1205.

23. Ku JH, Kim ME, Jeon YS, et al. Minimally invasive management of ureteral injuries Recognized later after obstetric and gynecologic surgery. Injury. 2003;34: 480–483.

24. Danuser H, Wille S, Zöscher G, Studer U. How to treat blunt kidney ruptures: Primary open surgery or conservative treatment with deferred surgery when necessary? Eur Urol. 2001;39:9–14.

25. Gomez RG, Ceballos L, Coburn M, et al. Consensus statement on bladder injuries. BJU Int. 2004;94:2732.

26. Morey AF, Iverson AJ, Swan A, et al. Bladder rupture after blunt trauma: Guidelines for diagnostic imaging. J Trauma. 2001;51:683–686.

27. Avey G, Blackmore CC, Wessells H, et al. Radiographic and clinical predictors of bladder rupture in blunt trauma patients with pelvic fracture. Acad Radiol. 2006;13:573–579.

28. Inaba K, McKenney M, Munera F, et al. Cystogram follow-up in the management of traumatic bladder disruption. J Trauma. 2006;60:23–28.

29. Corriere JN, Sandler CM. Management of the ruptured bladder: Seven years of experience with 111 cases. J Trauma. 1986;26:830–833.

30. Volpe MA, Pachter EM, Scalea TM, et al. Is there a difference in outcome when treating traumatic intraperitoneal bladder rupture with or without a suprapubic tube? J Urol. 1999;161:1103–1105.

31. Alli MO, Singh B, Moodley J, et al. Prospective evaluation of combined suprapubic and urethral catheterization to urethral drainage alone for intraperitoneal bladder injuries. J Trauma. 2003;55:1152–1154.

32. Elgammal MA. Straddle injuries to the bulbar urethra: Management and outcome in 53 patients. Int Braz J Urol. 2009;34:450–458.

33. Peng X, Guo H, Zhang X, Wang J. Straddle injuries to the bulbar urethra: What is the best choice for immediate management? J Trauma Acute Care Surg. 2019 Oct;87(4):892–897. doi: 10.1097/TA.0000000000002388. PMID: 31205218.

34. Park S, McAninch JW. Straddle injuries to the bulbar urethra: Management and outcomes in 78 patients. J Urol. 2004;171:722–725.

35. Ku JH, Kim ME, Jeon YS, et al. Management of bulbous urethral disruption by blunt external trauma: The sooner, the better? Urology. 2002;60:579–583.

36. Gong IH, Oh JJ, Choi DK, et al. Comparison of immediate primary repair and delayed urethroplasty in men with bulbous urethral disruption after blunt straddle injury. Kor J Urol. 2012;53:569–572.

37. Mouraview V, Coburn M, Santucci R. The treatment of posterior urethral disruption associated with pelvic fractures: Comparative experience of early realignment versus delayed urethroplasty. J Urol. 2005;173:873–876.

38. Phonsombat S, Master VA, McAninch JW. Penetrating external genital trauma: A 30-year single institution experience. J Urol. 2008;180:192–196.

39. Kunkle DA, Leed BD, Mydlo JH, et al. Evaluation and management of gunshot wounds of the penis: 20-year experience at an urban trauma center. J Trauma. 2008;64:1038–1042.

40. Koifman L, Barros R, Junior R, et al. Penile fracture: Diagnosis, treatment, and outcomes of 150 patients. Urology. 2010;76:1488–1492.

41. Zargooshi J. Penile fracture in Kermanshah, Iran: The long-term results of surgical treatment. BJU Int. 2002;89: 890–894.

42. Gamal WM, Osman MM, Hammady AH, et al. Penile fracture: Long-term results of surgical and conservative management. J Trauma. 2011;71:491–493.

43. El Atat R, Sfaxi M, Benslama MR, et al. Fracture of the penis: Management and long-term results of surgical treatment. Experience in 300 cases. J Trauma. 2008;64:121–125.

44. Mydlo JH. Surgeon experience with penile fracture. J Urol. 2001;166:526–529.

45. El-Assmy A, El-Tholoth HJ, Mohsen T, et al. Does timing of presentation of penile fracture affect outcome of surgical intervention? Urology. 2011;77:1388–1392.

37

Ileus and Small Bowel Obstruction

Vishal Kumar and John Hong

37.1 Postoperative Ileus

37.1.1 Introduction

Dysregulation of normal bowel movements in absence of obstruction is called ileus. It can be normal (physiologic) postoperative ileus that lasts for less than 3 days after any surgery or prolonged (paralytic) postoperative ileus which lasts greater than 3 days. The physiologic postoperative ileus is secondary to colonic dysmotility, as the colon is the last organ to recover (takes 48–72 hours), while the small bowel is the first to recover (takes 0–24 hours), and the paralytic ileus is secondary to small bowel dysmotility [1]. Symptoms of ileus include nausea, vomiting, inability to tolerate any oral intake, abdominal distension, abdominal pain, and obstipation. Physical exam findings include diffuse tympanic percussion, mild tenderness, and reduction of bowel sounds.

Any event that affects gastrointestinal motility can cause prolonged ileus, which can be surgical and nonsurgical. Risk factors for prolonged ileus include prolonged abdominal or pelvic surgery, open surgery, perioperative complications (abscess, leaks), peritonitis, sepsis, routine nasogastric tube (NGT) placements, delayed enteral nutrition, perioperative transfusion, aggressive resuscitation, electrolyte derangements, and opioid use [2–7]. Ileus is diagnosed clinically based on signs, symptoms, and duration. However, imaging can be performed to rule out other differential diagnoses. Plain abdominal radiographs are first obtained which show dilated loops of the bowel with air in the rectum and without any transition point. If the clinical picture is still unclear, the next step is to perform a computed tomography of the abdomen with oral contrast if possible, as it will distinguish ileus from a complete small bowel obstruction (SBO). The next study to perform may be upper gastrointestinal (GI) contrast study (enteroclysis) with water-soluble radio-opaque contrast material (e.g., Gastrografin) if the diagnosis is still in question. It is particularly useful for distinguishing the ileus from a partial SBO.

Management of ileus is conservative and supportive and includes correcting electrolytes, definitive source control of infection, starting the patient on a multimodal pain regimen, nutritional support, bowel rest, bowel decompression when excess vomiting is present, and serial abdominal exams. Resolution of ileus is assessed with a tolerance of diet; the passage of flatus/stool; return of bowel sounds; and decrease in nausea, vomiting, distension, and NGT output.

37.1.1.1 Does Epidural Block or Transversus Abdominis Plane Block Shorten the Duration of the Ileus?

Epidural catheter blocks are intended to block nociceptive spinal sensory afferents and sympathetic efferent outflow; they are placed at the mid-thoracic level to block nociceptive afferent signals. Guay et al. performed a database search where they included 128 trials with 8,754 participants in the review and 94 trials with 5,846 participants in the analysis comparing epidural local anesthetics with opioid-based regimens for adults undergoing abdominal surgery. They found an epidural containing a local anesthetic, with or without the addition of an opioid, accelerated the return of gastrointestinal transit by 17 hours (high quality of evidence). An epidural containing a local anesthetic with an opioid decreased pain after open and laparoscopic abdominal surgery (moderate quality of evidence), while for open surgery, an epidural containing a local anesthetic reduced the length of hospital stay (very low quality of evidence) [8]. Since there is a risk of bleeding, infection, and urinary retention with epidural catheters, trials came to compare them with transversus abdominis plane (TAP) blocks. Torgeson et al. performed a prospective randomized controlled trial comparing TAP and epidural blocks; they found that TAP block was associated with a 0.5-day reduction in length of stay (LOS) compared with epidural and a lower risk of urinary retention (15% versus 30%) but a higher risk of nausea and vomiting (33% versus 14%). The time to the first flatus was comparable between the two groups [9]. Another randomized controlled trial by Felling et al. found no significant differences in time to GI recovery, hospital LOS, and postoperative complications between TAP and epidural blocks with increased cost for the epidurals [10]. The choice between two blocks depends on multiple factors, anatomical or patient factors, institutional, and type of surgery. Factors that favor epidural include a long midline open incision (TAP block is most effective in the sub-umbilical region), complex hernia repair (which disrupts the fascial plane and renders TAP blocks less effective), a history of difficult pain control or opiate dependency, and a history of postoperative nausea/vomiting. While factors that favor TAP block include patients on anticoagulation (risk of epidural hematoma with epidurals), less extensive surgery (epidurals may be a hindrance to mobility and early discharge), and history of urinary retention (epidurals can cause urinary retention).

DOI: 10.1201/9781003316800-37

37.1.1.2 Does the Use of Perioperative Lidocaine Infusion Shorten the Duration of Ileus?

Weibel et al. reviewed 68 trials with 4,525 randomized participants and analyzed the effects of perioperative infusion of lidocaine. They found a very low quality of evidence to conclude that lidocaine increases the return of GI function [11]. Another study by Herroeder et al. found that perioperative lidocaine infusion decreased hospital stay and increased GI return [12]. Another study by Swenson et al. found no difference in pain control, hospital stay, and return of bowel function in patients undergoing systemic lidocaine infusion vs. epidural analgesia [13].

37.1.1.3 Does Laparoscopy Shorten the Duration of Ileus?

Schwenk et al. looked at a Cochrane review comparing laparoscopic with open colorectal surgery. They included 25 randomized controlled trials and found operative time was longer in laparoscopic surgery, but intraoperative blood loss was less than in conventional surgery. Laparoscopy also accelerated the passage of flatus or bowel movement by 0.9–1 day, which contributed to a 1.5-day shorter hospital stay compared with open surgery [14].

37.1.1.4 Does the Use of Selective Opiate Receptor Inhibitors Decrease the Duration of the Ileus?

Opioids worsen postoperative ileus through the activation of mu-opioid receptors. Taguchi et al. studied the effects of an investigational opioid antagonist with limited oral absorption that does not readily cross the blood–brain barrier on postoperative GI function and the length of hospitalization and found that it speeds recovery of bowel function and shortens the duration of hospitalization without compromising the analgesic effect of opioids [15]. Alvimopan is an oral peripherally acting mu-opioid receptor antagonist that is approved by the U.S. Food and Drug Administration (FDA) to treat postoperative ileus. Steele et al. performed a database propensity-score matched cohort study that included 18,559 patients undergoing bowel resection (BR) and found that the mean postoperative LOS was 4.62 days in alvimopan-treated patients compared with 5.24 days in control subjects ($p < 0.001$). Alvimopan-treated patients had lower rates of postoperative GI complication (12.15% vs. 16.50%; $p < 0.001$). The rates of urinary tract infections; other postoperative infections; and cardiovascular (CV), pulmonary, thromboembolic, and cerebrovascular events were also lower compared with the control subjects [16]. Several studies showed that alvimopan is associated with early bowel recovery after different surgeries.

Delaney et al. performed a retrospective matched-cohort study using a national inpatient database comparing in-hospital clinical outcomes after open and laparoscopic BR with or without alvimopan treatment. Each cohort included >3,500 patients with similar baseline characteristics. The alvimopan group had a lower incidence of mortality (0.4% vs. 1%), morbidities (i.e., GI, CV, pulmonary, infectious, thromboembolic), mean intensive care unit (ICU) stay (0.3 vs. 0.6 days), postoperative LOS (–1.1 days for all, –0.8 days for laparoscopic, and –1.8 days for open) and estimated direct costs (–$2,345 for all, –$1,382 for laparoscopic, and –$3,218 for open) compared to the non-alvimopan group [17].

Wolff et al. prospectively randomized 510 patients undergoing BR or radical hysterectomy to receive either alvimopan or placebo and demonstrated that the time to GI recovery was improved by 15–20 hours following doses of 6 mg and 22–28 hours following doses of 12 mg of alvimopan. The mean time to hospital discharge was 13 and 20 hours sooner for patients treated with the 6- or 12-mg doses, respectively [18]. Subsequently, Delaney et al. performed a pooled retrospective subset analysis of bowel resection patients in alvimopan phase III trials, where they randomized BR patients into the ones who received alvimopan 6 mg ($n = 397$), 12 mg ($n = 413$), or placebo ($n = 402$) ≥2 hours before surgery and twice daily until hospital discharge for ≤7 days. The primary endpoint of each trial was time to recovery of GI function. They found that alvimopan significantly accelerated GI recovery in BR patients with a decrease in postoperative morbidity rates, prolonged hospital stay, and rates of hospital readmission [19]. Despite the statistically significant improvement in recovery from postoperative ileus, the 13- to 20-hour improvement may not represent a clinically meaningful metric.

37.1.1.5 Do Prokinetics or Gastrografin Decrease the Duration of the Ileus?

Traut et al. performed an analysis of 39 randomized controlled trials with more than 4,500 patients and found that there is insufficient evidence to recommend the use of prokinetics (cholecystokinin-like drugs, erythromycin cisapride, dopamine antagonists, propranolol, or vasopressin) in reducing the duration of ileus [20]. Another study also showed no benefit of neostigmine on recovery from ileus [21]. A double-blinded, placebo-controlled, randomized trial by Vather et al. found no effect of Gastrografin on the duration of postoperative ileus [22].

RECOMMENDATION

Neither prokinetics nor Gastrografin affect the duration of ileus.

Grade of recommendation: A.

37.1.1.6 Does the Aggressive Fluid Resuscitation Increase the Duration of Ileus?

Corcoran et al. performed a meta-analysis that included about 5,000 patients from 35 randomized controlled trials comparing liberal vs. goal-directed fluid therapy and found an association between liberal fluid therapy and increased time to first bowel movement (2 days, 95% confidence interval [CI] 1.3–2.3) as well as prolonged duration of hospital stay (4 days, 95% CI 3.4–4.4) compared with restricted fluid therapy [23].

RECOMMENDATION

Goal-directed resuscitation decreases the duration of ileus and the hospital LOS.

Grade of recommendation: B.

37.1.1.7 Does Chewing Gum Shorten the Duration of Ileus?

Based on the evidence that early enteral feedings lessened the extent of ileus, Asao et al. examined the effect of gum chewing as an alternative approach to stimulate bowel function in the postoperative period. Gum is theorized to increase vagal tone, normally provided by food, and to stimulate the release of GI hormones associated with bowel motility. Their data showed an earlier return of bowel function in a small series of 19 patients who underwent laparoscopic colon resection for cancer who were prospectively randomized to either a gum-chewing or a control group. The first passage of flatus was about 24 hours sooner and the first defecation was approximately 2.7 days sooner in the gum-chewing group than in controls [24]. Short et al. performed a Cochrane review of 81 randomized trials with over 9,000 patients and found that chewing gum reduced time to flatus by 12.5 hours, time to

bowel movement by 18.1 hours, and length of hospital stay by 1 day compared with conventional postoperative care [25].

RECOMMENDATION

Gum chewing is a relatively inexpensive and safe intervention that can shorten the duration of ileus and hospital LOS in postoperative patients.

Grade of recommendation: B.

37.2 Intraabdominal Adhesions

37.2.1 Introduction

After any injury to endothelium or epithelium, scar forms, and adhesions are scars after peritoneal injury, i.e., violation, trauma, and surgery. They are common after abdominal surgery as an inflammatory response is provoked leading to activation of the coagulation cascade and fibrin deposition while simultaneously decreasing fibrinolytic activity by increasing levels of plasminogen activator inhibitors and reducing tissue oxygenation. This sequence of events leads to a fibrin gel matrix that may serve as the scaffolding for the development of mature adhesions. Adhesions contain inflammatory cells that include fibroblasts, macrophages, mast cells, eosinophils, red blood cells, and tissue debris. Over time the numbers of cells decrease and adhesions mature into fibrous bands composed of collagen and covered by mesothelium [26]. The most common cause of mechanical SBO in the western world is intraperitoneal adhesions, tumors, and complicated hernias [27]. Seventy percent of SBO cases in developed countries is caused by adhesions, and 80% of patients with adhesive SBO have a history of prior intraabdominal surgery [28].

Postoperative adhesions not only cause SBO but also increased operating time, inadvertent enterotomy, intraoperative bleeding, trocar injury, conversion from laparoscopy to laparotomy, surgical site infection, prolonged length of hospital stay, and chronic abdominal and pelvic pain [29]. Adhesion-related SBO requiring surgical treatment has a 33% risk of inadvertent enterotomy, and the presence of adhesions has a 19% risk of inadvertent enterotomy during a reoperative laparotomy [30]. Reviews of hospital admissions for adhesional SBO have identified a mortality rate of almost 10% [31], with the rate increasing to approximately 15% in patients undergoing small bowel resection [32]. There is also a 20–50% mortality rate in those patients who have an undetected bowel injury when undergoing an operation for adhesional SBO [31].

37.2.1.1 Which Is More Advantageous: Open or Laparoscopic Adhesiolysis?

SBO requiring adhesiolysis is a frequent problem in the United States resulting in increased morbidity, complication, and LOS. Open adhesiolysis has long been the established operation of choice. With the advent of laparoscopy, there has been a debate as to whether it provides a benefit when compared to open adhesiolysis. In a comparative analysis performed by Kelly,

9,619 patients with SBO were analyzed in which 14.9% of patients were performed laparoscopically. Patients undergoing laparoscopic procedures had shorter mean operative times (77.2 vs. 94.2 minutes) and decreased postoperative LOS (4.7 vs. 9.9 days). After controlling for comorbidities and surgical factors, patients undergoing laparoscopic adhesiolysis were less likely to develop major complications. Therefore, laparoscopic adhesiolysis demonstrated a benefit in 30-day morbidity and mortality [33]. Lombardo et al. compared the outcomes of 6,762 patients who underwent adhesiolysis and stratified patients into laparoscopically versus open laparotomy. They showed that laparoscopy was associated with significantly lower rates of any complications with an odds ratio (OR) of 0.41, including surgical site infections (OR 1.15) and shorter hospital stay (4 vs. 10 days) [34]. Li et al. performed a meta-analysis comparing laparoscopic and open surgery for SBO; they looked at the outcomes of a total of 334 patients enrolled in four retrospective comparative studies and found laparoscopic adhesiolysis was associated with a reduced overall complication rate, prolonged ileus rate, and pulmonary complication rate [35]. Patel et al. performed an analysis of American College of Surgeons National Surgical Quality Improvement Program (ACS NSQIP) data from the year 2005 to 2015; they analyzed over 24,000 patients who underwent surgery for SBO. Propensity matching found over 6,500 patients who underwent emergent surgery for SBO. They found that laparoscopic intervention decreased postoperative mortality, morbidity, and LOS compared to open surgery for the treatment of bowel obstruction with an adjusted OR 3.826 (95% CI 3.012–4.910, $p < 0.0001$) [36]. Of note, however, all of these retrospective reviews suffer from inherent selective bias: Adhesiolysis, when able to be performed laparoscopically, is almost certainly "easier" than those cases starting laparoscopically but requiring conversion to open.

RECOMMENDATION

Performing laparoscopic adhesiolysis in the hands of an experienced surgeon provides improved outcomes compared to those of conventional open adhesiolysis.

Grade of recommendation: B.

37.2.1.2 Should the Sun Set on an SBO?

It's an old saying that now the question of proper timing of operative planning depends on the patient's clinical presentation, which includes the patient's symptoms, radiological findings, and the presence of metabolic derangements, to name a few. If the patient has generalized peritonitis; other evidence of clinical deterioration such as fever, leukocytosis, tachycardia, metabolic acidosis, and continuous pain; or evidence of ischemia on imaging, they should undergo timely exploration once adequately resuscitated [37]. O'Leary et al. performed a retrospective review of 219 patients and found four readily evaluable clinical parameters that may be used to predict the need for early surgery that included persistent abdominal pain, abdominal distention, fever at 48 hours, and CT findings of

high-grade obstruction as factors that were predictive of nonoperative failure [38]. Schraufnagel et al. performed a large retrospective study that included 27,046 patients with SBO of which 4,826 required adhesiolysis. They found that complications, prolonged postoperative LOS, and death were more likely in patients for whom surgery was delayed 4 days or more. Patients on the fourth day or later had a 26% greater risk of staying more than 7 days postoperatively [39].

RECOMMENDATION

In the absence of hard signs such as intraabdominal sepsis, peritonitis, and strangulation, a patient can be observed with a complete SBO. There appears to be an increased risk of complications, LOS, and death in patients with complete SBO whose surgery is delayed by 4 or more days.

Grade of recommendation: A.

37.2.1.3 Should Patients with SBO in the Setting of a Virgin Abdomen Undergo Early Intervention?

The majority of SBOs are the result of adhesions caused by previous abdominal surgeries. Other causes of SBO include congenital bands, internal hernias, and malignancies. The thought of missing a malignant disease resulting in SBO prompted surgeons to approach SBO in the virgin abdomen (VA) more aggressively. Choi et al. performed a meta-analysis of six studies including 442 patients with SBO in the absence of prior abdominopelvic surgery; >50% of the patients underwent a trial of nonoperative management, which often failed. The most common etiology was de novo adhesion (54%), whereas malignancy was found in 7.7–13.4% of patients, most not suspected before surgery. However, if nonoperative management is successful, the prognosis is good [40]. Amara et al. reviewed seven original studies that included SBO in VA and found that adhesions were found to be the cause of the obstruction in approximately half of the reported cases of SBO in VA. A relatively high number of cases of SBO-VA were managed surgically, with studies reporting 39–83%. However, in cases where a trial of nonoperative management was started, this was generally successful [41]. Yvonne et al. performed a retrospective analysis of 72 patients presenting with SBO in VA and concluded that adhesions were the most common cause despite the absence of previous abdominopelvic surgery [42].

RECOMMENDATION

In the absence of aberrant laboratory values, evidence of strangulation, or intraabdominal sepsis, it appears safe to offer a trial of nonoperative management to patients with no previous history of intraabdominal surgery or a VA.

Grade of recommendation: B.

37.2.1.4 Are There Any Techniques/Agents that Have Been Shown to Decrease Intraabdominal Adhesion Formation Following Laparotomy?

Technical (minimizing injury), physical (introducing barriers between injured surfaces), and pharmacological methods can be used to decrease adhesion formation following surgery.

A variety of technical methods are used to minimize the formation of postoperative adhesions. One of the key surgical technical aspects is to reduce the amount of surgical trauma. Using electrocautery close to the bowel will cause adjacent tissue necrosis and contribute to robust adhesion formation as compared to sharp mechanical transection. The presence of foreign material that arises from gauze; sponges; starch powder; suture; and debris from surgical drapes, gowns, masks, and many other items can elicit a peritoneal inflammation and be found in postoperative adhesions, demonstrating a causal relationship between the presence of foreign material and formation of adhesions [43]. Kapustian et al. performed a prospective randomized trial of 533 patients undergoing primary cesarean sections. The peritoneum was left open in 256 patients, while 277 patients had closure of the peritoneum; subsequently, 50 in the nonclosure group and 47 in the closure group were analyzed at a repeat cesarean section, and they found that the nonclosure and closure groups were comparable in terms of the proportion of patients with adhesions at any site (60% vs. 51% $P = 0.31$). They concluded that closure or nonclosure of the peritoneum at cesarean section did not lead to large differences in the adhesion rate [44]. Closure of the peritoneum layer does not necessarily lead to an improved outcome overall. Closure of the fascia as a single layer, as opposed to the peritoneum as a separate layer, offered no difference in wound complications or dehiscence. Nonclosure of the peritoneum is safer, allowing the underlying viscera to remain under direct visualization during the closure and reducing operative time.

Krielen et al. performed a retrospective cohort study from 2009 to 2011 in which >50,000 patients underwent open abdominal or pelvic surgery and >21,000 patients underwent laparoscopic surgery. They followed the patients until 2017 and found that the laparoscopic approach was associated with a lower incidence of readmissions directly related to adhesions (1.7% versus 4.3%; $p < 0.0001$) [45]. This shows that laparoscopic surgery doesn't prevent adhesions but at least has less risk compared to open surgery.

There has been substantial investigation targeting a variety of mechanisms involved in adhesion formation. Use of nonsteroidal antiinflammatory drugs (NSAIDs), corticosteroids, anticoagulants like heparin, and low molecular weight heparin (LMWH) have reported success in preventing postoperative adhesions in animal studies; similar results in humans are lacking.

Barrier devices aim at keeping the damaged peritoneal surfaces separated for at least 5–7 days until re-epithelialization happens, thus ideally leading to decreased adhesion formations. A barrier ideally should provide unrestricted coverage of the affected peritoneum. Various forms of barriers include polymer solutions and solid membranes of polysaccharides such as hyaluronic acid, cellulose, dextran, or chitosan. Various barriers currently FDA-approved include regenerated cellulose (Interceed), expanded polytetrafluoroethylene (Preclude), hyaluronic acid–carboxymethylcellulose (Seprafilm), polylactide membrane (Surgiwrap), and icodextrin solution (Adept). Seprafilm is a nontoxic, nonimmunogenic, biocompatible material that was designed to reduce postoperative abdominal adhesion formation. It turns into a hydrophilic gel in approximately 24 hours after placement and provides a protective coating around traumatized tissues for up to 7 days during remesothelialization. Fazio et al. performed a prospective, randomized, multicenter, multinational, single-blind, controlled study and found that the incidence of overall bowel obstruction was unchanged in patients whether they receive Seprafilm or not; however, the incidence of adhesive SBO requiring reoperation was significantly lower for Seprafilm patients compared with no-treatment patients (1.8% vs. 3.4%, $P < 0.05$) [46]. Robb et al. performed a systematic review of 5 different antiadhesives in 24 studies with 17 being randomized and the rest being nonrandomized. They found that a hyaluronic acid/carboxymethylcellulose membrane reduces the incidence, extent, and severity of adhesions but without strong evidence of prevention of bowel obstruction. They are safe but should not be placed in close contact with a new anastomosis due to the higher frequency of anastomotic leaks (4% vs. 2%) [47].

RECOMMENDATION

A variety of methods can be used to decrease the formation of postoperative abdominal adhesions, such as utilizing sharp dissection and minimizing tissue trauma, reducing the amount of foreign body contamination within the surgical field, and employing minimally invasive surgical techniques if indicated. The use of barriers between the peritoneal layers seems logical; however, the improvement in postoperative adhesion formation observed has shown no impact on the rate of postoperative SBO.

Grade of recommendation: B.

37.3 Adhesional SBO

37.3.1 Introduction

As previously stated, the most common cause of SBO in the western world is scar tissue. If there are no warning signs as previously mentioned, SBO can undergo a trial of nonoperative management; however, the sepsis that results from bowel necrosis and perforation secondary to the strangulation is a devastating complication from adhesional SBO. Keenan et al. retrospectively studied the effect of incremental delays in surgery on the 30-day postoperative outcomes of patients undergoing surgery for uncomplicated adhesive SBO. Of the 9,297 patients included in the analysis, 46% received their operation after 3 days of hospitalization, while 22.5% received operation after 5 days. The 30-day postoperative mortality and overall morbidities were 4.4% and 29.6% respectively.

Preoperative length of hospital stay of 3 or more days was associated with a higher risk of 30-day postoperative morbidity with a greater length of postoperative management for adhesive SBO [48].

37.3.2 Diagnosis of SBO

37.3.2.1 What Does the Use of Water-Soluble Contrast Do?

Gastrografin (diatrizoate meglumine-diatrizoate sodium) is the most commonly used water-soluble contrast medium for the treatment of adhesive SBO. Each 100 mL of Gastrografin solution contains 10 g of sodium diatrizoate and 66 g of meglumine diatrizoate with an osmolarity of 2,150 mOsm/L (six times the osmolarity of extracellular fluid). Gastrografin acts by causing a movement of water into the bowel lumen via osmosis, decreasing the edema of the bowel wall that contributes to proximal bowel distension, leading to an increase in the pressure gradient across an obstructing region [49].

37.3.2.2 Is the Early Use of Water-Soluble Contrast Indicated in the Diagnosis/ Management of SBO?

Abbas et al. performed a meta-analysis of 10 studies and found that the presence of Gastrografin in the colon at 24 hours on x-ray has 97% sensitivity and 96% specificity in determining the resolution of adhesive SBO. It also showed that water-soluble contrast decreased the length of stay by 1.83 days but did not reduce the need for surgical intervention (OR 0.81, 95% CI 0.54–1.21) [50]. There have been multiple studies that demonstrate the utility of water-soluble contrast in accelerating the resolution of nonoperative SBOs without affecting the resolution rates of the SBOs that will eventually require surgery. However, it decreases hospital stay by increasing the resolution rate of nonoperative SBOs as well as pointing surgeons to intervene early in the SBOs that failed Gastrografin. It is important with any discussion of SBO to differentiate between partial and complete obstructions, as evidenced by clinical signs (e.g., ongoing flatus versus complete obstipation) or radiography (e.g., the presence of "distal" gas on kidney, ureters, bladder [KUB] or CT). Partial obstructions are much more likely to be successfully managed nonoperatively.

RECOMMENDATION

In the absence of alarming signs to operate emergently, the use of Gastrografin may be helpful to differentiate between obstructions that may resolve without surgical intervention versus those that require laparotomy and will not benefit from nonoperative observation. (Of note, the use of a high-osmolarity oral solvent such as Gastrografin, if aspirated, results in severe pneumonitis, which is of significant concern in elderly or other patients who may be more at risk of aspiration.)

Grade of recommendation: B.

37.3.2.3 Can CT Predict the Need for Operation in Patients with Incomplete or Partial SBO?

Abdominal radiographs can appear normal in patients with SBO and miss complete obstruction, closed-loop obstruction, and strangulated obstruction [51]. Plain abdominal radiographs have proven to be diagnostic of SBO in only 67–80% of patients [52]. CT scan has had a well-established role in the diagnosis of SBO since the first large published series showing its utility and efficacy [53]. CT findings of SBO include distended bowel loops proximal to collapsed loops, air–fluid levels, and a possible transition point. CT can also help delineate partial vs. complete obstruction [54]. Studies have since proved the value of CT in confirming the diagnosis and revealing the cause of SBO, with a sensitivity of 94–100% and an accuracy of 90–95% [55]. Further reviews have shown that CT is highly accurate for diagnosing ischemic bowel with a sensitivity of 83%, specificity of 92%, positive predictive value of 79%, and negative predictive value of 93% [56]. Many CT findings can point to strangulation, like high attenuation of the bowel wall, pneumatosis, hemorrhagic changes in the mesentery, gas in the portal vein, and poor or no enhancement of the bowel wall (the "target sign"), and engorgement of the mesenteric vasculature and mesenteric edema. Perhaps the most valuable information an abdominal CT scan can provide is more definitive differentiation between complete versus partial obstruction, as noted by the absence of gas in the colon. A study by Ha et al. found that the use of five highly specific findings, including poor enhancement of the bowel wall, a serrated beak, diffuse engorgement of mesenteric vasculature, an unusual course of mesenteric vasculature, and a large number of ascites, correctly identified 85% of patients with a strangulated SBO [57]. Scrima et al. performed a study of 179 patients with suspected SBO and found that CT findings were better predictors for surgical intervention compared to laboratory and clinical values [58].

RECOMMENDATION

If there is no free air on the x-ray that will require an emergent operation, the use of CT with IV contrast, if not contraindicated, can help with the diagnosis of obstruction, especially looking at the transition point, signs of strangulation, and the possible need for surgery.

Grade of recommendation: B.

37.3.2.4 Is There Any Difference between Stapled, Compression, or Hand-Sewn Techniques for Bowel Anastomosis?

Steger et al. performed a meta-analysis of 26 articles and concluded that all the techniques are more or less the same in terms of leakage, reoperation, mortality rates, tendency to cause bleeding, wound infections, abscesses, anastomotic hemorrhages, pulmonary embolisms, and fistulas. But the hand-suture technique has only a statistically significant superior outcome over stapling anastomoses concerning the occurrence of obstructions/strictures [59]. In the SHAPES study performed by Bruns et al. 595 patients from 15 institutions were prospectively analyzed. These patients underwent emergent bowel resection due to emergent pathology. This study found that emergency general surgery patients are already at higher risk of anastomotic failure; that's why there is no difference in leak rate between hand-sewn and stapled anastomosis [60]. In the absence of truly randomized prospective data, however, stapled anastomoses should not be attempted for highly edematous, inflamed, or friable bowel.

RECOMMENDATION

All anastomoses are the same in terms of complications; however, when making a stapled anastomosis, one has to be cautious not to narrow the lumen.

Grade of recommendation: B.

TABLE 37.1

Chapter Questions Followed by Level of Evidence and Selected References

Question	Answer	Grade	References
Does epidural block or transversus abdominis plane (TAP) block shorten the duration of the ileus?	Yes	B	[8–10]
Does the use of perioperative lidocaine infusion shorten the duration of ileus?	Yes	C	[11–13]
Does laparoscopy shorten the duration of ileus?	Yes	B	[14]
Does the use of selective opiate receptor inhibitors decrease the duration of postoperative ileus?	Yes	B	[15–19]
Do prokinetics/Gastrografin decrease the duration of ileus?	No	A	[20–22]
Does aggressive fluid resuscitation increase the duration of ileus?	Yes	B	[23]
Does chewing gum shorten the duration of postoperative ileus?	Yes	B	[24, 25]
Which is more advantageous: Open or laparoscopic adhesiolysis?	Performing laparoscopic adhesiolysis in the hands of an experienced surgeon provides improved outcomes compared to those of conventional open adhesiolysis.	B	[33–36]
Should the sun set on an SBO?	In the absence of hard signs such as intraabdominal sepsis, peritoneal examination findings, and strangulation, it is safe to say that there is an increased risk of complications, LOS, and death in patients whose surgery is delayed by 4 or more days.	A	[37–39]
Should patients with SBO in the setting of a virgin abdomen be intervened on sooner?	In the absence of aberrant laboratory values, strangulation, and intraabdominal sepsis, it is safe to offer a trial of nonoperative management to patients with no previous history of intraabdominal surgery or virgin abdomen.	B	[40–42]
Are there any techniques/agents that have been shown to decrease intraabdominal adhesion formation following laparotomy?	A variety of methods can be used to decrease the formation of postoperative abdominal adhesions, such as utilizing sharp dissection and minimizing tissue trauma, reducing the amount of foreign body contamination within the surgical field, and employing minimally invasive surgical techniques if indicated. The use of barriers between the peritoneal layers seems logical; however, the improvement in postoperative adhesion formation observed has shown no impact on the rate of postoperative SBO.	B	[43–47]
What does the use of water-soluble contrast do?	Gastrografin creates an osmotic gradient by influxing the fluid in the lumen and then creating a pressure gradient.	C	[49]
Is the early use of water-soluble contrast indicated in the diagnosis/management of SBO?	In the absence of alarming signs to operate emergently, a trial of Gastrografin will help to resolve the nonoperative SBO quickly or will give the insight to operate early on SBOs that fail Gastrografin.	B	[50]
Can CT predict the need for operation in patients with incomplete SBO?	If there is no free air on the x-ray that will require an emergent operation, the use of CT with IV contrast, if not contraindicated, can help with the diagnosis of obstruction, especially looking at the transition point, signs of strangulation, and the possible need for surgery.	B	[51–58]
Is there any difference between stapled or hand-sewn techniques for bowel anastomosis?	All anastomoses are the same in terms of complications; however, when making a stapled anastomosis, one has to be cautious not to narrow the lumen.	B	[59, 60]

Editor's Note

This chapter elegantly explores a treacherous area of great controversy in general surgery: The management of small bowel obstruction. There is a dearth of high-quality evidence to support our current protocols. There is little argument that an abdominal CT scan is an ideal method of diagnosing SBO, sometimes identifying the etiology (mass, hernia, foreign body) and differentiating complete from partial obstruction (air in the colon). Signs of mesenteric ischemia can be very subtle clinically and may be absent on imaging. Therefore, the surgeon is vigilant regarding observation of the patient with partial SBO (complete SBOs typically are explored early unless there are mitigating circumstances such as inflammatory bowel disease, carcinomatosis, or radiation). About 15% of partial SBO patients require operative intervention, which typically occurs after deterioration or failure to improve following a 48- to 72-hour trial of observation. The benefit of the "Gastrografin challenge" is questionable, as the supportive data utilize highly subjective endpoints (i.e., time to flatus) in nonblinded trials. The clinician must understand the potential risks of severe pneumonitis that may result from aspiration of hyperosmotic contrast agents in patients with intestinal obstruction. The usual cause of SBO, adhesions, can be often managed by laparoscopic surgery. The number and extent of prior operations, the ability of the patient to tolerate insufflation and a potentially longer procedure, and the skill of the operating surgeon are certainly important factors in selecting the operative technique. Finally, it is essential to mention concerns regarding the use of stapled anastomoses in highly edematous bowel. This practice should be condemned in my opinion.

REFERENCES

1. Livingston EH, Passaro EP. Postoperative ileus. Dig Dis Sci. 1990;35(1):121–132. doi:10.1007/bf01537233.
2. Nelson R, Edwards S, Tse B. Prophylactic nasogastric decompression after abdominal surgery. Cochrane Database Syst Rev. 2005 Jan 25;(1):CD004929. doi: 10.1002/14651858. CD004929.pub2. Update in: Cochrane Database Syst Rev. 2007;(3): CD004929. PMID: 15674971.
3. Inman BA, Harel F, Tiguert R, Lacombe L, Fradet Y. Routine nasogastric tubes are not required following cystectomy with a urinary diversion: A comparative analysis of 430 patients. J Urol. 2003 Nov;170(5):1888–1891. doi: 10.1097/01.ju.0000092500.68655.48. PMID: 14532800.
4. Porpiglia F, Renard J, Billia M, Scoffone C, Cracco C, Terrone C, Scarpa RM. Open versus laparoscopy-assisted radical cystectomy: Results of a prospective study. J Endourol. 2007 Mar;21(3):325–329. doi: 10.1089/end.2006.0224. PMID: 17444780.
5. Chapuis PH, Bokey L, Keshava A, Rickard MJ, Stewart P, Young CJ, Dent OF. Risk factors for prolonged ileus after resection of colorectal cancer: An observational study of 2400 consecutive patients. Ann Surg. 2013 May;257(5): 909–915. doi: 10.1097/SLA.0b013e318268a693. PMID: 23579542.
6. Böhm B, Milsom JW, Fazio VW. Postoperative intestinal motility following conventional and laparoscopic intestinal surgery. Arch Surg. 1995 Apr;130(4):415–419. doi: 10.1001/archsurg.1995.01430040077017. PMID: 7710343.
7. Artinyan A, Nunoo-Mensah JW, Balasubramaniam S, Gauderman J, Essani R, Gonzalez-Ruiz C, Kaiser AM, Beart RW Jr. Prolonged postoperative ileus-definition, risk factors, and predictors after surgery. World J Surg. 2008 Jul;32(7):1495–1500. doi: 10.1007/s00268-008-9491-2. PMID: 18305994.
8. Guay J, Nishimori M, Kopp S. Epidural local anaesthetics versus opioid-based analgesic regimens for postoperative gastrointestinal paralysis, vomiting and pain after abdominal surgery. Cochrane Database Syst Rev. 2016 Jul 16;7(7):CD001893. doi: 10.1002/14651858.CD001893.pub2. PMID: 27419911; PMCID: PMC6457860.
9. Torgeson M, Kileny J, Pfeifer C, Narkiewicz L, Obi S. Conventional epidural vs transversus abdominis plane block with liposomal bupivacaine: A randomized trial in colorectal surgery. J Am Coll Surg. 2018 Jul;227(1):78–83. doi: 10.1016/j.jamcollsurg.2018.04.021. Epub 2018 May 1. PMID: 29723578.
10. Felling DR, Jackson MW, Ferraro J, Battaglia MA, Albright JJ, Wu J, Genord CK, Brockhaus KK, Bhave RA, McClure AM, Shanker BA, Cleary RK. Liposomal bupivacaine transversus abdominis plane block versus epidural analgesia in a colon and rectal surgery enhanced recovery pathway: A randomized clinical trial. Dis Colon Rectum. 2018 Oct;61(10):1196–1204. doi: 10.1097/DCR.0000000000001211. PMID: 30192328.
11. Weibel S, Jelting Y, Pace NL, Helf A, Eberhart LH, Hahnenkamp K, Hollmann MW, Poepping DM, Schnabel A, Kranke P. Continuous intravenous perioperative lidocaine infusion for postoperative pain and recovery in adults. Cochrane Database Syst Rev. 2018 Jun 4;6(6):CD009642. doi: 10.1002/14651858.CD009642.pub3. PMID: 29864216; PMCID: PMC6513586.
12. Herroeder S, Pecher S, Schönherr ME, Kaulitz G, Hahnenkamp K, Friess H, Böttiger BW, Bauer H, Dijkgraaf MG, Durieux ME, Hollmann MW. Systemic lidocaine shortens the length of hospital stay after colorectal surgery: A double-blinded, randomized, placebo-controlled trial. Ann Surg. 2007 Aug;246(2):192–200. doi: 10.1097/SLA.0b013e31805dac11. Erratum in: Ann Surg. 2009 Apr;249(4):701. Dijkgraaf, Omarcel G W [corrected to Dijkgraaf, Marcel G W]. PMID: 17667496; PMCID: PMC1933564.
13. Swenson BR, Gottschalk A, Wells LT, Rowlingson JC, Thompson PW, Barclay M, Sawyer RG, Friel CM, Foley E, Durieux ME. Intravenous lidocaine is as effective as epidural bupivacaine in reducing ileus duration, hospital stay, and pain after open colon resection: A randomized clinical trial. Reg Anesth Pain Med. 2010 Jul-Aug;35(4): 370–376. doi: 10.1097/AAP.0b013e3181e8d5da. PMID: 20588151.
14. Schwenk W, Haase O, Neudecker J, Müller JM. Short-term benefits for laparoscopic colorectal resection. Cochrane Database Syst Rev. 2005 Jul 20;2005(3):CD003145. doi: 10.1002/14651858.CD003145.pub2. PMID: 16034888; PMCID: PMC8693724.

15. Taguchi A, Sharma N, Saleem RM, Sessler DI, Carpenter RL, Seyedsadr M, Kurz A. Selective postoperative inhibition of gastrointestinal opioid receptors. N Engl J Med. 2001 Sep 27;345(13):935–940. doi: 10.1056/NEJMoa010564. PMID: 11575284.

16. Steele SR, Brady JT, Cao Z, Baumer DL, Robinson SB, Yang HK, Delaney CP. Evaluation of healthcare use and clinical outcomes of alvimopan in patients undergoing bowel resection: A propensity score-matched analysis. Dis Colon Rectum. 2018 Dec;61(12):1418–1425. DOI: 10.1097/DCR.0000000000001181. PMID: 30312222.

17. Delaney CP, Craver C, Gibbons MM, Rachfal AW, VandePol CJ, Cook SF, Poston SA, Calloway M, Techner L. Evaluation of clinical outcomes with alvimopan in clinical practice: A national matched-cohort study in patients undergoing bowel resection. Ann Surg. 2012 Apr;255(4):731–738. doi: 10.1097/SLA.0b013e31824a36cc. PMID: 22388106.

18. Wolff BG, Michelassi F, Gerkin TM, Techner L, Gabriel K, Du W, Wallin BA; Alvimopan Postoperative Ileus Study Group. Alvimopan, a novel, peripherally acting mu opioid antagonist: Results of a multicenter, randomized, double-blind, placebo-controlled, phase III trial of major abdominal surgery and postoperative ileus. Ann Surg. 2004 Oct;240(4):728–734; discussion 734-5. doi: 10.1097/01.sla.0000141158.27977.66. PMID: 15383800; PMCID: PMC1356474.

19. Delaney CP, Wolff BG, Viscusi ER, Senagore AJ, Fort JG, Du W, Techner L, Wallin B. Alvimopan, for postoperative ileus following bowel resection: A pooled analysis of phase III studies. Ann Surg. 2007 Mar;245(3):355–363. doi: 10.1097/01.sla.0000232538.72458.93. PMID: 17435541; PMCID: PMC1877012.

20. Traut U, Brügger L, Kunz R, Pauli-Magnus C, Haug K, Bucher HC, Koller MT. Systemic prokinetic pharmacologic treatment for postoperative adynamic ileus following abdominal surgery in adults. Cochrane Database Syst Rev. 2008 Jan 23;(1):CD004930. doi: 10.1002/14651858.CD004930.pub3. PMID: 18254064.

21. Myrhöj T, Olsen O, Wengel B. Neostigmine in postoperative intestinal paralysis. A double-blind, clinical, controlled trial. Dis Colon Rectum. 1988 May;31(5):378–379. doi: 10.1007/BF02564889. PMID: 3284726.

22. Vather R, Josephson R, Jaung R, Kahokehr A, Sammour T, Bissett I. Gastrografin in Prolonged postoperative ileus: A double-blinded randomized controlled trial. Ann Surg. 2015 Jul;262(1):23–30. doi: 10.1097/SLA.0000000000001062. PMID: 25575258.

23. Corcoran T, Rhodes JE, Clarke S, Myles PS, Ho KM. Perioperative fluid management strategies in major surgery: A stratified meta-analysis. Anesth Analg. 2012 Mar;114(3):640–651. doi: 10.1213/ANE.0b013e318240d6eb. Epub 2012 Jan 16. PMID: 22253274.

24. Asao T, Kuwano H, Nakamura J, et al. Gum chewing enhances early recovery from postoperative ileus after laparoscopic colectomy. J Am Coll Surg. 2002;195:30–32.

25. Short V, Herbert G, Perry R, Atkinson C, Ness AR, Penfold C, Thomas S, Andersen HK, Lewis SJ. Chewing gum for postoperative recovery of gastrointestinal function. Cochrane Database Syst Rev. 2015 Feb 20;(2): CD006506. doi: 10.1002/14651858.CD006506.pub3. PMID: 25914904.

26. Maciver AH, Mc Call M, Shapiro AM. Intra-abdominal adhesions: Cellular mechanism and strategies for prevention. Int J Surg. 2011;9(8):589–594.

27. Miller G, Boman J, Shrier I, Gordon PH. Etiology of small bowel obstruction. Am J Surg. 2000 Jul;180(1):33–36. doi: 10.1016/s0002-9610(00)00407-4. PMID: 11036136.

28. Mullan CP, Siewert B, Eisenberg RL. Small bowel obstruction. AJR Am J Roentgenol. 2012 Feb;198(2):W105–W17. doi: 10.2214/AJR.10.4998. PMID: 22268199.

29. van Goor H. Consequences and complications of peritoneal adhesions. Colorectal Dis. 2007 Oct;9(Suppl 2):25–34. doi: 10.1111/j.1463-1318.2007.01358.x. PMID: 17824967.

30. Van Der Krabben AA, Dijkstra FR, Nieuwenhuijzen M, Reijnen MM, Schaapveld M, Van Goor H. Morbidity and mortality of inadvertent enterotomy during adhesiotomy. Br J Surg. 2000 Apr;87(4):467–471. doi: 10.1046/j.1365-2168.2000.01394.x. PMID: 10759744.

31. Menzies D, Parker M, Hoare R, et al. Small bowel obstruction due to postoperative adhesions: Treatment patterns and associated costs in 110 hospital admissions. Ann R Coll Surg Engl. 2001;83:40–46

32. Wysocki A, Pozniczek M, Kulawik J, et al. Peritoneal adhesions as a cause of small bowel obstruction. Przegl Lek. 2003;60:32–35.

33. Kelly KN 1, Iannuzzi JC, Rickles AS. Laparotomy for small-bowel obstruction: First choice or last resort for adhesiolysis? A laparoscopic approach for small-bowel obstruction reduces 30-day complications. Surg Endosc. 2014 Jan;28(1):65–73.

34. Lombaro S, Baum K, Filho JD. Should adhesive small bowel obstruction be managed laparoscopically? A National Surgical Quality Improvement Program propensity score analysis. J Trauma Acute Care Surg. 2014 Mar;76(3): 696–703.

35. Li MZ, Lian L, Xiao LB, Wu WH, He YL, Song XM. Laparoscopic versus open adhesiolysis in patients with adhesive small bowel obstruction: A systematic review and meta-analysis. Am J Surg. 2012 Nov;204(5):779–786. doi: 10.1016/j.amjsurg.2012.03.005. Epub 2012 Jul 12. PMID: 22794708.

36. Patel R, Borad NP, Merchant AM. Comparison of outcomes following laparoscopic and open treatment of emergent small bowel obstruction: An 11-year analysis of ACS NSQIP. Surg Endosc. 2018 Dec;32(12):4900–4911. doi: 10.1007/s00464-018-6249-2. Epub 2018 Jun 4. PMID: 29869083.

37. Maung AA, Johnson DC, Piper GL, et al. Evaluation, and management of small-bowel obstruction: An eastern association for the surgery of trauma practice management guideline. J Trauma Acute Care Surg. 2012;73(5 Suppl 4):362.

38. O'Leary EA, Desale SY, Yi WS, Fujita KA, Hynes CF, Chandra SK, Sava JA. Letting the sun set on small bowel obstruction: Can a simple risk score tell us when nonoperative care is inappropriate? Am Surg. 2014 Jun;80(6):572–579. PMID: 24887795.

39. Schraufnagel D, Rajaee S, Millham FH. How many sunsets? Timing of surgery in adhesive small bowel obstruction: A study of the Nationwide Inpatient Sample. J Trauma Acute Care Surg. 2013 Jan;74(1):181–187; discussion 187-9. doi: 10.1097/TA.0b013e31827891a1. PMID: 23271094.

40. Choi J, Fisher AT, Mulaney B, Anand A, Carlos G, Stave CD, Spain DA, Weiser TG. Safety of foregoing operation for small bowel obstruction in the virgin abdomen: Systematic review and meta-analysis. J Am Coll Surg. 2020 Sep;231(3):368–375.e1. doi: 10.1016/j.jamcollsurg.2020.06.010. Epub 2020 Jun 20. PMID: 32574687.

41. Amara Y, Leppaniemi A, Catena F, Ansaloni L, Sugrue M, Fraga GP, Coccolini F, Biffl WL, Peitzman AB, Kluger Y, Sartelli M, Moore EE, Di Saverio S, Darwish E, Endo C, van Goor H, Ten Broek RP. Diagnosis and management of small bowel obstruction in virgin abdomen: A WSES position paper. World J Emerg Surg. 2021 Jul 3;16(1):36. doi: 10.1186/s13017-021-00379-8. PMID: 34217331; PMCID: PMC8254282.

42. Ng YY, Ngu JC, Wong AS. Small bowel obstruction in the virgin abdomen: Time to challenge surgical dogma with evidence. ANZ J Surg. 2018 Jan;88(1–2):91–94. doi: 10.1111/ans.13714. Epub 2016 Aug 25. PMID: 27561369.

43. Saxen L, Myllarniemi H. Foreign material and postoperative adhesions. N Engl J Med. 1968;279:200–202.

44. Kapustian V, Anteby EY, Gdalevich M. Effect of closure versus nonclosure of peritoneum at the cesarean section on adhesions: A prospective randomized study. Am J Obstet Gynecol. 2012 Jan;206(1):56.

45. Krielen P, Stommel MWJ, Pargmae P, Bouvy ND, Bakkum EA, Ellis H, Parker MC, Griffiths EA, van Goor H, Ten Broek RPG. Adhesion-related readmissions after open and laparoscopic surgery: A retrospective cohort study (SCAR update). Lancet. 2020 Jan 4;395(10217):33–41. doi: 10.1016/S0140-6736(19)32636-4. Erratum in: Lancet. 2020 Jan 25; 395(10220):272. PMID: 31908284.

46. Fazio VW, Cohen Z, Fleshman JW, van Goor H, Bauer JJ, Wolff BG, Corman M, Beart RW Jr, Wexner SD, Becker JM, Monson JR, Kaufman HS, Beck DE, Bailey HR, Ludwig KA, Stamos MJ, Darzi A, Bleday R, Dorazio R, Madoff RD, Smith LE, Gearhart S, Lillemoe K, Göhl J. Reduction in adhesive small-bowel obstruction by Seprafilm adhesion barrier after intestinal resection. Dis Colon Rectum. 2006 Jan;49(1):1–11. doi: 10.1007/s10350-005-0268-5. PMID: 16320005.

47. Robb WB, Mariette C. Strategies in the prevention of the formation of postoperative adhesions in digestive surgery: A systematic review of the literature. Dis Colon Rectum. 2014 Oct;57(10):1228–1240. doi: 10.1097/DCR.0000000000000191. PMID: 25203381.

48. Keenan JE, Turley RS, McCoy CC, Migaly J, Shapiro ML, Scarborough JE. Trials of nonoperative management exceeding 3 days are associated with increased morbidity in patients undergoing surgery for uncomplicated adhesive small bowel obstruction. J Trauma Acute Care Surg. 2014 Jun;76(6):1367–1372. doi: 10.1097/TA.0000000000000246. PMID: 24854302.

49. Laerum F, Stordahl A, Aase S. Water-soluble contrast media compared with barium in enteric follow-through: Local effects and radiographic efficacy in rats with simple obstruction of the small bowel. Acta Radiol. 1988;29:603–610.

50. Abbas S, Bissett IP, Parry BR. Oral water soluble contrast for the management of adhesive small bowel obstruction. Cochrane Database Syst Rev. 2007 Jul 18;2007(3): CD004651. doi: 10.1002/14651858.CD004651.pub3. PMID: 17636770; PMCID: PMC6465054.

51. Gough IR. Strangulating adhesive small bowel obstruction with normal radiographs. Br J Surg. 1978;65:431–434.

52. Maglinte DD, Balthazar EJ, Kelvin FM, et al. The role of radiology in the diagnosis of small bowel obstruction. AJR. 1997;168:1171–1180.

53. Megibow AJ, Balthazar EJ, Cho KC, et al. Bowel obstruction: Evaluation with CT. Radiology. 1991;180:313–318.

54. Ten Broek RPG, Krielen P, Di Saverio S, Coccolini F, Biffl WL, Ansaloni L, Velmahos GC, Sartelli M, Fraga GP, Kelly MD, Moore FA, Peitzman AB, Leppaniemi A, Moore EE, Jeekel J, Kluger Y, Sugrue M, Balogh ZJ, Bendinelli C, Civil I, Coimbra R, De Moya M, Ferrada P, Inaba K, Ivatury R, Latifi R, Kashuk JL, Kirkpatrick AW, Maier R, Rizoli S, Sakakushev B, Scalea T, Søreide K, Weber D, Wani I, Abu-Zidan FM, De'Angelis N, Piscioneri F, Galante JM, Catena F, van Goor H. Bologna guidelines for diagnosis and management of adhesive small bowel obstruction (ASBO): 2017 update of the evidence-based guidelines from the world society of emergency surgery ASBO working group. World J Emerg Surg. 2018 Jun 19;13:24. doi: 10.1186/s13017-018-0185-2. PMID: 29946347; PMCID: PMC6006983.

55. Maglinte DD, Gage SN, Harmon BH, et al. Obstruction of the small intestine: Accuracy and role of CT in diagnosis. Radiology. 1993;188:61–64.

56. Mallo RD, Salem L, Lalani T, et al. Computed tomography of ischemia and complete obstruction in small bowel obstruction: A systematic review. J Gastrointest Surg. 2005; 9:690–694.

57. Ha HK, Kim JS, Lee MS et al. Differentiation of simple and strangulated small-bowel obstructions: Usefulness of known CT criteria. Radiology. 1997;204:507–512.

58. Scrima A, Lubner MG, King S, Pankratz J, Kennedy G, Pickhardt PJ. Value of MDCT and clinical and laboratory data for predicting the need for surgical intervention in suspected small-bowel obstruction. AJR Am J Roentgenol. 2017 Apr; 208(4):785–793. doi: 10.2214/AJR.16.16946. PMID: 28328258.

59. Steger J, Jell A, Ficht S, Ostler D, Eblenkamp M, Mela P, Wilhelm D. Systematic review and meta-analysis on colorectal anastomotic techniques. Ther Clin Risk Manag. 2022 May 4;18:523–539. doi: 10.2147/TCRM.S335102. PMID: 35548666; PMCID: PMC9081039.

60. Bruns BR, Morris DS, Zielinski M, Mowery NT, Miller PR, Arnold K, Phelan HA, Murry J, Turay D, Fam J, Oh JS, Gunter OL, Enniss T, Love JD, Skarupa D, Benns M, Fathalizadeh A Leung PS, Carrick MM, Jewett B, Sakran J, O'Meara L, Herrera AV, Chen H, Scalea TM, Diaz JJ. Stapled versus hand-sewn: A prospective emergency surgery study. An American Association for the Surgery of Trauma multi-institutional study. J Trauma Acute Care Surg. 2017 Mar;82(3):435–443. doi: 10.1097/TA.0000000000001354. PMID: 28030492.

38

Upper Gastrointestinal Bleeding

Christopher S. Thomas and Bruce A. Crookes

38.1 Introduction

Upper gastrointestinal (UGI) bleeding is a common cause of admission to the intensive care unit (ICU) and accounts for over 300,000 ICU admissions in the United States alone [1]. Optimal outcomes depend on both the rapid identification of the etiology of the hemorrhage and the subsequent implementation of appropriate pharmacologic and procedural therapies.

The majority (80–90%) of episodes of acute UGI bleeding are due to nonvariceal causes [2], with ulcer disease accounting for the majority of this category. Aside from ulcer disease, other etiologies of UGI bleeding include varices, Mallory–Weiss syndrome, vascular lesions, and inflammatory states of the UGI tract. Despite advances in pharmacology and endoscopic therapies over the last several decades, all-cause mortality has remained constant, ranging from 6% to 10% in most series [3] and up to 50% for variceal bleeding [4]. Medical comorbidities and the use of anticoagulants complicate treatment. Fortunately, over 80% of UGI bleeds stop spontaneously. However, when bleeding continues or when the bleeding occurs in the setting of a high-risk patient, prompt decisive management is required. Initial guidelines for the management of UGI bleeding were published almost 30 years ago. Since that time, significant advancements in treatment and prophylaxis have been developed. UGI bleeding mortality rates have significantly decreased in the last three decades, most significantly in patients more than 65 years of age. This chapter will review the current evidence, including practice guidelines, for the prevention and management of UGI bleeding.

38.2 What Is the Role of Medical Therapy in the Prevention of UGI Bleeds and How Successful Is It?

The type and use of medical prophylaxis are highly dependent on the etiology of a UGI bleed. In some cases, medical prophylaxis is the primary means of prevention, while in others, secondary prevention is the goal. As ulcer disease is the most common cause of UGI bleeds, providers must identify the etiology of the ulceration. There are three principal causes: Stress-related mucosal damage (SRMD), nonsteroidal antiinflammatory drug (NSAID) use, and *Helicobacter pylori* infection.

Patients who are critically ill have several causes of ulcer formation, including decreased mucous secretion, altered GI motility, and mucosal ischemia [5]. These factors are especially prevalent in patients with large burns, head injury, coagulopathy, or those patients who require mechanical ventilation. Traditionally, antacids, sucralfate, or histamine-2 receptor antagonists (H2RAs) have been used [5]. All have been shown to reduce bleeding episodes, but none are superior. Several studies have shown decreased mortality and pneumonia rates with sucralfate [5]. More recently, proton pump inhibitors (PPIs) have been studied for stress ulcer prophylaxis. These agents can keep gastric pH >4 by suppressing acid secretion [5]. Conrad et al. [6], in a randomized double-blind study, found omeprazole to be more effective than cimetidine in preventing GI bleeding for critically ill patients. Omeprazole reduced the rate of bleeding from 6.8% to 4.5%, although neither pneumonia nor mortality rates were improved.

How should the intensivist medically manage patients whose UGI bleed is associated with NSAID use? Fortunately, pharmacotherapy is beneficial for preventing bleeding related to NSAIDs used for pain relief or cardiovascular disease. For this reason, a review of the patient's current medications is paramount in the prevention of future UGI bleeds. Chan et al. [7], in a randomized placebo-controlled study, found that patients with a history of bleeding ulcers have less frequent bleeding when esomeprazole was added to aspirin as opposed to changing to clopidogrel (0.7% as compared to 8.6%). Alternative drugs, such as COX-2 inhibitors, also can be used when NSAIDs are used for pain control in arthritis. A case-control study of 1,600 patients who used NSAIDs, low-dose aspirin, antiplatelets, and anticoagulant medications within 2 weeks of endoscopy with endoscopically confirmed gastroduodenal ulcer disease showed that low-dose aspirin (odds ratio [OR] 1.8) and NSAIDs (OR 1.35) individually increased risk of bleeding, and a combination of low-dose aspirin and NSAIDs (OR 3.59) or low-dose aspirin and antiplatelet agents (OR 6.7) contributed to more profound bleeding rates [8]. Lai et al. [9] studied patients who were taking aspirin and were *H. pylori* positive. After eradication therapy, patients were randomized to lansoprazole or placebo while continuing aspirin. The PPI group had an ulcer complication rate of 1.6% compared to 14.8% with placebo. Other medications may put patients at higher risk of UGI bleeding: Retrospective data suggest that selective serotonin reuptake inhibitors used to treat various psychiatric disorders are associated with almost a twofold

DOI: 10.1201/9781003316800-38

increase in the risk of developing a UGI bleed, especially among patients with concurrent use of NSAIDs or antiplatelet drugs [10].

While acid suppression is the hallmark of prevention for ulcer-related bleeding, reduction in portal venous pressure is the mainstay for preventing esophageal bleeding. Beta-blockers are the primary class of drugs that are used to accomplish this goal, having first been used in the 1980s. Lebrec found that patients with large varices were significantly less likely to bleed when nadolol was added as therapy for variceal hemorrhage when compared with placebo [11]. Kiire similarly found that propranolol significantly reduced bleeding when used in secondary prevention [12]. Other authors have investigated the use of beta-blockers to prevent the formation and growth of varices: Merkel et al. [13] found that the risk of variceal growth was decreased from 21% to 7% and 51% to 20%, at 1 and 5 years follow-up, respectively.

Other drugs, such as isosorbide mononitrate (IM), have also been investigated in the prevention of variceal bleeding. Angelico et al. [14] found that propranolol and IM provided similar protection against variceal bleeding. Long-term use of nitrates, however, has been linked to increased mortality. A review by Talwalkar and Kamath [15] showed that beta-blockers provide a 9% absolute risk reduction for primary prophylaxis and a 21% reduction for secondary prevention.

RECOMMENDATIONS

1. PPIs should be used as stress ulcer prophylaxis in critically ill patients to prevent GI bleeding.
2. Risk of ulcer formation for patients taking NSAIDs is significantly reduced with PPI or H2RA prophylaxis.
3. Beta-blockers can be used safely for primary prophylaxis from variceal bleeding and may slow the growth of small varices.

Grade of recommendations: 1. A; 2. A; 3. B (Table 38.1).

TABLE 38.1

Upper GI Bleeds: Question Summary

No.	Question	Answer	Grade	References
1	What is the role of medical therapy in the prevention of UGI bleeds?	PPIs should be used as stress ulcer prophylaxis in critically ill patients to prevent GI bleeding.	A	[5, 6]
		The risk of ulcer formation for patients taking NSAIDs is significantly reduced with PPI or H2RA prophylaxis.	A	[7–10]
		Beta-blockers can be used safely for primary prophylaxis from variceal bleeding and may slow the growth of small varices.	B	[11–15]
2	What is the role of medical therapy in treating active UGI bleeds?	PPIs should be preferentially used over H2RAs to reduce rebleeding episodes after successful endoscopic therapy.	A	[16–18]
		In *H. pylori–positive* patients, eradication therapy should be employed.	B	[19, 20]
		Octreotide should be used to slow the rate of variceal bleeding until definitive endoscopic therapy can be implemented.	B	[21–23]
3	What is the role of endoscopy in treating or preventing UGI bleeds?	Endoscopic treatment should be used to stop active hemorrhage from ulcer disease and confers additional prevention of rebleeding episodes.	A	[1, 3, 24–29]
		Endoscopic banding ligation is the treatment of choice for acute variceal hemorrhage and should be undertaken as soon as possible.	A	[23, 30]
		Banding ligation is an effective means of preventing variceal bleeding and can be used when medical prophylaxis cannot be tolerated.	B	[31–35]
4	What is the role of interventional radiology in treating UGI bleeds?	Angiography is safe and should be used in patients with massive UGI bleeding who are too ill to undergo an operation.	C	[36–38]
5	Under what circumstances is an operation indicated for a bleeding peptic ulcer?	Surgery is indicated for peptic ulcer hemorrhage that is not controlled by endoscopic therapy or recurs following successful endoscopic therapy (5–20%).	A	[39, 40]
6	What surgical techniques are associated with the lowest rate of UGI rebleeding?	When used for peptic ulcer bleeding, combined partial gastric resection and vagotomy are associated with the lowest recurrence rate. However, this approach also has a higher rate of short-term and long-term postoperative complications. Vagotomy with oversewing of the ulcer is effective when combined with anti–*H. pylori* therapy in *H. pylori*–positive patients.	B	[41, 42]
7	What approach is preferred for the management of perforated PUD?	Nonoperative therapy can be used in selected patients who are found to have a sealed perforation in a contrast study. Patch closure is indicated in most patients. *H. pylori* should be eradicated when the infection is present. The laparoscopic approach is being used with increased frequency.	B	[43–50]

38.3 What Is the Role of Medical Therapy in Treating UGI Bleeds and How Effective Is It?

As mentioned earlier, most UGI bleeds stop spontaneously. However, clinicians should optimize patient outcomes through both pharmacologic and procedural interventions. UGI bleeds caused by ulcer disease are both prevented and treated with acid suppression. In the mid-1980s it was found that H2RA drugs decreased rates of surgery and death in certain populations of patients with UGI bleeding, marking the dawn of a new era in the treatment of what was then a common problem.

Over the next decade, however, PPIs were introduced. Lanas et al. [16] found that omeprazole was superior to ranitidine in decreasing rebleeding episodes. No differences were found in mortality or units of blood transfused. Khuroo et al. [17] found that PPIs reduced ongoing bleeding from 36.4% to 10.9% and reduced the need for surgery as compared to placebo. Lau et al. [18] also found that PPI treatment was superior in preventing rebleeding after endoscopic treatment of ulcer bleeding.

In addition to acid suppression, treating the etiology of the ulcer is imperative. This includes managing critical illness, limiting NSAID use, and treating *H. pylori* when appropriate. Riemann et al. [19] demonstrated that curative triple therapy with PPI was superior to maintenance therapy with H2RAs. Sung et al. [20], however, showed that medical therapy should not stand alone: This study found that patients treated with both endoscopy and PPI were much less likely to rebleed than PPI treatment alone (1.1% compared to 11.6%).

Medical treatment of variceal bleeding differs from ulcer bleeding in that the therapeutic agents used are different in their mechanisms of action: The mainstays of the pharmacologic treatment of active variceal bleeding are vasoconstrictive and vasoactive drugs. Vasopressin and terlipressin are vasoconstrictive agents that have been shown to decrease active variceal bleeding.

Octreotide is the main vasoactive drug used to treat variceal bleeding. It is a hormone analog of somatostatin that alters GI hormone signaling, decreases gastric and pancreatic secretions, and alters splanchnic blood flow. Multiple studies have demonstrated the superior efficacy of octreotide over vasopressin [21, 22] for stopping active bleeding and preventing rebleeds. Despite this, no mortality benefit has been shown. A meta-analysis by Gross et al. [23] found that vasoconstrictive therapy was only 68.7% successful as compared to vasoactive therapy, which was 75.9% successful. It should be kept in mind, however, that banding ligation is the most effective therapy and should be the primary intervention for stopping variceal bleeding [23].

RECOMMENDATIONS

1. PPIs should be preferentially used over H2RAs to reduce rebleeding episodes after successful endoscopic therapy.

2. In *H. pylori*–positive patients, eradication therapy should be employed.

3. Octreotide should be used to slow the rate of variceal bleeding until definitive endoscopic therapy can be implemented.

Grade of recommendations: 1. A; 2. B; 3. B (Table 38.1).

38.4 What Is the Role of Endoscopy in Treating or For Prophylaxis in UGI Bleeds and How Successful Is It?

Endoscopy is beneficial in UGI bleeds because it can be simultaneously diagnostic and therapeutic, particularly in patients with no prior history of bleeding. Of note, therapeutic endoscopy is required in only 6% of patients presenting with hematemesis requiring transfusion and, when performed, is over 90% successful [24]. Ulcer bleeding can be stopped or reduced with medical treatment, as discussed previously; however, multiple studies have shown that endoscopy confers further prevention of rebleeding [25]. Endoscopic findings of active bleeding or a visible vessel require treatment due to their high rates of rebleeding.

Ulcers with adherent clots are more controversial. Bini and Cohen [25] directly compared endoscopy with medical treatment in patients with adherent clots. These authors found that recurrent bleeding, mean hospital stay, transfusion requirements, and repeat endoscopy were significantly reduced with endoscopy.

Several methods are available to achieve endoscopic hemostasis, including adrenaline injection, laser therapy, and heater probes. No significant differences, however, have been found when these therapeutic modalities have been compared [3]. Similarly, Chung et al. [26] found that initial hemostasis was achieved equally by injection and heater probe. Yet for ulcers with "spurting" vessels, combination treatment (injection and heater probe) reduced the rate of surgery from 29.6% to 6.5%. Administration of prokinetics such as erythromycin before endoscopy for UGI bleeding has been shown to improve visualization of gastric mucosa and decrease the need for repeat endoscopy, blood transfusions, and duration of hospital stay [27].

Some patients fail endoscopic treatment, although this occurs in only 9% of patients [28]. Lau et al. [29] studied patients who had undergone successful initial endoscopic treatment and randomized them to surgery or repeat endoscopy upon rebleeding. Over one-quarter of patients who were randomized to have repeat endoscopy still required a salvage operation [29].

While endoscopy has no use in prophylaxis of ulcer disease, this intervention can be used for both the treatment of active bleeding and prophylaxis in patients with varices. Options for the endoscopic management of varices include injection sclerotherapy and banding ligation. While both techniques have been used for the control of acute hemorrhage, multiple studies have found that ligation is superior to sclerotherapy [30]. Banding has a lower rebleeding rate and reduced complications. A meta-analysis by Gross et al. [23] demonstrated the superiority of endoscopic banding ligation over medical therapy in the treatment of acute variceal bleeding.

While endoscopic banding is superior for the treatment of acute bleeding, the role of endoscopy and the type of prophylaxis treatment are discordant and more divisive. van Buuren et al. [31] found that there was no difference in the number of episodes of bleeding when sclerotherapy was compared with no treatment. Endoscopic banding has been widely studied for the prophylaxis of variceal bleeding. This technique is often compared with medical prophylaxis with beta-blockers alone or in combination with IM. A study by Wang et al. [32] found that combined medical (beta-blocker plus IM) and procedural therapies were equally effective for primary prophylaxis.

Conversely, Sarin et al. [33] showed that banding reduced initial bleeding risk from 43% to 15% as compared to beta-blocker alone. Lo et al. [34] published a series indicating that banding was better for secondary prevention but that combined medical therapy improved overall survival. A meta-analysis by Gluud et al. [35] showed that banding ligation reduced bleeding episodes as compared to beta-blockers without any difference in morality.

RECOMMENDATIONS

1. Endoscopic treatment should be used to stop active hemorrhage from ulcer disease and confers additional prevention of rebleeding episodes.

2. Endoscopic banding ligation is the treatment of choice for acute variceal hemorrhage and should be undertaken as soon as possible.

3. Banding ligation is an effective means of preventing variceal bleeding and can be used when medical prophylaxis cannot be tolerated.

Grade of recommendations: 1. A; 2. A; 3. B (Table 38.1).

38.5 What Is the Role of Interventional Radiology in Treating UGI Bleeds?

Angiography has been established as the primary therapy for many lower GI bleeds. Its role in UGI bleeding, however, is not as well defined. While there are many case reports of the use of angiography for the identification and control of bleeding from more obscure bleeding sources (such as small bowel diverticula or mesenteric aneurysms), the data for its use in the control of typical UGI hemorrhage are far from robust.

Defreyne et al. [36] published a series of patients with GI bleeding treated with angioembolization that showed patients with a UGI source had higher rates of rebleeding and a lower success rate when compared to lower GI sources. Carreira et al. [37], however, showed that embolization was successful 90% of the time in a study with predominately upper GI bleeds. A 10-year retrospective review of 98 hemodynamically unstable (systolic blood pressure [SBP] <90 mmHg) patients who underwent super-selective angioembolization for UGI bleeding demonstrated technical and clinical success rates of 98% and 71%, respectively, of the initial bleeding episode and a 20% rebleeding rate within 30 days requiring additional intervention [38]. Most of these studies indicate that embolization should be used in patients with

massive ongoing hemorrhage who cannot tolerate surgery due to medical comorbidities.

RECOMMENDATION

Angiography is safe and should be used as rescue therapy in patients with massive UGI bleeding who are too ill to undergo an operation.

Grade of recommendation: C (Table 38.1).

38.6 Under What Circumstances Is an Operation Indicated for a Bleeding Peptic Ulcer? What Techniques Are Associated with the Lowest Rate of Rebleeding?

Surgical therapy is indicated in patients whose bleeding is not controlled by nonoperative measures. The presence of exsanguinating hemorrhage or the lack of endoscopic support is a self-evident indication for emergency operations. Recurrent bleeding after endoscopy is a more common (albeit less precise) indication. Risk factors identified by logistic regression analysis as independent predictors of rebleeding or mortality include advanced age, shock, comorbidities, size of the ulcer, and presence of major stigmata of hemorrhage [39].

Importantly, most patients with rebleeding can benefit from a second-look endoscopy that provides additional hemostatic therapy or consultation with interventional radiology. In a randomized trial comparing endoscopic retreatment with surgery, control of recurrent bleeding was achieved endoscopically in 35 of the 48 patients (72.9%) with fewer complications experienced than in the surgery-alone group (7 vs. 16) [40]. Both selective and routine second-look endoscopy appears to favorably influence the outcome of peptic ulcer bleeding.

Unsuccessful endoscopic retreatment manifesting as persistent or recurrent bleeding should generally be addressed by operation. Unfortunately, the most appropriate procedure is difficult to delineate because high-grade evidence is rare. Therefore, widely divergent opinions as to the "correct" operation prevail. Millat et al. [41] compared ulcer oversewing and vagotomy with a more aggressive protocol of gastric resection and Billroth I or Billroth II anastomosis. The resection group had a significantly lower rate of recurrent bleeding. The authors concluded that gastric resection was the procedure of choice in the management of uncontrolled peptic bleeding. In contrast, a database audit of more than 900 patients from the Department of Veterans Affairs National Surgical Quality Improvement Program (NSQIP) demonstrated no differences in mortality, morbidity, or rebleeding rates when vagotomy and drainage were compared to vagotomy and gastric resection [42]. Notably, all operative techniques described in these studies were associated with a similar and relatively high mortality rate.

Taken together, such sparse data provide little guidance for the surgeon faced with treating a patient who presents with hemorrhage refractory to nonoperative therapies. Based on the available literature, the authors cannot recommend a single definitive operation for the patient with recurrent gastric bleeding—the procedure of choice should be the operation with which the surgeon is the most comfortable. Regardless of the operative approach, the patient should be tested for *H. pylori* infection and treated if positive. Eradication of the organism must be confirmed.

RECOMMENDATIONS

1. Surgery or transarterial embolization (TAE) is indicated for peptic ulcer hemorrhage that is not controlled by endoscopic therapy or that recurs following successful endoscopic therapy (5–20%).

2. When the operation is used for peptic ulcer bleeding, combined partial gastric resection and vagotomy are associated with the lowest recurrence rate. However, this approach also has a higher rate of short-term and long-term postoperative complications. Vagotomy with oversewing of the ulcer is effective when combined with anti–*H. pylori* therapy in *H. pylori*–positive patients.

Grade of recommendations: 1. B; 2. B (Table 38.1).

38.7 What Approach Is Preferred for the Management of Perforated Peptic Ulcer Disease?

Perforation is a potentially catastrophic complication of peptic ulcer disease (PUD) that is usually heralded by the abrupt and dramatic onset of severe, mid-epigastric, or generalized abdominal pain. Because the large majority of perforations occur on the anterior aspect of the stomach or duodenum, pneumoperitoneum is present in the majority of cases and is readily detectable on plain abdominal films or computed tomography scans.

The therapy of ulcer perforation should address three separate but related issues: The perforation itself, its underlying cause, and the resultant peritonitis and sepsis. In the latter regard, initial management should include rapid fluid resuscitation, nasogastric tube drainage, and systemic antibiotic administration. There is less unanimity about the respective roles of operative and nonoperative therapies for the actual perforation and its associated pathogenetic factors.

The use of nonoperative therapy for ulcer perforation remains controversial but appears to be gaining wider acceptance. Nonrandomized studies have generally indicated that nonoperative treatment of sealed perforations can result in lower morbidity and mortality than with conventional surgical therapy [43]. However, nonoperative treatment fails in 16–32% of perforated patients, necessitating emergency operations. In a controlled, randomized trial, Crofts et al. compared initial nonoperative therapy with early operation in 83 patients with perforation [44]. No difference was noted in

mortality (4.7% vs. 5.0%), but the hospital stay was 35% longer in the nonoperative group, and patients over 70 years of age were significantly less likely to respond to conservative measures. The mixed results with nonoperative therapy suggest that such an approach cannot be universally applied; however, its selective use, especially in high-risk patients, may be appropriate if a strict protocol and close follow-up can be ensured.

Specific operative strategies for the management of ulcer perforation have continued to evolve. Before the recognition of the pathogenic roles of *H. pylori* and NSAIDs, studies comparing simple closure with definitive operations (vagotomy with or without resection) demonstrated a lower recurrence rate following the more aggressive approach [45, 46]. The authors reported an operative mortality rate of 0.9% and a recurrence rate of 7.4%.

In the current *Helicobacter* era, pharmacotherapy has largely replaced definitive surgery in the management of ulcer perforation. Worldwide, the prevalence of *H. pylori* infection in patients with a perforated peptic ulcer is reported to range from 47% to 100% [47]. In a controlled, randomized trial comparing PPI therapy with anti-*Helicobacter* therapy following simple closure of the ulcer, the relapse rate was found to be significantly reduced in the anti-*Helicobacter* group after 1 year (4.8% vs. 38.1%) [48].

The data suggest that the majority of patients with perforated peptic ulcers can be treated with simple closure of the ulcer when the procedure is combined with appropriate medical measures such as anti-*Helicobacter* therapy, PPI administration, or NSAID modulation. More definitive surgical approaches may be reserved for patients with recurrent ulcer disease or for perforations that are associated with hemorrhage or obstruction.

Successful closure of perforations can be achieved with either open, laparoscopic, or robotic techniques. A recent meta-analysis of 1,113 patients from 15 selected studies found that the laparoscopic approach required longer operating times but was associated with less postoperative analgesic use, a shorter hospital stay, and fewer wound infections [49]. A Cochrane review of three randomized studies concluded that open and laparoscopic repairs are equally safe and effective [50].

RECOMMENDATIONS

Nonoperative therapy can be used in selected patients who are found to have a sealed perforation in a contrast study. Patch closure is indicated in most patients undergoing an operation. *H. pylori* should be eradicated when the infection is present. The laparoscopic approach is being used with increased frequency.

Grade of recommendation: B (Table 38.1).

Disclaimer

There were no sources of funding or conflicts of interest in the writing of this chapter.

Editor's Note

As the authors have nicely delineated, there is a great deal of quality data to inform us on the subject of upper gastrointestinal bleeding. In critically ill patients, proton pump inhibitors (PPIs) should be used to provide stress ulcer prophylaxis. The risk of ulcer formation for patients taking NSAIDs is significantly reduced with PPI or H2RA use. And beta-blockers should be employed as primary prophylaxis for variceal bleeding. For the treatment of upper GI bleeding, PPIs should be preferentially used over H2RAs to reduce rebleeding episodes after successful endoscopic therapy. In bleeding patients who are *H. pylori*-positive, eradication therapy should be employed. Octreotide should be used to slow the rate of variceal bleeding until definitive endoscopic therapy can be implemented.

While endoscopy is utilized in about half of patients presenting with active upper GI bleeding requiring transfusion, therapeutic endoscopic maneuvers are only required in 6%. Fortunately, they are successful more than 90% of the time. Endoscopic banding ligation is the treatment of choice for acute variceal hemorrhage and is an effective means of preventing variceal bleeding when medical prophylaxis cannot be tolerated. In the small number of patients who fail therapeutic endoscopy (3 in 1,000 patients presenting with GI bleeding), angioembolization or surgery must be considered.

If surgery is required for GI bleeding, the operative technique is best left to the experience of the surgeon, as no particular operation has been demonstrated to have better outcomes. Nonoperative management of perforated peptic ulcers is often successful in a stable patient with minimal symptoms. For those requiring surgery, the omental patch is commonly performed.

REFERENCES

1. Conrad SA. Acute upper gastrointestinal bleeding in critically ill patients: causes and treatment modalities. Crit Care Med 2002;30:S365–S8.
2. Khamaysi I, Gralnek IM. Acute Upper Gastrointestinal Bleeding (UGIB) - initial evaluation and management. Best Pract Res Clin Gastroenterol 2013;27:633–8.
3. Barkun A, Bardou M, Marshall JK. Consensus recommendations for managing patients with nonvariceal upper gastrointestinal bleeding. Ann Intern Med 2003;139:843–57.
4. Qureshi W, Adler DG, Davila R, et al. ASGE Guideline: the role of endoscopy in the management of variceal hemorrhage, updated July 2005. Gastrointest Endosc 2005;62: 651–5.
5. Cook DJ, Reeve BK, Guyatt GH, et al. Stress ulcer prophylaxis in critically ill patients. Resolving discordant meta-analyses. JAMA J Am Med Assoc 1996;275:308–14.
6. Conrad SA, Gabrielli A, Margolis B, et al. Randomized, double-blind comparison of immediate-release omeprazole oral suspension versus intravenous cimetidine for the prevention of upper gastrointestinal bleeding in critically ill patients. Crit Care Med 2005;33:760–5.
7. Chan FK, Ching JY, Hung LC, et al. Clopidogrel versus aspirin and esomeprazole to prevent recurrent ulcer bleeding. N Engl J Med 2005;352:238–44.
8. Kawasaki K, Kurahara K, Yanai S, Kochi S, Fuchigami T, Matsumoto T. Low-dose aspirin and non-steroidal anti-inflammatory drugs increase the risk of bleeding in patients with gastroduodenal ulcer. Dig Dis Sci 2014;60(4): 1010–1015.
9. Lai KC, Lam SK, Chu KM, et al. Lansoprazole reduces ulcer relapse after eradication of *Helicobacter pylori* in nonsteroidal anti-inflammatory drug users–a randomized trial. Aliment Pharmacol Ther 2003;18:829–36.
10. Jiang HY, Chen HZ, Hu XJ, et al. Use of selective serotonin reuptake inhibitors and risk of upper gastrointestinal bleeding: a systematic review and meta-analysis. Clin Gastroenterol Hepatol 2014;13(1):42–50.
11. Lebrec D, Poynard T, Capron JP, et al. Nadolol for prophylaxis of gastrointestinal bleeding in patients with cirrhosis. A randomized trial. J Hepatol 1988;7:118–25.
12. Kiire CF. Controlled trial of propranolol to prevent recurrent variceal bleeding in patients with non-cirrhotic portal fibrosis. BMJ 1989;298:1363–5.
13. Merkel C, Marin R, Angeli P, et al. A placebo-controlled clinical trial of nadolol in the prophylaxis of growth of small esophageal varices in cirrhosis. Gastroenterology 2004;127:476–84.
14. Angelico M, Carli L, Piat C, et al. Isosorbide-5-mononitrate versus propranolol in the prevention of first bleeding in cirrhosis. Gastroenterology 1993;104:1460–5.
15. Talwalkar JA, Kamath PS. An evidence-based medicine approach to beta-blocker therapy in patients with cirrhosis. Am J Med 2004;116:759–66.
16. Lanas A, Artal A, Blas JM, Arroyo MT, Lopez-Zaborras J, Sainz R. Effect of parenteral omeprazole and ranitidine on gastric pH and the outcome of bleeding peptic ulcer. J Clin Gastroenterol 1995;21:103–6.
17. Khuroo MS, Yattoo GN, Javid G, et al. A comparison of omeprazole and placebo for bleeding peptic ulcer. N Engl J Med 1997;336:1054–8.
18. Lau JY, Sung JJ, Lee KK, et al. Effect of intravenous omeprazole on recurrent bleeding after endoscopic treatment of bleeding peptic ulcers. N Engl J Med 2000;343:310–6.
19. Riemann JF, Schilling D, Schauwecker P, et al. Cure with omeprazole plus amoxicillin versus long-term ranitidine therapy in *Helicobacter pylori*-associated peptic ulcer bleeding. Gastrointest Endosc 1997;46:299–304.
20. Sung JJ, Chan FK, Lau JY, et al. The effect of endoscopic therapy in patients receiving omeprazole for bleeding ulcers with nonbleeding visible vessels or adherent clots: a randomized comparison. Ann Intern Med 2003;139: 237–43.
21. Hwang SJ, Lin HC, Chang CF, et al. A randomized controlled trial comparing octreotide and vasopressin in the control of acute esophageal variceal bleeding. J Hepatol 1992;16:320–5.
22. Jenkins SA, Baxter JN, Corbett W, Devitt P, Ware J, Shields R. A prospective randomised controlled clinical trial comparing somatostatin and vasopressin in controlling acute variceal haemorrhage. Br Med J 1985;290:275–8.
23. Gross M, Schiemann U, Muhlhofer A, Zoller WG. Meta-analysis: efficacy of therapeutic regimens in ongoing variceal bleeding. Endoscopy 2001;33:737–46.
24. Khoury L, Hill DMD, Panzo M, Chiappetta M, Tekade S, Cohn SM. The natural history of hematemesis in the 21st century. Cureus 2018;10:e3029.

25. Bini EJ, Cohen J. Endoscopic treatment compared with medical therapy for the prevention of recurrent ulcer hemorrhage in patients with adherent clots. Gastrointest Endosc 2003;58:707–14.

26. Chung SS, Lau JY, Sung JJ, et al. Randomised comparison between adrenaline injection alone and adrenaline injection plus heat probe treatment for actively bleeding ulcers. BMJ 1997;314:1307–11.

27. Theivanayagam S, Lim RG, Cobell WJ, et al. Administration of erythromycin before endoscopy in upper gastrointestinal bleeding: a meta-analysis of randomized controlled trials. Saudi J Gastroenterol 2013;19:205–10.

28. Khoury L, Tobin-Schnittger P, Champion N, et al. Natural history of patients undergoing therapeutic endoscopies for acute gastrointestinal bleeding. Am Surg 2019;85:1246–52.

29. Lau JY, Sung JJ, Lam YH, et al. Endoscopic retreatment compared with surgery in patients with recurrent bleeding after initial endoscopic control of bleeding ulcers. N Engl J Med 1999;340:751–6.

30. Gimson AE, Ramage JK, Panos MZ, et al. Randomised trial of variceal banding ligation versus injection sclerotherapy for bleeding oesophageal varices. Lancet 1993;342:391–4.

31. van Buuren HR, Rasch MC, Batenburg PL, et al. Endoscopic sclerotherapy compared with no specific treatment for the primary prevention of bleeding from esophageal varices. A randomized controlled multicentre trial [ISRCTN03215899]. BMC Gastroenterol 2003;3:22.

32. Wang HM, Lo GH, Chen WC, et al. Comparison of endoscopic variceal ligation and nadolol plus isosorbide-5-mononitrate in the prevention of first variceal bleeding in cirrhotic patients. JCMA 2006;69:453–60.

33. Sarin SK, Lamba GS, Kumar M, Misra A, Murthy NS. Comparison of endoscopic ligation and propranolol for the primary prevention of variceal bleeding. N Engl J Med 1999;340:988–93.

34. Lo GH, Chen WC, Lin CK, et al. Improved survival in patients receiving medical therapy as compared with banding ligation for the prevention of esophageal variceal rebleeding. Hepatology 2008;48:580–7.

35. Gluud LL, Klingenberg S, Nikolova D, Gluud C. Banding ligation versus beta-blockers as primary prophylaxis in esophageal varices: systematic review of randomized trials. Am J Gastroenterol. 2007;102:2842–8; quiz 1, 9.

36. Defreyne L, Vanlangenhove P, De Vos M, et al. Embolization as a first approach with endoscopically unmanageable acute nonvariceal gastrointestinal hemorrhage. Radiology 2001;218:739–48.

37. Carreira JM, Reyes R, Pulido-Duque JM, et al. Diagnosis and percutaneous treatment of gastrointestinal hemorrhage. Long-term experience. Rev Esp Enferm Dig 1999;91:684–92.

38. Mejaddam AY, Cropano CM, Kalva S, et al. Outcomes following "rescue" superselective angioembolization for gastrointestinal hemorrhage in hemodynamically unstable patients. J Trauma Acute Care Surg 2013;75:398–403.

39. Rockall TA, Logan RF, Devlin HB, Northfield TC. Risk assessment after acute upper gastrointestinal haemorrhage. Gut 1996;38:316–21.

40. Lau JY, Sung JJ, Lam YH, et al. Endoscopic retreatment compared with surgery in patients with recurrent bleeding after initial endoscopic control of bleeding ulcers. N Engl J Med 1999;340:751–6.

41. Millat B, Hay JM, Valleur P, Fingerhut A, Fagniez PL. Emergency surgical treatment for bleeding duodenal ulcer: oversewing plus vagotomy versus gastric resection, a controlled randomized trial. French Associations for Surgical Research. World J Surg 1993;17:568–73; discussion 74.

42. de la Fuente SG, Khuri SF, Schifftner T, Henderson WG, Mantyh CR, Pappas TN. Comparative analysis of vagotomy and drainage versus vagotomy and resection procedures for bleeding peptic ulcer disease: results of 907 patients from the Department of Veterans Affairs National Surgical Quality Improvement Program database. J Am Coll Surg 2006;202:78–86.

43. Marshall C, Ramaswamy P, Bergin FG, Rosenberg IL, Leaper DJ. Evaluation of a protocol for the non-operative management of perforated peptic ulcer. Br J Surg 1999;86:131–4.

44. Crofts TJ, Park KG, Steele RJ, Chung SS, Li AK. A randomized trial of nonoperative treatment for perforated peptic ulcer. N Engl J Med 1989;320:970–3.

45. Boey J, Branicki FJ, Alagaratnam TT, et al. Proximal gastric vagotomy. The preferred operation for perforations in acute duodenal ulcer. Ann Surg 1988;208:169–74.

46. Tsugawa K, Koyanagi N, Hashizume M, et al. The therapeutic strategies in performing emergency surgery for gastroduodenal ulcer perforation in 130 patients over 70 years of age. Hepatogastroenterology 2001;48:156–62.

47. Gisbert JP, Pajares JM. *Helicobacter pylori* infection and perforated peptic ulcer prevalence of the infection and role of antimicrobial treatment. Helicobacter 2003;8:159–67.

48. Ng EK, Lam YH, Sung JJ, et al. Eradication of *Helicobacter pylori* prevents recurrence of ulcer after simple closure of duodenal ulcer perforation: randomized controlled trial. Ann Surg 2000;231:153–8.

49. Lunevicius R, Morkevicius M. Comparison of laparoscopic versus open repair for perforated duodenal ulcers. Surg Endosc 2005;19:1565–71.

50. Sanabria A, Villegas MI, Morales Uribe CH. Laparoscopic repair for perforated peptic ulcer disease. Cochrane Database Syst Rev 2013;19(4):Cd004778.

39

Enterocutaneous Fistulas

Leah M. Pearl, Jordyn Baldwin, and Peter P. Lopez

Enterocutaneous fistulas (ECFs) represent a catastrophic problem for patients and continue to be complex and labor-intensive issues for healthcare providers. In addition to the many physiologic and mental stressors that patients must endure, the development of ECFs also strains healthcare systems, resulting in prolonged hospital stays, multiple readmissions, and increased resource consumption. Nutritional support, fluid and electrolyte management, wound care, frequent infections, chronic pain, and depression are just a few healthcare issues requiring significant investment when managing these patients. Up to one-third of ECFs will close spontaneously when medically optimized, but surgery becomes necessary for patients whose ECFs do not close spontaneously [1]. Unfortunately, definitive operative closure is only successful 75–85% of the time [1].

The management of ECFs has improved significantly, resulting in decreased mortality rates, from 50% in the 1950s to approximately 5–15% at present [2]. Despite overall improvements in the care of these patients with ECFs, sepsis and malnutrition remain the leading causes of death [3]. As many as 85% of ECFs present as a complication after abdominal surgery, providing further challenges to already compromised postoperative patients. Spontaneous fistulas usually result as a complication of inflammatory bowel disease, radiation, or cancer [2–5]. As a clinician involved in treating ECFs, it is essential to have a stepwise approach to the management of ECFs (Table 39.1). Treatment decisions for the management of ECFs must be based around reducing patient morbidity and mortality.

TABLE 39.1

Management Phases for Enterocutaneous Fistulas

Phase	Goal	Timing
Recognition/control of sepsis	• Septic source control. • Image-guided drainage vs. open drainage of abdominal wall abscess. • Broad-spectrum antibiotics. • *Resuscitation*: Crystalloid, colloid, and blood products	1–2 days
Stabilization	• Electrolyte homeostasis. • Control of fistula drainage. • Skin protection. • Maintaining adequate source control.	2–7 days
Nutritional support	• Parental nutrition should be started early and continued until full nutritional needs can be provided via an enteral source. • Nutritional marker monitoring. • Electrolyte monitoring.	Day 1–2 until fistula closure
Control of fistula output and wound care	• Pharmacologic agents. • Protective skin barriers and creative wound protection and collection devices. • VAC therapy.	2 days until fistula closure
Decision	• Investigation of the source of fistula. • Etiology, anatomy, drainage output. • Duration of nonoperative management.	7 days until fistula closure
Definitive therapy	• Planning operative approach. • Resection of fistula with the performance of anastomosis. • Secure abdominal wall closure. • Feeding tube if needed.	>4–5 months after fistula development
Healing	• Continuation of nutritional support. • Vitamin supplementation.	Postoperatively

Source: Modified from Everson, AR, and Fischer, JE, *J Gastrointest Surg*, 10, 455, 2006.

DOI: 10.1201/9781003316800-39

39.1 What Is the Definition of ECF?

An ECF is an abnormal connection between the gastrointestinal tract and the skin. Most ECFs develop from one of the following conditions: Extension of bowel disease to surrounding structures, an extension of disease of the surrounding structures to the bowel, unrecognized bowel injury, or breakdown of a gastrointestinal tract anastomosis [2]. ECFs can form after the repair of a ventral hernia with permanent mesh; fistula formation has been estimated as high as 10% from mesh erosion into the surrounding bowel [2]. ECFs can further be defined by their anatomical location, output amount, etiology, and complexity. Postoperative ECFs account for 75–85% of all fistulas, whereas spontaneous fistulas account for 15–25%. [2–7]. Cancer and inflammatory bowel disease are the two most common processes causing spontaneous ECF formation [2–7].

> **RECOMMENDATIONS**
>
> Postoperative ECFs are more common than spontaneous fistulas. They are often caused by unrecognized bowel injuries or anastomotic breakdown.
>
> Grade of recommendation: B.
>
> Permanent meshes have become more prevalent sources for ECF development, so careful surgical decision-making should guide their use.
>
> Grade of recommendation: C.

39.2 What Are the Risk Factors for Developing an ECF?

Multiple preoperative patient factors can increase the likelihood of ECF development. These factors include previous and active infection, inflammatory bowel disease especially active disease, uncontrolled diabetes, electrolyte abnormalities, smoking, malnutrition, anemia, hypothermia, poor oxygen delivery, and emergent procedures. These factors should be optimized for elective surgery, and tobacco use should be stopped before elective surgery. Ideally, albumin levels should be >3.3 g/dL, and glucose levels should be well controlled. Nutritional status should be optimized using enteral immune-enhancing diets, and, if needed, parenteral nutrition should be combined with enteral feeding to provide additional support [2, 7]. Cardiac output, electrolytes, and anemia should be examined and corrected. Controversy remains in the literature about preoperative bowel preparation (mechanical and antibiotic). The preparation will decrease the number of bacteria in the enteric contents, allowing for a cleaner anastomosis and less chance of postoperative infection and inflammation [8]. Last, intravenous antibiotics given within 1 hour of the incision will help decrease the rate of postoperative surgical site infections.

Optimizing these factors can be challenging in patients requiring urgent or emergent surgical intervention. Hypotensive patients should be resuscitated with intravenous fluids and an equal ratio of blood products. Goal-directed endpoints for fluid resuscitation should be used to avoid harmful side effects of fluid overload. Maintenance of cardiac output, temperature, and oxygenation will help improve overall outcomes.

Most important, however, is adherence to meticulous surgical technique. Hemostasis should be assured, and the bowel should be thoroughly inspected before abdominal wall closure. Recognized injuries should be repaired, as they represent areas of bowel weakness and a setup for ECF formation.

> **RECOMMENDATIONS**
>
> Multiple factors contribute to the formation of ECFs, such as poor nutritional status, diabetes, inflammatory bowel disease, and smoking, which should be optimized before surgery if possible.
>
> Grade of recommendation: B.
>
> Furthermore, attention to meticulous surgical technique will aid in better outcomes.
>
> Grade of recommendation: C.

39.3 How Are ECFs Classified?

ECFs are defined as a fistulous tract between the gastrointestinal tract and the outer surface of the body. ECFs have been classified according to anatomic location, etiology, and output volume. Anatomic location greatly influences mortality and spontaneous healing rates. ECF may be classified by location in the abdomen as superficial or deep. Esophageal, duodenal stump, and jejunal fistulas with enteric defects less than 1 cm and tracts longer than 2 cm are favorable, as they have higher spontaneous closure rates than gastric, lateral duodenal, ligament of Treitz, and ileal fistulas.

Furthermore, fistulas resulting from adjacent abscesses; complete disruption of intestinal continuity; exposed bowel; diseased, radiated, and strictured bowel or obstructed bowel; and involving foreign bodies are unlikely to close spontaneously. Understanding the anatomic makeup of the ECF is essential in the decision-making process. This information provides insight into the type and amount of intestinal fluid lost from an ECF and if surgical closure will be required.

ECFs can also be classified based on physiologic output. Fistulas may be classified as low-output (<200 mL daily), moderate-output (200–500 mL daily), or high-output (>500 mL daily) [2–7]. Thorough monitoring of fistula output helps determine appropriate nutritional support, as intestinal fluid is rich in minerals, electrolytes, and protein. Loss of intestinal fluid through the ECF results in dehydration, electrolyte imbalances, and malnutrition that require ongoing treatment until ECF resolution. Fistula output is also predictive of overall mortality [4]. Mortality rates of up to 54% for patients with high-output fistulas and 16–26% with low-output fistulas have been reported [4, 9]. Unfortunately, it is still a matter of debate whether or not fistula output is directly related to spontaneous closure. Some studies suggest low-output fistulas are two to three times more likely to close spontaneously, while others lack this evidence [4, 10, 11].

RECOMMENDATIONS

ECF has been classified according to anatomic location, etiology, and output volume. Anatomic location affects the amount of fistula output, which influences mortality and spontaneous healing rates.

Grade of recommendation: B.

Measures should be taken to aggressively monitor and replace lost volume and protein output to decrease patient morbidity and mortality.

Grade of recommendation: B.

39.4 How Do ECFs Present Clinically?

An ECF begins with disruption of bowel wall integrity, resulting in leakage of bowel contents into the abdominal cavity or from the surface of the body. Once this occurs, the postoperative clinical presentation follows a distinct pattern. The patient usually experiences a feeling of malaise and, overall, does not progress as predicted [2–5]. The patient develops a fever around postoperative days 3–5, along with leukocytosis [2–5]. An ileus with abdominal distension and pain develops when the normal postoperative ileus should be resolving [2–5]. A wound infection may develop at this point, presenting either as superficial, deep, or an intraabdominal abscess. The infection is drained by opening the previous incision, opening an abdominal wall abscess, or placing an intraabdominal drain. When drainage of enteral contents continues to manifest, the diagnosis of enterocutaneous fistula is confirmed.

RECOMMENDATIONS

A high suspicion of ECF development should be entertained if postoperative patients do not progress as predicted after surgery. Malaise, fever, ileus, leukocytosis, and an intraabdominal abscess or wound infection develop. The development of these signs and symptoms should lead a clinician to suspect the development of an ECF and promptly lead to a workup to exclude or find an ECF.

Grade of recommendation: C.

39.5 What Is the Best Method to Define ECF Anatomy?

If the patient is stable and if the fistula is matured to the point of supporting probing with a small catheter, typically 7–10 days after the recognition of the fistula, it is generally recommended

that the patient undergo fistulography with water-soluble contrast. Much information can be obtained by performing a fistulogram such as length and course of the fistula tract, its relationship to surrounding structures, the absence or presence of bowel continuity, the absence or presence of distal obstruction, and whether the bowel adjacent to the fistula is inflamed or strictured and the presence or absence of an abscess cavity communicating with the fistula [4]. Computed tomography (CT) can also identify abscesses within the abdominal cavity and show the relationship of the fistula to surrounding organs. Unfortunately, CT cannot always identify the fistula's exact location.

RECOMMENDATIONS

Fistulography coupled with CT scanning provides the most accurate evaluation of an ECF better to develop the overall management plan.

Grade of recommendation: C.

39.6 Medical Management

39.6.1 What Are the First Steps in ECF Management?

The management of ECFs is a complex problem that challenges even the most experienced clinicians. Not only can ECF lead to multiple hospitalizations, recurrent infections and sepsis, deep vein thrombosis, complex wound care issues, severe malnutrition, and extreme deconditioning, they are mentally and emotionally taxing on both patients and clinicians. When approaching this complex disease process, a detailed stepwise approach should be embraced (Table 39.1). A multidisciplinary team consisting of a surgeon, nutrition specialist or registered dietitian, pharmacist, wound care nurse/enterostomal therapist, social worker, and physical therapist should be assembled. The immediate goal is to control the fistula output and drainage, begin the replacement of fluid and electrolyte losses, and provide parenteral nutritional support. The aim for these patients is to eventually restore the continuity of the gastrointestinal tract while reducing morbidity and mortality.

ECFs are associated with a classic triad of complications, including sepsis, malnutrition, and fluid and electrolyte abnormalities. Initially, these patients require control of their septic source while undergoing appropriate resuscitation and stabilization. Once stabilized, the patient can start total parenteral nutrition (TPN) to correct malnutrition. Bowel contents outside the lumen lead to soft tissue infections, abscess formation, sepsis or peritonitis, and loss of skin integrity. Gaining control of fistula output and localized drainage of abscesses coupled with appropriate antibiotic selection is vital in the initial management of ECFs. Clinicians must ensure proper skin protection and control of the fistula output because the fistula effluent can be caustic to the surrounding skin. There is a 22-fold increase in mortality when an associated infectious complication accompanies an ECF [4, 10, 11].

The infectious source must be adequately controlled and drained, and source control must be maintained. CT scanning should be used liberally, assuring adequate drainage of abscesses. If deep abscesses are discovered, image-guided drainage can be utilized and closely monitored for the need for replacement with larger-caliber drains. Antibiotics alone are rarely sufficient in resolving the infectious abscess and should only be used as an adjunct to adequate drainage. Broad-spectrum empiric antibiotics should be administered and tailored to the specific identified pathogens [12]. Operative intervention for source control is often prohibited by the patient's hostile abdomen and physiologic condition. Operating during this phase can lead to additional enterotomies, complete disruption of a created anastomosis, or conversion of a contained abscess into widespread intraabdominal sepsis.

Septic patients further complicate the situation, as they are severely hypercatabolic and unable to achieve positive nitrogen balances. This is often the case regardless of adequate nutritional support. Studies demonstrated that ECF patients with uncontrolled sepsis lost 2% of body protein stores daily despite receiving TPN [4, 13]. Controlling sepsis while providing adequate nutritional support is essential for the management of ECF patients.

Restoration of intravascular volume and correction of multiple electrolyte deficiencies is also necessary. Aggressive crystalloid resuscitation may be required to account for septic third-spacing and continued fluid losses from the fistula. In the acute phase of resuscitation, a central venous catheter and arterial catheter placement can help guide fluid resuscitation [13]. These patients are usually dehydrated, anemic, malnourished, and have low serum oncotic protein levels. Continued resuscitation should be carefully guided to avoid fluid overload leading to bowel wall edema and other complications. TPN is essential in optimizing patients with malnutrition.

RECOMMENDATIONS

Initial recognition and control of the septic source in a timely fashion are crucial for ECF patients to improve mortality.

Grade of recommendation: B.

Adequate drainage coupled with appropriate antibiotics will provide the best resolution of the patient's sepsis and hypermetabolic state.

Grade of recommendation: B.

Surgical intervention should be avoided in the hostile abdomen. Aggressive intravascular volume resuscitation is required and should be carefully monitored to avoid the effects of fluid overload. TPN should be started early. Fistula effluent control to protect the surrounding skin is vitally important.

Grade of recommendation: C.

39.6.2 What Is the Best Way to Provide Nutritional Support to ECF Patients?

Nutritional support is imperative in caring for, stabilizing, and rehabilitating patients with ECFs. These patients are usually malnourished before ECF development due to their underlying disease process or surgical stressors. With the development of sepsis and an ECF, metabolic demands increase substantially. Baseline nutritional needs in nonseptic patients are 20 kcal/kg/day of carbohydrates and fat and 0.8 g/kg/day of protein. These requirements can increase to 30 kcal/kg/day and 2.5 g/kg/day, respectively, in the setting of sepsis and high-output fistulas [4, 5, 14–16]. Patients require a calorie–nitrogen ratio of 100:1 during severe catabolic states, and when more stable, the calorie–nitrogen ratio increases to 150:1 [2, 4, 14].

Once septic complications resolve, the external loss of protein-rich enteric contents contributes to further malnutrition. This fluid loss results in dehydration and extreme electrolyte abnormalities. Colonic fistulas tend to be low-output, whereas small bowel fistulas tend to be moderate- to high-output fistulas resulting in worse dehydration and protein loss. The location of ECFs also affects the composition and amount of output. Nearly all fistulas have output high in potassium resulting in hypokalemia.

The route for nutritional delivery is based on caloric needs, fistula tract anatomy, and fistula output. It has been long recognized that TPN is an integral part of ECF management, especially when first diagnosed. Starting TPN as soon as the patient is stabilized is important to help replete and prevent further nutritional losses. Often patients cannot tolerate enteral nutrition due to ileus, obstruction, or high fistula output [3, 11, 15]. Caution should be taken when utilizing TPN, as it is not without its risks and drawbacks. TPN can be very costly, as it must be made individually for the patient. This requires frequent lab work and long-term central venous access. If not carefully monitored, TPN can cause extreme electrolyte abnormalities, hyperglycemia, and bloodstream infections [16]. It is important to remember that the reintroduction of calories to patients who have severe malnutrition can lead to refeeding syndrome [5]. Refeeding syndrome results in metabolic, electrolyte, and arrhythmic abnormalities, usually present within 2 days of caloric renourishment [5]. The route for nutritional delivery is based on caloric needs, fistula tract anatomy, and fistula output. Once the fistula output and infectious source are controlled, then enteral feeding can begin, as it is physiologically preferred for nutritional support [2, 4]. A hybrid model of TPN and enteral nutrition can be introduced to the patient by slowly adding in enteral feeding while total caloric needs are supplemented with TPN. Over time the TPN is weaned as the patient tolerates full caloric enteral feeds. Enteral nutrition has been shown to maintain bowel integrity, speed healing and repletion of the bowel, promote hepatic protein synthesis, and improve the gut's hormonal function and immune function [5, 9].

Traditionally, the Harris–Benedict equation and patient stress factors have been used to provide a starting point for calculating the caloric and protein requirements for ECF patients. The caloric needs should be supplied through glucose and fat. Protein should not be used to meet basal metabolic requirements, but to replenish body protein needs and heal wounds

[3]. Consultation with a nutritional specialist can be beneficial, as it is essential to address nutritional deficits early, providing the best possible outcomes. Reversing the poor nutritional status of these patients depends on the ability to control the septic source and hypermetabolic state.

Nutritional status is an essential predictor of mortality in patients with ECFs [6, 7, 14]. Serum albumin is the best marker to examine overall nutritional status [2–4]. Albumin levels <2.5 g/dL have been associated with mortality rates as high as 42%, whereas those patients obtaining albumin levels ≥3.5 g/dL usually have lower mortality rates [17]. After fistula output and the infectious source are controlled, typically months down the line, patients may consider surgical treatment. For any patient undergoing surgical closure of their fistula, correcting malnutrition and maintaining their nutritional status will improve their wound healing, enhance their immune system, and preserve their lean cell mass. Subsequent surgical morbidity and mortality will be improved with good nutrition. Serum markers such as transferrin, retinol-binding protein, and thyroxin-binding prealbumin have also been associated with predicting mortality in ECF patients [2, 4].

RECOMMENDATIONS

TPN is the preferred source of initial nutritional support in patients with enterocutaneous fistula.

Grade of recommendation: B.

Once nutrition is optimized and fistula output is controlled, enteral nutrition should begin, as the gut is always the preferred route for nutritional support, if it is tolerated.

Grade of recommendation: B.

A hybrid model can be initiated with TPN, while slowly incorporating enteral calories into the patient's diet as tolerated.

Grade of recommendation: B.

Fistula patients should be closely monitored to adjust nutritional support.

Grade of recommendation: C.

39.6.3 What Is the Best Way to Decrease Fistula Output?

Several strategies have been used to decrease fistula output. Initially, patients are restricted to nothing by mouth, and TPN is initiated for nutrition optimization. Over time, liquids and food are cautiously introduced to help with nutritional and electrolyte support as long as fistula output does not substantially increase. Medications such as H2-receptor antagonists, proton pump inhibitors, and sucralfate are useful to decrease the volume and acidity of gastric secretions [2, 4]. Although these medications have never been shown to improve fistula closure rates, decreasing gastric acid secretion allows for better control of electrolyte and acid–base imbalances [2, 4]. Historically, nasogastric tubes have been used to help decrease fistula output. Unless the patient has an obstruction or prolonged ileus, this is now an undesirable treatment, as it can lead to other complications such as sinusitis, acid reflux, or esophageal strictures. Antidiarrheal medication and bulking agents, such as psyllium, can also help to control fistula output.

Somatostatin and its analog, octreotide, have frequently been utilized to help slow fistula output. Somatostatin inhibits the endocrine and exocrine secretion of many gastrointestinal hormones, including gastrin, cholecystokinin, secretin, insulin, glucagon, and vasoactive intestinal peptide [18]. Furthermore, somatostatin inhibits gastric acid secretion, intestinal and gallbladder motility, and contractility [18]. Theoretically, it makes sense that somatostatin would decrease ECF output and aid in the spontaneous closure of ECFs; however, multiple studies have failed to demonstrate this process [4, 19]. Occasionally, somatostatin may convert high-output fistulas to moderate- or low-output fistulas; however, there has been little success in using this medication to close ECFs [5]. Another meta-analysis of the use of somatostatin analogs for the treatment of ECFs concluded that these analogs appear to decrease the time to fistula closure and hospital length of stay but have no mortality benefit [20]. Caution should be taken when using somatostatin, as it can result in hyperglycemia, a significant rebound effect of fistula output when discontinued, and decreased blood supply to the gastrointestinal tract [4, 19]. Teduglutide is a glucagon-like peptide 2 (GLP-2) analog approved for treating adults with short bowel syndrome. The drug improves small bowel villus height, crypt depth, and enteral absorption [21]. A recent randomized controlled pilot study using teduglutide to treat low-output ECFs showed that the treatment was well tolerated and was associated with decreased ECF drainage [22]. In a patient with Crohn's disease who presents with a spontaneous ECF, a trial of biological therapy before surgery may allow spontaneous closure of the ECF [23].

RECOMMENDATIONS

Bulking agents and medications that reduce gastric acid production can help decrease fistula output and maintain acid–base balances.

Grade of recommendation: C.

Somatostatin analogs should be used cautiously, as they may decrease fistula output but are not without side effects.

Grade of recommendation: C.

Newer GLP-2 analogs may help with decreasing output and increasing absorption of enteral contents.

Grade of recommendation: C.

39.6.4 What Is the Best Way to Manage the ECF Wound?

Maintaining skin integrity surrounding the fistula is important in ECF management. Protecting or diverting the fistula output will decrease local irritation and infection and assure an intact abdominal wall, aiding in complete abdominal closure should surgery be required. Various methods have been reported for managing fistula drainage, including simple gauze dressings, skin barriers, pouches, and suction catheters. These methods work well for low-output fistulas, but for more complicated fistulas, Karaya powder or seal, Stomahesive, glycerin, or ion exchange resins may be required. Using a large wound manager can be very helpful in protecting the skin from large, complex fistulas. A highly experienced, creative, and skilled enterostomal therapist can significantly contribute to patient care and improve their overall quality of life.

Multiple studies have demonstrated that vacuum-assisted closure (VAC) dressings can help manage effluent drainage and promote wound healing through granulation tissue formation [4, 21]. Furthermore, VAC dressings can simplify care by decreasing the number of dressing changes. There are concerns associated with the use of VAC dressings, however. Effluent trapped under the VAC dressing could potentiate further skin breakdown and infection. It has also been reported that negative pressure dressings applied to granulating bowel can cause additional ECFs [4]. Despite these concerns, VAC therapy continues to be an encouraging management option.

One of the most dangerous types of ECF is the enteroatmospheric fistula (EAF). This is a fistula where the bowel drains not to an epithelized surface but to a granulation plate on an open abdomen. The optimal treatment is to avoid an open abdomen with exposed bowel, as this can lead to an EAF—all attempts to close the abdomen early should help prevent these fistulas. However, the principles remain the same after the development of an EAF with all resources used to control the output. Early skin grafting to assist in a bag or wound manager control is essential, but again may be difficult and may take multiple attempts at grafting. The grafting will help control the output and decrease the increased metabolic demands of the open abdomen.

RECOMMENDATIONS

Any method that will help control fistula effluent while protecting the skin should be utilized.

Grade of recommendation: C.

VAC dressing therapy is a promising management option and should be monitored closely when utilized.

Grade of recommendation: C.

39.7 Surgical Management

39.7.1 When Is the Best Time to Provide Surgical Closure of an ECF?

Spontaneous ECF closure only occurs in approximately 30% of patients. In this group of patients about 90–95% of fistulas will spontaneously resolve within the first 4–6 weeks [2, 4]. Fistulas of the stomach, ileum, and ligament of Treitz, as well as those associated with large abscesses, short fistula tracts, large openings in the bowel, damaged or strictured intestine, intestinal discontinuity, or distal obstruction are less likely to resolve spontaneously. Fistulas associated with cancer, inflammatory bowel disease, or radiation rarely close without surgical intervention.

Once the ECF has been appropriately investigated, planning for operative intervention begins. During this phase of care, the surgeon must balance the adequacy of nutritional support, the likelihood of spontaneous closure, and the technical feasibility of the procedure [2, 4]. The preoperative frailty of patients with ECF predicts poor postoperative outcomes [24]. One of the biggest challenges of ECF management is patients and their families who continually push clinicians to repair the ECF before surgery can safely be tolerated. Many elements must be considered at this stage, especially the timing of the operation [25]. Studies suggest that patients with an ECF who are reoperated on within 10 days of the initial surgery or whose reoperation is delayed beyond 120 days have mortality rates of approximately 10%. Those patients who are operated on between 10 and 120 days after the initial surgery have mortality rates of approximately 20% [2, 21]. Although mortality is decreased with early ECF operative intervention, it is wise to avoid operating during (7–120 days) this period, as the risks of causing additional enterotomies or disrupting the previously created anastomosis are too significant. Furthermore, the patient is rarely optimized at this time, specifically from a septic or nutritional standpoint. Instead, it is more prudent to stabilize the patient by controlling and eradicating sepsis, controlling fistula output, correcting fluid and electrolyte deficiencies, and correcting nutritional deficits. Furthermore, time is allotted to allow the fistula to close spontaneously, thus avoiding an operation. Before surgically addressing the ECF, the surgeon must have many open and honest discussions with the patient about the expected road ahead. Definitive surgical therapy cannot be achieved until the patient has been adequately optimized.

RECOMMENDATIONS

ECFs should not be surgically corrected for at least 4–5 months and sometimes longer to allow for potential spontaneous closure and to medically optimize these patients for the best possible outcomes if surgery is required.

Grade of recommendation: C.

39.7.2 What Is the Optimal Surgical Technique for ECF Resection?

The operation for resolving an ECF is extensive, requiring a significant time commitment and multiple resources. We recommend at least a 4- to 6-hour block of time for the surgery, especially if abdominal wall reconstruction is required. The patient and family should be adequately informed of the extensive nature of the surgery and the recovery time needed.

The abdomen should be entered through a new incision away from previous incisions. If the prior midline incision must be used to access the abdomen, it is recommended to make the incision above or below to avoid enterotomies. Once in the abdominal cavity, the viscera should be completely freed from each other through extensive lysis of adhesions. Taking the bowel down should be performed sharply with great care to avoid bowel injury, as this could create another ECF. Tediously working to free the entire bowel and fistula allows for resection;

once the bowel containing the ECF is removed, anastomosis of healthy bowel is performed. If multiple bowel loops are involved, the decision becomes whether to resect these multiple enterotomies as a single segment with one anastomosis or several segments with several anastomoses. The usual preference is to perform one resection with one anastomosis if this is possible without losing significant bowel length. The bowel anastomosis can be performed with success in either a stapled or handsewn fashion. Many studies have demonstrated that there is no significant difference between stapled and handsewn anastomosis; however, retrospective studies have shown increased anastomotic leak with stapled anastomosis [20]. Many institutions prefer the two-layer handsewn anastomosis technique to decrease rates of leak and stricture [20, 26–28]. Once the resection is completed, the bowel surface must be carefully inspected, making sure to repair any serosal tears and/or enterotomies [2, 4]. If these injuries are not appropriately repaired, they can become sources of recurrent ECFs.

Once the gastrointestinal portion of the operation is complete, the next challenge is closure and possible reconstruction of the abdominal wall. Often the fistula takedown requires full-thickness resection of a portion of the abdominal wall. If this resection is small, then primary fascial closure is usually adequate. However, if this resected portion is significant and primary closure is unattainable, a component separation can be performed to bring the abdominal fascia more midline to attain closure. The optimal approach for combined large ventral hernia and ECF repair has yet to be defined. Historically, multiple operations would be performed; the first procedure would be to take down the ECF or ECFs and close the hernia defect using a biological mesh or to reinforce the hernia closure. A second operation would require definitive closure of the large ventral hernia with some version of component separation with or without permanent mesh reinforcement. As component separation can only be done once, it is ideal to complete this portion of the operation on an elective basis during a second operation. One-stage ventral hernia repair with ECF takedown has been successfully done. However, the risks for hernia and fistula recurrence remain high [20]. A recent paper described higher complications such as wound infections, recurrent ventral hernia rates, and hematomas when performing a single-stage ventral hernia repair and ECF takedown [29].

Unfortunately, repaired bowel can break down, and ECFs can recur. Whether the ECF is closed spontaneously or operatively, nutritional support is essential for appropriate healing and prevention of recurrent ECFs. The TPN should typically be continued, or restarted, postoperatively until the patient's postoperative ileus has resolved. Once the patient has reached adequate daily oral caloric intake, the TPN is slowly weaned.

Various endoscopic techniques have been used to close some fistulas. Endoscopic over-the-scope techniques used to close various ECFs have been successful in closing up to 70% of highly selective cases [30]. More case reports and series on the use of these over-the-scope endoscopic techniques will help define who and when should be a candidate for these procedures in the future. This will allow clinicians to apply these endoscopic techniques more successfully for some patients with ECF [31].

RECOMMENDATIONS

Complete excision of the bowel containing the fistula must be performed and accompanied by either handsewn or stapled anastomosis of the healthy bowel.

Grade of recommendation: C.

During extensive lysis of adhesions, the surgeon must be careful to avoid further bowel injury and to preserve bowel length.

Grade of recommendation: C.

It is up to the primary surgeon's discretion to repair the ventral hernia as a staged operation or primarily with the fistula resection.

Grade of recommendation: C.

Patients should be well informed of the anticipated recovery and the possibility of ECF recurrence (Table 39.2).

Grade of recommendation: C.

TABLE 39.2

Summary of Recommendations for the Management of Enterocutaneous Fistulas

Question	Answer	Grade	References
What is the definition of ECF?	• Abnormal connection between gastrointestinal tract and skin. • More common in postoperative patients.	B, C	[2–7]
What are the risk factors for developing an ECF?	• Infection, electrolyte abnormalities, malnutrition, anemia, hypothermia, poor oxygen delivery, emergent procedures, and poor surgical technique.	B, C	[2, 7, 8]
How are ECFs classified?	• According to anatomic location and daily output (low, medium, or high).	B, C	[2–7, 9–11]
How do ECFs present clinically?	• Within 3–5 days from original abdominal surgery. • Patients will not follow the normal postoperative progress and develop a fever, leukocytosis, and wound infection.	C	[2–5]
What is the best method to define ECF anatomy?	• Fistulography with computed tomography.	C	[4]

(Continued)

TABLE 39.2 (Continued)

Summary of Recommendations for the Management of Enterocutaneous Fistulas

Question	Answer	Grade	References
What are the first steps in ECF management?	• Recognition and drainage of the septic source. • Antibiotic administration. • Intravascular volume restoration.	B, C	[3, 9–13]
What is the best way to provide nutritional support to ECF patients?	• Parenteral nutrition must be initiated promptly for nutritional support. • Once infection and output are controlled, enteral nutrition can be reintroduced. • Enteral nutrition is always preferred, but if inadequate or not tolerated, parenteral nutrition should be used to supplement.	B, C	[2–6, 9, 11, 15–17]
What is the best way to decrease fistula output?	• H_2 blockers, proton pump inhibitors, sucralfate, and bulking agents can help decrease fistula output. • Somatostatin analogs may decrease fistula output but are not without side effects.	C	[2–5, 18, 19]
What is the best way to manage an ECF wound?	• Any method to manage the effluent from the ECF while protecting the skin. • VAC therapy looks to be very promising.	C	[3, 4, 21]
When is the best time to provide surgical closure of an ECF?	• Surgical closure after 120 days is associated with better mortality rates compared to earlier closure. • This also allows for the potential spontaneous closure of the ECF.		[2–4, 24, 29–33]
What is the surgical technique for the definitive management of an ECF?	• Enter the virgin abdomen if possible. • Thoroughly inspect all bowels for injuries and repair. • Perform one anastomosis if possible. • Continue aggressive nutritional support postoperatively and inform the patient that recurrent ECFs are possible.	C	[2–4]

Editor's Note

Enterocutaneous fistula is, fortunately, an uncommon condition so no institution has developed a large experience. Thus, there are essentially no quality scientific data to guide our care of patients with this complication. The authors have nicely delineated the current standard of care in the management of enterocutaneous fistula and explained the basic philosophy of care. Unfortunately, none of these concepts are derived from high-quality data and are essentially all based on limited clinical experience.

REFERENCES

1 Owen RM, Love TP, Perez SD, et al. Definitive surgical treatment of enterocutaneous fistula. *JAMA Surg.* 2013;*148*(2):118–126.

2 Fischer JE, Everson AR. 2012. Chapter 146. In: *Gastrointestinal-Cutaneous Fistulas. Fischer's Mastery of Surgery*, 6th ed. Lippincott Williams & Wilkins: Philadelphia, PA, pp. 1564–1574.

3 Polk TM, Schwab CW. Metabolic and nutritional support of the enterocutaneous fistula patient: A three-phase approach. *World J Surg.* 2012;*36*:514–533.

4 Everson AR, Fischer JE. Current management of enterocutaneous fistulas. *J Gastrointest Surg.* 2006;*10*:455–464.

5 Manos LL, Wolfgang CL. 2014. The management of enterocutaneous fistulas. In: *Current Surgical Therapy*, 11th ed. Elsevier: Philadelphia, PA, pp. 142–145.

6 Martinez JL, Luque-de-Leon E, Blanco-Benavides R, et al. Factors predictive of recurrence and mortality after surgical repair of enterocutaneous fistula. *J Gastrointest Surg.* 2012;*16*:156–164.

7 Martinez JL, Luque-de-Leon E, Mier J, et al. Systematic management of postoperative enterocutaneous fistulas: Factors related to outcomes. *World J Surg.* 2008;*32*:436–443.

8 Zelhart MD, Hauch AT, Slakey DP, et al. Preoperative antibiotic colon preparation: Have we had the answer all along? *J Am Coll Surg.* 2014;*219*(5):1070–1077.

9 Levy E, Frileux P, Cugnenc PH, et al. High-output external fistulae of the small bowel: Management with continued enteral nutrition. *Br J Surg.* 1989;*76*:676–679.

10 Campos AC, Andrade DF, Campos GM. A multivariate model to determine prognostic factors in gastrointestinal fistulas. *J Am Coll Surg.* 1999;*188*:483–490.

11 Soeters PB, Ebeid AM, Fischer JE. Review of 404 patients with gastrointestinal fistulas: Impact of parenteral nutrition. *Ann Surg.* 1979;*190*:189–202.

12 Dellinger RP, Levy MM, Rhodes A, et al. Surviving sepsis campaign: International guidelines for management of severe sepsis and septic shock: 2012. *Crit Care Med.* 2013;*41*(2):580–637.

13 Hill GL, Bourchier RG, Witney GB. Surgical and metabolic management of patients with enteral fistulas of the small intestine associated with Crohn's disease. *World J Surg.* 1988;*12*:191–197.

14 Rose D, Yarborough MF, Canizaro PC, et al. One hundred and fourteen fistulas of the gastrointestinal tract are treated with total parenteral nutrition. *Surg Gynecol Obstet.* 1986;*163*:345–350.

15 Berlana D, Barraquer A, Sabin P, et al. Impact of paren-
    teral nutrition standardization on costs and quality in adult
    patients. *Nutr Hosp.* 2014;*30*(2):351–358.

16 Fazio VS, Coutsoftides T, Steiger E. Factors influencing
    the outcome of treatment of small bowel cutaneous fistula.
    World J Surg. 1983;*7*:481–488.

17 Alivizatos V, Felekis D, Zorbalas A. Evaluation of the effec-
    tiveness of octreotide in the conservative treatment of post-
    operative enterocutaneous fistulas. *Hepatogastroenterology.*
    2002;*49*:1010–1012.

18 Martineau P, Showed JA, Denis R. Is octreotide a new hope
    for enterocutaneous and external pancreatic fistulas clo-
    sure? *Am J Surg.* 1996;*172*:386–395.

19 De Leon JM. Novel techniques using negative pres-
    sure wound therapy for the management of wounds with
    enterocutaneous fistulas in a long-term acute care facil-
    ity. *J Wound Ostomy Continence Nurs.* 2013;*40*(5):
    481–488.

20 Lafti R Joeph B, Kulvatunyou N, et al. Enterocutaneous
    fistulas and a hostile abdomen: Reoperative surgical
    approaches. *World J Surg.* 2012;*36*:516–523.

21 Yeh DD, Vasileiou G, Jawad KA, et al. Teduglutide for
    the treatment of low-output enterocutaneous fistula – A
    pilot randomized controlled study. *Clin Nutr ESPEN.*
    2022;*50*:49–55.

22 O' Keefe SJ, Jeppesen PB, Gilroy R, et al. Safety and effi-
    cacy of teduglutide after 52 weeks of treatment in patients
    with short bowel intestinal failure. *Clin Gastroenterol
    Hepatol.* 2013;*11*(17):815–823.

23 Gefen R, Garoufalia Z, Zhou P, et al. Treatment of entero-
    cutaneous fistula: A systemic review and meta-analysis.
    Tech Coloproctol. 2022 Aug 1;*26*,863–874.

24. Alser O, Naar L, Christensen MA, et al. Preoperative frailty
    predicts postoperative outcomes in intestinal-cutaneous fis-
    tula repair. *Surgery.* 2021 May;*169*(5):1199–1205.

25 Coughlin S, Roth L, Lurati G, Faulhaber M. Somatostatin
    analogs for the treatment of enterocutaneous fistulas: A
    systemic review and meta-analysis. *World J Surg.* 2012;*36*:
    1016–1029.

26 Schecter WP, Hirschburg A, Chang DS, et al. Enteric fistu-
    las: Principles of management. *J Am Coll Surg.* 2009;*209*:
    484–491.

27 Neutzling CB, Lustosa SA, Proenca IM, et al. Stapled ver-
    sus handsewn methods for colorectal anastomosis surgery.
    Cochrane Database Syst Rev. 2012;*15*(2):CD003144.

28 Farrah JP, Lauer CW, Bray MS, et al. Stapled versus
    hand-sewn anastomoses in emergency general surgery: A
    retrospective review of outcomes in the unique patient pop-
    ulation. *J Trauma Acute Care Surg.* 2013;*74*:1187–1192.

29 Klifto KM, Othman S, Messa CA, et al. Risk factors,
    outcomes, and complications associated with a combined
    ventral hernia and enterocutaneous fistula single-staged
    abdominal wall reconstruction. *Hernia.* 2021;*25*:1537–1548.

30 Roy J, Sims K, Rider P, et al. Endoscopic technique for
    closure of enterocutaneous fistulas. *Surg Endosc.* 2019;*33*:
    3463–3468.

31 Monkemueller K, Martinez-Alcala A, et al. The use of the
    over-the-scope clips beyond its standard use: A pictorial
    description. *Gastrointest Endoscopy Clin N Am.* 2020;*30*:
    41–74.

32 Osborn C, Fischer JE. How I do it: Gastrointestinal cutane-
    ous fistulas. *J Gastrointest Surg.* 2009;*13*(*11*):2068.

33 Bhama AR. Evaluation and management of enterocutane-
    ous fistula. *Dis Colon Rectum.* 2019;*62*:906–991.

40

Paraesophageal Hernia Repair

Sebastian R. Eid and George Mazpule

40.1 Introduction

Hiatal hernias are characterized by the intrathoracic protrusion of elements of the abdominal cavity through a widened esophageal hiatus. They are anatomically classified into four types (I–IV). Types II–IV hernias are collectively referred to as paraesophageal hernias (PEHs). Characterized by the presence of a hernia sac, these are true hernias that protrude through a defect in the phrenoesophageal membrane with relative preservation of the posterolateral phrenoesophageal attachments around the gastroesophageal junction (GEJ) [1]. Types II–IV are considered paraesophageal hernias; they compromise between 5% and 15% of all hiatal hernias [2]. Of the paraesophageal hernias, more than 90% are type III.

40.1.1 Hiatal hernias are traditionally classified according to the position of the GEJ

- *Type I*: Classic sliding hiatal hernia in which the GEJ migrates cephalad through the esophageal hiatus due to a laxity in the phrenoesophageal membrane (which remains intact); accounts for >95% of hiatal hernias. Frequently associated with gastroesophageal reflux disease (GERD).
- *Type II*: True paraesophageal hernia in which the fundus herniates into the posterior mediastinum alongside a normally positioned GEJ.
- *Type III*: Combined or mixed type hiatal hernia, in which both the GEJ and the fundus herniate into the mediastinum through the hiatus.
- *Type IV*: Often described where all of the stomach and/or other viscera (i.e., colon, spleen, pancreas) herniate into the chest.

Although no consensus definition exists, it is widely accepted that giant PEHs are present when greater than 50% of the stomach resides within the chest.

Surgical repair is analogous to all types of hiatal hernias; however, paraesophageal hernias have a characteristic presentation and workup and carry the potential for an acute presentation that sets them apart from sliding hiatal hernias [3].

The diagnosis of PEHs seems to be encountered with increasing frequency, whether due to improved recognition or an actual increase in our aging population. Before the laparoscopic/robotic era, most of these hernias were repaired with an open abdominal approach, and the standard mantra was that the diagnosis of this lesion mandated operative treatment [4, 5] With the advent of minimally invasive procedures, a laparoscopic approach for repair has become much more common, and some would argue it should be the standard of care [6]. Several studies have demonstrated the efficacy and safety of this approach. However, except for the acceptance of laparoscopic repair, virtually all other aspects of PEH repair have some elements of controversy associated with them.

40.2 Should All Paraesophageal Hernias Be Repaired?

The natural history of PEHs is progressive enlargement such that eventually, the entire stomach herniates alongside the esophagus, with the pylorus juxtaposed to the gastric cardia, forming an intrathoracic upside-down stomach. The driving force for this progression is positive intraabdominal pressure combined with negative intrathoracic pressure [7]. As more stomach moves up into the thorax, respiratory symptoms may predominate secondary to pulmonary compression [8].

Sliding hiatal hernias most frequently present with symptoms of GERD; however, this is not a common presentation for PEHs. Most patients with PEHs are asymptomatic. In symptomatic patients, the most common finding is gastritis and gastric ulceration. Symptoms of postprandial fullness, epigastric discomfort, and dysphagia are not infrequent. Serious complications include acute gastric hemorrhage, volvulus, obstruction, strangulation, and perforation.

Acute incarceration, strangulation, or gastric volvulus with a PEH is a true surgical emergency, and early recognition and treatment are essential to prevent further morbidity and mortality [3, 9]. The most common cause of gastric volvulus in adults is PEH. This is when the stomach rotates more than 180 degrees, causing a closed obstruction. This happens in the organoaxial direction (longitudinal axis) or the mesenteroaxial direction (transverse axis). Ischemia and perforation of the stomach can result until the volvulus is reduced [10]. Borchardt's triad—(1) nonproductive vomiting, (2) severe lower chest and epigastric pain, and (3) inability to pass a nasogastric tube (NGT)—are associated with gastric volvulus and clinically diagnostic [9, 10].

NGT placement usually is effective in decompressing the stomach and may result in a spontaneous reduction in the case of gastric volvulus. The tube should, however, be placed with

DOI: 10.1201/9781003316800-40

fluoroscopic or endoscopic guidance to limit the risk of gastric perforation [9–11]. Once the stomach is decompressed, the NGT should remain in place and the patient optimized for repair during the index admission [11].

Traditionally, prophylactic repair of asymptomatic PEHs had been preferred secondary to a perceived high incidence of catastrophic complications (29%) and exceedingly high mortality associated with emergent repair (17%) [12].

More recent studies have shown that the occurrence of such complications is infrequent, thus advocating for a censored observation policy in asymptomatic cases. In 1993, Allen et al. reported a large retrospective chart review series from the Mayo Clinic. Out of 147 patients, 23 patients were managed nonoperatively; 4/23 developed progression of their symptoms [13].

Stylopoulos et al. designed a Markov Monte Carlo decision analytic model and used it to determine if elderly asymptomatic or minimally symptomatic patients benefit from elective PEH repair. The model examined existing literature regarding mortality and hernia progression rates in patients who were 65 years old and asymptomatic.

They concluded that the mortality rate of emergency repair of PEHs was overestimated by early studies, likely only 5.4% versus the 17% quoted previously. They also estimated that the mortality rate of elective PEH repair likely was 1.4%, whereas the annual likelihood of developing gastric complications from hernias was only 1.1%. This analysis found that fewer than 1 in 5 asymptomatic patients aged 65 years and older, and fewer than 1 in 10 asymptomatic patients aged 85 years and older, benefit from elective PEH repair. Therefore, even if an emergency operation is required, the burden of the procedure is not as severe as was previously thought [3, 14]. The same group recently repeated their analysis in 2018 and found that despite improvements in surgical options and medical care, 82% of patients would still benefit from a watchful waiting approach [15].

Based on these data, prophylactic PEH repair in the absence of symptoms is rarely indicated. There remains little debate, however, that all symptomatic patients who are medically operable should undergo surgical treatment, particularly those with acute obstructive symptoms or volvulus [16].

RECOMMENDATION

The decision to surgically repair a PEH is based on the patient's overall medical status, symptomatic complaints, and the chance of incarceration/strangulation [17]. All symptomatic patients who are medically operable should be surgically treated. Routine elective repair of asymptomatic or minimally symptomatic PEHs is not indicated.

Grade of recommendation: B.

40.3 What Is the Best Approach to Repair PEH When Indicated?

The preferred technique to repair a PEH has evolved over the past several years. Originally, PEHs were repaired via an open approach, via thoracotomy or laparotomy. However, advances in laparoscopy and robotic-assisted surgery have led to their increase in popularity [3].

Due to the proven increased morbidity with open approaches, they are now obsolete except in certain circumstances. Studies have shown increased length of stay, worse postoperative pain, and a higher incidence of pulmonary complications with a transthoracic PEH repair. However, esophageal mobilization is easier via this approach. Esophageal mobilization via the transabdominal approach is more difficult. The benefits of PEH repair via a laparotomy include the ability to perform a gastropexy, gastrostomy, and easier reduction of gastric volvulus. Outcomes between these two methods of PEH repair have shown to be equivalent [18].

Minimally invasive repair of PEH has become the standard of care. Initially with laparoscopy, and now with robotic assistance, outcomes have improved, including a short length of stay, less pain, less blood loss, and fewer pulmonary complications. Recent studies have shown the advantages of minimally invasive PEH repair over open repairs. The view via a laparoscopic or robotically assisted approach is superior to a transabdominal approach, which leads to an easier and more extensive esophageal mobilization [19].

The minimally invasive approach can also be done in emergent situations such as gastric volvulus with or without gastric ischemia. An open repair or conversion to open may be needed if there is gross peritoneal contamination [20].

Robotic-assisted laparoscopic PEH repair has several advantages over traditional laparoscopy. These include a stable camera platform, 3D high-definition magnified vision, long articulating instruments that may allow for more extensive esophageal mobilization, and the control of an assistant fourth "arm." While costs may be higher and operative times may be longer, the robotic platform may offer prevention of certain PEH repairs from being converted to open. A recent prospective study by Gerull et al. in 2021 compared 830 robotic PEH repairs to 1,024 done via conventional laparoscopy. The robotic cohort was found to have significantly less need for an esophageal-lengthening procedure, less conversion to open, and a lower length of stay. Intraoperative costs were shown to be similar [20].

Studies have shown that minimally invasive repairs of PEH have better outcomes than open repairs. The recurrence rate of laparoscopic PEH repairs has improved over the years [21].

In 2007, Rathore et al. published a meta-analysis of a nonrandomized series of laparoscopic PEH repairs. In 965 patients with follow-up beyond 6 months, the overall recurrence rate was 10.2%. Among those patients formally evaluated with a contrast esophagogram postoperatively, 25.5% had a recurrence. Lower recurrence rates were noticed in those who underwent an esophageal-lengthening procedure with a Collis–Nissen gastroplasty versus those who did not (0% vs. 12%) [22]. Given the high recurrence rates following laparoscopic PEH repair (25.5%), the authors recommended mandatory follow-up esophagograms at 1 year [22].

In 2011, Nguyen et al. retrospectively compared 2,069 laparoscopic and 657 open repairs of PEH. For elective procedures, utilization of laparoscopic repair was 81% and was associated with a shorter hospital stay (3.7 vs. 8.3 days, $p < 0.01$), less requirement for intensive care unit care, and lower overall complications. In patients presenting with obstruction or gangrene, utilization of laparoscopic repair was 57% and was similarly associated with improved outcomes compared with open repair [23].

RECOMMENDATION

Laparoscopic or robotically assisted PEH repair is the preferred approach for the majority of PEHs. It is as effective as open transthoracic or transabdominal repair, but it is associated with a reduced rate of perioperative morbidity and shorter hospital length of stay.

Grade of recommendation: C.

40.4 What Operative Strategies Have Been Shown to Minimize Recurrence Rates Following PEH Repair?

Several essential elements can lead to a successful and durable PEH repair. First, a significant esophageal mobilization leads to at least 3 cm of intraabdominal esophagus. Second, dissection of the hernia sac from within the mediastinum. Third, performing an antireflux procedure. And fourth, posterior reapproximation of the crura. The effectiveness of intraabdominal fixation of the stomach via gastropexy or gastrostomy tube is still debated [25].

40.4.1 Hernia Sac Resection

PEHs lead to the development of a mediastinal peritoneal hernia sac. It is essential to thoroughly dissect the peritoneal sac from its mediastinal attachments into the abdomen completely or as much as possible. This allows for tension to be released off the esophagus, increasing the amount of intraabdominal esophagus, which is known to reduce recurrence rates. The sac, if large, may need to be excised from the GEJ, so that a fundoplication can be performed. Edye et al. prospectively compared laparoscopic repair with and without excision of the hernia sac. About 5 of 25 operations without sac excision suffered hernia recurrence during a 38-month follow-up period. No recurrences were reported at the 15-month follow-up for the 30 patients whose PEH repair procedure included hernia sac excision [26].

40.4.2 Reinforced Crural Repair

The use of mesh reinforcement in PEH repair is still widely debated. There is no consensus on when or when not to use mesh. Though rare, synthetic mesh has the hypothetical risk of esophageal erosion. Also, the repair of a recurrent PEH with a prior mesh in place is much more difficult. However, numerous prospective trials have shown decreased short-term recurrence rates with the use of mesh reinforcement. Long-term data to date fail to prove a significant reduction in recurrence [27]. The first randomized controlled trial (RCT) studied patients

with hiatal defects >8 cm. With a mean follow-up of 3.3 years, radiographic recurrence was significantly higher in patients undergoing primary crural repair alone versus those whose crural repair was reinforced with an onlay polytetrafluoroethylene (PTFE) mesh (22% vs. 0%). No mesh-related complications during the study period were reported [28]. Similar findings were reported by another RCT in patients with hernia defects >5 cm (26% recurrence rate in patients undergoing primary crural repair vs. 8% mesh-reinforced crural repair) [28]. Oelschlägel et al. demonstrated similar short-term results using a bioprosthetic mesh with no mesh-related complications reported. This improvement in recurrence rates, however, was not seen at 4 years. The findings of the follow-up study must be interpreted with caution given a significant dropout rate and the lack of uniform radiographic evaluation [29].

The erosion of the mesh into the esophagus is what leads to the reluctance for its use. Mesh erosion may require an esophagectomy if indicated. Because of this, bioabsorbable meshes have been used, but studies have failed to show long-term benefits.

RECOMMENDATIONS

The peritoneal hernia sac involving the PEH should be dissected out of the mediastinum completely, if possible, and excised.

Grade of recommendation: C.

Current data fail to support a recommendation on when mesh should or should not be used.

Grade of recommendation: C.

40.5 Is There a Role for Esophageal-Lengthening Procedures during Paraesophageal Hernia Repair?

Decades of experience with open and laparoscopic PEH repairs have established certain principles as essential for a successful tension-free repair. One of these defining aspects is establishing a 2.5- to 3-cm intraabdominal esophagus. Extensive hernia sac resection, high mediastinal dissection, and esophageal mobilization may all be employed in bringing the GEJ at least 2.5 cm below the hiatus without tension. If such strategies are unsuccessful, most reports would agree that this constitutes a shortened esophagus, and a Collis gastroplasty should be attempted [30]. This technique creates a tube of neo-esophagus from a proximal portion of the stomach using a stapled technique [31].

Although the precise incidence of esophageal shortening in PEH is unknown, with reports ranging from 0% to 60%, its true burden is probably close to 10%. Intrinsic shortening of the esophagus is invariably encountered in the setting of GERD, where repeated cycles of acid or alkali injury result in chronic periesophageal inflammation and fibrosis. Longitudinal contraction of collagen in the fibrous tissue results in a shortened esophagus. Although certain preoperative findings may raise the index of suspicion for a short esophagus (e.g., giant hiatal hernia, long-standing GERD), no imaging or endoscopic modality is superior to surgeon assessment in predicting intraabdominal esophageal length intraoperatively [30]. At a median follow-up of 58 months, Oelschlager described a 54% radiologic recurrence rate even with the use of a biologic mesh. Only 5/108 (4.6%) patients in this group underwent a Collis gastroplasty [29].

At a median of 22 postoperative months, Luketich et al. reported a radiographic recurrence of 15.7% after 662 laparoscopic giant PEH repairs; interestingly 63% of these repairs included a Collis gastroplasty [32]. Although no prospective data exist, there is general agreement that a lengthening gastroplasty reduces the rate of recurrent herniation following repair of PEH when esophageal shortening is encountered [33, 34].

RECOMMENDATION

After the hiatal repair, the intraabdominal esophagus should measure at least 2.5–3 cm in length to decrease the risk of recurrence.

Grade of recommendation: C.

Although no prospective data exist, a lengthening gastroplasty reduces the rate of recurrent herniation when esophageal shortening is encountered.

Grade of recommendation: C.

40.6 Is There Evidence Supporting Routine Fundoplication in Patients Undergoing Laparoscopic PEH Repair?

Fundoplication during repair of a type 1 sliding hiatal hernia is considered standard of care [16]; however, high-level evidence supporting the practice of routine fundoplication in all PEH repairs is lacking; nevertheless, expert opinion suggests a fundoplication be performed when feasible.

The benefits of a fundoplication are thought to be twofold; they help reduce postoperative reflux and may decrease recurrence rates. The extensive dissection is necessary to fully mobilize the esophagus, and dissecting the hernia sac is thought to render the GEJ incompetent, resulting in postoperative reflux. This has been reported as high as 65% in patients who did not receive a fundoplication [35, 36]. A fundoplication may re-establish a "lower esophageal sphincter" mechanism. A fundoplication may also buttress the repair and anchor the stomach intraabdominally, theoretically reducing the likelihood of recurrence [16, 37]. As with fundoplication done for GERD, gas-bloat syndrome and dysphagia are the most frequent postoperative complications. These complications usually improve 3–6 months after surgery [38].

One recent case-controlled study of 46 patients compared laparoscopic PEH repair with and without fundoplication (laparoscopic Nissen over a 56 Fr bougie). Findings included

increased dysphagia with fundoplication and reflux symptoms in the group without fundoplication [16, 39]. Data in support of one fundoplication technique over another are likewise mixed. In general, complete wraps result in increased dysphagia, whereas partial wraps tend to have a higher incidence of GERD. In patients with PEHs, where dysphagia, as opposed to reflux, is the defining symptomatology and preoperative manometry is less reliable, an argument can be made that partial wraps are favorable [3].

RECOMMENDATION

High-level evidence supporting the practice of routine fundoplication is lacking; nevertheless, most surgeons consider it essential during PEH repair to reduce recurrence and minimize reflux symptoms.

Grade of recommendation: C.

40.7 What Are the Options for High-Risk Patients with Symptomatic PEH?

Formal PEH repair may not be suitable in high-risk symptomatic patients. In these cases, reduction of the PEH can be performed with endoscopy or laparoscopy. Gastropexy can be done to anchor the stomach in the abdomen via suture gastropexy, laparoscopic gastrostomy tube, or percutaneous endoscopic gastrostomy tube placement. More than one gastrostomy may be needed. While recurrence rates are high with this option, it can also act as a bridge to an elective formal repair of the PEH and prevent gastric volvulus [40].

RECOMMENDATIONS

Hernia reduction with gastropexy alone and no hiatal repair may be a safe alternative in high-risk patients but may be associated with high recurrence rates.

Grade of recommendation: C.

Laparoscopic-assisted endoscopic hernia reduction with PEG tube placement may be useful in symptomatic patients with prohibitive surgical risk.

Grade of recommendation: C.

Conclusions

PEHs represent a small portion of all hiatal hernias. When symptomatic, they are defined by symptoms of dysphagia, gastritis, early satiety, and epigastric pain rather than primarily GERD and have the propensity for acute presentation. Watchful waiting is a reasonable treatment option for most asymptomatic cases. Other than the benefits of minimally invasive approaches for their repair and the treatment in an

TABLE 40.1

Clinical Questions

Question	Answer	Level of Evidence	Grade of Recommendation	References
Should all paraesophageal hernias be repaired?	The decision to surgically repair a PEH is based on the patient's overall medical status, symptomatic complaints, and the chance of incarceration/ strangulation. All symptomatic patients who are medically operable should be surgically treated. Routine elective repair of asymptomatic or minimally symptomatic paraesophageal hernias is not indicated.	2B	B	[7–17]
What is the best approach to repair PEH when indicated?	Laparoscopic or robotically assisted PEH repair is the preferred approach for the majority of PEHs. It is as effective as open transthoracic or transabdominal repair, but it is associated with a reduced rate of perioperative morbidity and shorter hospital length of stay.	2C	C	[3, 18–23]
What operative strategies have been shown to minimize recurrence rates following PEH repair?	The peritoneal hernia sac involving the PEH should be dissected out of the mediastinum completely, if possible, and excised. Current data fail to support a recommendation on when mesh should or should not be used. The use of mesh reinforcement with large hiatal hernia repairs leads to decreased short-term recurrence rates. Long-term data on which to base a recommendation either for or against the use of mesh at the hiatus are lacking.	3B 2B	C C	[25–29]
Is there a role for esophageal-lengthening procedures during PEH repair?	After the hiatal repair, the intraabdominal esophagus should measure at least 2.5–3 cm in length to decrease the risk of recurrence. Although no prospective data exist, a lengthening gastroplasty reduces the rate of recurrent herniation when esophageal shortening is encountered.	3A	C C	[29–34]
Is there evidence supporting routine fundoplication in patients undergoing laparoscopic PEH repair?	High-level evidence supporting the practice of routine fundoplication is lacking; nevertheless, most surgeons consider it essential during PEH repair to reduce recurrence and minimize reflux symptoms.	4	C	[3, 16, 35–39]
What options are there for high-risk patients with symptomatic PEH?	Hernia reduction with gastropexy alone and no hiatal repair may be a safe alternative in high-risk patients but may be associated with high recurrence. Laparoscopic-assisted endoscopic hernia reduction with PEG tube placement may be useful in the symptomatic patient with prohibitive surgical risk.	4 4	C C	[40]

acute presentation, several controversies still exist regarding their ideal management. The data are still debated in regard to indications for surgery, sac excision, need for fundoplication, lengthening procedures, and need for mesh reinforcement. See Table 40.1 for a summary of the clinical questions with corresponding level of evidence and recommendations.

REFERENCES

1. Kahrilas PJ, Pandolfino JE. *Hiatus hernia.* GI Motility Online, 2006.
2. Siegal SR, Dolan JP, Hunter JG. Modern diagnosis and treatment of hiatal hernias. *Langenback's Arch Surg.* 2017 Dec;*402*(8):1145–1151.
3. Mazer L, Telem DA. Paraesophgeal hernia; current management. *Adv Surg.* 2021;*55*:109–122.
4. Hill LD. Incarcerated paraesophageal hernias: A surgical emergency. *Am J Surg.* 1973;*126*:206–209.
5. Geha AS, Massad MG, Snow NJ, Bave AE. A 32-year experience in 100 patients with giant paraesophageal hernia: The case for abdominal approach and selective antireflux repair. *Surgery.* 2000 October;*128*(4):623–630.
6. Metha S, Boddy A, Rhodes M. Review of outcome after laparoscopic paraesophageal hernia repair. *Surg Laparosc Endogc.* 2006;*16*:301–306.
7. Landreneau RJ, Del Pino M, Santos R. Management of paraesophageal hernias. *Surg Clin N Am.* 2005;*85*(*3*):411–432.
8. Low DE, Simchuk EJ. Effect of paraesophageal hernia repair on pulmonary function. *Ann Thorac Surg.* 2002;*74*(2):333–337; discussion 337.
9. Coleman C, Musgrove K, Bardes J, Dhamija A, Buenaventura P. Incarcerated paraesophageal hernia and gastric volvulus: Management options for the acute care surgeon. *J Trauma Acute Care Surg.* 2020;*88*(6):e146–e148.
10. Cardile AP, Heppner DS. Gastric volvulus, Borchardt's triad, and endoscopy: A rare twist. *Hawaii MED J.* 2011 Apr;*70*(4):80–82.

11. Wirsching A, El Lakis MA, Mohiuddin K, et al. Acute vs. elective paraesophageal hernia repair: Endoscopic gastric decompression allows semi-elective surgery in a majority of acute patients. *J Gastrointest Surg.* 2018;*22*:194–202.

12. Skinner DB, Belsey RH. Surgical management of esophageal reflux and hiatus hernia. Long-term results with 1,030 patients. *J Thorac Cardiovasc Surg.* 1967;*53(1)*:33–54.

13. Allen MS, Trastek VF, Deschamps C, et al. Intrathoracic stomach. Presentation and results of operation. *J Thorac Cardiovasc Surg.* 1993;*105(2)*:253–258; discussion 258–259.

14. Stylopoulos N, Gazelle GS, Rattner DW. Paraesophageal hernias: Operation or observation? *Ann Surg.* 2002;*236(4)*:492–500; discussion 500–501.

15. Jung JJ, Naimark DM, Behman R, et al. Approach to asymptomatic paraesophageal hernia: Watchful waiting or elective laparoscopic hernia repair? *Surg Endosc.* 2018;*32(2)*:864–871.

16. Kohn GP, Price RR, DeMeester SR et al. Guidelines for the management of hiatal hernia. *Surg Endosc.* 2013;*27(12)*: 4409–4428.

17. Sheff SR, Kothari SN. Repair of the giant hiatal hernia. *J Long Term Eff Med Implants.* 2010;*20(2)*:139–148.

18. Rogers MP, Velanovich V, DuCoin C. Narrative review of management controversies for paraesophageal hernia. *J Thorac Dis.* 2021 Jul;*13(7)*:4476–4483. DOI: 10.21037/jtd-21-720. PMID: 34422374; PMCID: PMC8339754.

19. Klinginsmith M, Jolley J, Lomelin D, Krause C, Heiden J, Oleynikov D. Paraesophageal hernia repair in the emergency setting: Is laparoscopy with the addition of a fundoplication the new gold standard? *Surg Endosc.* 2016 May;*30(5)*:1790–1795. DOI: 10.1007/s00464-015-4447-8. Epub 2015 Jul 21. PMID: 26194263.

20. Gerull WD, Cho D, Arefanian S, Kushner BS, Awad MM. Favorable peri-operative outcomes were observed in paraesophageal hernia repair with the robotic approach. *Surg Endosc.* 2021 Jun;*35(6)*:3085–3089. DOI: 10.1007/s00464-020-07700-7. Epub 2020 Jun 15. PMID: 32556775.

21. Cohn TD, Soper NJ. Paraesophageal hernia repair: Techniques for success. *J Laparoendosc Adv Surg Tech A.* 2017 Jan;*27(1)*:19–23. DOI: 10.1089/lap.2016.0496. Epub 2016 Nov 22. PMID: 27875096.

22. Rathore MA, Andrabi SI, Bhatti MI, Najfi SM, McMurray A. Metaanalysis of recurrence after laparoscopic repair of paraesophageal hernia. *JSLS.* 2007 Oct-Dec;*11(4)*:456–460. PMID: 18237510; PMCID: PMC3015848.

23. Nguyen NT, Christie C, Masoomi H, Matin T, Laugenour K, Hohmann S. Utilization and outcomes of laparoscopic versus open paraesophageal hernia repair. *Am Surg.* 2011 Oct;*77(10)*:1353–1357. PMID: 22127087

24. Zehetner J, Demeester SR, Ayazi S, Kilday P, Augustin F, Hagen JA, Lipham JC, Sohn HJ, Demeester TR. Laparoscopic versus open repair of paraesophageal hernia: The second decade. *J Am Coll Surg.* 2011 May;*212(5)*: 813–820. DOI: 10.1016/j.jamcollsurg.2011.01.060. Epub 2011 Mar 23. PMID: 21435915.

25. Arafat FO, Teitelbaum EN, Hungness ES. Modern treatment of paraesophageal hernia: preoperative evaluation and technique for laparoscopic repair. *Surg Laparosc Endosc Percutan Tech.* 2012 Aug;*22(4)*:297–303. DOI: 10.1097/SLE.0b013e31825831af. PMID: 22874677.

26. Edye M, Salky B, Posner A, Fierer A. Sac excision is essential to adequate laparoscopic repair of paraesophageal hernia. *Surg Endosc.* 1998 Oct;*12(10)*:1259–1263. DOI: 10.1007/s004649900832. PMID: 9745068.

27. Velanovich V. Practice-changing milestones in anti-reflux and hiatal hernia surgery: A single surgeon perspective over 27 years and 1200 operations. *J Gastrointest Surg.* 2021 Nov;*25(11)*:2757–2769. DOI: 10.1007/s11605-021-04940-3. Epub 2021 Feb 2. PMID: 33532979.

28. Frantzides CT, Madan AK, Carlson MA, Stavropoulos GP. A prospective, randomized trial of laparoscopic polytetrafluoroethylene (PTFE) patch repair vs simple cruroplasty for large hiatal hernia. *Arch Surg.* 2002 Jun;*137(6)*:649–652. DOI: 10.1001/archsurg.137.6.649. PMID: 12049534.

29. Oelschlager BK, Pellegrini CA, Hunter J, Soper N, Brunt M, Sheppard B, Jobe B, Polissar N, Mitsumori L, Nelson J, Swanstrom L. Biologic prosthesis reduces recurrence after laparoscopic paraesophageal hernia repair: A multicenter, prospective, randomized trial. *Ann Surg.* 2006 Oct;*244(4)*: 481–490. DOI: 10.1097/01.sla.0000237759.42831.03. PMID: 16998356; PMCID: PMC1856552.

30. R Horvath KD, Swanstrom LL, Jobe BA. The short esophagus: Pathophysiology, incidence, presentation, and treatment in the era of laparoscopic antireflux surgery. *Ann Surg.* 2000; *232(5)*:630–640.

31. Collis J. Gastroplasty. *Thorax.* 1961;*16*:197.

32. Luketich JD, Nason KS, Christie NA, et al. Outcomes after a decade of laparoscopic giant paraesophageal hernia repair. *J Thorac Cardiovasc Surg.* 2010;*139(2)*:395–404, 404.e1.

33. Darling G, Deschamps C. Technical controversies in fundoplication surgery. *Thorac Surg Clin.* 2005;*15(3)*:437–444.

34. Parekh KR, Iannettoni MD. 2007. Lengthening gastroplasty for managing giant paraesophageal hernia. In: *Difficult Decisions in Thoracic Surgery.* Springer: London, pp. 318–322.

35. Pearson F, Cooper JD, Ilves R, et al. Massive hiatal hernia with incarceration: A report of 53 cases. *Ann Thorac Surg.* 1983;*35(1)*:45–51.

36. Ponsky J, Rosen M, Fanning A et al. Anterior gastropexy may reduce the recurrence rate after laparoscopic paraesophageal hernia repair. *Surg Endosc Other Intervent Techniq.* 2003;*17(7)*:1036–1041.

37. Wu J, Dunnegan D, Soper N. Clinical and radiologic assessment of laparoscopic paraesophageal hernia repair. *Surg Endosc.* 1999;*13(5)*:497–502.

38. Richter JE. Gastroesophageal reflux disease treatment: Side effects and complications of fundoplication. *Clin Gastroenterol Hepatol.* 2013;*11(5)*:465–471.

39. Morris-Stiff G, Hassn A. Laparoscopic paraoesophageal hernia repair: Fundoplication is not usually indicated. *Hernia.* 2008;*12(3)*:299–302.

40. Shehzad K, Askari A, Slesser AAP, Riaz A. A safe and effective technique of paraesophageal hernia reduction using combined laparoscopy and nonsutured PEG gastropexy in high-risk patients. *JSLS.* 2019 Oct-Dec;*23(4)*:e2019.00041. DOI: 10.4293/JSLS.2019.00041. PMID: 31624456; PMCID: PMC6791400.

41

Lower Gastrointestinal Bleeding

Gregory J. Gallina, Alexander Fortgang, and Jessica Wassef

41.1 Introduction

Lower gastrointestinal bleeding (LGIB) is defined as bleeding originating distal to the ligament of Treitz. This section will focus on LGIB from a colonic source, as that is the predominant reason for surgical consultation in the hospital setting. Gastrointestinal (GI) bleeding is the most common cause of hospitalization related to GI disease in the USA. The true incidence of LGIB is likely underestimated as minor episodes may never present to a hospital. LGIB has varied presentations due to its heterogeneous causes, and the large anatomical range of the "lower GI" distribution can pose a challenge for clinicians, as it is difficult at times to pinpoint the source of the bleeding, and this is critical for optimal management.

Bleeding may present actively and acutely (even massively) or chronically. Acute LGIB is characterized by a sudden onset of hematochezia and/or melena and may even be associated with hemodynamic instability. Chronic LGIB is indolent and may be slow or intermittent. It usually presents as iron deficiency anemia and/or positive fecal occult blood testing. In up to 15% of patients, acute LGIB originates from the upper GI tract. Slower upper GI bleeding (UGIB) sources result in dark, tarry stools, or melena, due to oxidation of heme as it traverses the lower GI tract; thus with a presentation of melena, an upper GI source must be investigated first. However, brisk upper GI bleeds may transit the GI tract much more quickly, too fast to be converted into melena. Therefore, hematochezia associated with hemodynamic instability can be indicative of an upper GI source. A special note should be made for patients with post-procedural bleeding. Any patient that has undergone recent intervention via colonoscopy should have a repeat colonoscopy as the primary intervention.

The elderly are at an increased risk of both frequency and mortality from LGIB. The incidence of LGIB increased more than 200-fold in patients >80 years old compared to those who are 20 years old. This increase can be attributed to a higher incidence of diverticulosis and angiodysplasia with age [1].

The role of the history and physical exam is to clarify the source of bleeding. The amount, frequency, and duration of bleeding are informative. Physicians should inquire about upper GI symptoms, liver disease, recent endoscopic procedures, history of radiation, and/or inflammatory bowel disease (IBD). Symptoms such as diarrhea and abdominal pain can suggest an ischemic, inflammatory, or infectious etiology. Malignancy is a rare cause of acute significant LGIB but should be considered in patients with appropriate symptoms such as a change in bowel habits, weight loss, or pre-existing anemia. A review of medication history, especially the use of antiplatelet drugs, anticoagulants, or nonsteroidal anti-inflammatory drugs (NSAIDs), is imperative.

Initial assessment should include vital signs (including supine and orthostatic changes), an abdominal exam, and a rectal exam. Nasogastric lavage (with bile aspiration) and proctoscopy or anoscopy in the ER can quickly define an upper GI or anorectal source. UGIB should also be strongly considered if the blood urea nitrogen/creatinine (BUN/Cr) ratio is greater than 30:1 [2]. Recall that hemorrhoidal bleeding rarely will cause hemodynamic instability, and other sources must be promptly investigated in an unstable patient.

41.2 Has Computed Tomography Angiography (CTA) Replaced Technetium-99m (Tc-99m) Sulfur Colloid Injection or Tc-99m Tagged Red Cells as the Better Initial Test?

Nuclear scintigraphy was classically the standard in noninvasive testing of LGIB. It remains effective compared to CTA, especially in scenarios with intermittent or slow bleeding. But due to less predictable availability and length of time to obtain nuclear imaging results, CTA is preferably used today [3].

TC-99m tagged red cells were proven to detect slow bleeding rates. An early comparative study by Siddiqui and colleagues performed a comparison of Tc-99m sulfur colloid (SC) and Tc-99m tagged red blood cell (RBC) scintigraphy. They found far greater sensitivity in the tagged red cell group with 70% of the studies destined to be positive diagnoses in the first hour [4]. The majority of studies conclude that when compared to Tc-99m SC, Tc-99m-labeled RBCs are more sensitive, though less specific.

The limitation of scintigraphy studies lies in the ability to localize bleeding. Recent studies suggest that the rate of accurate localization of a bleeding site may vary from 39% to 48%. Rapid transit of tagged hemorrhaged red cells within the lumen of the colon is cited for this discrepancy. Gunderman found an increased diagnostic yield of 2.4× for arteriography with prior screening scintigraphy [5]. Angiographic yield could be further refined by selecting only patients whose scintigraphy is positive early after injection(level 4 evidence).

Alternatively, CTA has a sensitivity of 85–89% and a specificity of 85–92%. It also shows a higher sensitivity in patients with massive bleeding compared to those with the occult, slower GI bleeds. [6] (level 3 and level 4 evidence). It also remains predictive in determining positive angiography rates, about 86% [7]. Compared to scintigraphy, CT angiograms have a similar rate of detection of lower GI bleeds, but CTA is superior in the localization of bleeds [3]. Due to the increased availability of CTA compared to scintigraphy especially in the emergency setting, it has been advocated as a preferred alternative [6]. Still, TC-99m tagged RBC has increased sensitivity and may be useful in detecting slower bleeding.

RECOMMENDATIONS

CT angiography (CTA) and nuclear scintigraphy have similar sensitivity and specificity, but localization of hemorrhage sites by CTA is more precise and consistent with angiography findings. CT angiogram is advantageous in its speed and availability in the emergency setting and should be the first diagnostic test used in a patient with active LGIB.

Grade of recommendation: C.

41.3 How Should We Compare the Diagnostic Accuracy of Colonoscopy, Radionuclide Scanning, Computed Tomography Angiography (CTA), and Angiography in the Setting of LGIB?

Although radionuclide scanning is sensitive in picking up bleeds as slow as 0.05–0.1 mL/minute, it does not localize the bleeding accurately and surgical planning should never solely rely on such results [8]. Forty-two percent of patients could have an undesirable result if a limited surgical procedure was planned based on Tc-99m-labeled RBCs alone [9].

Computed tomography has been increasingly utilized to evaluate LGIB. It can detect bleeds as low as 0.3 mL/minute (1/3 less than radionuclide scanning). Several authors have studied CTA and found this method to be 85–89% sensitive with a specificity of 85–92%. for evaluating LGIB [8] (level 1 and level 4 evidence). In a prospective study of 26 patients for massive GI bleeding, Yoon demonstrated that arterial-phase CTA was about 90% sensitive and 99% specific with an overall accuracy rate of 88%. The negative predictive value was 98%, suggesting formal angiography would not be indicated in CTA-negative studies [10] (level 3 evidence). This test was found to be readily available and sufficiently sensitive to recommend CTA as the initial screen for LGIB, especially in light of its rapidity and noninvasiveness [11] (level 4 evidence). Wu performed a meta-analysis of 9 studies with 198 patients comparing the accuracy of CTA to other modalities including endoscopy, colonoscopy, angiography, and surgery and determined that CT is cost-effective and accurate at diagnosing the location of acute GI bleeding, with a pooled sensitivity of 89% and specificity of 85% [12] (level 3 evidence).

Colonoscopy is regarded as the initial procedure of choice for nearly all patients presenting with acute LGIB. The significant advantage of colonoscopy is its ability to identify the bleeding source and provide therapeutic intervention. The diagnostic yield of colonoscopy was recently reported at approximately 55% [13]. In a patient with hemodynamic instability, esophagogastroduodenoscopy (EGD) should be performed concomitantly just before colonoscopy. A colonoscopy should be performed within the first 24 hours of admission, with adequate bowel cleansing. Colonoscopy without adequate bowel preparation in the setting of LGIB is often unfruitful and should be avoided.

Angiography is less sensitive than radionuclide scanning and is used to detect bleeds greater than 0.5 mL/minute [14]. Angiography has been able to detect bleeding in 20–70% of cases [15] (level 2a evidence). It has been found to have a 42–86% sensitivity with close to 100% specificity [15] (level 3 evidence).

The utility of surgical site resection based on angiography is debatable. Angiography has guided segmental resections in 50–95% of positive diagnostic angiograms; however, 20–50% with negative studies still may require surgery [15]. Surgical site localization guided by angiography was noted to be low in a retrospective study by Cohn in 1998 [16] (level 4 evidence) where only 12% of the angiograms were useful in selecting the site of colon resection, noting an 11% complication rate from angiography. Similar complication rates of approx. 10% from angiography are recorded in the literature. These complications include infection, hematoma, dissection, contrast reaction, and thrombosis.

Angiography and panendoscopy have often been compared. Chaudhry studied 85 patients where unprepped colonoscopy was performed as the initial evaluation in cases of suspected LGIB. They concluded that this method was 95% sensitive and allowed for concomitant therapeutic control in 63% of the patients with active bleeding. In addition, they were able to diagnose that the source of bleeding was proximal to the ileocecal valve in 10% of the total patients studied [17] (level 4 evidence). Early colonoscopy is associated with shorter hospitalizations. Another Randomized Controlled Trial (RCT) shows that urgent colonoscopy when compared to expectant colonoscopy after imaging or angiography had higher rates of identification of the definitive source of LGIB, 42% and 22%, respectively, but did not show statistically significant differences in mortality, hospital stay, or surgical intervention (level 2b evidence) The diagnostic yield of colonoscopy ranges from 45% to 90% [18].

RECOMMENDATION

Colonoscopy when available is the most accurate method of diagnosing.

LGIB is the gold standard against which other studies are measured, offering control of bleeding from some lesions as well.

Grade of recommendation: C.

41.4 Is There an Ideal Single Test in the Setting of LGIB?

One critical purpose for performing diagnostic testing in LGIB is to rule out the presence of bleeding above the ileocecal valve which has been noted above to be as high as 15% of patients presenting for evaluation. Chaudhry and colleagues suggest that colonoscopy is an accurate single-stage evaluation for LGIB [19] (level 4 evidence). The diagnostic yield of colonoscopy can range from 42% to 90% [17]. The yield of colonoscopy is significantly improved with bowel prep and is recommended in hemodynamically stable patients. Additionally, a colonoscopy can help rule out bleeding above the ileocecal valve by intubating the terminal ileum. As an invasive procedure, a colonoscopy may not always be readily available.

CTA is highly effective at localizing LGIB as well. CTA is generally available more rapidly than colonoscopy, and therefore, a diagnosis can be obtained earlier in the patient's hospital course.

There is some evidence that the shock index (heart rate/systolic blood pressure) ≥1 may predict extravasation on CTA which can help predict patients in whom CTA will yield positive results. A three-phase CTA has a reported sensitivity of 85% and specificity of 92% for acute GIB. One benefit of early CTA is the ability to rapidly localize bleeding without bowel prepping, though the risk against contrast nephropathy needs to be weighed [7, 19].

The yield from catheter-based angiography for all comers is low and is best performed after a confirmatory study *unless* the patient is hemodynamically unstable [20] (level 4 evidence). Furthermore, in this potentially volume-depleted population, the incidence of complications from contrast angiography has been underappreciated [8] (level 4 evidence). The positive predictive value of either scintigraphy or CTA is sufficient to utilize either of these tests before angiography [21] (level 4 evidence). Nonetheless, a negative angiogram after a positive CTA is fairly common. The yield of angiogram can be increased with provocation (heparin, nitroglycerin, urokinase, or tPA) though this can increase the risk of uncontrolled bleeding and must be considered with caution. One randomized controlled trial comparing urgent colonoscopy to angiographic intervention with expectant colonoscopy found that though a definite source of bleeding was found more often in the urgent colonoscopy group, there was no difference in outcomes including mortality, hospital stay, transfusion requirement, and rebleeding [22] (level 1 evidence).

RECOMMENDATION

Colonoscopy with bowel prep is the ideal single test in the face of LGIB.

Compared to angiography, colonoscopy is better at identifying the source of the bleeding, though it may not improve clinical outcomes.

Grade of recommendation: B.

TABLE 41.1

Initial Treatment Modality

Colonoscopy	
Timing	Within 24 hours
Bowel preparation	Recommended—NGT can be placed to help facilitate
Rule out small bowel source	By intubating terminal ileum
Localization	Place tattoo in case of rebleed
Visualize entire mucosa	Use water-jet irrigation and a large working channel
CT Angiography	
High predictive value	0.3 cc–0.5 cc/minute of bleeding
	Shock index (SI) >1
	5U PRBC within 24 hours
Obtain three phases	Noncontrast, arterial, portal venous phase
Critical finding	Active extravasation
Subtle finding	The site of the clot can be visualized on maximum intensity projection [23]

41.5 What Is the Rationale for Timing of Colonoscopy for LGIB and the Clinical Outcomes?

Retrospective studies demonstrate that colonoscopy during hospitalization for LGIB is associated with an increased likelihood of discharge and that an early colonoscopy (within 24 hours of admission) predicted earlier hospital discharge [24] (level 2 evidence). A nationwide cross-sectional study also examined this issue and also demonstrated that colonoscopy within the first 24 hours of hospitalization is associated with a statistically significantly decreased length of hospital stay (2.9 vs. 4.6 days, $p < 0.001$), decreased need for blood transfusion (45% vs. 54%, $p < 0.001$), and decreased hospitalization costs ($22,123 vs. $28,749, $p < 0.001$), though no difference in mortality was observed [25] (level 4 evidence). A subsequent 2010 trial randomized 72 LGIB patients to either urgent (within 12 hours of presentation) or elective (36–60 hours after presentation) colonoscopy, and no differences in rebleeding, transfusions, length of stay, or hospital charges were observed; however, the small study size and suggestion of more severe bleeding in the urgent colonoscopy arm patients make it difficult to conclude this study [1] (level 2b evidence). Additionally, the rate of definitive diagnosis in a randomized trial of early colonoscopy (<8 hours from presentation) improved the rate of diagnosis (42% vs. 22%) [25].

If high-risk stigmata of bleeding are found (active bleeding, visible vessel, and adherent clot), then endoscopic interventions can be effective at preventing rebleeding. The highest benefit of endoscopic intervention is in patients with diverticulosis, angioectasias, and postpolypectomy bleeds. Ischemia, IBD, and cancer are less amenable to endoscopic hemostasis [25].

41.6 What Is the Appropriate Setting for Selective Transcatheter Embolization?

Mesenteric angiography and embolization are the sole radiographic modalities that allow for both localization and treatment of LGIB. The goal of angiographic embolization is to decrease arterial perfusion to the bleeding site and facilitate cessation. Superselective embolization is employed using microcatheters for arteries less than 1 mm in diameter. For angiography to be successful, the rate of bleeding must be >0.5 mL/minute and continuous [26]. Angiography has a higher success rate at localization in hemodynamically unstable patients who have required >5 units of blood in 24 hours and have a systolic blood pressure of <90 mm Hg. Success using embolization ranges from 65% to 81% with rebleeding rates reported at 19–35%. The incidence of bowel ischemia with microcatheters is approximately 1%, rising to close to 5% if a larger vessel is embolized [27, 28].

Even in cases where angiography fails to control the source of bleeding, it should assist in surgical planning directed at the specific source of bleeding so that segmental colectomy can be accomplished. Bowel ischemia with abdominal pain and a minimally symptomatic rise in lactic acid is occasional and most often self-limited, with major episodes of significant ischemia reported in approximately 5% of cases [29, 30].

41.7 What Are the Criteria for Surgical Intervention in LGIB and What Operation Should Be Done?

Being that 65–80% of cases of LGIB resolve spontaneously, and surgical resection is required in only 7–25% of patients, management of LGIB is challenging and often frustrating. Risk stratification using vital signs, patient factors, age, comorbidities, and laboratory data can determine whether the patient can be safely evaluated as an outpatient. The shock index is a good predictor of active extravasation and can be used to guide diagnostic evaluation [31]. Age is an independent predisposing factor for LGIB, and the most common causes in the elderly are diverticular disease and ischemia. Neoplasm and inflammatory disease should also be considered especially in the younger population.

Unfortunately, studies regarding immediate resuscitation, management of hemodynamically unstable patients, and transfusion guidelines for GI bleed have mostly been conducted in UGIB patients. For such patients, a transfusion threshold of up to 7 g/dL showed improved survival and decreased rebleeding compared to that of 9 g/dL. Patients excluded from these criteria included those with massive bleeding, acute coronary syndrome, symptomatic peripheral vascular disease, or a history of stroke or CVA. The precise indications for surgery in LGIB can be elusive and frustrating. Patients with persistent hemodynamic instability despite adequate resuscitative efforts warrant rapid surgical intervention.

Relative indications for surgery include patients who exceed the transfusion threshold (generally around 5U PRBC), rebleeding after successful embolization or endoscopic treatment (directed segmental colectomy), and persistent small bowel bleeding (especially if diagnosed with angiography or capsule endoscopy) [32]. Patients with recurrent clinically significant LGIB are at significant risk for repeated episodes and should be offered surgery, especially if localization has been accomplished.

Patients with surgically correctable conditions such as IBD and colorectal cancer with persistent bleeding also should be considered for prompt surgery. A special caveat exists for rectal cancer, however. All attempts should be made to temporize these patients with endoscopic methods to control hemorrhage until they can receive radiation treatment and all subsequent adjuvant oncologic therapy to optimize survival.

Regarding the specific surgical procedure, the advancement of localization studies as outlined above has resulted in a preponderance of segmental colectomy rather than the more traditional total abdominal colectomy for LGIB. In a recent review, 85% of patients underwent a partial colectomy, while 15% underwent a total colectomy. Total colectomy was more common in patients who received greater than 4 units of blood before surgery. Patients who had partial colectomy were more likely to have laparoscopic surgery (35.3% vs. 20.0%) and to have a stoma (20.6% vs. 1.6%). Total colectomy was associated with an increased risk of cardiac complications, renal complications, postoperative ileus, and mortality (all $p < 0.05$) but not with surgical site infection, anastomotic leak, return to the operating room, or readmissions [33] (Grade C recommendation).

41.8 Anticoagulant Use and Reversal in the Management of LGIB

Newer (Novel) oral anticoagulants (NOACs), non-vitamin K antagonist oral anticoagulants such as clopidogrel, and other oral anticoagulants that include thrombin inhibitor dabigatran and coagulation factor Xa inhibitors rivaroxaban, apixaban, edoxaban, and betrixaban are commonly prescribed for many cardiovascular and cerebrovascular conditions in the elderly population. NOACs have several benefits over warfarin, including faster time to effect, rapid onset of action, fewer food and drug interactions, and the lack of need for routine monitoring. However, a major disadvantage of these agents is the challenge of reversal in the event of acute hemorrhage or emergency surgery. The Food and Drug Administration (FDA) has approved two reversal agents for NOACs: idarucizumab for dabigatran and andexanet alfa for apixaban and rivaroxaban [34].

The American Heart Association/American College of Cardiology/Heart Rhythm Society (AHA/ACC/HRS) guidelines define major bleeding as all major bleeds that are associated with either hemodynamic compromise, bleeding in a critical organ site (e.g., intracranial and pericardial), a drop in hemoglobin >2 g/dL (when the baseline is unknown), or a need for 2 units of red cells [35]. Patients presenting with life-threatening bleeding, presenting with major uncontrolled bleeding, or requiring rapid anticoagulant reversal for emergent surgical procedures are candidates for the use of reversal agents.

Several nonspecific reversal agents are used for the reversal of NOAC anticoagulation. Disappointingly, fresh frozen plasma (FFP) has shown no improvement in bleeding outcomes. It is noteworthy to mention that the benefit of blood-component therapies or prohemostatic agents in the absence of coexisting coagulopathy remains unclear [36].

Tranexamic acid is used off-label as a hemostatic agent in major NOAC-associated bleeds. Prothrombin complex concentrate (PCC) is a mixture of three or four coagulation factors and is used off-label to reverse NOACs. Inactivated four-factor PCC (Kcentra®) may be used in cases of factor Xa inhibitor-associated bleeding. However, activated PCC (aPCC), factor VIII inhibitor bypassing agent (FEIBA®), is preferred for dabigatran.

The efficacy of PCCs on clinical outcomes in patients with NOACs and active bleeding is not yet established in a randomized control trial although observational studies are suggestive of efficacy in achieving hemostasis. In a randomized double-blinded placebo-controlled study by Erenberg et al., 50 IU/kg PCC immediately and completely reversed the anticoagulant effect of rivaroxaban but failed to reverse the anticoagulant action of dabigatran [37]. The European Heart Association recommends the use of PCC or aPCC in the absence of specific reversal agents in patients with major bleeding (Grade 2 recommendation). A dose of 50 IU PCC/kg or 50 IU activated PCC/kg is recommended. No renal or hepatic dose adjustments have been reported.

Idarucizumab is a humanized antibody fragment. It acts by binding directly to dabigatran to counteract its anticoagulant effect. To reverse dabigatran, two separate 2.5 g/50 mL vials (total of 5 g) are administered intravenously. A 2019 update of the 2014 AHA/ACC/HRS guidelines for the management of patients with atrial fibrillation showed that idarucizumab showed a rapid and complete reversal of dabigatran activity in 97.5% of patients presenting with GI bleeding who had an elevated dTT regardless of the GI bleeding location (Class I) [38].

Andexanet alfa is a recombinant modified factor Xa protein approved by the FDA to reverse apixaban and rivaroxaban in patients with life-threatening or uncontrolled bleeding. Andexanet alfa acts as a decoy and sequesters rivaroxaban or apixaban, inhibiting them from binding to natural factor Xa. Two dosing regimens (low and high) have their basis on which factor Xa inhibitor requires reversal when the patient received their last dose and the size of the dose. The low-dose protocol includes a bolus of 400 mg, given at a rate of 30 mg/minute, followed by an infusion of 4 mg/minute for up to 2 hours. The low-dose protocol is recommended for the following situations: (a) if the last dose of rivaroxaban was 10 mg or less and drug administration was less than 8 hours ago or unknown, (b) if the last dose of apixaban was 5 mg or less and drug administration was less than 8 hours ago or unknown, and (c) if the patient received the last dose of either drug 8 or more hours ago.

The high-dose protocol is 800 mg administered at 30 mg/minute and then an infusion at 8 mg/minute for up to 2 hours and is recommended for the following situations: (a) if the last dose of rivaroxaban was more than 10 mg or of an unknown amount and drug administration was less than 8 hours ago or unknown and (b) if the last dose of apixaban was more than 5 mg or unknown and drug administration was less than 8 hours ago or unknown. The AHA/ACC/HRS recommends andexanet alfa for the reversal of apixaban and rivaroxaban in patients with life-threatening or uncontrolled bleeding (Class IIa). Andexanet alfa does not currently have approval for the reversal of edoxaban, fondaparinux, or low-molecular-weight heparins [39].

Adverse effects include deep vein thrombosis, arterial thrombosis, pulmonary embolism, ischemic stroke, acute myocardial infarction, and death. Other effects include cardiogenic shock, heart failure exacerbations, urinary tract infections, pneumonia, acute respiratory failure, and infusion-related reactions. Drug effects are measurable by anti-Xa activity, free fraction of apixaban or rivaroxaban, and thrombin generation. Anti-Xa activity returns to placebo concentrations about 2 hours after a bolus or infusion, but tissue factor pathway inhibitors persist for about 22 hours after giving the drug. Patients should be monitored for signs and symptoms of thrombosis. It is crucial to re-initiate anticoagulation therapy as soon as clinically appropriate to reduce the risk of thrombosis after andexanet alfa therapy. Thrombosis may occur even after the re-initiation of anticoagulation.

RECOMMENDATION

Patients on NOAC (novel oral anticoagulants) may commonly experience LGIB. Challenges exist for reversal in the event of hemorrhage or emergent surgery. Several specific and nonspecific agents exist, but their efficacy is not well documented. They must be used with great caution, and consideration of risk of thrombosis must be weighed versus the potential benefit. As these drugs are more widely used, further evidence should be forthcoming.

Grade of recommendation: C.

TABLE 41.2

Question Summary

Question	Answer	Grade of Recommendation	Level of Evidence	References
What is the diagnostic accuracy of Tc-99 sulfur colloid injection versus Tc-99 tagged red cells?	Tc-99-labeled RBCs appear to demonstrate superior sensitivity to Tc-99 sulfur colloid injection in the detection of LGIB.	B	1b	[5]
	Angiography is not indicated when scintigraphy is negative.	C	4	[7–20]
	The utility of Tc-99-labeled RBC scanning is limited by the poor predictive value of the anatomic location of bleeding; therefore, positive scans should be followed up with further localization studies to improve anatomic accuracy.	C	4	[18–22]
What is the diagnostic accuracy of colonoscopy, radionuclide scanning, and angiography in the setting of LGIB?	Colonoscopy when available is the most accurate method of diagnosing LGIB and is the gold standard against which other studies are measured offering control of some lesions as well.	C	4	[26, 27, 29]
	Scintigraphy may offer valuable information for angiographic screening but is insufficient for operative planning alone.	C	4	[11–25]
	MDCT is highly sensitive and specific at detecting ongoing GI bleeding, and its rapidity, cost-effectiveness, and noninvasiveness make it an ideal first-line test to direct further management.	C	3a, 3b, 4, 5	[26, 35–37, 40]
What is the ideal single test in the setting of LGIB?	Colonoscopy is the ideal single test in the face of LGIB.	B	1b, 4	[20, 24, 27, 33, 38]
	Compared to angiography, an upfront colonoscopy is better at identifying a source of bleeding, though it may not improve clinical outcomes.			
	In the event, this is not available and an intervention is required, and scintigraphy or MDCT should be performed to rule out proximal sources in the small bowel prior to angiographic embolization/vasopressin or surgical resection.	C	4	[16–18, 25, 26, 33, 40]
What is the preferred timing of colonoscopy for LGIB and the effect on clinical outcomes?	Colonoscopy performed early in the clinical course may lead to decreased length of hospital stay and hospitalization costs; however, there is insufficient evidence to suggest that it has an impact on clinical outcomes.	C	2b, 4	[28, 39]
What is the clinical effectiveness of intra-arterial vasopressin infusion versus transcatheter embolization?	The major drawbacks of vasopressin therapy are coronary ischemia and rebleeding after cessation of therapy. Cessation of bleeding occurs in up to 90% of patients. Some studies have shown significant rebleeding after therapy is stopped.	No recommendations	4	
	On the other hand, embolic therapy shows a similar rate of initial hemorrhage control with less early rebleeding; however, there is about a 10% risk of significant colon ischemia. Super-selective embolism has not eliminated ischemia as a risk.		4	
	The late rebleeding risk is 10–15% with either technique.		4	

(Continued)

TABLE 41.2 (Continued)

Question Summary

Question	Answer	Grade of Recommendation	Level of Evidence	References
What are the criteria for surgical intervention in LGIB and what operation should be done?	Patients who bleed 2 or more units of blood should receive an evaluation to localize the source of bleeding expeditiously.	C	4	
	Stable patients without massive bleeding should not be considered for surgery as many of these episodes will resolve either spontaneously or with less invasive therapies such as barium enema.	C	4	
	Persistent bleeding with true anatomic localization may allow for segmental resection; otherwise, subtotal colectomy with ileorectostomy should be performed.	C	4	[29]
	If the transfusion requirement is approaching 10 units, surgery should be seriously considered. Other factors, such as hypotension on presentation, the presence of comorbidities, and localization of left-sided bleeding should prompt consideration for earlier operative therapy, as complications of urgent surgery may be unacceptably high.	C	4	

Abbreviations: LGIB: Lower gastrointestinal bleeding, RBC: Red blood cell, Tc-99: Technetium-99m.

Editor's Note

Much has changed over the past few decades in the diagnosis and management of LGIB. The initial diagnostic test for LGIB is now an abdominal pelvic CT angiogram which has a similar sensitivity and specificity as nuclear medicine scanning and is more accurate in locating the actual site of bleeding. Years ago, we showed that localizing the site of bleeding with an aim of segmental colectomy was of questionable value as there was a very high likelihood of requiring an additional intervention for a completion colectomy in the years following the initial procedure. In addition, there does not appear to be a mortality or morbidity difference between segmental and subtotal colectomy.

A colonoscopy is the ideal diagnostic intervention once upper GI sources have been ruled out with bilious nasogastric drainage or upper endoscopy, and anorectal pathology with anoscopy. A colonoscopy also gives the provider an opportunity to terminate bleeding during the procedure. The use of angiographic embolization is rarely required and can lead to ischemia mandating surgical excision. Recently, I cared for a complex medical patient who, despite hemodynamic stability and minimum transfusion requirements, underwent interventional radiologic embolization after abdominal CTA showed a small amount of extravasation. The resulting dead colon required emergency colectomy for colonic perforation related to multiple areas of ischemia. Very few patients with transfusion requiring LGIB have the need for therapeutic endoscopy (6%) and when indicated therapeutic endoscopy is successful in over 90% of cases [41]. Therefore, there is very little that surgery has to offer for acute LGIB today as operative intervention is only required in about 2 per 1,000 cases.

REFERENCES

1. Laine L, Yang H, Chang S-C, Datto C. Trends for incidence of hospitalization and death due to GI complications in the United States from 2001 to 2009. Am J Gastroenterol. 2012;107(8):1190–5.
2. Zia Ziabari SM, Rimaz S, Shafaghi A, Shakiba M, Pourkazemi Z, Karimzadeh E, Amoukhteh M. Blood urea nitrogen to creatinine ratio in differentiation of upper and lower gastrointestinal bleedings; a diagnostic accuracy study. Arch Acad Emerg Med. 2019 Jun 2;7(1):e30. PMID: 31432040; PMCID: PMC6637801.
3. Feuerstein JD, Ketwaroo G, Tewani SK, Cheesman A, Trivella J, Raptopoulos V, Leffler DA. Localizing acute lower gastrointestinal hemorrhage: CT angiography versus tagged RBC scintigraphy. AJR Am J Roentgenol. 2016 Sep;207(3):578–84. doi: 10.2214/AJR.15.15714. Epub 2016 Jun 15. PMID: 27303989.
4. Siddiqui AR, Schauwecker DS, Wellman HN, Mock BH. Comparison of technetium-99m sulfur colloid and in vitro labeled technetium-99m RBCs in the detection of gastrointestinal bleeding. Clin Nucl Med. 1985 Aug;10(8): 546–9. doi: 10.1097/00003072-198508000-00003. PMID: 3876189.

5. Gunderman R, Leef J, Ong K, Reba R, Metz C. Scintigraphic screening prior to visceral arteriography in acute lower gastrointestinal bleeding. J Nucl Med. 1998 Jun;39(6):1081–3. PMID: 9627348.

6. Kim J, Kim YH, Lee KH, Lee YJ, Park JH. Diagnostic performance of CT angiography in patients visiting emergency department with overt gastrointestinal bleeding. Korean J Radiol. 2015 May-Jun;16(3):541–9. doi: 10.3348/kjr.2015.16.3.541. Epub 2015 May 13. PMID: 25995683; PMCID: PMC4435984.

7. Clerc D, Grass F, Schäfer M, Denys A, Demartines N, Hübner M. Lower gastrointestinal bleeding-computed tomographic angiography, colonoscopy or both? World J Emerg Surg. 2017 Jan 3;12:1. doi: 10.1186/s13017-016-0112-3. PMID: 28070213; PMCID: PMC5215140.

8. Wortman JR, Landman W, Fulwadhva UP, Viscomi SG, Sodickson AD. CT angiography for acute gastrointestinal bleeding: what the radiologist needs to know. Br J Radiol. 2017 Jul;90(1075):20170076. doi: 10.1259/bjr.20170076. Epub 2017 Apr 26. PMID: 28362508; PMCID: PMC5594987.

9. Hunter JM, Pezim ME. Limited value of technetium 99m-labeled red cell scintigraphy in localization of lower gastrointestinal bleeding. Am J Surg. 1990 May;159(5):504–6. doi: 10.1016/s0002-9610(05)81256-5? PMID: 2334015.

10. Yoon W, Jeong YY, Shin SS, Lim HS, Song SG, Jang NG, Kim JK, Kang HK. Acute massive gastrointestinal bleeding: detection and localization with arterial phase multi-detector row helical CT. Radiology. 2006 Apr;239(1):160–7. doi: 10.1148/radiol.2383050175. Epub 2006 Feb 16. PMID: 16484350.

11. Lee HS, Kang SH, Rou WS, Eun HS, Joo JS, Kim JS, Lee ES, Moon HS, Kim SH, Sung JK, Lee BS, Jeong HY. Computed tomography versus lower endoscopy as initial diagnostic method for evaluating patients with hematochezia at emergency room. Medicine (Baltimore). 2020 May 29;99(22):e20311. doi: 10.1097/MD.0000000000020311. PMID: 32481401.

12. Wu LM, Xu JR, Yin Y, Qu XH. Usefulness of CT angiography in diagnosing acute gastrointestinal bleeding: a meta-analysis. World J Gastroenterol. 2010 Aug 21;16(31):3957–63. doi: 10.3748/wjg.v16.i31.3957. PMID: 20712058; PMCID: PMC2923771.

13. Mosli M, Aldabbagh A, Aseeri H, Alqusair S, Jawa H, Alsahafi M, Qari Y. The diagnostic yield of urgent colonoscopy in acute lower gastrointestinal bleeding. Acta Gastroenterol Belg. 2020 Apr–Jun;83(2):265–70. PMID: 32603045.

14. Ng DA, Opelka FG, Beck DE, Milburn JM, Witherspoon LR, Hicks TC, Timmcke AE, Gathright JB Jr. Predictive value of technetium Tc 99m-labeled red blood cell scintigraphy for positive angiogram in massive lower gastrointestinal hemorrhage. Dis Colon Rectum. 1997 Apr;40(4):471–7. doi: 10.1007/BF02258395. PMID: 9106699.

15. Whitaker SC, Gregson RH. The role of angiography in the investigation of acute or chronic gastrointestinal haemorrhage. Clin Radiol. 1993 Jun;47(6):382–8. doi: 10.1016/s0009-9260(05)81057-8. PMID: 8519143.

16. Cohn SM, Moller BA, Zieg PM, Milner KA, Angood PB. Angiography for preoperative evaluation in patients with lower gastrointestinal bleeding: are the benefits worth the risks? Arch Surg. 1998 Jan;133(1):50–5. doi: 10.1001/archsurg.133.1.50. PMID: 9438759.

17. Chaudhry V, Hyser MJ, Gracias VH, Gau FC. Colonoscopy: the initial test for acute lower gastrointestinal bleeding. Am Surg. 1998 Aug;64(8):723–8. PMID: 9697900.

18. ASGE Standards of Practice Committee, Pasha SF, Shergill A, Acosta RD, Chandrasekhara V, Chathadi KV, Early D, Evans JA, Fisher D, Fonkalsrud L, Hwang JH, Khashab MA, Lightdale JR, Muthusamy VR, Saltzman JR, Cash BD. The role of endoscopy in the patient with lower GI bleeding. Gastrointest Endosc. 2014 Jun;79(6):875–85. doi: 10.1016/j.gie.2013.10.039. Epub 2014 Apr 2. PMID: 24703084

19. Oakland K, Chadwick G, East JE, Guy R, Humphries A, Jairath V, McPherson S, Metzner M, Morris AJ, Murphy MF, Tham T, Uberoi R, Veitch AM, Wheeler J, Regan C, Hoare J. Diagnosis and management of acute lower gastrointestinal bleeding: guidelines from the British Society of Gastroenterology. Gut. 2019 May;68(5):776–89. doi: 10.1136/gutjnl-2018-317807. Epub 2019 Feb 12. PMID: 30792244

20. Expert Panel on Interventional Radiology, Karuppasamy K, Kapoor BS, Fidelman N, Abujudeh H, Bartel TB, Caplin DM, Cash BD, Citron SJ, Farsad K, Gajjar AH, Guimaraes MS, Gupta A, Higgins M, Marin D, Patel PJ, Pietryga JA, Rochon PJ, Stadtlander KS, Suranyi PS, Lorenz JM. ACR Appropriateness Criteria® radiologic management of lower gastrointestinal tract bleeding: 2021 update. J Am Coll Radiol. 2021 May;18(5S): S139–52. doi: 10.1016/j.jacr.2021.02.018. PMID: 33958109.

21. García-Blázquez V, Vicente-Bártulos A, Olavarria-Delgado A, Plana MN, van der Winden D, Zamora J, EBM-Connect Collaboration. Accuracy of CT angiography in the diagnosis of acute gastrointestinal bleeding: systematic review and meta-analysis. Eur Radiol. 2013 May;23(5):1181–90. doi: 10.1007/s00330-012-2721-x. Epub 2012 Nov 29. PMID: 23192375.

22. Green BT, Rockey DC, Portwood G, Tarnasky PR, Guarisco S, Branch MS, Leung J, Jowell P. Urgent colonoscopy for evaluation and management of acute lower gastrointestinal hemorrhage: a randomized controlled trial. Am J Gastroenterol. 2005 Nov;100(11):2395–402. doi: 10.1111/j.1572-0241.2005.00306.x. PMID: 16279891.

23. Steele SR, Hull TL, Hyman N, Maykel JA, Read TE, Whitlow CB (Ed). The ASCRS Textbook of Colon and Rectal Surgery, 4th edition. Springer Nature Switzerland AG. 2022.

24. Roshan Afshar I, Sadr MS, Strate LL, Martel M, Menard C, Barkun AN. The role of early colonoscopy in patients presenting with acute lower gastrointestinal bleeding: a systematic review and meta-analysis. Therap Adv Gastroenterol. 2018 Feb 19;11:1756283X18757184. doi: 10.1177/1756283X18757184. PMID: 29487627; PMCID: PMC5821297.

25. Navaneethan U, Njei B, Venkatesh PG, Sanaka MR. Timing of colonoscopy and outcomes in patients with lower GI bleeding: a nationwide population-based study. Gastrointest Endosc. 2014 Feb;79(2):297–306.e12. doi: 10.1016/j.gie.2013.08.001. Epub 2013 Sep 20. PMID: 24060518.

26. Ghassemi KA, Jensen DM. Lower GI bleeding: epidemiology and management. Curr Gastroenterol Rep. 2013 Jul;15(7):333. doi: 10.1007/s11894-013-0333-5. PMID: 23737154; PMCID: PMC3857214.

27. Aoki T, Hirata Y, Yamada A, Koike K. Initial management for acute lower gastrointestinal bleeding. World J Gastroenterol. 2019 Jan 7;25(1):69–84. doi: 10.3748/wjg.v25.i1.69. PMID: 30643359; PMCID: PMC6328962.

28. Senadeera SC, Vun SV, Butterfield N, Eglinton TW, Frizelle FA. Role of super-selective embolization in lower gastrointestinal bleeding. ANZ J Surg. 2018 Sep;88(9):E644–48. doi: 10.1111/ans.14441. Epub 2018 Mar 14. PMID: 29537132.

29. Tan KK, Strong DH, Shore T, Ahmad MR, Waugh R, Young CJ. The safety and efficacy of mesenteric embolization in the management of acute lower gastrointestinal hemorrhage. Ann Coloproctol. 2013 Oct;29(5):205–8. doi: 10.3393/ac.2013.29.5.205. Epub 2013 Oct 31. PMID: 24278859; PMCID: PMC3837086.

30. Bua-Ngam C, Norasetsingh J, Treesit T, Wedsart B, Chansanti O, Tapaneeyakorn J, Panpikoon T, Vallibhakara SA. Efficacy of emergency transarterial embolization in acute lower gastrointestinal bleeding: a single-center experience. Diagn Interv Imaging. 2017 Jun;98(6):499–505. doi: 10.1016/j.diii.2017.02.005. Epub 2017 Mar 22. PMID: 28341118.

31. Rassameehiran S, Teerakanok J, Suchartlikitwong S, Nugent K. Utility of the shock index for risk stratification in patients with acute upper gastrointestinal bleeding. South Med J. 2017 Nov;110(11):738–43. doi: 10.14423/SMJ.0000000000000729. PMID: 29100227.

32. Greco L, Zhang J, Ross H. Surgical options and approaches for lower gastrointestinal bleeding: when do we operate and what do we do? Clin Colon Rectal Surg. 2020 Jan;33(1):10–15. doi: 10.1055/s-0039-1693439. Epub 2020 Jan 7. PMID: 31915420; PMCID: PMC6946603.

33. Greco L, Koller S, Philp M, Ross H. Surgical management of lower gastrointestinal hemorrhage: an analysis of the ACS NSQIP database. J Curr Surg. 2017;7(1–2):4–6.

34. Mujer MTP, Rai MP, Atti V, Dimaandal IL, Chan AS, Shrotriya S, Gundabolu K, Dhakal P. An update on the reversal of non-vitamin K antagonist oral anticoagulants. Adv Hematol. 2020 Jan 27;2020:7636104. doi: 10.1155/2020/7636104. PMID: 32231703; PMCID: PMC7097770.

35. January CT, Wann LS, Calkins H, Chen LY, Cigarroa JE, Cleveland JC Jr, Ellinor PT, Ezekowitz MD, Field ME, Furie KL, Heidenreich PA, Murray KT, Shea JB, Tracy CM, Yancy CW. 2019 AHA/ACC/HRS focused update of the 2014 AHA/ACC/HRS guideline for the management of patients with atrial fibrillation: a report of the American College of Cardiology/American Heart Association Task Force on Clinical Practice Guidelines and the Heart Rhythm Society in Collaboration with the Society of Thoracic Surgeons. Circulation. 2019 Jul 9;140(2):e125–51. doi: 10.1161/CIR.0000000000000665. Epub 2019 Jan 28. Erratum in: Circulation. 2019 Aug 6;140(6):e285. PMID: 30686041.

36. Smith SR, Murray D, Pockney PG, Bendinelli C, Draganic BD, Carroll R. Tranexamic acid for lower GI hemorrhage: a randomized placebo-controlled clinical trial. Dis Colon Rectum. 2018 Jan;61(1):99–106. doi: 10.1097/DCR.0000000000000943. PMID: 29215478.

37. Eerenberg ES, Kamphuisen PW, Sijpkens MK, Meijers JC, Buller HR, Levi M. Reversal of rivaroxaban and dabigatran by prothrombin complex concentrate: a randomized, placebo-controlled, crossover study in healthy subjects. Circulation. 2011 Oct 4;124(14):1573–9. doi: 10.1161/CIRCULATIONAHA.111.029017. Epub 2011 Sep 6. PMID: 21900088.

38. Van der Wall SJ, Lopes RD, Aisenberg J, Reilly P, van Ryn J, Glund S, Elsaesser A, Klok FA, Pollack CV Jr, Huisman MV. Idarucizumab for dabigatran reversal in the management of patients with gastrointestinal bleeding. Circulation. 2019 Feb 5;139(6):748–56. doi: 10.1161/CIRCULATIONAHA.118.036710. Erratum in: Circulation. 2019 Feb 5;139(6):e36. PMID: 30586692.

39. Song Y, Wang Z, Perlstein I, Wang J, LaCreta F, Frost RJA, Frost C. Reversal of apixaban anticoagulation by four-factor prothrombin complex concentrates in healthy subjects: a randomized three-period crossover study. J Thromb Haemost. 2017 Nov;15(11):2125–37. doi: 10.1111/jth.13815. Epub 2017 Oct 9. PMID: 28846831.

40. Strate LL, Gralnek IM. ACG clinical guideline: management of patients with acute lower gastrointestinal bleeding. Am J Gastroenterol. 2016 Apr;111(4):459–74. doi: 10.1038/ajg.2016.41. Epub 2016 Mar 1. Erratum in: Am J Gastroenterol. 2016 May;111(5):755. PMID: 26925883; PMCID: PMC5099081.

41. Khoury L, Tobin-Schnittger P, Champion N, Sim V, Gave A, Hawkins S, Panzo M, Cohn S. Natural history of patients undergoing therapeutic endoscopies for acute gastrointestinal bleeding. Am Surg. 2019 Nov 1;85(11):1246–52.

42

Appendicitis

Emily A. Kerby, Danielle Collins, and Peter P. Lopez

42.1 Introduction

Acute appendicitis (inflammation of the vermiform appendix) remains the most common intraabdominal surgical emergency requiring operative intervention. The lifetime risk of developing appendicitis is around 7–9%. Men are more likely to develop acute appendicitis than women (1.4:1), and men are more likely to have a perforated appendix than women [1, 2]. Appendicitis can occur at any age but is most frequently seen in patients in their second and fourth decade of life, with a mean age of 31.3 and a median age of 22 years [1].

Early reports described a potentially lethal inflammatory disease process of the right lower quadrant (RLQ), known then as "perityphlitis." In 1886, Reginald Fitz first described this inflammatory process in the RLQ and coined the term "appendicitis," including the clinical sequelae of abscess formation and perforation. Even today, the diagnosis of acute appendicitis remains a challenging clinical entity. This condition is more difficult to diagnose at the extremes of age: In the very young and elderly because of a lack of history, late presentation, and often less-than-impressive physical examination. The diagnoses can also be challenging in women of childbearing age who have a wider differential for RLQ pain.

The timely and accurate recognition of patients requiring urgent surgical and nonsurgical management continues to be the overriding principle in the workup and treatment of patients with suspected appendicitis. Appendicitis can be either uncomplicated or complicated. Uncomplicated appendicitis is appendicitis with no clinical or radiographic signs of perforation (inflammatory mass, phlegmon, or abscess). Complicated appendicitis is defined as clinical or radiographic signs of perforation. Delays in the diagnosis and treatment of appendicitis can result in increased morbidity and mortality.

In this chapter, we try to answer a few common issues clinicians face when diagnosing and managing acute appendicitis. Important questions to consider in caring for a patient with appendicitis include how to make an accurate diagnosis, whether to treat the patient medically or surgically, and whether to proceed surgically with an open or laparoscopic approach. The answers to these questions are based on an evidence-based review of the literature.

42.2 What Clinical Signs and Symptoms Are Most Reliable to Rule In or Out Appendicitis?

History and physical examination continue to be the most reliable predictor for the diagnosis of appendicitis [3]. By performing a thorough history and physical examination, an experienced clinician can accurately diagnose acute appendicitis in most cases. However, only about 25% of patients who present with acute appendicitis do so with a classic presentation, leaving 75% who have an atypical presentation. A typical patient will present with vague abdominal pain (usually in the epigastric region) followed by anorexia, and nausea, with or without vomiting. The pain then shifts to the RLQ as the inflammation of the appendix progresses to involve the overlying peritoneum. Common symptoms of appendicitis include the following: Periumbilical abdominal pain and anorexia in nearly 100% of cases, nausea in 90%, and migration of pain from the periumbilical area to the RLQ around 50% of the time [4]. The most reliable symptom in making the diagnosis of appendicitis is the classic pattern of migratory abdominal pain from the periumbilical to the RLQ. Occasionally, patients will complain of dysuria, hematuria, urgency and frequent urination, diarrhea, or constipation from inflammation adjacent to the ureter, bladder, colon, and rectum. In practice, these clinical features are not entirely reliable. However, the history and physical examination continue to remain reliable indicators for the diagnosis of appendicitis. Most patients with appendicitis except the very young, very old, and those who are neurologically impaired will have some degree of tenderness on palpation of the abdomen. In more than 95% of patients with acute appendicitis, the sequence of symptoms was anorexia, followed by abdominal pain, and then vomiting. In 1996, a meta-analysis performed by Wagner et al. [5] reported the sensitivity, specificity, and positive likelihood ratio with a 95% confidence interval for findings on the clinical examination characteristic of appendicitis. They reported the sensitivity, specificity, and positive likelihood ratio for RLQ pain (0.81, 0.53, 7.31–8.46), fever (0.67, 0.79, 1.94), and anorexia (0.68, 0.36, 1.27). A 2010 article confirmed the continued reliability of history and physical exam in the diagnosis of acute appendicitis [6].

Physical examination findings are determined by the anatomic position of the inflamed appendix and whether it has

DOI: 10.1201/9781003316800-42

ruptured. A retrocecal appendix can give rise to tenderness in the right flank or right upper quadrant (RUQ), whereas a pelvic appendix can give rise to little abdominal tenderness but pain on rectal examination. A patient who presents with uncomplicated appendicitis may present with a low-grade temperature (elevated by 1°C or 1.8°F) and a slight elevation in heart rate; otherwise, vital signs are normal. Patients with peritonitis will prefer to lie still, as any motion will tend to worsen their pain. If the appendix lies in the classic anterior position, abdominal pain will be maximal at McBurney's point (one-third the distance from the anterior superior iliac spine to the umbilicus), with rebound tenderness elucidated in the RLQ [4]. Palpation of the left lower quadrant (LLQ) may cause RLQ pain, also known as Rovsing's sign.

Deviations from these commonly associated physical findings usually are related to the anatomic position of the inflamed appendix. The common anatomic locations of the appendix include paracolic (the appendix lies in the right paracolic gutter lateral to the cecum), retrocecal (the appendix lies posterior to the cecum and may be partially or totally extraperitoneal), preileal (the appendix is anterior to the terminal ileum), postileal (the appendix is posterior to the ileum), promontory (the tip of the appendix lies in the vicinity of the sacral promontory), pelvic (the tip of the appendix lies in or toward the pelvis), and subcecal (the appendix lies inferior to the cecum) [7]. Wakeley [8] performed a postmortem analysis of 10,000 cases and described the frequency of the location of the appendix as follows: Retrocecal, 65.3%; pelvic, 31%; subcecal, 2.3%; preileal, 1%; and right paracolic and postileal, 0.4%. When the appendix occupies an unusual location, the diagnosis of appendicitis can be more difficult and may contribute to delays in presentation, diagnosis, and treatment.

> **RECOMMENDATION**
>
> Abdominal pain localized to the epigastrium or periumbilical area with subsequent radiation to the RLQ and associated with anorexia and nausea are the most reliable diagnostic signs and symptoms for acute appendicitis.
>
> Grade of recommendation: B.

42.3 What Is the Best Laboratory Test to Help Make the Diagnosis of Appendicitis?

The use of laboratory values in diagnosing appendicitis has been disappointing, as no one test is highly sensitive and/or specific. The sensitivity of an elevated white blood cell (WBC) count above 10,000 cells/μL for acute appendicitis is 70–90%, but the specificity is very low [9]. A value greater than 18,000 cells/μL suggests complicated appendicitis with either gangrene or perforation. The diagnostic value of C-reactive protein (CRP) and erythrocyte sedimentation rate in diagnosing

appendicitis has been both controversial and disappointing. A recent paper by Yang et al. [10] found the use of WBC and CRP individually or together had a high sensitivity to differentiate patients with appendicitis but a very low specificity. A study in adults with normal WBC and normal CRP found these combined laboratory values to be highly predictive in excluding appendicitis [11]. Other studies have shown that inflammatory cytokines and acute-phase reaction proteins such as interleukin-6 (IL-6), tumor necrosis factor (TNF-alpha), lipopolysaccharide-binding protein, alpha-1-glycoprotein (alpha 1GP), and endotoxin are also elevated in patients with suspected appendicitis. The result of many of these studies is that these inflammatory markers are elevated in appendicitis (high sensitivity) but most of the inflammatory markers are not specific enough to reliably diagnose acute appendicitis [12]. A study by Lycopoulou et al. [13] reported the sensitivity and specificity of the use of WBC count >10 (75% and 76%), CRP >10 mg/L (62% and 94%), and serum amyloid protein (SSA) >45 mg/L (86% and 83%) in diagnosing acute appendicitis in children. Procalcitonin was found to be increased in rare cases of severe inflammation after appendiceal perforation and gangrenous appendicitis, but because of its low sensitivity, it cannot be recommended for confirming the diagnosis of acute appendicitis [14].

Recent research using the neutrophil-to-lymphocyte ratio (NLR) has helped clinicians predict those with acute appendicitis and helps predict who may have uncomplicated versus complicated appendicitis. A systemic review by Hajbandeh et al. [15] looked at 8,914 patients in 17 different studies, and their results were able to predict acute appendicitis and its severity. An NLR greater than 4.7 was a powerful independent predictor of acute appendicitis. If the NLR was greater than 8.8, it predicted complicated appendicitis.

> **RECOMMENDATION**
>
> Overall, laboratory markers of acute inflammation in acute appendicitis remain highly sensitive but relatively nonspecific when it comes to making the diagnosis of acute appendicitis. The use of the NLR has been found to help predict which patients have acute appendicitis and whether it is uncomplicated versus complicated appendicitis.
>
> Grade of recommendation: B.

42.4 Does Giving Pain Medicine to a Patient with Suspected Appendicitis Decrease the Ability of the Clinician to Make the Diagnosis of Acute Appendicitis?

Conventional teaching instructs that patients with abdominal pain should not receive narcotics for fear of masking a surgical condition and delaying the diagnosis of acute surgical conditions, such as appendicitis. A prospective randomized double-blind study of parenteral tramadol analgesic use versus placebo in 68 emergency department (ED) patients with RLQ pain resulted in significant levels of pain control without concurrent normalization of abdominal pain [16]. In another prospective, double-blind study in ED patients with undifferentiated abdominal pain, patients were randomized to receive a placebo or morphine sulfate (MS) [17]. Diagnostic accuracy, however, did not differ between MS and control groups (64.2% vs. 66.7%). These results support the practice of early provision of analgesia with narcotics to patients with undifferentiated abdominal pain. In the pediatric population, the findings were consistent as well. Another prospective randomized study performed in children with a presumptive diagnosis of appendicitis was randomized to receive parenteral MS or placebo [18]. The authors found no difference in the time to surgical decision and no decrease in pain at 30 minutes between morphine at a dose of 0.1 mg/kg and placebo.

RECOMMENDATION

Giving pain medicine to adults and children suspected of acute appendicitis does not adversely affect the ability to diagnose appendicitis. Analgesia should not be withheld pending clinical investigation in patients with suspected acute appendicitis.

Grade of recommendation: B.

42.5 What Is the Best Imaging Modality to Diagnose Acute Appendicitis?

Many different radiologic modalities have been used to diagnose acute appendicitis. The optimal radiologic technique used should be accurate, quick, safe, readily available, cost-efficient, and provide little risk or discomfort to the patient. The use of abdominal ultrasound (US) and computed tomography (CT) has proven extremely useful in diagnosing appendicitis. Despite the recent increase in their use, these tests have not consistently increased the diagnostic accuracy of making the diagnosis of acute appendicitis in all patient populations [3].

The use of plain radiography for diagnosing acute gastrointestinal diseases has been around since the early 1900s. The appearance of an opaque fecalith in the RLQ is often quoted as being the hallmark radiographic finding in acute appendicitis, but less than 5–8% of patients present with this finding [19]. Other common but nonspecific findings on plain films include localized paralytic ileus, loss of the cecal shadow, blurring of the right psoas muscle, and rightward scoliosis of the lumbar spine. In a recent study of 821 consecutive patients hospitalized for suspected appendicitis, no individual radiographic finding was highly sensitive or specific in ultimately making the diagnosis of appendicitis [20]. Plain abdominal radiographs may be indicated when other acute abdominal conditions, such as gastric or duodenal perforation, intestinal obstruction, or ureteral calculus, are part of the differential as the cause of RLQ

abdominal pain. Overall, plain abdominal radiographs are not cost-effective and lack both sensitivity and specificity in the diagnosis of appendicitis.

Deutsch and Leopold [21] first visualized the inflamed appendix using US in 1981. US has become a more frequently used radiologic test to rule out appendicitis in children and pregnant women because of concerns about exposure to ionizing radiation from CT scans. Its accuracy in diagnosing appendicitis has been hampered by the interference of the US image by overlying bowel gas, the slow development of a transducer with enough spatial resolution to pick up small structures such as the appendix, and the highly variable operator-dependent interpretation and technical expertise at individual hospitals. With the advancement in US technology and the use of the graded compression technique when scanning the RLQ, the ability to visualize the appendix has improved. The graded compression technique involves applying steady, gradual pressure to the RLQ to collapse the normal bowel and eliminate bowel gas in the area to visualize the appendix. The inflamed appendix when seen by US commonly includes the following findings: An appendix of 7 mm or more in the anteroposterior diameter; an immobile, thick-walled, noncompressible luminal structure seen in cross-section referred to as a target lesion; or the presence of an appendicolith, a blind-ending structure consisting of an anechoic lumen surrounded by mucosa and a hypoechoic thickened wall adjacent to the cecum [22].

US is most reliable when there is considerable experience using this modality to diagnose acute appendicitis. In a meta-analysis looking at the sensitivity and specificity of US in diagnosing appendicitis, in children, it had 88% sensitivity and 94% specificity, and in adults, 83% sensitivity and 93% specificity were reported [23]. In another study reporting on the sensitivity and specificity of US in making the diagnosis of appendicitis in adults and children, it reported an overall 83% sensitivity and 98% sensitivity [24]. The reported sensitivity and specificity of US in diagnosing acute appendicitis in pregnant patients were 66–100% and 95–96%, respectively [25]. However, it is recommended that if a US is negative or inconclusive in a pregnant patient with a suspected diagnosis of appendicitis, another imaging study such as CT or magnetic resonance imaging (MRI) should be performed [26].

CT has been used as a diagnostic modality for acute abdominal pain since it became available in the late 1970s. Helical CT scans have excellent resolution, are widely available, are operator-independent, and are easy to interpret, making them often the preferred diagnostic test to rule out appendicitis. Findings strongly suggestive of acute appendicitis on standard abdominal CT scan include (1) a thick wall (>2 mm), often with "targeting" (concentric thickening of the inflamed appendix wall); (2) increased diameter of the appendix (>7 mm); (3) an appendicolith; (4) a phlegmon or abscess; or (5) free fluid [26]. Stranding of the adjacent fatty tissues in the RLQ is also commonly associated. The top four CT findings suggestive of appendicitis are an enlarged appendix, appendiceal wall thickening, appendiceal wall enhancement, and periappendiceal fat stranding [27]. If air is seen in the appendix or if the appendiceal lumen is filled with contrast and there are no other abnormalities seen on CT, these findings virtually eliminate appendicitis as the diagnosis. Additionally, a recent study showed that nonvisualization of the appendix on a CT scan was negative for appendicitis in 98% of cases [28]. CT is also useful in diagnosing an appendiceal abscess and can be used to guide percutaneous drainage. CT can also help diagnose other causes of acute abdominal pain in patients suspected of acute appendicitis.

The performance of CT scans to evaluate RLQ pain has increased considerably since Rao et al. [29] reported an accuracy rate of 98% with the administration of rectal contrast in diagnosing acute appendicitis. Rao also reported that the use of CT at his institution decreased the rate of removal of a normal appendix from 20% before the introduction of CT scanning to 7% after [30]. In a retrospective review of CT use in the pediatric population suspected of appendicitis, a normal appendix was removed in 7% of children who underwent CT before appendectomy, 11% with the use of US before appendectomy, and an 8% negative appendectomy rate when no preoperative radiologic study was performed [31]. In a recent retrospective study, the use of preoperative CT scans only decreased the negative appendectomy rate for women of childbearing age (women 45 years and younger) [32]. Although many studies have found CT to be accurate in diagnosing acute appendicitis, there is still controversy regarding the optimal technique. Three common techniques used include a focused appendiceal CT using rectally administered contrast and the unenhanced or the use of oral and/or intravenous contrasted CT of the abdomen and pelvis. Every institution has its preference as to which version they prefer to use to diagnose appendicitis, all of which seem to have the same reported accuracy [33].

In a systemic review performed by van Redan et al. [34] comparing graded compression US to CT in the diagnosis of appendicitis, the authors found the respective mean sensitivities for CT and graded compression US were 91% (95% confidence interval [CI]: 84%, 95%) and 78% (95% CI: 67%, 86%) ($p < 0.017$) and the respective mean specificities for CT and graded compression US were as follows: 90% (95% CI: 85%, 94%) and 83% (95% CI: 76%, $-< 0.$ ($p < 0.037$). The authors concluded from their meta-analysis of head-to-head comparison studies in patient populations with a high prevalence of appendicitis that CT was found to have a better test performance than graded compression US in making the diagnosis. The authors recommend the use of CT in patients with suspected acute appendicitis.

Should CT be used routinely in the diagnostic evaluation of patients suspected of appendicitis? Because of the increasing reports of excellent accuracy rates of CT in diagnosing appendicitis, some have called for its routine use for all patients with possible appendicitis [35]. Others have questioned the need for routine use of CT for all patients, especially those with classic clinical presentations. McCay and Shepherd [36] recommend only ordering CT on patients presenting to the emergency room suspected of having appendicitis if their Alvarado score [37] is between 4 and 6. For a score of less than 3, no CT or US was recommended, as appendicitis was unlikely. The authors do, however, recommend a surgical consult for an Alvarado score of 7 or more. In a prospective randomized study of patients presenting to the emergency room for possible appendicitis comparing clinical assessment versus CT, the reported diagnostic accuracy was 90% for clinical assessment and 92%

for CT [38]. The authors concluded that clinical assessment unaided by CT reliably identifies patients with acute appendicitis who need an operation. These authors do not advocate for the routine use of CT for the diagnosis of suspected appendicitis. In a prospective randomized study performed on women of childbearing age who presented to the emergency room with the suspected diagnosis of appendicitis, each was randomized to the clinical assessment only arm or the CT arm [39]. In this study, the reported accuracy for the diagnosis of appendicitis was 93% for both clinical assessment and CT. The authors concluded that a CT scan is as good as clinical assessment alone and reliably identifies women of childbearing age who need an appendectomy. In a retrospective study of children reported by Martin et al. [40], the liberal use of CT scans did not decrease the negative appendectomy rate. In conclusion, the selective use of CT scans seems more appropriate in diagnosing suspected appendicitis. The use of CT scans should be reserved as an adjunct in clinical settings where the history, physical exam, and laboratory tests alone do not help make the diagnosis of appendicitis.

MRI for the evaluation of acute appendicitis has been performed more frequently recently to avoid the risks associated with ionizing radiation. MRI has become a frequently performed test in pregnant women and children with symptoms of appendicitis and the nondiagnostic US [41]. MRI has good resolution and is accurate in diagnosing acute appendicitis [42]. It is considered positive for acute appendicitis when the appendix is enlarged (>7 mm), the appendiceal wall is thicker than 2 mm, or there are signs of inflammatory changes surrounding the appendix, such as fat stranding, phlegmon, or abscess formation [43]. MRI is safe and reliable in diagnosing acute appendicitis in pregnant patients [44]. No IV contrast should be given to pregnant patients because gadolinium is a category C drug and potentially teratogenic.

In a recent multicenter diagnostic study of MRI in patients with suspected appendicitis, the authors suggest that MRI is found to be sufficiently accurate in the general population of patients with suspected appendicitis [45]. MRI could replace CT in some patients, as MRI limits or obviates ionizing radiation exposure and decreases the risk of contrast medium–induced nephropathy with CT. Limitations to the use of MRI are it is a more expensive test, it is not always widely available, images can be degraded by motion, and a specialist needs to interpret the MRI images. Until these limitations can be overcome, MRI should not be a first-line test to rule out appendicitis.

RECOMMENDATION

The most accurate radiographic imaging modality for making the diagnosis of appendicitis is CT. US and MRI can also be used to aid in the diagnosis of appendicitis in children and pregnant females. These studies should be reserved as an adjunct in clinical settings in which the physical exam and history alone are not sufficient to make the diagnosis of appendicitis.

Grade of recommendation: B.

42.6 Does Administration of Antibiotics to Patients with Appendicitis Who Undergo Appendectomy Decrease Postoperative Infectious Complications?

Appendicitis, once diagnosed, is typically treated with an appendectomy. Antibiotics should be given as soon as the diagnosis is suspected. The bacteria that populate the appendix are similar to the bacterial flora of the colon. The antibiotics chosen for patients with appendicitis should provide coverage for gram-negative and gram-positive aerobic and anaerobic bacteria, along with anaerobes. *Bacteroides fragilis* and *Escherichia coli* are the two most common organisms grown from peritoneal cultures after acute appendicitis.

Acute appendicitis is a polymicrobial infection. In 1938, William Altemeier isolated at least four different organisms per specimen in patients with perforated appendicitis [46]. More recent reports demonstrate on average up to 12 organisms per specimen from patients with gangrenous or perforated appendicitis [47]. Few bacteria are cultured from the peritoneal fluid of patients with acute appendicitis only; however, bacteria are recovered from peritoneal fluid in over 80% of patients with a gangrenous or perforated appendix. Two common postoperative complications following appendectomy are wound infections and intraabdominal abscesses.

All patients undergoing appendectomy for acute appendicitis should receive antibiotics preoperatively. Gorbach, in his review of antimicrobial prophylaxis for appendectomy, reported a reduction in the rate of postoperative infectious complications in all operations for acute appendicitis and especially in patients with perforated and/or gangrenous appendicitis [48]. In a study by Mui et al., a single dose of preoperative antibiotics was found to be adequate for the prevention of postoperative infective complications in patients with nonperforated appendicitis [49]. Another study also supported the fact that only one preoperative dose of antibiotic is needed to prevent postoperative infectious complications in patients with nonperforated appendicitis, and the use of any further postoperative antibiotics does not decrease the rate of surgical site infections (SSIs) [50]. Anderson et al. performed a meta-analysis of randomized or controlled clinical trials investigating the use of antibiotics versus placebo for patients with suspected appendicitis who underwent an appendectomy [51]. The authors evaluated 45 studies with 9,576 patients. Their outcome measures were wound infection, intraabdominal abscess, hospital length of stay, and mortality. They concluded that the use of antibiotics is superior to a placebo in preventing wound infection and intraabdominal abscesses in patients with acute, gangrenous, and perforated appendicitis. They were unable to determine from their analysis the optimal duration of antibiotic treatment for complicated cases.

A retrospective study included 266 patients, 78 with complicated and 188 with uncomplicated appendicitis. They concluded that antibiotic therapy postoperatively for uncomplicated appendicitis showed no significant advantage in preventing postoperative intraabdominal infections. They also concluded that prolonged postoperative IV antibiotics for complicated appendicitis that lasts beyond 5 days did not improve the incidence of intraabdominal infections [52]. A recent study evaluating the optimal length of postoperative antibiotic duration after laparoscopic appendectomy for complicated appendicitis showed 3 days may be sufficient to decrease infectious complications [53]. These findings are further supported by recent studies including the STOP-IT trial. According to this trial, in patients with an intraabdominal infection who have undergone an adequate source control procedure, there was no significant difference in outcome between patients treated with a 4-day course of antibiotics versus an 8-day course of antibiotics for complicated appendicitis [54]. Unfortunately, nearly 20% of the patients in the shorter antibiotic course group crossed over to receive a longer course of antibiotics, possibly invalidating the author's conclusions. Patients with perforated or complicated appendicitis can be treated initially with a shorter course of antibiotics—4 days if they undergo a source control procedure such as an appendectomy, washout, or abscess drainage. Continuation of antibiotics for a longer duration will be dependent on the patient's response to treatment.

A recent prospective study by Fraser et al. of pediatric patients with perforated appendicitis examined early transition to oral antibiotics in comparison to a traditional 5-day IV antibiotic course. Patients were transitioned to oral antibiotics as soon as they tolerated a diet and were discharged, to complete a total 7-day regimen of IV/PO antibiotics. This group had no increased morbidity compared to the group receiving 5 days of IV antibiotics [55].

RECOMMENDATION

Antibiotic prophylaxis is effective in preventing postoperative wound infections and intraabdominal abscesses. For nonperforated/uncomplicated appendicitis, the one-time preoperative dose of antibiotics seems to be sufficient to decrease infectious complications. The optimal duration of administration of antibiotics for complicated appendicitis seems to be 3–5 days.

Grade of recommendation: B.

42.7 What Operation Is Better for Treating Acute Appendicitis: Laparoscopic or Open Appendectomy?

The longtime treatment for acute appendicitis has been to perform an appendectomy through an RLQ incision since its introduction by McBurney [56] in 1894. The first laparoscopic appendectomy was performed by Semm [57] in 1983. This new surgical technique was slow to be accepted because the standard open technique provided excellent therapeutic efficacy combined with its low morbidity and mortality rates. The use of laparoscopic appendectomy varies considerably. It seems that the most important determinant of whether a patient will have an open versus laparoscopic appendectomy is the preference and experience of the treating surgeon, which may vary significantly even within an institution.

During the traditional open appendectomy technique performed through a muscle-splitting incision in the RLQ, the appendix is usually ligated with an absorbable suture. Inversion of the appendiceal stump has been advocated to prevent leakage and fistulization, but studies have shown no difference in complication rates between inversion and simple ligation of the appendiceal stump [58]. The peritoneal cavity is typically irrigated after an appendectomy. The skin incision is normally closed without complications, although if the wound is grossly contaminated, one may consider delayed primary closure or simply allow the wound to heal by secondary intention [59]. Leaving an intraperitoneal drain is not useful even in cases of a perforated appendix [60].

Is laparoscopic appendectomy better than open appendectomy? The answer to this question depends on the outcomes being measured. Over the last 20 years, various studies have looked at factors such as the duration of operation, cost of operation, cost of hospitalization, length of hospital stay, the time to return to work, and postoperative pain, often with conflicting results [61, 62]. Although many of the randomized controlled trials comparing laparoscopic and open appendectomy are plagued by several biases, they represent the best evidence available.

Two early meta-analyses of laparoscopic versus open appendectomy for acute appendicitis have confirmed the benefits of the laparoscopic approach in terms of less pain, a faster recovery, and a lower incidence of wound infections when compared to an open appendectomy [62, 63]. As surgeons have become more skilled with minimally invasive surgical techniques, the incidence of laparoscopic appendectomy has become more common [64]. Reported complications after laparoscopic appendectomy include injury to the bowel, bladder, and ureter; bleeding from epigastric vessels, iliac vessels, and mesentery; appendiceal stump leak; wound infection; and intraabdominal abscesses. Another reported complication of the laparoscopic technique is recurrent appendicitis. This entity, known as stump appendicitis, occurs when the surgeon fails to remove the appendix at the base of the cecum, thus leaving a stump of the appendix that can become infected, causing recurrent appendicitis [65].

A systematic Cochrane review of randomized clinical trials compared open (OA) versus laparoscopic appendectomy (LA) in 2018 [66] in adults and children. Other than a higher rate of intraabdominal abscesses after LA in adults, LA showed advantages over OA in terms of pain intensity, wound infections, length of hospital stay, and time until return to normal activity in adults. In contrast, LA showed advantages over OA in terms of wound infections and length of hospital stay in children. However, the quality of evidence ranged from very low to moderate, and some of the clinical effects of LA were small and of limited clinical relevance. The authors concluded that in clinical settings where surgical expertise and equipment are available and affordable, LA seems to hold various advantages over OA. They recommend LA be done for patients with suspected appendicitis, especially in young patients, female patients, obese patients, and employed patients.

The role of laparoscopy between male and female patients is an area that needs further exploration and strict protocols. The diagnosis of abdominal pain is variable between the sexes,

especially in females of childbearing age, where the differential includes but is not limited to ovarian cysts, pelvic infection, ectopic pregnancy, and appendicitis. A review was recently published which included 12 studies and 1,020 patients; 8 studies compared laparoscopy versus OA, and 4 compared laparoscopy with a "wait and see" approach. They concluded that laparoscopy was superior to both OA and a "wait and see" strategy in the ability to make a specific diagnosis before discharge, as well as attributing it to shorter hospital stays and earlier return to work in female patients of childbearing age [67]. Early laparoscopy in females with abdominal pain can lead to a more accurate diagnosis and allow for timely treatment and possible avoidance of other disease-associated complications.

Conversely, using the laparoscopic technique in males may not always be necessary. A 1996 study examined 100 males between 16 and 65 years old and randomized patients to laparoscopic and open appendectomy groups and compared them based on clinical parameters, postoperative complications, and length of stay. They reported that LA versus OA required longer anesthetic (72.5 vs. 55 minutes) and operative times (45 vs. 25 minutes), and no significant difference was found in the recovery of bowel function (24.7 vs. 21 hours) and length of stay (4.9 vs. 5.3 days). These authors concluded that there was no significant advantage to using the laparoscopic technique in males with the diagnosis of appendicitis and that the use of laparoscopy should be reserved for obese patients and males with an uncertain diagnosis [68].

Traditional OA performed on obese patients may require a larger skin incision, potentially resulting in more postoperative pain and a higher potential for wound complications. In obese individuals, LA is a potentially easier technique that avoids a large and deep incision and can lead to improved wound outcomes. It has been reported that laparoscopy is superior to OA for obese patients (body mass index $\geq$30) based on clinical outcomes, which include length of stay and wound complication rates [69]. A recently published review examined the outcomes of 13,330 patients with body mass index $\geq$30 who underwent either laparoscopic or open appendectomy. The laparoscopic technique was associated with a 57% reduction in overall morbidity (odds ratio [OR]: 0.43; 95% CI: 0.36–0.52), a 53% reduction in risk (OR: 0.47; 95% CI: 0.32–0.65), and a 1.2 days shorter length of stay (mean difference 1.2 days; 95% CI: 0.98–1.42). The authors concluded that for the obese population, LA is not only safe but also superior based on clinical outcomes [70].

In considering elderly patients, the differential diagnosis of abdominal pain is variable and extends to include perforated diverticulitis as well as neoplastic processes. There is also the difficulty in making an early and accurate diagnosis in elderly patients. One study retrospectively examined 10 years of data that included patients with appendicitis who were 60 years old and older. They reported that only 26% of elderly patients have typical symptoms and one-third delay seeking medical care [71]. When comparing age groups, elderly patients with acute appendicitis have significantly increased rates of perforation attributed to presentation delay and increased morbidity and mortality [72]. Given the fact that elderly patients with appendicitis have increased perforation rates that are likely attributable to a delay in presentation, a question is raised as to whether

LA has an advantage in the treatment of this patient population. One meta-analysis included six studies and a total of 4,398 laparoscopic and 11,454 open appendectomies in older patients. The laparoscopic technique was associated with significant reductions in postoperative mortality (pooled OR: 0.24; 95% CI: 0.15–0.37), postoperative complications (pooled OR: 0.61; 95% CI: 0.50–0.73), and length of hospital stay (−0.51 days; 95% CI: −0.64 to −0.37 days). When comparing operative time, postoperative wound infection, and intraabdominal collection, no significant difference was found between groups [73]. A second study examined elderly patients (65 and older) from the Nationwide Inpatient Database [74]: 65,464 patients were evaluated for the outcomes of laparoscopic versus open appendectomy for perforated and nonperforated appendicitis. In nonperforated appendicitis, laparoscopy had lower overall complication rates (15.82% vs. 23.49%), in-hospital mortality (0.39% vs. 1.31%), and mean length of stay (3.0 vs. 4.8 days) when compared with OA. Results were similar when comparing patients with perforated appendicitis. They reported that laparoscopy was associated with a lower overall complication rate (36.27% vs. 46.92%), in-hospital mortality (1.4% vs. 2.63%), and shorter mean length of stay (5.8 vs. 8.7 days, $p < 0.01$). The authors concluded that LA can be performed safely and has the advantages of shorter lengths of stay and decreased complications when compared with OA in elderly patients with appendicitis.

RECOMMENDATION

The data support performing either open or laparoscopic appendectomy for patients with known acute appendicitis. If surgical expertise and equipment are available, the literature supports the consideration of a laparoscopic approach, especially in female patients of childbearing age, obese patients, and elderly patients.

Grade of recommendation: B.

42.8 Is Interval Appendectomy Necessary?

Patients presenting with a periappendiceal mass or abscess diagnosed preoperatively by physical examination or imaging studies can be treated with antibiotics with the potential of having their periappendiceal abscess drained by an image-guided percutaneous catheter. With the increased use of CT in the workup of acute appendicitis, the ability to identify complicated appendicitis preoperatively has allowed for the utilization of initial nonoperative therapy. Generally, antibiotics for 7–14 days with or without catheter drainage have been necessary to treat complicated appendicitis. An interval appendectomy has been advocated after the abscess and surrounding inflammatory phlegmon have resolved, usually 6–8 weeks after initial nonoperative treatment to prevent recurrent appendicitis and to treat other tumor pathology of the cecum and appendix [75]. Alternative treatment options for complicated appendicitis have included early aggressive resection,

or initial conservative treatment with interval appendectomy only if symptoms recur. An immediate appendectomy may be technically demanding secondary to distorted anatomy and the challenges faced when closing an inflamed/necrotic appendiceal stump. Occasionally during immediate exploration for complicated appendicitis, the surgeon ends up performing an ileocecal resection or a right-sided hemicolectomy due to inflammation distorting the tissue planes or suspicion of malignancy. Following successful nonsurgical treatment of a periappendiceal mass, the need for interval appendectomy has been questioned, as the risk of recurrent appendicitis is relatively low (0.2–7%) [76].

In a retrospective study, it was found that children presenting with complicated appendicitis could be successfully treated with conservative treatment followed by interval appendectomy. Roach et al. [77] concluded from their data that for children who presented with prolonged symptoms and a discrete appendiceal abscess or phlegmon, drainage and performance of a delayed appendectomy should be the treatment of choice. In another study, children with complicated appendicitis were initially treated nonoperatively and then underwent an interval appendectomy. This study concluded that interval appendectomy could be safely performed and was associated with a shorter hospital stay, with minimal morbidity, analgesia, and scarring. These authors recommended that interval LA be routinely performed because it eliminates the risk of recurrent appendicitis and serves to excise undiagnosed carcinoid tumors [78]. A randomized prospective study compared initial LA versus initial nonoperative management and interval appendectomy for complicated appendicitis in children [79]. These authors found that the initial laparoscopic surgery took longer but that the overall days in the hospital, infection rates, and total costs did not differ between the two treatment strategies.

In a large retrospective study performed by Kaminski et al. [80], 32,938 patients were hospitalized with acute appendicitis. Emergency appendectomy was performed in 31,926 (97%) patients. Nonoperative treatment was used initially in 1,012 patients (3%). Of these, 148 (15%) had an interval appendectomy and the remaining 864 (85%) did not. In their study, only 39 patients (5%) had a recurrence of appendicitis after a median follow-up of 4 years. Males were more likely to have a recurrence of their symptoms than females. The median length of hospital stay was 4 days for the admission for recurrent appendicitis compared with 6 days for the interval appendectomy admission. The authors concluded that they could not justify the practice of routine interval appendectomy after initial successful nonoperative treatment of appendicitis based on these findings. In a similar retrospective study in children reported by Paupong et al. [81], there were 6,439 patients, of which 6,367 (99%) underwent initial appendectomy for acute appendicitis. Seventy-two (1%) patients were initially managed nonoperatively, and 11 patients had interval appendectomy. Of the remaining 61 patients without interval appendectomy, 5 (8%) developed recurrent appendicitis. The authors concluded that since recurrent appendicitis is rare in children after successful nonoperative treatment of perforated appendicitis, the performance of routine interval appendectomy is not necessarily indicated. Another study looking at the successful nonoperative treatment of appendiceal mass found the risk of recurrent appendicitis was 20.5% (95% CI, 14.3–28.4%). The incidence of complications after interval appendectomy (23 studies, $n = 1247$) were 3.4% (95% CI, 2.2–5.1), and the incidence of carcinoid tumor found at interval appendectomy (15 studies, $n = 955$) was 0.9% (95% CI, 0.5–1.8). The authors concluded that the data suggest that 80% of children with appendiceal mass may not need interval appendectomy [82].

Adult patients who present with complicated appendicitis and an appendiceal mass in the RLQ are commonly managed nonoperatively and then scheduled for an interval appendectomy following the resolution of the inflammatory process. This mass could represent a perforated appendix, complicated Crohn's disease, or perforated colon cancer. Tekin et al. [83] reported their experience with not performing routine interval appendectomy after successful treatment of an appendiceal mass. Four patients (4%) in their series had another diagnosis found for their appendiceal mass (two cecal cancers, one cecal diverticulitis, and one Crohn's disease). The recurrence rate of appendicitis in their series was 14.6%, with most recurrences happening in the first 6 months after the initial presentation. Patients who presented with recurrent symptoms underwent interval appendectomy. They concluded that routine interval appendectomy after initial successful conservative treatment is not justified, but they recommend that a protocol be developed for the management of patients presenting with an appendiceal mass. Similar recommendations were reported by Lai et al. [84]. In their study, five patients were found to have colon cancer, and the rate of recurrent appendicitis was 25.5% with 83% of patients presenting with recurrent symptoms within 6 months of their initial presentation. They recommend that adult patients who recover from the nonoperative treatment of an appendiceal mass undergo a colonoscopy to detect any underlying disease, and interval appendectomy should only be offered to patients who present with recurrent symptoms.

Stevens and de Vries [85] reported on their experience of performing an interval appendectomy only after symptoms developed rather than routinely offering it to their patients with complicated appendicitis. They concluded that the rate of appendectomies performed dropped by 63% and the total length of hospital stay also decreased by 4 days. A group from China reported that performing an interval appendectomy only after symptoms develop was more cost-effective than performing a routine interval appendectomy [86]. In their study, the authors showed that the performance of routine interval appendectomy would increase the cost per patient by 38% compared with follow-up and appendectomy after the recurrence of symptoms. It is important to also consider patients, such as military personnel, who have undergone nonoperative management of appendicitis and who will, in the future, be in an environment with limited access to medical and surgical care. With recurrent symptoms, these patients risk future development of complications and even death; therefore, this select population may benefit from routine interval appendectomy.

In one systematic review of the nonsurgical treatment of appendiceal abscess or phlegmon, the need for an interval appendectomy was evaluated [87]. Findings from the meta-analysis included the following: Nonsurgical treatment fails in 7.2% of cases (CI: 4.0–10.5), the risk of recurrent symptoms

is 7.4% (CI: 3.7–11.1), the risk of finding malignant disease is 1.2% (CI: 0.6–1.7), and the risk of finding an important benign disease is 0.7% (CI: 0.2–11.9) during follow-up. From their meta-analysis (mainly from retrospective studies), the authors support the practice of nonsurgical treatment without interval appendectomy in patients with appendiceal abscess or phlegmon. Another systematic review has confirmed that nonoperative management of complicated appendicitis will be successful in most cases with a low incidence of recurrent symptoms. As a result, the authors suggest that the routine use of interval appendectomy may no longer be justified in all patients [88].

However, the incidence of finding a neoplasm in complicated appendicitis is significantly higher than in uncomplicated appendicitis (12.6% vs. 1.2%) [89]. In a recent study by Mallinen et al., patients ages 18–60 had appendiceal abscess initially successfully treated with antibiotics and percutaneous drainage. The study planned to randomize 120 patients to interval appendectomy or continued nonoperative management. The trial was prematurely terminated after interim analysis demonstrated an unexpectedly high rate of appendiceal neoplasm of 17%. Patients who were initially randomized to nonoperative management were then offered appendectomy, and this led to a 20% overall rate of neoplasm [90]. The likelihood of discovering an incidental neoplasm in complicated appendicitis increases with age. Colonoscopy should be performed in most adult patients, especially those greater than 30 with complicated appendicitis who were managed nonoperatively. In adult patients with complicated appendicitis, interval appendectomy should be encouraged, especially for those at increased risk for colon cancer.

RECOMMENDATION

The routine performance of interval appendectomy after nonoperative treatment of uncomplicated acute appendicitis is not supported for all patients. Patients presenting with an appendiceal abscess or mass managed nonoperatively should undergo further workup to rule out other pathology. The age of the patient and the risk of finding a neoplasm should be considered for each patient, and an interval appendectomy should be performed in those at increased risk for neoplasm, especially those older than 40.

Grade of recommendation: B.

42.9 Should Antibiotic Treatment Replace Appendectomy for Uncomplicated Acute Appendicitis?

In 1995, Eriksson and Granstrom [91] reported a randomized controlled trial of appendectomy versus antibiotics alone in 40 patients suspected to have appendicitis who presented with abdominal pain for less than 72 hours. Twenty patients underwent surgery, and 20 patients received IV antibiotics for 2 days, followed by an 8-day course of oral antibiotics. The authors concluded that antibiotic treatment in patients with acute appendicitis was as effective as surgery. However, they reported a 15% negative appendectomy rate for the surgery group and a 40% recurrence rate of appendicitis that led to appendectomy within 1 year of treatment in the nonoperative group.

The APPAC randomized clinical trial reported by Salminen in 2015 was a multicenter trial in which 530 patients from Finland were randomized to OA or nonoperative management with antibiotics. Overall, 70 (27.3%) of the antibiotic-only patients required appendectomy within 12 months and 72.7% (186) of antibiotic-only patients were successfully treated without operative intervention [92].

The CODA trial was another multicenter study with 1,552 patients with uncomplicated appendicitis who were randomized to appendectomy (96% laparotomy) versus nonoperative management with 10 days of antibiotics. Forty-seven percent of the nonoperative management arm did not require hospitalization. At 90 days 29% of the nonoperative management patients underwent appendectomy. The rate of appendectomy was higher in those nonoperative management patients with appendicolith (41% with vs. 25% without) [93]. Interestingly, all the differences between those patients with and without fecalith were noted in the first 48 hours of hospitalization, raising concerns regarding bias by the treating surgeons.

The COMMA trial by O'Leary et al. [94] randomized 186 patients to antibiotic-only vs. appendectomy. Twenty-three patients (25.3%) randomized to antibiotics alone experienced a recurrence of symptoms within a year. Quality-of-life scores were significantly better in the surgery group. The mean total cost was higher in patients who underwent surgery.

A recent meta-analysis of randomized controlled trials confirmed earlier findings that uncomplicated appendicitis can be successfully treated with antibiotics. [95] The authors also reported no difference in major adverse events between operative and nonoperative management. However, in the nonoperative group, the length of stay was significantly longer. The reported cumulative incidence of recurrent appendicitis was 18%. The continued lifetime risk of, and the associated morbidity and mortality of nonoperative treatment with antibiotics only for uncomplicated acute appendicitis, continue to be investigated. Currently, antibiotics-alone treatment as an alternative to the surgical management of uncomplicated acute appendicitis appears to be an acceptable option in comparison to appendectomy in about 30% of patients. Those patients who present with an appendicolith may have a higher failure rate of nonoperative management with antibiotics alone.

RECOMMENDATION

Although antibiotics may be used as the primary treatment for selected patients with uncomplicated appendicitis, surgery continues to remain the primary treatment option for the management of acute appendicitis in the United States. Patients with uncomplicated appendicitis may be offered nonoperative treatment and should have a thorough understanding of the risks and benefits of nonoperative therapy.

Grade of recommendation: B.

TABLE 42.1

Clinical Questions Summary

Question	Answer	Level of Evidence	Grade of Recommendation	References
What clinical signs and symptoms are most reliable to rule in or out appendicitis?	Abdominal pain localized to the epigastrium or periumbilical area radiating to the right lower quadrant and associated with anorexia and nausea are the most reliable diagnostic symptoms for acute appendicitis.	4	B	[3–8]
What is the best laboratory test to help make the diagnosis of appendicitis?	Overall laboratory markers of inflammation in acute appendicitis remain highly sensitive but relatively nonspecific when it comes to making the diagnosis of acute appendicitis. No one test is both highly sensitive and specific for acute appendicitis.	2B	B	[9–14]
Does giving a patient with suspected appendicitis pain medicine decrease the ability to make the diagnosis of appendicitis?	Giving pain medicine to adults and children suspected of acute appendicitis does not adversely affect the ability to diagnose appendicitis. Analgesia should not be withheld pending clinical investigation with suspected acute appendicitis.	3B	B	[15–18]
What is the best diagnostic imaging modality to diagnose acute appendicitis?	The most accurate imaging modality for making the diagnosis of appendicitis is CT. The routine use of performing CT on all patients suspected of appendicitis cannot be recommended.	2B	B	[3, 19–45]

(Continued)

TABLE 42.1 (Continued)

Clinical Questions Summary

Question	Answer	Level of Evidence	Grade of Recommendation	References
Does giving antibiotics to patients with appendicitis who undergo appendectomy decrease postoperative complication rates?	Antibiotic prophylaxis is effective in preventing postoperative wound infections and intraabdominal abscesses. For nonperforated appendicitis, the one-time preoperative dose of antibiotics seems to be sufficient to decrease infection complications. The optimal duration of administration of antibiotics for complicated appendicitis seems to be 5–7 days but needs to be further evaluated.	2B	B	[46–55, 91–93]
What operation is better for treating acute appendicitis: Laparoscopic or open appendectomy?	The data support performing both open and laparoscopic appendectomy for patients with acute appendicitis if surgical expertise and equipment are available. The laparoscopic approach is preferred in female patients of childbearing age, obese patients, and elderly patients. An open appendectomy may be the preferred method of appendectomy in males aged 18–65 with a BMI of less than 30.	2B	B	[57–74]
Is interval appendectomy necessary?	The routine performance of interval appendectomy after nonoperative treatment of uncomplicated acute appendicitis is not supported. Interval appendectomy should be performed when patients present with recurrent symptoms. Patients presenting with an appendiceal mass managed conservatively should undergo further workup to rule out other pathology for their mass before definitive surgery, and interval appendectomy should be strongly considered, particularly over age 30.	3B	B	[75–90]
Should antibiotic treatment replace appendectomy for acute appendicitis?	Antibiotics may be used as the primary treatment for selected patients with uncomplicated appendicitis.	3B	B	[91–95]

Editor's Note

The management of acute appendicitis has changed dramatically over the last few decades. First, the use of CT scans replaced the history and physical exam in patients with acute abdominal pain in many emergency centers, simplifying the diagnosis for surgeons. Second, the primary operation in the United States changed from open appendectomy to a laparoscopic approach today in more than 95% of adults and children. Most recently, the use of antibiotics alone for uncomplicated appendicitis has been recognized as an effective option. Interval appendectomy should be performed in all adults over 40 who are managed nonoperatively to exclude malignancy.

REFERENCES

1. Moris D, Paulson EK, Pappas TN. Diagnosis and management of acute appendicitis in adults: A review. *JAMA.* 2021 Dec 14;*326*(22):2299–2311. doi:10.1001/jama.2021.20502. PMID: 34905026.
2. Golz RA, Flum DR, Sanchez SE, et al. Geographical association between the incidence of acute appendicitis and socioeconomic status. *JAMA Surg.* 2020;*155*(4):330–338.
3. Lee SL. Computed tomography and ultrasonography do not improve and may delay the diagnosis and treatment of acute appendicitis. *Arch Surg.* 2001;*136*(5):556. doi:10.1001/archsurg.136.5.556.
4. Silen W. 1996. *Cope's Early Diagnosis of the Acute Abdomen,* 19th edn. Oxford University Press: New York.
5. Wagner J, McKinney WP, Carpenter JL. Does this patient have appendicitis? *JAMA.* 1996;*276*:1589.
6. Howell JM, Eddy OL, Lukens TW, Thiessen MEW, Weingart SD, Decker WW. Clinical policy: Critical issues in the evaluation and management of emergency department patients with suspected appendicitis. *Ann Emerg Med.* 2010;*55*(1):71–116. doi:10.1016/j.annemergmed.2009.10.004.
7. Prystowsky JP, Pugh CM, Nagle AP. Current problems in surgery. Appendicitis. *Curr Prob Surg.* 2005;*42*(10):685–742.
8. Wakeley CP. The position of the vermiform appendix was ascertained by an analysis of 10,000 cases. *J Anat.* 1933;*67*:277–283.
9. Hoffmann J, Rausmussen O. Aids in the diagnosis of acute appendicitis. *Br J Surg.* 1989;*76*:774.
10. Yang HR, Wang YC, Chung PK, et al. Laboratory tests in patients with acute appendicitis. *ANZ J Surg.* Jan–Feb 2006;*76*(1–2):71–74.

11. Sengupta A, Bax G, Paterson-Brown S. White blood cell count and C-reactive protein measurement in patients with possible appendicitis. *Ann R Coll Surg Engl.* Sep 2009; *91(2)*:113–115.

12. Yildirim O, Solak C, Kocer B, et al. The role of serum inflammatory markers in acute appendicitis and their success in preventing negative laparotomy. *J Invest Surg.* 2006; *19(6)*:345–352.

13. Lycopoulou L, Mamoulakis C, Hantzi E, et al. Serum amyloid A protein levels as a possible aid in the diagnosis of acute appendicitis in children. *Clin Chem Lab Med.* 2005;*43(1)*:49–53.

14. Sand M, Trullen XV, Bechara FG, et al. A prospective bicenter study investigating the diagnostic value of procalcitonin in patients with acute appendicitis. *Eur Surg Res.* 2009;*43(3)*:291–297.

15. Hajibandeh S, Hajibandeh S, Hobbs N, Moustafa M. AM J Surg. 2020.

16. Manadevan M, Graff L. Prospective randomized double-blind study of analgesic use for ED patients with right lower quadrant abdominal pain. *Am J Emerg Med.* 2000;*18*:753–756.

17. Thomas SH, Silen W, Cheema F, Reisner A, Aman S, Goldstein JN, Kumar Am, Stair TO. Effects of morphine analgesia on diagnostic accuracy in emergency department patients with abdominal pain: A prospective, randomized trial. *J Am Coll Surg.* 2003;*196*:18–31.

18. Bailey B, Bergeron S, Gravel J, Bussieres JF, Bensoussan A. Efficacy and impact of intravenous morphine before surgical consultation in children with right lower quadrant pain suggestive of appendicitis: A randomized controlled trial. *Ann Emerg Med.* 2007;*50*:371–378.

19. Old JL, Dusing RW, Yap W, Dirks J. Imaging for suspected appendicitis. *Am Fam Phys.* 2005;*71*:71–78.

20. Graffeo CS, Counselman FL. Appendicitis. *Emerg Med Clin North Am.* 1996;*14*:653–671.

21. Deutsch A, Leopold GR. Ultrasonic demonstration of the inflamed appendix: Case report. *Radiology.* 1981;*140*: 163–164.

22. Adams DH, Fine C, Brooks DC. High-resolution real-time ultrasonography. A new tool in the diagnosis of acute appendicitis. *Am J Surg.* 1988;*155*:93–97.

23. Doria AS, Moineddin R, Kellenberger CJ, et al. US or CT for diagnosis in children and adults? A meta-analysis. *Radiology.* Oct 2006;*241(1)*:83–94.

24. Johansson EP, Rydh A, Rilund KA. Ultrasound, computed tomography, and laboratory findings in the diagnosis of appendicitis. *Acta Radiol.* Apr 2007;*48(3)*:267–273.

25. Patel SJ, Reede DL, Katz DS, et al. Imaging the pregnant patient for nonobstetric conditions: Algorithms and radiation dose considerations. *Radiographics.* 2007;*27(6)*: 1705–1722.

26. Parks NA, Schroeppel TJ. Update on imaging for acute appendicitis. *Surg Clin N Am.* 2011;*91*:141–154.

27. Choi D, Park H, Lee YR, Kook SH, Kim SK, Kwag HJ, Chung EC. The most useful findings for diagnosing acute appendicitis in contrast-enhanced helical CT. *Acta Radiol.* 2003;*44*:574–582.

28. Ganguli S, Raptopoulos V, Komlos F, Siewert B, Kruskal J. Right lower quadrant pain: Value of the non-visualized appendix in patients at multidetector CT. *Radiology.* 2006; *241(1)*:175–180.

29. Rao PM, Rhea JT, Novelline RA, et al. Effect of computed tomography of the appendix on treatment of patients and use of hospital resources. *N Engl J Med.* 1998;*338*:141–146.

30. Rao PM, Rhea JT, Rattner DW, et al. Introduction of appendiceal CT: Impact on negative appendectomy and appendiceal perforation rates. *Ann Surg.* 1999;*229*:339–344.

31. Patrick DA, Janik JE, Janik JS Bensard DD, Karrer FM. Increased CT scan utilization does not improve the diagnostic accuracy of appendicitis in children. *J Pediatr Surg.* 2003;*38*:659–662.

32. Coursey CA, Nelson RC, Patel MB, et al. Making the diagnosis of acute appendicitis: Do more preoperative scans mean fewer negative appendectomies? A 10-year study. *Radiology.* 2010;*254(2)*:460–468.

33. Guiliano V, Guiliano C, Pinto F, et al. CT method for visualization of the appendix using fixed oral dosage of diatrizoate clinical experience in 525 cases. *Emerg Radiol.* 2005; *190*:1300–1306.

34. Van Randen A, Bipat S, Zwindermann AH, Ubbink DT, Stoker J, Boermeester MA. Acute appendicitis: Meta-analysis of diagnostic performance of CT and graded compression US related to prevalence of the disease. *Radiology.* 2008. Aug 5 Epub ahead of print.

35. Morris KT, Kavanagh M, Hansen P, Whiteford MH, Deveney K, Standage B. The rational use of computed tomography scans in the diagnosis of appendicitis. *Am J Surg.* 2002;*183*:547–550.

36. McKay R, Shepherd J. The use of the clinical scoring system by Alvardo in the decision to perform computed tomography for acute appendicitis in the ED. *Am J Emerg Med.* 2007;*25*:489–493.

37. Alvarado A. A practical score for early diagnosis of acute appendicitis. *Ann Emerg Med.* 1986;*15*:557–565.

38. Hong JJ, Cohn SM, Ekeh AP, et al. A prospective randomized study of clinical assessment versus computed tomography for the diagnosis of acute appendicitis. *Surg Infect (Larchmt).* 2003;*3*:231–239.

39. Lopez PP, Cohn SM, Popkin CA, et al. The use of computed tomography scan to rule out appendicitis in women of childbearing age is as accurate as clinical exam: A prospective randomized trial. *Am Surg.* 2007;*73*:1232–1236.

40. Martin AE, Vollman D, Adler B, Caniano DA. CT scans may not reduce the negative appendectomy rate in children. *J Pediatr Surg.* 2004;*39*:886–890.

41. Singh A, Danrad R, Hahn PF, et al. MR imaging of the acute abdomen and pelvis: Acute appendicitis and beyond. *Radiographics.* 2007;*27*:1419–1431.

42. Cobben L, Groot I, Kingma L, et al. A simple MRI protocol in patients with clinically suspected appendicitis: Results in 138 patients and effect on the outcome of appendectomy. *Eur Radiol.* 2009;*19*:1175–1183.

43. Tkacz JN, Anderson SA, Soto J. MR imaging in gastrointestinal emergencies. *Radiographics.* 2009;*29*:1767–1780.

44. Beddy P, Keogan MT, Sala E, Griffin N. Magnetic resonance imaging for the evaluation of acute abdominal pain in pregnancy. *Semin Ultrasound CT MR.* 2010;*31*: 433–441.

45. Leeuwenburgh MM, Lameris W, van Randen A et al. Optimizing imaging in suspected appendicitis (OPTIMAP-Study): A multicenter diagnostic accuracy study of MRI in patients with suspected acute appendicitis. *Study protocol BMC Emerg Med.* 2010;*20*:10–19.

46. Altmeier WA. The bacterial flora of acute perforated appendicitis with peritonitis. A bacteriological study based upon a hundred cases. *Ann Surg.* 1938;*107*:517–528.

47. Bennion RS, Thompson JE, Jr., Baron EJ, Finegold SM. Gangrenous and perforated appendicitis with peritonitis: Treatment and bacteriology. *Clin Ther.* 1990;*12(Suppl C)*:31–44.

48. Gorbach SL. Antimicrobial prophylaxis for appendectomy and colorectal surgery. *Rev Infect Dis.* Sept-Oct 1991; *13(Suppl 10)*:15–20.

49. Mui LM, Ng CS, Wong SK, et al. Optimum duration of prophylactic antibiotics in acute non-perforated appendicitis. *ANZ J Surg.* Jun 2005;*75(6)*:425–428.

50. Le D, Rusin W, Hill B, Langell J. Post-operative antibiotic use in non-perforated appendicitis. *Am J Surg.* Dec 2009; *198(6)*:748–752.

51. Andersen BR, Kallehave FL, Andersen HK. Antibiotics versus placebo for prevention of postoperative infection after appendectomy. *Cochrane Database Syst Rev.* 2005;*2005(3)*: CD001439.

52. Hughes MJ, Ewen H, Simon P-B. Post-operative antibiotics after appendectomy and post-operative abscess development: A retrospective analysis. *Surg Infect.* 2013;*14(1)*: 56–61.

53. Van Rossem CC, Schreinemacher MHF, Van Geloven AAW, Bemelman WA. Antibiotic duration after laparoscopic appendectomy for acute complicated appendicitis. *JAMA Surg.* 2016;151(4):323. doi:10.1001/jamasurg.2015.4236.

54. Sawyer RG, Claridge JA, Nathens AB, et al. Trial of short-course antimicrobial therapy for intraabdominal infection. *N Engl J Med.* 2015;372(21):1996–2005. doi:10.1056/nejmoa1411162.

55. Fraser JD, Aguayo P, Leys CM, et al. A complete course of intravenous antibiotics vs a combination of intravenous and oral antibiotics for perforated appendicitis in children: A prospective, randomized trial. *J Ped Surg.* Jun 2010; *45(6)*:1198–1202.

56. McBurney C. The incision made in the abdominal wall in cases of appendicitis, with a description of a new method of operating. *Ann Surg.* 1894;*20*:38.

57. Semm K. Endoscopic appendectomy. *Endoscopy.* 1983; *15*:59–64.

58. Street D, Bodai BI, Owens LJ, et al. Simple ligation vs. stump ligation in appendectomy. *Arch Surg.* 1988;*123*:689.

59. Cohn SM, Giannotti G, Ong AW, et al. Prospective randomized trial of two wound management strategies for dirty abdominal wounds. *Ann Surg.* 2001;*233*:409–413.

60. Greenall MJ, Evans M, Pollack AV. Should you drain a perforated appendix? *Br J Surg.* 1978;*65*:880.

61. Hellberg A, Rudberg C, Kullman E, et al. Prospective randomized multicenter study of laparoscopic versus open appendectomy. *Br J Surg.* 1999;*86*:48–53.

62. Sauerland S, Lefering R, Holthausen U, et al. 1998. A meta-analysis of studies comparing laparoscopic with conventional appendectomy. In: Krahenbuhl L, Frei E, Klaiber Ch, et al., eds., *Acute Appendicitis: Standard Treatment or Laparoscopic Surgery?* Karger: Basel, Germany, pp. 109–114.

63. Golub R, Siddiqui F, Pohl D. Laparoscopic versus open appendectomy: A meta-analysis. *J Am Coll Surg.* 1998;*186*: 545–553.

64. Paterson HM, Qadan M, de Luca SM, et al. Changing trends in surgery for acute appendicitis. *Br J Surg.* 2008; *95*:363–368.

65. Milne AA, Bradbury AW. "Residual" appendicitis following incomplete laparoscopic appendicectomy. *Br J Surg.* 1996;*83*:

66. Jaschinski T, Mosch CG, Eikermann M, Neugebauer EA, Sauerland S. Laparoscopic versus open surgery for suspected appendicitis. *Cochrane Database Syst Rev.* 2018;*2018*(11). doi:10.1002/14651858.cd001546.pub4.

67. Gaitán HG, Ludovic R, Cindy F. Laparoscopy for the management of acute lower abdominal pain in women of childbearing age. *Cochrane Database Syst Rev.* 2011;*1*.

68. Mutter D, Vix M, Bui A, et al. Laparoscopy not recommended for routine appendectomy in men: Results of a prospective randomized study. *Surgery.* 1996;*120(1)*:71–74.

69. Corneille MG, Steigelman MB, Myers JG, et al. Laparoscopic appendectomy is superior to open appendectomy in obese patients. *Am J Surg.* 2007;*194(6)*:877–881.

70. Mason RJ, Moazzez A, Moroney JR, Katkhouda N. Laparoscopic vs open appendectomy in obese patients: Outcomes using the American College of Surgeons National Surgical Quality Improvement Program database. *J Am Coll Surg.* 2012;*215*:88–99; discussion 99–100.

71. Storm-Dickerson TL, Horattas MC. What have we learned over the past 20 years about appendicitis in the elderly? *Am J Surg.* 2003;*185(3)*:198–201.

72. Kraemer M, Franke C, Ohmann C, Yang Q. Acute Abdominal Pain Study Group. Acute appendicitis in late adulthood: Incidence, presentation, and outcome: Results of a prospective multicenter acute abdominal pain study and a review of the literature. *Langenbecks Arch Surg.* 2000;*385(7)*:470–481.

73. Southgate E, Vousden N, Karthikesalingam A, Markar SR, Black S, Zaidi A. Laparoscopic vs open appendectomy in older patients. *Arch Surg.* 2012;*147*:557–562.

74. Masoomi H, Mills S, Dolich MO, Ketana N, Carmichael JC, Nguyen NT, Stamos MJ. Does laparoscopic appendectomy impart an advantage over open appendectomy in elderly patients? *World J Surg.* 2012;*36*:1534–1539.

75. Nitecki S, Assalia A, Schein M. Contemporary management of Appendiceal mass. *Br J Surg.* 1993;*30*:18.

76. Andersson RE, Petzhold MG. Nonsurgical treatment of appendiceal abscess or phlegmon: A systematic review and meta-analysis. *Ann Surg.* 2007;*246*:741–748.

77. Roach JP, Patrick DA, Bruny JL, Allshouse MJ, Karrer FM, Ziegler MM. Complicated appendicitis in children: A clear role for drainage and delayed appendectomy. *Am J Surg.* 2007;*194*:769–772.

78. Owen A, Moore O, Marven S, Roberts J. Interval laparoscopic appendectomy in children. *J Laparoendosc Adv Surg Tech A.* 2006;*16*:308–311.

79. St Peter SD, Aguayo P, Fraser JD, et al. Initial laparoscopic appendectomy versus initial nonoperative management and interval appendectomy for perforated appendicitis with abscess: A prospective, randomized trial. *J Pediatr Surg.* Jan 2010;*45(1)*:236–240.

80. Kaminski A, Liu IL, Appelbaum H, Lee SL, Haigh PI. Routine interval appendectomy is not justified after initial nonoperative treatment of acute appendicitis. *Arch Surg.* 2005;*140(9)*:897–901.

81. Paupong D, Lee SL, Haigh PI, Kaminski A, Lui IL, Applebaum H. Routine interval appendectomy in children is not indicated. *J Pediatr Surg.* 2007;*42(9)*:1500–1503.

82. Hall NJ, Jones CE, Eaton S, Stanton MP, Burge DM. Is interval appendicectomy justified after successful non-operative treatment of an appendix mass in children? A systematic review. *J Pediatr Surg.* 2011;*46(4)*:767–771. doi:10.1016/j.jpedsurg.2011.01.019.

83. Tekin A, Kurtoglu HC, Can I, Oztan S. Routine interval appendectomy is unnecessary after conservative treatment of appendiceal mass. *Colorectal Dis.* Jun 2008;*10(5)*: 465–468.

84. Lai HW, Loong CC, Chiu JH, et al. Interval appendectomy after conservative treatment of an appendiceal mass. *World J Surg.* Mar 2006;*30(3)*:352–357.

85. Stevens CT, de Vries JE. Interval appendectomy as indicated rather than as routine therapy: Fewer operations and shorter hospital stays. *Ned Tijdschr Geneeskd.* Mar 2007; *151(13)*:759–763.

86. Lai HW, Loong CC, Wu CW, Lui WY. Watchful waiting versus interval appendectomy for patients who recovered from acute appendicitis with tumor formation: A cost-effectiveness analysis. *J Chin Med Assoc.* Sep 2005;*68(9)*:431–434.

87. Andersson RE, Petzold MG. Nonsurgical treatment of appendiceal abscess or phlegmon: A systemic review and meta-analysis. *Ann Surg.* 2007;*246*:741–748.

88. Deakin DE, Ahmed I. Interval appendectomy after resolution of adult inflammatory appendix mass—Is it necessary? *Surgeon.* 2007;*5*:45–50.

89. Son J, Park YJ, Lee SR, et al. Increased risk of neoplasms in adult patients undergoing interval appendectomy. *Ann Coloproctol.* 2020;*36(5)*:311.

90. Mallinen J, Rautio T, Gronroos J, et al. Risk of appendiceal neoplasm in periappendicular abscess in patients treated with interval appendectomy vs follow-up with magnetic resonance imaging: 1-year outcomes of the peri-appendicitis acute randomized clinical trial. *JAMA Surg.* 2019;*154(3)*:200–207.

91. Eriksson S, Granstrom L. Randomized controlled trial of appendectomy versus antibiotic therapy for acute appendicitis. *Br J Surg.* 1995;*82*:166–169.

92. Salminen P, Paajanen H, Rautio T, et al. Antibiotic therapy vs appendectomy for treatment of uncomplicated acute appendicitis: The APPAC randomized clinical trial. *JAMA.* Jun 16, 2015;*313(23)*:2340–2348.

93. CODA Collaborative; Flum DR, Davidson GH, Monsell SE, et al. A randomized trial comparing antibiotics with appendectomy for appendicitis. *N Engl J Med.* Nov 12, 2020;*383(20)*:1907–1919.

94. O'Leary DP, Walsh SM, Bolger J, et al. A randomized clinical trial evaluating the efficacy and quality of life of antibiotic-only treatment of acute uncomplicated appendicitis: Results of the COMMA Trail. *Ann Surg.* Aug 1, 2021;*274(2)*:240–247.

95. De Almeida Leite RM, Seo DJ, Gomez-Eslava B, et al. Nonoperative vs operative management of uncomplicated acute appendicitis. *JAMA Surg.* 2022;*157(9)*:828. doi:10.1001/jamasurg.2022.2937.

43

Diverticular Disease of the Colon

Akpofure Peter Ekeh and Mary Stuever

43.1 Introduction

Diverticular disease of the colon is a common condition, predominant in Western societies, that generates a significant socioeconomic burden. The prevalence of diverticulosis is age-related in Western societies, affecting only 5% of individuals less than 40 years of age, but involving two-thirds of adults over the age of 65 [1]. Recent U.S. population-based studies reveal that diverticular disease is the sixth most frequent outpatient gastrointestinal diagnosis, with 2.6 million emergency department visits annually. It represents the most common inpatient gastrointestinal diagnosis with 283,355 yearly hospitalizations for 2.7 billion dollars [2]. Acute diverticulitis is the most frequent complication arising from the presence of colonic diverticula. The incidence of diverticulitis in patients with diverticulosis has historically ranged from 10% to 25% with the sigmoid colon being affected in 95% of cases. Acute diverticulitis is classified into uncomplicated and complicated diseases. Patients with the uncomplicated disease typically present with abdominal pain, fever, nausea, and vomiting. These cases are routinely managed nonoperatively, often in the outpatient setting, with bowel rest and antibiotics. Most patients recover without further episodes. Approximately one-third of patients treated for acute diverticulitis will experience a second attack, and a third attack will occur in roughly another third of this population. A 2013 study by Shahedi et al. at the Los Angeles Veterans Healthcare System that followed over 2,000 patients with diverticulosis over 11 years determined that only a small proportion of individuals with diverticulosis went on to develop acute diverticulitis—4% in this series.

Complicated diverticulitis refers to cases in which patients present with an abscess, perforation, stricture, fistula formation, or sepsis. Approximately 22% of patients admitted for diverticulitis will undergo surgery for the management of their complicated disease [3].

The methods of management of diverticulitis in both acute and elective settings have evolved over the last few decades. Several of the commonly accepted standards and guidelines have required revision as larger studies, randomized trials, and the increasing use of laparoscopic surgery are changing the landscape.

We will review the existing evidence in the literature regarding the management of colonic diverticular disease, including indications for elective operative management, the role of the patient's age in operative decision-making, optimal operative management in the acute setting, the role of laparoscopy in the acute setting, and the prevention of recurrent attacks.

43.2 What Is the Appropriate Indication for Elective Sigmoid Resection after Uncomplicated Diverticulitis?

Surgical intervention in complicated diverticulitis (abscess, perforation, peritonitis, fistula, or obstruction) remains the mainstay for treatment in most of these situations. Controversy exists in determining the most appropriate indications for surgery after uncomplicated acute diverticulitis. Both the American Society of Colon and Rectal Surgeons (ASCRS) and the European Association for Endoscopic Surgery in the 1990s, based on available literature at the time, recommended elective colon resection for patients who had two or more attacks of uncomplicated diverticulitis, and even sooner in younger patients (<50 years) after a single attack [4, 5]. This strategy, which reflected prevailing clinical practice patterns at the time, was predicated on the assumption that diverticular disease is a progressive process, with worsening symptoms with increasing numbers of attacks. It was also believed that subsequent diverticulitis episodes would be more "virulent" in younger patients. Over time, studies have, however, revealed that most patients admitted with acute diverticulitis respond positively to nonoperative treatment. Recurrence rates have been noted to be 13–33% with low rates of complicated diseases that need surgical intervention [6]. Additionally, complications presented more often in patients who had just one or two attacks, and patients with more than two episodes were not at increased risk for poorer outcomes, nor did they more often require emergent surgery. While the incidence of diverticulitis is increasing in younger patients, the risk of requiring surgery has remained similar between older and younger patients, 22% and 24%, respectively. Broderick et al. reported that in a subset of 2,551 patients treated with nonoperative management, over 8.9 years, 2,366 (92.7%) did not require a colectomy [7].

The discussion of surgical indications in diverticular disease has evolved from hard recommendations to a more individualized patient-specific approach. The 2014 and 2020 ASCRS guidelines recommend elective surgery on an individualized, case-by-case basis. This will involve evaluating patients for modifiable risk factors, quality-of-life scores, minimizing costs, and appropriate risk stratification associated with recurrent diverticulitis compared with inherent risks of surgical morbidity and mortality. Elective resection offers the advantage to the surgeon and patient of a time to optimize for surgery and any modifiable risk factors.

DOI: 10.1201/9781003316800-43

Immunosuppressed patients with diverticular disease deserve special mention. Older data suggested this population to be more prone to morbidity if not operated on early. This led to the previous ASCRS recommendations indicating a low threshold for proceeding with elective surgery after uncomplicated diverticulitis episodes. More recent studies have demonstrated that even in this population, the decision to offer colectomy after recovery from uncomplicated acute diverticulitis can similarly be individualized. Al-Khamis et al., using data from the National Surgical Quality Improvement Program (NSQIP), noted that immunosuppressed and immunocompetent patients who underwent elective sigmoid colectomy had similar mortality rates although worse morbidity and wound dehiscence rates [8]. Biondo et al., following patients medically managed after acute diverticulitis for almost 7 years, showed a comparable recurrence rate in immunosuppressed and immunocompetent patients (21.5% vs. 20.5%; $p = 0.82$) as well as similar rates of requiring emergency surgery after recurrent attacks [9].

While there has been a move away from mandatory operations after just a few episodes of diverticulitis, some prospective trials have highlighted the quality-of-life advantages that patients who undergo elective surgery have in the case of multiple recurrences. The DIRECT trial was a multicenter randomized controlled study that followed patients with recurrent diverticulitis or chronic abdominal symptoms attributed to diverticular disease. The study compared 53 patients who underwent sigmoidectomy with 56 patients who were nonoperatively managed. The gastrointestinal quality-of-life index (GIQLI) was used as a primary endpoint. The operative resection group had significantly better scores at 6 months [10]. These better scores persisted in a 5-year follow-up where the surgical resection cohort had improved pain scores, mental well-being, and SF-36 physical scores. Of note, however, in the operatively treated patients, 11% of patients had anastomotic leakage, and reinterventions were required in 15% [11]. This trade-off further supports the need for individualized consideration with the patient being part of the decision-making process (Table 43.1).

> **RECOMMENDATION**
>
> The decision to proceed with elective sigmoid resection after uncomplicated diverticulitis should be individualized. Factors such as immune status, modifiable patient risk factors, and patient lifestyle choices should be considered.
>
> Level of evidence: 2. Grade of recommendation: B.

43.3 Should Younger Patients (<50 Years) Undergo Elective Sigmoid Colon Resection after a Single Attack of Diverticulitis?

Patients younger than 50 years of age may present with attacks of acute diverticulitis, ranging from uncomplicated to more complicated. Previous clinical practice and expert guidelines advocated for elective sigmoid colectomy after a single attack of uncomplicated diverticulitis in patients less than 40 years of

age. This recommendation was based on multiple case series and retrospective studies demonstrating more recurrences and subsequent virulent presentations in younger patients [12, 13].

Contemporary practice has abandoned this former trend of "early" surgical management based on newer data. More recent studies confirm that younger patients tend to have a higher recurrence rate of acute diverticulitis following initial episodes. These recurrences are, however, not necessarily more complicated, nor do they result in worse outcomes than those in older patients. Furthermore, younger patients were shown to have a higher rate of readmission although a similar risk of requiring emergency operations when compared to their older counterparts [14, 15]. In a metanalysis from the Netherlands in 2013 which included eight studies with over 20,000 patients, van de Wall et al. showed that younger patients (<50) had a higher incidence of recurrent diverticulitis [16]. The ASCRS updated guidelines (2020), based on available data, concluded on this subject that "elective resection based on a younger age at presentation is not recommended" [17].

> **RECOMMENDATION**
>
> There is no evidence that younger patients should be managed differently than older patients based on age alone.
>
> Level of evidence: 2A. Grade of recommendation: B. (Table 43.1)

43.4 Do Lifestyle Changes Such as Increased Fiber Intake, Increased Physical Activity, Weight Loss, Tobacco Cessation, and Reduced Red Meat Intake Reduce the Risk of Diverticulitis? Is the Practice of Prohibiting the Intake of Nuts, Seeds, Popcorn, etc., after an Acute Episode Valid?

After the first attack of acute diverticulitis, patients are often given advice centering on lifestyle and dietary modification aimed at reducing the likelihood of future attacks. Are these admonitions based on clear scientific evidence? Some of these are discussed next.

43.4.1 Fiber Intake

The progression of colonic diverticular disease has paralleled the drop in dietary fiber consumption in the United States, Europe, and Asia. Several studies have highlighted the benefits of fiber intake in the prevention and recurrence of diverticular disease. The original observations of the effect of fiber were published decades ago by Burkitt, based on his experiences in rural Eastern Africa. He compared colonic transit times and stool weight in three populations with low-, mixed-, and high-residue diets. Colonic transit time was decreased, and stool weight was increased in patients with high-residue diets. He further obtained epidemiological data from various countries, noting the very low prevalence of diverticular disease in populations with high-residue diets compared to those with low- and mixed-residue diets [18].

A prospective cohort study involving 47,033 people by Crowe et al. in 2011 demonstrated that higher fiber intake was a factor associated with a decreased risk of hospitalization for diverticular disease. This study had a mean follow-up time of 11.6 years [19]. An earlier prospective cohort study with a 4-year follow-up by Aldoori et al. evaluated the effect of various diets on the incidence of diverticular disease. Participants who consumed diets high in fruit and vegetable fiber had a significantly lower incidence of symptomatic diverticulitis. Diets high in fat and red meat were also noted to augment the risk [20]. Aldoori et al. also determined that the insoluble component of fiber was inversely associated with the risk of diverticular disease. This was particularly strong for cellulose [21]. These findings are consistent with a Greek study which showed that patients with diverticulitis had a lower intake of fiber and a higher intake of red meat [22]. All of this gives further credence to earlier studies from the 1970s that highlighted the beneficial role of fiber in diverticular disease [23, 24].

43.4.2 The Role of Other Dietary and Lifestyle Changes

The consumption of a high-fiber diet is often intricately linked to other healthy practices such as low red meat consumption. Two recent studies have highlighted the contrast in the development of diverticular disease between persons who consume a "Western-type diet"—typically replete with red meat, processed grains, and high-fat dairy as opposed to a healthier diet (high in fruits, vegetables, and whole grains. Strate et al. concluded that a Western dietary pattern increase, and a prudent dietary pattern decrease the risk and incidence of diverticulitis. Their study was a questionnaire-based prospective cohort study using data from the Health Professionals Follow-Up Study that tracked over 46,000 subjects over 4 years. Red meat and fiber were attributed to the highest associations with diverticulitis [25]. These findings were supported by a different study by Liu et al. in which they examined the association between a "low-risk lifestyle" and the risk of developing diverticulitis. A low-risk lifestyle was defined as an average red meat intake of <51 g per day, dietary fiber intake of about 23 g per day, vigorous physical activity (roughly 2 hours of exercise weekly), normal body mass index (BMI) between 18.5 and 24.9 kg m^{-2}, and never-smoker. There was an inverse linear relationship between several low-risk lifestyle factors and diverticulitis incidence [26] (Table 43.1).

43.4.3 The Role of Tobacco Cessation

As in several other disease processes, tobacco use has been shown to have deleterious associations with the onset and outcomes related to diverticular disease of the colon. Aune et al., in a large meta-analysis of several studies, concluded that smoking was associated with a higher relative risk for developing acute diverticulitis when compared with nonsmokers. Former smokers similarly had a heightened risk, though less than active ones. The meta-analysis also demonstrated a

higher risk of complications from diverticular disease (perforations or abscesses) in smokers [27].

43.4.4 Popcorn, Seeds, and Nuts

The advice given against the consumption of popcorn, seeds, and nuts in an attempt to prevent obstruction of colonic diverticula and prevent inflammation has no basis in the medical literature. Strate et al., in a prospective cohort study of male health professionals in 2008, demonstrated that dietary nuts, corn, and seeds were not associated with an increased risk of diverticulitis or diverticular bleeding [28].

RECOMMENDATIONS

Dietary fiber can play a role in both the prevention of initial and recurrent attacks of diverticulitis. Patients should be advised to increase the fiber content in their diet after a bout of uncomplicated diverticulitis. Additionally, healthy lifestyle choices such as lower red meat consumption, smoking cessation, and weight loss have associations with the initial incidence and subsequent attacks of diverticulitis.

Level of evidence: 2A. Grade of recommendation: A.

43.5 What Is the Optimal Operation for Patients Requiring Surgery for Acute Complicated Diverticulitis? Is Performing a Primary Anastomosis an Option?

Acute complicated diverticulitis is distinguished by the presence of abscess formation, free perforation, stricture, or the presence of fistulas. In his classic 1978 paper on the treatment of diverticulitis based on intraoperative findings, Hinchey described acute complicated diverticulitis in four stages, with worse clinical features and mortality with each successive stage. These were described as follows: Stage I, localized pericolic abscess; stage II, large mesenteric abscess; stage III, free perforation with purulent peritonitis; and stage IV, free perforation with feculent peritonitis [29]. This staging system has been widely adopted to provide a standard for comparison of the severity of the disease. In more recent years, with the increased utilization and improved quality of CT imaging, a modified Hinchey classification has been introduced [30].

The operative management of complicated acute diverticulitis has evolved. Historically, staged operations were commonly performed involving the initial closure of the perforation with a proximal diversion (ileostomy or transverse colostomy) with subsequently delayed resection of the diseased portion and anastomosis. This approach has been replaced by the Hartmann procedure (HP)—resection of the acutely inflamed bowel, including the perforated portion of the colon and a proximal end colostomy. Currently, about 25% of patients with acute diverticulitis require emergency intervention [31].

While HP has been the mainstay of management for patients with purulent and feculent peritonitis over the last few decades, recent studies have explored the use of colon resection with primary anastomosis (PA) with or without a diverting proximal ostomy and have demonstrated certain distinct advantages this approach confers.

Oberkoffer et al. conducted a multicenter randomized controlled trial comparing PA with diverting ileostomy to HP. This study, which had 62 patients divided equally into both groups, showed no differences in morbidity or mortality between both cohorts. The stoma reversal rate was higher after PA with ileostomy (90% vs. 58% $p = 0.005$). Serious complications (0% vs. 20%, $p = 0.046$), operating time (73 vs. 183 minutes, $p < 0.001$), hospital stay (6 vs. 9 days, $p = 0.016$), and in-hospital costs ($16,717 vs. $24,014) were reduced in the PA group. Total overall complications (80% HP vs. 84% PA) were similar, confirming that perforated Hinchey III and IV diverticulitis carries high morbidity regardless of the approach [32].

The DIVERTI trial, a French multicenter randomized controlled trial, was designed to compare PA with diverting ostomy to HP, with a primary endpoint of mortality rate at 18 months. Secondary outcomes were postoperative complications, operative time, length of stay, rate of definitive stoma, and morbidity. One hundred and two patients with Hinchey III or IV diverticulitis were randomized to the PA arm or HP arm. Overall mortality did not differ between HP and PA (7.7% vs. 4%) and morbidity was also comparable (39% HP vs. 44% PA). At 18 months, 96% of PA patients had stoma reversal versus 65% of the HP patients ($p = 0.0001$). This study was ended prematurely due to difficulties with patient enrollment [33].

The LADIES trial, a multicenter, multiarm, randomized controlled European trial, had one arm of the trial (DIVA) specifically designed to assess outcomes after HP versus sigmoidectomy with PA, with or without defunctioning ileostomy, for Hinchey III or IV diverticular disease. A total of 130 patients were randomly assigned to HP (66 patients) or PA (64 patients). The 12-month stoma-free survival was significantly better for the PA group compared with HP (94.6% vs. 71.7% $p < 0.0001$). There were no significant differences in short-term morbidity and mortality after the index procedure for HP with PA morbidity (44% vs. 39%; $p = 0.60$) or mortality (3% vs. 6%; $p = 0.44$). The authors concluded that in hemodynamically stable, immunocompetent patients younger than 85 years, PA is preferable to HP as a treatment for perforated diverticulitis [34]. These results continued to stand at a 3-year follow-up with two additional findings: More parastomal hernias in the HP group (HP 16% vs. PA 2%; $p = 0.009$) and fewer mean total in hospital days in the PA group (PA 14 days vs. HP 17 days, $p = 0.025$) [35].

RECOMMENDATIONS

Primary resection of the inflamed colon (with or without PA) is the optimal method of treating complicated sigmoid diverticulitis. PA with or without a diverting ostomy should be considered in immunocompetent patients, as it has comparable morbidity and mortality and is associated with a higher rate of stoma reversal and fewer postoperative stomal site hernias.

Level of evidence: 1B. Grade of recommendation: A.

43.6 Is There a Role for Laparoscopic Lavage in Acute Complicated Diverticulitis?

Since originally described in 1996, laparoscopic lavage (LL) has been touted as a potential alternative to acute sigmoid resection, especially in patients with purulent diverticulitis (Hinchey III). Three randomized controlled trials have been performed to date addressing the role of LL in acute complicated diverticulitis. These three studies, all arising in Europe, were DILALA (Diverticulitis – Laparoscopic Lavage versus resection), SCANDIV, and the aforementioned LADIES trials [36–38]. Each of these studies utilized different protocols and endpoints, making it difficult to directly compare results.

The DILALA trial was a prospective, randomized controlled trial of LL versus HP after diagnostic laparoscopy for Hinchey staging. In this study, 39 patients were randomized to LL and 36 to HP. No difference was found in morbidity, mortality, reoperation, or further intervention. The authors concluded that LL was a viable alternative for this group of patients. Their results held after a 2-year follow-up [36].

The LADIES trial was a large multicenter randomized trial that set up two arms after diagnostic laparoscopy was performed and a diagnosis of purulent peritonitis was established. One of the objectives of this study was to determine whether LL and drainage are safe and effective treatments for patients with purulent peritonitis. In the arm of interest to this discussion, patients were randomized into LL or surgical resection. The trial was ended prematurely due to a higher complication rate in the LL arm found on interim analysis. (39% vs. 19%). Additionally, over 10% of patients in the LL arm required surgical reintervention for feculent peritonitis, raising concerns for possible misdiagnosis. They concluded that LL is not superior to sigmoidectomy for the treatment of purulent perforated diverticulitis in terms of major morbidity and mortality at 12 months. Although the acute reintervention rate was higher after lavage, in more than three-quarters of these patients, the sepsis was controlled [37].

The Scandinavian Diverticulitis (SCANDIV) trial was performed in Sweden and Norway, an open-labeled randomized, clinical study. This study aimed to compare outcomes in patients who underwent either LL or resection. After 1 year, there was no difference in mortality or serious complications in both groups. However, LL was associated with more deep surgical site infections (32% vs. 13%; $P = 0.006$) but fewer superficial surgical site infections (1% vs. 17%; $P = 0.001$). More patients in the lavage group underwent unplanned reoperations (27% vs. 10%; $P = 0.010$. They concluded that the advantages of LL should be weighed against the risk of secondary intervention (if sepsis is unresolved) [38]. The results held consistent after 5 years, where a follow-up analysis concluded that "recurrence of diverticulitis after laparoscopic lavage was more common, often leading to sigmoid resection." The authors indicated that this must be considered against the lower stoma prevalence in this LL group and highlighted the importance of shared decision-making between surgeons and their patients [39].

Penna et al., in a meta-analysis incorporating all three studies and including four others with a total of 589 patients, concluded that the preservation of diseased bowel by LL is associated with approximately a three times greater risk of persistent peritonitis, intraabdominal abscesses, and the need for emergency surgery compared with resection [40].

RECOMMENDATIONS

LL in acute complicated diverticulitis has an equivalent complication profile to surgical resection but is associated with more unplanned reoperations, intraabdominal abscesses, and the need for reinterventions. For these reasons, it should not be routinely utilized.

Level of evidence: 1B. Grade of recommendation: A. (Table 43.1)

43.7 Are Minimally Invasive Approaches for Colectomy for Diverticular Disease Preferred to Open Operations? What Place Do Robotic Approaches Have in Elective Colon Operations for Diverticular Disease?

From a historical perspective, a clear role for a laparoscopic approach in the management of colon cancer was established by a multi-institutional randomized prospective trial demonstrating noninferiority in recurrence rates as well as a shorter length of stay and less use of parenteral narcotics in the laparoscopic group by the COST trial [41]. These findings were appropriately extrapolated to laparoscopic surgery for diverticular disease. Further establishing the benefits of laparoscopic surgery in the management of complicated diverticulitis, the SIGMA trial compared laparoscopic with open colon resection. This study demonstrated that laparoscopic resections had less intraoperative blood loss, less postoperative pain, shorter length of stay, fewer major complications at 30 days (9.6% vs. 25.0%; $P = 0.038$), and better postoperative quality of life on SF-36 questionnaires [42]. These findings held in a 6-month follow-up of the same population [43]. Further studies through the years have echoed distinct advantages of the minimally invasive approach for elective sigmoid colectomy for diverticular disease, including decreased length of stay, quicker return to diet, quicker postoperative recovery, and earlier return to baseline activities [44–46]. Keller et al., reviewing the Premier Prospective Database for colorectal surgery for the year 2013, concluded that compared with open surgery, laparoscopic colorectal surgery was associated with significantly shorter length of stay (mean 5.78 vs. 7.80 days, $p < 0.0001$), lower readmission rates (5.82 vs. 7.68%, $p < 0.0001$), fewer complications (32.60 vs. 42.28%, $p < 0.0001$), and lower mortality rates (0.52 vs. 1.28%,

$p < 0.0001$). Additionally, the overall cost was significantly lower in laparoscopic than in open procedures (mean \$17,269 vs. \$20,552, $p < 0.0001$) [47]. A recent randomized prospective study from Finland by Santos et al. comparing outcomes of patients who underwent laparoscopic sigmoid colectomy for diverticular disease with those who underwent observation alone showed an improved quality of life in patients with recurrent, complicated, or persistent painful diverticulitis; however, this was accompanied by a 10% risk of major complications [48].

All of this has contributed to the recent recommendation by the ASCRS stating that "when expertise is available, a minimally invasive approach to colectomy for diverticulitis is preferred."[17]

No discussion of minimally invasive surgery for diverticular disease of the colon is complete without mentioning the role of robotic surgery. Robotic approaches have gained increasing popularity over the last decade for a variety of abdominal procedures, including colonic surgery. There is a paucity of randomized prospective data comparing the traditional laparoscopic to the robotic approaches. Several individual studies and recent meta-analysis have, however, uniformly come to similar conclusions. Robotic surgery is associated with a lower risk of conversion to open surgery and a shorter hospital stay. It is associated with higher operative costs and longer operative time, however. In a meta-nalysis of nine studies with over 4,000 patients, Giuliani et al. showed that patients undergoing robotic-assisted colectomy for diverticular disease had a significantly lower rate of conversion into an open procedure (7.4% vs. 12.5%, $p < 0.00001$), a shorter hospital stay ($p < 0.0001$), and longer operating time ($p < 0.00001$) [49]. A similar meta-analysis by Solaini et al., which included all left-sided colectomies for benign and malignant disease, came to similar conclusions. Reviewing 11 articles with over 52,000 patients, they similarly found robotic surgery was associated with a lower rate of conversion to open surgery (risk ratio [RR] 0.5, 0.5–0.6; $p < 0.001$) and longer operative times ($p = 0.002$). Overall complications (RR 0.9, 0.8–0.9, $p < 0.001$), anastomotic leaks (RR 0.7, 0.7–0.8; $p < 0.001$), and superficial wound infection (RR 3.1, 2.8–3.4; $p < 0.001$) were less common in the robotic group [50].

RECOMMENDATION

Laparoscopic colon resection is a safe and effective approach for the elective treatment of patients with diverticular disease, demonstrating no increased morbidity and a shorter hospital stay, quicker resumption of bowel function, and reduced blood loss and should be the preferred approach if the expertise is available. Robotic-assisted colectomy for diverticular disease is associated with longer operations and increased operative costs but a lower conversion rate to open surgery and shorter length of hospital stay.

Level of evidence: 2B. Grade of recommendation: B. (Table 43.1)

TABLE 43.1

Clinical Questions

Question	Answer	Grade of Recommendation	References
What is the appropriate indication for elective sigmoid resection after uncomplicated diverticulitis?	The decision to proceed with elective sigmoid resection after uncomplicated diverticulitis should be individualized.	C	[8–11]
Should younger patients (<40–50 years) undergo elective sigmoid colon resection after a single attack of acute diverticulitis?	As with the rest of this population, individualized decisions based on the patient's circumstance will need to be made before proceeding with surgery. There is no evidence that younger patients should be managed differently than older patients based on age alone.	C	[14–16]
Do lifestyle changes (increased fiber intake, increased physical activity, weight loss, tobacco cessation, and reduced red meat intake) reduce the risk of diverticulitis?	Dietary fiber can help prevent initial and recurrent attacks of diverticulitis. Healthy lifestyle choices (lower red meat consumption, smoking cessation, and weight loss) have associations with the initial incidence and subsequent attacks of diverticulitis.	B	[19–27]
Is the practice of prohibiting the intake of nuts, seeds, popcorn, etc., after an acute episode valid?	There is no basis for prohibiting these items to aid in the prevention of diverticulitis.	B	[28]
What is the optimal operation for patients requiring surgery for acute complicated diverticulitis?	Primary resection of the inflamed colon (with or without primary anastomosis) is the optimal treatment for complicated sigmoid diverticulitis.	A	[31–35]
Is performing a primary anastomosis an option?	Primary anastomosis with or without a diverting ostomy should be considered in immunocompetent patients.		
Is there a role for laparoscopic lavage or laparoscopic resection in the emergent setting?	Laparoscopic lavage in acute complicated diverticulitis has an equivalent complication profile to surgical resection but is associated with more unplanned reoperations, intraabdominal abscesses, and the need for reinterventions.	A	[36–40]
Are minimally invasive approaches for colectomy for diverticular disease preferred to open operations?	Laparoscopic colon resection is a safe and effective approach for the elective treatment of diverticular disease, with a shorter hospital stay, quicker resumption of bowel function, and reduced blood loss. It should be the preferred approach if the expertise is available.	B	[41–48]
What place do robotic approaches have in elective colon operations for diverticular disease?	Robotic-assisted colectomy is associated with longer operations and increased operative costs, but shorter hospital length of stay and a lower conversion rate to open surgery.	C	[49, 50]

TABLE 43.2

Levels of Evidence

Subject	Year	Reference	Level of Evidence	Strength of Recommendation	Findings
Indication for elective colectomy after uncomplicated diverticulitis	2017	[10]	II	B	Medical management of recurrent is appropriate; however, GI quality of life index (GIQLI) scores are improved in patients who had operative resection.
Elective colectomy in younger patients	2013	[15]	IIb	B	Age is not associated with more severe disease, although there is a higher incidence of recurrence.
Dietary fiber intake and risk of diverticulitis	2017	[25]	IIb	B	Diets high in fiber and healthy lifestyle choices are associated with a lower incidence of symptomatic diverticulitis.
PA for sigmoid diverticulitis	2022	[35]	II	A	Primary resection and anastomosis (with/without diverting ostomy) have equivalent morbidity and mortality to Hartmann procedure and a higher stoma reversal rate.
Laparoscopic lavage for acute complicated diverticulitis	2021	[39]	I	A	Laparoscopic lavage is associated with a three times greater risk of persistent peritonitis, intraabdominal abscesses, and the need for emergency surgery compared with resection.

Editor's Note

There is a considerable amount of quality scientific evidence to support our current care of diverticulitis. The treatment of uncomplicated diverticulitis rarely involves colonic resection today, irrespective of the patient's age, medical condition, immunologic status, or number of episodes.

A diet high in fiber can reduce the likelihood of developing diverticulitis or having a recurrent episode. (I have found this to be most easily achievable by having patients add two heaping tablespoons of Metamucil to their daily regimen.)

For acute perforated diverticulitis, the Hartman procedure should be avoided whenever possible and primary anastomosis, with or without fecal diversion, be performed. This has been clearly shown to minimize patient morbidity. Laparoscopic lavage should generally be avoided in acute complicated diverticulitis, as the results are inferior to colonic resection.

For elective resection of sigmoid diverticulitis, a minimally invasive approach appears safe and may lower morbidity.

These comments are based on multiple randomized clinical trials and are therefore grade A or B recommendations.

REFERENCES

1. Parks TG. Natural history of diverticular disease of the colon. Clin Gastroenterol. 1975; 4:53–69.
2. Peery AF, Sandler RS. Diverticular disease: Reconsidering conventional wisdom. Clin Gastroenterol Hepatol. 2013; 11:1532–1537.
3. Morris AM, Regenbogen SE, Hardiman KM, Hendren S. Sigmoid diverticulitis: A systematic review. JAMA. 2014; 311:287–297. Review.
4. Roberts P, Abel M, Rosen L, Cirocco W, Fleshman J, Leff E, Levien D, Pritchard T, Wexner S, Hicks T, et al. Practice parameters for sigmoid diverticulitis. The Standards Task Force American Society of Colon and Rectal Surgeons. Dis Colon Rectum. 1995; 38:125–132.
5. Köhler L, Sauerland S, Neugebauer E. Diagnosis and treatment of diverticular disease: Results of a consensus development conference. The Scientific Committee of the European Association for Endoscopic Surgery. Surg Endosc. 1999; 13:430–436.
6. Hall JF, Roberts PL, Ricciardi R, Read T, Scheirey C, Wald C, Marcello PW, Schoetz DJ. Long-term follow-up after an initial episode of diverticulitis: What are the predictors of recurrence? Dis Colon Rectum. 2011; 54:283–288.
7. Broderick-Villa G, Burchette RJ, Collins JC, Abbas MA, Haigh PI. Hospitalization for acute diverticulitis does not mandate routine elective colectomy. Arch Surg. 2005 Jun; 140(6):576–581.
8. Al-Khamis A, Abou Khalil J, Demian M, Morin N, Vasilevsky CA, Gordon PH, Boutros M. Sigmoid colectomy for acute diverticulitis in immunosuppressed vs immunocompetent patients: Outcomes from the ACS-NSQIP database. Dis Colon Rectum. 2016 Feb; 59(2):101–109.
9. Biondo S, Borao JL, Kreisler E, Golda T, Millan M, Frago R, Fraccalvieri D, Guardiola J, Jaurrieta E. Recurrence and virulence of colonic diverticulitis in immunocompromised patients. Am J Surg. 2012; 204:172–179.
10. van de Wall BJM, Stam MAW, Draaisma WA, et al. Surgery versus conservative management for recurrent and ongoing left-sided diverticulitis (DIRECT trial): An open-label, multicentre, randomised controlled trial. Lancet Gastroenterol Hepatol. 2017; 2(1):13–22.
11. Bolkenstein HE, Consten, ECJ, van der Palen J, van de Wall BJM, Broeders Ivo AMJ, Bemelman WA, Lange JF, Boermeester MA, Draaisma WA. Dutch Diverticular Disease (3D) Collaborative Study Group. Long-term outcome of surgery versus conservative management for recurrent and ongoing complaints after an episode of diverticulitis: 5-year follow-up results of a multicenter randomized controlled trial (DIRECT-Trial). Ann Surg. 2019; 269: 612–620.
12. Cunningham MA, Davis JW, Kaups KL. Medical versus surgical management of diverticulitis in patients under age 40. Am J Surg. 1997; 174:733–735.
13. Minardi AJ, Jr., Johnson LW, Sehon JK, Zibari GB, McDonald JC. Diverticulitis in the young patient. Am Surg. 2001; 67:458–461.
14. Li D, de Mestral C, Baxter NN, et al. Risk of readmission and emergency surgery following nonoperative management of colonic diverticulitis: A population-based analysis. Ann Surg. 2014; 260:423–430.
15. Katz LH, Guy DD, Lahat A, Gafter-Gvili A, Bar-Meir S. Diverticulitis in the young is not more aggressive than in the elderly, but it tends to recur more often: Systematic review and meta-analysis. J Gastroenterol Hepatol. 2013; 28:1274–1281.
16. van de Wall BJ, Poerink JA, Draaisma WA, Reitsma JB, Consten EC, Broeders IA. Diverticulitis in young versus elderly patients: A meta-analysis. Scand J Gastroenterol. 2013; 48:643–651.
17. Hall J, Hardiman K, Lee S, Lightner A, Stocchi L, Paquette IM, Steele SR, Feingold DL; Prepared on Behalf of the Clinical Practice Guidelines Committee of the American Society of Colon and Rectal Surgeons. The American society of colon and rectal surgeons clinical practice guidelines for the treatment of left-sided colonic diverticulitis. Dis Colon Rectum. 2020; 63:728–747.
18. Burkitt DP, Walker AR, Painter NS. Effect of dietary fibre on stools and the transit-times, and its role in the causation of disease. Lancet. 1972; 7792:1408–1412.
19. Crowe FL, Appleby PN, Allen NE, Key TJ. Diet and risk of diverticular disease in Oxford cohort of European Prospective Investigation into Cancer and Nutrition (EPIC): Prospective study of British vegetarians and non-vegetarians. BMJ. 2011 Jul 19; 343:d4131.
20. Aldoori WH, Giovannucci EL, Rimm EB, Wing AL, Trichopoulos DV, Willett WC. A prospective study of diet and the risk of symptomatic diverticular disease in men. Am J Clin Nutr. 1994; 60:757–764.
21. Aldoori WH, Giovannucci EL, Rockett HR, Sampson L, Rimm EB, Willett WC. A prospective study of dietary fiber types and symptomatic diverticular disease in men. J Nutr. 1998; 128:714–719.
22. Manousos O, Day NE, Tone A, Papadimitriou C, Kapetanakis A, Polychronopoulou-Trichopoulou A, Trichopoulos D. Diet and other factors in the aetiology of diverticulosis: An epidemiological study in Greece. Gut. 1985; 26:544–549.

23. Brodribb AJ. Treatment of symptomatic diverticular disease with a high-fiber diet. Lancet. 1977; 1:664–666.
24. Taylor I, Duthie HL. Bran tablets and diverticular disease. Br Med J. 1976; 24:988–990.
25. Strate LL, Keeley BR, Cao Y, Wu K, Giovannucci EL, Chan AT. Western dietary pattern increases, and prudent dietary pattern decreases, risk of incident diverticulitis in a prospective cohort study. Gastroenterology. 2017; 152:1023–1030.e2.
26. Liu PH, Cao Y, Keeley BR, Tam I, Wu K, Strate LL, Giovannucci EL, Chan AT. Adherence to a healthy lifestyle is associated with a lower risk of diverticulitis among men. Am J Gastroenterol. 2017 Dec; 112(12):1868–1876.
27. Aune D, Sen A, Leitzmann MF, Tonstad S, Norat T, Vatten LJ. Tobacco smoking and the risk of diverticular disease—A systematic review and meta-analysis of prospective studies. Colorectal Dis. 2017; 19:621–633.
28. Strate LL, Liu YL, Syngal S, Aldoori WH, Giovannucci EL. Nut, corn, and popcorn consumption and the incidence of diverticular disease. JAMA. 2008; 300:907–914.
29. Hinchey EJ, Schaal PG, Richards GK: Treatment of perforated diverticular disease of the colon. Adv Surg. 1978; 12:85–109.
30. Klarenbeek BR, de Korte N, van der Peet DL, Cuesta MA. Review of current classifications for diverticular disease and a translation into clinical practice. Int J Colorectal Dis. 2012; 27:207–214.
31. Abbas S. Resection and primary anastomosis in acute complicated diverticulitis, a systematic review of the literature. Int J Colorectal Dis. 2007; 22:351–357.
32. Oberkofler CE, Rickenbacher A, Raptis DA, et al. A multicenter randomized clinical trial of primary anastomosis or Hartmann's procedure for perforated left colonic diverticulitis with purulent or fecal peritonitis. Ann Surg. 2012; 256:819–826.
33. Bridoux V, Regimbeau JM, Ouaissi M, Mathonnet M, Mauvais F, Houivet E, Schwarz L, Mege D, Sielezneff I, Sabbagh C, Tuech JJ. Hartmann's procedure or primary anastomosis for generalized peritonitis due to perforated diverticulitis: A prospective multicenter randomized trial (DIVERTI). J Am Coll Surg. 2017; 225:798–805.
34. Lambrichts DPV, Vennix S, Musters GD, Mulder IM, Swank HA, Hoofwijk AGM, Belgers EHJ, Stockmann HBAC, Eijsbouts QAJ, Gerhards MF, van Wagensveld BA, van Geloven AAW, Crolla RMPH, Nienhuijs SW, Govaert MJPM, di Saverio S, D'Hoore AJL, Consten ECJ, van Grevenstein WMU, Pierik REGJM, Kruyt PM, van der Hoeven JAB, Steup WH, Catena F, Konsten JLM, Vermeulen J, van Dieren S, Bemelman WA, Lange JF; LADIES Trial Collaborators. Hartmann's procedure versus sigmoidectomy with primary anastomosis for perforated diverticulitis with purulent or faecal peritonitis (LADIES): A multicentre, parallel-group, randomised, open-label, superiority trial. Lancet Gastroenterol Hepatol. 2019; 8:599–610.
35. Edomskis PP, Hoek VT, Stark PW, Lambrichts DPV, Draaisma WA, Consten ECJ, Bemelman WA, Lange JF; LADIES Trial Collaborators. Hartmann's procedure versus sigmoidectomy with primary anastomosis for perforated diverticulitis with purulent or fecal peritonitis: Three-year follow-up of a randomised controlled trial. Int J Surg. 2022; 98:106221.
36. Kohl A, Rosenberg J, Bock D, Bisgaard T, Skullman S, Thornell A, Gehrman J, Angenete E, Haglind E. Two-year results of the randomized clinical trial DILALA comparing laparoscopic lavage with resection as treatment for perforated diverticulitis. Br J Surg. 2018; 105:1128–1134.
37. Vennix S, Musters GD, Mulder IM, Swank HA, Consten EC, Belgers EH, van Geloven AA, Gerhards MF, Govaert MJ, van Grevenstein WM, Hoofwijk AG, Kruyt PM, Nienhuijs SW, Boermeester MA, Vermeulen J, van Dieren S, Lange JF, Bemelman WA; Ladies Trial Collaborators. Laparoscopic peritoneal lavage or sigmoidectomy for perforated diverticulitis with purulent peritonitis: A multicentre, parallel-group, randomised, open-label trial. Lancet. 2015; 386:1269–1277.
38. Schultz JK, Wallon C, Blecic L, Forsmo HM, Folkesson J, Buchwald P, Kørner H, Dahl FA, Øresland T, Yaqub S; SCANDIV Study Group. One-year results of the SCANDIV randomized clinical trial of laparoscopic lavage versus primary resection for acute perforated diverticulitis. Br J Surg. 2017; 104:1382–1392.
39. Azhar N, Johanssen A, Sundström T, Folkesson J, Wallon C, Kørner H, Blecic L, Forsmo HM, Øresland T, Yaqub S, Buchwald P, Schultz JK; SCANDIV Study Group. Laparoscopic lavage vs primary resection for acute perforated diverticulitis: Long-term outcomes from the Scandinavian diverticulitis (SCANDIV) randomized clinical trial. JAMA Surg. 2021; 156:121–127.
40. Penna M, Markar SR, Mackenzie H, Hompes R, Cunningham C. Laparoscopic lavage versus primary resection for acute perforated diverticulitis: Review and meta-analysis. Ann Surg. 2018; 2(67):252–258.
41. Clinical Outcomes of Surgical Therapy Study Group. A comparison of laparoscopically assisted and open colectomy for colon cancer. N Engl J Med. 2004; 350:2050–2059.
42. Klarenbeek BR, Veenhoff AA, Bergamaschi R, et al. Laparoscopic sigmoid resection for diverticulitis decreases major morbidity rates: A randomized control trial: Short-term results of the Sigma Trial. Ann Surg. 2009; 249:39–44.
43. Klarenbeek BR, Bergamaschi R, Veenhof AA, van der Peet DL, van den Broek WT, de Lange ES, Bemelman WA, Heres P, Lacy AM, Cuesta MA. Laparoscopic versus open sigmoid resection for diverticular disease: Follow-up assessment of the randomized control Sigma trial. Surg Endosc. 2011; 25:1121–1126.
44. Dwivedi A, Chahin F, Agrawal S, Chau WY, Tootla A, Tootla F, Silva YJ. Laparoscopic colectomy vs open colectomy for sigmoid diverticular disease. Dis Colon Rectum. 2002; 45:1309–1314.
45. Alves A, Panis Y, Slim K, Heyd B, Kwiatkowski F, Mantion G; Association Français de Chirurgie. French multicentre prospective observational study of laparoscopic versus open colectomy for sigmoid diverticular disease. Br J Surg. 2005; 92:1520–1525.
46. Königsrainer A. Acute and elective laparoscopic resection for complicated sigmoid diverticulitis: Clinical and histological outcome. J Gastrointest Surg. 2013; 17:1966–1971.
47. Keller DS, Delaney CP, Hashemi L, Haas EM. A national evaluation of clinical and economic outcomes in open versus laparoscopic colorectal surgery. Surg Endosc. 2016; 30:4220–4228.

48. Santos A, Mentula P, Pinta T, Ismail S, Rautio T, Juusela R, Lähdesmäki A, Scheinin T, Sallinen V. Comparing laparoscopic elective sigmoid resection with conservative treatment in improving quality of life of patients with diverticulitis: The laparoscopic elective sigmoid resection following diverticulitis (LASER) randomized clinical trial. JAMA Surg. 2021; 156:129–136.

49. Giuliani G, Guerra F, Coletta D, Giuliani A, Salvischiani L, Tribuzi A, Caravaglios G, Genovese A, Coratti A. Robotic versus conventional laparoscopic technique for the treatment of left-sided colonic diverticular disease: A systematic review with meta-analysis. Int J Colorectal Dis. 2022; 37:101–109.

50. Solaini L, Bocchino A, Avanzolini A, Annunziata D, Cavaliere D, Ercolani G. Robotic versus laparoscopic left colectomy: A systematic review and meta-analysis. Int J Colorectal Dis. 2022; 3(7):1497–1507.

44

Large Bowel Obstruction

Josh Cassedy and John J. Hong

Large bowel obstruction is a potentially life-threatening condition that can present as a result of a variety of mechanisms. The breadth of causes can complicate management and treatment decisions. Knowledge of anatomy, physiology, surgical treatment options, and critical care are all vital in managing this disease entity. Since patients can present with significant physiologic derangements, early identification followed by prompt intervention is necessary. Bowel obstructions can be classified in several ways, but the treatment philosophy is the same regardless of what classification system is used: Resuscitation and supportive measures followed by definitive therapy, most often in the form of surgery (unlike the typical management of small bowel obstruction). Surgical decision-making can sometimes be challenging, given the paucity of Level 1 evidence. Ogilvie's syndrome, or acute colonic pseudo-obstruction, presents with similar symptoms and is initially managed the same; however, in contrast to large bowel obstruction, nonoperative management remains the mainstay of treatment. This chapter presents the most up-to-date and applicable research. Recent review articles were also used to support some of the points presented in other retrospective and prospective evaluations.

44.1 How Does Colonic Obstruction Present?

The presentation of colonic obstruction depends on the degree of intestinal luminal narrowing, duration of the obstruction, and etiology of the obstruction. The inciting pathologic process will often dictate the patient's presentation. Common symptoms include abdominal distention, nausea and vomiting, and crampy or colicky abdominal pain. They may present with constipation, obstipation, or diarrhea. The presence and severity of symptoms are related to the level of obstruction and may be widely variable. Other symptoms such as hypotension and tachycardia may be present secondary to dehydration or sepsis (from perforation, bowel ischemia, etc.).

In a prospective observational study of 150 adult patients admitted with acute mechanical bowel obstruction to a surgical specialty hospital in Greece over 2 years, it was noted that 24% of these patients had a large bowel obstruction. Overall, admissions for large bowel obstruction represent about 2–4% of all surgical admissions [1].

RECOMMENDATION

Absence of passage of flatus (90%) and/or feces (80.6%) and abdominal distension (65.3%) were the most common symptoms and physical findings. These percentages are for all patients admitted with mechanical bowel obstruction.

Grade of recommendation: C.

44.2 What Are the Causes of Large Bowel Obstruction?

A variety of classification schemes have been derived to organize the causes of large bowel obstruction. Given the initial similarity in presentation between Ogilvie's syndrome and large bowel obstruction, the first branching point delineates between mechanical and functional obstruction. Within the mechanical arm of obstruction, a comprehensive and simple outline is illustrated in *Current Therapy in Colon and Rectal Surgery* [2]. Categories include (1) lesions extrinsic to the bowel wall, (2) lesions intrinsic to the bowel wall, (3) lesions within the bowel lumen, and (4) bowel torsion. Lesions extrinsic to the bowel include compression due to extraluminal tumor or abscess, hernia, and postoperative adhesions. Lesions intrinsic to the bowel wall would encompass intramural tumors, inflammatory bowel disease, endometriosis, ischemia, or stricture. Lesions within the bowel lumen would comprise foreign bodies, gallstone obstruction, intussusception, or fecal impaction. Bowel torsion essentially refers to volvulus, usually cecal or sigmoidal, with transverse colon and splenic flexure being less common sites.

By far, neoplasm represents the most common cause of colonic obstruction despite continuing efforts to promote rational screening tests such as colonoscopy. The incidence of mechanical obstruction in patients with colorectal cancer ranges between 14% and 34% based on multiple studies. Sigmoid cancer accounted for 15 (75%) of the 20 patients with obstruction due to large bowel cancer in the study by Markogiannakis et al. [3], whereas 2 (10%) patients had an ascending colon cancer, 1 (5%) had a descending colon cancer, and 1 (5%) had rectal cancer. Ovarian cancer has a similarly high reported incidence.

DOI: 10.1201/9781003316800-44

Hernias account for less than 3% of patients who present with a large bowel obstruction. However, hernias causing obstruction do have a significant clinical impact, since they are associated with ischemia, necrosis, and perforation at a higher rate than other causes of obstruction [3]. Hernias comprise one of the main causes of extrinsic large bowel obstruction.

Diverticulitis and associated stricture remain the third cause of large bowel obstruction. Partial obstruction in acute diverticulitis is more commonly encountered than a complete obstruction and may be due to severe colonic wall edema combined with intramural or extraluminal abscess formation. Differentiating an obstructing neoplasm from diverticulitis with associated abscess or phlegmon can be challenging in such cases based on CT alone. Standard initial nonoperative treatment of diverticulitis may reduce the edema substantially enough to permit further evaluation before an operation. In a retrospective review of patients diagnosed with acute diverticulitis who later underwent colonoscopy, 2.2% of them were diagnosed with colon cancer, with an odds ratio of 24.43 if obstruction and localized mass were noted on CT. The increased risk of recurrence of diverticulitis with incomplete resection also highlights the importance of interval colonoscopy given its capability to more fully evaluate the extent of diverticular disease [4]. The sequela of repeated or severe diverticulitis and fibrosis of the bowel wall can cause an obstructing stricture. Given the association of malignancy with stricture, resection is typically indicated. Additionally, the severity of the stricture may preclude further colonoscopic evaluation of the remaining colon, thus potentially hiding an upstream synchronous neoplasm even if the stricture itself is benign [2]. Stent placement has been considered as a bridge to surgery and to permit a complete colonoscopic evaluation, outside of the acute inflammatory setting. However, presumably due to the chronic inflammation, there is an associated high complication rate, and it is not generally recommended [5, 6].

Colonic volvulus is responsible for roughly 5% of large bowel obstructions in the United States. This occurs when part of the colon rotates on its mesentery, leading to colonic obstruction and subsequent venous congestion and obstruction of arterial inflow. Sigmoid volvulus is most common, accounting for up to 75% of all colonic volvulus cases, followed by cecal volvulus then transverse colon and splenic flexure volvulus.

Colonic pseudo-obstruction, or Ogilvie's syndrome, should be viewed as a separate disease entity. It involves massive colonic dilation without true mechanical obstruction. The etiology is thought to be related to an autonomic imbalance leading to a disturbance of the efferent parasympathetic output of the sacral spinal segments S2–S4 to the distal colon, but there is no direct evidence for this. The most common predisposing conditions are trauma (34%), cardiac disease (10–18%), and infection (10%) [7, 8]. Initial therapy is similar to mechanical obstruction with fluid resuscitation, nil per os (NPO), and possibly decompression in the form of nasogastric suction and/or rectal tube decompression. However, it is imperative to exclude true colonic obstruction, as the subsequent management strategies can vary widely.

RECOMMENDATION

Large bowel cancer, adhesions, retroperitoneal tumors, and hernias were the most common causes of large bowel obstruction. Hernias, adhesions, diverticulitis, strictures, endometriosis, ingested foreign bodies, phytobezoars, gallstones, and rectal foreign bodies have all been found to cause large bowel obstruction. The less commonly encountered acute colonic pseudo-obstruction remains an important clinical entity given the poorly understood cause and notably different management.

Grade of recommendation: C.

44.3 What Is the Proper Diagnostic Evaluation?

A thorough laboratory evaluation is useful in determining the patient's overall clinical status and may suggest intestinal ischemia, necrosis, or perforation. Although no Level 1 evidence can be found to support the routine ordering of certain laboratory tests, it is well known that patients with colonic obstruction often present with multiple metabolic derangements requiring correction before surgical intervention. A basic metabolic panel and complete blood count should be done to evaluate for electrolyte imbalances, anemia, and leukocytosis. Lactate may help in evaluating for ischemia and gauging the urgency of an operation, while a coagulation panel assists in preoperative preparation. Given that the most common cause of large bowel obstruction is cancer, a baseline carcinoembryonic antigen level may be reasonable. A single upright chest radiograph may be useful to screen for free air if there is a high suspicion of perforation.

In terms of options for confirming a radiographic diagnosis of large bowel obstruction, several studies have been used. Often, a plain abdominal radiograph can confirm the diagnosis and is said to have 84% sensitivity and 72% specificity in diagnosing large bowel obstruction [5].

A water-soluble contrast enema is another option that may be utilized to establish a diagnosis. This has a sensitivity of 96% and a specificity of 98% [5]. However, CT scanners are now readily available in most hospitals and can usually be performed in a timely fashion. In a single-institution review over 7 years, it was noted that multidetector CT imaging was more accurate in making the diagnosis of large bowel obstruction than was contrasted enema. Beneficially, CT imaging was also evaluated for other disease processes—metastatic disease in the case of neoplasm—and was more readily available [9]. In contrast, Cappell and Batke [5] state that the sensitivity and specificity of abdominopelvic CT in diagnosing large bowel obstruction is 90%. The combination of a contrast enema and CT imaging provides an even better evaluation. For functional obstruction, evaluation is much the same given that mechanical obstruction must be ruled out before a diagnosis of Ogilvie's.

44.4 Management

Following diagnosis, treatment starts with resuscitation, correction of electrolyte derangements, NPO status (with the
placement of a nasogastric tube or with a colorectal tube in
some cases if needed for decompression), and mechanical
relief of the obstruction, typically operatively. There is Level 2
evidence that hydration of over 1 L/day may be associated with
less nausea, based on a randomized trial of 15 patients with
inoperable malignant bowel obstructions [1]. Additionally,
adequate hydration corrects the typical dehydration present,
often with concomitant metabolic abnormalities. Careful
attention to antibiotic and prophylactic (deep venous thrombosis and gastrointestinal) regimens is needed [2].

While initial management is similar, colonic pseudo-
obstruction typically resolves with nonoperative management
in contrast to mechanical causes. However, perforation and
ischemia with particularly severe dilation warrant operation.
The risk of spontaneous perforation is low at 3%, but the mortality rate in ischemia or perforation is between 40% and 50%,
compared to 15% without [7, 8, 10–12]. Such a risk seems to
increase with the duration of symptoms, progression of the
disease process, and cecal diameter greater than 12 cm. In a
retrospective review of 400 patients, mortality increased twofold when the cecal diameter was 14 cm or more [10]. Multiple
studies have shown up to 96% resolution with nonoperative
measures alone [13–19]. These measures include nasogastric
tube placement, correction of electrolyte abnormalities, serial
abdominal examinations and radiographs, removal of potentiating drugs, rectal tube placement, optimal body positioning,
and enemas [14]. Potassium and magnesium are particularly
important to correct. To assist in passing flatus, optimal body
positioning is either prone with hips elevated or knees to chest
with hips high.

In the case of Ogilvie's, essentially all studies attempt at
least 24–48 hours of noninterventional treatment. Given the
preponderance of data, absent signs of peritonitis or pneumoperitoneum, a trial of nonoperative management carries
a grade A recommendation. Regarding mechanical obstruction, there is little Level 1 evidence comparing one operative
approach to another. With the gaining popularity and capabilities of colonic stents, it is feasible that fewer large bowel
obstructions will be taken emergently to the operating room
(OR). However, the local capabilities for endoscopic intervention, the patient's underlying disease process, and the clinical
presentation should be carefully considered. If there is a concern for ischemia or perforation, the patient has not clinically
improved, or the cecal diameter continues to increase, laparotomy should be performed [4]. Since most cases of colonic
obstruction are due to colon cancer, we will elaborate more
thoroughly on this topic. In any case, it is incumbent upon the
operating surgeon to thoroughly evaluate the remaining colon
for synchronous lesions.

44.5 What Is the Preferred Operative Approach?

44.5.1 Operative Management of Obstructing Colon Cancer

The debate over management in obstructing colorectal cancer
centers on two issues: Nonoperative management using stents
and whether to perform a primary anastomosis. The role of
stenting in colonic obstruction will be covered later in the
chapter. In right-sided colon cancer, a right hemicolectomy
should be performed [5]. The distal resection margin may
include the right branch of the middle colic, especially if the
cancer is located at the hepatic flexure [2]. In stable patients,
this can be done with primary anastomosis. Unstable patients,
who have perforation with peritonitis or have a very distended
bowel, should have an ileostomy performed or temporary
abdominal closure [5]. An article by Stoyanov et al. [7] looked
at 232 cases of obstructing colorectal cancer requiring urgent
surgical intervention. One hundred and sixty tumors were in
the colon and the remaining 72 had obstructing rectal lesions.
In this group, there was a 25% mortality rate. It was noted that
there was a higher mortality rate in the primary anastomosis
group [18]. A second series retrospectively reviewed the
records of 23 patients with obstructing lesions of the left colon
[16]. The patients underwent different surgical procedures:
14 underwent one-stage colonic resection with intraoperative
colonic lavage ($n = 10$) or subtotal colectomy ($n = 4$), which
comprised the resection and primary anastomoses group. Nine
patients underwent staged resection with either Hartmann's
or loop colostomy and comprised the staged resection group.
There was one case of anastomotic dehiscence in the resection and primary anastomoses group and two cases in the
staged resection group. The authors concluded that a one-
stage procedure is safe and may be indicated for the management of most cases [8]. With disseminated disease, a palliative
resection should be considered, while for recurrent obstructive disease, a bypass procedure or proximal stoma is most
appropriate [5].

44.5.2 Operative Management of Other Causes of Large Bowel Obstruction

Benign strictures can be treated by segmental resection. Preoperative screening colonoscopy is warranted to rule out malignancy. However, this may not be feasible in cases of complete or near-complete obstruction. Although radiation history does not entirely exclude a primary anastomosis, a diverting colostomy must be strongly considered in the case of a radiation-induced stricture [5]. There is also literature that supports the use of endoscopic balloon dilation for the treatment of benign strictures, either from inflammatory bowel disease or surgical anastomoses. This is most successful when the stricture length is equal to or less than 4 cm [20]. However, the presence of malignancy must be thoroughly evaluated.

Operative management of volvulus depends on the type. Sigmoid volvulus is ideally treated with endoscopic decompression followed by semi-elective surgery in the form of sigmoidectomy and primary anastomosis. Surgical detorsion is associated with a 40–60% recurrence rate, with similar results for extraperitoneal fixation, and is therefore not recommended [21, 22]. Patients with cecal volvulus, on the other hand, classically go directly to the OR secondary to the high failure rate of colonic decompression [20]. Right hemicolectomy is the standard operative choice. For an extremely debilitated patient with extensive comorbidities in which operative risk is prohibitive, a cecostomy is an option. In cases with extensive peritoneal contamination or nonviable bowel, an end colostomy is the safest option.

> **RECOMMENDATION**
>
> Since colonic obstruction is overwhelmingly due to colon cancer, the approach must use standard oncologic operative techniques. A diverting ostomy is indicated in the setting of hemodynamic compromise, gross peritonitis, grossly overdistended bowel, palliative operations, and prior radiation. If none of these conditions are met, performing a primary anastomosis is reasonable. On the table, colonic lavage does not appear to add any benefit.
>
> Grade of recommendation: C.

44.6 What Is the Role of Laparoscopy in the Treatment of Large Bowel Obstruction?

Gash et al. did a prospective electronic database review between April 2001 and June 2009 looking at the outcomes in consecutive patients presenting with large bowel obstruction who were treated with laparoscopic resectional surgery. In their study, 24 patients underwent laparoscopic surgery secondary to cancer [11] and diverticulosis [12]. There were two conversions. The transition time to a normal diet was 24 hours, and the median hospital stay was 3 days. There were complications in 25% of the patients. For volvulus, in particular, the distention and lack of colonic fixation intrinsic to the disease process worsened laparoscopic exposure, making an open

approach the generally preferred method. Comparative studies suggest no difference in outcomes between either an open or laparoscopic approach [23].

> **RECOMMENDATION**
>
> Based on these results, the authors concluded that laparoscopic surgery in acute colonic obstruction is safe and feasible.
>
> Grade of recommendation: C.

44.7 Are There Any Nonoperative Options?

Great advances have been made in the nonoperative treatment of large bowel obstruction. Traditionally surgery was the treatment of choice. The current widespread use and technical advancements of endoscopy have expanded the available armamentarium to treat this disease. The current options for nonoperative management include photodynamic therapy, electrocoagulation, laser coagulation, and balloon dilatation.

However, the self-expanding endoluminal stent has made the most significant impact on the nonoperative treatment of colonic obstruction. Given that patients with large bowel obstruction have significant morbidity and mortality from diverting colostomy (16% and 5%, respectively), stents have become an acceptable treatment option for those patients with inoperable disease and for those who are poor surgical candidates [10, 14, 15]. As such, Level 1 evidence to justify the use of laser coagulation and the other aforementioned methods is scarce. Articles are now appearing frequently on the benefits of colonic stents. We will explore the indications, applications, and complications here. Outcomes for colonic stenting will be covered in the next section.

The minimally invasive nature of colonic stents makes them a perfect adjunct for treating large bowel obstruction in poor surgical candidates and those needing palliative treatment from obstructing cancer. Benign strictures are also being treated by stenting [10]. Some tout the widespread applicability of colonic stenting [10]. To these authors, colonic stenting is indicated in all patients when technically feasible, thus allowing a one-stage procedure while also allowing full evaluation of disease extent [10, 16].

The most recent series published in *Colorectal Disease* highlights 63 patients referred for large bowel obstruction [8]. A prospective database was evaluated. Sixty-three patients had 71 stenting procedures performed. Thirty-two patients had metastatic disease discovered during their evaluation. Extrinsic compression caused seven strictures. The indication for stenting was palliation in 56 patients and served as a bridge to a one-stage procedure in 7 patients. Technical success was achieved 91% of the time. Obstructive symptoms were relieved in 89%. Twenty-four percent of the patients had complications including overgrowth (8%), migration (6%), fistulation (4%), stent fracture (3%), tenesmus (3%), and fecal urgency (1%). No procedure-related deaths occurred, and there were no technical failures for lesions proximal to the descending colon. The authors concluded that a combination of endoscopic/fluoroscopic colorectal stenting is effective and safe [8]. Dauphine et al. [17] retrospectively reviewed 26 patients with malignant obstruction who underwent colonic stenting. The indications, success, and complication rates are mirrored in other studies. Fourteen patients had palliative procedures performed. Twelve patients had colonic stents placed as a bridge to surgery. The first attempts were successful in 22 patients. Of the remaining four individuals, three required emergency surgery, and one was successfully stented at the second attempt. Seventy-five percent of patients in the bridge-to-surgery group went on to elective colon resection. There was a 29% reobstruction rate and one (9%) stent migration. Patency was maintained in nine (64%) patients who underwent palliative treatment. Based on this, the authors concluded that colonic stents achieve immediate nonoperative decompression that is both safe and effective. Stenting is also a useful adjunct allowing a semi-elective resection in the majority of resectable cases [8]. A Cochrane review article published by Trompetas [18] found that colonic stenting is the best option for palliation or as a bridge to surgery. Using stents reduces morbidity, mortality, and colostomy rates. Stenting, depending on the healthcare system, is likely to be cost-effective [18]. The literature focuses on descending colon, sigmoid, and rectal obstruction. As such, more information is needed on the applicability of stenting with regard to right colon and transverse lesions.

Colonic stenting is the most widely accepted method of nonoperative treatment. However, its use is limited by the small number of trained physicians and centers performing the procedure, and its utility, at this point, seems to be most pronounced in treating rectal, sigmoid, left, and distal transverse colon lesions. Some technical considerations limit the use of stenting, such as the length of the stricture. Stenting allows for the relief of obstruction, for a full evaluation of the primary process, and for a one-stage procedure. The complication rate is very low. Stenting is particularly helpful in those where treatment is palliative and for patients who are stable and can undergo resuscitation and primary disease evaluation as a bridge to a single operation [8, 10, 18].

RECOMMENDATION

Colonic stenting can be used as a bridge to surgery or as a palliative option. The success rate for relieving obstruction is around 90%. Three-quarters of patients in which colonic stents are used as a bridge to surgery will go on to elective resection.

Grade of recommendation: B.

44.8 What Is the Preferred Management for Colonic Pseudo-Obstruction: Observation versus Medical or Endoscopic Decompression?

A functional disorder of the colon, colonic pseudo-obstruction, or Ogilvie's syndrome, involves significant colonic dilation without true mechanical obstruction. Initial therapy is similar to mechanical obstruction: Fluid resuscitation; NPO; enteric decompression; and minimization of contributing factors such as morphine derivatives, medications with anticholinergic properties, and calcium channel antagonists. Additionally, electrolyte derangements, renal insufficiency, hypothyroidism, and infection can all contribute to the syndrome. Supportive measures, correction of any offending agents, and observation should be the initial treatment in all colonic pseudo-obstruction patients according to a review by Saunders and Kimmey [19]. Further intervention in the form of pharmacologic or endoscopic decompression should be considered in patients who are not showing signs of improvement after 72 hours or have significant cecal dilation (over 10 cm) persisting to 72 hours. In a pooled literature review and retrospective analysis of 400 patients, Vanek and Al-Salti correlated the two most relevant factors in prognosticating morbidity and mortality. These are cecum diameter and time to decompression. A diameter of at least 12 cm was associated with a mortality of 7%, which doubled to 14% at a diameter greater than 14 cm. Time of colonic dilation before decompression of fewer than 4 days was associated with a 15% mortality, while delaying past 7 days had a mortality of 73% [10]. Therefore, if a patient has failed supportive treatment with persistent symptoms at 72 hours or is at high risk of perforation with increasing cecal diameter greater than 10 cm, decompressive therapy should be pursued per guidelines from both the European Society of Gastrointestinal Endoscopy and the American Society for Gastrointestinal Endoscopy [24–26].

After supportive measures, the two established therapies are medication and endoscopic decompression [27]. Generally, the first therapy of choice is neostigmine. Neostigmine is a reversible acetylcholinesterase inhibitor that indirectly stimulates muscarinic and nicotinic receptors, thus increasing colonic activity and motility. In a randomized, double-blind, placebo-controlled trial by Ponec et al., patients with acute colonic pseudo-obstruction with a cecal diameter greater than 10 cm and no response after 24 hours of conservative therapy were given either 2 mg of neostigmine or saline infusion over 3–5 minutes. Clinical response was observed in 91% of patients who received neostigmine compared to 0% of those receiving the saline infusion. There was an associated recurrence rate of about 11% in this study [6]. If the first dose of neostigmine has been ineffective, a second dose is recommended [28–30] (grade B recommendation).

Colonic decompression has been reserved for those who have cecal distension greater than 10 cm without improvement after 72 hours of supportive therapy and those who have contraindications to neostigmine. Those include renal insufficiency (serum creatinine greater than 3 mg/dL), uncontrolled cardiac arrhythmias, severe bronchospasm, and pregnancy. Although there are no randomized controlled trials to date establishing the efficacy of colonoscopic decompression, the available data show that up to 95% of patients experienced initial and sustained decompression [31, 32]. Repeat colonoscopy can be required given an approximate recurrence rate risk of 40% [33]. In cohort studies, there are contradicting data on whether leaving a decompression tube in place reduces recurrence [32, 34–37]. However, prospective randomized data from an admittedly small study does support the use of polyethylene glycol to reduce recurrence after decompression [28]. Two retrospective trials evaluating colonoscopy versus neostigmine found colonoscopic decompression superior to neostigmine with equivalent perforation rates and no difference in outcomes for patients later requiring an operation [37, 38]. In other studies, the two treatment methods have been found equivalent [39]. One other controversial issue is whether mucosal ischemia is a contraindication to colonic decompression. Traditionally, mucosal ischemia identified on endoscopy has been an indication to proceed with surgery. To date, however, there is no Level 1 evidence to support or contest this. There are case reports of patients with mucosal ischemia being managed successfully with endoscopic decompression [21]. Given the lack of evidence, this should be reserved for patients who have no evidence of peritonitis and who are poor operative candidates (grade C recommendation).

Surgical treatment of colonic pseudo-obstruction is typically reserved for patients with perforation, mucosal ischemia with peritonitis, or those who fail decompressive therapy. Cecostomy may be performed for patients without perforation or ischemia, with segmental resection or subtotal colectomy being options for the latter depending on the extent of the disease [21]. Surgical mortality rates are high given the typical indications, reaching 44% for patients with ischemia or perforation; therefore, nonoperative management should be first-line and started early enough to avert these outcomes [10].

RECOMMENDATION

Initial management is supportive, followed by pharmacologic decompression. Neostigmine should be considered first-line therapy with colonoscopic decompression as an alternative only for those with contraindications to medical therapy. The evidence on the placement of a decompressive rectal tube after colonoscopic decompression is limited but is recommended. Operative management is reserved for peritonitis, perforation, or failure of the previous therapies.

Grade of recommendation: B.

44.9 What Are the Outcomes?

The outcomes for patients presenting with large bowel obstruction vary depending on the cause and whether or not the patient has compromised bowel at the time of operation. Outcomes for some causes of large bowel obstruction were alluded to in their corresponding section. Mortality rates for those presenting with large bowel obstruction from colon cancer range from 5% to 25%. The mortality rates for those needing urgent operative Hartmann's procedure are similar [13, 19]. The mortality rate increases with findings of necrosis and perforation. Incarcerated hernias are more likely to cause necrosis or perforation [3]. A study by Zorcolo et al. [27] retrospectively reviewed the records of 323 patients who presented acutely and underwent surgery over 10 years. The etiology of obstruction was left-sided colorectal cancer and diverticular disease. The review aimed to identify a difference in the outcome of resection and primary anastomosis with Hartmann's procedure. Primary anastomosis was performed in 176 (55.7%) patients with a 30-day mortality of 5.7%. Nine (5.1%) patients had an anastomotic breakdown. Hartmann's resection was associated with a higher incidence of systemic and surgical morbidity (39.5% and 24.3%, respectively). Mortality from primary anastomosis (5.7%) compared favorably with those undergoing Hartmann's resections (20.4%). As mentioned previously, colonic stenting can convert an emergency procedure to an elective procedure with the ability to have a colon preparation and evaluate the patient for other systemic diseases.

RECOMMENDATION

Mortality rates for patients presenting with large bowel obstruction are 20–25%. If colonic stenting is available, the mortality rate can be significantly reduced.

Grade of recommendation: B.

TABLE 44.1

Clinical Question Summary

Question	Answer	Grade	References
How does colonic obstruction present?	Absence of passage of flatus (90%) and/or feces (80.6%) and abdominal distension (65.3%) were the most common symptoms and physical findings, respectively.	C	[3]
What are the causes of large bowel obstruction?	Large bowel cancer, adhesions, retroperitoneal tumors, and hernias were the most common causes of large bowel obstruction. Hernias, adhesions, strictures, endometriosis, ingested foreign bodies, phytobezoars, gallstones, and rectal foreign bodies have all been found to cause large bowel obstruction.	C	[2, 3, 24, 25, 40]
What is the proper diagnostic evaluation?	CT imaging is more accurate in making the diagnosis of large bowel obstruction than contrast enema. CT imaging also allows for the evaluation of other disease processes and is more readily available.	C	[9]
What is the preferred operative approach?	Stomas are preferred for patients with recurrent disease or palliative resections. A primary anastomosis can be performed for obstructing colon lesions.	C	[5, 22, 23]
What is the role of laparoscopy in large bowel obstruction?	Laparoscopic surgery in large bowel obstruction is safe and feasible and may reduce the hospital length of stay.	C	[13]

(Continued)

TABLE 44.1 (Continued)

Clinical Question Summary

Question	Answer	Grade	References
Are there any nonoperative options?	Colonic stenting can be used as a bridge to surgery or as a palliative option. The success rate for relieving obstruction is around 90%. Three-quarters of patients in which colonic stents are used as a bridge to surgery will go on to elective resection.	B	[16–18, 27]
What is the preferred management for colonic pseudo-obstruction?	Initial management is supportive, followed by either pharmacologic or endoscopic decompression. Surgery is reserved for peritonitis, perforation, or failure of the earlier therapies.	B	[6, 14, 21]
What are the outcomes?	Mortality rates for patients presenting with large bowel obstruction are 20–25%. If colonic stenting is available, the mortality rate can be significantly reduced.	B	[7, 16, 23, 26]

Editor's Note

The diagnosis of large bowel obstruction has changed considerably in the last 30 years related to the availability and accuracy of CT scans. When pseudo-obstruction is found, conclusive evidence from over 20 years ago demonstrated a greater than 90% success rate with the administration of neostigmine. I have noted an overuse of colonoscopic decompression without even attempts at neostigmine, which may be related to the financial rewards for proceduralists in our current fee-for-service environment. Stenting of colonic obstruction has been highly effective in lowering morbidity and mortality by reducing the need for operative intervention in debilitated patients and also can represent a bridge to elective colonic resection. Finally, the need to abbreviate laparotomy is now well established in the hemodynamically unstable or coagulopathic patient undergoing emergency colonic procedures.

REFERENCES

1. Mercadante S Ripamonti C, Casuccio A Zecca E, Groff L. Comparison of octreotide and hyoscinebutylbromide in controlling gastrointestinal symptoms due to malignant inoperable bowel obstruction. *Support Care Cancer.* May 2000;*8(3)*:188–191.
2. Fazio V, Church J, Delaney C. 2004. *Current Therapy in Colon and Rectal Surgery.* 2nd ed. Mosby: St. Louis, MO.
3. Markogiannakis H, Messaris E, Dardamanis D, et al. Acute mechanical bowel obstruction: Clinical presentation, etiology, management, and outcome. *World J Gastroenterol.* 2007;*13*:432–437.
4. Lopez-Kostner F Hool GR, Lavery IC Management and causes of acute large bowel obstruction. *Surg Clin North Am.* 1997;*77*:1265–1290.
5. Cappell MS Batke M. Mechanical obstruction of the small bowel and colon. *Med Clin North Am.* 2008;*92*:575–597.
6. Ponec RJ, Saunders MD, Kimmey MB. Neostigmine for the treatment of acute colonic pseudo-obstruction. *N Engl J Med.* 1999;*341(3)*:137–141.
7. Stoyanov H Julianov A, Valtchev D, et al. Results of the treatment of colorectal cancer complicated by obstruction. *Wien Klin Wochenschr.* 1998;*110*:262–265.
8. Finan PJ Campbell S, Verma R, et al. The management of malignant large bowel obstruction: ACPGBI position statement. *Colorectal Dis.* 2007;*9(4)*:1–17.
9. Jacob SE, Lee SH, Hill J. The demise of the instant/unprepared contrast enema in large bowel obstruction. *Colorectal Dis.* November 12, 2007 [Epub ahead of print].
10. Raveenthiran V. Restorative resection of unprepared left colon in gangrenous vs viable sigmoid volvulus. *Int J Colorectal Dis.* 2004;*19*:258–263.
11. Chueng HYS, Chung CC, Chieng WW, Wong JCH, Yau KKK, Li MKW. Endolaparoscopic approach vs conventional open surgery in the treatment of obstructing leftsided colon cancer. *Arch Surg.* 2009;*144(12)*:1127–1132.
12. De Giorgio R, Knowles CH. Acute colonic pseudoobstruction. *Br J Surg.* 2009;*96*:229–239.
13. Gash K, Chambers W, Ghosh A, Dixon AR. The role of laparoscopic surgery for the management of acute large bowel obstruction. *Colorectal Dis.* March 2011;*13(3)*: 263–266.
14. Lopera JE, Ferral H, Wholey M, et al. Treatment of colonic obstructions with metallic stents: Indications, technique, and complications. *Am J Roentgenol.* 1997;*169*:1285–1290.
15. Seymour K, Johnson R, Marsh R, Corson J. Palliative stenting of malignant large bowel obstruction. *Colorectal Dis.* 2002,*4*:240–245.
16. Baraza W, Lee F, Brown S, Hurlstone DP. Combination endoradiological colorectal stenting: A prospective 5-year clinical evaluation. *Ann Surg Oncol.* 2002;*9*:574–579.
17. Dauphine CE, Tan P, Beart RW, Jr., Vukasin P, Cohen H, Corman ML. Placement of self-expanding stents for acute malignant large-bowel obstruction: A collective review. *Ann Surg Oncol.* July 2002;*9(6)*:574–579.
18. Trompetas V. Emergency management of malignant acute left-sided colonic obstruction. *Ann R Coll Surg Engl.* April 2008;*90(3)*:181–186.
19. Saunders MD, Kimmey MD. Systematic review: Acute colonic pseudo-obstruction. *Aliment Pharmacol Ther.* 2005; *22*:917–925.
20. Small AJ Young-Fadok TM, Baron TH. Expandable metal stent placement for benign colorectal obstruction: Outcomes for 23 cases. *Surg Endosc.* 2008;*22*:454–462.
21. Florto JJ, Schoen RE, Brandt LF. Pseudo-obstruction associated with colonic ischemia: successful management with colonoscopic decompression. *Am J Gastroenterol.* 1991; *86*:1472–1476.
22. De Aguilar-Nascimento JE, Caporossi C, Nascimento M. Comparison between resection and primary anastomosis and staged resection in obstructing adenocarcinoma of the left colon. *Arq Gastroenterol.* 2002;*39*:240–245.

23. Zorcolo L Covotta L, CarloMagno N, et al. Safety of primary anastomosis in emergency colorectal surgery. *Colorectal Dis.* 2003;5:262–269.

24. Varras M, Kostopanagiotou E, Katis K, et al. Endometriosis causes extensive intestinal obstruction simulating carcinoma of the sigmoid colon: A case report and review of the literature. *Eur J Gynaecol Oncol.* 2002;23:353–357.

25. Efrati Y, Freud E, Serour F, Klin B. Phytobezoar-induced ileal and colonic obstruction in childhood. *J Pediatr Gastroenterol Nutr.* 1997;25:214–216.

26. Hennekine-Mucci S, Tuech JJ, Brehant O, et al. Management of obstructed left colon carcinoma. *Hepatogastroenterology.* 2007;54:1098–1101.

27. Harrison ME, Anderson M, Appalaneni V, et al. The role of endoscopy in the management of patients with known and suspected colonic obstruction and pseudoobstruction. *GI Endosc.* 2010;71(4):669–679.

28. Wegener M, Borsch G. Acute colonic pseudo-obstruction (Ogilvie's syndrome). Presentation of 14 of our own cases and analysis of 1027 cases reported in the literature. *Surg Endosc.* 1987;1(3):169–174.

29. Rex DK. Acute colonic pseudo-obstruction (Ogilvie's syndrome). *Gastroenterologist.* 1994;2(3):233–238.

30. Rex DK. Colonoscopy and acute colonic pseudo-obstruction. *Gastrointest Endosc Clin N Am.* 1997;7(3):499–508.

31. Shen SH, Chen JD, Tiu CM, et al. Differentiating colonic diverticulitis from colon cancer: The value of computed tomography in the emergency setting. *J Chin Med Assoc.* 2005;68:411–418. doi: 10.1016/S1726-4901(09)70156-X.

32. Venara A, Toqué L, Barbieux J, Cesbron E, Ridereau-Zins C, Lermite E, Hamy A. Sigmoid stricture associated with diverticular disease should be an indication for elective surgery with lymph node clearance. *J Visc Surg.* Sep 2015;152(4):211–215. doi: 10.1016/j.jviscsurg.2015.04.001. Epub 2015 May 6. PMID: 25958304.

33. Eskarous H, Krishnamurthy M, Habtesilassie E. Colon stenting in benign diverticular stricture - A case report and review of literature. *J Community Hosp Intern Med Perspect.* Nov 15, 2021;11(6):863–865. doi: 10.1080/20009666.2021.1969079. PMID: 34804408; PMCID: PMC8604465.

34. Johnson WR, Hawkins AT. Large bowel obstruction. *Clin Colon Rectal Surg.* Jul 2021;34(4):233–241. doi: 10.1055/s-0041-1729927. Epub 2021 Jul 20. PMID: 34305472; PMCID: PMC8292000.

35. Taourel P, Kessler N, Lesnik A, Pujol J, Morcos L, Bruel JM. Helical CT of large bowel obstruction. *Abdom Imaging.* 2003;28:267–275.

36. Elmi A, Hedgire SS, Pargaonkar V, Cao K, McDermott S, Harisinghani M. Is early colonoscopy beneficial in patients with CT-diagnosed diverticulitis? *Am J Roentgenol.* 2013;200:1269–1274.

37. Batke M, Cappell MS. Adynamic ileus and acute colonic pseudo-obstruction. *Med Clin North Am.* 2008;92(3):649–670, ix.

38. Wells CI, O'Grady G, Bissett IP. Acute colonic pseudo-obstruction: A systematic review of aetiology and mechanisms. *World J Gastroenterol.* Aug 14, 2017;23(30):5634–5644. doi: 10.3748/wjg.v23.i30.5634. PMID: 28852322; PMCID: PMC5558126.

39. Vanek VW, Al-Salti M. Acute pseudo-obstruction of the colon (Ogilvie's syndrome). An analysis of 400 cases. *Dis Colon Rectum.* 1986;29(3):203–210.

40. Jenkins JT, Taylor AJ Behrns KE. Secondary causes of intestinal obstruction: Rigorous preoperative evaluation is required. *Am Surg.* 2000;66:662–666.

41. Sloyer AF, Panella VS, Demas BE, et al. Ogilvie's syndrome. Successful management without colonoscopy. *Dig Dis Sci.* 1988;33(11):1391–1396.

42. Eisen GM, Baron TH, Dominitiz JA et al. Acute colonic pseudo-obstruction. *Gastrointest Endosc.* 2002;56(6):789–792.

43. Wanebo H, Mathewson C, Conolly B. Pseudo-obstruction of the colon. *Surg Gynecol Obstet.* 1971;133(1):44–48.

44. Meyers MA. Colonic ileus. *Gastrointest Radiol.* 1977;2(1):37–40.

45. Bachulis BL, Smith PE. Pseudoobstruction of the colon. *Am J Surg.* 1978;136(1):66–72.

46. Baker DA, Morin ME, Tan A et al. Colonic ileus. Indication for prompt decompression. *JAMA.* 1979;241(24):2633–2634.

47. Hutchinson R, Griffiths C. Acute colonic pseudoobstruction: A pharmacological approach. *Ann R Coll Surg Engl.* 1992;74(5):364–367.

48. Catena F, De Simone B, Coccolini F, et al. Bowel obstruction: A narrative review for all physicians. *World J Emerg Surg.* 2019;14:20. doi: 10.1186/s13017-019-0240-7

49. Halabi WJ, Jafari MD, Kang CY, et al. Colonic volvulus in the United States: trends, outcomes, and predictors of mortality. *Ann Surg.* 2014;259:293–301.

50. Bhatnagar BN, Sharma CL. Nonresective alternative for the cure of nongangrenous sigmoid volvulus. *Dis Colon Rectum.* 1998;41:381–388.

51. Basato S, Lin Sun Fui S, Pautrat K, et al. Comparison of two surgical techniques for resection of uncomplicated sigmoid volvulus: Laparoscopy or open surgical approach? *J Visc Surg.* 2014;151:431–434.

52. Weusten BL, Barret M, Bredenoord AJ, Familiari P, Gonzalez JM, van Hooft JE, et al. Endoscopic management of gastrointestinal motility disorders – part 2: European Society of Gastrointestinal Endoscopy (ESGE) Guideline. *Endoscopy.* Jul 2020;52(7):600–614.

53. Naveed M, Jamil LH, Fujii-Lau LL, Al-Haddad M, Buxbaum JL, Fishman DS, et al. American Society for Gastrointestinal Endoscopy guideline on the role of endoscopy in the management of acute colonic pseudo-obstruction and colonic volvulus. *Gastrointest Endosc.* Feb 2020;91(2):228–235.

54. Harrison ME, Anderson MA, Appalaneni V, Banerjee S, Ben-Menachem T, Cash BD, et al.; ASGE Standards of Practice Committee. The role of endoscopy in the management of patients with known and suspected colonic obstruction and pseudo-obstruction. *Gastrointest Endosc.* Apr 2010;71(4):669–679.

55. Loftus CG, Harewood GC, Baron TH. Assessment of predictors of response to neostigmine for acute colonic pseudo-obstruction. *Am J Gastroenterol.* Dec 2002;97(12):3118–3122.

56. Saunders MD. Acute colonic pseudo-obstruction. *Best Pract Res Clin Gastroenterol.* 2007;21(4):671–687. doi: 10.1016/j.bpg.2007.03.001

57. Geller A, Petersen BT, Gostout CJ. Endoscopic decompression for acute colonic pseudo-obstruction. *Gastrointest Endosc.* 1996;*44*(2):144–150. doi: 10.1016/s0016-5107(96)70131-1

58. Harig JM, Fumo DE, Loo FD, Parker HJ, Soergel KH, Helm JF, Hogan WJ. Treatment of acute nontoxic megacolon during colonoscopy: Tube placement versus simple decompression. *Gastrointest Endosc.* 1988;*34*(1):23–27. doi: 10.1016/s0016-5107(88)71224-9

59. Lavignolle A, Jutel P, Bonhomme J, Cloarec D, Cerbelaud P, Lehur PA, Galmiche JP, Le Bodic L. Syndrome d'Ogilvie: Résultats de l'exsufflation endoscopique dans une série de 29 cas [Ogilvie's syndrome: Results of endoscopic exsufflation in a series of 29 cases]. *Gastroenterol Clin Biol.* Feb 1986;*10*(2):147–151. French. PMID: 3754523.

60. Tsirline VB, Zemlyak AY, Avery MJ, Colavita PD, Christmas AB, Heniford BT, Sing RF. Colonoscopy is superior to neostigmine in the treatment of Ogilvie's syndrome. *Am J Surg.* 2012;*204*(6):849–855. doi: 10.1016/j.amjsurg.2012.05.006

61. Sgouros SN. Effect of polyethylene glycol electrolyte balanced solution on patients with acute colonic pseudo obstruction after resolution of colonic dilation: A prospective, randomised, placebo controlled trial. *Gut.* 2006;*55*(5): 638–642. doi: 10.1136/gut.2005.082099

62. Peker KD, Cikot M, Bozkurt MA, Ilhan B, Kankaya B, Binboga S, Seyit H, Alis H. Colonoscopic decompression should be used before neostigmine in the treatment of Ogilvie's syndrome. *Eur J Trauma Emerg Surg.* 2016. *43*(4):557–566. doi: 10.1007/s00068-016-0709-y

63. Bernardi M.-P, Warrier S, Lynch AC, Heriot AG. Acute and chronic pseudo-obstruction: A current update. *ANZ J Surg.* 2015;*85*(10), 709–714. doi: 10.1111/ans.13148

64. Mehta, R. A. J. I. V, et al. Factors predicting successful outcome following neostigmine therapy in acute colonic pseudo-obstruction: A prospective study. *J Gastroenterol Hepatol.* 2006;*21*(2):459–461. doi: 10.1111/j.1440-1746.2005.03994.x

45

Acute and Chronic Mesenteric Ischemia

Abdul Q. Alarhayem, Sungho Lim, and Zaid Alirhayim

45.1 Introduction

Acute mesenteric ischemia (AMI) is a challenging and potentially fatal condition that requires a high index of suspicion, early diagnosis, and prompt restoration of blood flow to avoid fulminant bowel necrosis and death. Delays in diagnosis have been associated with a mortality of up to 80% [1, 2]. Intestinal ischemia is broadly categorized according to the segment of the bowel to which blood flow is compromised and the acuity of onset. The presentation, management strategies, and outcomes of these entities vary widely; an accurate diagnosis is thus paramount.

Whereas colonic ischemia (ischemic colitis) is limited to the colon, mesenteric ischemia primarily affects the small bowel. Patients with chronic mesenteric ischemia (CMI) exhibit episodic or recurrent intestinal angina and "food fear" and can be managed less urgently [3].

AMI requires immediate intervention. Thrombotic or embolic occlusion of the superior mesenteric artery is the most common cause of AMI [4]. Less frequent etiologies include mesenteric venous thrombosis and nonocclusive mesenteric ischemia (NOMI).

45.2 What Is the Ideal Mode of Imaging in the Diagnosis of Acute or Chronic Mesenteric Ischemia?

The initial presentation of patients with AMI is vague and nonspecific, making timely diagnosis challenging. Severe periumbilical pain or "pain out of proportion with physical examination" associated with vomiting should raise suspicion.

Unlike other vascular disorders, AMI primarily affects women; more than 70% of patients are female. Tenderness on examination suggests bowel necrosis causing peritoneal irritation. As the disease progresses and bowel ischemia sets in, lactic acidosis and signs of shock may ensue. The clinician should not wait for severe leukocytosis or lactic acidosis to intervene, as these often are markers of severe ischemia or irreversible bowel injury [1].

High-resolution computed tomography (CT) angiography is the diagnostic modality of choice for AMI. With a sensitivity and specificity of 95%, not only does it establish the diagnosis, but it can also distinguish embolic from thrombotic or nonocclusive etiologies as well as aid in therapeutic decision-making [5, 6].

Duplex ultrasound is not particularly useful in the setting of AMI. Visualization beyond the main branches is limited under normal circumstances, and even more challenging in patients with AMI with extensive bowel gas and patient discomfort. In patients with CMI, a peak systolic velocity (PSV) of ≥275 cm/second in the superior mesenteric artery (SMA) and ≥200 cm/second in the celiac artery (CA) are predictive of >70% stenosis [7].

In the setting of AMI, MRA is of limited value. In patients with CMI, MRA can provide accurate imaging; however, CTA is superior due to faster acquisition times, better resolution, and the improved ability to visualize flow through metallic stents [8].

Angiographic evaluation is both diagnostic and therapeutic for AMI and CMI. Given its invasive nature, it is often performed after the diagnosis is confirmed with CTA.

RECOMMENDATION

In AMI, CTA or diagnostic angiography is the diagnostic modality of choice. For CMI, duplex ultrasound, CTA, MRA, and angiography offer diagnostic accuracy in detecting mesenteric disease

Level IIIb evidence in CMI; Grade of recommendation: B.

45.3 Can Endovascular Therapy Be Recommended for Acute Thromboembolic Mesenteric Ischemia?

The goal of the intervention is focused on expeditious restoration of visceral perfusion. In patients with embolic disease, this is achieved via midline laparotomy and open Fogarty catheter embolectomy.

In patients with thrombotic disease, however, thrombectomy alone is unlikely to be effective or durable, as the underlying disease process causing thrombosis is not being addressed. Mesenteric bypass, classically considered the "gold standard," constructs a graft from the aorta or iliac artery to a site distal to the occlusion. It offers excellent relief and is remarkably durable. However, it can be prohibitive in patients in shock or those with extensive cardiovascular comorbidities [9].

Endovascular treatment, typically using mechanical thrombectomy and angioplasty +/– stenting, may be as effective as traditional surgical approaches while eliminating the need for aortic cross-clamping, thus minimizing physiologic insult [10–12].

A hybrid approach, retrograde open mesenteric stenting, involves endarterectomy with patch angioplasty of the SMA followed by retrograde stenting and treatment of the inflow [13]. Following revascularization, the abdomen should be explored and the necrotic bowel resected. Marginal-appearing bowel should be observed; a second-look laparotomy in 24–48 hours to reevaluate the bowel is often necessary. Bowel anastomosis should not be performed in patients with questionable bowel viability or hemodynamic instability.

While no head-to-head comparisons are comparing open surgery to endovascular treatment, patients managed with an endovascular first approach have been found to have a high success rate with lower in-hospital mortality versus traditional open surgery [14–16].

RECOMMENDATION

No head-to-head comparison exists comparing open surgery with endovascular treatment for acute thromboembolic mesenteric ischemia. Endovascular treatment may be attempted first, mandating postprocedure observation for signs of intestinal infarction.

Grade of recommendation: C.

45.4 Does Evidence Favor Open Bypass or Catheter-Based Endovascular Intervention for Chronic Mesenteric Ischemia?

The management of CMI has undergone considerable evolution over the last several decades. Endovascular treatment has emerged as an effective alternative to open surgical bypass and is now the primary treatment modality for these lesions, independent of patients' surgical risk. It is associated with a significant reduction in mortality and length of stay when compared to open reconstruction [17–19]. Technical success can be achieved in the majority of patients, and multiple vessels can be treated simultaneously. Long-term patency rates; however, have remained a primary concern [20, 21]. Despite the lower overall patency of stents compared to surgical bypass, the majority of reinterventions required for restenosis or stent occlusion can be managed endovascularly [22].

Open mesenteric bypass, traditionally the "gold-standard" therapy in CMI, remains a durable option with relatively low reintervention rates. Mortality rates of less than 3% have been reported at high-volume centers in select patients [11].

Overall, however, open revascularization can be associated with significant morbidity in CMI patients, who are often chronically malnourished and harbor extensive cardiovascular comorbidities. Mesenteric bypass may be best reserved for patients who have failed a percutaneous intervention in the setting of multiple recurrent in-stent stenosis or occlusions and in patients with extensive disease, especially long-segment or flush calcific occlusions (occlusion of the artery at its origin with severe calcific disease).

Open and endovascular therapeutic options should thus be viewed as complementary rather than competing modalities.

RECOMMENDATION

Percutaneous angioplasty and stenting is the primary treatment modality of CMI. Long-term patency remains a concern. Mesenteric bypass may be best reserved for patients who have failed a percutaneous intervention.

Grade of recommendation: B.

45.5 Should Open Revascularization for CMI Include Single or Multiple-Vessel Reconstruction?

The surgical approach to revascularization in patients with CMI is dictated by the patient's overall pathology and physiological condition. Patients with an overall higher atherosclerotic disease burden may benefit from both celiac and SMA revascularization. In multiple retrospective case series, no statistically significant difference in either primary patency or mortality has been shown between single (SMA) and multiple vessel reconstruction [23].

RECOMMENDATION

The data are inconclusive. The choice of open revascularization technique may be tailored to the patient.

Grade of recommendation: C.

45.6 What Is the Ideal Treatment for Acute Mesenteric Venous Thrombosis?

The mainstay of treatment of mesenteric venous thrombosis is systemic anticoagulation with observation for signs of development of intestinal infarction, which would mandate surgical exploration and resection of the involved bowel [24]. In cirrhotic patients (and those with varices), treatment is first directed toward the varices, and once addressed, patients should then be treated with anticoagulation. Anticoagulation therapy reduces mortality and the recurrence of symptoms [25].

RECOMMENDATION

Systemic anticoagulation with serial observation for signs of bowel infarction.

Grade of recommendation: C.

45.7 What Is the Ideal Treatment for Nonocclusive Mesenteric Ischemia?

NOMI is most frequently encountered in patients in shock and those with low-flow states (congestive heart failure [CHF], post–myocardial infarction [MI], end-stage kidney disease [ESKD]

on hemodialysis [HD]). It is exacerbated by vasopressors or medications associated with mesenteric vasospasm (cocaine, digitalis, etc.) and can occur in the absence of underlying atherosclerotic lesions. Vigorous treatment of the underlying cause of low cardiac output while avoiding agents that may exacerbate gut ischemia remains the cornerstone of treatment [26, 27].

RECOMMENDATION

In patients with NOMI who do not respond to systemic supportive therapy, early angiography with an intraarterial infusion of vasodilators (typically papaverine) and selective laparotomy for gut infarction are recommended.

Grade of recommendation: C.

TABLE 45.1

Clinical Questions

Question	Answer	Grade of Recommendation	References
What is the ideal mode of imaging in CMI and AMI?	AMI—CTA, angiogram CMI—duplex, CTA, angiogram	B	[5–8]
Endovascular therapy for AMI?	Thrombectomy ± stenting of underlying lesions	C	[9–12]
Open or endovascular treatment for CMI?	*Embolic*: Open embolectomy *Thrombotic*: Endovascular/Bypass *Laparotomy*: Assess bowel viability	B	[11–15]
Single or multivessel open reconstruction?	Equivalent. May be tailored to the patient	Can't	[12, 15, 16]
How to treat mesenteric venous thrombosis?	Anticoagulation ± surgery for peritonitis. Catheter-directed thrombolysis may be safe	C	[24, 25]
How to treat NOMI?	Resuscitation, wean off pressors Catheter-directed vasodilators ± surgery for peritonitis	C	[26, 27]

TABLE 45.2

Levels of Evidence

Subject	References	Level of Evidence	Strength of Recommendation	Findings
Duplex vs. angiography in CMI	[5, 6]	Ib	B	Duplex sensitivity/specificity is 92% and 96% for SMA and 87% and 80% for CA
CT angiography	[5, 6]	IIIb	B	Improved sensitivity/specificity when examining a constellation of findings
MRA for CMI	[8]	IIIb	B	CTA is superior to MRA in the diagnosis of mesenteric ischemia
Thrombolysis for AMI	[9–12]	IV	C	Thrombolysis +/– laparotomy may be attempted for thromboembolic AMI
OR vs. PAS for CMI	[12–15]	IIIB	B	OR more durable, higher M&M
Single or multivessel open reconstruction	[12, 16]	IV	C	No difference between single and multiple vessel open reconstruction
Anticoagulation for MVT	[24, 25]	IV	C	Anticoagulant treatment is safe and effective in most patients with MVT
Vasodilator therapy for NOMI	[26, 27]	IV	C	Case series describe vasodilator therapy for NOMI

Editor's Note

Fortunately, mesenteric ischemia is unusual. Unfortunately, this means that a single institution has limited experience with the entity, and therefore, there is little high-quality evidence supporting our current management protocols. Acute mesenteric ischemia typically presents in the emergency situation in elderly patients with significant comorbidity, which further complicates investigation. The major development of the last few decades is the employment of endovascular techniques to the restoration of blood flow in specific circumstances to improve bowel viability.

REFERENCES

1. Clair DG, Beach JM. Mesenteric ischemia. New England Journal of Medicine. 2016;374(10):959–68.
2. Mamode N, Pickford I, Leiberman P. Failure to improve outcome in acute mesenteric ischaemia: seven year review. The European Journal of Surgery. 1999;165(3):203–8.
3. Boley S, Freiber W, Winslow P, Gliedman M, Veith F. Circulatory responses to acute reduction of superior mesenteric arterial flow. Physiologist. 1969;12:180.
4. Acosta S, Ögren M, Sternby N-H, Bergqvist D, Björck M. Clinical implications for the management of acute thromboembolic occlusion of the superior mesenteric artery: autopsy findings in 213 patients. Annals of Surgery. 2005; 241(3):516.
5. Kim AY, Ha HK. Evaluation of suspected mesenteric ischemia: efficacy of radiologic studies. Radiologic Clinics. 2003;41(2):327–42.
6. Huber TS, Björck M, Chandra A, Clouse WD, Dalsing MC, Oderich GS, et al. Chronic mesenteric ischemia: clinical practice guidelines from the Society for Vascular Surgery. Journal of Vascular Surgery. 2021;73(1):87S–115S.
7. Mitchell EL, Moneta GL. Mesenteric duplex scanning. Perspectives in Vascular Surgery and Endovascular Therapy. 2006;18(2):175–83.
8. Laissy J, Trillaud H, Douek P. MR angiography: noninvasive vascular imaging of the abdomen. Abdominal Imaging. 2002;27(5):488–506.
9. Oderich GS. Current concepts in the management of chronic mesenteric ischemia. Current Treatment Options in Cardiovascular Medicine. 2010;12(2):117–30.
10. Oderich GS, Bower TC, Sullivan TM, Bjarnason H, Cha S, Gloviczki P. Open versus endovascular revascularization for chronic mesenteric ischemia: risk-stratified outcomes. Journal of Vascular Surgery. 2009;49(6):1472–9.e3.
11. Oderich GS, Gloviczki P, Bower TC. Open surgical treatment for chronic mesenteric ischemia in the endovascular era: when it is necessary and what is the preferred technique? Seminars in Vascular Surgery. 2010;23(1):36–46.
12. Oderich GS, Malgor RD, Ricotta JJ, 2nd. Open and endovascular revascularization for chronic mesenteric ischemia: tabular review of the literature. Annals of Vascular Surgery. 2009;23(5):700–12.
13. Wyers MC, Powell RJ, Nolan BW, Cronenwett JL. Retrograde mesenteric stenting during laparotomy for acute occlusive mesenteric ischemia. Journal of Vascular Surgery. 2007;45(2): 269–75.
14. Roussel A, Castier Y, Nuzzo A, Pellenc Q, Sibert A, Panis Y, et al. Revascularization of acute mesenteric ischemia after creation of a dedicated multidisciplinary center. Journal of Vascular Surgery. 2015;62(5):1251–6.
15. Roy T, Forbes T, Wright G, Dueck A. Burning bridges: Mechanisms and implications of endovascular failure in the treatment of peripheral artery disease. Journal of Endovascular Therapy: An Official Journal of the International Society of Endovascular Specialists. 2015; 22(6):874–80.
16. Sivamurthy N, Rhodes JM, Lee D, Waldman DL, Green RM, Davies MG. Endovascular versus open mesenteric revascularization: immediate benefits do not equate with short-term functional outcomes. Journal of the American College of Surgeons. 2006;202(6):859–67.
17. Schermerhorn ML, Giles KA, Hamdan AD, Wyers MC, Pomposelli FB. Mesenteric revascularization: management and outcomes in the United States, 1988–2006. Journal of Vascular Surgery. 2009;50(2):341–8.e1.
18. Becquemin J. Management of the diseases of mesenteric arteries and veins: clinical practice guidelines of the European Society for Vascular Surgery (ESVS). European Journal of Vascular and Endovascular Surgery. 2017;53(4): 455–7.
19. Lim S, Halandras PM, Bechara C, Aulivola B, Crisostomo P. Contemporary management of acute mesenteric ischemia in the endovascular era. Vascular and Endovascular Surgery. 2019;53(1):42–50.
20. Atkins MD, Kwolek CJ, LaMuraglia GM, Brewster DC, Chung TK, Cambria RP. Surgical revascularization versus endovascular therapy for chronic mesenteric ischemia: a comparative experience. Journal of Vascular Surgery. 2007; 45(6):1162–71.
21. Kasirajan K, O'Hara PJ, Gray BH, Hertzer NR, Clair DG, Greenberg RK, et al. Chronic mesenteric ischemia: open surgery versus percutaneous angioplasty and stenting. Journal of Vascular Surgery. 2001;33(1):63–71.
22. Tallarita T, Oderich GS, Macedo TA, Gloviczki P, Misra S, Duncan AA, et al. Reinterventions for stent restenosis in patients treated for atherosclerotic mesenteric artery disease. Journal of Vascular Surgery. 2011;54(5):1422–9. e1.
23. Park WM, Cherry KJ, Jr., Chua HK, Clark RC, Jenkins G, Harmsen WS, et al. Current results of open revascularization for chronic mesenteric ischemia: a standard for comparison. Journal of Vascular Surgery. 2002;35(5):853–9.
24. Salim S, Zarrouk M, Elf J, Gottsäter A, Ekberg O, Acosta S. Improved prognosis and low failure rate with anticoagulation as first-line therapy in mesenteric venous thrombosis. World Journal of Surgery. 2018;42(11):3803–11.
25. Ageno W, Riva N, Schulman S, Beyer-Westendorf J, Bang SM, Senzolo M, et al. Long-term clinical outcomes of splanchnic vein thrombosis: results of an international registry. JAMA Internal Medicine. 2015;175(9):1474–80.
26. Miyazawa R, Kamo M. What affects the prognosis of NOMI patients? Analysis of clinical data and CT findings. Surgical Endoscopy. 2020;34(12):5327–30.
27. Stahl K, Rittgerodt N, Busch M, Maschke SK, Schneider A, Manns MP, et al. Nonocclusive mesenteric ischemia and interventional local vasodilatory therapy: a meta-analysis and systematic review of the literature. Journal of Intensive Care Medicine. 2020;35(2):128–39.

46

Hemorrhoids

Clarence E. Clark and Adatee Okonkwo

46.1 Introduction

In the United States, the prevalence of symptomatic hemorrhoids has ranged from a rate of 4.4% (or 10 million people) to 40% [1–3]. Nearly 3.2 million ambulatory care visits and over 300,000 hospitalizations are reported per year for hemorrhoids in the United States, making this condition a significant healthcare issue [4].

Hemorrhoids are classified as internal, external, or mixed. Internal hemorrhoids (IHs) are vascular cushions found above the dentate line, and external hemorrhoids (EHs) are found below the dentate line [5]. IHs are further classified based on their symptoms: Grade I hemorrhoids are those that cause bleeding but do not prolapse; grade II hemorrhoids prolapse out of the anal canal during defecation and spontaneously return to their anatomical position; grade III hemorrhoids prolapse and require digital replacement; and grade IV hemorrhoids are prolapsed and cannot be reduced [5].

Evaluation starts with a history and physical exam, paying close attention to complaints of anal bleeding, itching, discharge, discomfort, pain, or prolapse. Anoscopy is included to help classify the type of hemorrhoids in question.

Because this disease is commonly seen in general and colorectal surgical practices, evidence-based data are essential for guiding nonoperative and operative treatment decisions. Conservative measures (topical agents, stool softeners, and dietary/lifestyle modifications) are effective first-line treatments, but the focus of this chapter will be recent evidence-based data on the treatment of hemorrhoids after the failure of conservative management. Details of techniques for the listed interventions will not be discussed in this chapter and can be found in their original articles.

46.2 Management of Internal Hemorrhoids

46.2.1 Observation for Symptomatic Internal Hemorrhoids

Observation of symptomatic IHs still has a place in clinical practice, but comparative outcomes studies demonstrate a limited role. For example, in a prospective randomized trial, Jensen et al. compared rubber band ligation (RBL) to observation alone in patients with their first episode of symptomatic grade II hemorrhoids [6]. The median follow-up was 48 months. The need to treat patients for recurrent symptoms with excisional hemorrhoidectomy favored the RBL group compared to the observation group (29.6% versus 40.2%, respectively). In addition, relief of symptoms after initial therapy was 48% in the RBL group compared to 19.8% in the observation group. Lastly, the authors noted a significant difference in actuarial recurrence rates at 48 months favoring RBL over observation (33% versus 61%, $p < 0.05$).

> **RECOMMENDATION**
>
> Observation alone significantly increases the risk of developing symptomatic hemorrhoids requiring surgery. Intervention should be considered early in these patients given the clear benefit of symptom relief. Early intervention with RBL is superior to the observation of grade II internal hemorrhoids:
>
> Level of evidence: Ib. Grade of recommendation: A.

46.2.2 Nonexcisional Management Strategies for the Treatment of Symptomatic Hemorrhoids

Hemorrhoid embolization, anal dilation, injection sclerotherapy (IS), cryotherapy, infrared coagulation, laser therapy, diathermy coagulation, and RBL have been described as outpatient, nonexcisional options for treating symptomatic IHs [7–15]. Here, we will discuss the evidence-based data of these treatment modalities.

46.2.2.1 Hemorrhoid Embolization

In 2014, Vidal et al. published a novel treatment modality for symptomatic hemorrhoids using endovascular embolization coined "emborrhoid" [15]. This approach allows the interventionalist to identify the arterial branches of the hemorrhoidal cushions for embolization while reducing trauma seen in excisional approaches. Since Vidal's publication, several observational studies have reported the use of polyvinyl alcohol particles, tris-acryl gelatin particles, and coils to occlude arterial branches to bleeding hemorrhoids [15–21]. This modern approach to hemorrhoids has a reported clinical success rate of 63–97% [15–21]. Further randomized trials comparing this approach to gold-standard nonoperative and operative treatment options are needed with long-term data before the universal adoption of this endovascular strategy.

46.2.2.2 Anal Dilation

A randomized prospective study in Europe with a 17-year follow-up compared anal dilation to surgical hemorrhoidectomy for grade II–III hemorrhoids [7]. Three groups were assigned: Group A underwent Milligan hemorrhoidectomy (41 patients), group B underwent the original Lord's six-finger dilation with a dilator (46 patients), and group C underwent anal dilation as described previously without a dilator (51 patients). More patients were symptom-free in group A (52%) versus group B (23%) and group C (27%) after treatment. The recurrence of hemorrhoids was lower for the hemorrhoidectomy group. Fecal incontinence was the major complication found during follow-up for groups B and C (52% of the total patients).

46.2.2.3 Rubber Band Ligation, Sclerotherapy, and Infrared Photocoagulation

A meta-analysis by MacRae et al. compared several of the nonoperative treatment methods to surgical hemorrhoidectomy [8]. Overall, patients undergoing hemorrhoidectomy had a significantly better response to treatment than did patients treated with RBL ($p = 0.001$), although this was at a cost of a significantly greater risk of complications ($p = 0.02$) and pain ($p < 0.0001$). For grade III hemorrhoids alone, no difference was shown. RBL was shown to be significantly better than IS in response to treatment ($p = 0.005$). This difference was shown for both grade I and II hemorrhoids ($p = 0.007$) and grade III hemorrhoids ($p = 0.042$), with no significant difference in the complication rate. Patients treated with RBL were less likely to require further therapy than those treated with either IS ($p = 0.031$) or infrared photocoagulation ($p = 0.0014$). Despite this trend, the pain was significantly more likely to occur following RBL. No difference was found between IS and infrared photocoagulation for any of the outcomes. Therefore, the authors concluded that RBL is the therapy of choice for grade I–II hemorrhoids and the first-line treatment for grade III prolapsing hemorrhoids, reserving hemorrhoidectomy for patients whose symptoms are not relieved with this modality.

46.2.2.4 Doppler-Guided Laser Therapy

Giamundo et al. randomized 60 patients with grades II and III hemorrhoids to either RBL or Doppler-guided laser therapy (also known as the hemorrhoidal laser procedure or HeLP) [9]. Immediate postprocedural pain and reduction of postprocedural analgesics were improved in the HeLP group ($p < 0.001$ and $p = 0.038$, respectively). In addition, the downgrading of IHs by at least one grade ($p < 0.001$) and resolution of symptoms at 6 months ($p < 0.001$) were noticed in the HeLP group. The authors concluded that both RBL and the HeLP procedures are effective for grades II and III hemorrhoids but favor the HeLP procedure over RBL in treating symptomatic hemorrhoids due to the overall improvement of immediate postprocedural pain [9].

46.2.2.5 Rubber Band Ligation Compared to Excisional Hemorrhoidectomy

A meta-analysis of randomized controlled trials (RCTs) comparing RBL to excisional hemorrhoidectomy (closed or open) [10] found RBL to be as effective for grade II hemorrhoids. For grade III hemorrhoids, the recurrence rate was improved with hemorrhoidectomy. Symptoms (incontinence, anal stenosis, sepsis, and significant bleeding), time from intervention to return to work, and complications were higher for excisional hemorrhoidectomy.

RECOMMENDATION

RBL is the therapy of choice for grade I and II IHs. RBL should be the first-line treatment for grade III prolapsing hemorrhoids, reserving hemorrhoidectomy for patients whose symptoms are not relieved. Laser therapy is another viable nonoperative option for grade II and III IHs. Anal dilation should be abandoned due to the significant morbidity associated with this treatment modality.

Level of evidence: Ib. Grade of recommendation: A.

46.2.3 Recent Advances in Nonoperative Management of Internal Hemorrhoids

Multiple approaches to the nonoperative, in-office management of IHs have been described. Traditional approaches include RBL, sclerotherapy, and energy ablation, including infrared photocoagulation and bipolar diathermy. RBL was first described by Blaisdel in 1954 and subsequently popularized with the demonstration of increased efficacy by Barron in 1963 [22, 23]. The traditional technique involves the placement of a rubber band on the hemorrhoid column, which leads to subsequent strangulation and necrosis. Recently, Jin et al. described and evaluated modified rubber band ligation (MRBL) using an elastic coil in the management of grade III IHs [24]. A total of 120 patients were randomly assigned to MRBL (60 patients) or open excisional hemorrhoidectomy (60 patients). Recurrence at 1 year, defined as recurrent bleeding or symptomatic recurrence, was similar in the two groups (4 vs. 2 patients, $p = 0.39$). Secondary outcomes, including postoperative pain, bleeding, and urinary retention, were significantly less in the MRBL group ($p < 0.05$). At 1 month follow-up, resting anorectal pressure (RAP) remained unchanged in the MRBL group. In the hemorrhoidectomy cohort, RAP was significantly increased compared to baseline values ($p < 0.01$) and compared to postoperative MRBL values ($p < 0.01$). (Increased RAP may result in postoperative defecatory dysfunction and increase the risk of anal canal stenosis.)

A BANANA-Clip (BC), designed to reduce the incidence of delayed bleeding and rectal stenosis, has also been described for treating IHs [25]. The BC, named after its curvilinear shape, is a nonabsorbable polymer clip designed to facilitate ligation and necrosis with minimal foreign body reaction. Kang et al. compared the use of BC vs. RBL in patients with grade I–III hemorrhoids [25]. A total of 632 patients were enrolled and assigned to BC or RBL (316 patients each). Most patients in the RBL group were grade II hemorrhoids (50%) vs. grade III in the BC group (56%, $p < 0.001$). The number of triple ligations in one session was significantly higher in the BC group (29% vs. 3.8% RBL, $p < 0.001$). Delayed bleeding, defined as bleeding requiring operative intervention within 2 weeks of the procedure, only occurred in the RBL group (11 patients, 3.5% $p < 0.001$). There was no difference in minor complications, including minor bleeding, pain, band slippage, or urinary retention. Success was defined as the absence of relapsing symptoms, including pain, bleeding, and prolapse. The 1-year success rate was significantly higher in the BC group (99.7 vs. 95.9%, $p = 0.005$). Early data support the use of the BC as an alternative to traditional RBL, with reduced incidence of delayed bleeding and an increased 1-year success rate.

RECOMMENDATION

These methods, MRBL and BC, are investigational. Early data support baseline safety and feasibility. Further data are needed to establish efficacy and examine long-term outcomes.

Level of evidence: IIb. Strength of recommendation: B.

46.2.4 Which Invasive Operative Strategies Have More Favorable Outcomes When Managing Symptomatic Hemorrhoids?

Surgical intervention is usually reserved for patients who fail nonoperative management. Excisional hemorrhoidectomy has long been considered the mainstay operation; however, the approach to excision has dramatically evolved to include the use of stapling and energy devices. More recently, the introduction of transanal hemorrhoidal dearterialization (THD) has emerged as a novel approach that omits excision altogether.

46.2.4.1 Open versus Closed Hemorrhoidectomy

Excisional hemorrhoidectomy may be performed in an open (Milligan-Morgan technique) or closed (Fergueson technique) fashion. The Fergueson technique was first described in the early 1950s and remains the most common approach for hemorrhoidectomy in the United States [26, 27]. Current literature evaluating the open and closed techniques has struggled to identify one as superior. Bhatti et al. sought to resolve this debate through a systematic analysis of RCTs [28]. Eleven RCTs, for a total of 1,326 patients with grade III or IV hemorrhoids, were analyzed. Six hundred and sixty-three

patients underwent closed hemorrhoidectomy (CH) and 663 patients underwent open hemorrhoidectomy (OH). It is important to note that there was significant heterogeneity among the included trials, with five trials considered to be of poor quality due to lack of adequate randomization, absence of blinding, lack of power calculations, and inadequate methods of concealment. CH demonstrated less postoperative pain (standardized mean difference [SMD] −0.36, $p = 0.01$), earlier wound healing (odds ratio [OR] 0.08, $p < 0.0001$), and decreased risk of postoperative bleeding (OR 0.50, $p < 0.02$). CH was associated with longer operative times (SMD 6.10, $p < 0.001$). There was no significant difference in additional variables: Pain on defecation, length of hospital stay, postoperative complications, risk of recurrence, and risk of surgical site infection. These data support the clinical safety and efficacy of the closed and open technique, while CH offers the advantages of lower postoperative pain, decreased postoperative bleeding, and improved wound healing.

46.2.4.2 Use of Energy Devices

Excisional hemorrhoidectomy has been long considered the "gold standard" of hemorrhoidectomy, upon which newer techniques are evaluated against. Modified approaches to hemorrhoidectomy employ energy sources, including bipolar diathermy and ultrasonic shears. The use of a bipolar electrothermal sealing device (Ligasure) achieves sealing and hemostasis before the excision of hemorrhoidal tissue [29]. A 2009 Cochrane review comparing Ligasure hemorrhoidectomy to conventional techniques, open and closed hemorrhoidectomy, found a significant reduction in early postoperative pain with no difference in postoperative complications. The pain score was significantly less in the Ligasure group; however, this reduction diminished at 14 days [29]. Improved short-term outcomes, including intraoperative blood loss, postoperative pain, and earlier return to work, have been demonstrated in subsequent studies [30, 31]. The use of the harmonic scalpel has shown similar improvements in short-term outcomes. A 2014 meta-analysis demonstrated significantly less postoperative pain and earlier return to work following harmonic scalpel hemorrhoidectomy compared to conventional techniques [32].

46.2.4.3 Stapled Hemorrhoidopexy

Stapled hemorrhoidopexy, introduced by Longo in 1998, uses a circular stapling device to excise circumferential IHs and create a mucosa-to-mucosa anastomosis proximal to the dentate line [33]. This technique, also known as the procedure for prolapsing hemorrhoids (PPH), results in the excision of redundant tissue and cephalad relocation of the anal cushions, thus restoring normal anatomy. Longo reported shorter operative time and improved postoperative pain compared to conventional hemorrhoidectomy [33]. Nisar et al. performed a meta-analysis of 15 RCTs, for a total of 1,077 patients, comparing stapled hemorrhoidopexy with conventional hemorrhoidectomy [34]. Disease severity varied, while the majority evaluated grade III and IV hemorrhoids, three trials recruited a total of 51 patients with second-degree hemorrhoids.

Follow-up ranged from 6 weeks to 37 months. Meta-analysis favored PPH regarding postoperative pain, with significantly less pain at 24 hours (four trials), at 1 and 2 weeks (six trials), and at 6 weeks (two trials). PPH demonstrated a significantly shorter operative time (–12.82 minutes, $P = 0.01$), shorter inpatient stay (–1.02 days, $P = 0.0001$), and earlier return to normal activity (–4.03 days, $P = 0.007$). The overall complication rate was only reported in three trials with no significant differences; however, the meta-analysis did demonstrate a higher recurrence rate after PPH (OR 3.64, $P = 0.008$). A subsequent meta-analysis of 27 RCTs, 2,279 patients, similarly reported less postoperative pain but significantly higher recurrence (OR 4.34, $P = 0.003$) and a higher need for reintervention for prolapse (OR 5.78, $P = 0.002$) [35]. The authors concluded that stapled hemorrhoidopexy is a less painful yet less effective alternative to conventional hemorrhoidectomy. Further, they identified the need for long-term outcomes to evaluate the unique complications of this approach [34].

In a systematic review, Porrett et al. sought to better elucidate the long-term sequelae of stapled hemorrhoidopexy [36]. The search identified 92 articles, 29 RCTs, 7 comparative studies, 23 noncomparative studies, and 21 case reports, for a total of 14,245 patients undergoing PPH. All patients had grade II–IV hemorrhoids. The primary endpoint was early and late complications, defined as complications occurring within or after 7 days, respectively. Patient follow-up ranged from 1 month to 7 years. The median early complication rate was 16.1% (range 2.3–52.5%). Bleeding was the most common early and late complication. Early complications unique to PPH included failure of the stapling gun, urosepsis, and pelvic sepsis. All 16 cases of sepsis required hospitalization and surgical reintervention, with one patient requiring diversion. Four deaths were identified, all associated with rectal perforation and subsequent sepsis. Cases of rectovaginal fistula and rectal stricture were also reported. The median late complication was 23.7% (range 2.5–80%). Proctitis was a unique late complication to PPH, and tenesmus was more commonly reported following PPH, with an occurrence rate of up to 40%.

RECOMMENDATION

Traditional excisional hemorrhoidectomy has long been considered the gold standard, to which newer methods of hemorrhoidectomy are compared. Conventional hemorrhoidectomy may be performed in an open or closed fashion. The closed technique offers the advantages of decreased postoperative pain and improved wound healing. The use of energy devices has not been proven superior to conventional hemorrhoidectomy, but their use may improve early short-term outcomes. PPH may also offer improvement in postoperative pain, albeit at the expense of decreased efficacy and unique complications. Conventional hemorrhoidectomy and hemorrhoidectomy employing energy devices are superior to PPH.

Level of evidence: Ia. Strength of recommendation: A.

46.2.5 What Are the More Recent Advances in Operative Management of Internal Hemorrhoids?

THD is a recent innovative approach to the management of IHs. This approach involves the targeted ligation of hemorrhoidal arteries using an anoscope fashioned with a Doppler probe. THD can be combined with subsequent mucopexy and plication of the redundant mucosa and submucosa, resulting in the restoration of normal anatomy [37]. In a 2016 meta-analysis of randomized control trials, Xu et al. aimed to analyze the outcomes of THD with mucopexy against open hemorrhoidectomy [38]. Four RCTs, including 316 patients with grade II–IV hemorrhoids, were analyzed. Follow-up ranged from 12 to 43 months. There was no significant difference in total complications (OR 0.69; $p = 0.14$). Further, there was no difference in bleeding (OR 0.41, $p = 0.06$), gas or fecal incontinence (OR 0.14, $p = 0.07$), recurrent prolapse (OR 3.15, $p = 0.07$), or urinary retention (OR 0.59, $p = 0.30$). There was no significant difference in postoperative pain 7 days after surgery. One trial demonstrated no difference at 1, 3, 4, and 14 days after surgery. There was a significant difference in return to convalescence, favoring THD (OR –11.06, $p < 0.00001$). The authors determined THD with mucopexy and open hemorrhoidectomy to be equally effective.

Current literature supports THD as a noninferior approach to hemorrhoidectomy, compared to stapled hemorrhoidopexy and vessel-sealing device hemorrhoidectomy (VSH) [39, 40]. In a subsequent 2019 meta-analysis, Xu et al. investigated clinical outcomes of stapled hemorrhoidopexy and THD [39]. Their analysis included nine RCTs for a total of 1,077 patients, of which 533 underwent stapled hemorrhoidopexy and 542 underwent THD. Again, there was no difference in total or individual complications, postoperative bleeding, residual skin tag or prolapse, or urinary retention. There was no difference in postoperative pain or return to work. In a different meta-analysis of six RCTs involving 554 patients (THD = 280; VSH = 274), Emile et al. detected a significant difference in early postoperative pain, defined as within 24 hours from surgery (2.9 ± 1.5 versus 3.3 ± 1.6, $p = 0.002$) [41]. There was no difference in total complications or average return to work.

In a multicenter RCT, Trenti et al. compared THD with mucopexy with Ligasure hemorrhoidectomy [40]. Eighty patients met the inclusion criteria (39 patients undergoing THD versus 41 VSH). The primary outcome was the mean postoperative number of days in which patients required nonsteroidal antiinflammatory drugs (NSAIDs). The number of patients taking NSAIDs in the second postoperative week was significantly higher in the VSH group (87.8% vs. 53.8%, $p = 0.002$). Similarly, the average number of days patients required pain medication was higher in the VSH group (15.2 vs. 10.1 days, $p = 0.006$). Secondary outcomes included 30-day morbidity, use of laxatives, fecal continence status, patient satisfaction, and quality of life. There was no difference demonstrated in secondary outcomes.

46.3 Management of Thrombosed External Hemorrhoids

46.3.1 What Is the Best Management Strategy for Symptomatic External Hemorrhoids?

IHs and EHs are differentiated by their location, in addition to differences in innervation and sensation. IHs are proximal to the dentate line with overlying anal mucosa, while EHs are distal to the dentate line with overlying anoderm. Differences in innervation and sensation explain typical symptomology. EHs have somatic innervation, resulting in the classic symptom of acute anal pain in the setting of acute thrombosis. The exact etiology of thrombosis remains undefined but has been linked with increased intravenous pressure within the hemorrhoidal plexus that leads to rupture of the endothelial lining and subsequent thrombosis [42–44]. Thrombosed external hemorrhoids (TEHs) may be managed surgically with excision, incision, or nonoperatively with conservative measures. There is a paucity of data in the literature comparing nonoperative and operative approaches.

46.3.2 Conservative Management

A variety of interventions have been proposed for the nonoperative management of TEHs, including dietary modification, sitz baths, and analgesics. Gebbensleben et al. questioned the need for surgical intervention in the management of TEHs in a prospective cohort study [45]. A total of 72 patients were enrolled and managed with a strict conservative management approach, limited to gentle dry cleaning with smooth toilet paper after defecation. Follow-up information was obtained at 6 months by phone questionnaire. Only 48 out of 72 patients completed the questionnaire. Compliance was reported at more than 1 week (37.5%), 1 week (25%), and not at all or unknown (37.5%). The majority of patients (45 patients) described themselves as "healed" or "ameliorated," while 3 patients reported symptoms as "unchanged." Nearly half of respondents (22 patients, 45.8%) reported at least one symptom, of which itching was the most common (18.8%). Recurrence was suspected in 13.9% (10/72 patients); however, 25 patients did not answer this question and 3 patients did not know. Therapy following suspected recurrence varied: Surgery (2 patients), ointments or suppository (2 patients), and reinstitution of proposed anal cleaning policy (13 patients). Despite limitations, including a small patient cohort and patient-based reporting, the authors concluded that a strict conservative policy can be successful. Further study with randomization and longer follow-up is needed.

Perotti et al. aimed to evaluate the utility of topical nifedipine in addition to conservative measures for the management of TEHs [46]. Patients were prospectively recruited and randomized to local application of 0.3% nifedipine and 1.5% lidocaine ointment twice daily for 2 weeks versus 1.5% lidocaine alone. Conservative measures, a high-fiber diet, bulk laxatives, and sitz baths were utilized in both groups. A total of 98 patients were recruited, 50 patients with nifedipine and 48 patients without. Results were obtained by questionnaire on day 7 and day 14. After 7 days of therapy, complete pain relief was significantly higher in the nifedipine group (86% vs. 50% of patients, $p < 0.01$). Total remission after completion of therapy was achieved in 92% of nifedipine cases compared to 45.8% of the control group ($p < 0.01$). No systemic side effects were observed with the use of nifedipine. Four patients in the nifedipine cohort required further therapy, one prolonged nifedipine therapy, and three were treated by hemorrhoidectomy. In the control group, delayed healing was demonstrated at 4 weeks (7 patients) and 6 weeks (4 patients). Fifteen patients (31.2%) required hemorrhoidectomy by 6 months follow-up. These data favor the use of nifedipine in the conservative management of TEHs.

46.3.3 Operative Management

Greenspoon et al. sought to evaluate recurrence after conservative or surgical management in a retrospective review of all patients treated for TEHs between 1990 and 2002 at their institution [47]. A total of 231 patients were identified, of which 119 patients (51.5%) were initially treated conservatively and 112 (48.5%) patients were treated surgically. Conservative management included dietary modifications, stool softeners, sitz baths, localized hygiene, and oral and topical analgesics. The majority of surgically treated patients underwent excision (109, 97.3% vs. incision 3, 2.7%). The mean follow-up was 7.6 months, with a higher rate of follow-up for the surgical group (82.1% vs. 37.8%). The overall incidence of recurrence for all patients was 15.6%. The frequency of recurrence was significantly higher for patients managed conservatively (25.4% vs. 6.3%, $p < 0.0001$). The mean time to recurrence was significantly higher in the conservative group (7.1 vs. 25 months, $p < 0.0001$). Subsequent logistic regression analysis of multiple factors, including obesity, prior TEH, constipation, and straining, was performed to identify predictors of recurrence. No variable was identified as a significant predictor of recurrence. However, patients managed conservatively were less likely to have a prior history (38.1 vs. 51.3%, $p < 0.05$) but were more likely to recur ($p < 0.0001$). The authors concluded that surgical intervention results in a lower incidence of recurrence and a longer time to recurrence.

TABLE 46.1

Clinical Questions

Question	Answer	Grade of Recommendation	References
Is observation alone a viable option for symptomatic internal hemorrhoids (IHs)?	No. The clear benefit of intervention for grade II and greater hemorrhoids is apparent.	A	[6]
Is there a clear advantage of one nonexcisional management strategy over the others for the treatment of symptomatic hemorrhoids?	Yes. Rubber band ligation (RBL) is superior to anal dilation, sclerotherapy, and infrared photocoagulation. RBL is just as effective as Doppler-guided laser therapy for grade II and III hemorrhoids.	A	[7–9]
What are the more recent advances in the nonoperative management of IHs?	MRBL and BC are safe and feasible approaches to IHs. Further data are needed to establish long-term outcomes and efficacy.	B	[24–25]
Which invasive operative strategies have more favorable outcomes when managing symptomatic hemorrhoids?	Conventional hemorrhoidectomy and hemorrhoidectomy employing energy devices are superior to PPH.	A	[34–36]
What are the more recent advances in the operative management of IHs?	THD is a noninferior alternative to excisional hemorrhoidectomy with the additional benefit of decreased postoperative pain.	A	[38–40]
What is the best management strategy for symptomatic external hemorrhoids (EHs)?	Operative management is superior to nonoperative management of TEHs, with the advantage of improved symptom control and decreased recurrence.	B	[44–47]

TABLE 46.2

Levels of Evidence

Subject	Year	Reference	Level of Evidence	Strength of Recommendation	Findings
First-line treatment of IHs	2005	[10]	Ib	A	RBL is the first-line therapy followed by hemorrhoidectomy if symptoms persist or grade IV
The open or closed technique	2016	[28]	IIb	B	Both are acceptable operative strategies with no significant difference in outcomes
Conventional hemorrhoidectomy or PPHs	2009	[35]	Ia	A	Conventional hemorrhoidectomy is superior to PPHs
Conventional hemorrhoidectomy or HAL with Doppler guidance (THD)	2016	[38]	Ib	A	THD has similar outcomes to conventional hemorrhoidectomy with less pain and narcotic use
Management of symptomatic EHs	2004	[47]	IIb	B	Excision is superior to topical agents and incision of EHs

Editor's Note

Unlike most areas of surgery, there are considerable high-quality data upon which to base clinical decisions regarding the care of hemorrhoids. Internal hemorrhoids that are asymptomatic can be observed. Symptomatic internal hemorrhoids are typically treated with rubber band ligation if grade I–III. Recurrent high-grade hemorrhoids respond best to surgical hemorrhoidectomy. External hemorrhoids are optimally managed with excision. These recommendations are grade A.

REFERENCES

1. Johanson JF, Sonnenber A. The prevalence of hemorrhoids and chronic constipation: An epidemiologic study. *Gastroenterology.* 1990;*98*.

2. Janicke DM, Pundt MR. Anorectal disorders. *Emerg Med Clin North Am.* 1996;*14*.

3. Ohning GV, Machicado GA, Jensen DM. Definitive therapy for internal hemorrhoids; new opportunities and options. *Rev Gastrenterol Disord.* 2009;*9*.

4. Everhart JE. 2008. The Burden of Digestive Diseases in the United States. National Institute of Diabetes and Digestive and Kidney Diseases, U.S. Department of Health and Human Services: Bethesda, MD.

5. Kaidar-Person O, Person B, Wexner S. Hemorrhoidal disease: A comprehensive review. *J Am Coll Surg.* Jan 2007;*204(1)*:102–117.

6. Jensen S, Harling H, Arseth-hansen P, et al. The natural history of symptomatic hemorrhoids. *Int J Colorectal Dis.* 1989;*4(1)*:41–44.

7. Konsten J, Baeten C. Hemorrhoidectomy vs Lord's method: 17-year follow-up of a prospective, randomized trial. *Dis Colon Rectum.* Apr 2000;*43(4)*:503–206.

8. MacRae H, McLeod R. Comparison of hemorrhoidal treatment modalities: A meta-analysis. *Dis Colon Rectum.* 1995;*38(7)*:687–694.

9. Giamundo P, Salfi R, Geraci M, et al. The hemorrhoid laser procedure technique vs rubber band ligation: A randomized trial comparing 2 mini-invasive treatments for second- and third-degree hemorrhoids. *Dis Colon Rectum.* 2011;*34*:693–698.

10. Shanmugam V, Thaha M, Rabindranath K, et al. Rubber band ligation versus excisional haemorrhoidectomy for haemorrhoids. *Cochrane Database Syst Rev.* 2005;*2005(1)*: Art. No.: CD005034.

11. Ono T, Goto K, Takagi S. Sclerosing effect of OC-108, a novel agent for hemorrhoids, is associated with granulomatous inflammation induced by aluminum. *J Pharmacol Sci.* 2005;*99*:353–363.

12. Ponsky J, Mellinger J, Simon I. Endoscopic retrograde hemorrhoidal sclerotherapy using 23.4% saline, a preliminary report. *Surg Today.* 2011;*41*:806–809.

13. Hachiro Y, Kunimoto M, Abe T, et al. Aluminum potassium sulfate and tannic acid (ALTA) injection as the mainstay of treatment for internal hemorrhoids. *Surg Today.* 2011;*41*:806–809.

14. Abe T. Distal hemorrhoidectomy with ALTA injection: A new method for hemorrhoid surgery. *Int Surg.* 2014;*99*:295–298.

15. Vidal V, Sapoval M, Sielezneff Y, et al. Emborrhoid: A new concept for the treatment of hemorrhoids with arterial embolization: The first 14 cases. *Cardiovasc Interv Radiol.* 2014;*38*:72–78.

16. Zakharchenko A, Kaitoukov Y, Vinnik Y, et al. Safety and efficacy of superior rectal artery embolization with particles and metallic coils for the treatment of hemorrhoids (Emborrhoid Technique). *Diagn Interv Imaging.* 2016;*97*:1079–1084.

17. Tradi F, Louis G, Giorgi R, et al. Embolization of the superior rectal arteries for hemorrhoidal disease: Prospective results in 25 patients. *J Vasc Interv Radiol.* 2018;*29*:884–892.

18. Giurazza F, Corvino F, Cavaglià E, et al. Emborrhoid in patients with portal hypertension and chronic hemorrhoidal bleeding: Preliminary results in five cases with a new coiling release fashion "Spaghetti Technique". *Radiol Med.* 2020;*125*:1008–1011.

19. El Tawab KA, Salem AA, Khafagy R. New technique of embolization of the hemorrhoidal arteries using embolization particles alone: Retrospective results in 33 patients. *Ara J Interv Radiol.* 2020;*4*:27–31.

20. Küçükay MB, Küçükay F. Superior rectal artery embolization with tri-acryl-gelatin microspheres: A randomized comparison of particle size. *J Vasc Interv Radiol.* 2021 Jun;*32(6)*:819–825.

21. Moussa N, Sielezneff I, Sapoval M, et al. Embolization of the superior rectal arteries for chronic bleeding due to haemorrhoidal disease. *Colorectal Dis.* 2016;*19*:194–199.

22. Blaisdell PC. Prevention of massive hemorrhage secondary to hemorrhoidectomy. *Surg Gynecol Obstet.* 1958 Apr; *106(4)*:485–488.

23. Barron J. Office ligation treatment of hemorrhoids. *Dis Colon Rectum.* 1963 Mar-Apr;*6*:109–113.

24. Jin L, Yang H, Qin K, et al. Efficacy of modified rubber band ligation in the treatment of grade III internal hemorrhoids. *Ann Palliat Med.* 2021 Feb;*10(2)*:1191–1197.

25. Kang DW, Kim BS, Kim JH, et al. A comparative study of rubber band ligation versus BANANA-clip in grade 1 to 3 internal hemorrhoids. *Ann Coloproctol.* 2021 Dec 9.

26. Ferguson JA, Mazier WP, Ganchrow MI, et al. The closed technique of hemorrhoidectomy. *Surgery.* 1971 Sep;*70(3)*:480–484.

27. Lohsiriwat V. Treatment of hemorrhoids: A coloproctologist's view. *World J Gastroenterol.* 2015 Aug 21;*21(31)*:9245–952.

28. Bhatti MI, Sajid MS, Baig MK. Milligan-Morgan (Open) versus Ferguson haemorrhoidectomy (Closed): A systematic review and meta-analysis of published randomized, controlled trials. *World J Surg.* 2016 Jun;*40(6)*:1509–1519.

29. Ng KS, Holzgang M, Young C. Still a case of "No Pain, No Gain"? An updated and critical review of the pathogenesis, diagnosis, and management options for hemorrhoids in 2020. *Ann Coloproctol.* 2020 Jun;*36(3)*:133–147.

30. Bakhtiar N, Moosa FA, Jaleel F, et al. Comparison of hemorrhoidectomy by Ligasure with conventional Milligan Morgan's hemorrhoidectomy. *Pak J Med Sci.* 2016 May-Jun;*32(3)*:657–661.

31. Xu L, Chen H, Lin G, et al. Ligasure versus Ferguson hemorrhoidectomy in the treatment of hemorrhoids: A meta-analysis of randomized control trials. *Surg Laparosc Endosc Percutan Tech.* 2015 Apr;*25(2)*:106–110.

32. Mushaya CD, Caleo PJ, Bartlett L, et al. Harmonic scalpel compared with conventional excisional haemorrhoidectomy: A meta-analysis of randomized controlled trials. *Tech Coloproctol.* 2014 Nov;*18(11)*:1009–1016.

33. Longo A. Treatment of hemorrhoids disease by reduction of mucosa and hemorrhoidal prolapse with a circular suturing device: a new procedure. In: Proceedings of the 6th World Congress of Endoscopic Surgery, June 3–6, 1998, Rome, Italy. Monduzzi Editore, Bologna, 1998:777–784.

34. Nisar PJ, Acheson AG, Neal KR, et al. Stapled hemorrhoidopexy compared with conventional hemorrhoidectomy: A systematic review of randomized, controlled trials. *Dis Colon Rectum.* 2004 Nov;*47(11)*:1837–1845.

35. Burch J, Epstein D, Sari AB, et al. Stapled haemorrhoidopexy for the treatment of haemorrhoids: A systematic review. *Colorectal Dis.* 2009 Mar;*11(3)*:233–243; discussion 243.

36. Porrett LJ, Porrett JK, Ho YH. Documented complications of staple hemorrhoidopexy: A systematic review. *Int Surg.* 2015 Jan;*100(1)*:44–57.

37. Ratto C. THD Doppler procedure for hemorrhoids: The surgical technique. *Tech Coloproctol.* 2014 Mar;*18(3)*:291–298.

38. Xu L, Chen H, Lin G, et al. Transanal hemorrhoidal dearterialization with mucopexy versus open hemorrhoidectomy in the treatment of hemorrhoids: A meta-analysis of randomized control trials. *Tech Coloproctol.* 2016 Dec;*20(12)*:825–833.

39. Xu L, Chen H, Gu Y. Stapled hemorrhoidectomy versus transanal hemorrhoidal dearterialization in the treatment of hemorrhoids: An updated meta-analysis. *Surg Laparosc Endosc Percutan Tech.* 2019 Apr;*29(2)*:75–81.

40. Trenti L, Biondo S, Kreisler Moreno E, et al; THDLIGA-RCT Study Group. Short-term outcomes of transanal hemorrhoidal dearterialization with mucopexy versus vessel-sealing device hemorrhoidectomy for grade III to IV hemorrhoids: A prospective randomized multicenter trial. *Dis Colon Rectum.* 2019 Aug;*62(8)*:988–996.

41. Emile SH, Elfeki H, Sakr A, et al. Transanal hemorrhoidal dearterialization (THD) versus stapled hemorrhoidopexy (SH) in treatment of internal hemorrhoids: A systematic review and meta-analysis of randomized clinical trials. *Int J Colorectal Dis.* 2019 Jan;*34(1)*:1–11.

42. Wronski K. Etiology of thrombosed external hemorrhoids. *Postepy Hig Med Dosw (Online).* 2012;*66*:41–44.

43. Gebbensleben O, Hilger Y, Rohde H. Aetiology of thrombosed external haemorrhoids: A questionnaire study. *BMC Res Notes.* 2009;*2*:216.

44. Picciariello A, Rinaldi M, Grossi U, Verre L, De Fazio M, Dezi A, Tomasicchio G, Altomare DF, Gallo G. Management and treatment of external hemorrhoidal thrombosis. *Front Surg.* 2022 May 3;*9*:898850.

45. Gebbensleben O, Hilger Y, Rohde H. Do we at all need surgery to treat thrombosed external hemorrhoids? Results of a prospective cohort study. *Clin Exp Gastroenterol.* 2009; *2*:69–74.

46. Perrotti P, Antropoli C, Molino D, De Stefano G, Antropoli M. Conservative treatment of acute thrombosed external hemorrhoids with topical nifedipine. *Dis Colon Rectum.* 2001 Mar;*44(3)*:405–409.

47. Greenspon J, Williams S, Young H, et al. Thrombosed external hemorrhoids: Outcome after conservative or surgical management. *Dis Colon Rectum.* 2004 Sep;*47(9)*: 1493–1498.

47

Anal Fissure, Fistula, and Abscess

Varun Krishnan

47.1 Introduction

Anorectal complaints are common, but often poorly understood. More often than not, a referral for "hemorrhoids" is often vague and can refer to any number of perianal abnormalities. Proper treatment depends on the correct diagnosis.

Once an accurate assessment is made, therapy can be based on evidence-based guidelines for the treatment of anorectal abscesses, fistula, and fissures. This chapter covers anal abscess, anal fissure, and fistula-in-ano (Table 47.1). Hemorrhoids and pilonidal disease are covered in other chapters.

TABLE 47.1

Overall Evidence Table

Question	Answer	Levels of Evidence	Grade of Recommendation	References
How do nonoperative medical therapies (nitroglycerin, calcium channel blockers, and botulinum toxin) compare with placebo and lateral internal sphincterotomy in the treatment of anal fissures?	Nonsurgical therapies are superior to placebo but inferior to lateral internal sphincterotomy for healing anal fissures.	Ia	A	[1–6]
What is the impact of the technique on the outcomes of patients undergoing surgery for anal fissures?	Lateral internal sphincterotomy (open or closed) is the surgical treatment of choice for chronic anal fissures.	Ia	A	[1, 7–12]
What is the healing and incontinence rate for fistulotomy for simple fistula-in-ano?	Fistulotomy is appropriate for simple fistula-in-ano with high rates of healing and low rates of incontinence.	Ib	A	[13, 14]
What is the healing and incontinence rate for more complex fistulas treated with fibrin glue, fistula plug, or a seton?	Treatment of complex fistula-in-ano by fibrin glue and fistula plug is generally not recommended. Cutting seton may be used in carefully selected patients, but success and incontinence rates vary.	IIb–IIc	C	[13–22]
What is the healing and incontinence rate for more complex fistulas treated with an endorectal advancement flap?	Complex fistula-in-ano may be successfully treated with an endorectal advancement flap. Recurrent fistula-in-ano may be treated by endorectal advancement flap with modest success rates. Incontinence is infrequent.	Ib	B	[14, 23–25]
What is the role of ligation of intersphincteric fistula tract (LIFT) in the management of fistula-in-ano?	Transsphincteric fistula-in-ano may be successfully treated with LIFT. Incontinence is infrequent.	Ib	B	[14, 26–29]
Is there any role for minimally invasive approaches to fistula-in-ano?	Minimally invasive treatments for cryptoglandular fistula-in-ano have reasonable short-term healing rates with unknown long-term healing and recurrence rates. No recommendation due to the paucity of long-term follow-up data.	IIIa	C	[14, 30–32]
Are antibiotics unnecessary for most patients undergoing routine incisions and drainage of perirectal abscesses?	Antibiotics are unnecessary for most patients following adequate drainage and should be used for patients with extensive cellulitis, systemic sepsis, or immunosuppression. It is unclear whether antibiotics have an effect on fistula formation after incision and drainage of an anal abscess.	IIb	C	[14, 33, 34]

DOI: 10.1201/9781003316800-47

47.2 How Do Nonoperative Medical Therapies (Nitroglycerin, Calcium Channel Blockers, and Botulinum Toxin) Compare with Placebo and Lateral Internal Sphincterotomy in the Treatment of Anal Fissures?

Multiple randomized prospective trials have examined the role of various nonoperative therapies in the treatment of anal fissures. All effective modalities are aimed at decreasing the hypertonicity found in the internal anal sphincter of fissure patients. Therapies that do not lower sphincter pressures have been uniformly found to be no better than placebo. Most studies focus on chronic fissures [1].

Glyceryl trinitrate (GTN) and its derivatives are smooth muscle relaxants that have been shown to decrease internal anal sphincter pressures. In controlled trials, the application of these nitric oxide products is associated with a greater than 50% fissure healing rate, compared with only 30–35% for placebo. A recent Cochrane review combining 15 studies showed a statistically better healing rate with GTN (49% vs. 37%). Headache is the principal adverse event with GTN use, causing about a quarter of patients to stop therapy; incontinence was not observed in any study. Interestingly, one small study showed no difference between anal application and distant transdermal delivery. In studies with follow-up periods of more than 1 year, recurrence after cessation of therapy approached 50% [2].

Calcium channel blockers, given either topically or orally, have been shown to heal fissures in 65–95% of patients. Comparisons to GTN show similar results. Headache is less frequently reported with topical use, but oral administration has more side effects and less efficacy [2].

Botulinum toxin (Botox) induces a temporary "chemical sphincterotomy" that initially heals approximately two-thirds of fissures with a single application. There is little consensus on dosing, injection sites, or repeated use. Transient incontinence to flatus and minor stool leakage are reported in up to 10% of patients. At 1 year, fissure recurrence rates are 40–50% [2]. Adding topical GTN to patients treated with Botox does not improve healing rates but does have significant side effects, primarily headaches [4].

Surgical sphincterotomy outperforms all medical therapies in numerous randomized controlled trials with an overall healing rate greater than 90%. A minor incontinence rate of less than 10% compares favorably with topical therapy [4–6].

> ### RECOMMENDATION
>
> Nonsurgical therapies are superior to placebo but inferior to lateral internal sphincterotomy for healing anal fissures.
>
> Level of evidence: Ia. Grade of recommendation: A.

47.3 What Is the Impact of Technique on the Outcomes of Patients Undergoing Surgery for Anal Fissure?

Surgical options for the treatment of anal fissures include anal stretch, open or closed lateral internal sphincterotomy (LIS), and posterior sphincterotomy, with or without papillae excision or dermal flap coverage [1]. Meta-analysis of stretch versus LIS clearly favors LIS for both recurrence (odds ratio [OR] = 3.08, 95% confidence interval [CI] 1.26–7.54) and incontinence (OR = 4.22, 95% CI 1.89–9.42). Randomized trials of surgical techniques may suffer from performance variations. Nevertheless, multiple trials comparing open LIS to closed LIS show no difference in either recurrence or incontinence. Posterior sphincterotomy is inferior to LIS for both persistence of the fissure and incontinence [7]. Additional procedures such as papillae excision and dermal flap coverage show a trend toward increased patient satisfaction in small trials [8, 9]. Overall, the risk of incontinence is low and patient satisfaction following LIS is high, even in those patients with minor continence disturbances [10]. Sphincter-sparing fistulectomy, combined with either concomitant Botox injection [11] or angioplasty [12], shows promise in small observational series.

> ### RECOMMENDATION
>
> LIS (open or closed) is the surgical treatment of choice for chronic anal fissures.
>
> Level of evidence: Ia. Grade of recommendation: A.

47.4 What Is the Healing and Incontinence Rate for Fistulotomy for Simple Fistula-in-Ano?

Anal fistulas vary in complexity from short, straight tracts involving primarily the internal sphincter to branching complexes through a large amount of the external sphincter. In patients with normal sphincter function and simple fistulas, fistulotomy is effective, with recurrence rates of less than 10% and minor incontinence rates of 0–17%. Risk factors for postoperative complications include high or complex fistulas, recurrent fistula, preoperative fecal incontinence, and women with anterior fistulas with or without birth trauma [14]. While recurrence rates are similar, fistulectomy is inferior to fistulotomy due to longer healing times and a greater risk of incontinence. Marsupialization of the wound edges following fistulotomy has been shown to speed final healing and decrease bleeding. Most functional problems following surgery for simple fistulas improve in 1–2 years [13, 14].

> ### RECOMMENDATION
>
> Fistulotomy is appropriate for simple fistula-in-ano with high rates of healing and low rates of incontinence.
>
> Level of evidence: Ib. Grade of recommendation: A.

47.5 What Is the Healing and Incontinence Rate for More Complex Fistulas Treated with Fibrin Glue, Fistula Plug, or a Seton?

Fistulotomy alone is contraindicated when the division of a significant amount of external sphincter is required, due to an increased risk of permanent incontinence [13, 14]. Several surgical treatment modalities have been developed to increase the likelihood of durable fistula closure while reducing the risk of postoperative functional problems.

Utilizing fibrin glue to obliterate fistula tracts was initially considered an attractive option as no sphincter muscle is divided. The early series were encouraging; however, more recent data have been disappointing [14]. Similarly, a bioabsorbable xenograft fistula plug made from lyophilized porcine intestinal submucosa (Surgisis®, Cook Surgical, Inc., Bloomington, IN) was developed as a sphincter-sparing fistula treatment. Early studies demonstrated an overall success rate of 83% with a median follow-up of 12 months [15]. The results of subsequent studies have been highly variable, with success rates of 25–81%, dependent on the length of follow-up and fistula complexity, with simple fistulas faring better [16–20]. In a more recent retrospective review, Sugrue et al. reviewed 462 patients between 2005 and 2015 who underwent sphincter-preserving procedures for cryptoglandular anal fistula. Fistula plugs were associated with a healing rate of 24%, and fibrin glue was associated with a healing rate of 18%. Fistula plugs were more likely to have recurrence when compared to endorectal advancement flap and ligation of intersphincteric fistula tract (LIFT) [20].

A seton is a flexible foreign body placed through a fistula and secured to itself to keep the tract open, preventing subsequent abscess formation, It may be draining or cut, depending on how it is used. The fibrosis induced is thought to lessen subsequent incontinence. Draining setons are used to manage sepsis and as a bridge to a definitive fistula procedure at a later date, with healing rates depending on the specific definitive procedure used [21]. Cutting setons are left in place and tightened sequentially, allowing for the slow division of the fistula tract as well as the anal sphincter. It is thought that by doing this over time, the incontinence risk is minimized with successful healing of the fistula. A pooled analysis of 1,460 patients who underwent cutting seton revealed a wide variety of success rates and fecal incontinence (0–67%) based on the specific fistula type and definition of incontinence used [22].

RECOMMENDATION

Treatment of complex fistula-in-ano by fibrin glue and fistula plug is generally not recommended. Cutting seton may be used in carefully selected patients, but success and incontinence rates vary.

Levels of evidence: IIb–II2c. Grade of recommendation: C.

47.6 What Is the Healing and Incontinence Rate for More Complex Fistulas Treated with an Endorectal Advancement Flap?

An endorectal advancement flap treats fistula-in-ano by curettage of the fistula tract, suture closure of the internal opening, and covering the closed internal opening with a well-vascularized and -mobilized flap of the healthy rectum. Numerous small case series demonstrate successful fistula closure in 55–98% of patients, with low rates of major continence disturbance (<10%). Success rates decrease with increasing fistula complexity, Crohn's disease, radiation, and recurrent fistulas [14]. Retrospective studies and meta-analyses have shown healing rates upwards of 66% [14]. A meta-analysis by Ali et al. showed healing rates for cryptoglandular fistulas after endorectal advancement flap to be as high as 87% with incontinence rates of 13.7% [23]. Additionally, an endorectal advancement flap can be used after a prior failed flap or LIFT with modest healing rates [14, 24, 25].

RECOMMENDATION

Complex fistula-in-ano may be successfully treated with an endorectal advancement flap. Recurrent fistula-in-ano may be treated by endorectal advancement flap with modest success rates. Incontinence is infrequent.

Level of evidence: Ib. Grade of recommendation: B.

47.7 What Is the Role of Ligation of the Intersphincteric Fistula Tract in the Treatment of Fistula-in-Ano?

LIFT is a sphincter-sparing procedure that may prove useful in the management of high transsphincteric anal fistulas [14]. Rojanasakul showed a 94% healing rate after 3 months of follow-up [26]. Subsequent reports of LIFT have shown success rates from 57% to 89%, with variable follow-up durations [27]. Adjuncts such as an interposed piece of a biologic sheet [28] have been investigated in small trials with modest improvements in healing rates. A meta-analysis of 1,378 LIFT operations by Emile et al. has demonstrated a success rate of 76% with a complication rate of 14%. The pooled incontinence rate was 1.4%. Risk factors for failure of LIFT were Crohn's disease, horseshoe fistula, and history of fistula operations [29].

RECOMMENDATION

Transsphincteric fistula-in-ano may be successfully treated with LIFT. Incontinence is infrequent.

Level of evidence: IB. Grade of recommendation: B.

47.8 Is There Any Role for Minimally Invasive Approaches (i.e., Video-Assisted or Laser Closure) in the Management of Fistula-in-Ano?

There are two minimally invasive treatments for cryptoglandular fistula-in-ano: Video-assisted anal fistula treatment (VAAFT) and fistula laser tract closure (FiLaC). VAAFT involves using a small scope to perform a fistuloscopy via the external opening, ultimately definitively identifying the internal opening. Next, the internal opening is closed with sutures, staples, or mucosal advancement flap, and the tract is obliterated with thermal energy as the scope is withdrawn [14]. The theoretical advantages of this approach are that the fistula tract can be visualized and fistula branches can be identified and obliterated [14, 30]. Studies on this treatment are preliminary and short-term. Garg et al. performed a meta-analysis that examined eight studies with 786 patients who underwent VAAFT. They found a 76.01% success rate and a 16.2% complication rate. Notably, none of these studies found worsening incontinence [31].

FiLaC involves passing a probe with a radially emitting laser through the fistula tract, which, in theory, ablates the epithelium and causes obliteration of the fistula tract [14, 30]. Elfeki et al. performed a meta-analysis of seven studies involving 454 patients who underwent FiLaC. They found a healing rate of 67.3% at 24 months of follow-up, with a 4% complication rate and a 1% incontinence rate [32].

RECOMMENDATION

Minimally invasive treatments for cryptoglandular fistula-in-ano have reasonable short-term healing rates with unknown long-term healing and recurrence rates.

Level of evidence: IIIa. Grade of recommendation: None due to the paucity of long-term data.

47.9 Are Antibiotics Unnecessary for Most Patients Undergoing Routine Incision and Drainage of Perirectal Abscesses?

Neither time to complete healing nor recurrence rates is improved by treating patients with antibiotics following incision and drainage of uncomplicated perirectal abscesses. However, antibiotics may be used in patients who have extensive cellulitis, systemic illness, or immunosuppression [14]. Antibiotic use and subsequent fistula development have been studied with conflicting results. Ghahramani et al. performed a single-blind randomized controlled trial where 309 patients were randomized to receiving antibiotics vs. no antibiotics after incision and drainage of a simple anal abscess. At a 3 months follow-up, antibiotic use was significantly associated with decreased odds of fistula formation in regression analysis (OR = 0.371, CI = 0.196–0.703) [33]. However, other studies

have shown the opposite. Sozener et al. performed a double-blinded, placebo-controlled randomized clinical trial where patients were randomized to receive antibiotic vs. placebo after incision and drainage of an anal abscess. They found that antibiotics did not protect against fistula formation after incision and drainage [34].

RECOMMENDATION

Antibiotics are unnecessary for most patients following adequate drainage and should be used for patients with extensive cellulitis, systemic sepsis, and immunosuppression. It is unclear whether antibiotics have an effect on fistula formation after incision and drainage of an anal abscess.

Level of evidence: IIb. Grade of recommendation: C.

Editor's Note

This area of surgery has been extensively studied and the high quality of the data has enabled the clinician to practice patient care with excellent scientific support. Anal fissures can be best managed by lateral internal sphincterotomy. Fistulotomy is the best treatment for simple fistula-in-ano. The management of less common, complex anal fistulae ranges from the simple injection of fibrin glue to laser therapy. Management of these wounds is still under investigation due to the scarcity of these lesions, the lack of success in avoiding recurrence, and the higher complication rates (incontinence) often encountered.

REFERENCES

1. Perry WB, Dykes SL, Buie WD, et al. Practice parameters for the management of anal fissures (3rd Revision). *Dis Colon Rectum*. 2010;*53(8)*:1110–1115.
2. Nelson R. Nonsurgical therapy for anal fissure. *Cochrane Database Syst Rev*. 2006;*4*:CD003431.
3. Asim M, Lowrie N, Stewart J, et al. Botulinum toxin versus botulinum toxin with low-dose glyceryl trinitrate for healing of the chronic anal fissure. *N Z Med J*. 2014;*127(1393)*: 80–86.
4. Arsian K, Erenoglu B, Dogru O, et al. Lateral internal sphincterotomy versus 0.25% isosorbide dinitrate ointment for chronic anal fissures: A prospective randomized controlled trial. *Surg Today*. 2013;*43(5)*:500–505.
5. Nicholls J. Anal fissure; surgery is the best treatment. *Colorectal Dis*. 2008;*10(5)*:529–530.
6. Nasr M, Ezzat H, Elsbae M. Botulinum toxin injection versus lateral internal sphincterotomy in the treatment of chronic anal fissure: A randomized controlled trial. *World J Surg*. 2010;*34(11)*:2730–2734.
7. Nelson R. Operative procedures for fissure in ano. *Cochrane Database Syst Rev*. 2005;*2*:Art No. CD002199.
8. Gupta PJ, Kalaskar S. Removal of hypertrophied anal papillae and fibrous anal polyps increases patient satisfaction after anal fissure surgery. *Tech Coloproctol*. 2003;*7(2)*: 155–158.

9. Leong AF, Seow-Choen F. Lateral internal sphincterotomy compared with anal advancement flap for chronic anal fissure. *Dis Colon Rectum.* 1995;*38(1)*:69–71.

10. Hyman N. Incontinence after lateral internal sphincterotomy: A prospective study and quality of life assessment. *Dis Colon Rectum.* 2004;*47(1)*:35–38.

11. Witte ME, Klaase JM, Koop R. Fissurectomy combined with botulinum toxin A injection for medically resistant chronic anal fissures. *Colorectal Dis.* 2010;*12*(7 online):e163–e169.

12. Abramowitz L, Bouchard D, Souffran M et al. Sphincter-sparing anal-fissure surgery: A 1-year prospective, observational, multicenter study of fissurectomy with anoplasty. *Colorectal Dis.* 2013;*15(3)*:359–367.

13. Bokhari S, Lindsey I. Incontinence following sphincter division for treatment of anal fistula. *Colorectal Dis.* 2010; *12*(7 online):e135–e139.

14. Gaertner WB, Burgess PL, Davids JS, et al. The American Society of Colon and Rectal Surgeons clinical practice guidelines for the management of anorectal abscess, fistula-in-ano, and rectovaginal fistula. *Dis Colon Rectum.* 2022;*65*:964–985.

15. Champagne BJ, O'Connor LM, Ferguson M, et al. Efficacy of anal fistula plug in closure of cryptoglandular fistulas: Long term follow-up. *Dis Colon Rectum.* 2006;*49(10)*:1817–1821.

16. van Koperen PJ, D'Hoore A, Wolthuis AM, et al. Anal fistula plug for closure of difficult anorectal fistula: A prospective study. *Dis Colon Rectum.* 2007;*50(12)*:2168–2172.

17. Ky AJ, Sylla P, Steinhagen R, et al. Collagen fistula plug for the treatment of anal fistulas. *Dis Colon Rectum.* 2008; *51(6)*:838–843.

18. El-Gazzaz G, Zutshi M, Hull T. A retrospective review of chronic anal fistulae treated by anal fistulae plug. *Colorectal Dis.* 2010;*12(5)*:442–447.

19. Ellis CH, Rostas JW, Greiner FG. Long-term outcomes with the use of bioprosthetic plugs for the management of complex anal fistulas. *Dis Colon Rectum.* 2010;*53(5)*:798–802.

20. Sugrue J, Mantilla N, Abcarian A, Kochar K, Marecik S, Chaudhry V, Mellgren A, Nordenstam J. Sphincter-sparing anal fistula repair: Are we getting better? *Dis Colon Rectum.* 2017 Oct;*60(10)*:1071–1077.

21. Tyler KM, Aarons CB, Sentovich SM. Successful sphincter-sparing surgery for all anal fistulas. *Dis Colon Rectum.* 2007 Oct;*50(10)*:1535–1539.

22. Ritchie RD, Sackier JM, Hodde JP. Incontinence rates after cutting seton treatment for anal fistula. *Colorectal Dis.* 2009 Jul;*11(6)*:564–571.

23. Soltani A, Kaiser AM. Endorectal advancement flap for cryptoglandular or Crohn's fistula-in-ano. *Dis Colon Rectum.* 2010 Apr;*53(4)*:486–495.

24. Podetta M, Scarpa CR, Zufferey G, Skala K, Ris F, Roche B, Buchs NC. Mucosal advancement flap for recurrent complex anal fistula: A repeatable procedure. *Int J Colorectal Dis.* 2019 Jan;*34(1)*:197–200.

25. Wright M, Thorson A, Blatchford G, Shashidharan M, Beaty J, Bertelson N, Aggrawal P, Taylor L, Ternent CA. What happens after a failed LIFT for anal fistula? *Am J Surg.* 2017 Dec;*214(6)*:1210–1213.

26. Rojansakul A, Pattanaarun J, Sahakitrungruang C, et al. Total anal sphincter saving technique for fistula-in-ano: The ligation of the intersphincteric fistula tract. *J Med Assoc Thai.* 2007;*90(8)*:581–586.

27. Vegara-Fernandez O, Espino-Urbina LA. Ligation of the intersphincteric fistula tract: What is the evidence in a review? *World J Gastroenterol.* 2013;*19(40)*:6805–6813.

28. Ellis CN. Outcomes with the use of bioprosthetic grafts to reinforce the ligation of the intersphincteric fistula tract (BioLIFT procedure) for the management of complex anal fistulas. *Dis Colon Rectum.* 2010;*53(10)*:1361–1364.

29. Emile SH, Khan SM, Adejumo A, Koroye O. Ligation of intersphincteric fistula tract (LIFT) in treatment of anal fistula: An updated systematic review, meta-analysis, and meta-regression of the predictors of failure. *Surgery.* 2020; *167*:484–492.

30. Steele SR, Hull TL, Hyman N, Maykel JA, Read TE, Whitlow CB. *The ASCRS Textbook of Colon and Rectal Surgery.* 4th Ed. Springer, 2022.

31. Garg P, Singh P. Video-Assisted Anal Fistula Treatment (VAAFT) in Cryptoglandular fistula-in-ano: A systematic review and proportional meta-analysis. *Int J Surg.* 2017 Oct; *46*:85–91.

32. Elfeki H, Shalaby M, Emile SH, Sakr A, Mikael M, Lundby L. A systematic review and meta-analysis of the safety and efficacy of fistula laser closure. *Tech Coloproctol.* 2020 Apr; *24(4)*:265–274.

33. Ghahramani L, Minaie MR, Arasteh P, et al. Antibiotic therapy for prevention of fistula in-ano after incision and drainage of simple perianal abscess: A randomized single-blind clinical trial. *Surgery.* 2017 Nov;*162(5)*:1017–1025.

34. Sözener U, Gedik E, Kessaf Aslar A, Ergun H, Halil Elhan A, Memikoğlu O, Bulent Erkek A, Ayhan Kuzu M. Does adjuvant antibiotic treatment after drainage of anorectal abscess prevent development of anal fistulas? A randomized, placebo-controlled, double-blind, multicenter study. *Dis Colon Rectum.* 2011 Aug;*54(8)*:923–929.

48

Acute Cholecystitis and Cholangitis

Brian I. Shaw and Suresh K. Agarwal

48.1 History and Epidemiology

Surgeons are often involved in the management of benign biliary diseases, including cholecystitis and cholangitis. Surgical treatment of cholecystitis was first described in 1882 by Langenbuch, while the first laparoscopic cholecystectomy was performed in 1985, leading to the widespread adoption of the laparoscopic technique thereafter [1]. Presently, up to 25% of Americans have gallstones and nearly one-third will become symptomatic [2]. Cholangitis was described by Charcot in 1877, and acute bacterial cholangitis accounts for nearly 250,000 hospitalizations in the United States each year with a significant mortality rate (~6%) [3]. Both acute cholecystitis and cholangitis have several etiologies; however, they are often linked by the common cause of cholelithiasis. In the following chapter, we will explore the presentation, diagnosis, and management of both entities, focusing on the diseases caused by gallstones.

48.2 Anatomy, Physiology, and Pathophysiology

The biliary anatomy is quite variable and contributes to the diagnostic and therapeutic difficulty of both acute cholecystitis and cholangitis. The textbook-like structure of the biliary tree with "classic" cystic duct drainage anatomy is only noted in about 17% of patients undergoing cholecystectomy [4]. Indeed, the fact that the minority of patients have "standard" anatomy combined with limited dissection leads to visual perceptions of "biased confirmation" and ultimately bile duct injury [5, 6]. In more than 50% of patients, cholelithiasis is thought to be the etiology of acute cholecystitis [7].

In acute cholangitis, an increase in intrabiliary pressure may lead to disruption of the tight junctions of the bile canalicular cells and also impairment in the phagocytic function of the Kupffer cell. It is also thought that diversion of bile from the gastrointestinal tract due to obstruction could lead to altered endogenous gut flora and loss of gut mucosal integrity, thereby promoting bacterial translocation [8–10].

48.3 Initial Evaluation and Diagnosis

In diagnosing both acute cholecystitis and cholangitis, the gold standard scoring rubric is the Tokyo Guidelines, last updated in 2018 [11]. Acute cholecystitis includes local signs of inflammation (Murphy's sign, right upper quadrant pain, mass, or tenderness), systemic signs of inflammation (fever, elevated white blood cell count, and elevated C-reactive protein), and imaging findings characteristic of cholecystitis. The diagnosis can be suspected with one local and one systemic sign, while imaging is considered definitive. In a retrospective review of 227 patients with pathology-confirmed acute cholecystitis, these criteria had a sensitivity and specificity of 91.2% and 96.9%, respectively [12].

With regard to acute cholangitis, the Tokyo Guidelines similarly have diagnostic criteria, which are defined by the presence of systemic inflammation, jaundice, and imaging findings characteristic of acute cholangitis. A probable diagnosis of acute cholangitis requires only systemic inflammation and either jaundice or supportive imaging findings, while a definitive diagnosis mandates all three characteristics. Of note, the severity of acute cholecystitis and cholangitis is graded on Tokyo Guidelines from 2018 based on the presence of dysfunction of other organ systems [13].

RECOMMENDATION

1. No single clinical criterion is sufficient to predict or rule out acute cholecystitis; however, in the presence of one local and systemic sign of inflammation, the diagnosis should be strongly suspected.

   Grade of recommendation: B.

2. No single clinical criterion is sufficient to predict or rule out acute cholangitis but should be strongly suspected in the setting of systemic inflammation and either jaundice or supportive imaging.

   Grade of recommendation: B.

48.3.1 What Is the Role of Imaging Studies for the Diagnosis of Acute Cholecystitis and Cholangitis?

Ultrasound remains the initial study of choice for most patients [14]. Though a CT scan may be noninferior [15], examination of the whole abdomen may introduce unnecessary diagnostic uncertainty. In cases in which a diagnosis of acute cholecystitis is challenging, the most helpful test with the highest sensitivity and specificity is cholescintigraphy (HIDA scan) [16]. Of special note, a patient must have eaten in the past 24 hours

DOI: 10.1201/9781003316800-48

to avoid a false-positive study, and the use of provocative morphine studies (to constrict the sphincter of Oddi and allowing filling of the gallbladder) may be helpful in some patients [17]. This test is most appropriate in the case where treatment of acute cholecystitis is complicated by critical illness.

In acute cholangitis, imaging of the common bile duct (CBD) via either ultrasound (US) (as part of a right upper quadrant US) or magnetic resonance cholangiopancreatography (MRCP) allows for the determination of CBD dilation, as well as potentially defining the cause of that dilation in advance of a potentially therapeutic endoscopic retrograde cholangiopancreatography (ERCP). Indeed, MRCP has had as high as 100% negative predictive value (NPV) in some studies [18]. The types and utilization of imaging, however, are nuanced and should be determined on a per-patient basis.

RECOMMENDATION

1. US remains the preferred initial study in acute cholecystitis and will correctly diagnose most patients. If US is equivocal or does not correlate with the medical history, cholescintigraphy (HIDA scan) is an appropriate next step. Abdominal CT should be reserved for patients in whom the entire abdomen requires evaluation.

   Grade of recommendation: B.

2. The exact imaging modality used should be tailored to the clinical situation in acute cholangitis.

   Grade of recommendation: C.

48.4 Management

48.4.1 Should Laparoscopic, Robotic, or Open Cholecystectomy Be Performed in Acute and Complicated Acute Cholecystitis?

Laparoscopy was originally contraindicated in the setting of acute cholecystitis and reserved for purely elective procedures in the setting of biliary colic. This is no longer the case. In 2009, the Society of American Gastrointestinal and Endoscopic Surgeons published its guidelines on indications, operative techniques, and management of complications for laparoscopic cholecystectomy based on a literature review. Of 219 abstracts reviewed, 38 articles were evaluated as pertinent, and the society concluded that laparoscopy should be the preferred approach for acute cholecystitis [19].

Additionally, Boo et al. [20] studied inflammatory markers in patients randomized to open versus laparoscopic cholecystectomy in acute cholecystitis. Using blood samples obtained preoperatively and 24 and 72 hours postoperatively, they found that laparoscopy patients had a faster normalization of C-reactive protein and a less marked reduction in postoperative monocyte count and production of tumor necrosis factor (TNF)-alpha, suggesting reduced immunosuppression with the laparoscopic approach.

In 2008, Borzellino et al. completed a meta-analysis of outcomes for patients undergoing laparoscopic cholecystectomy for severe acute cholecystitis, defined by the presence of empyema or emphysematous gallbladder. Seven studies totaling 1,408 patients were analyzed comparing surgery for severe versus nonsevere acute cholecystitis and found a higher risk of conversion and overall complications (risk ratio [RR] 3.2, confidence interval [CI] 2.5–4.2 and RR 1.6, CI 1.2–2.2, respectively) [21]. However, the authors were unable to find any studies comparing outcomes after urgent laparoscopy with urgent open cholecystectomy and concluded that one should have a lower threshold for conversion when operating on patients with severe cholecystitis.

The da Vinci Platform has described and implemented robotic assistance for cholecystectomy. A paucity of articles exists comparing robotic-assisted with conventional laparoscopic cholecystectomy. Pilot studies demonstrate that the outcomes are equivalent concerning mortality, length of stay, and complications; however, the length of operation is higher for the robot-assisted group. Additionally, robotic cholecystectomy may be associated with a higher incisional hernia rate [22]. It has been suggested that the rate of bile spillage may be lower with robotic approaches [23].

The approach in a patient with Mirizzi's syndrome, where a large stone impacted in the neck of the gallbladder causes extrinsic compression or fistula into the CBD, remains a controversial topic. The current literature suggests that the laparoscopic approach has a significantly higher rate of conversion [24–26], and the standard of care has not been definitively established.

RECOMMENDATION

Laparoscopic cholecystectomy should be the initial approach of choice in the vast majority of cases.

Grade of recommendation: B.

Robotic assistance adds little benefit to the performance of cholecystectomy.

Grade of recommendation: D.

The best approach to Mirizzi's syndrome is unknown.

Grade of recommendation: C.

48.4.2 What Should the Timing of Surgical/Procedural Intervention Be?

As early as 2013, a systematic review of randomized trial data concluded that early cholecystectomy—defined as within 7 days of symptom onset—was associated with a shorter length of stay by 4 days without an increase in morbidity or mortality. Additionally, patients undergoing delayed operations had a nearly 20% chance of experiencing recurrent symptoms in that interval. Given this, they recommended that early cholecystectomy was preferable [27]. Even among patients with longer symptom duration (i.e., >72 hours), there are now data from randomized clinical trials showing that patients undergoing early cholecystectomy have lower morbidity, shorter length of stay, and shorter duration of antibiotic therapy [28] (Table 48.1). However, this is a nuanced judgment that should be driven by individual patient factors and surgeon experience.

In acute cholangitis, there is a need for immediate decompression due to the potential progression of infection to sepsis and septic shock. Indeed, increasing the time between diagnosis and intervention is associated with longer hospital stays and increased need for interventions such as the use of vasopressors [29]. In patients with cholangitis, it is also appropriate to pursue early cholecystectomy, as multiple retrospective single-institution reviews note an increase in postoperative complications with delayed surgery. However, there are limitations to this interpretation, as one study defined as early as on the index admission [30] while the other defined early as within 6 weeks of admission [31]. Additionally, a large retrospective database analysis using administrative data found a decrease in recurrent biliary complications (including pancreatitis, cholangitis, and biliary colic) without a concomitant increase in mortality for early cholecystectomy after ERCP [32]. In the severely debilitated patient, cholecystectomy may be deferred. In the special case of gallstone pancreatitis, there is a decreased length of stay with early cholecystectomy [33] and up to a 10% risk of recurrence at 1 year in the absence of cholecystectomy [34].

RECOMMENDATION

Early cholecystectomy is the preferred approach in acute cholecystitis and after clinical resolution of gallstone pancreatitis or acute cholangitis.

Grade of recommendation: B.

Early ERCP for acute cholangitis should be pursued where clinically feasible.

Grade of recommendation: B.

48.4.3 What Are the Indications and Outcomes for Percutaneous Cholecystostomy?

Some patients with acute cholecystitis are severely ill and have a high perioperative risk due to comorbid illness. Though cholecystostomy placement has been well described, it is unclear which patients are most appropriate.

With regard to slightly less sick patients, the CHOCOLATE trial showed that early cholecystectomy in high-risk patients—defined as APACHE II score between 7 and 15—had superior outcomes compared with percutaneous cholecystostomy tube in place across a wide variety of metrics in the setting of a randomized clinical trial. Patients undergoing immediate cholecystectomy had lower rates of reintervention, lower rates of recurrent biliary disease, and shorter hospital stays (when including readmissions) [35]. Of special note, the authors did exclude 10 patients deemed too sick for the study with APACHE scores greater than or equal to 15.

In sicker patients, percutaneous cholecystectomy is indeed the preferred treatment. However, data from administrative review do show that the use of percutaneous cholecystostomy tubes generally increases readmissions, as well as long-term (30- and 60-day) costs in patients with acute cholecystitis [36]. Further randomized studies are required to determine patients appropriate for percutaneous cholecystectomy. One cohort where this should be more thoroughly studied is among patients with *acalculous* cholecystitis, who teleologically are at lower risk for subsequent biliary complications, though administrative studies have found no difference in relevant outcomes [36].

Finally, among patients who undergo percutaneous cholecystostomy tubes, it is unclear when the optimal interval for subsequent cholecystectomy is. In severe debilitated patients, removal may be quite delayed or not pursued entirely depending on the overall clinical trajectory. One recent study attempted to determine this question by utilizing a mix of center-level and national retrospective observational data. Overall, they conclude that intervention before 4 weeks is

---

TABLE 48.1

Summarized Results of a Systematic Review of Early versus Delayed Cholecystectomy for Acute Cholecystitis

	Number of Trials	Number of Patients	Favors	Effect Size of Early Cholecystectomy
Mortality	5	438	Neither—there were no deaths in any studies	Not applicable
Biliary injury	5	438	Early cholecystectomy	Odds ratio 0.49 95% CI [0.05–4.72] $p = 0.54$
Other serious complication	5	438	Delayed cholecystectomy	Risk ratio 1.29 95% CI [0.61–2.72] $p = 0.50$
Conversion to open cholecystectomy	6	488	Early cholecystectomy	Risk ratio 0.89 95% CI [0.63–1.25] $p = 0.50$
Hospital length of stay	4	373	Early cholecystectomy	Mean difference (days): −4.12 95% CI [−5.22 to −3.03] $p < 0.0001$
Operative time	6	488	Early cholecystectomy	Mean difference (minutes): −1.22 95% CI: [−3.07 to −0.64] $p = 0.20$

Source: Gurusamy, K et al., *Cochrane Database Syst Rev*, Issue 6, Art. No. CD005440, 2013.

associated with increased operative complications, whereas interventions later than 8 weeks are associated with an increase in cholecystostomy tube–related complications (including the need for tube exchange) [37].

RECOMMENDATION

Early cholecystostomy may be preferred to conservative management in patients who are unable to undergo cholecystectomy (grade D recommendation), though cholecystectomy is preferred in patients who will tolerate the procedure (grade B recommendation). Among patients undergoing cholecystostomy tube placement, interval removal should be planned between 4 and 8 weeks after intervention.

Grade of recommendation: C.

48.4.4 What Are the Indications for Intraoperative Cholangiogram?

Surgeons must determine which, if any, of their patients should undergo intraoperative cholangiography (IOC) with cholecystectomy. In 2012, Ford et al. [38] published a systematic review of randomized controlled trials published in the literature between 1980 and 2011 comparing routine, selective, or no IOC, ultimately evaluating eight trials with 1,715 patients. These authors were unable to conclude if there was a benefit of routine IOC in patients with a low risk of biliary obstruction.

Further studies utilizing U.S. administrative data showed that surgeons who used routine IOC did not have a decreased incidence of bile duct injury but did have increased complications compared to those that selectively performed IOC [39]. However, a meta-analysis that included observational studies and performed by a Swedish group did show that there was a decrease in bile duct injury with routine IOC that met

generally accepted criteria for being cost-effective [40]. A further Cochrane review is underway to try and further address this exact question but has not yet been published [41]. With regard to the diagnosis of choledocholithiasis, both ERCP and IOC are sensitive and specific, though direct comparisons are limited [42]. In general, the authors prefer aggressive use of preoperative ERCP (due to its ubiquity and ease) to IOC in order to prove common duct patency.

RECOMMENDATION

There are little data to recommend for or against routine IOC. IOC and ERCP may be used to diagnose CBD stones.

Grade of recommendation: C.

Surgeons should be facile in IOC should the need for IOC be apparent in a given case.

Grade of recommendation: D.

48.4.5 What Are the Indications for Drain Placement?

Gurusamy et al. assessed the use of routine abdominal drainage for uncomplicated open cholecystectomy in a systematic review for the Cochrane database in 2007 [43]. Included were 28 open cholecystectomy trials (3,659 patients) of which 20 trials evaluated the comparison of "no drain placement" vs. "drain placement" and 12 trials evaluated one drainage method versus another (closed suction vs. Penrose). No significant differences were encountered for intraabdominal fluid collections; however, wound and chest infections were more frequent with drain placement [43].

In 2013, the same authors updated a separate review focusing on laparoscopic cholecystectomy (Table 48.2) [44]. In a meta-analysis of 12 randomized clinical trials totaling

TABLE 48.2

Summarized Results of a Systematic Review of Routine Drainage During Laparoscopic Cholecystectomy

	Number of Trials	Number of Patients	Favors	Effect Size of Drain
Mortality	10	1681	Drain	Risk ratio 0.41 95% CI [0.04–4.37] $p = 0.46$
Serious adverse events (proportion of patients)	7	1143	No drain	Risk ratio 2.12 95% CI [0.61–7.40] $p = 0.24$
Serious adverse events (total number)	8	1286	No drain	Risk ratio 1.60 95% CI [0.66–3.87] $p = 0.30$
Quality of life	1	93	Drain	Standard mean difference: 0.22 95% CI [−0.19 to 0.63]
Hospital length of stay	5	449	No drain	Mean difference (days): 0.22 95% CI [−0.06 to 0.50] $p = 0.31$
Operative time	7	775	No drain	Mean difference (minutes): 4.97 95% CI: [2.70–7.25] $p < 0.0001$

Source: Gurusamy, KS et al., *Cochrane Database Syst Rev*, Issue 9, Art. No. CD006004, 2013.

1,831 patients consisting largely of patients undergoing elective cholecystectomy, there were no significant differences in serious adverse events, short-term mortality, hospital length of stay, or quality of life between patients who did and did not receive a drain. Drain recipients had a mean operative time that was reported as 5 minutes longer than the nondrain patients (CI 2.6–7.3 minutes) [29].

A separate meta-analysis by Antoniou et al. of six randomized trials found higher pain scores 6–12 hours postoperatively in patients receiving prophylactic drain placement, with no differences in 30-day morbidity or wound infections [45].

RECOMMENDATION

Routine drain placement does not appear to provide any benefit and may be associated with an increased frequency of infections. Routine drain placement should not be pursued.

Grade of recommendation: B.

48.4.6 Which Antibiotic Therapy Is Warranted?

The use of appropriate antibiotic prophylaxis in acute cholecystitis is of special concern due to the incidence of the operation and the potential for the acquisition of antibiotic resistance. Indeed, prior guidelines state that for patients undergoing elective cholecystectomy for mild-to-moderate community-acquired acute cholecystitis, it was appropriate to omit prophylaxis [46]. However, recent randomized data from the PEANUTS II trial showed that omission of perioperative antibiotics failed to meet noninferiority criteria [47], suggesting that perioperative antibiotics are necessary in acute cholecystitis. Additionally, there are randomized data to suggest that there is no benefit to extending antibiotic therapy past a prophylactic dose in patients with mild acute cholecystitis [48].

With regard to acute cholangitis, the Tokyo Guidelines from 2018 suggest a duration of 4–7 days of antibiotics once source control has been achieved, based on low-quality evidence

(Level C) [49]. Some recent studies have challenged this dogma, with a meta-analysis showing that there is no difference between 3 days and greater than 3 days of antimicrobial therapy after biliary drainage [50]. Additional randomized controlled trials are now planned based on these findings and should report soon [51].

RECOMMENDATION

A single dose of prophylactic antibiotics is appropriate for all patients with acute cholecystitis.

Grade of recommendation: A.

Extended duration of antibiotics for mild acute cholecystitis is not indicated.

Grade of recommendation: A.

Three days of antibiotics after biliary drainage are likely sufficient in uncomplicated cases of acute cholangitis.

Grade of recommendation: B.

48.5 Discussion

Biliary disease remains a common problem in general surgical practice. Many aspects of diagnosis, management, and postoperative care have not been rigorously evaluated with the gold standard of randomized controlled trials (Table 48.3). Uncertainty remains for many interventions; however, further information is especially needed around complex patients such as those requiring percutaneous cholecystostomy tubes and the appropriate use of biliary imaging methodologies for the diagnosis of CBD stones in acute cholecystitis. Overall, there has been a shift toward less therapy (be it the routine use of IOC, drains, antibiotic therapy, or the use of percutaneous cholecystostomy tubes) in the modern era. Many randomized trials are underway that will further elucidate optimal management of these common clinical scenarios.

TABLE 48.3

Summary of Recommendations and Level of Evidence

Question	Answer	Level of Evidence	Grade of Recommendation	References
What are the clinical criteria required for the diagnosis of acute cholecystitis?	No one clinical criterion is sufficient to predict or rule out acute cholecystitis; however, in the presence of one local and systemic sign of inflammation, the diagnosis should be strongly suspected.	III	B	[10, 11]
What are the clinical criteria required for the diagnosis of acute cholangitis?	No one clinical criterion is sufficient to predict or rule out acute cholangitis but should be strongly suspected in the setting of systemic inflammation and either jaundice or supportive imaging.	III	B	[12]

(Continued)

TABLE 48.3 (Continued)

Summary of Recommendations and Level of Evidence

Question	Answer	Level of Evidence	Grade of Recommendation	References
What is the value of imaging studies for the diagnosis of acute cholecystitis?	Ultrasound remains the preferred initial study and will correctly diagnose most patients. If ultrasound is equivocal or does not correlate with the medical history, cholescintigraphy is an appropriate next step. Abdominal CT should be reserved for patients in whom the entire abdomen requires evaluation.	IV	B	[13–15]
What imaging modality is most appropriate in the evaluation of acute cholangitis?	The exact imaging modality used should be tailored to the clinical situation in acute cholangitis.	IV	C	[16]
Should laparoscopic or open cholecystectomy be performed in acute and complicated acute cholecystitis?	Laparoscopic cholecystectomy should be the initial approach of choice in the vast majority of cases.	II	B	[17–19]
What is the role of robotic surgery in cholecystectomy?	Robotic assistance adds little benefit to the performance of cholecystectomy.	IV	D	[20, 21]
What is the best approach to Mirizzi's syndrome?	The best approach to Mirizzi's syndrome is unknown.	IV	D	[22–24]
What should the timing of surgical intervention be?	Early cholecystectomy is the preferred approach in acute cholecystitis, after gallstone pancreatitis, and after acute cholangitis.	I	B	[25–32]
What is the appropriate timing of ERCP for acute cholangitis?	Early ERCP for acute cholangitis should be pursued.	III	B	[27]
What is the indication for cholecystostomy tube placement?	Early cholecystostomy may be preferred to conservative management in patients who are unable to undergo cholecystectomy and is preferred in patients who will tolerate the procedure.	III	D	[33, 34]
When should the cholecystostomy tube be removed?	Among patients undergoing cholecystostomy tube placement, interval removal should be planned between 4 and 8 weeks after intervention.	IV	C	[35]
What are the indications for intraoperative cholangiogram?	There are little data to recommend for or against routine IOC.	II	D	[36–40]
What are the indications for drain placement?	Routine drain placement does not appear to provide any benefit and may be associated with an increased frequency of infections. Routine drain placement should not be pursued.	I	B	[41–43]
Which antibiotic therapy is warranted?	A single dose of prophylactic antibiotics is appropriate for all patients with acute cholecystitis.	I	A	[45]
	Antibiotic therapy greater than 24 hours is not indicated.	I	A	[46]
What is the duration of antibiotics needed after biliary drainage in acute cholangitis?	Three days of antibiotics after biliary drainage are likely sufficient in uncomplicated cases of acute cholangitis.	II	B	[47–49]

Editor's Note

The clinician needs to be aware of the fact that gallstones are ubiquitously occurring in about a quarter of the population, but only about 25% ever have attributable symptoms requiring medical management. The diagnosis of acute cholecystitis is usually fairly straightforward, with many patients presenting with classic symptoms and signs and typical findings on ultrasound imaging. In patients with atypical presentation or equivocal ultrasound studies, the HIDA scan can be confirmatory. This nuclear medicine study requires that the patient not be starving for 24 hours to avoid a false nonvisualization of the gallbladder (abnormal test). In this situation, a dose of morphine (constricting the sphincter of Oddi) is effective in helping fill the gallbladder, converting an abnormal to a normal study.

In acute cholecystitis, early cholecystectomy appears prudent. However, in patients presenting with more than 72 hours of symptoms, it is the editor's experience that one can expect a much more difficult operation. Whether a cholecystectomy is performed in the setting of acute cholangitis after ERCP drainage and stenting is determined based on the clinical status of the patient. Many of these individuals are quite debilitated, and observation is prudent. In the medically unstable patient who cannot undergo cholecystectomy and a cholecystostomy tube is placed, the timing of subsequent cholecystectomy is controversial. As these patients are quite complicated, many clinicians delay operation for long periods. The cholecystectomy procedure is much more difficult after tube placement, as the posterior aspect of the gallbladder is often quite adherent to the liver surface due to inflammation.

Intraoperative cholangiogram should be performed very selectively in this era of aggressive preoperative ERCP. Drains have no place in routine cholecystectomy. Antibiotics are typically used for short perioperative periods and should include drugs with a spectrum aimed at community-acquired organisms. These recommendations have moderate levels of evidence to support them and are mostly grade B.

REFERENCES

1. Polychronidis A, Laftsidis P, Bounovas A, Simopoulos C. Twenty years of laparoscopic cholecystectomy: Philippe Mouret–March 17, 1987. *JSLS*. Jan-Mar 2008;12(1):109–11.
2. Everhart JE, Khare M, Hill M, Maurer KR. Prevalence and ethnic differences in gallbladder disease in the United States. *Gastroenterology*. Sep 1999;117(3):632–9. doi:10.1016/s0016-5085(99)70456-7
3. McNabb-Baltar J, Trinh QD, Barkun AN. Biliary drainage method and temporal trends in patients admitted with cholangitis: a national audit. *Can J Gastroenterol*. Sep 2013;27(9):513–8. doi:10.1155/2013/175143
4. Berci G. Biliary ductal anatomy and anomalies. The role of intraoperative cholangiography during laparoscopic cholecystectomy. *Surg Clin North Am*. Oct 1992;72(5):1069–75. doi:10.1016/s0039-6109(16)45832-9
5. Way LW, Stewart L, Gantert W, et al. Causes and prevention of laparoscopic bile duct injuries: analysis of 252 cases from a human factors and cognitive psychology perspective. *Ann Surg*. Apr 2003;237(4):460–9. doi:10.1097/01.SLA.0000060680.92690.E9
6. Hugh TB. New strategies to prevent laparoscopic bile duct injury–surgeons can learn from pilots. *Surgery*. Nov 2002;132(5):826–35. doi:10.1067/msy.2002.127681
7. Stewart L, Griffiss JM, Jarvis GA, Way LW. Gallstones containing bacteria are biofilms: bacterial slime production and ability to form pigment solids determines infection severity and bacteremia. *J Gastrointest Surg*. Aug 2007;11(8):977–83; discussion 983-4. doi:10.1007/s11605-007-0168-1
8. Huang T, Bass JA, Williams RD. The significance of biliary pressure in cholangitis. *Arch Surg*. May 1969;98(5):629–32. doi:10.1001/archsurg.1969.01340110121014
9. Sheen-Chen SM, Chau P, Harris HW. Obstructive jaundice alters Kupffer cell function independent of bacterial translocation. *J Surg Res*. Dec 1998;80(2):205–9. doi:10.1006/jsre.1998.5467
10. Diamond T, Dolan S, Thompson RL, Rowlands BJ. Development and reversal of endotoxemia and endotoxin-related death in obstructive jaundice. *Surgery*. Aug 1990;108(2):370–4; discussion 374-5.
11. Okamoto K, Suzuki K, Takada T, et al. Tokyo Guidelines 2018: flowchart for the management of acute cholecystitis. *J Hepatobiliary Pancreat Sci*. Jan 2018;25(1):55–72. doi:10.1002/jhbp.516

12. Yokoe M, Takada T, Strasberg SM, et al. New diagnostic criteria and severity assessment of acute cholecystitis in revised Tokyo guidelines. *J Hepatobiliary Pancreat Sci*. Sep 2012;19(5):578–85. doi:10.1007/s00534-012-0548-0
13. Miura F, Okamoto K, Takada T, et al. Tokyo Guidelines 2018: initial management of acute biliary infection and flowchart for acute cholangitis. *J Hepatobiliary Pancreat Sci*. Jan 2018;25(1):31–40. doi:10.1002/jhbp.509
14. Expert Panel on Gastrointestinal I, Peterson CM, McNamara MM, et al. ACR Appropriateness Criteria((R)) right upper quadrant pain. *J Am Coll Radiol*. May 2019;16(5S):S235–S43. doi:10.1016/j.jacr.2019.02.013
15. Hiatt KD, Ou JJ, Childs DD. Role of ultrasound and CT in the workup of right upper quadrant pain in adults in the emergency department: a retrospective review of more than 2800 cases. *AJR Am J Roentgenol*. Jun 2020;214(6):1305–10. doi:10.2214/AJR.19.22188
16. Kiewiet JJ, Leeuwenburgh MM, Bipat S, Bossuyt PM, Stoker J, Boermeester MA. A systematic review and meta-analysis of diagnostic performance of imaging in acute cholecystitis. *Radiology*. Sep 2012;264(3):708–20. doi:10.1148/radiol.12111561
17. Hung BT, Traylor KS, Wong CY. Revisiting morphine-augmented hepatobiliary imaging for diagnosing acute cholecystitis: the potential pitfall of high false positive rate. *Abdom Imaging*. Jun 2014;39(3):467–71. doi:10.1007/s00261-013-0067-8
18. Chang JH, Lee IS, Lim YS, et al. Role of magnetic resonance cholangiopancreatography for choledocholithiasis: analysis of patients with negative MRCP. *Scand J Gastroenterol*. Feb 2012;47(2):217–24. doi:10.3109/00365521.2011.638394
19. Overby DW, Apelgren KN, Richardson W, Fanelli R. SAGES guidelines for the clinical application of laparoscopic biliary tract surgery. *Surg Endosc*. Oct 2010;24(10):2368–86. doi:10.1007/s00464-010-1268-7
20. Boo YJ, Kim WB, Kim J, et al. Systemic immune response after open versus laparoscopic cholecystectomy in acute cholecystitis: a prospective randomized study. *Scand J Clin Lab Invest*. 2007;67(2):207–14. doi:10.1080/00365510601011585
21. Borzellino G, Sauerland S, Minicozzi AM, et al. Laparoscopic cholecystectomy for severe acute cholecystitis. A meta-analysis of results. *Surg Endosc*. Jan 2008;22(1):8–15. doi:10.1007/s00464-007-9511-6
22. Han C, Shan X, Yao L, et al. Robotic-assisted versus laparoscopic cholecystectomy for benign gallbladder diseases: a systematic review and meta-analysis. *Surg Endosc*. Nov 2018;32(11):4377–92. doi:10.1007/s00464-018-6295-9
23. Han DH, Choi SH, Kang CM, Lee WJ. Propensity score-matching analysis for single-site robotic cholecystectomy versus single-incision laparoscopic cholecystectomy: a retrospective cohort study. *Int J Surg*. Jun 2020;78:138–142. doi:10.1016/j.ijsu.2020.04.042
24. Antoniou SA, Antoniou GA, Makridis C. Laparoscopic treatment of mirizzi syndrome: a systematic review. *Surg Endosc*. Jan 2010;24(1):33–9. doi:10.1007/s00464-009-0520-5
25. Lledó JB, Barber SM, Ibañez JC, Torregrosa AG, Lopez-Andujar R. Update on the diagnosis and treatment of mirizzi syndrome in laparoscopic era: our experience in 7 years. *Surg Laparosc Endosc Percutan Tech*. Dec 2014;24(6):495–501. doi:10.1097/sle.0000000000000079

26. Erben Y, Benavente-Chenhalls LA, Donohue JM, et al. Diagnosis and treatment of mirizzi syndrome: 23-year mayo clinic experience. *J Am Coll Surg.* Jul 2011;213(1):114–9; discussion 120-1. doi:10.1016/j.jamcollsurg.2011.03.008

27. Gurusamy KS, Davidson C, Gluud C, Davidson BR. Early versus delayed laparoscopic cholecystectomy for people with acute cholecystitis. *Cochrane Database Syst Rev.* Jun 30 2013;(6):Cd005440. doi:10.1002/14651858.CD005440.pub3

28. Roulin D, Saadi A, Di Mare L, Demartines N, Halkic N. Early versus delayed cholecystectomy for acute cholecystitis, are the 72 hours still the rule?: a randomized trial. *Ann Surg.* Nov 2016;264(5):717–22. doi:10.1097/SLA.0000000000001886

29. Hou LA, Laine L, Motamedi N, Sahakian A, Lane C, Buxbaum J. Optimal timing of endoscopic retrograde cholangiopancreatography in acute cholangitis. *J Clin Gastroenterol.* Jul 2017;51(6):534–38. doi:10.1097/MCG.0000000000000763

30. Discolo A, Reiter S, French B, et al. Outcomes following early versus delayed cholecystectomy performed for acute cholangitis. *Surg Endosc.* Jul 2020;34(7):3204–10. doi:10.1007/s00464-019-07095-0

31. Li VK, Yum JL, Yeung YP. Optimal timing of elective laparoscopic cholecystectomy after acute cholangitis and subsequent clearance of choledocholithiasis. *Am J Surg.* Oct 2010;200(4):483–8. doi:10.1016/j.amjsurg.2009.11.010

32. Elmunzer BJ, Noureldin M, Morgan KA, Adams DB, Cote GA, Waljee AK. The impact of cholecystectomy after endoscopic sphincterotomy for complicated gallstone disease. *Am J Gastroenterol.* Oct 2017;112(10):1596–1602. doi:10.1038/ajg.2017.247

33. Gurusamy KS, Nagendran M, Davidson BR. Early versus delayed laparoscopic cholecystectomy for acute gallstone pancreatitis. *Cochrane Database Syst Rev.* Sep 2 2013;(9):CD010326. doi:10.1002/14651858.CD010326.pub2

34. Hwang SS, Li BH, Haigh PI. Gallstone pancreatitis without cholecystectomy. *JAMA Surg.* Sep 2013;148(9):867–72. doi:10.1001/jamasurg.2013.3033

35. Loozen CS, van Santvoort HC, van Duijvendijk P, et al. Laparoscopic cholecystectomy versus percutaneous catheter drainage for acute cholecystitis in high risk patients (CHOCOLATE): multicentre randomised clinical trial. *BMJ.* Oct 8 2018;363:k3965. doi:10.1136/bmj.k3965

36. Fleming MM, DeWane MP, Luo J, Liu F, Zhang Y, Pei KY. A propensity score matched comparison of readmissions and cost of laparoscopic cholecystectomy vs percutaneous cholecystostomy for acute cholecystitis. *Am J Surg.* Jan 2019;217(1):83–9. doi:10.1016/j.amjsurg.2018.10.047

37. Woodward SG, Rios-Diaz AJ, Zheng R, et al. Finding the most favorable timing for cholecystectomy after percutaneous cholecystostomy tube placement: an analysis of institutional and national data. *J Am Coll Surg.* Jan 2021;232(1):55–64. doi:10.1016/j.jamcollsurg.2020.10.010

38. Ford JA, Soop M, Du J, Loveday BP, Rodgers M. Systematic review of intraoperative cholangiography in cholecystectomy. *Br J Surg.* Feb 2012;99(2):160–7. doi:10.1002/bjs.7809

39. Ragulin-Coyne E, Witkowski ER, Chau Z, et al. Is routine intraoperative cholangiogram necessary in the twenty-first century? A national view. *J Gastrointest Surg.* Mar 2013;17(3):434–42. doi:10.1007/s11605-012-2119-8

40. Rystedt JML, Wiss J, Adolfsson J, et al. Routine versus selective intraoperative cholangiography during cholecystectomy: systematic review, meta-analysis and health economic model analysis of iatrogenic bile duct injury. *BJS Open.* Mar 5 2021;5(2). doi:10.1093/bjsopen/zraa032

41. Kleinubing DR, Riera R, Matos D, Linhares MM. Selective versus routine intraoperative cholangiography for cholecystectomy. *Cochrane Database Syst Rev.* 2018;(2). doi:10.1002/14651858.CD012971

42. Gurusamy KS, Giljaca V, Takwoingi Y, et al. Endoscopic retrograde cholangiopancreatography versus intraoperative cholangiography for diagnosis of common bile duct stones. *Cochrane Database Syst Rev.* Feb 26 2015;(2):CD010339. doi:10.1002/14651858.CD010339.pub2

43. Gurusamy KS, Samraj K. Routine abdominal drainage for uncomplicated open cholecystectomy. *Cochrane Database Syst Rev.* Apr 18 2007;2007(2):Cd006003. doi:10.1002/14651858.CD006003.pub2

44. Gurusamy KS, Koti R, Davidson BR. Routine abdominal drainage versus no abdominal drainage for uncomplicated laparoscopic cholecystectomy. *Cochrane Database Syst Rev.* Sep 3 2013;(9):Cd006004. doi:10.1002/14651858.CD006004.pub4

45. Antoniou S, Koch O, Antoniou G, et al. Routine versus no drain placement after elective laparoscopic cholecystectomy: meta-analysis of randomized controlled trials. *Minerva Chir.* Jun 2014;69(3):185–94.

46. Bratzler DW, Dellinger EP, Olsen KM, et al. Clinical practice guidelines for antimicrobial prophylaxis in surgery. *Am J Health Syst Pharm.* Feb 1 2013;70(3):195–283. doi:10.2146/ajhp120568

47. van Braak WG, Ponten JEH, Loozen CS, et al. Antibiotic prophylaxis for acute cholecystectomy: PEANUTS II multicentre randomized non-inferiority clinical trial. *Br J Surg.* Feb 24 2022;109(3):267–73. doi:10.1093/bjs/znab441

48. Loozen CS, Kortram K, Kornmann VN, et al. Randomized clinical trial of extended versus single-dose perioperative antibiotic prophylaxis for acute calculous cholecystitis. *Br J Surg.* Jan 2017;104(2):e151–e57. doi:10.1002/bjs.10406

49. Gomi H, Solomkin JS, Schlossberg D, et al. Tokyo Guidelines 2018: antimicrobial therapy for acute cholangitis and cholecystitis. *J Hepatobiliary Pancreat Sci.* Jan 2018;25(1):3–16. doi:10.1002/jhbp.518

50. Haal S, Wielenga MCB, Fockens P, et al. Antibiotic therapy of 3 days may be sufficient after biliary drainage for acute cholangitis: a systematic review. *Dig Dis Sci.* Dec 01 2021;66(12):4128–39. doi:10.1007/s10620-020-06820-3

51. Iwata K, Doi A, Oba Y, et al. Shortening antibiotic duration in the treatment of acute cholangitis: rationale and study protocol for an open-label randomized controlled trial. *Trials.* Jan 17 2020;21(1):97. doi:10.1186/s13063-020-4046-4

49

Acute Pancreatitis

Stephen W. Behrman

Acute pancreatitis (AP) is responsible for over one-quarter of a million hospital admissions in the United States annually, and its incidence is increasing in the United States and Europe [1]. While most cases are self-limiting, about 10–20% of patients will develop severe inflammation of the pancreas requiring intensive diagnostic and therapeutic intervention. Care pathways for AP continue to evolve, are often dynamic, and, in many instances, remain controversial and topics of much debate even at present. These evolving paradigm shifts in the treatment of those with AP represent an opportunity to enhance patient outcomes by reducing infection-related morbidity and mortality while delivering care in a more cost-effective manner and with a reduction in hospital length of stay (LOS).

49.1 What Is the Role (If Any) of Magnetic Resonance Cholangiopancreatography in Suspected Choledocholithiasis in Those with Acute Biliary Pancreatitis?

Magnetic resonance cholangiopancreatography (MRCP) is a noninvasive technique that is more sensitive than ultrasound and computed tomography (CT) as a modality to diagnose choledocholithiasis. This advantage, however, is encumbered by higher financial costs and a potential delay in more invasive therapeutic intervention. Furthermore, MRCP as a "screening" tool to identify candidates for preoperative endoscopic retrograde cholangiopancreatography (ERCP) is often overutilized and remains controversial. Finally, concerning acute biliary pancreatitis (ABP), the need for MRCP in the absence of cholestasis remains debatable since the vast majority of stones will pass spontaneously in this cohort. Given the high cost of this diagnostic test, it should be reserved only if there is a reasonable risk of choledocholithiasis and if it can be proven to have acceptable sensitivity and specificity. If so, it could prove to be advantageous in reducing the need for ERCP with its inherent risks of bleeding, perforation, and pancreatitis. In contrast, indiscriminate use of MRCP in those with little risk of retained common bile duct (CBD) stones is unnecessary and increases costs, whereas in those with predicted high risk for choledocholithiasis, proceeding to immediate ERCP (avoiding MRCP) would not only reduce costs but decrease LOS.

Mofidi et al. retrospectively reviewed the clinical course of 249 patients admitted with ABP (diagnosis not defined) before and after the introduction of MRCP at their institution [2].

Ninety-six patients with a nondilated CBD (<10 mm) and normal or resolving liver function tests within 48 hours went directly to cholecystectomy (CCY) with intraoperative cholangiography (IOC). Eight of 96 had CBD stones—the timing of cholangiography in this cohort was not reported. Preoperative diagnostic testing was utilized for nonresolving cholestasis or evidence of a dilated CBD by ultrasound examination in 106 patients. MRCP (n = 49) was used to identify candidates for ERCP after its introduction. The incidence of choledocholithiasis in up-front ERCP vs. MRCP was 17.5% and 14.2%, respectively (p = NS). Three of 57 patients having ERCP suffered procedure-related complications. Those having MRCP had a significantly shorter LOS, and the sensitivity and specificity of MRCP for CBD stones were 100 and 96%, respectively. The authors conclude that MRCP should be used selectively, preferential to ERCP, in those with the clinical suggestion of retained CBD stones.

Liu et al. assessed 440 patients eligible for laparoscopic CCY and analyzed the results of a selective approach toward up-front ERCP and the need for preoperative MRCP based on risk stratification developed utilizing clinical presentation along with preoperative chemistry and ultrasound criteria [3]. Patients (n = 27) with a CBD >5 mm and elevated liver function tests in the absence of acute cholecystitis or ABP were triaged to up-front ERCP, 93% of whom had choledocholithiasis. Patients (n = 37) with similar criteria but *also* with either acute cholecystitis or pancreatitis had screening MRCP and, if positive, underwent preoperative ERCP. Thirty-two percent had CBD stones, and there was an excellent correlation between MRCP and ERCP. Twenty-six patients in this group that had a negative MRC had intraoperative cholangiography, only one of whom had a CBD stone. A third group (n = 52) with cholecystitis or pancreatitis, a CBD <5 mm, and elevated liver function tests had up-front laparoscopic CCY with attempted cholangiography that was completed in 48. Two (3.8%) had choledocholithiasis. The last group (n = 324) had biliary colic or cholecystitis but not pancreatitis, a CBD <5 mm, and normal liver chemistries. Cholangiography was utilized in <1%, and only three (0.9%) were found to have CBD stones on follow-up evaluation. This study suggests that MRCP can be avoided in those without pancreatitis or cholecystitis but with radiographic and chemical aberrations suggesting choledocholithiasis, allowing a more efficient progression to early ERCP. MRCP can help predict CBD stones in those with cholecystitis and pancreatitis with hard signs by ultrasound and chemistries but can be avoided in those with discordant radiographic and laboratory studies.

DOI: 10.1201/9781003316800-49

Telem et al. retrospectively analyzed 144 patients with ABP (defined as elevated pancreatic enzymes with ultrasound evidence of cholelithiasis) and through a multivariate analysis identified the five most important variables and their "cut-off" points predictive of retained CBD stones [4]. These include CBD ≥9 mm, alkaline phosphatase ≥250 U/I, gamma-glutamyl transferase ≥350 U/I, total bilirubin ≥3 mg/dL, and direct bilirubin ≥2 mg/dL. The presence of four to five of these variables within 72 hours of admission was highly predictive of a retained CBD stone, and this population can proceed directly to ERCP without MRCP. In contrast, in the absence of any variables, patients may proceed directly to CCY with or without cholangiography, as the risk of persistent CBD stones was minimal. Those with one to three variables may benefit from initial MRCP on a selective basis to avoid ERCP, if possible, as 22% of these patients had a positive exam. The importance of a selective approach toward biliary imaging based on these "hard criteria" is highlighted by the fact that 62% and 60% of patients in this study had negative MRCP and ERCP, respectively.

In a follow-up study from this same institution, Prigoff et al. used the same predictive scoring system as proposed by Telem and, utilizing a decision analytic model, prospectively assessed the financial and clinical outcomes of those presenting with ABP and whether patients were managed per protocol (73) or not (32) [5]. Following the predetermined protocol resulted in a cost savings of $2,176/patient for procedural costs and reduced mean LOS by 2.1 days for a reduction of $3,444/patient resulting in a total cost savings of 19% versus those with protocol violation—a direct result of avoiding MRCP in low- and high-risk groups for choledocholithiasis, thus proceeding to earlier CCY and ERCP in these groups, respectively.

Finally, it should be noted that MRCP has its shortcomings relative to ERCP and cannot be relied upon as a definitive examination to exclude biliary pathology when radiologic and laboratory findings suggest otherwise and thus should *not* be used as a bridge to ERCP. Aydelotte et al. identified 81 patients over 6 years having ERCP preceded within 48 hours by MRCP [6]. Twenty-eight "normal" MRCPs were followed by ERCP mostly commonly for a dilated CBD, a poor-quality MRCP, or stones found on IOC. Thirteen of the 28 had clinically important pathology identified on the follow-up ERCP. The negative predictive value of MRCP for the stone disease was only 64%.

RECOMMENDATION

In conclusion, a selective approach that combines abnormal liver function tests and screening ultrasound criteria seems prudent to identify a population presenting with ABP appropriate for early up-front CCY or ERCP, eliminating the need for MRCP and reducing LOS. When utilized more conservatively, MRCP can avoid the need for invasive preoperative ERCP or the need for intraoperative IOC. Adherence to these evidence-base protocols represents an avenue to reduce costs and LOS while eliminating unnecessary expensive MRCP in certain circumstances and enhancing its efficacy in others.

Grade of recommendation: B.

49.2 What Is the Role of Early Endoscopic Retrograde Cholangiopancreatography in Acute Biliary Pancreatitis?

The need for and timing of ERCP in biliary pancreatitis has been a controversial subject in both gastroenterology and the surgical literature. The vast majority of stones will pass spontaneously into the duodenum and thus will neither aggravate ensuing pancreatitis nor present a risk for the development of concurrent cholangitis. Indeed, early ERCP may exacerbate pancreatitis. However, the development of cholangitis in the face of severe AP would most certainly contribute substantially to morbidity and mortality, favoring early endoscopic evaluation. Perhaps more controversial is the role of early ERCP in ameliorating the degree of pancreatitis and the ensuing inflammatory cascade. Several randomized controlled studies and meta-analyses have addressed these issues.

Fan et al. studied the role of ERCP in AP of all causes (predominantly biliary in this Oriental population) in a prospective randomized trial of 197 patients [7]. The purpose of this study was to compare the efficacy of early (<24 hours) ERCP with papillotomy if stones were identified versus initial conservative treatment with ERCP +/− papillotomy reserved for those with clinical deterioration. Indications of clinical deterioration included rising fever, tachycardia, worsening leukocytosis, and/or an increase in bilirubin. The outcome was assessed based on local and systemic complications as well as death. Severe pancreatitis was defined as a Ranson score of 4 or more. Impacted stones were found in 37 of 97 (38%) patients having early ERCP. In contrast, 27 of 98 patients initially followed conservatively required ERCP for deterioration, with stones found in the CBD or ampulla in only 12 (12%), confirming that the vast majority of stones pass spontaneously. Complications were higher in those with initial conservative treatment (29 versus 18%), but this difference was not significant (p = 0.07). Except for those developing cholangitis in the conservative group (8 versus 0 patients), other complications did not differ dramatically. Mortality was higher in those treated conservatively (9 versus 5 patients) but did not reach statistical significance. All deaths occurred in those with severe pancreatitis—the vast majority of whom had no stone found on endoscopic evaluation. Early ERCP did not seem to either worsen or improve the progression of pancreatitis. The authors, surprisingly, conclude that emergency ERCP is indicated in all patients with AP, although their data seem to suggest otherwise.

Folsch et al. conducted a prospective, randomized, multicenter study comparing early ERCP (<72 hours) vs. conservative management in those with ABP *without* evidence of obstructive jaundice [8]. Disease severity was measured by the modified Glasgow criteria (>3 severe). Indications for ERCP in the conservatively managed group were similar to those described by Fan et al. [8] Fifty-eight of 126 patients undergoing early ERCP had documented bile duct stones versus 13 of 112 in the conservative group. Of note, 22 of 112 patients in the conservatively managed group developed indications for ERCP, and the incidence of choledocholithiasis in this group was 60%. Overall, morbidity and mortality did not differ between groups, including the risk of developing pancreatic-related complications such as pseudocyst and necrosis. The authors conclude that early ERCP is not indicated in those with acute biliary pancreatitis in the absence of clinical evidence of biliary obstruction or sepsis.

In a more recent study, Oria et al. examined the role of early (<48–72 hours) ERCP in those presenting with acute gallstone pancreatitis *and* evidence of biliopancreatic obstruction, defined as a CBD >8 mm or serum bilirubin >1.2 mg/dL [9]. Importantly, patients with clinical evidence of cholangitis (Charcot's triad) were excluded, as this condition was felt to mandate early ERCP in this randomized, prospective study. Severe pancreatitis was defined as an APACHE-II score >6. The specific aims of this study were to determine if early ERCP could reduce the severity of pancreatitis and thereby limit organ failure and complications of pancreatitis. The safety of early endoscopy was also assessed. Fifty-one of 103 patients were randomized to early ERCP, with choledocholithiasis noted on 47 (72%) successful cannulations with minimal complications. When comparing the two groups, early clearance of the common duct did not reduce organ failure, local complications of the pancreas, or mortality in either mild or severe pancreatitis. The authors concluded that early ERCP did not alter the course of acute gallstone pancreatitis and was not indicated in the absence of cholangitis.

In a prospective *observational* multicenter study from the Netherlands, the role of early ERCP in predicting severe ABP was examined in 153 patients [10]. Those with cholangitis were excluded, but those with cholestasis or radiographic suggestion of choledocholithiasis (n = 78) were not. Severe pancreatitis was defined as an APACHE-II score ≥8, or Imrie score ≥3, or a C-reactive protein (CRP) >150 mg/dL within 72 hours of admission. A similar time frame defined "early" ERCP that was performed at the discretion of the treating physician. Early ERCP was successful in 70/91 patients in whom it was attempted, and stones were found in 41 (29/52 in those with cholestasis). Overall complications (but not mortality) were reduced in those patients with cholestasis that received early ERCP (n = 52), primarily by a reduction in the extent of pancreatic necrosis. However, the incidence of multiorgan failure and/or the need for pancreas-related therapeutic intervention was not different between treatment groups. Those without cholestasis did not derive the same benefit from early ERCP (n = 29). The authors concluded that early ERCP did not alter the course of acute gallstone pancreatitis and was not indicated in the absence of cholangitis.

Three meta-analyses have yielded the same conclusions while recognizing the heterogeneity of patient populations, enrollment criteria, the arbitrary assignment of mild and severe pancreatitis, and the definition of "early" ERCP [11–13].

RECOMMENDATION

In conclusion, ERCP has proven to be safe when performed in the face of ABP. If performed early, the incidence of choledocholithiasis is substantially higher than if ERCP is performed selectively when there is evidence of persistent biliary obstruction based on routine radiologic and chemical analysis. However, in the studies to date, early clearance of the CBD has not correlated with a reduction in organ failure, pancreatic-related complications, or mortality. For these reasons, in the absence of cholangitis or radiographic or laboratory evidence of biliary obstruction, early ERCP in gallstone pancreatitis is not recommended.

Grade of recommendation: A.

49.3 Should Patients Have Early or Delayed Cholecystectomy Following Acute Biliary Pancreatitis?

Acute biliary pancreatitis (ABP) is the most common etiology of AP worldwide and can vary from mild self-limited disease to severe pancreatitis that may lead to pancreatic necrosis and death. Within this spectrum includes patients who may require prolonged hospitalization and/or are at risk for delayed pancreatic pathology such as pseudocyst formation. Practically, it would be advantageous to perform CCY early and with minimally invasive techniques if the anticipation of AP complications is limited *and* if the inflammatory response is minimized to the extent that one could predict a successful laparoscopic approach. Further, it would help to avoid the need for more than one surgical intervention—i.e., performing gallbladder surgery when it might be anticipated that future surgery for pancreas-related disease would be necessary. Determining the optimal timing of CCY to prevent disease recurrence is therefore not clear-cut.

What is clear, however, is that prolonged delay in CCY is associated with a significant recidivism rate for not only gallstone-related diseases but also recurrent pancreatitis. Burch et al. compared outcomes of patients with similar degrees of pancreatitis that had a CCY during their index admission for ABP vs. those discharged and scheduled for elective surgery [14]. Morbidity and mortality were similar between these two groups. However, 29 of the 65 (44%) patients followed after discharge were represented with either recurrent pancreatitis or biliary tract disease before definitive CCY—most within 3 months. Cameron et al. noted a 25% incidence of hospital readmission when CCY was delayed beyond 4 weeks vs. 6% when the surgery occurred within that period following presentation for biliary pancreatitis [15]. Complications resulting in readmission included cholecystitis, biliary colic, and recurrent pancreatitis.

Studies have examined the results of early versus delayed CCY most often in those with mild to moderate pancreatitis.

Falor et al. compared early (<48 hours) vs. delayed CCY for ABP in a two-institution study for 5 years [16]. Exclusion criteria included >3 Ranson criteria, cholangitis, or high suspicion of a retained CBD stone. Approximately 40% (117/303) of patients had early CCY, and groups were well matched. CCY was accomplished laparoscopically in all with no procedure-related mortality. Median LOS was significantly decreased in the early cohort (3 vs. 6 days). Morbidity and readmission rates did not differ between treatment groups. The need for postoperative ERCP was equivalent (~10%).

A randomized prospective trial from yet this same group was subsequently performed with mild pancreatitis similarly defined [17]. Forty-nine well-matched patients were randomized to laparoscopic CCY within 48 hours of admission or a delayed procedure until clinical and laboratory evidence of pancreatitis had resolved. Exclusion criteria were similar to their prior study. Patients in the delayed group had surgery performed at a mean of 77.8 vs. 35.1 hours in those having early surgery. Laparoscopic CCY was completed in all, and there was no difference in the number requiring postoperative ERCP. LOS was significantly reduced in those with early surgery (median 3 vs. 4 days), and no procedure-related morbidity occurred in either group. The need for postoperative ERCP was equivalent, and there were no readmissions in either study arm.

Noel et al. randomized 66 patients to either early or delayed CCY for mild ABP [18]. Early CCY was defined as within 48 hours, assuming a stable or improved clinical status. Mild pancreatitis was defined by the absence of persistent organ failure and "local" complications at 48 hours. Patients with concurrent cholangitis or ongoing cholestasis requiring therapeutic intervention were excluded. The median time to delayed CCY was 50 days. There was a statistically significant higher rate of gallstone-related events in the delayed group (nine, including five with recurrent pancreatitis, vs. 1). There was no significant difference in CBD stones discovered during surgery or CCY complications between groups. A meta-analysis confirmed the safety of CCY within 48 hours in those with mild ABP [19].

In contradistinction to those presenting with mild disease, patients with severe ABP are not uncommonly hemodynamically unstable, may develop multiple organ failures, and are at risk for necrotizing pancreatitis or pseudocyst formation. Surgeons have been reluctant to proceed with early CCY under these circumstances due to patient instability, difficulty with successful laparoscopic removal, and the potential need for a second operation to address pancreas-specific complications arising from the inflammatory insult. Furthermore, early CCY might contaminate an otherwise sterile pancreatic fluid collection if one exists. There has been a paucity of literature examining early vs. delayed CCY in severe AP. Nealon et al. reported on 187 patients with moderate to severe pancreatitis as defined by 5 or more Ranson criteria, 151 of whom had peripancreatic fluid collections equally distributed between those who had early and delayed CCY (defined as surgery deferred until a fluid collection resolved or required surgical intervention) [20]. Seventy-eight patients had "early" (unfortunately *not* defined in this study) CCY. The number of patients

having attempted laparoscopic removal in the early group was not reported. Forty-four percent suffered postoperative complications, and 49 patients in this group required reoperation following CCY for definitive management of a pancreatic pseudocyst. Of the 109 patients having delayed CCY, all required only one operation for definitive management, including 56 who had successful laparoscopic CCY as their sole procedure and 53 who had combined CCY and internal pseudocyst drainage. Postoperative morbidity was 5%.

RECOMMENDATION

In summary, early CCY in mild to moderate ABP can be safely performed at the index admission following clinical improvement and can most often be accomplished laparoscopically, even if clinical symptoms have not completely abated and/or laboratory examinations normalized. Such a strategy results in a low risk of procedure or disease-related morbidity or the need for hospital readmission due to repeat gallstone-related complications. In contrast, a lower level of evidence suggests that CCY should be delayed in those with severe pancreatitis to allow sepsis and multiorgan failure to resolve and to assess for pancreas-related complications that may require surgical intervention.

Grade of recommendation: A.

49.4 What Is the Role of Prophylactic Antibiotics in Severe Acute Pancreatitis?

Severe pancreatitis, defined by any grading system, is associated with a substantial risk for the development of pancreatic fluid collections and/or pancreatic necrosis. If these processes remain sterile, there is a good probability that patients will recover without the need for operative intervention. In contrast, secondary pancreatic infections mandate the need for therapeutic intervention and debridement, markedly increase hospital LOS, and are associated with significant morbidity and mortality. In theory, prophylactic antibiotics in those with severe AP might prevent the progression of a sterile process into an infected milieu. Questions remain if this mode of therapy is chosen. When should antimicrobial therapy be initiated and for how long? What antibiotic best penetrates pancreatic tissue? Finally, there may be a price to pay for such a strategy, including antibiotic-associated colitis and the potential selection of resistant or fungal organisms given prolonged therapy that may augment, rather than protect against, the risk for mortality.

A review of antimicrobial agents with satisfactory tissue concentrations in the pancreatic bed is appropriate. In a classic study, Buchler et al. measured the tissue (not serum) concentrations of 10 different antibiotics in 89 patients having *elective* pancreatic surgery [21]. Antimicrobial agents with the highest tissue concentrations as well as bactericidal activity included ciprofloxacin, ofloxacin, and imipenem. Further work from Bassi et al. examined the utility of these favored antibiotics in the face of human necrotizing pancreatitis [22]. Tissue (not serum) levels of antimicrobials were obtained by needle biopsy, samples obtained at the time of surgery, or from surgically placed drains in 12 patients. In this study, fluoroquinolones and metronidazole had concentrations in pancreatic tissue higher than the minimal inhibitory concentration (MIC) for the most commonly cultured organisms. Carbapenem concentrations in necrotic tissue did not always exceed the MIC for common pathogens. The liposolubility of these agents proved to be a common trait, and repeated administration enhanced their penetration in necrotic pancreatic tissue. In common with the study by Buchler, aminoglycosides proved inadequate, presumably due to their limited liposolubility. Thus, fluoroquinolones and carbapenems have formed the basis of clinical studies investigating the role of antimicrobial prophylaxis in severe pancreatitis.

A study supporting antibiotic prophylaxis was reported from seven Norwegian hospitals on 73 antibiotic-naive patients, with severe AP defined as a CRP >120 mg/L and evidence of necrosis by CT imaging [23]. Patients were randomized to imipenem for 5–7 days or control in a nonblinded fashion. While overall infectious complications were significantly reduced in those who received prophylaxis, the incidence of organ failure, peripancreatic infection, need for pancreas-specific therapeutic intervention, and death was not different between treatment groups. While admitting the study was underpowered, the authors surprisingly conclude that the utilization of antimicrobial prophylaxis in severe AP is recommended.

In a study from Lithuania, the impact of antibiotic prophylaxis instituted within 72 hours of presentation on the clinical course of 210 well-matched patients with severe AP defined as CRP >120 mg/:, APACHE II score >7, and evidence of >30% pancreatic necrosis by CT imaging was assessed [24]. Results were analyzed based on two time periods: 2 years during which prophylaxis was employed (ciprofloxacin 800 mg/day, metronidazole 1,500 mg/day for 14 days) and 1 subsequent year when it was withdrawn (103 and 107 patients, respectively). There was no difference in the incidence of infected necrosis, the need for necrosectomy, organ failure, LOS, or mortality between treatment groups.

Isenmann et al. performed a multicenter, randomized, placebo-controlled, double-blind study on the effect of ciprofloxacin and Flagyl, administered for a minimum of 14 days, in preventing infected pancreatic necrosis and thereby reducing mortality [25]. One hundred and fourteen patients with severe acute pancreatitis defined as a CRP >150 mg/L and/or the presence of pancreatic necrosis on contrast-enhanced CT and entering within 72 hours of admission were studied. Study patients were converted to open antibiotic therapy if extrapancreatic or de novo pancreatic sepsis was documented, multiple organ failure developed, or CRP levels increased. The etiology of pancreatitis was predominantly biliary and alcohol-related. Of the 58 patients randomized to treatment, only 16 required conversion to open antimicrobial administration versus 26 in the placebo group—a significant difference. However, the incidence of secondary and extrapancreatic infections was not different, nor was the mortality rate. Approximately one-half

of the isolates in both groups with infected necrosis were gram-positive organisms. However, it was not noted how these isolates were obtained—open versus percutaneous. Thus, while empiric antibiotic treatment did not lead to the development of resistant or fungal organisms, it failed to prevent pancreatic and systemic infections and it did not reduce mortality in this study. It should be noted, however, that the initial power analysis called for a study population of 200 patients, assuming an incidence of pancreatic infection of 40%. Surprisingly, this study was terminated after an interim analysis because the authors stated that infected pancreatic necrosis occurred in 7/53 treated patients versus 5/52 receiving placebo and this was a reverse trend. Certainly, it could be argued that study recruitment should have continued.

Dellinger et al. reported a multicenter similarly designed study and patient population to that of Isenmann comparing prophylactic meropenem infusion to placebo in 40 patients, each within 5 days of onset of severe AP and delivered for 7–21 days [26]. In contrast to the study by Isenmann, most patients in this study had documented pancreatic necrosis >30%, consistent with severe disease. The incidence of developing a pancreatic infection, the number of operative interventions on the pancreas, and the mortality rate were not different between groups. The utilization of prophylaxis did not increase the incidence of resistant organisms, with gram-positive and negative flora predominating. The authors concluded that antibiotic prophylaxis did not reduce septic pancreatic infections in those with severe AP. This study again did not reach its desired power analysis, assuming an incidence of pancreatic infection of 40%, and it was not continued to reach the desired number of patients due to a "restriction of resources."

A final single-center double-blind randomized controlled trial (RCT) studied imipenem vs. placebo in 98 antibiotic-naïve patients, each with AP and a calculated APACHE II score of 8 or greater [27]. Infectious complications occurred in 20 vs. 25%, respectively, and were not different between groups, nor was the development of infected pancreatic necrosis, organ failure, and mortality. The incidence of multidrug-resistant organisms, but not fungal infections, was found in the group receiving imipenem. A meta-analysis confirmed that prophylactic antibiotics have no impact on the development of infectious sequelae in severe AP [28]. Unfortunately, despite this evidence-based recommendation, real-world data suggest antibiotics are still utilized in over 50% of patients with severe AP [29].

RECOMMENDATION

To summarize, the utilization of prophylactic antibiotics in severe necrotizing pancreatitis is well tolerated but may alter the flora recovered if infection ensues, as well as lead to the development of resistant organisms. Although not an absolute contraindication, the routine use of antibiotic prophylaxis in those with severe pancreatitis and significant necrosis should be discouraged.

Grade of recommendation: B.

49.5 Is Enteral Nutrition Safe and Superior to Total Parenteral Nutrition in Severe Acute Pancreatitis?

Nutritional support in severe AP is vital due to the local and systemic inflammatory response that increases metabolic demands resulting in hypercatabolism [30]. In an attempt to "rest" the pancreas and not worsen its severity, hyperalimentation has traditionally provided the backbone of therapy to meet nutritional needs. In addition, severe pancreatitis is often associated with gastric stasis and/or intestinal ileus, limiting enteral feeding, and many patients are simply too ill to consume adequate calories. It has long been recognized that enteral nutrition (EN) is superior to the parenteral route in terms of immune competence, metabolic homeostasis, and reducing catheter-related sepsis, as well as the overall cost of support, and its utilization in other areas of surgical care has been well-established [31]. Most recently, the paradigm that EN in severe pancreatitis exacerbates the disease or will not be tolerated has been challenged. The utilization of this mode of nutritional support, however, must not present its own set of complications *and* it must prove superior outcomes to standard therapy with total parenteral nutrition (TPN).

In the setting of severe AP, the utilization of jejunal nutrition has its inherent limitations and potential associated complications beyond just intolerance secondary to disease-associated ileus. Nasojejunal (NJ) tube placement typically requires either radiologic or endoscopic advancement, either of which can be problematic in an unstable intensive care unit patient. Bedside placement can be utilized but is cumbersome and time-consuming. In addition, jejunal feedings in the hypotensive patient, those with large volume fluid requirements, and patients with clinical evidence of an ileus have been associated with the development of catastrophic small bowel necrosis [32]. With these caveats in mind, jejunal feedings have been successfully implemented in AP in several comparison studies with TPN.

Windsor et al. investigated the impact of EN on decreasing the acute-phase response, and thereby the disease severity, of AP when compared with TPN in a randomized trial of 34 patients [33]. Severe pancreatitis was defined as an Imrie score >3, and NJ tubes were placed under radiographic guidance. Enrollment was within 48 hours of admission, and the influence of nutritional support was assessed after 7 days of implementation. Patients were followed clinically for the development of systemic inflammatory response syndrome, intraabdominal sepsis, multiple organ failure, the need for operative intervention, and mortality. Four of 16 patients in the EN group required a temporary reduction in their goal rate due to intolerance. The EN group had a significant reduction in CRP levels and APACHE II scores—a trend *not* found in the TPN group. EN significantly reduced measured inflammatory mediators vs. TPN. The clinical parameters assessed demonstrated a superior trend favoring EN. The authors conclude that EN is superior to TPN in attenuating the acute-phase response of pancreatitis, which may translate to an improved clinical course.

A well-performed randomized study of 38 patients with severe pancreatitis was reported by Kalfarentzos et al. [34]. Severe pancreatitis was defined as three or more Imrie criteria or an APACHE II score >8 combined with a CRP concentration >120 mg/L within 48 hours of admission and grade D or E findings by Balthazar CT criteria. All patients received antibiotic prophylaxis with imipenem. The 18 patients randomized to EN had a nasoenteric tube placed fluoroscopically within 48 hours of admission (2 patients had unsuccessful placement and were excluded from analysis). Feedings were initiated immediately thereafter in resuscitated "stable" patients. There was no difference in the clinical course of either group concerning the need for operation, LOS, and mortality. Target nutritional goals were reached and nitrogen balance improved progressively and equally in both groups. The mean number of infections per patient as well as the overall complication rate was significantly less in those receiving EN; however, few pancreatic infections were noted. EN was significantly less expensive. The authors conclude that early EN in those with severe pancreatitis is safe and preferential to TPN.

Petrov et al. examined the impact of EN on reducing secondary pancreatic infections and mortality in a randomized trial of 69 well-matched patients presenting with severe AP defined as an APACHE II score >8 and/or a CRP concentration >150 mg/dL [35]. Nutritional support was initiated within 72 hours of presentation, with enteral catheters positioned radiologically. The hemodynamic stability, or lack thereof, of patients receiving EN was not reported. Prophylactic antibiotics were routinely utilized in both groups. When compared with TPN, EN was associated with a statistically significant reduction in pancreatic and extrapancreatic septic morbidity. Since pancreatic infection mandated operative intervention, the need for surgery was significantly reduced in those receiving EN as well. Mortality from pancreatic sepsis and/or multiple organ failure was significantly worse in those receiving TPN. The need for additional feeding tube positioning, abdominal bloating, diarrhea, and a reduction in the rate of administration of support were all more common in those receiving EN. The authors conclude that EN could be an important adjunct in reducing pancreatic infectious complications, and thereby mortality, in those with severe AP.

A study from Poland assessed the impact of early (<48 hours) versus delayed (*n* = 100) EN (3–7 days after admission) on infectious complications and clinical outcomes in 197 well-matched patients with predicted severe AP [36]. The diagnosis of severe AP was similar to that in other studies. Exclusion criteria included those admitted after 72 hours of the onset of symptoms. The authors make no mention of withholding feedings in hemodynamically unstable patients. NJ tube placement was made by a "medical staff," while endoscopy was reserved for those who had a failure of bedside placement. The need for surgical intervention for pancreas-related complications was not different between treatment groups (7 early, 11 delayed). The incidence of infected peripancreatic collections and mortality was higher in those with delayed EN. Except for respiratory failure, systemic complications were not different between treatment groups. The authors conclude that early EN should be instituted following admission for severe AP. Caution, however, needs to be utilized in those with hemodynamic instability to reduce the risk of bowel infarction.

RECOMMENDATION

In conclusion, when compared with TPN, careful utilization of EN is well tolerated, reduces the inflammatory response of AP, reduces infectious morbidity, and is less expensive. Data demonstrating a clinical improvement concerning the need for operative intervention, a shorter hospital LOS, and disease-related mortality when EN is utilized remain sparse but promising due to the small number of patients reported in comparative studies to date. While further study is needed and with the acknowledged difficulty in feeding tube placement, EN in the hemodynamically stable patient with severe pancreatitis is favored with close monitoring of tolerance.

If jejunal feeding is not tolerated due to hemodynamic instability or ileus, TPN remains an important therapy.

Grade of recommendation: A.

49.6 Is Gastric Feeding Safe and Equivalent to Jejunal Feeding in Acute Pancreatitis?

With the aforementioned benefits of jejunal feedings, a reasonable extrapolation would be to simplify the limitations of tube placement by feeding directly into the stomach. As previously noted, such a management scheme may be associated with its inherent complications, specifically intolerance due to gastric stasis, the possibility of aspiration in those without airway protection, and an exacerbation of pancreatitis due to stimulation of the pancreas. Several clinical trials have compared these routes of administration.

Eatock et al. randomized 49 well-matched patients with severe AP defined as an Imrie score >3 and APACHE II score >6 or a CRP >150 mg/dL to nasogastric (NG) vs. endoscopically placed NJ feedings beginning within 72 hours of the onset of symptoms [37]. All but one patient tolerated the enteral route, and the majority of patients in both groups were receiving at least 75% of goal calories within 48 hours of initiation of feedings. Groups did not differ concerning follow-up APACHE II scores, CRP levels, or pain analog scales, and mortality was not statistically different (24.5% of the study population). Gastrointestinal complications were equivalent between groups. One patient required a repeat endoscopy to replace an NJ tube. The authors conclude that NG feeding is simpler, less expensive, and equivalent to the NJ route.

Kumar et al. randomized 31 evenly matched patients with severe AP defined as organ failure and an APACHE II score >8 or Balthazar score >7 to NG ($n = 15$) or NJ (placed endoscopically) feedings [38]. Importantly, patients in shock (systolic blood pressure <90 mmHg) were appropriately excluded, and feedings were gradually increased over 7 days. Patients were assessed for study accrual up to 4 weeks after the onset of symptoms—a delay in initiation that might allow better tolerance of feedings. No patient required TPN once the goal rate of feeding was achieved (day 7). When compared with the NJ route, NG feedings were associated with similar rates of pancreatic infection and operative intervention, and the LOS and mortality were not different between groups. Anthropometric and nutritional parameters declined regardless of the route of administration, and complications were similar. Neither modality exacerbated pancreatitis. The authors conclude that both routes of administration, when gradually delivered, are well tolerated but fail to reverse the catabolism associated with the disease.

Eckerwall et al. compared NG feedings to TPN in 48 well-matched patients with severe AP defined as an APACHE II score >8 and/or a CRP level >150 mg/dL [39]. The goal of the study was to assess the impact of nutrient delivery on the inflammatory response of AP during the first 10 days of illness. Nutritional support was started within 24 hours of admission with a target goal reached in 66% of the entire population with no difference between groups. No patient receiving NG feeds had aspiration. A measure of inflammation decreased equally in both groups during the study period. Only one patient in the entire series required operative pancreatic surgery. The authors concluded that NG feedings were tolerated well in those with predicted severe AP but did not attenuate the inflammatory response associated with the disease when compared with TPN.

Finally, Singh et al. randomized 78 well-matched patients with severe AP defined as organ failure, APACHE II score >8, or a CT Balthazar score >7 to NG or NJ feedings [40]. Patients in shock were excluded. The NJ tube was placed endoscopically, and feedings were initiated within 48 hours and aimed at achieving the nutrient goal within 3–4 days, which was successful in all study patients. Diarrhea occurred in three and four patients with NJ and NG feedings, respectively. There were fewer overall infectious complications, including those within the pancreatic bed, in the group receiving NG feeds. However, four and two patients in the NG and NJ pathways required surgery for infected necrosis. The authors claim that some with infected necrosis were treated with antibiotics alone; however, this would seem exceptional in terms of definitive treatment. In addition, the total number of patients with infected necrosis was not clearly stated. Measures of intestinal permeability and endotoxemia were not different between groups. Given these limitations, their data would support their conclusion that NG feeding was not inferior to that provided by the NJ route.

RECOMMENDATION

In summary, these studies suggest that NG feeding seems to be tolerated as well as NJ feeding in those with severe AP in the hemodynamically stable patient without exacerbating the disease process provided a close assessment of tolerance is made.

The relationship of NG feedings to a decline in secondary pancreatic infections and disease-related mortality has yet to be ascertained.

Grade of recommendation: A.

49.7 Is the Step-Up Approach toward the Management of Pancreatic Necrosis Superior to Up-Front Open Pancreatic Necrosectomy?

Severe AP may result in pancreatic necrosis. While most often self-limited and sterile, necrotic debris may become secondarily infected, necessitating necrosectomy for control of sepsis. Management over the last two decades has shifted from aggressive early operative intervention to supportive care and a delayed approach even in the face of organ failure to allow the demarcation of necrotic debris from viable retroperitoneal tissues. Most recently, attention has focused on therapeutic techniques that may avoid open laparotomy or at least temporize source control until physiologic status allows a more optimal environment to proceed to surgery. While in theory, these nonoperative approaches are appealing, questions regarding this step-up approach toward necrosectomy need to be entertained, including the following: How many nonoperative therapeutic interventions might be required for complete necrosectomy and over what period? What if bleeding ensues? Could failure with this approach lead to outcomes inferior to initial operative necrosectomy? Thus, a critical review of the literature is important.

The importance of delayed management of pancreatic necrosis has been highlighted in many studies and expert consensus guidelines [41]. A recent University of Minnesota study challenging a delayed approach supports its importance (despite this paper's opposite conclusions) [42]. In a nonrandomized fashion 305 patients with collections resulting from necrotizing pancreatitis and who received an endoscopically centered step-up approach utilizing both endoscopic and/or percutaneous drainage were divided into those receiving treatment <4 weeks vs. those with delayed management. Those with early drainage more frequently suffered organ failure, perhaps prompting earlier intervention. However, there was a significantly increased LOS, need for salvage open necrosectomy, and mortality in the early intervention group. While unrelenting septic shock, progressive organ failure, and physiologic decline warrant early intervention, a delayed approach even in the face of stable organ dysfunction leads to improved patient outcomes and more definitive, initial debridement.

A look at percutaneous catheter drainage (PCD) as a sole therapeutic intervention for necrotizing pancreatitis was reported in a systemic review by van Baal et al. inclusive of 11 studies (384 patients) [43]. The success rate (percentage of patients surviving without surgical necrosectomy) was 56%. Of the five series reporting, final drain removal occurred from 16 to 98 days. Two or more catheters were necessary for the seven studies reporting, but the mean number of procedures and imaging required were *not* captured and reported. Twenty-one percent suffered one or more complications, the most frequent being pancreaticocutaneous fistula. The chronicity and management of this complication were not reported. Surgical necrosectomy was still required in 133 patients with an interval between PCD and operation ranging between 1 and 600 days—most occurring greater than 1–2 months into the disease process. Overall mortality was approximately 17% and was not different in those with sterile or infected necrosis.

Transgastric necrosectomy by endoscopic, minimally invasive, or open techniques has received significant attention in the last decade. The advantages of this method include avoidance of pancreatic fistula if a persistent pancreatic leak or disconnected pancreatic duct syndrome occurs as a result of the necrotizing process. The disadvantages are the potential need for multiple procedures due to limited access and the fact that this approach may not allow complete debridement if the necrotizing process extends down the paracolic gutters to the base of the mesentery. A multi-institutional series assessing the results of surgical transgastric necrosectomy in 178 patients were reported by Driedger et al [44]. Procedures were performed at a median of 60 days following the onset of pancreatitis. Postoperative morbidity and mortality were 23% and 2%, respectively. Repeat surgery and intervention were necessary for 10% and 13%, respectively. The median LOS was 14 days, and 20% required readmission. Ultimate symptom recovery occurred in 91%.

Analysis of up-front open necrosectomy in the current era is lacking due to a shift toward less invasive management. More historical publications (before a delayed management approach was appreciated) reported significant morbidity, including reoperation, bleeding, pancreatic fistula, erosion into hollow viscus, and hernia formation. A report from the Indiana group offers a modern appraisal of this approach [45]. Eighty-six patients by a single surgeon were accumulated over 12 years, and 40 patients were initially managed in a step-up manner. Twenty-eight percent required necrosectomy in an "urgent/emergent" manner due to clinical deterioration. The median time for surgical necrosectomy was 64 days. Postoperative organ dysfunction occurred in 40% and 35% required further intervention, 50% of whom required reoperation. The median LOS was 11 days. Ninety-day morbidity and mortality rates were 70% and 2%, respectively. The authors suggest open necrosectomy in a delayed manner results in a marked decrease in mortality when compared to historical reports even though this technique was applied in often high-risk clinical scenarios. They suggest open necrosectomy needs to be considered in the multidisciplinary approach to pancreatic necrosis.

In a large multicenter trial by van Santvoort et al., 88 patients with suspected or confirmed infected necrosis during 3 years were randomized to open necrosectomy versus a minimally invasive step-up approach [46]. The primary endpoint was the development of major complications or death. The emphasis was to delay any intervention for at least 4 weeks after the initial onset of the disease. The step-up approach consisted of initial percutaneous or endoscopic drainage progressing to further percutaneous drains, followed by video-assisted retroperitoneal debridement. Of those randomized to open necrosectomy, the median number of operations was 1 (range 1–7) and 42% required repeat laparotomy for further necrosectomy or complications, while 33% required postoperative percutaneous drainage. In the minimally invasive group, 35% eradicated disease with either percutaneous or endoscopic drainage and two patients died before further intervention could occur.

Sixty percent proceeded to video-based necrosectomy with only two patients requiring an operative approach. Patients in this group underwent a median of 1 (range 1–3) video-assisted necrosectomies, and 33% and 27% required further surgery or postoperative percutaneous drainage, respectively. While major complications occurred more frequently in those with open necrosectomy, mortality was not different between groups.

It is worth noting that percutaneous drainage and the "step-up" approach toward pancreatic necrosectomy are not without their own set of inherent complications. In a single-center study of 171 patients with necrotizing pancreatitis that was managed most often by a step-up approach (*n* = 158) from the University of California, a median of seven CT examinations and seven fluoroscopic procedures were performed, with a median cumulative effective dose (CED) of 274 mSv [47]. Thirty percent had more than 500 mSv, which carries a 5% lifetime risk of developing cancer, and the need for these excessive procedures was associated with infected necrosis and endoscopic necrosectomy. Gupta et al. reviewed a single-institution experience of 707 PCDs in 314 patients with necrotizing pancreatitis [48]. Enteric communication occurred in 8.9% and bleeding in 7.3%. Twenty percent of those with hollow viscus involvement required operative intervention. Bleeding complications required angioembolization and surgical intervention in ~20% and 35%, respectively.

RECOMMENDATION

Cumulatively, these data suggest one approach toward the management of pancreatic necrosis is not superior to another and that all strategies toward treatment carry an inherent risk of morbidity and mortality given this difficult disease. Treatment often requires multiple avenues for therapeutic intervention and multidisciplinary care to completely eradicate the disease. Thus, these approaches should be viewed as complementary rather than mutually exclusive. The sole RCT comparing the step-up approach to open necrosectomy suggests decreased complications when the former is utilized and implies this patient population is best managed by regional centers of expertise.

Grade of recommendation: B.

TABLE 49.1

Summary of evidence and recommendations

Question	Answer	Levels of Evidence	Grade of Recommendation	References
What is the role (if any) of MRCP in suspected choledocholithiasis in those with acute biliary pancreatitis?	Routine use is discouraged. A selective approach based on ultrasound and liver profile to identify candidates for preoperative ERCP or up-front surgery is recommended.	II-2	B	[2–5]
What is the role of ERCP in acute biliary pancreatitis?	Only if evidence of cholangitis or biliary obstruction exists.	I	A	[6–12]
Should patients have early or delayed cholecystectomy following acute biliary pancreatitis?	Early in mild to moderate disease. Delay in those with severe AP.	II-1	B	[13–19]
What is the role of prophylactic antibiotics in severe AP?	Studies do not show a routine benefit. Reasonable in those with multiorgan failure.	II-1	B	[20–28]
Is EN safe and superior to TPN in severe AP?	Safe and less expensive, but clinical benefits are unclear.	I	A	[29–35]
Is gastric feeding safe and equivalent to jejunal feeding in SAP?	Safe in hemodynamically stable patients if tolerated.	I	A	[36–39]
Is a step-up approach toward the management of pancreatic necrosis superior to up-front open necrosectomy?		II-3	B	[40–47]

Abbreviations: AP: Acute pancreatitis, EN: Enteral nutrition, ERCP: Endoscopic cholangiopancreatography, MRCP: Magnetic resonance cholangiopancreatography, SAP: Severe acute pancreatitis, TPN: Total parenteral nutrition.

Editor's Note

Acute pancreatitis (AP) is one of the few areas in general surgery where there is a considerable amount of quality research to guide our management. In the past, antibiotics, nasogastric suction, and early cholecystectomy were proven to be unnecessary in patients with AP. In the setting of gallstones, the issue of diagnostic imaging required in patients with elevated liver function tests or ductal dilatation remains controversial. The majority of the high-quality scientific literature does not support early ERCP in this setting. MRCP misses nearly half of the common duct stones, is expensive, and delays management. In my opinion, trending the clinical status of the patient as well as liver function tests avoids the need for unnecessary imaging. Improvement leads directly to cholecystectomy, while lack of resolution of symptoms should be dealt with using ERCP. The timing of cholecystectomy has been well studied and supports at least a short delay (48 hours) to allow for the manifestation of the development of severe disease before proceeding to operation. Antibiotics should be avoided in AP, even severe pancreatitis, as they do not improve outcomes and lead to resistance. As stated earlier, there is high-level evidence (grade A recommendations) for aggressive, appropriate use of ERCP in biliary ductal obstruction and for enteral feedings via gastric approach in severe pancreatitis.

REFERENCES

1. Iannuzi JP, King JA, Leong JH, et al. Global incidence of acute pancreatitis is increasing over time: a systematic review and meta-analysis. Gastroenterology. 2022;162:122–34.
2. Mofidi R, Lee AC, Madhavan KK, et al. The selective use of magnetic resonance cholangiopancreatography in the imaging of the axial biliary tree in patients with acute gallstone pancreatitis. Pancreatology. 2008;8:55–60.
3. Liu TH, Consorti ET, Kawahima A, et al. Patient evaluation and management with selective use of magnetic resonance cholangiography and endoscopic retrograde cholangiopancreatography before laparoscopic cholecystectomy. Ann Surg. 2001;234:33–40.
4. Telem DA, Bowman K, Hwang J, et al. Selective management of patients with acute biliary pancreatitis. J Gastrointest Surg. 2009;13:2183–88.
5. Prigoff JG, Swain GW, Divino CM. Scoring system for the management of acute gallstone pancreatitis: cost analysis of a prospective study. J Gastrointest Surg. 2016;20:905–13.
6. Aydelotte JD, Ali J, Huynh PT, et al. Use of magnetic resonance cholangiopancreatography in clinical practice: not as good as we once thought. J Am Coll Surg. 2015;221:215–19.
7. Fan S, Lai E, Mok F, et al. Early treatment of acute biliary pancreatitis by endoscopic papillotomy. N Engl J Med. 1993;328:228–32.
8. Folsch UR, Nitsche R, Ludtle R, et al. Early ERCP, and papillotomy compared with conservative treatment for acute biliary pancreatitis. The German Study Group on acute biliary pancreatitis. N Engl J Med. 1997;336:237–42.
9. Oria A, Cimmino D, Ocampo C, et al. Early endoscopic intervention versus early conservative management in patients with acute gallstone pancreatitis and biliopancreatic obstruction: a randomized clinical trial. Ann Surg. 2007;245:10–7.
10. Van Santvoort HC, Besselink MG, de Vries AC, et al. Early endoscopic retrograde cholangiopancreatography in predicted severe acute biliary pancreatitis. Ann Surg. 2009;250:68–75.
11. Behrns KE, Ashley SW, Hunter JG, et al. Early ERCP for gallstone pancreatitis: for whom and when? J Gastrointest Surg. 2008;12:629–33.
12. Petrov MS, van Santvoort HC, van der Heijden GJ, et al. Early endoscopic retrograde cholangiopancreatography versus conservative management in acute biliary pancreatitis: a meta-analysis of randomized trials. Ann Surg. 2008;247:250–7.
13. Uy MC, Daez ML, Sy PP, et al. Early ERCP in acute gallstone pancreatitis without cholangitis: a meta-analysis. JOP. 2009;10:299–305.
14. Burch JM, Feliciano DV, Mattox KL, et al. Gallstone pancreatitis. Arch Surg. 1990;125:853–60.
15. Cameron DR, Goodman AJ. Delayed cholecystectomy for gallstone pancreatitis: re-admissions and outcomes. Ann R Coll Engl. 2004;86:358–62.
16. Falor AE, de Virgilio C, Stabile BE, et al. Early laparoscopic cholecystectomy for mild gallstone pancreatitis. Arch Surg. 2012;147:1031–5.
17. Aboulian A, Chan T, Yaghoubian A, et al. Early cholecystectomy safely decreases hospital stay in patients with mild gallstone pancreatitis. Ann Surg. 2010;251:615–9.
18. Noel R, Amelo U, Lundell L, et al. Index versus delayed cholecystectomy in mild gallstone pancreatitis: results of a randomized controlled trial. HPB. 2018;20:932–8.
19. Perez LJR, Parra JF, Dimas GA. The safety of early laparoscopic cholecystectomy (<48h) for patients with mild gallstone pancreatitis: a systematic review of the literature and meta-analysis. Cir Esp. 2014;92:107–13.
20. Nealon WH, Bawduniak J, Walser EM. Appropriate timing of cholecystectomy in patients who present with moderate to severe gallstone-associated acute pancreatitis with peripancreatic fluid collections. Ann Surg. 2004; 239:741–51.
21. Buchler M, Malfertheiner P, Friess, H et al. Human pancreatic tissue concentration of bactericidal antibiotics. Gastroenterology. 1992;103(6):1902–8.
22. Bassi C, Pederzoli P, Vesentini S, et al. Behavior of antibiotics during human necrotizing pancreatitis. Antimicrob Agents Chemother. 1994;38(4):830–6.
23. Rokke O, Harbitz TB, Liljedal J, et al. Early treatment of severe pancreatitis with imipenem: a prospective randomized clinical trial. Scan J Gastroenterol. 2007;42: 771–6.
24. Ignatavicius P, Vitkauskiene A, Pundzius J, et al. Effects of prophylactic antibiotics in acute pancreatitis. HPB. 2012; 14:396–402.
25. Isenmann R, Runzi M, Kron M, et al. Prophylactic antibiotic treatment in patients with predicted severe acute pancreatitis: a placebo-controlled, double-blind trial. Gastroenterology. 2004;126(4):997–1004.
26. Dellinger EP, Tellado JM, Soto NE, et al. Early antibiotic treatment for severe necrotizing pancreatitis: a randomized, double-blind, placebo-controlled study. Ann Surg. 2007;245(5):674–83.
27. Poropat G, Radovan A, Peric M, et al. Prevention of infectious complications in acute pancreatitis: results of a single-center, randomized, controlled trial. Pancreas. 2019;48:1056–1060.
28. Wittau M, Mayer B, Scheele J, et al. Systemic review and meta-analysis of antibiotic prophylaxis in severe acute pancreatitis. Scand J Gastroenterol. 2011;46:261–70.
29. Vlada AC, Schmit B, Perry A, et al. Failure to follow evidence-based best practice guidelines in the treatment of severe acute pancreatitis. HPB. 2013;15:822–7.
30. Dickerson RN, Vehe KL, Mullen JL, et al. Resting energy expenditure in patients with pancreatitis. Crit Care Med. 1991;19(4):484–90.
31. Kudsk KA. The beneficial effect of enteral nutrition. Gastrointest Endosc Clin N Am. 2007;17(4):647–62.
32. Schunn CD, Daly JM. Small bowel necrosis associated with postoperative jejunal tube feeding. J Am Coll Surg. 1995;180(4):410–16.
33. Windsor A, Kanwar S, Li A, et al. Compared with parenteral nutrition, enteral feeding attenuates the acute-phase response and improves disease severity in acute pancreatitis. Gut. 1998;42(3):431–5.

34. Kalfarentzos F, Kehagias J, Mead N, et al. Enteral nutrition is superior to parenteral nutrition in severe acute pancreatitis: results of a randomized prospective trial. Br J Surg. 1997; 84(12):1665–9.

35. Petrov MS, Kukosh MV, Emelyanov NV. A randomized controlled trial of enteral versus parenteral feeding in patients with predicted severe acute pancreatitis shows a significant reduction in mortality and infected pancreatic complications with total enteral nutrition. Dig Surg. 2006;23(5–6):336–45.

36. Wereszczynska-Siemiatkowska U, Swidnicka-Siergiejko A, Siemiatkowski A, et al. Early enteral nutrition is superior to delayed enteral nutrition for the prevention of infected necrosis and mortality in acute pancreatitis. Pancreas. 2013; 42:640–6.

37. Eatock F, Chong P, Menezes N, et al. A randomized study of early nasogastric versus nasojejunal feeding in severe acute pancreatitis. Am J Gastroenterology. 2005;100(2):432–9.

38. Kumar A, Singh N, Prakash S, et al. Early enteral nutrition in severe acute pancreatitis: a prospective randomized controlled trial comparing nasojejunal and nasogastric routes. J Clin Gastroenterol. 2006;40(5):431–4.

39. Eckerwall G, Axelsson J, Andersson R. Early nasogastric feeding in predicted severe acute pancreatitis: a clinical randomized study. Ann Surg. 2006;244(6):959–67.

40. Singh N, Sharma B, Sharma M, et al. Evaluation of early enteral feeding through a nasogastric and nasojejunal tube in severe acute pancreatitis. Pancreas. 2012;41:153–9.

41. Baron TH, Dimaio CJ, Wang AY, et al. American gastroenterological association clinical practice update: management of pancreatic necrosis. Gastroenterology. 2020;158:67–75.

42. Trikudanathan G, Tawfik P, Amateau SK, et al. Early (<4 weeks) versus standard (≥4 weeks) endoscopically centered step-up interventions for necrotizing pancreatitis. Pancreas. 2018;113:1550–58.

43. van Baal MC, van Santvoort HC, Bollen TL, et al. Systematic review of percutaneous catheter drainage as primary treatment for necrotizing pancreatitis. Br J Surg. 2011;98:18–27.

44. Driedger M, Zyromski NJ, Visser BC, et al. Surgical transgastric necrosectomy for necrotizing pancreatitis. Ann Surg. 2020;271:163–68.

45. Maatman TK, Flick KF, Roch AM, et al. Operative pancreatic debridement: contemporary outcomes in changing times. Pancreatology. 2020;20:968–75.

46. van Santvoort HC, Besselink MG, Bakker OJ, et al. A step-up approach or open necrosectomy for necrotizing pancreatitis. NEJM. 2010;362:1491–502.

47. Thiruvengadam NR, Miranda J, Kim C, et al. Burden of ionizing radiation in the diagnosis and management of necrotizing pancreatitis. Clin Transl Gastroenterol. 2021; 12:1–8.

48. Gupta R, Kulkarni A, Babu R, et al. Complications of percutaneous drainage in step-up approach for management of pancreatic necrosis: experience of 10 years from a tertiary care center. J Gastrointest Surg. 2020;24:598–609.

50

Pancreatic Pseudocysts

Zachary E. Stiles and Stephen W. Behrman

Pancreatic pseudocysts (PPs) are common sequelae of acute and chronic pancreatitis. Large pseudocysts are often symptomatic due to compression of surrounding hollow viscera and may, over time, lead to more dreaded complications such as infection, bleeding, and rupture resulting in pancreatic ascites. Assessing the need for any intervention of PP is often based on the dynamic interplay of symptomatology, size, and resolution or expansion over time. Treatment of PP may involve surgery, endoscopy, percutaneous drainage (PD), or a combination of these therapeutic interventions. While commonly encountered, algorithms for the therapeutic management of PP under a variety of clinical scenarios have surprisingly been infrequently assessed in head-to-head comparisons and in some instances, rarely at all. This chapter will attempt to frame best practice management for these problematic lesions that frequently lead to a prolonged course of disability and recovery.

50.1 Does the Size of a Pancreatic Pseudocyst Predict the Likelihood of Resolution Following Acute Pancreatitis?

Rates of PP resolution with conservative management have varied widely in the literature [1]. Multiple factors have been postulated to be associated with PP resolution, most notably the size of the collection. Most of the evidence for this association has been based on historic, retrospective, single-institutional series.

Several retrospective studies were published in the 1980s and 1990s evaluating the natural history and management of peripancreatic fluid collections and PP. In 1983, Aranha et al. evaluated the use of abdominal ultrasound for the imaging of pancreatic cystic lesions over 7 years [2]. While this study included diagnoses other than PP, they did note the mean diameter was 8.7 +/– 0.7 cm for cystic lesions that did not resolve and that only 15.4% of cysts greater than 6 cm resolved over the course of the study. Beebe et al. noted that among 10 patients with PPs smaller than 4 cm, 9 resolved with nonoperative management [3]. Andersson et al. retrospectively analyzed 68 patients with PPs treated over 18 years (1969–1987) at a university hospital system in Sweden [4]. The nine PPs treated conservatively in this study had a median size of 4 cm (range 2.5–5 cm) and

resolved ($n = 8$) or were unchanged ($n = 1$) after the study, whereas patients treated surgically ($n = 37$) or via percutaneous drainage ($n = 22$) had median diameters of 11 cm (range 3–25 cm) and 9 cm (range 2–15 cm), respectively. In the United States, a retrospective analysis of 75 patients with PP documented via computed tomography (CT) by Yeo et al. (1990) also described an association between PP size and the need for surgical intervention [5]. In this study, 67% of patients with PP greater than 6 cm underwent an operation, while only 40% of patients with PP less than 6 cm required a surgical procedure.

At least one study has been published in which the authors concluded cyst size was not predictive of successful conservative management. Cheruvu et al. retrospectively examined 36 patients with PPs treated at a single hospital in the United Kingdom over 11 years [6]. The median size of PP treated successfully conservatively was 7 cm (range 4–15 cm), which was deemed similar by the authors to those treated with surgical cyst-enteric drainage (9 cm, range 5–16 cm). It is worth noting, however, that no statistical analysis was performed in this comparison, as the authors felt the sample sizes were too small.

Much of the previous literature has focused on predicting the resolution of PP following episodes of acute pancreatitis. However, some authors have also attempted to analyze this question among patients with chronic pancreatitis. Gouyon et al. retrospectively analyzed 90 patients with chronic pancreatitis and PP formation, and similar to the studies of patients with acute pancreatitis, the authors noted that PP size was associated with successful nonoperative management [7]. Among the 45 patients with PP that regressed spontaneously or were asymptomatic, only 29% were larger than 4 cm. But for patients requiring drainage (both surgical and image-guided), over 70% had cysts greater than 4 cm in size.

There have been two studies that have prospectively examined the natural history of PP. London et al. followed 102 patients admitted with acute pancreatitis and underwent serial CT imaging [8]. PPs, when found, were assessed by determining the product of the anteroposterior and transverse dimensions of the cyst, what the authors termed the "pseudocyst size index." Among the 14 patients found to have PPs, the authors noted that all PPs requiring treatment had a size index of 15 cm² or greater. While the study does represent the first modern prospective study of a large cohort of patients with pancreatitis and PP, the rather short follow-up interval of 6 weeks may limit the inferences that can be made about PPs, as most modern definitions do not consider peripancreatic fluid collections to be a PP until at least 4 weeks following an episode of pancreatitis. In 1999, Maringhini et al. published a large prospective analysis of 926 consecutive patients admitted with acute pancreatitis [9]. Eighty-three patients were noted to have fluid collections, of which 48 were found to have PPs. Among multiple factors analyzed about the need for subsequent treatment, only a PP diameter less than 5 cm and cyst location in the pancreatic tail was associated with spontaneous resolution.

Overall, the literature on this subject displays significant variability. The previously mentioned studies took place over multiple decades of patient care, and the definitions of pancreatic fluid collection and PP have changed over time. These studies also comprise a heterogeneous group of patients from multiple centers and with different etiologies for their pancreatitis. Some studies also included variable amounts of patients with chronic pancreatitis. While the evidence to suggest a size cutoff for the outcomes of PP is largely retrospective and based on single-institutional series, there does appear to be a consensus on the data at hand.

RECOMMENDATION

In the absence of other complications of pancreatitis and peripancreatic fluid collections, it seems reasonable to manage PPs less than 4–6 cm expectantly with supportive care given that a significant number of these collections will resolve without intervention. Ultimately, size is likely just one factor at play in these cases, and other clinical and patient factors (etiology, number of cysts, location of PP, patient condition, etc.) should be considered as well.

Grade of recommendation: C.

50.2 How Can Complicated Pancreatic Pseudocysts Best Be Managed?

50.2.1 Pseudocyst Drainage in the Face of Portal Hypertension

The inflammatory reaction from pancreatitis and pancreatic pseudocyst may lead to thrombosis of the splenic vein (sinistral portal hypertension) or include the portal venous system. Thrombosis of these major portal venous branches leads to the development of gastric varices. These engorged varices often represent a contraindication for external drainage and may prove problematic when PP is drained internally by an endoscopic or surgical approach. Surprisingly little data exist regarding the safest approach to PP drainage in this scenario. Laique et al. reported on 30 patients receiving self-expandable metal stents by endoscopic ultrasound (EUS) for either

pseudocyst or walled-off necrosis [10]. Five of 30 patients were cirrhotic and 2 died (vs. 0 in the noncirrhotic group), though neither death was attributable to venous bleeding. A group from India reported on eight patients with chronic pancreatitis and varices that had EUS-guided drainage to avoid vessel disruption [11]. Six of eight had evidence of portal hypertension by ultrasound surveillance. Only one of eight had bleeding from the cyst following stent deployment that resolved spontaneously. Marino et al. reported on nine patients with portal hypertension having surgical drainage— eight with isolated splenic vein thrombosis [12]. Surgical drainage was accomplished by Roux-en-Y cystjejunostomy to the base of the transverse mesocolon in seven, thus avoiding the gastric varices entirely. Two patients underwent cyst-gastrostomy without the need for a blood transfusion. These data suggest that safe internal drainage of PP may be accomplished even in the face of portal hypertension and gastric varices. If performed endoscopically, EUS-guided drainage is vital to avoid varices. Open surgery offers the advantage to avoid varices altogether.

50.2.2 Infected Pancreatic Pseudocysts

PPs may become secondarily infected during observation, either spontaneously or by seeding during an episode of bacteremia from other sites. Infection may also be introduced by previous instrumentation such as PD of PP. Infection within a PP may be suspected by an elevated white blood cell count, fever, and/or air within the pseudocyst. Controversy exists on the best management of this population of patients, who are often quite ill. It is controversial whether patients with infected PP are candidates for internal drainage. Gerzof et al. reported on 10 patients with 11 infected pancreatic "pseudocysts" undergoing PD [13]. Nine of 11 resolved after 11–37 days of drainage. One patient died from overwhelming pancreatic sepsis. Six of 10 patients had a "pseudocyst," with a known age of fewer than 7 days likely representing an acute pancreatic fluid collection rather than infection within an established PP. van Sonnennberg et al. reported the results of PD on 51 infected PPs [14]. The definition of PP was not reported. The authors reported success in 48 with a mean length of catheter drainage of 16.7 days. Three patients ultimately required partial pancreatectomy, presumably for persistent pancreaticocutaneous fistula. The size and maturity of these PPs were not reported. A study from Turkey detailed the results of PD on 30 infected PPs with a mean size of 12.4 cm [15]. Eighteen occurred as a result of acute pancreatitis and 11 were associated with chronic pancreatitis. There was one treatment failure that required surgical intervention. The length of catheter drainage was not reported. The study by Marino reported 11 patients with infected PP having internal drainage [12]. Three of these patients had prior PD of pseudocysts, and four patients developed infected PP within 4 days of a central line infection. Five of these cysts had extensions beyond the lesser sac. Eight patients had Roux-en-Y drainage and three had cystgastrostomy. Adjunctive postoperative PD was necessary for three for definitive resolution. The current limited literature suggests safe drainage of infected PP may be safely accomplished by either the open (and thus likely endoscopic) or PD approach. Adjunctive postprocedure imaging and therapeutic intervention must be anticipated.

50.2.3 Multiple Pancreatic Pseudocysts and Cysts Located Outside the Lesser Sac

While uncommon, pseudocysts may occur outside the lesser sac, and one PP may be sequestered from another. These complicated scenarios are most often not amendable to a single drainage procedure, but rather require an innovative, multidisciplinary approach for ultimate PP resolution. In a very early study, Goulet et al. reported on 13 patients (14%) with multiple pseudocysts in a series of 91 patients with PP captured over 3 years at a single institution [16]. Four of seven had two separate direct enteric drainage procedures and one had all cysts drain through a single Roux-en-Y cystojejunostomy. Fedorak et al. analyzed 29 (18.5%) patients with multiple pseudocysts among 157 patients with PP over a 2-decade period at two institutions [17]. Multiple internal drainage procedures were performed in 19 patients for definitive management. A combination of internal and external drainage was required in six. Resection and internal drainage were performed in the balance of patients. Complications occurred in 20%, with pancreaticocutaneous fistula being the most common following external drainage. All resolved nonoperatively. Up-front PD in this population was identified as a predictor of failure. Marino et al. studied 24 patients over a 10-year time period that extended beyond or occurred outside the lesser sac, including the base of the mesentery and/or the paracolic gutters [12]. All but two patients had at least one drainage via Roux-en-Y cystojejunostomy to maximize dependent drainage. Five patients had two anastomoses. Five patients required adjunct PD for definitive resolution. These data suggest that PD is unlikely to successfully manage patients with multiple pseudocysts and/or pseudocysts located outside the lesser sac. Though not reported, it seems logical that an endoscopic approach is not feasible as well. Creative utilization of internal drainage is necessary, but the surgeon must anticipate the need for postoperative PD for definitive resolution.

RECOMMENDATIONS

There is a paucity of data regarding the management of complicated PP; however, inferences can be made. Patients with portal/splenic venous occlusion can be safely managed by endoscopic or surgical drainage, with the latter offering the advantage of avoiding gastric varices altogether. Infected PP may be safely managed by internal drainage of any method. Multiple PPs, including those located outside the lesser sac, are best managed surgically with the potential need for multiple cyst-enteric anastomoses and postoperative need for PD. Management of complicated pseudocysts should be determined in a multidisciplinary fashion.

Grade of recommendation: C.

50.3 Is Surgical or Endoscopic Drainage of Pancreatic Pseudocysts Superior?

Historically, surgical drainage (both open and, more recently, laparoscopic/robotically) was the standard practice for persistent, larger, symptomatic PPs. However, in recent years there has been increased interest in less invasive drainage by endoscopic means [18]. Proponents of endoscopic drainage cite the purported lower morbidity of the procedure and the ability to avoid general anesthesia in many cases. But the durability and success of endoscopic PP drainage have been questioned by those who favor traditional operative intervention.

Several single-institutional, retrospective studies comparing surgical and endoscopic drainage have been published over the past 20 years [19–23]. Studies by Johnson et al., Varadarajulu et al., and Saul et al. all found similar rates of PP resolution and treatment success between operative and endoscopic drainage [19, 20, 22]. In a comparison of 45 patients undergoing endoscopic drainage and 38 patients undergoing surgical drainage (16 laparoscopic/22 open), Melman et al. noted a greater primary success rate for surgical procedures compared to endoscopic drainage (84.2% vs. 35.5%) [21]. However, the authors also found that the rate of overall success for both drainage techniques was not different after further endoscopic procedures and, less frequently, salvage surgical drainage. In 2017, Redwan et al. also noted a lower primary success rate for endoscopic decompression compared to operative drainage, albeit higher than rates previously published in the study by Melman (82.9% vs. 100%) [23]. They also noted high rates of overall success for endoscopic procedures, as over 90% of patients were successfully treated after repeat endoscopic drainage.

Due to the limited size of existing studies and the overall paucity of literature on the subject, several meta-analyses have been published comparing surgical and endoscopic drainage in an attempt to pool the available data. Farias et al. compiled the results from six previously published retrospective comparisons and noted no significant difference between the two treatment modalities regarding treatment success rates, adverse events, and PP recurrence [24]. However, they did note that endoscopic PP drainage was associated with improved length of hospital stay and reduced overall hospital stay. Hao et al. also performed a meta-analysis of six studies comparing operative and endoscopic PP drainage but focused specifically on patients undergoing laparoscopic surgical drainage [25]. This pooled analysis included four studies out of China in addition to two of the retrospective studies included in the investigation by Farias et al. Once again, there was no difference in the rates of treatment success, adverse events, or PP recurrence between the two groups, but endoscopic drainage was found to be associated with reduced operative time, blood loss, and hospital length of stay (LOS).

Two randomized controlled trials have been published to date examining the optimal drainage technique. However, in the trial published by Garg et al., more than 80% of patients had walled-off necrosis rather than pure PPs, making it difficult to extrapolate these results to the question at hand [26]. Conversely, the 2013 randomized trial by Varadarajulu et al. focused solely on patients with well-formed PPs [27]. In this study, patients were randomized to either endoscopic ($n = 20$) or surgical cystgastrostomy ($n = 20$). Rates of treatment success (95% vs. 100%), complications (0% vs. 10%), and need for reintervention (5% vs. 5%) were similar between groups. LOS was shorter for the endoscopic treatment arm, and the authors also found endoscopic drainage was associated with a significantly reduced mean hospital cost.

Despite the successful outcomes for endoscopic drainage, there likely remains a continued need for surgical drainage in patients requiring more dependent drainage due to the anatomic position of the PP or in cases of PP away from the lesser sac [21]. In these patients, cystjejunostomy is often more appropriate. Operative intervention is therefore required in these instances in all but the most advanced endoscopic centers.

RECOMMENDATIONS

Endoscopic drainage of PPs appears to be safe and has similar outcomes when compared to surgical drainage with the added benefit of reduced LOS and cost [27, 28]. Treatment failure after endoscopic drainage can typically be managed with repeat endoscopic procedures, but these data have been limited to high-volume centers with expertise in these procedures. The literature also supports the use of EUS during drainage as opposed to conventional endoscopy with blind transmural drainage, as EUS is associated with a greater success rate [29]. Obviously, the applicability of nonsurgical drainage techniques will vary between institutions, depending on the experience of endoscopists and institutional expertise, and this should be considered when determining treatment plans for individual patients in a multidisciplinary fashion.

Grade of recommendation: C.

50.4 What Are the Implications of Failed Up-Front Nonsurgical Drainage of Pancreatic Pseudocysts?

Percutaneous and endoscopic drainage of PPs have gained traction as initial modalities to avoid surgical drainage and are frequently considered as initial management, often without surgical evaluation as part of multidisciplinary care. While these modalities may often result in initial early success, complications may ensue, including stent occlusion with subsequent sepsis, stent migration, bleeding, and pancreaticocutaneous fistula. Furthermore, these nonsurgical modalities frequently involve multiple procedures and imaging studies,

increasing the overall cost of care. Finally, if these nonoperative drainage procedures fail and surgical rescue is necessary, there may be a price to pay in terms of increased morbidity and mortality.

Chawla et al. analyzed 3,235 patients having PP drainage by PD, with both endoscopic and laparoscopic means, from the 2017 National Inpatient Sample database [30]. Patients having initial open surgical drainage were excluded, as more recently this mode of therapy has been reserved as a salvage procedure. Equal numbers underwent PD and laparoscopic drainage, with only 375 having endoscopic drainage. Laparoscopic drainage procedures were more commonly performed at large academic centers. On propensity score-matched analysis, PD was associated with a higher rate of septic shock when compared to laparoscopic drainage and a longer LOS when compared with endoscopic drainage. PD was associated with a lower rate of routine disposition when compared with both alternative drainage modalities. The authors conclude that PD is inferior to the internal drainage of PP.

Similar findings about PD were noted by Heider et al. in a single-institution study comparing 66 patients with this mode of therapy to a similar number having open surgical drainage over 11 years [31]. Compared to those having open surgical drainage, those having PD of PP had higher rates of complication, longer LOS, and greater mortality. In particular, infectious complications were more common in those having PD, especially in those in which this modality failed. Multiple regression analysis failed to identify predictors of successful PD, although the factors chosen for this model were not reported. Most patients who failed PD required open surgical salvage therapy.

More granularity relative to operative outcomes following failed initial nonsurgical management of PP was reported by the group from Loyola University [32]. Over 7 years, the authors assessed the results of 52 patients who had surgical drainage and 18 who had at least one attempt at nonoperative drainage that ultimately required surgical intervention. The number of patients undergoing successful nonoperative drainage of PP during this same period was not noted. Of the 18 failures, 15 had PD, 2 had endoscopic drainage, and 1 patient had both interventions. Mortality was similar between groups but there was a trend toward greater morbidity in the nonsurgical group related to an intraabdominal abscess. The average time from initial therapy to cyst resolution was five times higher in the nonsurgical drainage group (104 vs. 20 days); however, the average time from open surgical drainage until a resolution was similar between groups (21 vs. 20 days).

Nealon and Walser reported on 79 patients with complications related to PD ($n = 53$), endoscopic drainage ($n = 26$) of PP, or both ($n = 17$) (most referred from outside institutions) for 11 years and compared outcomes to 100 consecutive patients having surgery at their campus [33]. Again, the number of successful nonoperative drainage of PP was not known. Sixty-six (84%) of 79 patients initially having nonoperative management required subsequent operative intervention. Thirteen with complications had a management that was managed nonoperatively—nine of whom had initial endoscopic drainage. Indications for surgery in this group included sepsis, hemorrhage, or persistent drainage, and urgent operation was necessary for 41%. Fifty-seven of 66 had evidence of ductal disruption on magnetic resonance cholangiopancreatography (MRCP) or endoscopic retrograde cholangiopancreatography (ERCP). Forty-two percent required nonoperative procedures for stabilization before operative intervention. Salvage surgery entailed cyst-jejunostomy, tract-jejunostomy, and distal pancreatectomy with no mortality. When compared with up-front operative drainage, those with complications related to nonoperative drainage had a marked increase in episodes of sepsis, persistent pancreatic fistula, renal and respiratory failure, need for intensive care unit admission, and LOS (42.7 vs. 6.1 days).

> ### RECOMMENDATIONS
>
> The incidence of nonoperative drainage of PP has increased dramatically and offers the opportunity to avoid surgery if successful. However, operative intervention is frequently necessary and often more complicated if these modalities are unsuccessful. Management of those with failed nonoperative therapy is associated with greater morbidity and markedly increases the time to the ultimate resolution of PP disease. Failure of nonoperative management of PP can frequently be predicted based on pancreatic ductal anatomy. Thus, a multidisciplinary approach to this disease, including surgical expertise, is strongly encouraged.
>
> Grade of recommendation: C.

TABLE 50.1

Summary of evidence and recommendations

Question	Answer	Levels of Evidence	Grade of Recommendation	References
Does the size of a pancreatic pseudocyst predict the likelihood of resolution following acute pancreatitis?	Size likely is associated with the probability of pseudocyst resolution. Ultimately, this is multifactorial and other factors play a role.	IV	C	[1–9]
How can complicated pancreatic pseudocysts best be managed?	Internal drainage for portal venous occlusion and infection. A multidisciplinary approach with surgery as the anchor for PP located outside the lesser sac.	IV	C	[10–17]
Is surgical or endoscopic drainage of pancreatic pseudocysts superior?	Similar outcomes and safety profiles in experienced hands. Endoscopy is associated with lower costs and length of stay.	IIB	C	[18–29]
What are the implications of failed up-front nonsurgical drainage of pancreatic pseudocysts?	Failure leads to excessive morbidity and mortality and can be predicted based on pancreatic ductal anatomy.	IV	C	[30–33]

Editor's Note

Much of the quality data on pancreatic pseudocysts seems to come from large centers with tremendous expertise where care is regionalized (like in some European countries). Therefore, this information may not be applicable to hospitals in the United States, where these cases are rare and experience is limited. So, it is even more important to emphasize the need for a multidisciplinary approach to these complicated patients.

REFERENCES

1. Andren-Sandberg A, Dervenis C. Pancreatic pseudocysts in the 21st century. Part II: a natural history. JOP. 2004;5(2):64–70.
2. Aranha GV, Prinz RA, Esguerra AC, Greenlee HB. The nature and course of cystic pancreatic lesions diagnosed by ultrasound. Arch Surg. 1983;118(4):486–8.
3. Beebe DS, Bubrick MP, Onstad GR, Hitchcock CR. Management of pancreatic pseudocysts. Surg Gynecol Obstet. 1984;159(6):562–4.
4. Andersson R, Janzon M, Sundberg I, Bengmark S. Management of pancreatic pseudocysts. Br J Surg. 1989; 76(6):550–2.
5. Yeo CJ, Bastidas JA, Lynch-Nyhan A, Fishman EK, Zinner MJ, Cameron JL. The natural history of pancreatic pseudocysts is documented by computed tomography. Surg Gynecol Obstet. 1990;170(5):411–7.
6. Cheruvu CV, Clarke MG, Prentice M, Eyre-Brook IA. Conservative treatment as an option in the management of pancreatic pseudocyst. Ann R Coll Surg Engl. 2003; 85(5):313–6.
7. Gouyon B, Levy P, Ruszniewski P, Zins M, Hammel P, Vilgrain V, et al. Predictive factors in the outcome of pseudocysts complicating alcoholic chronic pancreatitis. Gut. 1997;41(6):821–5.
8. London NJ, Neoptolemos JP, Lavelle J, Bailey I, James D. Serial computed tomography scanning in acute pancreatitis: a prospective study. Gut. 1989;30(3):397–403.
9. Maringhini A, Uomo G, Patti R, Rabitti P, Termini A, Cavallera A, et al. Pseudocysts in acute nonalcoholic pancreatitis: incidence and natural history. Dig Dis Sci. 1999;44(8):1669–73.

10. Laique S, Franco MC, Bhatt A, et al. Clinical outcomes of endoscopic management of pancreatic fluid collections in cirrhotics vs non-cirrhotics: a comparative study. World J Gastrointest Endosc. 2019;11(6):403–12.

11. Sriram PVJ, Kaffes AJ, Rao GV, et al. Endoscopic ultrasound-guided drainage of pancreatic pseudocysts complicated by portal hypertension or by intervening vessels. Endoscopy. 2005;37(3):231–5.

12. Marino KA, Hendrick LE, Behrman SW. Surgical management of complicated pancreatic pseudocysts. Am J Surg. 2016;211(1):109–14.

13. Gerzof SG, Johnson WC, Robbins AH, et al. Percutaneous drainage of infected pancreatic pseudocysts. Arch Surg. 1984;119:888–93.

14. vanSonnenberg E, Wittich GR, Casola G, et al. Percutaneous drainage of infected and noninfected pancreatic pseudocysts: experience in 101 cases. Radiology. 1989;170:757–61.

15. Cantasdemir M, Kara B, Kantarci F, Mihmanli I, et al. Percutaneous drainage for treatment of infected pancreatic pseudocysts. S Afr Med J. 2003;96(2):136–40.

16. Goulet RJ, Goodman J, Schaffer R, et al. Multiple pancreatic pseudocyst disease. Ann Surg. 1984;199(1):6–13.

17. Fedorak IJ, Rao R, Prinz RA. The clinical challenge of multiple pancreatic pseudocysts. Am J Surg. 1994;168:22–8.

18. Agalianos C, Passas I, Sideris I, Davides D, Dervenis C. Review of management options for pancreatic pseudocysts. Transl Gastroenterol Hepatol. 2018;3:18.

19. Johnson MD, Walsh RM, Henderson JM, Brown N, Ponsky J, Dumot J, et al. Surgical versus nonsurgical management of pancreatic pseudocysts. J Clin Gastroenterol. 2009;43(6):586–90.

20. Varadarajulu S, Lopes TL, Wilcox CM, Drelichman ER, Kilgore ML, Christein JD. EUS versus surgical cystgastrostomy for management of pancreatic pseudocysts. Gastrointest Endosc. 2008;68(4):649–55.

21. Melman L, Azar R, Beddow K, Brunt LM, Halpin VJ, Eagon JC, et al. Primary and overall success rates for clinical outcomes after laparoscopic, endoscopic, and open pancreatic cystgastrostomy for pancreatic pseudocysts. Surg Endosc. 2009;23(2):267–71.

22. Saul A, Ramirez Luna MA, Chan C, Uscanga L, Valdovinos Andraca F, Hernandez Calleros J, et al. EUS-guided drainage of pancreatic pseudocysts offers similar success and complications compared to surgical treatment but with a lower cost. Surg Endosc. 2016;30(4):1459–65.

23. Redwan AA, Hamad MA, Omar MA. Pancreatic pseudocyst dilemma: cumulative multicenter experience in management using endoscopy, laparoscopy, and open surgery. J Laparoendosc Adv Surg Tech A. 2017;27(10):1022–30.

24. Farias GFA, Bernardo WM, De Moura DTH, Guedes HG, Brunaldi VO, Visconti TAC, et al. Endoscopic versus surgical treatment for pancreatic pseudocysts: Systematic review and meta-analysis. Medicine (Baltimore). 2019;98(8):e14255.

25. Hao W, Chen Y, Jiang Y, Yang A. Endoscopic versus laparoscopic treatment for pancreatic pseudocysts: a systematic review and meta-analysis. Pancreas. 2021;50(6):788–95.

26. Garg PK, Meena D, Babu D, Padhan RK, Dhingra R, Krishna A, et al. Endoscopic versus laparoscopic drainage of pseudocyst and walled-off necrosis following acute pancreatitis: a randomized trial. Surg Endosc. 2020;34(3):1157–66.

27. Varadarajulu S, Bang JY, Sutton BS, Trevino JM, Christein JD, Wilcox CM. Equal efficacy of endoscopic and surgical cystogastrostomy for pancreatic pseudocyst drainage in a randomized trial. Gastroenterology. 2013;145(3):583–90 e1.

28. Quinn PL, Bansal S, Gallagher A, Chokshi RJ. Endoscopic versus laparoscopic drainage of pancreatic pseudocysts: a cost-effectiveness analysis. J Gastrointest Surg. 2022;26(8):1679–85.

29. Varadarajulu S, Christein JD, Tamhane A, Drelichman ER, Wilcox CM. Prospective randomized trial comparing EUS and EGD for transmural drainage of pancreatic pseudocysts (with videos). Gastrointest Endosc. 2008;68(6):1102–11.

30. Chawla A, Afridi F, Prasath V, et al. Analysis of pancreatic pseudocyst drainage procedural outcomes: a population based study. Surg Endosc. 2023;37(1):156–164.

31. Heider R, Meyer AA, Galanko JA, et al. Percutaneous drainage of pancreatic pseudocysts is associated with a higher failure rate than surgical treatment in unselected patients. Ann Surg. 1999;229(6):781–9.

32. Rao R, Fedorak I, Prinz RA. Effect of failed computed tomography-guided and endoscopic drainage on pancreatic pseudocyst management. Surgery. 1993;114(4):843–7.

33. Nealon WH, Walser E. Surgical management of complications associated with percutaneous and/or endoscopic management of pseudocyst of the pancreas. Ann Surg. 2005;241(6):948–60.

51

Diagnosis and Treatment of Variceal Hemorrhage Due to Cirrhosis

Zoe Guzman, Harsimran Panesar, Gregory Simonian, and David O'Connor

51.1 Introduction

The most common cause of cirrhosis is alcoholic fatty liver disease, hepatitis B or C, and nonalcoholic fatty liver disease. After repetitive liver injury, the parenchyma becomes cirrhotic and develops irreversible, extensive scarring with nodular regeneration due to the activated stellate cells. The accumulated fibrosis results in crisscrossing banding that contracts the liver, distorting the architect and its function. Leading to impaired protein synthesis, ineffective detoxification, and impedance of blood flow. A major clinical problem in cirrhosis is portal hypertension, which is elevated pressure within the blood vessels entering the liver. Variceal hemorrhage is a common and serious complication of portal hypertension, with mortality rates as high as 50% with the initial episode [1]. Presented are practice guidelines that have been developed and endorsed by the American Association for the Study of Liver Disease and reviewed at the most recent international Billroth III and Baveno VI consensus conferences.

51.2 Pathophysiology

Cirrhosis is a heterogeneous disease, and it is classified based on the presence or absence of clinically evident decompensating events such as ascites, variceal hemorrhage, and hepatic encephalopathy. Portal hypertension develops because of both increased resistance to portal blood flow and increased portal blood flow. It is defined as a hepatic venous pressure gradient (HVPG, gradient between portal and central venous pressure, of >10 mmHg. Increased resistance to portal blood flow is due not only to architectural fibrotic distortion but also to vasoconstriction in the liver. This is mediated by contractile stellate cells responding both to decreased production of nitric oxide by adjacent hepatic endothelial cells and increased response to several endogenous vasoconstrictors, including endothelin, norepinephrine, angiotensin II, vasopressin, leukotrienes, and thromboxane A2. Portal hypertension also occurs due to increased splanchnic arterial flow from decreased systemic vascular resistance, increased cardiac output, and direct splanchnic arteriolar vasodilation mediated by multiple vasoactive agents [2].

51.3 Reliable Predictors of Visceral Hemorrhage Development in Patients with Cirrhosis

Risk stratification is done through the Child-Pugh-Turcotte (CPT) classification, where CPT-A class is compensated and CPT-B/C class is mostly decompensated. Portal hypertension is typically the first and main manifestation of cirrhosis, and it is responsible for many of its complications.

51.3.1 Value of the Hepatic Vein Pressure Gradient

Compared to liver biopsy, measuring the portal pressure (PP) via HVPG is better at predicting the development of complications of cirrhosis in patients with chronic liver disease. Since portal hypertension may occur before establishment of a formal anatomical diagnosis of cirrhosis. Compensated cirrhosis is asymptomatic and is the longest stage. Mild portal hypertension is defined as HVPG >5 but <10 mmHg, whereas clinically significant portal hypertension (CSPH) is defined as ≥10 mmHg. CSPH is associated with an increased risk of varices; overt clinical decompensation such as ascites, visceral hemorrhage, and hepatic encephalopathy; hepatocellular carcinoma; and postsurgical decompression [3]. It is important to note that CSPH is present in approximately 50–60% of patients with compensated cirrhosis without gastroesophageal varices (GEV) [4]. Since patients with GEV have a worse prognosis, it is important to substage patients with CSPH.

HVPG is measured utilizing a catheter into the hepatic vein to measure the wedge hepatic vein pressure (WHVP) (balloon inflated) and the free hepatic vein pressure (FHVP) (balloon deflated). The HVPG is WHVP – FHVP. Normal HVPG is 3–5 mmHg, and in portal hypertension, the HVPG is >5 mmHg (Table 51.1).

There is strong evidence that reduction in HVPG with pharmacological intervention reduces the risk of variceal hemorrhage. Reduction in HVPG ("responders") can include HVPG ≤12 mmHg or HVPG ≥20% from baseline, regardless of final HVPG. Despite the strong correlation, the use of HVPG measurements is criticized because of the variability and the lack of feasibility. Two large meta-analyses determined that the risk of variceal hemorrhage and liver-related mortality were lower

TABLE 51.1

HVPG Thresholds with Prognostic Significance in Patients with Cirrhosis [22]

HVPG Threshold (mmHg)	Prognostic Significance
<5	Normal or noncirrhotic portal hypertension
>5	Portal hypertension
>10	Clinically significant portal hypertension and is predictive of decompensation
>12	Variceal hemorrhage
>16	Variceal rebleeding
>20	Failure to control active hemorrhage, high mortality
>30	Spontaneous bacterial peritonitis

$$\text{Fibrosis-4-Index} = \frac{\text{Patient's age (years)} \times \text{AST}}{\text{Platelet count} \times \sqrt{\text{ALT}}}$$

FIGURE 51.1 Formula to calculate fibrosis-4-index (FIB-4).

in patients who achieved HVPG reduction [5]. Another study involving 71 cirrhotics confirmed that propranolol ± isosorbide mononitrate significantly reduced the 8-year cumulative probability of no variceal hemorrhage to 90% in responders vs. 45% in nonresponders, but there were no significant differences in liver-related mortality [6, 22]. Patients with HVPG ≥20 mmHg had greater failure to control variceal hemorrhage (29% vs. 83%), earlier recurrent hemorrhage, longer intensive care unit and hospital stays, more transfusion requirements, and worse 1-year mortality (20% vs. 64%) [7].

51.3.2 Noninvasive Blood Markers

It is important to recognize that although portal hypertension and varices formation help stage the cirrhosis, measuring the HVPG is not always feasible. The Model for End-Stage Liver Disease (MELD) score, CPT score, Fibrosis-4-Index (FIB-4), and additional noninvasive serum markers may be utilized as independent predictors of decompensation. A non-invasive means to monitor the patient with cirrhosis and their risk for developing a complication such as a variceal bleed/rebleed is important.

FIB-4: FIB-4 is recommended and validated by the World Health Organization guidelines for evaluating hepatic fibrosis (Figure 51.1). In a retrospective study FIB-4 was found to be an independent predictor of esophageal bleed, area under the receiver operating characteristics (AUROC) = 0.64 ($p < 0.05$) [8]. A prospective study followed 139 newly diagnosed cirrhotic patients (CPT of at least 5–13) with no incidences of variceal bleed measured that identified FIB-4 as the strongest predictor of esophageal varices development (odds ratio [OR]: 1.57, 95% confidence interval [CI]: 1.15–2.14, $p = 0.005$). A cutoff value of 3.23 for FIB-4 was a significant predictor of esophageal varices, with a sensitivity of 72%, a specificity of 58%, and a proportion of area under the curve (AUC) of 66% ($P = 0.01$) [9]. Another prospective study demonstrated that FIB-4 scores were significant in the group with bleeding ($p < 0.001$). However, when it came to predicting the power of variceal bleeding using ROC analysis, it was determined to be significant but weak (AUC = 0.63) [10].

CPT score: The CPT score was developed to predict mortality in cirrhosis patients to help identify which patient would benefit from portal decompression (Table 51.2). The sensitivity, specificity, positive predictive value (PPV), and negative predictive value (NPV) for predicting in-hospital rebleeding using the CPT were 74.6%, 63.9%, 34.5%, and 90.8%, respectively. CPT scoring systems could effectively discriminate and predict the occurrence of in-hospital adverse versus an in-hospital rebleed outcome in cirrhotic patients with variceal bleeding, AUROC = 0.717 ($p < 0.001$) [16]. Child Pugh class B/C was also independently associated with the presence of large esophageal varices (OR, 3.8; 95% CI, 2.3–6.5) [13].

MELD score: The MELD score was initially developed to predict the 6-week survival following transjugular intrahepatic portosystemic shunt but was also found to be an

TABLE 51.2

Child-Pugh-Turcotte Scoring System and Prognostic Indicators

Parameter	1 Point	2 Points	3 Points
Ascites	None	Mild	Moderate to severe
Hepatic encephalopathy	None	Grade I–II	Grade III–IV
Total bilirubin (mg/dL)	<2	2–3	>3
Serum albumin (g/dL)	>3.5	2.8–3.5	<2.8
Prothrombin time (sec)	<4.0	4.0–6.0	>6.0
INR	<1.7	1.7–2.3	>2.3

Prognostic Indicator of Child-Pugh Score			
Points	Class	1-Year Survival	2-Year Survival
5–6	A	100%	85%
7–9	B	81%	57%
10–15	C	45%	35%

MELD score formula: $9.57 \times \log_e$ (creatinine) $+ 3.78 \times \log_e$ (total bilirubin) $+ 11.2 \times \log_e$ (INR) $+ 6.43$

FIGURE 51.2 Formula to calculate Model for End-Stage Liver Disease (MELD) score.

accurate predictor of mortality among patients with end-stage liver disease and help with liver transplant allocation (Figure 51.2). Compared with the CPT scoring system, three of the four parameters utilized in the calculation of a MELD score are objective laboratory values. In a meta-analysis, the MELD score was better at predicting mortality in variceal hemorrhage patients within 3 months compared to the CPT score. The AUROC of MELD was higher than that of the CPT score (0.88 vs. 0.76) in variceal hemorrhage patients [17]. When it came to predicting in-patient mortality following acute variceal bleeding, MELD was not superior to the commonly used CPT score. Both had a high predictive rate >0.8 [16, 18].

Serum albumin: There is no significant difference in serum albumin levels among patients with esophageal variceal bleeding and those without esophageal variceal bleeding: 3.25 ± 0.38 versus 3.17 ± 0.72 ($p = 0.689$), respectively [9]. Using the serum-ascites albumin gradient (SAAG) in cirrhotic patients with ascites can be considered an indirect parameter for the detection of esophageal varices (Image 51.3). A SAAG of >1.1 g/dL is 97% accurate in detecting portal hypertension [10]. Patients with SAAG values >1.75 g/dL demonstrated esophageal varices with a sensitivity and specificity of 78.4% and 83.3%, respectively. SAAG values >1.8 g/dL were associated with the risk of large esophageal varices with an AUC of 0.856, sensitivity of 88.24%, and specificity of 50.79%. The correlation coefficient (r) between SAAG and esophageal varices was 0.429, which was statistically significant ($p < 0.001$) [11].

Serum aspartate transaminase/alanine transaminase (AST/ALT): There is no evidence of any significant association of esophageal varices with AST/ALT ratio (OR: 1.15, 95% CI:0.84–1.57). In addition, there was no significant difference between the AST/ALT ratio values between the patients who did have esophageal variceal bleeding versus those who did not 2.23 ± 1.57 versus 2.17 ± 1.64 ($p = 0.628$), respectively. Using the cutoff value of 1.71 for the AST/ALT ratio to predict esophageal variceal bleeding, the sensitivity was determined to be 59% and specificity 54% with AUC = 0.53 (0.42–0.64) ($p = 0.628$) [9]. AST value was also independently associated with HVPG grade (OR 1.033, 1.031–1.034 95% CI, $p = 0.005$) [12].

Serum platelet count: Many studies have demonstrated a correlation between low platelet count and higher grades of esophageal varices in patients with liver cirrhosis. In a cross-sectional study, the mean platelet count was $213,884.62/mm^3$ in patients with grade I varices, whereas it was $119,518.52/mm^3$, $58,386.49/mm^3$, and $21,600.00/mm^3$ in patients with grade II, III, and IV varices, respectively ($p \leq 0.0001$) [14]. Platelet count was also independently associated with HVPG

grade (OR 0.993, 0.990–0.995 95% CI, $p = 0.002$) and presence of large esophageal varices (OR, 2.7; 95% CI, 1.4–5.2) [12, 13]. A prospective study that found that the number of platelets (PLT) was significantly lower in the group with bleeding ($p < 0.001$). It was observed that the values of PLT ≤ 66.5 $10^9/L$ were better than other parameters (sensitivity, 62%; specificity 70%; positive likelihood ratio, 2.03; PPV, 64.3%; NPV, 67.18; OR, 3.74) [15].

RECOMMENDATION

Noninvasive serum liver fibrosis indexes exhibited modest diagnostic accuracy for portal hypertension in cirrhotic patients. These indexes may not be able to replace HVPG measurements for the diagnosis of portal hypertension but may be used as a first-line screening method for CSPH in cirrhosis patients. HVPG is still the preferred method to assess portal pressure, and HVPG >10 mmHg is the gold-standard method to assess the presence of CSPH.

Grade of recommendation: A.

51.4 Diagnosis and Workup of a Patient with a Visceral Bleed

In addition to measuring HVPG and noninvasive serum markers, imaging and upper endoscopy help with further risk stratification of patients with a cirrhotic liver.

51.4.1 Role of Upper Endoscopy in Esophageal Varices

Endoscopy is the gold-standard for diagnosing the presence of gastroesophageal varices and identifying risk signs of bleeding (large size; red signs). The disadvantages of esophagogastroduodenoscopy (EGD) include the complications associated with endoscopy, especially the need for intravenous sedation. In the last 10 years, increasing evidence regarding noninvasive methods (especially transient elastography) accumulated and proved useful for stratifying the risk of carrying varices. Endoscopy remains needed to identify other signs of portal hypertension such as hypertensive gastropathy that is often the cause of minor bleeding in patients with cirrhosis. Noninvasive methodologies do not screen for varices, and EGD is required if the patient needs treatment for their gastroesophageal varices [26].

SAAG = (albumin concentration of serum) − (albumin concentration of ascitic fluid)

IMAGE 51.3 Formula to calculate the serum-ascites albumin gradient (SAAG).

51.4.2 Imaging

Portocollateral circulation on any imaging (ultrasound, computed tomography [CT], or magnetic resonance imaging) has a very high specificity for CSPH and is enough to diagnose it.

i. *Transient elastography* (TE) to assess liver stiffness has proven to be an accurate means to discriminate patients with or without CSPH. The liver stiffness (LS) is a physical property of the liver parenchyma and correlates with the amount of fibrosis. In a meta-analysis, the AUROC was found to be 0.93. TE is considered the backbone of the noninvasive diagnosis of portal hypertension [24]. A cutoff to detect CSPH is LS >20–25 kPa and has a diagnostic accuracy over 90%. Two separate measurements of LS by TE of 15 kPa or more are highly suggestive of compensated advanced chronic liver disease [25, 35]. In a prospective study, HVPG >10 mmHg was equivalent to LS >21 kPa and was equally effective in predicting decompensation [27, 28].

ii. *Ultrasound* provides a safe and inexpensive way to assess the morphology of the cirrhotic liver and assess evidence of portal hypertension. In addition to evidence of portocollateral circulation, dilatation of the portal vein and the reduction of portal vein velocity are also indicative of portal hypertension. In a prospective study of 30 patients with liver cirrhosis 66.6% those that had an esophageal bleed had a portal vein dilatation >13 mm. A cutoff point of >13 mm had a strong correlation with the presence of esophageal varices ($p < 0.01$) with 100% sensitivity and 90% specificity and 95.24% PPV [23].

iii. CT allows the direct visualization of esophageal varices after intravenous contrast administration. It is not only better tolerated but allows simultaneous screening for hepatic carcinoma. Compared to EGD, the pooled sensitivity is approximately 87–89.6% and specificity is 72.3–80% [29, 30]. CT is a feasible alternative for detecting and monitoring varices in cirrhotic patients. In addition, CT can be used to measure the spleen diameter since portal hypertension leads to congestion of the intrasplenic blood flow and hence spleen enlargement. CT has been shown to have a high sensitivity and specificity in identifying splenomegaly [31]. The major drawback of this imaging modality is the radiation exposure, but the benefit likely outweighs the risk of radiation-induced carcinogenesis.

iv. *Magnetic resonance imaging*, when used for the detection of esophageal varices, is more challenging than CT given the movement artifacts. The reported accuracy is not as high, with a sensitivity of less than 81%, and appears to be inferior to the accuracy of CT [32].

Magnetic resonance elastography (MRE) has been used to grade the severity of cirrhosis and help calculate LS. The sensitivity is 88.9% and 96% and specificity is 56.4% and 60% with and without contrast, respectively [33, 34].

RECOMMENDATION

CSPH can be identified by noninvasive tests LS >20–25 kPa, alone or combined with PLT count and spleen size. Patients with LS <20 kPa and a PLT count >150,000/mm³ (Baveno VI criteria) were very unlikely to have high-risk varices (<5%), and endoscopy could be safely avoided in them. The presence of portosystemic collaterals on imaging is sufficient to diagnose CSPH. EGD remains the gold standard to risk-stratify patients with medium/large varices.

Grade of recommendation: A.

51.5 Management

Variceal hemorrhages are a decompensating event with the rate of bleeding with known varices being 12–15% per year [19]. The mortality rate with each variceal bleed episode is 15–20% [20]. The risk of rebleeding within 1 year of the initial bleed is approximately 60% [21]. Therefore, those that survive a variceal bleed episode should be started on prophylactic therapy to prevent future bleeds. Treatment of portal hypertension differs based on the stage of cirrhosis since the prognosis and mechanism of disease (and therefore therapeutic targets) are different. In addition, every effort should be taken to remove the aggravating factors such as alcohol, obesity, and drug-induced liver injury. Nonselective beta-blockers (NSBBs) such as propranolol, timolol, nadolol, and carvedilol are splanchnic vasoconstrictors and help decrease the portal venous inflow. On the other hand, endoscopic variceal ligation (EVL) has no effect on portal circulation and acts locally to obliterate varices. Compared to NSBB, EVL has lower overall rates of adversity, 2–6% of interventions, but if adverse events occur, they are more severe and life-threatening [49]. Information is summarized in Table 51.3.

A. **Patients with compensated cirrhosis and mild portal hypertension** are asymptomatic with the lowest risk of clinical decompensation. The objective of therapy in patients at an early stage is to prevent the development of advanced stages. The mechanism leading to portal hypertension is increased intrahepatic resistance. NSBB will be ineffective in this sub-stage given that the hyperdynamic circulatory state is not fully developed [19, 35]. Surveillance endoscopy to detect high risk varices in patients with compensated cirrhosis is recommended every 1–3 years or when decompensation occurs [37].

B. **Patients with compensated cirrhosis and CSPH**, but without varices, are defined as HVPG ≥10 mmHg. The objective of therapy should be to prevent

TABLE 51.3

Summary of Prophylaxis Treatment Based on Staging of Patient

	Treatment	Goal of Therapy
Pre–primary prophylaxis	No treatment, surveillance endoscopy	Prevent the development of advanced stages
Compensated cirrhosis with CSPH	No specific treatment	Prevent decompensation and prevent elevation in HVPG
Primary prophylaxis		Prevent the first episode of variceal hemorrhage
Small varices (<5 mm)	NSBB for high-risk EV *Alternative*: Follow-up endoscopy annually if decompensated cirrhosis or every 1–2 years in decompensated cirrhosis until the varices are treated or eradicated	
Medium to large varices (>5 mm, red spots signs, or CPT Class C)	NSBB *Alternative*: EVL	
Secondary prophylaxis	NSBB and EVL *Alternatives*: NSBB + isosorbide mononitrate TIPS BRTO (gastric varices)	Prevent further decompensation and death

decompensation and prevent elevation in HVPG. A large, multicenter, randomized controlled trial demonstrated that there is no difference between placebo and NSBB in the development of esophageal varices despite lowering the HVPG. Decrease in HVPG >10% from baseline showed no clinical significance in preventing bleeding episodes [4]. No specific portal pressure–reducing treatment to prevent formation of varices has been identified.

C. **Patients with compensated cirrhosis and gastro-esophageal varices proven by EGD** are defined as HVPG 10–12 mmHg. The objective of therapy should be to prevent the first episode of variceal hemorrhage. Utilization of NSBB to reduce HVPG to ≤12 mmHg or ≥20% from baseline was shown to be protective against the development of variceal hemorrhage [38]. The use of shunt surgery and sclerotherapy has been abandoned for primary prevention due to the high rate of complications [39, 40]. It is also recommended that HVPG not be routinely monitored since the NSBB goes beyond their portal pressure–reducing effects. Even among patients with ascites, where the line of evidence indicates that NSBBs were associated with higher mortality, NSBBs are not necessarily contraindicated. Primary prophylaxis should be initiated in patients with (1) medium/large varices, (2) small varices with red signs, or (3) decompensated patients with small varices.

a. *Medium/large varices:* Current guidelines recommend either NSBB or EVL for prevention of first variceal bleeding in patients with medium to large varices [19]. Given NSBB is noninvasive and less expensive, it tends to be a more preferred treatment. Compared to other NSBBs, carvedilol has shown a more efficient reduction in portal

pressure, mostly likely due to the additional anti-α-1-adrenergic activity [41, 44, 45] and is recommended as first line in some guidelines [46]. However, it should be noted that doses higher than 12.5 mg/day do not lead to further reduction in portal pressure. In addition, carvedilol has been shown to work in 58% of patients who did not respond to propranolol [41]. There are mixed reviews on whether EVL is superior to NSBB. EVL is just as effective as NSBB and has been shown to reduce the episodes of variceal bleed but has no impact on mortality [47, 48, 68]. Even when EVL and NSBB are utilized together and compared to EVL alone, there were no differences in the incidence of bleeding or death between groups [70]. When EVL is chosen for primary prophylaxis, it should be repeated every 2–4 weeks until varices are completely eradicated. Surveillance endoscopy should be repeated after 6 and 12 months [19, 35].

b. *Small varices*: Little high-quality evidence is available regarding treatment of patients with small and low-risk varices in primary prophylaxis. Hence, current guidelines do not specifically recommend treatment for small varices due to the lack of decisive studies [19, 35]. Some studies demonstrate no significant effect of NSBB on the incidence of first variceal bleeding [41], whereas other studies demonstrated carvedilol is an effective treatment to prevent progression to large varices [42]. The PREDESCI trial demonstrated a decrease in the rate of decompensation if treated with NSBB (hazard ratio [HR]: 0.51, CI 95%: 0.26–0.97, $p = 0.041$), resulting in a longer complication-free period [43].

RECOMMENDATION

NSBBs, carvedilol, or EVL should be used to prevent initial hemorrhage in cirrhotics with medium/large varices (Ia/A). NSBBs reduce the risk of first variceal hemorrhage in patients with large varices (Ia/A). Propranolol is the drug of choice, but carvedilol is an attractive alternative, especially in patients who are nonresponders to propranolol (Ib/A). EVL is probably more effective than NSBBs to reduce the risk of first variceal hemorrhage in these patients, but it may not improve survival and carries a risk of more severe adverse events (Ia/A). EVL should be recommended when these patients have contraindications, intolerance, or unresponsiveness to β-blockers (Ia/A). No data suggest that sclerotherapy or shunt therapy should be used in primary prophylaxis of medium/large varices (III/A–Ia/A).

51.6 Intervention for Acute Variceal Hemorrhage

The three main pillars for acute variceal bleeding treatment are fluid resuscitation, pharmacological treatment, and endoscopy/endoscopic band ligation. Patients at this stage are considered decompensated, with the 5-year mortality rate dependent on the presence of cirrhosis (20% mortality rate) and other complications (over 80% mortality rate). In addition, HVPG ≥20 mmHg within the first 24 hours of admission is a strong predictor of rebleed and death [7]. Granted, at this stage patients are critical and HVPG will not be measured, but more than 80% of patients in the CTP-C class have an HVPG ≥20 mmHg. The objective of therapy should be to control the bleeding, prevent early recurrence (within 5 days), and prevent 6-week mortality.

Initial management includes airway assessment/protection and placement of large peripheral venous catheters for blood volume resuscitation. Airway protection with a cuffed endotracheal tube prior to endoscopy is crucial to avoid aspiration. Replacement of blood loss should be done promptly but cautiously, often with colloid infusion to maintain hemodynamic stability and with packed red cells to maintain a hemoglobin of 7–8 g/dL. Retaining the hemoglobin in a conservative range has been associated with a significant decrease in mortality compared to liberal transfusion, maintaining hemoglobin at 9–11 g/dL [43]. Overzealous blood transfusion can lead to increased portal hypertension and persistent hemorrhage. A randomized controlled trial showed a lower rate of recurrent variceal hemorrhage and a survival advantage when restrictive transfusion strategies were employed. Saline solutions should generally be avoided due to their potential to increase portal pressure and to cause extravascular fluid accumulation in cirrhotics. Transfusions of fresh-frozen plasma and platelets can be considered in patients with significant coagulopathy and thrombocytopenia, but data are limited. Randomized controlled trials of recombinant and platelets have not shown clear benefit [52, 53].

Patients with cirrhosis presenting with gastrointestinal hemorrhage are at a high risk of bacterial infections. Bacterial overgrowth and translocation from the gastrointestinal tract, combined with increased susceptibility to infection, mainly due to reticuloendothelial system dysfunction, predispose cirrhotics to spontaneous bacterial peritonitis and bacteremia—both of which can lead to septic shock, multiorgan dysfunction, and death. Endotoxins released during bacterial infections cause contraction of hepatic stellate cells, resulting in increased intrahepatic vascular resistance and portal pressure. Endotoxins also inhibit platelet aggregation through nitric oxide and prostaglandin I2 release, increasing bleeding tendency. The use of antibiotic prophylaxis has been shown to decrease the development of infection, recurrent hemorrhage, and death [54, 55]. The specific antibiotic recommended is based on the patient's risk characteristics and the local antimicrobial resistance. The first choice in patients with advanced cirrhosis is ceftriaxone (1 g/24 hours) and should be administered before endoscopic treatment. The duration of prophylaxis antibiotic is short term, for a maximum of 7 days [3].

RECOMMENDATION

Prompt but careful resuscitation of blood loss from variceal hemorrhage should occur with colloid to maintain hemodynamic stability and with packed cells to maintain hemoglobin 7–8 g/dL (Ib/B–Ia/A). Data regarding the management of coagulopathy and thrombocytopenia are limited (V/D). Short-term (<7 days) prophylactic antibiotics should begin at hospital admission for all cirrhotics who present with acute variceal hemorrhage (Ia/A). Oral norfloxacin (400 mg BID) or intravenous ciprofloxacin (when oral administration is contraindicated) are the recommended antibiotics (Ib/A). Intravenous ceftriaxone can be considered in hospital settings with high rates of quinolone-resistant infections (Ib/A).

51.6.1 Pharmacological Intervention in Acute Variceal Hemorrhage

To counter active bleeding, vasoactive drugs such as vasopressin, terlipressin, somatostatin, and octreotide have been shown to reduce portal pressure and help decrease mortality rate. Vasoactive medication promotes systemic and portal vasoconstriction, allowing a reduction in both the portal and systemic blood flow. The duration of treatment is short-term, up to 5 days. β-blockers should not be administered with active variceal hemorrhage because they drop systolic blood pressure and mask tachycardia that occurs as a normal response to blood loss. NSBBs can be initiated once vasoactive drugs are discontinued. Pharmacological therapy alone controls acute variceal hemorrhage in most cases. A meta-analysis of 17 trials reported that pharmacological therapy (vasopressin and its analogs and somatostatin and its analogs) was equivalent to sclerotherapy and had much fewer severe side effects, suggesting that pharmacological intervention should be the first-line therapy in the control of acute variceal hemorrhage [56]. In a meta-analysis of 30 trials involving 3,111 cirrhotics with acute variceal hemorrhage, the use of vasoactive agents in acute variceal hemorrhage was associated with significantly lower transfusion requirements, improved hemostasis, shorter hospitalization, and lower 7-day all-cause mortality [57].

   a. *Vasopressin* is a potent splanchnic vasoconstrictor that decreases portal venous inflow, thus reducing portal pressure. Vasopressin is administered as a continuous infusion at 0.2–0.4 U/minute and can be increased to a maximal rate of 0.8 U/minute. Because vasopressin can cause cardiac, intestinal, and peripheral ischemia, it should not be used beyond 24 hours; because of these ischemic consequences, its use has dropped out of favor for the treatment of acute variceal hemorrhage. Nitroglycerin can be used as a continuous infusion to counteract these ischemic side effects [3]. Seven studies in a recent meta-analysis demonstrated that terlipressin, a synthetic analogue of vasopressin with longer biological activity and significantly fewer side effects, is useful in the control of variceal hemorrhage but offers no survival benefit [57].

   b. *Octreotide*, currently the only somatostatin analog available in the United States, causes splanchnic vasoconstriction by suppressing the release of vasodilatory gastrointestinal hormones such as glucagon. Octreotide is administered as an initial 50-mcg bolus followed by a continuous 50-mcg/hour infusion. This agent is relatively safe compared to vasopressin and can be used for 5 continuous days or more, allowing treatment during a period when the risk of recurrent hemorrhage is greatest. Because of its rare risk of tachyphylaxis, octreotide should not be used alone, but appears to be most beneficial when administered in conjunction with endoscopic therapy [19]. A Cochrane review of 21 trials involving 2,588 cirrhotics with acute variceal hemorrhage noted that octreotide decreased the number of patients who failed initial control of hemorrhage and the number of blood transfusions, but did not reduce the number of patients with recurrent variceal hemorrhage or mortality rates [58].

51.6.2 Endoscopic Intervention in Acute Variceal Hemorrhage

EVL is the gold standard of endoscopic treatment after hemodynamic stabilization. It should ideally be performed within the first 6–12 hours of admission when esophageal variceal bleeding is suspected or detected [58]. Erythromycin should be administered ideally 30–120 minutes before endoscopy to improve visualization during the procedure by promoting gastric emptying. In a meta-analysis of eight trials in 939 cirrhotics with acute variceal hemorrhage, this combined approach vs. endoscopic therapy alone improved initial control

of variceal hemorrhage and continuous 5-day hemostasis, although severe adverse side effects and 5-day mortality rates were equal [60]. A meta-analysis of 10 trials in 404 cirrhotics with acute variceal hemorrhage reported better initial control of variceal hemorrhage with EVL vs. sclerotherapy [61]. Consensus guidelines recommend EVL as the preferred endoscopic technique for hemorrhage control, and sclerotherapy is used only when EVL is technically difficult or not feasible.

   a. Refractory bleeding after failed EBL control is treated with transjugular intrahepatic portosystemic shunt (TIPS) implantation e.g., Rescue-TIPS. The method achieves bleeding control in 90–100% and has rebleeding rates of 15% [59]. Yet despite the encouraging result, the utilization of TIPS in an acute setting is limited by technical challenges and availability.

51.6.3 Rescue Intervention in Acute Variceal Hemorrhage

   a. *Sengstaken–Blakemore and Linton–Nachlas tube* is a method of balloon tamponade that is most commonly used in the treatment of refractory bleeding. The mechanical compression allows the bleeding in up to 90% of cases, but almost half the patients have rebleeding events post-deflation of the balloon [19]. In addition, there is a high rate of life-threatening complications associated with this procedure, including perforation, esophageal ulceration, aspiration pneumonia, and pressure-induced ulcers. The mortality rate is 20%.

   b. *Esophageal stent* is an alternative, given the high rates of complication with balloon tamponade. This device can be deployed without endoscopic guidance and left in situ for 7 days, unlike the balloon, which can only be used for 48 hours due to the risk of pressure-induced ulcers. The success rate ranges from 70% to 100%, with lower complication risks than balloon tamponade but no improvement in mortality rates [62–64]. Both balloon tamponade and esophageal stent are used as bridging therapy to more definitive treatment such as TIPS implant or surgical shunt.

   c. *TIPS* is a type of surgical shunt therapy and is known to quickly lower the portal pressure and effectively reach hemostasis. Observational studies compared preemptive TIPS (within 72 hours) to EVL+ vasoactive drugs in patients with Child-Pugh C or Child Pugh B cirrhosis with active bleeding [65, 66]. Compared to standard of care with medication and endoscopic treatment, early TIPS placement significantly reduced treatment failure and rebleeding in both Child-Pugh C and Child-Pugh B patients. This translated into a significantly lower mortality rate in Child-Pugh C patients, but Child-Pugh B patients had no changes in mortality rate compared to standard of care. It should be noted that TIPS is not recommended in patients to prevent the first variceal hemorrhage, given the higher rate of encephalopathy and a tendency for a higher mortality [51].

RECOMMENDATION

Pharmacological therapy should be initiated as soon as variceal hemorrhage is suspected, even before endoscopic confirmation (Ib/A–Ia/A). Vasoactive drugs should be used in conjunction with upper endoscopy (Ia/A). Upper endoscopy should be performed promptly to confirm the diagnosis and to control variceal hemorrhage, preferably with EVL. Sclerotherapy is used only when EVL is technically difficult or not feasible (Ib/A). Early rehemorrhage should prompt a second endoscopic attempt before considering rescue therapy with TIPS or surgical shunt (IIb/B). Persistent or severe recurrent hemorrhage despite combined pharmacological and endoscopic therapy is best treated by TIPS (I/C–IIb/B). Early use of TIPS may be warranted (Ib/A). Balloon tamponade should only be used as a temporizing measure to definitive therapy (TIPS/surgical shunt) (Ib/B–V/D).

51.7 Prevention of Recurrence: Secondary Prophylaxis

Patients who survive the first variceal episode carry a high risk of recurrent hemorrhage (60% in the first year) and mortality up to 33% [3]. Therefore, patients who recover from variceal hemorrhage should receive secondary prophylaxis soon after the first variceal episode to prevent recurrent hemorrhage. Patients who require rescue therapy with TIPS or surgical shunt do not need secondary prophylaxis. The patency of TIPS should be assessed by Doppler ultrasound every 6 months, which is also required for hepatocellular carcinoma surveillance. If suitable candidates otherwise, all of these patients should be referred to liver transplant centers early. The objective of secondary prophylaxis is to prevent additional complications such as variceal rebleeds and death.

The first-line treatment for patients who have not received a TIPS implementation is NSBBs + EVL. A meta-analysis comparing NSBBs + EVL to either modality alone reported that combination therapy significantly reduced the risk of recurrent variceal hemorrhage but not overall mortality [67]. Patients who are unable or unwilling to have EVL should have combination therapy with NSBBs and isosorbide mononitrate. The combination of NSBBs and isosorbide mononitrate has a greater portal pressure–reducing effect but has higher rates of side effects such as headaches and lightheadedness [68]. If β-blockers are not tolerated, then patients should be considered for TIPS during the acute episode as rescue therapy [19]. In a recent randomized controlled trial, patients treated with TIPS using covered stents compared to NSBBs + EVL had a significantly lower rebleed rate (0% vs. 29%). There was no

difference in survival or higher incidence of early encephalopathy in the TIPS group [69].

Sclerotherapy uses injections of ethanolamine oleate, absolute alcohol, or tetradecyl sulfate to induce endothelial damage and thrombosis. This is no longer recommended in the secondary prophylaxis of variceal hemorrhage. Compared to sclerotherapy, EVL shows superior results in relation to rates of recurrent variceal hemorrhage, mortality, and esophageal stricture [3].

RECOMMENDATION

For cirrhotics who recover from acute variceal hemorrhage, data support a combination of β-blockers and EVL for secondary prophylaxis (Ia/A). Patients who fail combined therapy should be considered for TIPS or surgical shunt (IIb/B–Ia/A). TIPS can be used as a bridge to transplantation (IV/C), and suitable candidates should be referred to liver transplant centers early (IIb/B). Sclerotherapy is no longer recommended for secondary prophylaxis of variceal hemorrhage.

51.8 Special Consideration for Gastric Varices

Gastric varices (GV) are attributed to about 20% of all variceal bleeds in cirrhotic patients. They are associated with more risk of uncontrolled bleeds, higher transfusion requirements, and higher rates of rebleed compared to esophageal bleeds. Sarin's classification is the most commonly used for risk stratification and management of GV (Table 51.4) [51]. The main factors associated with higher risk of bleeding are localization (IGV1 > GOV2 > GOV1), larger size, presence of red spots, and advanced liver cirrhosis. Cardiofundal varices (GOV2 and IGV1) are associated with portal vein or splenic vein thrombosis, and imaging should be conducted to investigate the presence of such thromboses.

Given the limited evidence on the management of GV, the recommendations are less robust. A trial on the primary prevention of gastric variceal hemorrhage contained 89 patients with large (>10 mm) GOV2 and IGV1 randomized to GV obturation (GVO) with *N*-butyl-2-cyanoacrylate

TABLE 51.4

Sarin's Classification of Gastric Varices

Type	Location	Prevalence
GOV type 1 (GOV1)	Extension of esophageal varices below the cardia into the lesser curvature	75% Most common of GV
GOV type 2 (GOV2)	Extension of esophageal varices into the fundus	21%
Isolated GV type 1 (IGV1)	Gastric varices present in the fundus	4–8%
Isolated GV type 2 (IGV2)	Gastric varices present in other areas of the stomach besides the fundus	2% Extremely infrequent

or isobutyl-2-cyanoacrylate injection, NSBBS, or observation. Patients who underwent cyanoacrylate injection were associated with lower bleeding rates (10%) than NSBBs (38%) and observation (53%). Survival was higher in the cyanoacrylate group (93%) compared to observation (74%), but no different from those on NSBBs (83%) [71]. Another study demonstrated GVO offers a success rate close to 95% and prevents rebleeding in 92% of patients [72]. No studies have assessed primary prevention of bleeding from GOV1 varices. These are commonly managed following guidelines for EV [3]. In a retrospective study of 210 patients with cirrhosis of the liver with GV, 34% underwent GVO, 20% underwent balloon-occluded retrograde transvenous obliteration (BRTO), and 46% were observed. The BRTO group had the lowest rate of GV bleed, 7.4%, compared to GVO (19.4%) and observation (35.1%). Even though the lower rate of GV bleeding in BRTO was not significant compared to the GVO group, the BRTO group had higher rates of complete GV eradication [73]. When comparing BRTO to TIPS, a meta-analysis found no statistically significant difference between the two methods for technical success, hemostasis, and complication rates. However, rebleed and hepatic encephalopathy were greater in TIPS [74].

The initial treatment of acute GV hemorrhage is the same as EV hemorrhage, fluid resuscitation, vasoactive medications, and antibiotics before diagnostic endoscopy. In cases of massive bleed, balloon tamponade can serve as a bridge to other treatments. Given the larger balloon capacity (600 mL), Linton–Nachal tubes are preferred in GV bleeds [19]. Inflating only the gastric balloon and anchoring it against the gastroesophageal junction should produce adequate tamponade. Endoscopic treatment includes GVO or EVL. One should note that EVL has limited ability to control GV bleeding. It should only be performed on small GV in which both the mucosal and contralateral wall of the vessel can be suctioned into the ligator in order to prevent the band from falling off and inducing ulceration with rebleeding [19]. Randomized controlled trials comparing band ligation with cyanoacrylate injection demonstrated that band ligation had lower initial hemostasis and higher rebleeding rates, 63% and 72% at 2-and 3-year intervals. Variceal band ligation should only be considered first-line treatment if cyanoacrylate is unavailable or for GOV1 [19, 35, 75]. The GVO is more effective in achieving variceal obturation, with a higher initial hemostasis and less need for surgery than sclerotherapy [35]. GVO is superior to band ligation for acute GV bleeding with higher initial hemostasis and lower rebleeding rates. The rebleeding rate of GVO

remains high, and if the patient is unresponsive to the initial endoscopic treatment, a second attempt should be made [36]. If the bleeding continues, the rescue therapy of choice is TIPS. In a randomized controlled trial, TIPS was shown to be more effective than GVO in preventing rebleeding with a hemostasis rate of 92.3% and post-TIPS encephalopathy occurring in 4–16% of patients [76].

The higher volume of blood flow in GV hemorrhage leads to rapid flushing of sclerosant into the bloodstream, requiring large dosages. The reported rebleeding from sclerotherapy to treat GV bleeding was up to 90%, and complications rates varied from 24% to 82% [50]. Considering the high rates of rebleed and complications, sclerotherapy is not recommended as the first-line treatment for GV bleeding.

Patients who survive the first variceal episode carry a high risk of recurrent hemorrhage. The first-line secondary prophylaxis is repeated GVO. In randomized controlled trials, injection of cyanoacrylate was superior to NSBB—in fact, even adding NSBB to cyanoacrylate injections did not improve rebleeding or mortality rate [77, 78]. On the other hand, in patients recovering from cardiofundal varices (GOV2 and IGV1) TIPS is more effective than glue injection in preventing rebleeding. BRTO is also effective in managing fundal variceal bleeding, given the large concentration of gastro-/splenorenal collaterals [79]. Table 51.5 summarizes the management of gastric varices depending on Sarin's classification.

RECOMMENDATION

For prevention of a first GV bleed from GOV2 or IGV1, NSBBs can be used (IIb/B). Prevention of a first bleed from GOV1 varices may follow the recommendation of EV (Ia/A). Initial treatment of acute GV hemorrhage is the same as EV hemorrhage: Fluid resuscitation, vasoactive medications, and antibiotics before diagnostic endoscopy. Patients with GOV1 bleed should undergo EVL or GVO with cyanoacrylate glue injection (IIb/B). TIPS is recommended for those bleeding from GOV2 or IGV1 (IIb/B). In patients recovering from GOV1 hemorrhage, it is recommended to undergo NSBBs + EVL (or cyanoacrylate injection) as the first-line therapy for secondary prophylaxis (Ia/A). In patients recovering from GOV2 or IGV1 hemorrhage, first-line secondary prophylaxis is TIPS or BRTO (Ia/A).

TABLE 51.5

Management for Gastric Varices

Type	Primary Prophylaxis	Acute Variceal Bleed	Secondary Prophylaxis
GOV type 1 (GOV1)	Same as EV	Cyanoacrylate glue injection Alternative: EVL	Cyanoacrylate glue injection +/– NSBBs
GOV type 2 (GOV2)	NSBB	TIPS or BRTO	TIPS or BRTO
Isolated GV type 1 (IGV1)	NSBB	TIPS or BRTO	TIPS or BRTO
Isolated GV type 2 (IGV2)	Same as EV	Cyanoacrylate glue injection Alternative: EVL	Cyanoacrylate glue injection +/– NSBBs

TABLE 51.6

Evidence-Based Diagnosis and Treatment of Variceal Hemorrhage

Question	Answer	Level of Evidence	References
In cirrhotics what is the most reliable prediction of variceal development?	HVPG*	A	[3, 4, 5, 7, 38]
What is the best diagnostic test to identify esophageal varices?	UEGD*	A	[3, 26]
In cirrhotics who have no varices by upper endoscopy, what is the best treatment to prevent the development of varices?	No preventive measures have been demonstrated. Patients should undergo regular surveillance.	Ib/A1	[3, 4]
In cirrhotics who have small varices, what is the best treatment to prevent the first variceal hemorrhage?	Current guidelines do not specifically recommend treatment for small varices due to a lack of decisive studies.	Ib/A–III/B	[19, 35, 41]
In cirrhotics who have medium/large varices, what is the best treatment to prevent the first variceal hemorrhage? In cirrhotics who have acute variceal hemorrhage, what specific resuscitative fluids should be given?	NSBB* or EVL for prevention of first variceal bleeding in patients with medium to large varices. Prompt but careful resuscitation of blood loss from variceal hemorrhage should occur with colloid to maintain hemodynamic stability and with packed cells to maintain Hg 7–8 g/dL	Ia/A Ib/B–I1b/A	[19, 68, 47, 48] [43]
In cirrhotics who have acute variceal hemorrhage, what is the role of prophylactic antibiotics?	Short-term (<7 days) prophylactic antibiotics should begin at hospital admission for all cirrhotics who present with acute variceal hemorrhage.	Ia/A	[3, 54, 55]
In cirrhotics who have acute variceal hemorrhage, what is the best treatment to control hemorrhage?	Pharmacological therapy should be initiated as soon as variceal hemorrhage is suspected. Upper endoscopy should be performed promptly to confirm the diagnosis and to control variceal hemorrhage, preferably with EVL.	Ia/A	[38, 57, 58]
In cirrhotics who recover from acute variceal hemorrhage, what is the best treatment to prevent recurrence?	NSBB and EVL for secondary prophylaxis. Patients who fail combined therapy should be considered for TIPS or surgical shunt. TIPS can be used as a bridge to transplantation, and suitable candidates should be referred to liver transplant centers early.	Ia/A, IIb/B–Ia/A, IVC, IIb/B	[3, 19, 69]

* *Gold standard.*

51.9 Conclusion

The results from evidenced-based protocols have clearly changed the treatment of variceal hemorrhage. HVPG measurement has become the most reliable predictor of variceal development, and screening upper endoscopy remains the best tool to detect varices. No medical therapy is available to prevent the formation of varices, but NSBBs and EVL are equivalent therapies to prevent a first variceal hemorrhage in patients with medium or large varices. Acute variceal hemorrhage requires prompt but careful resuscitation, and prophylactic antibiotic therapy is critical to prevent bacterial infections. A combination of immediate pharmacological therapy followed by prompt endoscopic therapy appears to be the most reasonable approach for acute variceal hemorrhage. For patients who fail optimal medical therapy for acute variceal hemorrhage, rescue techniques (Sengstaken–Blakemore tube placement, TIPSS, and esophageal stents) should be carefully considered. A combination of β-blockers and EVL appears to be the most effective approach in the prevention of recurrent variceal hemorrhage, and TIPS and operative shunts are reserved for patients who fail secondary prophylaxis. TIPS can be used as a bridge to liver transplantation, and suitable patients should be referred to specialized liver transplant centers early. Recommendations are summarized in Tale 51.6.

REFERENCES

1. La Mura V, Nicolini A, Tosetti G, Primignani M. Cirrhosis and portal hypertension: The importance of risk stratification, the role of hepatic venous pressure gradient measurement. World J Hepatol. 2015 Apr 8;7(4):688–95. doi: 10.4254/wjh.v7.i4.688. PMID: 25866605; PMCID: PMC4388996.

2. Garbuzenko DV, Arefyev NO, Belov DV. Mechanisms of adaptation of the hepatic vasculature to the deteriorating conditions of blood circulation in liver cirrhosis. World J Hepatol. 2016 Jun 8;8(16):665–72.

3. Garcia-Taso G, Abraldes JG, Berzigotti A, Bosch J. Portal hypertensive bleeding in cirrhosis: Risk stratification, diagnosis, and management: 2016 practice guidance by the American Association for the Study of Liver Diseases. Hepatology. 2017;65(1):331–335.

4. Groszmann RJ, Garcia-Tsao G, Bosch J, Grace ND, Burroughs AK, Planas R, et al. Beta-blockers to prevent gastroesophageal varices in patients with cirrhosis. N Engl J Med. 2005;353:2254–61.

5. D'Amico G, Garcia-Pagan JC, Luca A, Bosch J. Hepatic vein pressure gradient reduction and prevention of variceal bleeding in cirrhosis: A systematic review. Gastroenterology. 2006;131(5):1611–24.

6. Turnes J, Garcia-Pagan JC, Abraldes JG, Hernandez-Guerra M, Dell'Era A, Bosch J. Pharmacological reduction of portal pressure and long-term risk of first variceal bleeding in patients with cirrhosis. Am J Gastroenterol. 2006;101(3):506–12.

7. Moitinho E, Escorsell A, Bandi JC, et al. Prognostic value of early measurements of portal pressure in acute variceal bleeding. Gastroenterology. 1999;117(3):626–31.

8. Zhang F, Liu T, Gao P, Fei S. Predictive value of a noninvasive serological hepatic fibrosis scoring system in cirrhosis combined with oesophageal varices. Can J Gastroenterol Hepatol. 2018;2018:7671508.

9. Kraja B, Mone I, Akshija I, Koçollari A, Prifti S, Burazeri G. Predictors of esophageal varices and first variceal bleeding in liver cirrhosis patients. World J Gastroenterol. 2017 Jul 14;23(26):4806–14.

10. Chiejina M, Kudaravalli P, Samant H. Ascites. [Updated 2022 Aug 8]. In: StatPearls [Internet]. Treasure Island (FL): StatPearls Publishing; 2022 Jan.

11. Thong VD, Anh HTV. Prediction of esophageal varices based on serum-ascites albumin gradient in cirrhotic patients. Gastroenterol Insights. 2021;12(2):270–77.

12. Wang L, Feng Y, Ma X, Wang G, Wu H, Xie X, Zhang C, Zhu Q. Diagnostic efficacy of noninvasive liver fibrosis indexes in predicting portal hypertension in patients with cirrhosis. PLoS ONE. 2017 Aug 18;12(8):e0182969.

13. Cherian JV, Deepak N, Ponnusamy RP, Somasundaram A, Jayanthi V. Non-invasive predictors of esophageal varices. Saudi J Gastroenterol. 2011 Jan-Feb;17(1):64–8.

14. Afsar A, Nadeem M, Shah SAA, Hussain H, Rani A, Ghaffar S. Platelet count can predict the grade of esophageal varices in cirrhotic patients: a cross-sectional study. F1000Res. 2021 Nov 24;10:101.

15. Cifci S, Ekmen N. Evaluation of non-invasive fibrosis markers in predicting esophageal variceal bleeding. Clin Endosc. 2021 Nov;54(6):857–63.

16. Tantai XX, Liu N, Yang LB, Wei ZC, Xiao CL, Song YH, Wang JH. Prognostic value of risk scoring systems for cirrhotic patients with variceal bleeding. World J Gastroenterol. 2019 Dec 7;25(45):6668–80.

17. Wu SL, Zheng YX, Tian ZW, Chen MS, Tan HZ. Scoring systems for prediction of mortality in decompensated liver cirrhosis: A meta-analysis of test accuracy. World J Clin Cases. 2018 Dec 6;6(15):995–1006.

18. Chalasani N, Kahi C, Francois F, Pinto A, Marathe A, Bini EJ, Pandya P, Sitaraman S, Shen J. Model for end-stage liver disease (MELD) for predicting mortality in patients with acute variceal bleeding. Hepatology. 2002 May;35(5):1282–4.

19. Garcia-Tsao G, Abraldes JG, Berzigotti A, Bosch J. Portal hypertensive bleeding in cirrhosis: Risk stratification, diagnosis, and management: 2016 practice guidance by the American Association for the study of liver diseases. Hepatology. 2017;65:310–35.

20. Fleming KM, Aithal GP, Card TR, West J. All-cause mortality in people with cirrhosis compared with the general population: a population-based cohort study. Liver Int. 2012 Jan;32(1):79–84.

21. Haq I, Tripathi D. Recent advances in the management of variceal bleeding. Gastroenterol Rep (Oxf). 2017;5:113–26.

22. Bochnakova T. Hepatic venous pressure gradient. Clin Liver Dis (Hoboken). 2021 Apr 13;17(3):144–48.

23. Uppalapati S, Lokesh S. Correlation of portal vein diameter with the presence of oesophageal varices in chronic liver disease: A prospective study. Int J Adv Med Sci. 2018 July;5(4):859–64.

24. Shi KQ, Fan YC, Pan ZZ, Lin XF, Liu WY, Chen YP, et al. Transient elastography: A meta-analysis of diagnostic accuracy in evaluation of portal hypertension in chronic liver disease. Liver Int. 2013;33:62–71.

25. Augustin S, Millan L, Gonzalez A, Martell M, Gelabert A, Segarra A, et al. Detection of early portal hypertension with routine data and liver stiffness in patients with asymptomatic liver disease: A prospective study. J Hepatol. 2014;60:561–69.

26. Richardson E, Arastu S, Halegoua-DeMarzio D. PRO: Esophagogastroduodenoscopy is the preferred modality to screen for the diagnosis of esophageal and gastric varices when the diagnosis of cirrhosis is made. Clin Liver Dis. 2020;16:43–7.

27. Robic MA, Procopet B, Metivier S, Peron JM, Selves J, Vinel JP, et al. Liver stiffness accurately predicts portal hypertension related complications in patients with chronic liver disease: A prospective study. J Hepatol. 2011;55:1017–24.

28. Karatzas A, Konstantakis C, Aggeletopoulou I, Kalogeropoulou C, Thomopoulos K, Triantos C. Non-invasive screening for esophageal varices in patients with liver cirrhosis. Ann Gastroenterol. 2018 May-Jun;31(3):305–314.

29. Tseng YJ, Zeng XQ, Chen J, Li N, Xu PJ, Chen SY. Computed tomography in evaluating gastroesophageal varices in patients with portal hypertension: A meta-analysis. Dig Liver Dis. 2016;48:695–702.

30. Deng H, Qi X, Guo X. Computed tomography for the diagnosis of varices in liver cirrhosis: A systematic review and meta-analysis of observational studies. Postgrad Med. 2017;129:318–328.

31. Karatzas A, Triantos C, Kalafateli M, et al. Multidetector computed tomography versus platelet/spleen diameter ratio as methods for the detection of gastroesophageal varices. Ann Gastroenterol. 2016;29:71–78.

32. Lipp MJ, Broder A, Hudesman D, et al. Detection of esophageal varices using CT and MRI. Dig Dis Sci. 2011;56:2696–2700.

33. Shin SU, Lee JM, Yu MH, et al. Prediction of esophageal varices in patients with cirrhosis: Usefulness of three-dimensional MR elastography with echo-planar imaging technique. Radiology. 2014;272:143–53.

34. Sun HY, Lee JM, Han JK, Choi BI. Usefulness of MR elastography for predicting esophageal varices in cirrhotic patients. J Magn Reson Imaging. 2014;39:559–66.

35. de Franchis R Baveno VI Faculty. Expanding consensus in portal hypertension: Report of the Baveno VI consensus workshop: Stratifying risk and individualizing care for portal hypertension. J Hepatol. 2015;63:743–52.

36. Maggio D, Barkun AN, Martel M, Elouali S, Gralnek IM. Reason Investigators. Predictors of early rebleeding after endoscopic therapy in patients with nonvariceal upper gastrointestinal bleeding secondary to high-risk lesions. Can J Gastroenterol. 2013 Aug;27(8):454–8.

37. Jakab SS, Garcia-Tsao G. Screening and surveillance of varices in patients with cirrhosis. Clin Gastroenterol Hepatol. 2019 Jan;17(1):26–9. doi: 10.1016/j.cgh.2018.03.012. Epub 2018 Mar 15. Erratum in: Clin Gastroenterol Hepatol. 2019 Apr;17(5):1009.

38. D'Amico G, Garcia-Pagan JC, Luca A, Bosch J. HVPG reduction and prevention of variceal bleeding in cirrhosis. A systematic review. Gastroenterology. 2006;131:1611–24.

39. van Buuren HR, Rasch MC, Batenburg PL, Bolwerk CJ, Nicolai JJ, van der Werf SD, Scherpenisse J, Arends LR, van Hattum J, Rauws EA, et al. Endoscopic sclerotherapy compared with no specific treatment for the primary prevention of bleeding from esophageal varices. A randomized controlled multicentre trial [ISRCTN03215899] BMC Gastroenterol. 2003;3:22.

40. Peter B. Gregory, Pamela Hartigan, Donald J. Amodeo, Richard A. Baum, Daniel S. Camara, Donald R. Campbell, Henry Colcher, Pamela L. Garjian, et. al. Prophylactic sclerotherapy for esophageal varices in men with alcoholic liver disease. A randomized, single-blind, multicenter clinical trial. The Veterans Affairs Cooperative Variceal Sclerotherapy Group. N Engl J Med. 1991;324:1779–84.

41. Reiberger T, Bucsics T, Paternostro R, Pfisterer N, Riedl F, Mandorfer M. Small Esophageal varices in patients with cirrhosis-should we treat them? Curr Hepatol Rep. 2018;17:301–15.

42. Bhardwaj A, Kedarisetty CK, Vashishtha C, Bhadoria AS, Jindal A, Kumar G, Choudhary A, Shasthry SM, Maiwall R, Kumar M, Bhatia V, Sarin SK. Carvedilol delays the progression of small oesophageal varices in patients with cirrhosis: A randomised placebo-controlled trial. Gut. 2017; 66:1838–43.

43. Villanueva C, Albillos A, Genescà J, Garcia-Pagan JC, Calleja JL, Aracil C, Bañares R, Morillas RM, Poca M, Peñas B, Augustin S, Abraldes JG, Alvarado E, Torres F, Bosch J. β blockers to prevent decompensation of cirrhosis in patients with clinically significant portal hypertension (PREDESCI): A randomised, double-blind, placebo-controlled, multicentre trial. Lancet. 2019;393:1597–1608.

44. Schwarzer R, Kivaranovic D, Paternostro R, Mandorfer M, Reiberger T, Trauner M, Peck-Radosavljevic M, Ferlitsch A. Carvedilol for reducing portal pressure in primary prophylaxis of variceal bleeding: a dose-response study. Aliment Pharmacol Ther. 2018;47:1162–69.

45. Reiberger T, Ulbrich G, Ferlitsch A, Payer BA, Schwabl P, Pinter M, Heinisch BB, Trauner M, Kramer L, Peck-Radosavljevic M Vienna Hepatic Hemodynamic Lab. Carvedilol for primary prophylaxis of variceal bleeding in cirrhotic patients with haemodynamic non-response to propranolol. Gut. 2013;62:1634–41.

46. Reiberger T, Püspök A, Schoder M, Baumann-Durchschein F, Bucsics T, Datz C, Dolak W, Ferlitsch A, Finkenstedt A, Graziadei I, Hametner S, Karnel F, Krones E, Maieron A, Mandorfer M, Peck-Radosavljevic M, Rainer F, Schwabl P, Stadlbauer V, Stauber R, Tilg H, Trauner M, Zoller H, Schöfl R, Fickert P. Austrian consensus guidelines on the management and treatment of portal hypertension (Billroth III) Wien Klin Wochenschr. 2017;129:135–58.

47. Shah HA, Azam Z, Rauf J, Abid S, Hamid S, Jafri W, Khalid A, Ismail FW, Parkash O, Subhan A, Munir SM. Carvedilol vs. esophageal variceal band ligation in the primary prophylaxis of variceal hemorrhage: A multicentre randomized controlled trial. J Hepatol. 2014;60:757–64.

48. Sharma M, Singh S, Desai V, Shah VH, Kamath PS, Murad MH, Simonetto DA. Comparison of therapies for primary prevention of esophageal variceal bleeding: A systematic review and network meta-analysis. Hepatology. 2019;69:1657–75.

49. Drolz A, Schramm C, Seiz O, Groth S, Vettorazzi E, Horvatits T, Wehmeyer MH, Goeser T, Roesch T, Lohse AW, Kluwe J. Risk factors associated with bleeding after prophylactic endoscopic variceal ligation in cirrhosis. Endoscopy. 2021;53:226–34.

50. Sarin SK, Wadhawan M, Agarwal SR, Tyagi P, Sharma BC. Endoscopic variceal ligation plus propranolol versus endoscopic variceal ligation alone in primary prophylaxis of variceal bleeding. Am J Gastroenterol. 2005;100:797–804.

51. Villanueva C, Colomo A, Bosch A, Concepcion M, Hernandez-Gea V, Aracil C, et al. Transfusion strategies for acute upper gastrointestinal bleeding. N Engl J Med. 2013;368:11–21.

52. Bosch J, Thabut D, Bendtsen F, et al. Recombinant factor VIIa for upper gastrointestinal bleeding in patients with cirrhosis: A randomized, double-blind trial. Gastroenterology. 2004;127(4):1123–30.

53. Bosch J, Thabut D, Albillos A, Carbonell N, Spicak J, Massard J, et al. Recombinant factor VIIa for variceal bleeding in patients with advanced cirrhosis: A randomized, controlled trial. Hepatology. 2008;47:1604–14.

54. Bernard B, Grange JD, Khac EN, Amiot X, Opolon P, Poynard T. Antibiotic prophylaxis for the prevention of bacterial infections in cirrhotic patients with gastrointestinal bleeding: A meta-analysis. Hepatology. 1999;29: 1655–61.

55. Chavez-Tapia NC, Barrientos-Gutierrez T, Tellez-Avila F, Soares-Weiser K, Mendez-Sanchez N, Gluud C, et al. Meta analysis: Antibiotic prophylaxis for cirrhotic patients with upper gastrointestinal bleeding—an updated Cochrane review. Aliment Pharmacol Ther. 2011;34:509–18.

56. D'Amico G, Pietrosi G, Tarantino I, Pagliaro L. Emergency sclerotherapy versus vasoactive drugs for variceal bleeding in cirrhosis: A Cochrane meta-analysis. Gastroenterology. 2003;124(5):1277–91.

57. Wells M, Chande N, Adams P, et al. Meta-analysis: Vasoactive medications for the management of acute variceal bleeds. Aliment Pharmacol Ther. 2012;35(11):1267–78.

58. Gotzsche PC, Hrobjartsson A. Somatostatin analogues for acute bleeding oesophageal varices. Cochrane Database Syst Rev. 2008;(3):CD000193.

59. Vangeli M, Patch D, Burroughs AK. Salvage tips for uncontrolled variceal bleeding. J Hepatol. 2002;37:703–04

60. Banares R, Albillos A, Rincon D, et al. Endoscopic treatment versus endoscopic plus pharmacologic treatment for acute variceal bleeding: A meta-analysis. Hepatology. 2002;35(3):609–15.

61. Garcia-Pagan JC, Bosch J. Endoscopic band ligation in the treatment of portal hypertension. Nat Clin Pract Gastroenterol Hepatol. 2005;2(11):526–35.
62. Zehetner J, Shamiyeh A, Wayand W, Hubmann R. Results of a new method to stop acute bleeding from esophageal varices: Implantation of a self-expanding stent. Surg Endosc. 2008;22:2149–152.
63. Escorsell A, Bosch J. Self-expandable metal stents in the treatment of acute esophageal variceal bleeding. Gastroenterol Res Pract. 2011;2011:910986.
64. Escorsell À, Pavel O, Cárdenas A, Morillas R, Llop E, Villanueva C, Garcia-Pagán JC, Bosch J Variceal Bleeding Study Group. Esophageal balloon tamponade versus esophageal stent in controlling acute refractory variceal bleeding: A multicenter randomized, controlled trial. Hepatology. 2016;63:1957–1967.
65. Hernández-Gea V, Procopet B, Giráldez Á, Amitrano L, Villanueva C, Thabut D, Ibañez-Samaniego L, et al. International variceal bleeding observational study group and Baveno cooperation. Preemptive-TIPS improves outcome in high-risk variceal bleeding: An observational study. Hepatology. 2019;69:282–93.
66. Garcia-Pagan JC, Caca K, Bureau C, et al. Early use of TIPS in patients with cirrhosis and variceal bleeding. N Engl J Med. 2010;362(25):2370–79.
67. Puente A, Hernandez-Gea V, Graupera I, Roque M, Colomo A, Poca M, et al. Drugs plus ligation to prevent rebleeding in cirrhosis: an updated systematic review. Liver Int 2014; 34:823–33.
68. Gluud LL, Langholz E, Krag A. Meta-analysis: Isosorbide-mononitrate alone or with either beta-blockers or endoscopic therapy for the management of oesophageal varices. Aliment Pharmacol Ther. 2010;32:859–71.
69. Holster IL, Tjwa ET, Moelker A, Wils A, Hansen BE, Vermeijden JR, et al. Covered transjugular intrahepatic porto-systemic shunt versus endoscopic therapy 1 beta-blocker for prevention of variceal rebleeding. Hepatology. 2016;63:581–89.
70. Sarin SK, Lahoti D, Saxena SP, Murthy NS, Makwana UK. Prevalence, classification and natural history of gastric varices: A long-term follow-up study in 568 portal hypertension patients. Hepatology. 1992;16:1343–49.

71. Mishra SR, Sharma BC, Kumar A, Sarin SK. Primary prophylaxis of gastric variceal bleeding comparing cyanoacrylate injection and beta-blockers: A randomized controlled trial. J Hepatol. 2011;54:1161–67.
72. Al-Ali J, Pawlowska M, Coss A. Endoscopic management of gastric variceal bleeding with cyanoacrylate glue injection: safety and efficacy in a Canadian population. Can J Gastroenterol. 2010;24:593–96.
73. Choe JW, Yim HJ, Lee SH, Chung HH, Lee YS, Kim SY, et al. Primary prophylaxis of gastric variceal bleeding: Endoscopic obturation, radiologic intervention, or observation? Hepatol Int. 2021;15:934–45.
74. Wang YB, Zhang JY, Gong JP, Zhang F, Zhao Y. Balloon-occluded retrograde transvenous obliteration versus transjugular intrahepatic portosystemic shunt for treatment of gastric varices due to portal hypertension: A meta-analysis. J Gastroenterol Hepatol. 2016;31:727–33.
75. Tan PC, Hou MC, Lin HC, Liu TT, Lee FY, Chang FY, et al. A randomized trial of endoscopic treatment of acute gastric variceal hemorrhage: *N*-butyl-2-cyanoacrylate injection versus band ligation. Hepatology. 2006;43:690–97.
76. Lo GH, Liang HL, Chen WC, Chen MH, Lai KH, Hsu PI, et al. A prospective, randomized controlled trial of transjugular intrahepatic portosystemic shunt versus cyanoacrylate injection in the prevention of gastric variceal rebleeding. Endoscopy. 2007;39:679–85.
77. Mishra SR, Chander SB, Kumar A, Sarin SK. Endoscopic cyanoacrylate injection versus beta-blocker for secondary prophylaxis of gastric variceal bleed: A randomized controlled trial. Gut. 2010;59:729–35.
78. Hung HH, Chang CJ, Hou MC, Liao WC, Chan CC, Huang HC, et al. Efficacy of non-selective beta-blockers as adjunct to endoscopic prophylactic treatment for gastric variceal bleeding: A randomized controlled trial. J Hepatol. 2012;56:1025–32.
79. Fukuda T, Hirota S, Sugimura K. Long-term results of balloon-occluded retrograde transvenous obliteration for the treatment of gastric varices and hepatic encephalopathy. J VascInterv Radiol. 2001;12:327–36.

52

Acute Arterial Embolus

Boulos Toursarkissian

Peripheral arterial embolization is associated with a high risk of limb loss ranging from 5% to 40% [1–5]. A mortality rate of up to 25% is reported [3]. Patients with acute peripheral embolus are often a medically disadvantaged population. Frequently they have a cardiogenic nidus for the embolus, most often a clot from the left atrium due to atrial fibrillation. The next most common cause is a myocardial thrombus that occurs within several weeks of myocardial infarction.

The five "Ps" of acute limb ischemia—pain, paresthesia, pallor, paralysis, and pulselessness—characterize acute arterial ischemia. Ischemia will initially affect the sensory nerves, which will lead to pain, paresthesia, and loss of proprioception. More prolonged or intense ischemia will cause loss of gross sensation and motor function. Impaired motor function is a precursor to irreversible tissue loss, and paralysis indicates severe, likely irreversible muscle death. Evaluation of function is more important than the absolute elapsed time following the development of the inciting embolus [4]. Prevention of thrombus propagation by initiating anticoagulation and revascularization of the ischemic, but still salvageable, limb is strongly recommended [6, 7]. Viability is classified into categories (Rutherford classification). Categories of viability include viable (I), threatened (IIa and IIb), and irreversible (III) [8]. Articles report that 45% of limbs present as viable, 45% present as threatened (marginally or immediately), and 10% present with irreversible ischemia [6].

History and physical examination aid in sorting causes of the ischemia. Complaints of claudication or an abnormal examination on the opposite leg suggest thrombosis instead of an embolus in the presenting extremity. Differentiating between acute thrombosis due to atherosclerotic disease or a peripheral aneurysm versus an acute embolus can be difficult [5]. The difference is crucial as it does impact diagnostic testing and treatment.

Treatment options for acute arterial embolus range from observation to primary amputation. Anticoagulation is typically employed [6, 7]. Restoration and maintenance of blood flow often require intervention, which can involve open surgical revascularization, endovascular intraarterial pharmacologic and mechanical thrombectomy and thrombolysis, or a combined approach with thrombolysis and open revascularization. Three questions are essential in this situation: Embolic versus thrombotic etiology, anticoagulation strategy, and choice of revascularization approach.

52.1 Is It Possible to Diagnose an Embolic versus Thrombotic Etiology for Acute Limb Ischemia Based on History and Physical Examination?

Retrospective reviews of consecutive patient cohorts and one prospective study provide information on the subject. A retrospective review[3] examined patients treated with surgical embolectomy for acute limb ischemia. All patients had a preoperative diagnosis of acute arterial embolism. The analysis defined a group of patients misdiagnosed with arterial embolism instead of acute thrombosis. A diagnosis of arterial embolus was made if an embolic source was discovered (atrial fibrillation and myocardial infarction), the event was acute in onset, and the patient had no history of chronic arterial insufficiency (intermittent claudication). The main criteria for arterial thrombosis diagnosis were an absence of a cardiovascular source for the embolus, a rapid (not sudden) onset of symptoms with less than 7 days' duration, and a history of symptomatic peripheral arterial disease. Twenty-five percent of the patients were misdiagnosed with an embolic etiology for their ischemia (Level IV). Twenty-six percent of patients had an etiology of acute limb ischemia that was not identifiable in a more recent cohort (Level IIb) [2]. In 1984, Cambria and Abbott established that the diagnosis of embolus was wrong in 17% of their patients [9]. The presence of atrial fibrillation was the only distinguishing feature between the two groups. Forty percent of thrombotic patients had preceding symptoms of arterial insufficiency (Level IIIb). A 1-year prospective study of patients treated for acute limb ischemia based on examination alone demonstrated an incorrect diagnosis in 9% of patients. However, no impact on the outcome was seen due to misdiagnosis [1] (Level IIb).

RECOMMENDATION

In conclusion, it is often possible to distinguish between embolic versus thrombotic etiologies based on history and examination. However, the error rate can be as high as 25% (grade C recommendation).

Grade of recommendation: C.

DOI: 10.1201/9781003316800-52

52.2 Is Perioperative Anticoagulation Necessary in the Treatment of Acute Limb Ischemia?

Anticoagulation is an essential treatment for the prevention of the propagation of thrombus. Stasis created by the initial occlusive event can lead to thrombosis and loss of collateral flow via secondary occlusion from thrombus propagation [6, 7] (Level V). Surgical embolectomy can be delayed if anticoagulation alone is administered and there is no evidence of impending muscle loss [1, 2, 4, 5, 9]. However, this is not always an acceptable measure, as 50% of patients require immediate revascularization [2].

Patients undergoing revascularization without anticoagulants and receiving anticoagulants before surgery, during, and after revascularization were reviewed at one center [10]. Patients with temporary anticoagulation and those with incomplete records were omitted. Patients receiving anticoagulation were twice as likely to have a "good result," defined as amputation-free survival at 4 months. No difference in hospital deaths was found, but patients receiving anticoagulation had significantly more bleeding complications. Recurrence rates at 36 months were not different (Level IV). One hundred and eighteen patients with acute limb ischemia randomized to anticoagulation or no anticoagulation and thrombo-embolectomy were prospectively studied at multiple centers.

Anticoagulation with heparin was then transitioned to Coumadin. Results were evaluated at 30 days. No significant difference was found in amputation-free survival, mortality, or reoperation [11] (Level IIb).

RECOMMENDATION

In conclusion, consensus panels recommend perioperative anticoagulation without definitive evidence.

Grade of recommendation: C.

52.3 Is Percutaneous Endovascular Treatment the Preferred Initial Treatment over Surgical Revascularization?

Initial nonsurgical treatment of peripheral emboli evolved from heparin usage to systemic lytic agents such as urokinase and tissue plasminogen activator (tPA). Catheter-directed delivery of lytic agents was the next step. Catheter-directed lysis has fewer bleeding complications and improved clot resolution than systemic thrombolysis [12]. It is believed that thrombolytic therapy allows for enhanced clearance of thrombus from vessels too small for traditional embolectomy catheters and can diagnose underlying pathology (such as stenoses) in the angiography suite. This comes at the cost of increased time to reperfusion, medical costs, hospital resource use, hemorrhage, and distal embolization.

Endovascular treatment of peripheral arterial embolization has evolved over the last few years from a purely catheter-directed intraarterial thrombolysis therapy approach to a more encompassing mechanical and pharmaco-mechanical approach whereby the offending embolus or clot is aspirated and removed by a variety of means with or without adjunctive use of thrombolytic agents. This has resulted in shorter treatment times and faster re-establishment of flow, thereby enabling the treatment of many patients with immediately threatened limbs (class IIb) who would otherwise have required open surgical thrombo-embolectomy.

In several prospective randomized trials, surgical therapy has been compared with percutaneous thrombolysis (not including mechanical or pharmaco-mechanical approaches). Several single-center trials found no differences in limb salvage [14–16] (Level IIb). The Thrombolysis Or Peripheral Arterial Surgery (TOPAS) trial was a randomized, multi-center prospective trial comparing thrombolysis or surgery in patients with <2 weeks of acute ischemia. There was no difference in 1-year mortality or amputation-free survival. Forty-six percent of patients needed no further surgical revascularization following thrombolysis (Level IIb) [17]. Five hundred and forty-eight patients were evaluated in phase II. The primary endpoint was amputation-free survival, and there was no difference between the two groups. Bleeding complications were significantly higher in the thrombolysis group. There was no demonstrable difference between limbs treated for thrombotic etiology versus embolic etiology. The major conclusion is a decreased need for open surgical revascularization and a reduced magnitude of the surgery. Still, there is a higher rate of bleeding with thrombolytic therapy (Level IIb). A recently updated Cochrane Database meta-analysis [17] examined five randomized trials including 1,292 patients and confirmed many of these results. No differences in limb salvage, amputation, or death were noted at 30 days, 6 months, or 1 year (Level Ib due to bias and heterogeneity). Another Cochrane review [18] compared standard catheter-directed lysis to ultrasound-assisted lysis (the so-called EKOS system) and found no significant difference in outcomes between the two techniques.

When comparing pharmaco-mechanical endovascular approaches to open surgery, there have been several prospective and retrospective studies but no randomized prospective trials. The INDIAN trial looked at the efficacy of a vacuum-assisted device (Penumbra) for acute limb ischemia at several sites, demonstrating an 82% primary patency and a low reintervention rate of 7.3% [19]. Other single-center series with the same device have shown a lower success rate, around 50% [20]. The efficacy of an endovascular first approach to acute limb ischemia was also recently demonstrated in a single-center series with an 87% 30-day survival rate and 88% limb salvage rate [21].

Intraarterial endovascular techniques as initial therapy for acute limb ischemia appear to be in equipoise relative to open surgical treatment for achieving limb salvage and may reduce mortality (Level II data). The endovascular approach may

TABLE 52.1

Clinical Questions

Question	Answer	Levels of Evidence	Grade of Recommendation	References
Is it possible to diagnose embolus versus thrombus by history and physical?	Yes, but many patients will require further testing.	IIb, IIIb, IV	C	[1, 2, 3, 9]
Is preoperative anticoagulation indicated?	Yes, consensus panels support this.	V, IV, IIb	C	[1, 2, 4, 5, 9, 10]
Is percutaneous thrombectomy preferred over surgical revascularization?	No, they are fairly similar in obtaining limb salvage.	IIb, Ia	B	[6, 12–14, 17, 18]

further decrease surgical revascularization in some patients. However, there is an increased risk of significant bleeding, stroke, and distal embolization, especially with pure pharmacologic approaches. Pharmaco-mechanical approaches appear to be the dominant current modality. Careful patient selection is paramount.

RECOMMENDATION

In the treatment of acute embolic ischemia, intraarterial endovascular techniques as initial therapy for acute limb ischemia have similar outcomes when compared to open surgical treatment for achieving limb salvage.

Level of evidence: II data. Grade of recommendation: B (Table 52.1).

Editor's Note

Unfortunately, there is little high-quality data to guide our treatment of acute arterial embolus. While it is often possible to distinguish between embolic versus thrombotic etiologies based on history and examination, the error rate remains as high as 25%. Similarly, there is insufficient research on perioperative anticoagulation, which is currently recommended by clinician consensus.

The use of intraarterial endovascular techniques as initial therapy for acute limb ischemia has been extensively investigated but does not confer a significant advantage over surgical intervention in achieving limb salvage.

REFERENCES

1. McPhail N, Fratesi SJ, Barger GG, Scobie TK. Management of acute thromboembolic limb ischemia. *Surgery.* 1983;*93*: 381–385.
2. Jivegard L, Arfvidsson B, Holm J, Schersten T. Selective conservative and routine early operative treatment in critical limb ischemia. *Br J Surg.* 1987;*74*:798–801.
3. Jivegard L, Holm J, Schersten T. The outcome of arterial thrombosis is misdiagnosed as arterial embolism. *Acta Chir Scand.* 1986;*152*:251–256.
4. Dale W. Differential management of acute peripheral arterial ischemia. *J Vasc Surg.* 1984;*1*:269–278.
5. Blaisdell F, Steele M, Allen RE. Management of acute lower extremity arterial ischemia due to embolism and thrombosis. *Surgery.* 1978;*84*:822–834.
6. Norgren LHW, Dormandy JA, Nehler MR, Harris KA, Fowkes FGR. Inter-societal consensus for the management of peripheral arterial disease (TASC II). *J Vasc Surg.* 2007;*45*:S1–S67.
7. Clagett G.P.S.M., Jackson MR, Lip GYH, Tangelder M, Verhaeghe R. Antithrombotic therapy in peripheral arterial occlusive disease: The Seventh ACCP Conference on antithrombotic and thrombolytic therapy. *Chest.* 2004;*126*: 609–626.
8. Rutherford R, Baker JD, Ernst C et al. Recommended standards for reports dealing with lower extremity ischemia: Revised version. *J Vasc Surg.* 1997;*26*:517–538.
9. Cambria R, Abbott WM. Acute arterial thrombosis of the lower extremity. *Arch Surg.* 1984;*119*:784–787.
10. Jivegard LHJ, Schersten T. Arterial thromboembolectomy—Should anticoagulants be administered? *Acta Chir Scand.* 1986;*152*:493–497.
11. Jivegard L, Holm J, Bergqvist D et al. Acute lower limb ischemia: Failure of anticoagulant treatment to improve one-month results of arterial thromboem- lectomy. A prospective randomized multi-center study. *Surgery.* 1991;*109*: 610–616.
12. Berridge D, Gregson RHS, Hopkinson BR et al. Randomized trial of intra-arterial recombinant tissue plasminogen activator, intravenous recombinant tissue plasminogen activator and intra-arterial streptokinase in peripheral arterial thrombolysis. *Br J Surg.* 1991;*78*:988–995.
13. Poursina O, Elizondo-Adamchik H, Montero-Baker M et al. Safety and efficacy of an endovascular first approach to acute limb ischemia. *J Vasc Surg.* 2021;*73*(5): 1741–1749.
14. Ouriel K, Shortell CK, DeWeese JA et al. A comparison of thrombolytic therapy with operative revascularization in the initial treatment of acute peripheral arterial ischemia. *J Vasc Surg.* 1994;*19*:1021–1030.
15. Nilsson L, Albrechtsson U, Jonung T et al. Surgical treatment versus thrombolysis in acute arterial occlusion: A randomised controlled study. *Eur J Vasc Surg.* 1992;*6*: 189–193.
16. Ouriel K, Veith FJ, Sasahara AA et al. Thrombolysis or peripheral arterial surgery: Phase I results. *J Vasc Surg.* 1996;*23*:64–73.

17. Ouriel K, Veith FJ, Sasahara AA et al. A comparison of recombinant urokinase with vascular surgery as initial treatment for acute arterial occlusion of the legs. *N Engl J Med.* 1998;*338*:1105–1111.

18. Darwood R, Berridge DC, Kessel D et al. Surgery versus thrombolysis for initial management of acute limb ischemia. *Cochrane Database Syst Rev.* 2018;*8(8)*:CD002784.

19. Aranjo ST, Moreno DH, Cacione DG. Standard lysis vs. ultrasound-assisted lysis. *Cochrane Database Syst Rev.* 2020;*1*:CD013486.

20. deDonato G, Pasqui E, Spona M et al. Safety and efficacy of vacuum-assisted thrmbo-aspiration in patients with acute lower limb ischemia. The INDIAN trial. *Eur J Vasc Endovasc Surg.* 2012;*61(5)*:820–828.

21. Lopez R, Yamashita TS, Neisen M et al. Single center experience with Indigo aspiration thrombectomy for acute lower limb ischemia. *J Vasc Surg.* 2020;*72(1)*:226–232.

53

Ruptured Aortic Aneurysm

Boulos Toursarkissian

A ruptured abdominal aortic aneurysm (rAAA) is a life-threatening surgical emergency. Despite many advances in anesthesia and critical care medicine, it ranks among the 15 leading causes of death in the United States.

Essential considerations in the care of a patient with rAAA include preoperative resuscitation goals and methods; criteria used to select patients for surgery (i.e., survival prediction); the nature of imaging studies needed before surgical intervention; and the impact of delays in treatment, the type of intervention to be performed, the use of anticoagulants intraoperatively, and the need to monitor patients for frequent postoperative complications. Patients with rAAA are prone to the development of complications, including ischemic colitis (IC), paraplegia from spinal cord ischemia, renal failure, peripheral atheroembolic problems, and abdominal compartment syndrome (ACS) (Tables 53.1 and 53.2). The Society for Vascular Surgery has published clinical guidelines for patients with rAAA.

53.1 What Are the Optimal Resuscitation Goals and Methods to Be Used in Patients with Ruptured Aneurysms?

As far as resuscitation goals and measures are concerned, only expert opinions and prospective cohort studies are available in the literature (Level IV and V evidence). The suggestions are based on extrapolations from the trauma literature. However, one of the main limitations to be kept in mind is that trauma patients are usually younger and healthier than patients with rAAA. One prospective trial evaluated 90 patients requiring emergency surgery for trauma; patients were randomized to either intraoperative hypotensive resuscitation (mean arterial pressure of 50 mmHg) or standard fluid resuscitation (target mean arterial pressure of 65 mmHg). Patients in the low-pressure arm required less fluids and blood, had less coagulopathy, and had lower mortality in the early postoperative period [1] (Level I evidence).

Many experts suggest that it is acceptable to tolerate a systolic blood pressure under 100 mmHg or even lower (down to 70 mmHg) in patients with rAAA as long as adequate mentation is maintained (grade C recommendation). The rationale presented is that a higher pressure may exacerbate the tendency for retroperitoneal hemorrhage and convert what was otherwise a contained rupture into a free one. The added fluids required for a higher pressure goal may also exacerbate postoperative coagulopathy. A retrospective study of 248 patients with rAAA over 10 years suggested that aggressive volume resuscitation before proximal aortic control predicted an increased perioperative risk of death, which was independent of systolic blood pressure [2] (Level IIb evidence). On the other hand, a retrospective analysis of data from the British IMPROVE trial [3; see later] suggests that a systolic pressure under 70 mmHg was independently associated with increased mortality (51% vs. 34%). Although there are no definitive studies on patients with rAAA, it seems intuitive to recommend avoiding overt hypertension [4].

The nature of fluids for resuscitation purposes in the perioperative period in patients with rAAA has been the subject of at least one prospective cohort study (Level IIa evidence). In this Danish study, 55 patients with rAAA were proactively administered fresh-frozen plasma and platelet concentrate immediately when rAAA was diagnosed [5]. Thirty-day survival improved to 66% compared to a 44% survival for the 93 patients treated by conventional means in the preceding 2-year period. All patients in the study group were treated with an open aneurysm surgery. Another prospective cohort study from Denmark used a "transfusion package" of red cells (five units), plasma (five units), and platelets (two units) combined with thromboelastography to guide transfusion, resulting in a decrease in mortality at 30 days from 56% in historical controls to 34% in treated patients [6]. A recent 2021 systematic review found a survival benefit for rAAA patients undergoing surgery when the ratio of red cells to plasma was close to 1 [7]; from these studies, it appears that an aggressive approach toward the use of blood products appears justified (grade B recommendation)—the use of products such as hypertonic saline, albumin, or hetastarch does not seem to offer any benefits.

> ### RECOMMENDATION
>
> Moderate hypotension is acceptable, and blood products should be used early.
>
> Grades of recommendation: B and C.

53.2 Can Mortality from rAAA Be Predicted?

Mortality after repair of rAAA remains high. One of the factors that has been associated with increased mortality in several studies is advanced age, especially when comparing patients over the age of 80 years to younger individuals

DOI: 10.1201/9781003316800-53

(Level IIIb evidence). However, an age cutoff beyond which survival is unlikely has never been identified (as a single variable), and survival rates over 50% have been reported by some octogenarians [8]. Therefore, age alone cannot be used as a contraindication to attempting surgical repair of an rAAA (grade B recommendation).

There is no preoperative parameter to indicate whether or not a patient with an rAAA will survive a surgical attempt to repair the rAAA. Many models have been developed to help predict mortality and survival. The Glasgow Aneurysm Score is equal to the age in years, plus 17 points for the presence of shock, plus 7 points for a prior myocardial infarction or ongoing angina, plus 10 points for any prior stroke or transient ischemic attack (TIA), plus 14 points for renal insufficiency [9]. A retrospective nationwide survey in Finland [10] found the Glasgow score predictive of mortality, with a score greater than 98 associated with an 80% postoperative mortality (Level IIIb evidence). The Hardman index is another such model and gives 1 point for age greater than 76 years, creatinine over 190 μmol/L, hemoglobin less than 9 g/dL, myocardial ischemia on ECG, and a history of loss of consciousness after arrival in hospital. The presence of 3 or more points was reported as uniformly fatal in one study [11, 12]. The Glasgow score and the Hardman index have been reported as poor predictors of survival in at least one retrospective study from Scotland [13]. On the other hand, the Harborview score has been shown to have good predictability. It is based on four criteria: Age over 76, creatinine over 2, serum pH under 7.2, and systolic blood pressure under 70 mmHg at any one time. Patients with all four criteria had a uniform 100% mortality [14]. Other than for this cluster of criteria, it appears that there are currently no scores to allow reliable prediction of mortality (grade B recommendation).

While preoperative predictors of survival may be poor, some formulas use postoperative data to predict short-term mortality. For instance, in patients alive 48 hours after surgery, the Sequential Organ Failure Assessment (SOFA) score is predictive of mortality. The SOFA score evaluates respiratory, coagulation, hepatic, cardiovascular, renal, and neurologic function, with a value from 0 to 4 [15]. In one retrospective study, a 48-hour SOFA score greater than 11 predicted mortality with 93% specificity (Level IIIb evidence).

> **RECOMMENDATION**
>
> Neither age nor any available formulas are accurate enough to allow mortality prediction.
>
> Grade of recommendation: B.

53.3 Do Delays in Reaching an Operating Room Affect Outcomes?

Controversy continues as to whether delays in reaching an operating room affect the ultimate mortality of patients with rAAA. Studies have been published with completely conflicting results [16–18]. However, all these studies are retrospective cohort studies (Level III evidence). Many, but not all, exclude

patients who do not survive until hospital arrival, thereby creating a clear selection bias. Given the overall risks and benefit ratios (grade B recommendation), it appears relatively intuitive to minimize any delays in accessing an operating room.

The question of delay in getting to surgery has become particularly relevant with the increasing use of endovascular repair (EVAR) for treating rAAA (see later). A CT scan of the abdomen and pelvis is usually needed to allow proper EVAR planning. With spiral CT units, the time required for an abdomen scan has diminished. In a study of time-to-death patients with rAAA not operated upon, 87.5% of patients admitted to the hospital with rAAA died more than 2 hours after admission [19], with most not being treated aggressively. Data from the British IMPROVE trial (see the following text) suggest that there is sufficient time for most patients to obtain a CT scan and that the resulting delay is minimal [20]. Therefore, it appears reasonable to consider a CT angiogram of the abdomen and pelvis in all except the most unstable patients (grade B recommendation).

The other reason why delays may be critical is the possible need to regionalize the care of patients with rAAAs. Increasing data show that high-volume surgeons in high-volume facilities with subspecialty training may produce better results for patients with rAAAs (Level IIb evidence) [21]. Other data suggest that large centers that can more rapidly mobilize ample resources may produce better outcomes for rAAA [22]. A recent 2021 meta-analysis of effects following rAAA repair found that high institutional volume may reduce perioperative mortality following surgery for rAAA. This perioperative survival advantage is more pronounced for open surgery than EVAR. Individual surgeon caseload was not found to have a significant impact on outcomes [23]. The transfer may be time-consuming, although data from both the British IMPROVE and Amsterdam trials [24] (see later) suggest that such transfers do not affect outcomes. However, a selection bias may be present because only more robust patients may survive a transfer.

> **RECOMMENDATION**
>
> The data are controversial. However, getting a CT scan is reasonable in most cases.
>
> Grade of recommendation: B.
>
> Regionalization of care for rAAA is gaining increasing momentum.
>
> Grade of recommendation: B.

53.4 Is Endovascular Repair Preferred in Patients with rAAA?

An rAAA is usually a fatal condition unless treated surgically. There are two primary choices of surgical intervention: Open repair and stent graft placement or EVAR. A decade ago, the EVAR1 trial compared open repair to EVAR in patients undergoing elective repair of a nonruptured AAA [25]. The group undergoing EVAR had lower early mortality and fewer complications. Given this finding and given that open repair for rAAA continued to have a high mortality rate, EVAR started getting applied to patients presenting with rAAA.

Numerous retrospective studies have suggested that EVAR for rAAA may be beneficial over open repair. The most significant retrospective single-institution review published was a study of 283 cases over 10 years at Albany Medical Center. It showed a decreased 30-day and 5-year mortality rate in patients treated with EVAR instead of open repair (24% vs. 44% at 30 days). They did note an increased reintervention rate for the EVAR patient group [26]. A Vascular Quality Initiative (VQI database)–based propensity-matched analysis of 4,929 cases showed a reduced 30-day mortality of 18% with EVAR instead of 32% with open and fewer complications and shorter length of stay [27]. All such studies suffer from an inherent selection bias in that more stable patients with less complicated anatomy may be selected for EVAR instead of open repair. VQI studies have also shown that the 5-year survival after EVAR for rAAA has improved over time, whereas the survival for open repair for rAAA has remained the same [28].

Two randomized prospective trials have tried to address the question of EVAR vs. open repair for rAAAs [3, 24]. The Amsterdam trial [24] randomized 116 patients with rAAA who had anatomy suitable for EVAR and open repair. EVAR used an aortouniiliac graft configuration with a crossover femoral-femoral bypass. All rAAA care in the Amsterdam area was centralized to three participating centers. Overall, 20% of patients presented with systolic pressures under 90 mmHg. The most significant reason for exclusion among the 520 potential patients was unsuitable anatomy for EVAR. The 30-day mortality rate was 21% in patients assigned to EVAR vs. 25% in those set to open repair (no difference; intention to treat). Crossover from EVAR to open repair was 14%. Hospital stay, intensive care unit (ICU) stay, and estimated blood loss was lower in patients assigned to EVAR. Mortality in the nonrandomized cohort treated was 30% lower than seen in other studies; the centralization of care and protocols may explain this. Interestingly, a subsequent analysis of the Dutch Surgical Aneurysm Audit published in 2020 found improved survival for rAAA in hospitals that followed an EVAR-first approach [29].

The British IMPROVE trial [3] had a different design in that it randomized patients with suspected rAAA to either an endovascular strategy (CT scan followed by EVAR if anatomically suitable) or an immediate open surgery (with CT scan optional). Six hundred and twenty-three patients were randomized out of 1,275 possible at 30 centers. One-half of the patients had a systolic blood pressure of less than 90 mmHg. Of the 316 patients randomized to an endovascular approach, 87% had ruptures confirmed, and 36% of those were not suitable for EVAR. EVAR was attempted in 154 patients and open repair in 112 cases in the endovascular strategy group. Of the 297 randomized to an open approach, 88% had a confirmed rupture, and open repair was attempted in 220. The 30-day mortality in patients with confirmed rAAA was the same in both groups (36.4% and 40.6%). In women, the endovascular strategy seemed beneficial for 30-day mortality (37% vs. 57%). ICU and hospital lengths of stay were shorter in the endovascular strategy group. However, the mortality was lower with

EVAR than with open repair (25% vs. 38%) when looking at the treatment received. Several points can be made from reviewing all these studies.

Note: Even with versatile devices and the use of aortomonoiliac configurations (with crossover femoral-femoral bypass), there is still a significant proportion of patients with rAAA who have anatomy not suitable for EVAR [30]. The ratio of ineligible patients is higher than seen in patients presenting for elective repair. Emergency EVAR is also likely to be more technically challenging and requires adjunctive techniques such as the placement of temporary aortic occlusion balloons.

The use of local anesthesia may be beneficial in patients undergoing EVAR for rAAA. The British IMPROVE trial showed that patients treated under local anesthesia had a fourfold survival advantage compared to those treated with EVAR under general anesthesia [20]. A recent meta-analysis found locoregional anesthesia for EVAR for rAAA associated with a lower 30-day mortality [31]. This may also explain the benefits reported by some on using a totally percutaneous approach to EVAR for rAAA (as opposed to femoral cutdown) [32].

We conclude that EVAR for rAAA is a viable therapeutic option when offered by an experienced surgeon in a center familiar with elective EVAR therapy and quick access to various stent graft sizes.

RECOMMENDATION

EVAR is an acceptable treatment method.

Grade of recommendation: A.

53.5 Should Anticoagulation Be Used Intraoperatively?

Heparin anticoagulation before aortic clamping is routinely done in elective AAA surgery. Patients with rAAA have already lost large volumes of blood and may be coagulopathic and hypothermic. It seems, therefore, reasonable in those cases to avoid full anticoagulation. There are no good studies on the subject, and only expert opinion is available (Level V evidence). The data from Albany [26] recommend avoidance of anticoagulation in EVAR for rAAA. The decision to use anticoagulants must be individualized.

In patients who develop coagulopathy intraoperatively, abdominal packing is an option. A retrospective series of 23 patients identified from a prospective surgical database (Level III evidence) had a 48% survival but a 22% incidence of early or late infectious complications [33]. Even vacuum-assisted closure and mesh-mediated fascial traction are still associated with a risk of infectious issues and fistulas [34]. Therefore, packing should be very selective (grade C recommendation).

Intraoperative hypothermia is correlated with increased mortality in a retrospective review of 100 consecutive patients treated for rAAA at one institution [35] (Level IIb evidence). Therefore, every effort should avoid hypothermia starting in the preoperative period (grade B recommendation). The room should be warmed, blankets used, and fluids and gas administered should be heated.

The final issue relates to the level of aortic clamping for cases done via an open approach. Again, no prospective or retrospective data on the subject have been published, and only expert opinion is available (Level V evidence). Infrarenal clamping appears desirable when possible, as it avoids renal and mesenteric ischemia. However, this is often not possible, as a large hematoma with a large rAAA may obscure the planes and mandate a supraceliac clamp.

RECOMMENDATION

No data are available regarding intraoperative anticoagulation, and a decision must be individualized. Hypothermia should be avoided.

Grade of recommendation: C.

53.6 Can Paraplegia Be Avoided?

Spinal cord ischemia can be caused by shock, massive atheroembolization, interruption of flow to the artery of Adamkiewicz, and interruption of flow to the hypogastric arteries. The incidence with open repair of rAAA is between 1% and 2% [36]. One retrospective review of 35 patients with rAAA treated with EVAR noted an 11.5% incidence [37]; a statistical association was noted with occlusion of one or more hypogastric arteries with the stent graft (Level III evidence). Other reports have not suggested as high an incidence. Prevention should focus on maintaining spinal cord perfusion pressure by maintaining blood pressure and avoiding collateral disruption. It seems prudent to maintain flow to at least one hypogastric artery during stent graft placement for rAAA (grade B recommendation). Cerebrospinal fluid drainage in elective settings is useful but not practical for emergencies. However, it can be placed postoperatively if symptoms develop and may result in the reversal of symptoms.

RECOMMENDATION

Paraplegia cannot always be avoided. Try to maintain flow to at least one hypogastric artery.

Grade of recommendation: B.

53.7 Should Sigmoidoscopy Be Performed Routinely in the Postoperative Period?

IC after repair of rAAA is a common occurrence. It may be related to hypotension, embolization, or flow interruption to the inferior mesenteric and hypogastric arteries. Earlier studies showed that endoscopically verified IC after open repair of rAAA may be present in as many as 42% of cases [38] (Level I evidence). More recent studies have shown a lesser incidence of 22%, and most cases are mild [39]. This is similar to the incidence reported after EVAR for rAAA [40]. Unfortunately, there are no predictive parameters, and even patients with transmural ischemia may fail to show early laboratory anomalies. Retrospective data suggest that early IC detection may be associated with improved survival (Level III evidence). Consequently, many surgeons advocate for routine flexible sigmoidoscopy 24 hours after surgery for rAAA (grade C recommendation).

RECOMMENDATION

IC is frequent enough that sigmoidoscopy should be performed with any clinical suspicion.

Grade of recommendation: C.

53.8 Should Patients Be Monitored for Abdominal Compartment Syndrome?

ACS can affect 4–12% of patients following open repair of rAAA. A recent meta-analysis found a 9% incidence of ACS after EVAR for rAAA with a 56% mortality rate (versus 19.8% in those without) [41]. In retrospective series, several risk factors for ACS have been identified, including coagulopathy, massive transfusion, and the need for an aortic occlusion balloon for hypotension [41] (Level IIb evidence). Early recognition of ACS via bladder pressure monitoring and aggressive management appears to decrease mortality and appears reasonable (grade B recommendation).

RECOMMENDATION

ACS is frequent enough that bladder monitoring should be performed.

Grade of recommendation: B.

TABLE 53.1

Clinical Questions

Question	Answer	Grade of Recommendation	References
What are the optimal resuscitation goals?	Low-grade hypotension is acceptable	C	[1, 2]
What are the preferred resuscitation fluids?	Blood products are preferred	B	[5, 6]
Should a CT scan be obtained in patients with suspected rAAA?	Yes, except in most extreme cases	B	[20]
Should care for rAAA be regionalized?	Yes	B	[23]
Should EVAR be used in patients with rAAA, if possible?	Yes	A B	[3, 24]
What can be done to avoid paraplegia and ischemic colitis?	Try to maintain flow to at least one hypogastric artery	B	[35]

TABLE 53.2

Levels of Evidence

Subject	Year	References	Level of Evidence	Strength of Recommendation	Findings
Choice of fluids for resuscitation	2010	[5, 6]	IIb	B	Early administration of blood products may be beneficial.
Imaging before treatment	2014	[20]	IIb	B	Spiral CT scanning is a reasonable test for most patients.
Regionalization of care	2021	[23]	II	B	If possible, do rAAA in high-volume institutions.
Repair technique	2013–2014	[3, 24]	I	A	EVAR is an acceptable alternative to open repair.
Ischemic colitis post–rAAA repair	2013	[37]	IIb	B	Ischemic colitis is frequent, and vigilance is required for early detection.

Editor's Note

Unfortunately, there is little high-quality data to answer the essential questions related to the management of ruptured abdominal aortic aneurysms (AAA). There is a paucity of information to guide our resuscitation and little to guide us on the need for imaging and how quickly to intervene surgically. There are no validated predictors of outcomes after ruptured AAA that could aid in individual patient management. Practitioners need guidance to help decide when the potential benefits of care in high-volume tertiary centers outweigh the risks incurred by the time delays inherent in transfers from outlying community programs. There is also little information to guide decisions regarding intraoperative anticoagulation in the setting of a ruptured AAA. While all clinicians aim to avoid paraplegia, the data in support of the various creative management schemes are weak. Monitoring for the development of abdominal compartment syndrome and ischemic colitis is easy and inexpensive and therefore appears prudent.

It is only in the comparison of open versus endovascular repair of ruptured AAA that we have substantial investigations upon which to base our opinions. In this subset of patients who have a ruptured aneurysm amenable to endovascular stenting and where the surgeon has the skill set to perform the procedure, these patients appear to have improved outcomes when compared to individuals undergoing open abdominal aortic aneurysm repair.

REFERENCES

1. Morrison CA, Carrick MM, Norman MA, et al. Hypotensive resuscitation strategy reduces transfusion requirements and severe postoperative coagulopathy in trauma patients with hemorrhagic shock: Preliminary results of a randomized controlled trial. *J Trauma Injury Infect Crit Care.* 2011;*70(3)*:652–663.
2. Dick F, Erdoes G, Opfermann P, et al. Delayed volume resuscitation during initial management of ruptured abdominal aortic aneurysm. *J Vasc Surg.* 2013;*57*:943–950.
3. Improve Trial Investigators. Endovascular or open repair strategy for ruptured abdominal aortic aneurysms: 30-day outcomes from IMPROVE randomized trial. *Br Med J.* 2014;*348*:7661.
4. Piffaretti G, Caronno R, Tozzi M, et al. Endovascular versus open repair of ruptured abdominal aortic aneurysms. *Expert Rev Cardiovasc Ther.* 2006;*4(6)*:839–852.
5. Johansson PI, Stensballe J, Rosenberg I, et al. Proactive administration of platelets and plasma for patients with a ruptured abdominal aortic aneurysm: Evaluating a change in transfusion practice. *Transfusion.* 2007;*47*:593–598.
6. Johansson PI. Goal-directed hemostatic resuscitation for massively being patients: The Copenhagen concept. *Transfusion Apheresis Sci.* 2010;*43*:401–405.
7. Phillips AR, Tran L, Foust JE, et al. Systematic review of plasma/packed red blood cell ratio on survival in ruptured abdominal aortic aneurysms. *J Vasc Surg.* 2021;*73(4)*: 1438–1444.
8. Chiesa R, Setacci C, Tshomba Y, et al. Ruptured abdominal aortic aneurysm in the elderly patient. *Acta Chir Belg.* 2006;*106*:508–516.
9. Samy AK, Murray G, MacBain G. Glasgow aneurysm score. *Cardiovasc Surg.* 1994;*2*:41–44.
10. Korhonen SJ, Ylonen K, Biancari F, et al. Glasgow aneurysm score as a predictor of immediate outcome after surgery for ruptured abdominal aortic aneurysm. *Br J Surg.* 2004;*91*:1449–1452.
11. Prance SE, Wilson YG, Cosgrove CM, et al. Ruptured abdominal aortic aneurysms: Selecting patients for surgery. *Eur J Vasc Endovasc Surg.* 1999;*17*:129–132.
12. Tambyraja AL, Fraser SCA, Murie JA, et al. Validity of the Glasgow aneurysm store and the Hardman Index in predicting outcome alter ruptured abdominal aortic aneurysm repair. *Br J Surg.* 2005;*92*:570–573.
13. Kniemayer HW, Kessler T, Reber PU, et al. Treatment of ruptured abdominal aortic aneurysm, a permanent challenge or a waste of resources? Prediction of outcome using a multi-organ-dysfunction score. *Eur J Vasc Endovasc Surg.* 2000;*19*:190–196.
14. Hemingway JF, French B, Caps M, et al. Preoperative risk score accuracy confirmed in a modern ruptured abdominal aortic aneurysm experience. *J Vasc Surg.* 2021;*74(5)*: 1508–1518.
15. Laukontaus SJ, Lepantalo M, Hynninen M, et al. Prediction of survival after 48 hours of intensive care following open surgical repair of ruptured abdominal aortic aneurysm. *Eur J Vasc Endovasc Surg.* 2005;*30*:509–515.

16. DeSouza VC, Strachan DP. Relationship between travel time to the nearest hospital and survival from ruptured abdominal aortic aneurysms: Record linkage study. *J Public Health*. 2005;*27(2)*:165–170.

17. Hames H, Forbes TL, Harris JR, et al. The effect of patient transfer on outcomes after rupture of an abdominal aortic aneurysm. *Can J Surg*. 2007;*50(1)*:43–47.

18. Salhab M, Farmer J, Osman I. Impact of delay on survival of patients with a ruptured abdominal aortic aneurysm. *Vascular*. 2006;*14(1)*:38–42.

19. Lloyd GM, Bown MJ, Norwood MGA et al. Feasibility of preoperative computer tomography in patients with ruptured abdominal aortic aneurysm: A time-to-death study in patients without operation. *J Vasc Surg*. 2004;*39*:788–791.

20. Powell JT and the Improve Trial Investigators. Observations from the IMPROVE trial concerning the clinical care of patients with ruptured abdominal aortic aneurysm. *Br J Surg*. 2014;*101(3)*:216–224.

21. Dueck AD, Kucey DS, Johnston KW, et al. Survival after ruptured abdominal aortic aneurysm: Effect of patient, surgeon and hospital factors. *J Vasc Surg*. 2004;*39*:1253–1260.

22. Utter GH, Maier RV, Rivara FP, et al. Outcomes after ruptured abdominal aortic aneurysms: The halo effect of trauma center designation. *J Am Coll Surg*. 2006;*203*:498–505.

23. Kontopodis N, Galanakis N, Akoumianakis E, et al. Systematic review and meta-analysis of the impact of institutional and surgeon procedure volume on outcomes after ruptured abdominal aortic aneurysm repair. *Eur J Vasc Endovasc Surg*. 2021 Sep;*62(3)*:388–398.

24. Reimerink JJ, Hoornweg LL, Vahl AC, et al. Endovascular repair versus open repair of ruptured abdominal aortic aneurysms: A multicenter randomized controlled trial. *Ann Surg*. 2013;*258(2)*:248–256.

25. EVAR Trial Participants. Endovascular aneurysm repair versus open repair in patients with abdominal aortic aneurysm (EVAR trial 1): Randomized controlled trial. *Lancet*. 2005;*365*:2187–2192.

26. Mehta M, Byrne J, Darling RC, et al. Endovascular repair of ruptured infrarenal abdominal aortic aneurysm is associated with lower 30-day mortality and better 5-year survival rates than open surgical repair. *J Vasc Surg*. 2013;*57*: 368–375.

27. Wang LJ, Locham S, Al-Nouri O, et al. Endovascular repair of ruptured abdominal aortic aneurysm is superior to open repair: Propensity-matched analysis in the vascular quality initiative. *J Vasc Surg*. 2020;*72(2)*:498–507.

28. Varkevisser RRB, Swerdlow NJ, De Guerre LEVM, et al. Five year survival following endovascular repair of ruptured abdominal aortic aneurysms is improving. *J Vasc Surg*. 2020;*72(1)*:105–113.

29. Karthaus EG, Lijftogy N, Vahl A, et al. Patients with a ruptured abdominal aortic aneurysm are better informed in hospitals with an EVAR -preferred strategy: An instrumental variable. Analysis of the Dutch surgical aneurysm audit. *Ann Vasc Surg*. 2020;69:332–344.

30. Hoornweg LL, Wisselink W, Vahl A, et al. The Amsterdam Acute Aneurysm trial: Suitability and application rate for endovascular repair of ruptured abdominal aortic aneurysms. *Eur J Vasc Endovasc Surg*. 2007;*33*:679–683.

31. Deng J, Liu J, Rong D, et al. A meta-analysis of locoregional anesthesia versus general anesthesia in endovascular repair of ruptured abdominal aortic aneurysm. *J Vasc Surg*. 2021;*73(2)*:700–710.

32. Lee YH, Su TW, Su IH, et al. Comparison between totally percutaneous approach and femoral artery cutdown in endovascular aortic repair or ruptured abdominal aortic aneurysms in a single hospital. *Ann Vasc Surg*. 2021;*74*:141–147.

33. Adam DJ, Fitridge RA, Raptis S. Intra-abdominal packing for uncontrollable hemorrhage during ruptured abdominal aortic aneurysm repair. *Eur J Vasc Endovasc Surg*. 2005;*30*:516–519.

34. Sorelius K, Wanhainen A, Acosta S, et al. Open abdomen treatment after aortic aneurysm repair with vacuum-assisted wound closure and mesh mediated fascial traction. *Eur J Vasc Endovasc Surg*. 2013;*45(6)*:588–594.

35. Janczyk RJ, Howells GA, Blar HA, et al. Hypothermia is an independent predictor of mortality in ruptured abdominal aortic aneurysms. *Vasc Endovasc Surg*. 2004;*38*:37–42.

36. Peppelenbosch AG, Vermulen Windsant IC, Jacobs MJ, et al. Open repair for ruptured abdominal aortic aneurysm and the risk of spinal cord ischemia: Review of the literature and risk factor analysis. *Eur J Vasc Endovasc Surg*. 2010;*40(5)*:589–595.

37. Peppelenbosch N, Cuypers PWM, Vahl AC, et al. Emergency endovascular treatment for ruptured abdominal aortic aneurysm and the risk of spinal cord ischemia. *J Vasc Surg*. 2005;*42*:608–614.

38. Champagne BJ, Darling RC, Daneshmand M, et al. Outcome of aggressive surveillance colonoscopy in ruptured abdominal aortic aneurysm. *J Vasc Surg*. 2004;*39*:792–796.

39. Tottrup M, Fedder AM, Jensen RH, et al. The value of routine flexible sigmoidoscopy within 48 hours after surgical repair of ruptured abdominal aortic aneurysms. *Ann Vasc Surg*. 2013;*27(6)*:714–718.

40. Champagne BJ, Lee EC, Valerian B, et al. Incidence of colonic ischemia after repair of the ruptured abdominal aortic aneurysm with endograft. *J Am Coll Surg*. 2007;*204*: 597–602.

41. Sa P, Oliveira-Pinto J, Mansilha A. Abdominal compartment syndrome after r-EVAR: A systematic review with meta-analysis on incidence and mortality. *Inter Angiol*. 2020;*39(5)*:411–421.

42. Chaikof EL, Dalman RL, Eskandari M, et al. The society for vascular surgery practice guidelines on the care of patients with an abdominal aortic aneurysm. *J Vasc Surg*. 2018;*67(1)*:2–77.

54

Venous Thromboembolism: Deep Venous Thrombosis and Pulmonary Embolism

Steven Satterly, Suresh K. Agarwal, and George C. Velmahos

54.1 Deep Venous Thrombosis

54.1.1 Introduction

Deep venous thrombosis (DVT) is a major health problem with an annual incidence of 0.5–1 per 1,000 [1]. The main short-term complication of DVT is pulmonary embolism (PE), while the long-term complication is postthrombotic syndrome [2]. Multiple evidence-based reviews of the diagnosis and treatment of DVT [3–5] and practice guidelines [6–8] have been published. This chapter reviews venous thromboembolism (VTE) and addresses the topics of DVT and PE treatment.

54.2 What Are the Optimal Preventative Strategies for DVT?

Heparin binds to antithrombin III, inhibiting a cascade of procoagulation factors. Low-molecular-weight heparin (LMWH) is a fractionated heparin with fewer pentasaccharide chains. LMWH is more expensive than heparin, although its advantages include once-daily dosing. Current recommendations are that major trauma patients receive either heparin or LMWH [9].

Direct thrombin inhibitors (DTIs) are the newest agents for prophylaxis. In contrast to other agents, they do not require a plasma cofactor; rather, they bind to thrombin and block its enzymatic activity. DTIs are utilized for therapeutic and prophylactic anticoagulation. Patients with heparin-induced thrombocytopenia use DTIs for prophylaxis. DTI use is becoming more common although still limited by the recent advent of expensive reversal agents.

Lower-extremity compression devices minimize the effect of immobilization and circulatory stasis. Mechanical prophylaxis is only recommended for patients who are at low risk for DVT or for those in whom pharmacologic prophylaxis is contraindicated (risk for bleeding, traumatic brain injury, etc.). Intermittent pneumatic compression (IPC) devices are the preferred mechanical prophylaxis devices [9].

There are several ongoing areas of research in DVT prophylaxis, and recommendations are often changing. There is evidence of decreased VTE rates when LMWH is titrated based on anti–factor Xa levels [10]. Clinical trials are underway to examine the utility of using thromboelastography [11] to guide prophylaxis regimens. Improved prophylaxis regimens may decrease VTE rates in high-risk patients; however, more studies are needed.

> **RECOMMENDATION**
>
> Current optimal prophylaxis is with LMWH (grade 1B) over no prophylaxis.
>
> Level of evidence: Ib. Grade of recommendation: A.
>
> Adding mechanical prophylaxis with elastic stockings or IPC to pharmacologic prophylaxis is suggested.
>
> Level of evidence: IIc. Grade of recommendation: B.

54.3 How Is DVT Diagnosed?

Duplex ultrasonography (US) is the most widely used method for diagnosing DVT and has the same sensitivity and specificity value of 98% [12]. The advantages of the US include the following: Rapid employment, cost-effectiveness, no radiation exposure, and noninvasive. The US uses hypersonic sound waves to identify flow and patency within a vein. Utilizing the basics of the compression technique, the US probe directly compresses the lumen of a vein if it is patent, and upon release subsequent flow can be seen. However, in the presence of a thrombus, a vein will not compress and there isn't subsequent flow on the inducing of compression. This is diagnostic for a DVT. The compression technique is not sensitive in diagnosing DVT below the knee [13]. The sensitivity of US is also lower in patients with asymptomatic DVA. Symptomatic patients have a higher distribution of DVT in the calf veins [14]. US screening has been effective in high-risk trauma patients [15]; however, controversy remains, and routine US screening is not currently recommended [16].

> **RECOMMENDATION**
>
> Duplex US for the diagnosis of DVT. Surveillance in high-risk patients is not currently recommended.
>
> Level of evidence: IIc. Grade of recommendation: B.

DOI: 10.1201/9781003316800-54

54.4 What Is the Best Initial Treatment for Venous Thromboembolism?

Traditionally, a newly diagnosed DVT was treated with intravenous unfractionated heparin (UFH) until a therapeutic level of oral anticoagulation was achieved with vitamin K antagonists (VKAs). However, frequent lab tests with the adjustment of the UFH dose are necessary due to variable clinical effects. On the other hand, the effects of LMWH are more predictable and do not require routine lab testing [17]. Multiple randomized controlled trials have been performed comparing the efficacy and safety of UFH versus LMWH and have been summarized in evidence-based reviews [3, 4, 7, 17, 18] and society-sponsored practice guidelines [6, 7].

A Cochrane review [18] performed an analysis of 22 randomized trials with a total of 8,867 patients. The primary outcome of recurrence of symptomatic VTE using the pooled data revealed a significant reduction using LMWH during the initial treatment (odds ratio [OR] 0.68; 95% confidence interval [CI] 0.48–0.97) and at the end of follow-up (OR 0.68; 95% CI 0.55–0.84) compared to UFH. Secondary outcomes of reduction in major hemorrhage during the initial treatment (OR 0.57; 95% CI 0.39–0.83) and lower overall mortality at the end of follow-up (OR 0.76; 95% CI 0.62–0.92) also favored the LMWH group.

LMWH has the advantage of providing predictable anticoagulation levels in patients using weight-adjusted dosing without laboratory monitoring in most patients. However, clinical situations such as renal failure or pregnancy may require dose adjustment using plasma anti–factor Xa levels [7]. Furthermore, LMWH use provides the convenience of once-daily administration.

Another Cochrane review [19] examined five studies with a total of 1,508 participants. The pooled data showed no significant difference in recurrent VTE between the two treatment regimens (OR 0.82; 95% CI 0.49–1.39; $p = 0.47$). A comparison of major hemorrhagic events (OR 0.77; 95% CI 0.40–1.45; $p = 0.41$), improvement of thrombus size (OR 1.41; 95% CI 0.66–3.01; $p = 0.38$), and mortality (OR 1.14; 95% CI 0.62–2.08; $p = 0.68$) also showed no significant differences between the two treatment regimens. The review concluded that once-daily treatment with LMWH is as effective and safe as twice-daily treatment with LMWH.

For DVT of the upper extremity, treatment is similar to DVT of the leg [20]. For DVT of the distal lower extremity, treatment with anticoagulants is only indicated if severely symptomatic [20].

RECOMMENDATION

LMWH is the preferred initial treatment for DVT compared to UFH in most patients.

Level of evidence: Ia. Grade of recommendation: A.

54.5 Is Home Therapy for Venous Thromboembolism Safe and Effective Compared to Inpatient Care?

Multiple trials have been performed comparing the safety of DVT treatment at home with LMWH with the safety of hospitalization and treatment with UFH or LMWH; these trials have been summarized in several evidence-based reviews [4, 7, 21, 22]. A Cochrane review [22] performed an analysis of six randomized trials containing 1,708 participants. VTE recurrence was significantly lower in the LMWH patients treated at home (relative risk [RR, fixed] 0.6; 95% CI 0.42–0.90) compared to hospitalized patients. In addition, patients treated at home exhibited lower mortality and fewer major bleeding complications but were more likely to have minor bleeding complications compared to patients treated in the hospital; however, these differences were not significant. Home therapy was also deemed to be cost-effective and preferred by patients.

These studies had multiple limitations, mostly with variability between home and inpatient therapy, such as using UFH in the hospital but LMWH for home treatment [4, 21, 22]. Furthermore, strict criteria for patients considered for home treatment were used and may affect the generalizability of the studies to patients seen in clinical practice [21, 22].

More recently, the viability of home therapy has been extended to PE in consensus studies [23]. Randomized trials, as well as other studies, have supported outpatient management of PE in selected patients and circumstances [24, 25].

RECOMMENDATION

Home therapy for DVT with LMWH is safe and cost-effective in carefully chosen patients. PE can be treated on an outpatient basis in select patients.

Level of evidence: Ib. Grade of recommendation: A.

54.6 What Is the Optimal Oral Starting Dose of Vitamin K Antagonist Therapy?

Vitamin K–dependent clotting factors have circulating half-lives ranging from 6 to 60 hours. Factor II has the longest circulating half-life of 60 hours. The full anticoagulant effect of a VKA such as warfarin may be delayed by a week or more. Furthermore, initiation of VKA therapy can result in a transient hypercoagulable state. While a VKA is reaching therapeutic levels, lower levels of anticoagulant protein C and protein S increase a prothrombotic state due to shorter half-lives. Thus, UFH or LMWH therapy is initiated and maintained for several days until oral VKA therapy is therapeutic, as measured by an international normalized ratio (INR) with values generally between 2 and 3 [26]. Achieving a therapeutic INR with warfarin as soon as possible is important because this minimizes the duration of parenteral medication necessary to attain immediate anticoagulation, and it potentially decreases the cost and inconvenience of treatment. Although a 5-mg loading-dose nomogram tends to prevent excessive anticoagulation, a 10-mg loading-dose nomogram may achieve a therapeutic INR more quickly.

Six prospective randomized trials [27–32] compared starting doses of 5 or 10 mg of warfarin therapy. These trials have been previously reviewed [7, 26, 33], and guidelines for the initial dosing of VKA have been published by several societies [7, 33, 34]. Two small trials randomized 49 patients [29] and 53 patients [28] to receive an initial dose of 5 or 10 mg of warfarin and measured the time necessary to attain therapeutic INR. Harrison et al. [29] determined that at 36 hours, significantly more patients were therapeutic in the 10-mg group (44% versus 8%, $p = 0.005$) compared to the 5-mg group. In contrast, Crowther et al. [28] determined that significantly more patients in the 5-mg group exhibited a therapeutic INR on days 1–5 of therapy (66% versus 24%, $p < 0.003$) compared to the 10-mg group. The 10-mg group in both studies exhibited an increased risk of excessive anticoagulation [28, 29], and there was a faster rate of decrease in protein C levels in the first 36 hours of treatment with the 10-mg group [29]. The authors speculated that the 5-mg warfarin dose may be less likely to induce a hypercoagulable state. Both studies recommended using a 5-mg dose for the initiation of warfarin therapy.

Kovacs et al. [27] randomized 210 patients to receive 5 or 10 mg initial doses of warfarin; the study was powered to detect a 0.5-day difference in the time necessary to reach a therapeutic INR. Patients receiving 10 mg of warfarin achieved a therapeutic INR 1.4 days faster than patients receiving 5 mg (4.2 ± 1.1 vs. 5.6 ± 1.4 days, $p < 0.001$) with no significant increase in excessive anticoagulation. However, this study excluded patients at high risk for bleeding.

A recent Cochrane review [33] involving four of these trials [27, 30–32] found that no difference was observed in recurrent VTE (RVTE) at 90 days when the warfarin nomogram of 10 mg was compared with the warfarin nomogram of 5 mg (RR 1.48; 95% CI 0.39–5.56). No difference was observed in major bleeding at 14 days (RR 1.69; 95% CI 0.22–13.04) and 90 days (RR 0.62; 95% CI 0.10–3.78). No difference was observed in minor bleeding at 14–90 days (RR 0.32; 95% CI 0.15–1.83) or in the length of hospital stay (mean difference 2.30 days; 95% CI 7.96–3.36).

54.7 What Is the Optimal Length of Oral VKA Treatment for DVT?

Currently, the most frequently used secondary treatment for patients with VTE consists of VKA targeted at an INR of 2.5 (range 2.0–3.0). However, the discussion on the proper duration of treatment with VKA for these patients is ongoing. The risk of bleeding and recurrent VTE is well established with VKA therapy. Multiple trials have evaluated the duration of therapy with VKA on VTE; these trials have been summarized in several evidence-based reviews [4, 7, 35, 36] and society-sponsored practice guidelines [6, 7]. A recent Cochrane review [36] performed an analysis of 11 randomized trials with a total of 3,716 patients. A consistent and strong reduction in the risk of recurrent VTE events was observed during prolonged treatment with VKA (RR 0.20; 95% CI 0.11–0.38) independent of the period elapsed since the index thrombotic event. A statistically significant "rebound" phenomenon (i.e., an excess of recurrences shortly after cessation of prolonged treatment) was not found (RR 1.28; 95% CI 0.97–1.70). In addition, a substantial increase in bleeding complications was observed for patients receiving prolonged treatment during the entire period after randomization (RR 2.60; 95% CI 1.51–4.49). No reduction in mortality was noted during the entire study period (RR 0.89; 95% CI 0.66–1.21, $p = 0.46$). Thus, the authors concluded that the efficacy of VKA therapy decreased over time and that the optimal duration of therapy would vary between different groups of patients, dependent on balancing risk/benefit profiles [36].

Segal et al. [4] identified 10 trials that included 4,240 patients that utilized objective radiologic documentation of VTE and used INR to monitor VKA therapy. The duration of VKA therapy was evaluated in multiple trials. Only one randomized blinded trial [37] compared 1 versus 3 months of therapy for DVT associated with a transient event, such as surgery. Treatment for 1 month resulted in increased rates of RVTE with similar bleeding complications compared to 3 months of therapy. The trial was stopped because of slow patient accrual and was only able to randomize 165 patients of the estimated 390 patients needed to provide conclusive results.

RECOMMENDATION

In patients with acute VTE (DVT or PE), considerable uncertainty surrounds the use of a 10-mg or a 5-mg loading dose for initiation of VKA. There is currently no consensus on the optimal starting dose of VKA. Clinicians should consider patient-specific factors for determining the optimal starting dose. Patients at low risk for bleeding may safely tolerate a 10-mg loading dose if appropriate nomograms are strictly followed.

Level of evidence: IIb. Grade of recommendation: B.

RECOMMENDATION

Extended therapy with VKA is warranted to prevent RVTE. The risks of bleeding versus recurrence of VTE for individual patients may alter the optimal duration of therapy.

Level of evidence: Ia. Grade of recommendation: A.

DVT associated with a transient event may be effectively treated with 3 months of VKA.

Level of evidence: IIb. Grade of recommendation: B.

54.8 Does Catheter-Directed Thrombolysis Decrease DVT Recurrences and Incidence of Postthrombotic Syndrome?

The goal of catheter-directed thrombolysis is to rapidly dissolve the thrombus, thereby reducing the incidence and severity of postthrombotic syndrome and potentially preserving venous valvular function. A recent Cochrane review evaluated catheter-directed thrombolysis and anticoagulation compared to anticoagulation alone for acute DVT [38]. It consisted of 17 studies with 1,103 participants. Complete lysis of a clot was more often achieved in those with catheter-directed thrombolysis in both early (up to 1 month) and intermediate (after 6 months) follow-ups (RR 4.91, 95% CI 1.66–14.53, and $p = 0.004$ and RR 2.37, 95% CI 1.48–3.80, and $p = 0.0004$, respectively). Similarly, postthrombotic syndrome occurred less in the catheter-directed thrombolysis group (RR 0.64; 95% CI 0.52–0.79, $p < 0.001$). However, catheter-directed thrombolysis was associated with significantly more bleeding complications than anticoagulation alone (RR 2.23, 95% CI 1.41–3.52, $p = 0.0006$). There was no significant difference in mortality at early or intermediate follow-ups. PE and recurrent DVT data were inconclusive.

A randomized controlled trial by Enden et al. evaluated 103 participants aged 18–75 years with iliofemoral DVT to assess if additional catheter-directed thrombolysis versus anticoagulation alone improved iliofemoral patency after 6 months [39]. Patency in the catheter-directed thrombolysis group was 64% compared to 35.8% in the anticoagulation group, equivalent to an absolute risk reduction of 28.2%, 95% CI 9.7–46.7, and $p = 0.004$. Venous obstruction was seen in 20.0% with catheter-directed thrombolysis compared to 49.1% (absolute risk reduction of 29.1%, 95% CI 20.0–38.0, and $p = 0.004$). There was no difference in femoral vein insufficiency. Enden et al. [40] performed another analysis using iliofemoral DVT treated with catheter-directed thrombolysis and anticoagulation versus anticoagulation alone. Of 189 participants assessed after 24-month follow-up, a significant increase in postthrombotic syndrome was observed in 41.1% of the catheter-directed thrombolysis group compared to 55.6% in the anticoagulation alone group ($p = 0.047$, which corresponded to an absolute risk reduction of 14.4%, 95% CI 0.2–27.9). Patency after 6 months was higher in the catheter-directed thrombolysis group (65.9% versus 47.4%, $p = 0.012$). However, 20 bleeding complications were noted in the catheter-directed thrombolysis group.

Strict eligibility criteria to reduce the risk of bleeding complications are needed, and these limit the general use of catheter-directed thrombolysis [38]. Other interventions that combine chemical lysis with mechanical or ultrasound energy clot removal have been reviewed [41]. There is a randomized trial that is ongoing with promising midterm results (TORPEDO trial) [42]. Thus far, the authors have shown that these percutaneous endovenous interventions combined with systemic anticoagulation are superior to anticoagulation alone regarding the reduction of VTE and postthrombotic syndrome. Care should be taken with thrombolysis in perioperative patients and those with recent bleeding episodes, particularly intracranial hemorrhage.

RECOMMENDATION

Catheter-directed venous thrombolysis results in significantly increased venous patency and decreased incidence of postthrombotic syndrome. The therapeutic benefit should be clinically weighed due to elevated bleeding complications.

Level of evidence: Ia. Grade of recommendation: A.

54.9 Do Compression Stockings Reduce the Long-Term Complication of Postthrombotic Syndrome?

Historical data support the use of compression stockings to reduce the incidence of postthrombotic syndrome. A Cochrane review in 2004 included three randomized controlled trials to evaluate the role of compression therapy versus no intervention [43]. At 2 years, compression therapy was associated with a significantly decreased incidence of postthrombotic syndrome (OR, 0.31, 95% CI 0.20–0.48). In severe postthrombotic syndrome, the OR was 0.39 (95% CI 0.20–0.76). There was also a reduction in swelling, pain, and clinical scores observed in those undergoing compression therapy ($p < 0.05$), with no serious adverse events.

A subsequent meta-analysis expanded on these results [44] by including five randomized controlled trials. There was a reduction in the incidence of postthrombotic syndrome. Overall, compression therapy was associated with a postthrombotic syndrome incidence of 26% compared to 46% in the control group (RR 0.54). Mild-to-moderate postthrombotic syndrome occurred in 22% of the compression stocking group versus 37% in the control group (RR 0.52). When evaluating severe postthrombotic syndrome, the incidence was 5% with compression therapy, while it was 12% without compression therapy (RR 0.38).

However, there has been a recent paradigm shift. Kahn et al. [45] performed the first multicenter, randomized, placebo-controlled trial assessing compression stockings (30–40 mm Hg) compared to placebo (<5 mm Hg at the ankle) for 2 years. Stockings were initiated within 2 weeks of DVT diagnosis and were replaced every 6 months or sooner if they were torn or leg size changed. With 806 participants, this is the largest trial to date. The authors found that the incidence of postthrombotic syndrome was not significantly different between treatment and control groups (14.2% versus 12.7%, respectively, with a center-adjusted hazard ratio of 1.13, 95% CI 0.73–1.76, and $p = 0.58$). There was no difference in rates of RVTE, ipsilateral DVT, ipsilateral venous valvular reflux at 12 months, or death. There were also similar generic and disease-specific quality-of-life scores between the two groups. No differences were observed on subgroup analyses by age, body mass index, or extent of DVT, though sex showed a marginal benefit for women ($p = 0.047$). There were no serious adverse events.

RECOMMENDATION

Routine use of compression stockings to reduce post-thrombotic syndrome is not supported.

Level of evidence: Ib.

54.10 Pulmonary Embolism

54.10.1 Introduction

PE is a national health problem, claiming over 50,000 lives in the United States. It has been found in 32% of surgical patients who had an autopsy, and in about half of these cases, PE was thought to be the causing or contributing factor for death [46]. Although the sample of patients in that study was not representative of the entire surgical population and was subject to variable thromboprophylaxis practices, the high figures indicate the importance of the problem. Currently, the PE rates are estimated to be overall lower but vary significantly (0.3–30%) due to the inconsistent screening and diagnosis among centers. The exact percentage of fatal PE is unknown for the same reasons.

The pathogenesis of PE is based on the theory of clot dislodgment from a lower extremity or pelvic DVT. Neck and upper extremity veins contribute on occasion. However, there is a consistent disconnect in the literature between DVT and PE. Although one would expect that a lower extremity or pelvic DVT would be found in patients with PE, this is only infrequently the case. In the past, this discrepancy was explained by the inaccuracy of available diagnostic methods to detect DVT, particularly of pelvic origin. With the development of CT venography and high-definition ultrasonography, this is no longer the case. These tests evaluate accurately the pelvic and proximal extremity veins and frequently fail to discover DVT associated with an existing PE. Therefore, the original theory of PE pathogenesis may be incorrect. It is possible that PE does not always originate from peripheral veins but may be formed de novo in the pulmonary circulation [47]. There are more unknowns than standards in PE. The optimal diagnosis, prevention, and treatment are under constant debate.

54.11 Risk Factors

54.11.1 Who Is at Risk for PE?

The classic Virchow's triad places the surgical patient at risk for PE, but the exact level of risk that allows intelligent risk-to-benefit calculations and decisions about the administration of potentially harmful thromboprophylaxis is unknown. Multiple risk factors have been suggested: Obesity, immobility, cancer, major abdominal or pelvic operations, trauma, oral contraceptives, increasing age, previous thromboembolism, pregnancy and the postpartum period, smoking, coagulation abnormalities, and acute medical illness, including heart, renal, and respiratory failure. There is poor evidence documenting the impact of each one of these risk factors on the pathogenesis of PE, and contradictory studies are common. For example, it is unknown which exact level of obesity, exact duration and level of immobility, exact age, type and stage of cancer, or severity of medical illness predisposes the patient to PE. A systematic review and meta-analysis of the existing literature among trauma patients underscore precisely this inconsistency [48]. Although gender, head injuries, spinal fractures, spinal cord injuries, long-bone fractures, and pelvic fractures were examined as possible risk factors among studies of trauma patients, only spinal fractures and spinal cord injuries were found in pooled analysis to affect the incidence of venous thromboembolism (Level IIb evidence). The study also found that the likelihood of VTE increases with older age and a higher Injury Severity Score, and the threshold at which the rate of the outcome increases significantly could not be determined by the available literature.

The seventh American College of Chest Physicians (ACCP) conference created a stratification of risk according to the presence of risk factors [49]. This stratification makes clinical sense but is based on variable levels of evidence (typically Level III) and therefore should be considered with caution. Patients younger than 40 years, with no other risk factors, and minor surgery are at low risk for PE. Patients at moderate risk have only one of the following: Age 40–60 years, major surgery, or a major preexisting risk factor. Patients at high risk are those who are either older than 60 years or older than 40 years but with major surgery and a major preexisting risk factor present. At the highest risk are patients who are older than 40 years of age and have major surgery *and* one of the following: Previous thromboembolic event, cancer, or hypercoagulable condition; major trauma; spinal injury; hip/knee arthroplasty; and hip surgery. Major surgery was considered a thoracic or abdominal operation under general anesthesia lasting over 30 minutes. Multiple preexisting risk factors have been examined with variable degrees of certainty about their effect on PE, including obesity, prior episodes of thromboembolism, oral contraceptive use, and cancer, among others. The authors' calculated risk is 2–4% for PE and 0.4–1% for fatal PE in patients at high risk and 4–10% for PE and 0.5–5% for fatal PE in patients at the highest risk.

RECOMMENDATION

There is inconsistent evidence about the exact risk factors that predispose to PE. It seems that major trauma—and particularly spinal injuries—older age, major surgery, previous history of thromboembolism, and cancer increase the risk of PE. The effect of other factors, such as immobility, obesity, and medical illness, is ill-defined.

Grade of recommendation: B.

54.12 Diagnosis

54.12.1 What Is the Optimal Diagnostic Test for PE?

The ventilation-perfusion (V-P) scan and pulmonary angiography (PA) have been the main tests for the diagnosis of PE for more than 20 years. The prospective investigation of a PE diagnosis study [50] showed that a V-P scan is 96% sensitive when the index of clinical suspicion is high. However, 75% of the patients belong to the intermediate category in which the V-P scan is less sensitive. PA may remain the standard of reference but is invasive and requires significant time spent in the angiography suite, a major setback for critically ill patients.

Over the past 10 years, computed tomographic pulmonary angiography (CTPA) has evolved to become the preferred diagnostic method for PE in surgical patients. In a meta-analysis of the diagnostic performance of CTPA and V-P scan, Hayashino et al. [51] examined 12 studies from 1985 to 2003, which were selected according to the following three criteria: The tests were performed for the diagnosis of acute PE; PA was used as the standard of reference; and absolute numbers of true-positive, true-negative, false-positive, and false-negative findings were given. Based on these studies, a random effects model found CTPA to have 86% sensitivity (95% CI: 80.2%, 92.1%) and 93.7% specificity (95% CI: 91.1%, 96.3%). V-P scan was found to have low sensitivity (39%) and high specificity (97.1%) with a high probability threshold but high sensitivity (98.3%) and low specificity (4.8%) with the normal threshold. The authors concluded that although V-P scan and CTPA have similar diagnostic ability for patients with a high probability of PE, CTPA has higher discriminatory power than V-P scan for patients with normal and near-normal probability (Level Ib evidence).

In another systematic review of the literature, Quiroz et al. [52] examined the clinical validity of a negative CTPA for suspected PE. Of particular concern was the alleged low sensitivity of CTPA for peripheral PE. To calculate the overall negative likelihood ratio of PE after a negative or inconclusive CTPA, the authors included PE, which was confirmed by another diagnostic test within 3 months of CTPA. Fifteen studies with a total population of 3,500 patients were included from 1994 to 2002. Single-slice, multidetector, and electron-beam scanners were used in the different studies. The negative predictive value of a normal CTPA was 99.7% (95% CI: 98.7%, 99.5%), and the negative likelihood ratio of a PE after a normal CTPA was 0.7 (95% CI: 0.05, 011). There was no difference in the risk of PE based on the different types of computed tomographic scanners. The authors concluded that the clinical validity of CTPA to rule out PE is similar to that reported for conventional PA (Level Ib evidence). This study shows that even if the diagnosis of peripheral PE is the principal limitation of CTPA, undiagnosed peripheral PE (which can exist in as many as 30% of "normal" CTPAs) is usually not clinically significant and does not cause subsequent clinically detectable PE or death from PE.

Finally, a meta-analysis of different diagnostic strategies for PE by Roy et al. [53] included 48 of the 1,012 articles examined from 1990 to 2003. The study attempted to determine the clinical application of each test according to the pretest clinical probability. Patients with a high pretest probability, a high-probability V-P scan, a positive CTPA, and a positive lower extremity venous ultrasound were associated with a higher than 85% posttest probability of PE. Patients with an intermediate or low pretest probability, a normal or near-normal V-P scan, a normal CTPA in combination with normal lower extremity venous ultrasound, and a D-dimer concentration of less than 500 µg/L measured by quantitative enzyme-linked immunosorbent assay were associated with a less than 5% posttest probability of PE. CTPA, magnetic resonance angiography, a low-probability V-P scan, and a quantitative latex or hemagglutination D-dimer test could only exclude PE in patients with low pretest probability. The authors concluded that the accuracy of the different tests varies significantly according to the pretest clinical probability for PE (Level II evidence). At this time, CTPA is established as the optimal test for PE diagnosis. Using a prediction algorithm to limit CTPA to those patients with a reasonable degree of probability in the diagnosis is claimed to make CTPA cost-effective too.

RECOMMENDATION

CTPA is convenient, safe, and accurate for the diagnosis of clinically significant PE. It is the preferred diagnostic method for most emergency surgery and trauma patients.

Grade of recommendation: A.

54.13 Prevention

54.13.1 Are Heparin and Compression Devices Adequate for PE Prophylaxis?

The use of low-dose UFH, usually administered subcutaneously, for the prevention of PE was established in the mid-1970s by the seminal study of Kakkar et al. [54]. That study included only elective surgery patients; emergency surgery and trauma patients were excluded. Despite this fact, thromboprophylaxis by UFH became common practice for all surgical patients. An overview of randomized trials of general, orthopedic, and urologic surgery patients concluded that UFH reduced symptomatic PE rates from 2% to 1.3% and fatal PE rates from 0.8% to 0.3%, but the risk of perioperative bleeding increased from 3.8% to 5.9% [55]. However, the evidence about UFH in trauma is controversial, and the evidence about UFH in emergency nontraumatic general surgery patients simply does not exist. LMWH, also administered subcutaneously, has shown increased stability and bioavailability compared to UFH, with benefits possibly associated with improved effectiveness and safety. There are multiple randomized studies and meta-analyses in general surgery patients documenting equivalence or superiority of LMWH over UFH [56, 57], but again, this evidence is only modestly applicable to the emergency surgery population because the majority of included patients had elective operations.

Sequential compression devices (SCDs) have been used extensively based on the assumption that they promote blood flow, stimulate muscle function, and trigger the release of fibrinolytic agents from the vascular endothelium. The evidence of their effectiveness is also questionable, and at least two studies document poor compliance [58, 59]. This could be the ultimate drawback of their use, as it gives the physician a false sense of security, while the patient receives no benefit from the prescribed treatment.

There are several noncontrolled studies and a few prospective randomized trials in trauma patients. Knudson et al. [60] produced three randomized trials (Level Ic evidence). In 1992, the authors randomized 113 trauma patients to UFH or SCD and found no significant difference in thromboembolic complications (5 patients with DVT, 4 with PE, and 3 with DVT and PE) between the two groups. In 1994, the authors compared patients receiving UFH, SCD, or no treatment and found similar DVT rates in the three groups, except for a mild advantage of SCD over no treatment in neurosurgical patients [61]. There were only two documented PEs, one in an SCD patient and one in a patient who received no thromboprophylaxis. In 1996, they randomized 181 patients to LMWH or SCD and failed to find any significant difference in DVT [62]. There were no documented cases of PE in any of the randomized groups.

In a study of LMWH against SCD in head and spinal trauma, 60 patients were randomized to LMWH and 60 to SCD [63]. The incidence of PE was not different between the two groups, with 7% in the LMWH group and 3% in the SCD group. This high incidence of PE could indicate a poor thromboprophylaxis effect of LWMH and SCD (Level Ic evidence). In another randomized study, spinal cord injury patients received either UFH with SCD or LMWH and showed no difference in proximal DVT or PE rates [64]. The total number of thromboembolic events was very high and almost identical in the two groups (65.5% for LMWH and 63.3% for UFH with SCD, $p = 0.81$), placing again in doubt the effectiveness of these regimens (Level Ic evidence).

The likely two best-designed randomized trials in trauma patients examined LMWH vs. SCD [65] or LMWH vs. UFH [66]. In both, DVT and not PE (or total thromboembolic events) was the principal outcome. In the study by Ginzburg et al. [65], the DVT rates were similar between LMWH and SCD. There was one PE in each group. There was no difference in thromboembolic events when a subanalysis of patients with an Injury Severity Score higher than 19 was undertaken. The rate of bleeding was not different either (Level Ib evidence). In the study by Geerts et al. [66], LMWH was associated with lower DVT rates compared to UFH. There was only one patient with documented PE (a high-probability V-P scan), and he belonged to the LMWH group. The rate of major bleeding was not different (0.6% vs. 2.9%, $p = 0.12$), but of the six documented episodes, one was in the UFH group and five in the LMWH group (Level Ib evidence). Two systematic reviews of the existing evidence in trauma confirmed the low level of evidence that exists about UFH, SCD, and LMWH and the uncertainty about their exact profile of effectiveness and safety [67, 68] (Level Ib evidence).

> ### RECOMMENDATION
>
> Although general surgery patients with elective operations seem to benefit from the current thromboprophylaxis methods, the effectiveness of UFH, LMWH, and SCD in emergency surgery and trauma patients remains uncertain. An individual risk-to-benefit assessment should be made for each such patient at risk of PE. LMWH is probably more effective than UFH or SCD.
>
> Grade of recommendation: B.

54.13.2 Are PE and Mortality from PE Reduced by IVC Filters?

The effectiveness of inferior vena cava (IVC) filters relies on their ability to capture clots originating from the lower extremity or pelvic veins. Three scenarios may hamper this ability. First, a misplaced or tilted filter may not function adequately. A tilt of as little as 10 degrees in relationship with the IVC axis has been reported to compromise optimal function [69]. Second, the capture of a primary clot at the apex of the filter may force blood circulation toward the periphery of the vessel and recurrent clots to escape in this way. Third, clots may originate from the upper extremity or neck veins [70] or, even possibly, form de novo in the pulmonary circulation [47], in which case, a device in the IVC is obviously of no use. One can argue that a filter is never used therapeutically, as its effect never involves a PE that has already occurred but only the embolus that may follow. The use of IVC filters in patients with "breakthrough" PE (occurring while the patient is fully anticoagulated) or with primary PE and inability to anticoagulate is well-accepted. Other criteria are more controversial and include a contraindication for prophylactic anticoagulation in the presence of high risk for PE. This controversy exists with added prophylaxis in patients at very high risk for PE even if prophylactic anticoagulation is feasible. Further debate exists about added prophylaxis in patients who have already sustained a significant PE and are therapeutically anticoagulated but would be at risk of death if a breakthrough PE occurred [71] (Level IIIb evidence).

Currently, retrievable filters have replaced temporary filters for most indications. Unless it is deemed that a filter needs to remain in place for life, as may happen with spinal cord injury patients or very old patients with significant comorbidities, most trauma and emergency surgery patients have only a finite period of risk and therefore do not need a permanent device. Unfortunately, a multicenter study [72] has shown that only 19% of these filters are being removed, and therefore, most are left permanently, even if not designed for this purpose (Level IIIa evidence).

There is not a single prospective randomized study on the use of IVC filters in trauma and emergency surgery patients. Decousous et al. [73] randomized a mixed population of 200 predominantly medical patients with DVT into an IVC filter versus no filter. After a 2-year follow-up, those with filters had a significant decrease in PE but a significant increase in DVT. There was no difference in mortality. When this population was followed up for 8 years [74], the results remained unchanged: The IVC filter group had a lower incidence of PE (6.2% vs. 15.1%, *p* = 0.008), higher incidence of DVT (35.7% vs. 27.5%, *p* = 0.042), and no difference in mortality compared to the no filter group (Level Ib evidence). Studies of trauma patients have failed to consistently prove that the insertion of IVC filters resulted in a decrease in PE or death from PE [75–77] (Level IIIb evidence).

IVC filters are not complication free. Morbidity related to access (bleeding, thrombosis, arterial damage), catheter advancement (vessel damage), contrast material (anaphylaxis, renal failure), and the filter itself (vessel wall perforation, migration, IVC thrombosis, DVT, misplacement) are detected in approximately 4–7% of the cases, although the variability in rates among studies is great [71] (Level IIIa evidence). A new class of complications is now related to the removal of retrievable filters, including all of the aforementioned problems as well as dislodgement of the clot captured by the filter, damage of the IVC wall, and inability to retrieve.

Most importantly, the theory of "de novo" formation of clots in the pulmonary circulation, which contradicts the traditional theory of clot embolization from the deep venous system of the extremities, may in large part defy the logic behind IVC filter use. If clots form directly into the pulmonary arteries and do not travel from the legs, then the placement of an IVC filter to interrupt the course of such travel is obsolete. In an elegant study of 99 patients with proven PE, Van Langevelde et al. [78] performed total-body magnetic resonance imaging to identify venous clots. No thrombus was found in 55 patients, and of the 44 patients who had venous thrombi, 12 had isolated calf thrombosis and 5 had isolated superficial vein thrombosis. In the end, only 44% were presumed to have a peripheral venous origin of PE, and only slightly over 27% had it at the major deep venous system. In other words, an IVC filter could be unable to prevent PE in more than half of the patients.

54.14 Treatment

54.14.1 Is LMWH as Safe and Effective as UFH for the Treatment of PE?

Dose-adjusted intravenous UFH is used for the treatment of PE. However, subcutaneous LMWH at therapeutic doses presents significant benefits over UFH, as monitoring is not required and treatment can be self-administered at home. There are multiple randomized studies in the literature, and all of them include either exclusively or predominantly medical patients. Therefore, the evidence on emergency surgery and trauma patients is poor. A meta-analysis of 12 randomized studies [79] found that LMWH was associated with a nonsignificant decrease in symptomatic PE (1.7% vs. 2.3%) and asymptomatic PE (1.2% vs. 3.2%), while offering a nonsignificant advantage in decreasing bleeding (1.3% vs. 2.1%), compared to UFH (Level Ia evidence). The authors concluded that LMWH was at least as safe and effective as UFH for the initial treatment of PE. It is expected that in emergency surgery and trauma patients, the rates of the aforementioned outcomes—and specifically of bleeding—may be different, but there is little reason to believe that the equivalence between the two groups will not be maintained. However, concerns about the inability to reverse LMWH effectively by protamine if a high-risk patient were to bleed may still create discomfort in consistently using LMWH over UFH. In the ninth edition of the ACCP guidelines, LMWH is recommended over UFH for the acute management of PE, and if LMWH is to be given, a one-dose daily regimen is preferred over the two doses. Patient convenience and cost-effectiveness have been considered in these recommendations. In the same document, it is also recommended to start coumadin early, when possible, with a target INR of 2.0–3.0, before discontinuing parenteral anticoagulation [80].

RECOMMENDATION

There is no convincing evidence that in emergency surgery and trauma patients, IVC filters reduce the incidence of PE and mortality from PE. The use of IVC filters should be made based on an individual patient-by-patient risk-to-benefit analysis.

Grade of recommendation: C.

RECOMMENDATION

LMWH is as safe and effective as UFH for the treatment of PE. It may be the preferred treatment in patients at lower risk of bleeding based on the convenience of outpatient self-administration, and there is no need for monitoring

Grade of recommendation: A (Table 54.1).

TABLE 54.1

Summary of Clinical Questions and Evidence-Based Answers

Question	Answer	Grade	References
1. What are the optimal preventative strategies for DVT?	LMWH is optimal prophylaxis. LMWH is superior to UFH when able. UFH is superior to SCD. All are superior to nothing.	A	[9, 60–62, 65, 66]
2. Is LMWH as safe and effective as UFH for the treatment of PE?	Yes	A	[78]
3. How is DVT diagnosed?	Duplex US for diagnosis, yet surveillance in high-risk patients is not currently recommended.	B	[12]
4. What is the best initial treatment for VTE?	LMWH is the preferred initial treatment for DVT compared to unfractionated heparin in most patients.	A	[3, 4, 6, 7, 17–20]

(Continued)

TABLE 54.1 (Continued)

Summary of Clinical Questions and Evidence-Based Answers

Question	Answer	Grade	References
5. Is home therapy for VTE safe and effective compared to inpatient care?	Home therapy for DVT with LMWH is safe and cost-effective in carefully chosen patients.	A	[4, 7, 21, 22]
6. What is the optimal oral starting dose of VKA?	There is no consensus on the optimal starting dose of warfarin. Clinicians should consider patient-specific factors for determining a warfarin dose. Patients at low risk for bleeding may safely tolerate a 10-mg loading dose.	B	[7, 33, 34]
7. What is the optimal length of oral VKA treatment for DVT?	Extended therapy with VKA is warranted to prevent RVTE. Risks of bleeding versus recurrence of VTE for individual patients may alter the optimal duration of therapy.	A	[4, 6, 7, 35, 36]
	DVT associated with a transient event may be effectively treated with 3 months of VKA.	B	[4, 37]
8. Does catheter-directed thrombolysis decrease DVT recurrences and incidence of postthrombotic syndrome?	While catheter-directed thrombolysis results in increased venous patency and decreased incidence of postthrombotic syndrome, bleeding complications limit the routine use of this technology.	A	[38–40]
9. Do compression stockings reduce the long-term complication of postthrombotic syndrome?	Graded compression stockings do not reduce the incidence of postthrombotic syndrome.	A	[43–45]
10. Who is at risk for PE?	Patients with spinal injuries, older age, major surgery or trauma, previous history of thromboembolism, and cancer.	B	[48, 49]
11. What is the optimal diagnostic test for PE?	CTPA	A	[51–53]
12. Are heparin and compression devices adequate for PE prophylaxis?	The effectiveness of heparin and compression devices in trauma and emergency surgery patients is unclear. LMWH seems to perform better than UFH.	B	[56–68]
13. Are PE and mortality from PE reduced by IVC filters?	The effectiveness of IVC filters in reducing PE and mortality from PE in trauma and emergency surgery patients is unclear.	C	[73–77]

Abbreviations: CTPA: Computed tomographic pulmonary angiography, DVT: Deep venous thrombosis, IVC: Inferior vena cava, LMWH: Low-molecular-weight heparin, PE: Pulmonary embolism, RVTE: Recurrent venous thromboembolism, SCD: Sequential compression device, UFH: Unfractionated heparin, US: Ultrasound, VKA: Vitamin K antagonist, VTE: Venous thromboembolism.

Editor's Note

Unlike multiple topics in this book, venous thrombosis has been extensively studied and there are facets of care that have high-quality evidence to support our management. There are, however, numerous topics in the field that remain controversial. For example, the timing of the administration of venous thromboprophylaxis after major surgery or trauma is unknown. This is a particular issue in the setting of closed head trauma or brain surgery. Also, it is unclear when to stop full anticoagulation prior to major surgery. Accumulating data have shown that IVC filters are associated with postthrombotic syndrome and fail to alter fatal outcomes, which should diminish their use. Of course, in surgery we always have an ongoing conflict between the risk of thrombosis and the potential for bleeding.

REFERENCES

1. Fowkes FJ, Price JF, Fowkes FG. Incidence of diagnosed deep vein thrombosis in the general population: Systematic review. *Eur J Vasc Endovasc Surg.* 2003;*25(1)*:1–5.

2. Brandjes DP, Buller HR, Heijboer H, et al. Randomised trial of effect of compression stockings in patients with symptomatic proximal-vein thrombosis. *Lancet.* 1997; *349(9054)*:759–762.

3. Segal JB, Eng J, Jenckes MW, Tamariz LJ, Bolger DT, Krishnan JA, Streiff MB, Harris KA, Feuerstein CJ, Bass EB. Diagnosis and treatment of deep venous thrombosis and pulmonary embolism. *Evid Rep Technol Assess (Summ).* 2003 Jan:*(68)*:1–6.

4. Segal JB, Streiff MB, Hofmann LV, Thornton K, Bass EB. Management of venous thromboembolism: A systematic review for a practice guideline. *Ann Intern Med.* 2007;*146(3)*:211–222.

5. Segal JB, Eng J, Tamariz LJ, Bass EB. Review of the evidence on diagnosis of deep venous thrombosis and pulmonary embolism. *Ann Fam Med.* 2007;*5(1)*:63–73.

6. Snow V, Qaseem A, Barry P, et al. Management of venous thromboembolism: A clinical practice guideline from the American College of Physicians and the American Academy of Family Physicians. *Ann Intern Med.* 2007;*146(3)*:204–210.

7. Buller HR, Agnelli G, Hull RD, Hyers TM, Prins MH, Raskob GE. Antithrombotic therapy for venous thromboembolic disease: The seventh ACCP conference on antithrombotic and thrombolytic therapy. *Chest.* 2004;*126(3 Suppl)*:401S–428S.

8. Qaseem A, Snow V, Barry P, et al. Current diagnosis of venous thromboembolism in primary care: A clinical practice guideline from the American Academy of Family Physicians and the American College of Physicians. *Ann Intern Med.* 2007;*146(6)*:454–458.

9. Gould MK, Garcia DA, Wren SM, et al. Prevention of VTE in nonorthopedic surgical patients: Antithrombotic Therapy and Prevention of Thrombosis, 9th ed: American College of Chest Physicians Evidence-Based Clinical Practice Guidelines. *Chest.* 2012;*141(2 Suppl)*:e227S–e277S.

10. Lin H, Faraklas I, Saffle J, Cochran A. Enoxaparin dose adjustment is associated with low incidence of venous thromboembolic events in acute burn patients. *J Trauma.* 2011;*71(6)*:1557–1561.

11. Harrington RA, Becker RC, Cannon CP, et al. Antithrombotic therapy for non-ST-segment elevation acute coronary syndromes: American College of Chest Physicians Evidence-Based Clinical Practice Guidelines, 8th ed. *Chest.* 2008;*133(6 Suppl)*:670S–707S.

12. Kearon C, Julian JA, Newman TE, Ginsberg JS. Noninvasive diagnosis of deep venous thrombosis. McMaster diagnostic imaging practice guidelines initiative. *Ann Intern Med.* 1998;*128(8)*:663–677.

13. Wicky J, Bongard O, Peter R, Simonovska S, Bounameaux H. Screening for proximal deep venous thrombosis using B-mode venous ultrasonography following major hip surgery: Implications for clinical management. *VASA Zeitschrift fur Gefasskrankheiten.* 1994;*23(4)*:330–336.

14. Kearon C. Noninvasive diagnosis of deep vein thrombosis in postoperative patients. *Semin Thromb Hemost.* 2001;*27(1)*:3–8.

15. Thorson CM, Ryan ML, Van Haren RM, et al. Venous thromboembolism after trauma: A never event? *Crit Care Med.* 2012;*40(11)*:2967–2973.

16. Bates SM, Jaeschke R, Stevens SM, et al. Diagnosis of DVT Antithrombotic Therapy and Prevention of Thrombosis, 9th ed: American College of Chest Physicians Evidence-Based Clinical Practice Guidelines. *Chest.* 2012; *141(2)*:E351s–E418s.

17. Krishnan JA, Segal JB, Streiff MB, et al. Treatment of venous thromboembolism with low-molecular-weight heparin: A synthesis of the evidence published in systematic literature reviews. *Respir Med.* 2004;*98(5)*:376–386.

18. van Dongen CJ, van den Belt AG, Prins MH, Lensing AW. Fixed dose subcutaneous low molecular weight heparins versus adjusted dose unfractionated heparin for venous thromboembolism. *Cochrane Database Syst Rev.* 2004 Oct 18;*(4)*:CD001100.

19. Bhutia S, Wong PF. Once versus twice daily low molecular weight heparin for the initial treatment of venous thromboembolism. *Cochrane Database Syst Rev.* 2013;*7*:CD003074.

20. Kearon C, Akl EA, Comerota AJ, et al. Antithrombotic therapy for VTE disease: Antithrombotic Therapy and Prevention of Thrombosis, 9th ed: American College of Chest Physicians Evidence-Based Clinical Practice Guidelines. *Chest.* 2012;*141(2 Suppl)*:e419S–e494S.

21. Segal JB, Bolger DT, Jenckes MW, et al. Outpatient therapy with low molecular weight heparin for the treatment of venous thromboembolism: A review of efficacy, safety, and costs. *Am J Med.* 2003;*115(4)*:298–308.

22. Othieno R, Abu Affan M, Okpo E. Home versus inpatient treatment for deep vein thrombosis. *Cochrane Database Syst Rev.* 2007 July 18;*(3)*:CD003076.

23. Wells PS, Forgie MA, Rodger MA. Treatment of venous thromboembolism. *JAMA.* 2014;*311(7)*:717–728.

24. Aujesky D, Roy PM, Verschuren F, et al. Outpatient versus inpatient treatment for patients with acute pulmonary embolism: An international, open-label, randomised, noninferiority trial. *Lancet.* 2011;*378(9785)*:41–48.

25. Erkens PM, Gandara E, Wells P, et al. Safety of outpatient treatment in acute pulmonary embolism. *J Thromb Haemost: JTH.* 2010;*8(11)*:2412–2417.

26. Eckhoff CD, Didomenico RJ, Shapiro NL. Initiating warfarin therapy: 5 mg versus 10 mg. *Ann Pharmacother.* 2004;*38(12)*:2115–2121.

27. Kovacs MJ, Rodger M, Anderson DR, et al. Comparison of 10-mg and 5-mg warfarin initiation nomograms together with low-molecular-weight heparin for outpatient treatment of acute venous thromboembolism. A randomized, double-blind, controlled trial. *Ann Intern Med.* 2003;*138(9)*:714–719.

28. Crowther MA, Ginsberg JB, Kearon C, et al. A randomized trial comparing 5-mg and 10-mg warfarin loading doses. *Arch Intern Med.* 1999;*159(1)*:46–48.

29. Harrison L, Johnston M, Massicotte MP, Crowther M, Moffat K, Hirsh J. Comparison of 5-mg and 10-mg loading doses in initiation of warfarin therapy. *Ann Intern Med.* 1997;*126(2)*:133–136.

30. Farahmand S, Saeedi M, Seyed Javadi HH, Khashayar P. High doses of warfarin are more beneficial than their low doses in patients with deep vein thrombosis. *Am J Emerg Med.* 2011;*29(9)*:1222–1226.

31. Kovacs MJ, Cruickshank M, Wells PS, et al. Randomized assessment of a warfarin nomogram for initial oral anticoagulation after venous thromboembolic disease. *Haemostasis.* 1998;*28(2)*:62–69.

32. Quiroz R, Gerhard-Herman M, Kosowsky JM, et al. Comparison of a single end point to determine optimal initial warfarin dosing (5 mg versus 10 mg) for venous thromboembolism. *Am J Cardiol.* 2006;*98(4)*:535–537.

33. Garcia P, Ruiz W, Loza MC. Warfarin initiation nomograms for venous thromboembolism. *Cochrane Database Syst Rev.* 2013;*7*:CD007699.

34. Hirsh J, Fuster V, Ansell J, Halperin JL. American Heart Association/American College of Cardiology Foundation guide to warfarin therapy. *J Am Coll Cardiol.* 2003;*41(9)*:1633–1652.

35. Hutten BA, Prins MH. Duration of treatment with vitamin K antagonists in symptomatic venous thromboembolism. *Cochrane Database Syst Rev.* 2006 Jan 25;*(1)*:CD001367.

36. Middeldorp S, Prins MH, Hutten BA. Duration of treatment with vitamin K antagonists in symptomatic venous thromboembolism. *Cochrane Database Syst Rev.* 2014;*8*:CD001367.

37. Kearon C, Ginsberg JS, Anderson DR, et al. Comparison of 1 month with 3 months of anticoagulation for a first episode of venous thromboembolism associated with a transient risk factor. *J Thromb Haemost: JTH.* 2004;*2(5)*:743–749.

38. Watson L, Broderick C, Armon MP. Thrombolysis for acute deep vein thrombosis. *Cochrane Database Syst Rev.* 2014;*1*:CD002783.

39. Enden T, Klow NE, Sandvik L, et al. Catheter-directed thrombolysis vs. anticoagulant therapy alone in deep vein thrombosis: Results of an open randomized, controlled trial reporting on short-term patency. *J Thromb Haemost: JTH.* 2009;*7(8)*:1268–1275.

40. Enden T, Haig Y, Klow NE, et al. Long-term outcome after additional catheter-directed thrombolysis versus standard treatment for acute iliofemoral deep vein thrombosis (the CaVenT study): A randomised controlled trial. *Lancet.* 2012;*379(9810)*:31–38.

41. McLafferty RB. Endovascular management of deep venous thrombosis. *Perspect Vasc Surg Endovasc Ther.* 2008;*20(1)*: 87–91.

42. Sharifi M, Bay C, Mehdipour M, Sharifi J, Investigators T. Thrombus Obliteration by Rapid Percutaneous Endovenous Intervention in Deep Venous Occlusion (TORPEDO) trial: Midterm results. *J Endovasc Ther Offic J Int Soc Endovasc Spec.* 2012;*19(2)*:273–280.

43. Kolbach DN, Sandbrink MW, Hamulyak K, Neumann HA, Prins MH. Non-pharmaceutical measures for prevention of post-thrombotic syndrome. *Cochrane Database Syst Rev.* 2004;*(1)*:CD004174.

44. Musani MH, Matta F, Yaekoub AY, Liang J, Hull RD, Stein PD. Venous compression for prevention of post-thrombotic syndrome: A meta-analysis. *Am J Med.* 2010;*123(8)*:735–740.

45. Kahn SR, Shapiro S, Wells PS et al. Compression stockings to prevent post-thrombotic syndrome: A randomised placebo-controlled trial. *Lancet.* 2014;*383(9920)*:880–888.

46. Lindblad B, Eriksson A, Bergqvist D. Autopsy-verified pulmonary embolism in a surgical department. Analysis of the period from 1951 to 1988. *Br J Surg.* 1991;*78*:849–852.

47. Velmahos GC, Spaniolas K, Tabbara M, et al. The relationship of pulmonary embolism and deep venous thrombosis in trauma. Are they really related? *Arch Surg.* October 2009;*144(10)*:928–932.

48. Velmahos GC, Kern J, Chan LS, Oder D, Murray JA, Shekelle P. Prevention of venous thromboembolism after injury: An evidence-based report–part II: Analysis of risk factors and evaluation of the role of vena caval filters. *J Trauma.* 2000;*49(1)*:140–144.

49. Geerts WH, Pineo GF, Heit HA, et al. Prevention of venous thromboembolism: The seventh ACCP conference on antithrombotic and thrombolytic therapy. *Chest.* 2004; *126(3 Suppl)*:338S–400S.

50. The PIOPED Investigators. Value of the ventilation/perfusion scan in the diagnosis of pulmonary embolism: Results of the prospective investigation for pulmonary embolism diagnosis (PIOPED). *JAMA.* 1990;*263*;2753–2759.

51. Hayashino Y, Goto M, Noguchi Y, Fugul T. Ventilation-perfusion scanning and helical CT in suspected pulmonary embolism: Meta-analysis of diagnostic performance. *Radiology.* 2005;*234*:740–748.

52. Quiroz R, Kucher N, Zou KH, et al. Clinical validity of a negative computed tomography scan in patients with suspected pulmonary embolism. A systematic review. *JAMA.* 2005;*293*:2012–2017.

53. Roy PM, Colombet I, Durieux P, Chatellier G, Sors H, Meyer G. Systematic review and meta-analysis of strategies for the diagnosis of suspected pulmonary embolism. *Br Med J.* 2005;*331*:1–9.

54. Kakkar VV, Corrigan TP, Fossard DP, et al. Prevention of fatal postoperative pulmonary embolism by low doses of heparin. An international multicentre trial. *Lancet.* 1975; *2(7924)*:45–51.

55. Collins R, Scrimgeour A, Yusuf S, Peto R. Reduction in fatal pulmonary embolism and venous thrombosis by perioperative administration of subcutaneous heparin. Overview of results of randomized trials in general, orthopedic, and urologic surgery. *N Engl J Med.* 1988;*318*:1162–1173.

56. Koch A, Bouges S, Ziegler S, et al. Low molecular weight heparin and unfractionated heparin in thrombosis prophylaxis after major surgical intervention: Update of previous meta-analyses. *Br J Surg.* 1997;*84*:750–759.

57. Mismetti P, Laporte S, Darmon JY, et al. Meta-analysis of low molecular weight heparin for the prevention of venous thromboembolism in general surgery. *Br J Surg.* 2001;*88*:913–930.

58. Cornwell EE, Chang D, Velmahos G, et al. Compliance with sequential compression device prophylaxis in at-risk trauma patients: A prospective analysis. *Am Surg.* 2002;*68*:470–473.

59. Comerota AJ, Katz ML, White JV. Why does prophylaxis with external pneumatic compression for deep vein thrombosis fail? *Am J Surg.* 1994;*164*:265–268.

60. Knudson MM, Collins JA, Goodman SB, McCrory DW. Thromboembolism following multiple trauma. *J Trauma.* 1992;*32*:2–11.

61. Knudson MM, Lewis FR, Clinton A, Atkinson K, Megerman J. Prevention of venous thromboembolism in trauma patients. *J Trauma.* 1994;*37*:480–487.

62. Knudson MM, Morabito D, Paiement GD, Shackford S. Use of low molecular weight heparin in preventing thromboembolism in trauma patients. *J Trauma.* 1996;*41*:446–459.

63. Kurtoglou M, Yanar H, Bilsel Y, et al. Venous thromboembolism prophylaxis after head and spinal trauma: Intermittent pneumatic compression devices versus low molecular weight heparin. *World J Surg.* 2004;*28*:807–811.

64. Merli G and the Spinal Cord Injury Thromboprophylaxis Investigators. Prevention of venous thromboembolism in the acute treatment phase after spinal cord injury: A randomized, multicenter trial comparing low-dose heparin plus intermittent pneumatic compression with enoxaparin. *J Trauma.* 2003;*54*:1116–1126.

65. Ginzburg E, Cohn SM, Lopez P, et al. Randomized clinical trial of intermittent pneumatic compression and low molecular weight heparin in trauma. *Br J Surg.* 2003;*90*:1338–1344.

66. Geerts WH, Jay RM, Code KI, et al. A comparison of low-dose heparin with low-molecular-weight heparin as prophylaxis against venous thromboembolism after major trauma. *N Engl J Med.* 1996;*335*:701–707.

67. Velmahos GC, Kern J, Chan LS, Oder D, Murray JA, Shekelle P. Prevention of venous thromboembolism after injury: An evidence-based report—part I: Analysis of risk factors and evaluation of the role of vena caval filters. *J Trauma.* 2000;*49(1)*:132–138.

68. Rogers FB, Cipolle MD, Velmahos GC, Rozycki G, Luchette FA. Practice management guidelines for the prevention of venous thromboembolism in trauma patients: The EAST practice management guidelines work group. *J Trauma.* 2002;*53*:142–164.

69. Rogers FB, Strindberg G, Schackford GR, et al. Five-year follow-up of prophylactic vena cava filters in high-risk trauma patients. *Arch Surg.* 1998;*133*:406–411.

70. Hingorani A, Ascher E, Lorenson E, et al. Upper extremity deep venous thrombosis and its impact on morbidity and mortality rates in a hospital-based population. *J Vasc Surg.* 1997;*26(5)*:853–860.

71. Martin MJ, Salim A. Vena cava filters in surgery and trauma. *Surg Clin N Am.* 2007;*87*:1229–1252.

72. Karmy-Jones R, Jurkovich G, Velmahos GC, et al. Practice patterns and outcomes after retrievable vena cava filters in trauma patients: A AAST multicenter study. *J Trauma.* 2007;*62*:17–25.

73. Decousous A, Leizorovicz S, Parent F et al. for the PREPIC Study Group. A clinical trial of vena cava filters in the prevention of pulmonary embolism in patients with deep vein thrombosis. *N Engl J Med.* 1998;*338*:409–415.

74. The PREPIC study group. Eight-year follow-up of patients with permanent vena cava filters in the prevention of pulmonary embolism. *Circulation.* 2005;*112*:416–422.

75. Antevil JL, Sise MJ, Sack DI, et al. Retrievable vena cava filters for preventing pulmonary embolism in trauma patients: A cautionary tale. *J Trauma.* 2006;*60*:35–40.

76. Rogers FB, Shackford SR, Ricci MA, Wilson JT, Parsons S. Routine prophylactic vena cava filter insertion in severely injured trauma patients decreases the incidence of pulmonary embolism. *J Am Coll Surg.* 1995;*180*:641–647.

77. McMurtry AL, Owings JT, Anderson JT, Battistella FD, Gosselin R. Increased use of prophylactic vena cava filters in trauma patients failed to decrease the overall incidence of pulmonary embolism. *J Am Coll Surg.* 1999;*189*: 314–320.

78. Van Langevelde K, Sramek A, Vincken PWJ, van Rooden JK, Rosendaal FR, Cannegieter SC. Finding the origin of pulmonary emboli with a total-body magnetic resonance direct thrombus imaging technique. *Haematologica.* 2013; *98*:309–315.

79. Quinlan DJ, McQuillan AM, Eikelbloom JW. Low-molecular-weight heparin compared with intravenous unfractionated heparin for treatment of pulmonary embolism. *Ann Intern Med.* 2004;*140*:175–183.

80. Kearon C, Alk EA, Comerota AJ, et al. Antithrombotic therapy for VTE disease. *Chest.* 2012;*141(2 Suppl)*: e419S–e494S.

55

Necrotizing Soft Tissue Infections

Mark D. Sawyer

55.1 Introduction and Definitions

Necrotizing soft tissue infections (NSTIs) are a subject that would seem to lend itself poorly to a textbook of evidence-based surgery. Such uncommon and highly lethal disease processes make quality large, prospective, randomized trials extremely difficult to design and implement. Further complicating the picture is that a large proportion of current practice is, by necessity, based on individual observations and deductions concerning the disease. Thus, one might expect to engender strong biases, which at times seem to be in inverse proportion to available evidence. As a result, an evidence-based discussion of questions concerning NSTIs may have more the appearance of a photographic negative—deciding which tentative conclusions are likely, not justified because there is no quality evidence to support them, rather than raising to the fore those conclusions best supported by solid statistical evidence. This also points out the need for a larger, cooperative effort to glean more substantial evidence from the 3,800–5,800 cases per year that occur [11].

While NSTIs comprise a wide variety of clinical scenarios as reflected by the bewildering array of terms utilized in the literature, a simple division—predominantly fascial versus predominantly muscular involvement—categorizes these infections reasonably well both in terms of their behavior and a pragmatic approach to empiric treatment [6, 7]. Although anyone may be affected, the immunocompromised and debilitated—most commonly those with advancing age and diabetes mellitus—are disproportionately represented both in terms of acquiring the disease and suffering poorer outcomes.

55.2 Necrotizing Fasciitis

55.2.1 The Disease

Necrotizing fasciitis is an infection involving the investing fascia of muscle, primarily the superficial layer, and may secondarily involve a modest amount of juxtaposed fat and muscle. It has a predilection for the immunocompromised, which is more morbid and lethal as well. Originally described as a streptococcal or streptococcal-predominant infectious process [1, 2], it is usually a polymicrobial infection, although monomicrobial forms of the disease (*Vibrio, Pseudomonas, Klebsiella*, and others) exist as well. Studies carefully culturing the tissues may show a mix of gram-positive, gram-negative, and anaerobic bacteria, as well as candidal species in some.

Necrotizing fasciitis has been described as a rapidly progressive process, but at least some patients may describe a relatively indolent period before seeking medical attention, with subsequent decompensation giving the outward appearance of rapid progression [3, 4]. These patients are primarily those with the polymicrobial form of the disease. The monomicrobial forms of the disease—group A *Streptococcus*, certain toxin-producing strains of methicillin-resistant *Staphylococcus aureus* (MRSA), clostridial species (perfringens, septicum, novyi type A, and sordellii), and marine gram-negative organisms such as *Vibrio vulnificans*—are rapidly progressive, extraordinarily lethal disease processes.

55.2.2 Diagnosis

Early incision and exploration of suspected tissues to explore for NSTI is the most important element in both diagnosis and treatment and should not be delayed for other diagnostic studies. The use of biopsy and frozen section—once the standard of care—probably adds little to diagnosis and the extent of resection, both of which are generally clear without histopathology. If it does not delay surgical exploration, radiographic studies such as CT scans can provide useful data regarding the location and extent of the disease.

55.3 Mainstay Therapy

Two cornerstones of initial therapy are expeditious and complete debridement and broad-spectrum antimicrobial therapy. Immediate initiation of empiric broad-spectrum antimicrobial therapy based on an antistreptococcal component is key; awaiting culture or even Gram stain data to guide therapy would constitute an unnecessary and potentially dangerous delay. With one study utilizing careful culture techniques showing *Candida* species in a majority of patients and the dangers of superinfection following potent broad-spectrum

DOI: 10.1201/9781003316800-55

TABLE 55.1

Treatment of Necrotizing Infections of the Skin, Fascia, and Muscle

Type of Infection	First-Line Antimicrobial Agent	Adult Dosage	Pediatric Dosage Beyond the Neonatal Period	Antimicrobial Agent for Patients with Severe Penicillin Hypersensitivity
Mixed infections	Piperacillin-tazobactam plus vancomycin	3.375 g every 6–8 hours IV	60–75 mg/kg/dose of the piperacillin component every 6 hours IV	Clindamycin or metronidazole with an aminoglycoside or fluoroquinolone
	Imipenem-cilastatin	30 mg/kg/dose in 2 divided doses	10–13 mg/kg/dose every 8 hours IV	N/A
	Meropenem Ertapenem Cefotaxime plus metronidazole or clindamycin	1 g every 6–8 hours IV 1 g every 8 hours IV 1 g daily IV 2 g every 6 hours IV 500 mg every 6 hours IV 600–900 mg every 8 hours IV	N/A 20 mg/kg/dose every 8 hours IV 15 mg/kg/dose every 12 hours IV for children 3 months to 12 years 50 mg/kg/dose every 6 hours IV 7.5 mg/kg/dose every 6 hours IV 10–13 mg/kg/dose every 8 hours IV	N/A
Streptococcus	Penicillin plus clindamycin	2–4 million units every 4–6 hours IV (adult) 600–900 mg/every 8 hours IV	60,000–100,000 units/kg/dose every 6 hours IV 10–13 mg/kg/dose every 8 hours IV	Vancomycin, linezolid, quinupristin/dalfopristin, daptomycin
Staphylococcus aureus	Nafcillin	1–2 g every 4 hours IV	50 mg/kg/dose every 6 hours IV	Vancomycin, linezolid, quinupristin/dalfopristin, daptomycin
	Oxacillin Cefazolin Vancomycin (for resistant strains) Clindamycin	1–2 g every 4 hours IV 1 g every 8 hours IV 30 mg/kg/ dose in 2 divided doses IV 600–900 mg every 8 hours IV	50 mg/kg/dose/every 6 hours IV 33 mg/kg/dose every 8 hours IV 15 mg/kg/dose every 6 hours IV 10–13 mg/kg/dose every 8 hours IV	Bacteriostatic; potential cross-resistance and emergence of resistance in erythromycin-resistant strains; inducible resistance in MRSA
Clostridium species	Clindamycin plus penicillin	600–900 mg every 8 hours IV 2–4 million units every 4–6 hours IV (adult)	10–13 mg/kg/dose every 8 hours IV 60,000–100,000 units/kg/dose every 6 hours IV	N/A
Aeromonas hydrophila	Doxycycline plus ciprofloxacin or ceftriaxone	100 mg every 12 hours IV 500 mg every 12 hours IV 1–2 g every 24 hours IV	Not recommended for children but may need to use in life-threatening situations	N/A
Vibrio vulnificus	Doxycycline plus ceftriaxone or cefotaxime	100 mg every 12 hours IV 1 g QID IV 2 g TID IV	Not recommended for children but may need to use in life-threatening situations	N/A

Abbreviations: IV: Intravenous, MRSA: Methicillin-resistant *Staphylococcus aureus*, N/A: Not applicable, QID: Four times daily, TID: Three times daily.

antimicrobial therapy, many would advocate empiric therapy with an antifungal agent as well, although this is not considered standard of care. The Infectious Disease Societies of America have recently published an update to their evidence-based recommendations for antimicrobial choices for skin and soft tissue infections, including necrotizing fasciitis and myositis (Table 55.1). As with other evidence-based recommendations for NSTIs, the recommendations are strong, but with weak evidence.

The other unequivocal cornerstone of therapy is expeditious and complete excision of the infected and necrotic fascia to prevent further progression and begin the healing process. Although some have advocated for staged resections in the past, it would seem more logical to remove as much of the involved fascia as the patient will tolerate at the first resection. Regardless of the initial philosophy, returning to the operating room for "second look" procedures to at least assess, if not complete, the resection process is ubiquitous. This "second look" is typically performed about 24 hours after the initial operation and then every 24 hours until debridement is no longer required. At that point, we typically lengthen the interval between exploration. In the event the patient fails to respond appropriately to the initial procedure such as nonresponse, worsening physiology, or other signs of ongoing sepsis, an early return to the operating room is indicated. Necrotizing fasciitis is a progressive disease, and assuring that progression has been halted is mandatory. Though excision and debridement can be debilitating and disfiguring, completeness is essential to halt the progression of the disease and maximize survival. Following the initial phase, a prolonged healing convalescent phase is usual in survivors, with the care of open wounds that may constitute a large percentage of the patient's body surface area. In addition to standard techniques for dressing and closing such wounds, newer technologies such as vacuum-assisted wound closure devices may be helpful.

55.4 Supplemental Therapy

Several therapies have been utilized in NSTIs to try and improve outcomes, such as hyperbaric oxygen and antistreptococcal immunoglobulin administration. The rationale for the former had its genesis in the treatment of anaerobic NSTIs such as clostridial necrotizing myositis, and the latter as an attempt to improve the treatment of aggressive group A streptococcal infections and their complications such as streptococcal toxic shock syndrome. While theoretically attractive, neither has definitively proven itself as a mainstay of treatment in NSTIs. Unfortunately, these therapies have not been shown to improve outcomes.

55.5 Necrotizing Myositis

The most common synonyms for necrotizing muscle infections are gas gangrene, clostridial/streptococcal myonecrosis, and necrotizing myositis. The latter term is simple, descriptive, and alliteratively associates the disease process with its fascial counterpart. The infection infects, spreads, and necroses entire muscle compartments with celerity; it is rapidly progressive and, in contradistinction to necrotizing fasciitis, has no recognized indolent variants. Pragmatically, this means that exceptionally aggressive surgery such as proximal amputation may be required to gain control of the disease process before the patient succumbs, which may occur within hours of presentation. In further contradistinction to necrotizing fasciitis, necrotizing myositis is usually a monomicrobial infection, most commonly a toxin-producing *Clostridium* or *Streptococcus* species.

55.6 Diagnosis: Is Open Fascial Exploration and Biopsy Still the Standard for Diagnosis of NSTI, or Has It Been Supplanted by Radiographic Studies?

The standard of diagnosis in NSTIs is a clinical diagnosis, confirmed by open incision, examination of the tissues, and optionally obtaining a biopsy with a frozen section, although the latter is increasingly thought of as no longer necessary [12–14]. For imaging modalities to confer a benefit beyond this clinical standard, they would need to provide some additional benefit, either in providing more timely positive support of the diagnosis and thus shortening the time to definitive surgical therapy, or definitively ruling out the diagnosis, obviating the need for diagnostic surgery. This second benefit would

be more difficult to provide, as the negative predictive value would need to approach perfection; a missed diagnosis due to an imperfect prediction would delay surgery and increase mortality.

Imaging modalities—CT, MRI, and ultrasound—have all developed increasingly finer resolution, software sophistication, and in the case of ultrasound portability allowing for point-of-care use. The CT characteristics of NSTIs are well delineated, but are not specific, as exemplified by elements such as fascial thickening and edema without asymmetry. Other more specific findings, such as gas within soft tissues, are not ubiquitous; therefore, their absence does not rule out the disease [13, 14]. If it does not delay definitive surgical therapy, CT may help in planning a thorough surgical intervention by showing the extent of the disease, but should not be relied upon to rule in or out the diagnosis of NSTI.

MRI would be thought to be an ideal instrument in the circumstance of NSTIs, as its strength is in the delineation of soft tissue pathology, and it has been propounded as such by some authors [22, 23]. However, findings are not any more specific than CT; one author found the MRI findings similar between necrotizing fasciitis, dermatomyositis, and posttraumatic muscle injury [15]. While it has been shown that necrotizing infectious fasciitis can at times be differentiated from noninfectious necrotizing fasciitis, there remains some diagnostic uncertainty and interobserver variation—and therefore imperfect negative predictive value. MRI is not as rapidly obtained as a CT scan and does not seem to convey any significant additional diagnostic advantage over CT. Its role in NSTIs is therefore very limited.

Point-of-care ultrasound is a rapidly expanding field, especially in the field of emergency medicine. There have been recent interesting reports and limited case series utilizing point-of-care ultrasound to assess soft tissue infections [19–21]. While interesting, these do not as yet provide compelling evidence for their routine use, nor should they be relied upon as a substitute for a surgical consultation. It may be that they could shorten the time of surgical consultation by being able to be used at the point of care, but predictive values have yet to be established.

RECOMMENDATION

The standard for diagnosis in NSTI is clinical, with confirmation by open exploration and inspection of the tissues with biopsy and frozen section if the diagnosis is still uncertain.

Grade of recommendation: C.

55.6.1 Diagnosis: Is the Laboratory Risk Indicator for Necrotizing Fasciitis Score Clinically Useful in NSTIs?

The Laboratory Risk Indicator for Necrotizing Fasciitis (LRINEC) score, first proposed in 2004, has points for

C-reactive protein, white blood cell (WBC) count, hemoglobin, serum sodium, creatinine, and glucose, with gradations of points awarded to the total score based on the degree of derangement. A score of ≥6 denotes patients at high risk for NSTI, specifically necrotizing fasciitis. While it has been shown to correlate with necrotizing fasciitis, it has not been validated as a sole predictor in subsequent studies, It is a collection of nonspecific tests that, when elevated, indicate overall physiologic derangement, not necessarily due to an NSTI. It is not of sufficient sensitivity to rule out necrotizing fasciitis; patients with a low score still have a risk of disease that can only be ruled out by operative examination of the tissue. A review of studies performed between the original paper and 2018 showed that the LRINEC score had a wide range of sensitivity (43–80%), positive predictive value (57–64%), and negative predictive value (42–86%).

RECOMMENDATION

The LRINEC score has not been adequately shown to be a valuable adjunct in the diagnosis of NSTI, as the score does not impact whether or not a patient should undergo an operation. Patients with a low LRINEC but clinical suspicion of NSTI will still need operative exploration, and patients with a high LRINEC score and suspicion of NSTI will already need operative exploration.

Grade of recommendation: C.

55.7 Mainstay Therapy: Which Is a Better Approach to Initial Resection in NSTI: Staged or "Complete"?

There has been little in the literature to suggest a standardized approach to NSTI. Certainly, the objective is to remove all necrotic and infected tissue as quickly as possible. However, whether or not this may be achieved in one operative intervention depends heavily on the patient's ability to tolerate extended, aggressive resection. Regardless of whether the first procedure is considered complete, nearly all patients will require at least one second-look procedure to ensure a lack of disease progression. Recently, Wong et al. have advocated a standardized approach to resection, involving a complete resection in the first procedure, with second-look operations to follow [37]. While the approach seems sensible to those who will tolerate their complete approach to the initial procedure, it is not based on prospective randomized data, but the authors considered an approach to the problem. It is, as noted earlier, a logical approach to the disease process, with the caveat that it would seem prudent to halt the procedure once the patient's tolerance for operative intervention is reached and return when they have been further resuscitated and stabilized.

RECOMMENDATION

Complete an initial resection as the patient will tolerate.

Grade of recommendation: C.

55.8 Supplemental Therapy: Is There Convincing Evidence for the Use of Hyperbaric Oxygen Therapy in the Treatment of Necrotizing Soft Tissue Infections?

Hyperbaric oxygen (HBO) therapy was originally devised as a way to treat decompression sickness after deep underwater diving ("the bends"). At many atmospheres of depth, more nitrogen is solubilized in the bloodstream, and too-rapid ascent results in nitrogen desolubilizing out of the bloodstream as bubbles, which then cause gas emboli. The use of HBO is currently unregulated, and usage ranges from legitimate and proven (treating decompression sickness) to therapeutic and experimental use in medicine such as carbon monoxide poisoning and NSTIs, to "oxygen bar"–like operations hawking sessions for their purported general health benefits.

HBO therapy is a theoretically attractive potential therapy for NSTIs, utilizing oxygen as a direct toxin to combat anaerobic bacteria [29]. What comparative studies exist generally are not randomized, and controls may be historical. One recent comparative but nonrandomized study on a small number of patients showed a shorter length of treatment when utilizing HBO [27]. Most studies of NSTIs are observational in nature [25, 26, 28, 30]; there are synergistic factors that make randomized controlled trials in NSTIs difficult to complete. The first is the rarity of the infections; it can take a single center decades to accrue a few dozen cases, making adequate statistical analysis difficult as well as weakening any conclusions by the rapid general advances made in medicine over such a long period—the longer the study, the less comparable the first patients entered into such a study are to the last. The second factor is the zeal with which proponents of HBO therapy for NSTIs maintain despite any solid statistical evidence to support its use in these infections. Some have gone so far as to say that randomized controlled trials of its use are "unethical" because they believe it is so beneficial. This attitude may be compounded by a long time between patients, and in fact, there are studies spanning decades that use the "prehyperbaric chamber" era as a historical control for the "posthyperbaric chamber" era. A further potential bias is inherent in the purchase of these expensive chambers; having spent millions of dollars for one such, two questions must be asked: (1) Would such an expensive piece of equipment have been purchased if it was not thought to be efficacious *a priori* and (2), having invested, how objective can one be regarding its supposed benefits in the absence of the objective evidence of a randomized controlled trial? Two recent studies bear mention. First, the authors queried the

University Health Consortium database from 2008 to 2010 for NSTIs in centers with HBO capabilities. They found that the most direly ill patients with necrotizing fasciitis who underwent HBO therapy had significantly improved mortality (4% vs. 26%, $p < 0.01$) and fewer complications (45% vs. 66%, $p < 0.01$) with NSTIs [32]. However, only 7% of patients received HBO, and these 117 patients were stratified into four small groups based on the severity of illness, increasing the risk of a type I error. The nature of the database did not allow for a more granular analysis, such as which patients were selected for HBO therapy, a critical element for comparison. While the results are promising, confirmation with other studies would be important in that particular group of patients; to date, the extant literature has not shown a preponderance of evidence for HBO being of benefit for the population of NSTIs as a whole. In another database study, the Nationwide Inpatient Sample was queried for NSTIs from 1998 to 2010 and found that the use of HBO therapy had decreased from 1.6% to 0.8% over the epoch studied ($p < 0.0001$), while the overall survival of patients with NTSIs improved from 9.0% to 4.9% ($p < 0.0001$) [31]. These findings were in the face of worsening patient acuity and increasing complication rates. While no direct correlation between HBO and mortality trends in this study can be made, it does suggest that the overall gestalt of current treatment has increased patient survival and that survival is not correlated with the use of HBO.

RECOMMENDATION

HBO should not be part of the standard treatment for NSTIs. More rigorous trials are needed.

Grade of recommendation: C.

55.9 Supplemental Therapy: Is Immunoglobulin Therapy Part of Standard Care for Necrotizing Soft Tissue Infections?

As streptococcal species have been strongly implicated in NSTIs since their initial description and immunoglobulin has been utilized in the treatment of *Streptococcus pyogenes*

(group A *Streptococcus*) and streptococcal toxic shock syndrome, it is reasonable to examine whether or not immunoglobulin therapy has any salutary effect on NSTIs [24–26]. Polyclonal/polyvalent immunoglobulin products are heterogeneous and confer passive and nonspecific immunity. Because of their nature, their composition and effect will vary between manufacturing batches. While case reports and observational studies have been somewhat encouraging, the efficacy of gamma globulin in streptococcal toxic shock syndrome has not been confirmed by randomized studies. A recent meta-analysis showed a statistically significant mortality benefit, but only when all five pooled studies were considered; none of the individual studies—one randomized, four nonrandomized—achieved statistical significance on their own.

RECOMMENDATION

Intravenous immunoglobulin treatment has not been convincingly proven to improve outcomes.

Grade of recommendation: C.

55.10 Conclusions

NSTIs are uncommon, highly lethal diseases requiring rapid diagnosis and treatment to achieve optimal outcomes. With only a thousand or so cases a year across the United States, however, prospective randomized trials are difficult, and in the case of a single institution, near impossible. With agreement on the basics of therapy—aggressive surgical debridement and broad-spectrum antimicrobials—the important questions at present involve secondary therapies that remain unproven at best. To obtain quality data for questions such as the use of HBO and polyclonal immunoglobulin administration, multicenter studies and databases will almost certainly be required to obtain a level of evidence sufficient to recommend their use with confidence. The recent study utilizing a multicenter database to gather data is encouraging and is a novel manner in which to address the difficulties of researching a rare disease. The success in caring for patients with these difficult infections has improved, but secondary therapies, for now, remain unproven (Table 55.2).

TABLE 55.2

Evidence

Question	Answer	Grade	References
What is the standard for diagnosis in NSTIs?	Clinical; confirmation by open biopsy.	C	[5–10]
What is the best approach to initial resection?	As complete as the patient will tolerate.	C	[21]
Should hyperbaric oxygen be part of the standard treatment for NSTIs?	No. More rigorous trials are needed.	C	[14–20]
Should intravenous immunoglobulin be part of the standard treatment for NSTIs?	No, it has not been proven to improve outcomes.	C	[11–13]

Editor's Note

Necrotizing soft tissue infection is an unusual entity, making randomized clinical trials difficult to perform. There is general agreement, based only on clinical experience, that a combined approach of targeted antibiotics and aggressive operative eradication of these infections should be employed early in the course of the disease. The patients are typically returned to the operating room daily until the wound no longer requires debridement.

We recently participated in a large multicenter trial involving an immune modulator. During the first 2 years of the trial, over 175 patients with the diagnosis of NSTI were seen at our facility but only 2 met the rigorous inclusion standards for entry into the study. Performing rigorous investigations on this topic remains very challenging, and this contributes to the lack of quality evidence to support our current management protocols.

Unfortunately, in the United States, with limited access to healthcare for a substantial proportion of our population, many individuals present late, with extensive soft tissue infections that could have been easily managed with antibiotics initially. NSTI appears to be rarely seen in developed countries other than the United States.

REFERENCES

General

1. Meleny FL. Hemolytic streptococcus gangrene. *Arch Surg.* 1924;*9*:317–364.
2. Wilson B. Necrotizing fasciitis. *Am Surg.* 1952;*18*:416.
3. Wong CH, Tan SH. Subacute necrotizing fasciitis. *Lancet.* 2004;*364*:1376.
4. Wong CH, Wang YS. What is subacute necrotizing fasciitis? Proposed clinical diagnostic criteria. *J Infection.* 2006;*52*:415–419.
5. Cainzos M, Gonzalez-Rodriguez FJ. Necrotizing soft tissue infections. *Curr Opin Crit Care.* 2007;*13*:433–439.
6. Sawyer MD, Dunn DL. Deep soft tissue infections. *Curr Opin Infect Dis.* 1991;*4*:649–654.
7. Dunn DL, Sawyer MD. Deep soft-tissue infections. *Curr Opin Infect Dis.* 1990;*3*:691–696.
8. Hakkarainen T. Necrotizing soft tissue infections: Review and current concepts in treatment, systems of care, and outcomes. *Curr Prob Surg.* 2014;*51*:344–362.
9. Stevens D, Bisno A, Chambers H, Dellinger E, Goldstein E, Gorbach S, Hirschmann J, Kaplan S, Montoya J, Wade J. Practice guidelines for the diagnosis and management of skin and soft tissue infections: 2014 update by the infectious diseases Society of America. *CID.* 2014;*59*:47–159.
10. Ustin J, Malangoni M. Necrotizing soft-tissue infections. *Crit Care Med.* 2011;*39(9)*:2156–2162.
11. Psoinos C, Flahive J, Shaw J, YouFu L, Sing Chau N, Tseng J, Santry H. Contemporary trends in necrotizing soft tissue infections in the United States. *Surgery.* 2013;*153*:819–827.

Diagnosis: Imaging, Open Biopsy, and LRINEC score

12. Stamenkovic I, Lew PD. Early recognition of potentially fatal necrotizing fasciitis: The use of frozen section biopsy. *N Engl J Med.* 1984;*310*:1689–1693.
13. Maeski JA, Majeski E. Necrotizing fasciitis: Improved survival with early recognition by tissue biopsy and aggressive surgical treatment. *South Med J.* 1997;*90*:1065–1068.
14. Wong CH, Wag YS. The diagnosis of necrotizing fasciitis. *Curr Opin Infect Dis.* 2005;*18*:101–106.
15. Levenson RB, Singh AK, Novelline RA. Fournier gangrene: Role of imaging. *Radiographics.* 2008;*28*:519–528.
16. Wysoki MG, Santora TA, Sha RM, Friedman AC. Necrotizing fasciitis: CT characteristics. *Radiology.* 1997;*203*:859–863.
17. Arslan A, PierreJerome C, Borthne A. Necrotizing fasciitis: Unreliable MRI findings in the preoperative diagnosis. *Eur J Radiol.* 2000;*36*:139–143.
18. Malghem J, Lcouvet FE, Omoumi P, et al. Necrotizing fasciitis: Contribution and limitations of diagnostic imaging. *Joint Bone Spine.* 2013 March;*80(2)*:146–154.
19. Oelze L, Wu S, Carnell J. Emergency ultrasonography for the early diagnosis of necrotizing fasciitis: A case series from the ED. *Am J Emerg Med.* 2013;*31*:632, e5–e7.
20. Kehrl T. Point-of-care ultrasound diagnosis of necrotizing fasciitis missed by computed tomography and magnetic resonance imaging. *J Emerg Med.* 2014;*47(2)*:172–175.
21. Castleberg E, Jenson N, Dinh VA. Diagnosis of necrotizing fasciitis with bedside ultrasound: The STAFF exam. *Western J Emerg Med.* 2014;*15(1)*:111–113.
22. Rahmouni A, Chosidow O, Mathieu D, Gueroguieva E, Jazaerli N, Radier C, Faivre J, Roujeau J, Vasile N. MR imaging in acute infectious cellulitis. *Radiology.* 1994;*192*: 493–496.
23. Kim K, Yeo J, Lee J, Kim Y, Park S, Lim M, Suh C. Can necrotizing infectious fasciitis be differentiated from nonnecrotizing infectious fasciitis with MR imaging? *Radiology.* 2011;*259(3)*:816–824.

The LRINEC (Laboratory Risk Indicator for Necrotizing Fasciitis) score: a tool for distinguishing necrotizing fasciitis from other soft tissue infections

24. Wong CH, Khin LW, Heng KS, Tan KC, Low CO. *Crit Care Med.* 2004 July;*32(7)*:1535–1541. doi: 10.1097/01. ccm.0000129486.35458.7d.

Reliability of the Laboratory Risk Indicator in Necrotising Fasciitis (LRINEC) score

25. Abdullah M, McWilliams B, Khan SU. *Surgeon.* 2019 Oct;*17(5)*:309–318. doi: 10.1016/j.surge.2018.08.001. Epub 2018 Aug 27.

Use of Immunoglobulin/Streptococcal Toxic Shock

26. Stevens DL. Streptococcal toxic shock syndrome is associated with necrotizing fasciitis. *AnnuRev Med.* 2000; *51*:271–28.
27. Barry W, Hudgins L, Donta S, Pesanti E. Intravenous immunoglobulin therapy for toxic shock syndrome. *JAMA.* 1992;*267*:3315–3316.
28. Kaul R, McGeer A, Norrby-Teglund A, et al. Intravenous immunoglobulin therapy for streptococcal toxic shock syndrome—A comparative observational study. *Clin Infect Dis.* 1999;*28*:800–807.

29. Polyspecific Intravenous Immunoglobulin in Clindamycin-treated Patients With Streptococcal Toxic Shock Syndrome: A Systematic Review and Meta-analysis

30. Tom P, Clare W, Nigel C, Anna NT, Shiranee S. *Clin Infect Dis.* 2018 November:67(9):1434–1436. doi: 10.109/cid/ciy401

Hyperbaric Oxygen

31. Jallali N, Withey MS, Butler PE. Hyperbaric oxygen as adjuvant therapy in the management of necrotizing fasciitis. *Am J Surg.* 2005;*189*:462–466.

32. Sugihara A, Watanabe H, Oohashi M, Kato N, Murakami H, Tsukazaki S, Fujikawa K. The effect of hyperbaric oxygen therapy on the bout of treatment for soft tissue infections. *J Infect.* 2004;*48*:330–333.

33. Kornonen K. Hyperbaric oxygen therapy in acute necrotizing infections with special reference to the effects on tissue gas tensions. A clinical and experimental study. *Ann Chirurg Gynaecol Suppl.* 2000;*214*:3–36.

34. Kornonen K, Klossner J, Hirn M, Niinkoski J. Management of Clostridial gas gangrene and the role of hyperbaric oxygen. *Ann Chrurg Gynae.* 1999;*88*:19–12.

35. Massey P, Akram J, Mills A, Sarani B, Aufhauser D, Sims C, Pascual J, Kelz R, Holena D. Hyperbaric oxygen therapy in necrotizing soft tissue infections *J Surg Res.* 2012;*177*:16–151.

36. Saw JJ, Psoinos C, Emhoff TA, Shah SA, Santry HP. Not just full of hot air: Hyperbaric oxygen therapy increases survival in cases of necrotizing soft tissue infections. *Surg Infect (Larchmt).* 2014 June;*15(3)*:328–335.

Operative Approach

37. Wong CH, Yam AKT, Tan ABH, Song C. Approach to debridement in necrotizing fasciitis. *Am J Surg.* 2008 September;*196(3)*:e19–e24.

56

Incarcerated Hernias

Rachel E. Beard and Steven D. Schwaitzberg

56.1 Introduction

An incarcerated hernia is one of the more common emergencies for the general surgeon. There are several important questions to consider when dealing with this entity. Emergent imaging, though not essential, has become increasingly ubiquitous and seems to replace physical examination in several settings such as the emergency department before surgical consultation. In addition, hernia repair has evolved over the last decade with several new options and paradigms to consider. Certain dilemmas remain unchanged such as determining the viability of incarcerated intestine. Finally, the age-old dilemma of what to do when the incarcerated hernia turns out to be a strangulated hernia with contamination remains a formidable challenge.

56.1.1 What Are the Appropriate Physical Examination and Imaging Evaluations Necessary to Diagnose Incarcerated Hernias?

There are no randomized trials in the literature comparing physical examination alone to imaging in securing the diagnosis of incarcerated abdominal wall hernia. However, there are numerous case reports and short retrospective series that offered testimonial benefits to the use of computed tomography (CT) or ultrasound (US) in the diagnosis of abdominal wall incarcerated hernia [1, 2] (Level IV evidence). Imaging appeared to be of the greatest benefit in three categories: Obese patients, Spigelian hernias, and obturator hernias [3–9] (Level IV and V evidence; grade C recommendation). The literature also describes an unusual case of small bowel obstruction (SBO) following the open repair of an incarcerated inguinal hernia caused by intestine trapped in a hernia sac that was protruding into the preperitoneal space and ultimately required laparotomy for repair. The authors pointed out the diagnostic difficulty and the need for a CT scan in this case [10] (Level V evidence). Aside from these unusual circumstances, the vast majority of inguinal and ventral hernias appear to be diagnosed clinically. One large nationwide retrospective study from Sweden, which included more than 100,000 patients, demonstrated that patients who lacked a well-documented physical examination of the groin (37%) were more likely to undergo preoperative imaging ($p < 0.001$), resulting in an unnecessary delay in surgery [11] (Level IIB evidence). A thorough physical examination is mandatory, and there is no evidence that a diagnosis made on physical examination requires imaging confirmation (grade B recommendation). Finally, US may be useful in the evaluation of incarcerated umbilical hernia. Case reports of using real-time US to guide fluid aspirations in the hernia sac enabling reduction are common [12, 13] (Level V evidence).

> **RECOMMENDATION**
>
> A thorough physical examination is mandatory and, except in rare cases, is acceptable for the diagnosis of most incarcerated hernias. Adjunctive imaging, usually CT or US, is acceptable in specific clinical scenarios where the diagnosis is difficult, such as Spigelian, obturator, certain umbilical hernias, or if obesity limits physical examination. But routine imaging in all potential hernias can lead to delay in surgical management.
>
> Grade of recommendation: C.

56.1.2 What Are the Technical Considerations for Treating Incarcerated Hernia that Influence the Choice of Repair?

Before the mid-1980s, the choices for elective and emergent hernia repairs were simple. Primary tissue repairs were exclusively performed. The introduction of the first polypropylene mesh and then expanded polytetrafluoroethylene (PTFE) changed the face of elective hernia repairs almost completely by the mid-1990s. The use of mesh for elective hernia repairs is well established now [14–17] (Level IV evidence). Laparoscopic repairs were added to the elective hernia repair options in the early 1990s, and all utilize some form of prosthesis. It was inevitable that these options would be considered for urgent/emergent repairs as well.

A few small prospective trials have been performed to determine the optimal repair of incarcerated hernias with cohort sizes ranging from 40 to 54 patients [18–20] (Level IIB evidence), as well as a few retrospective studies [21, 22] (Level IV evidence). Karatepe et al. concluded that preperitoneal repair with mesh for strangulated hernias is superior to Lichtenstein mesh-only repair because it allows for bowel resection if needed and avoids the need for an additional incision, which was significantly associated with increased morbidity ($p = 0.003$) in their patient population [18]. Elsebae et al. concluded that Lichtenstein mesh repair also decreased recurrence when compared to repair with the Bassini technique, without increasing complication rates. This study, however, excluded patients with peritonitis and who underwent bowel resection from mesh repair [19]. Derici et al.'s retrospective study included 113 patients and suggests that Lichtenstein repair with mesh is preferred in incarcerated inguinal hernias because it significantly lowers recurrence rates when compared to primary repair ($p = 0.036$) without increasing complications [21]. Papaziogas et al. included 75 patients in their comparative study and concluded that a tension-free mesh repair did not increase complication rates or lead to mesh removal when compared to a modified Bassini repair, even in the setting of bowel resection [22]. Lastly, Abdel-Baki et al. randomized patients with incarcerated paraumbilical hernias to either prosthetic repair with a polypropylene mesh only or tissue repair and concluded that prosthetic repair significantly reduced recurrence rates ($p < 0.05$) without increasing complications [20]. The studies indicate that mesh repair is not contraindicated for strangulated hernias even if bowel resection is needed. For inguinal hernias, Lichtenstein repair reduces recurrence rates as compared to tissue repairs, though there is some suggestion that a preperitoneal approach may better allow for bowel resection if needed.

Laparoscopic repair as an option for the repair of incarcerated hernia continues to be studied. It is well established that operator experience will influence the outcome in laparoscopic repairs, though the breadth of laparoscopic experience among surgeons is likely narrowing, as it is increasingly an integral part of surgical training [23] (Level IIB evidence). There are several retrospective series and case reports indicating success in repairing inguinal, femoral, and ventral hernias with Lichtenstein repairs, transabdominal laparoscopic repairs (TAPs), and totally extraperitoneal laparoscopic repairs (TEPs) [24–29] (Level IV evidence). As with the aforementioned studies that examined open mesh repairs, these studies concluded that laparoscopic repair with mesh is not contraindicated for incarcerated and strangulated hernias and also suggested that the TAP approach is preferable for strangulated inguinal hernias, as it allows for good visualization of abdominal contents and bowel resection if needed. Robotic repair has been reported in 19 patients with no recurrences and mostly minor complications. Robotic incisional hernia repair is also reported, but with a higher incidence of major complications [30, 31] (Level IV evidence]

RECOMMENDATION

Repair with mesh is not contraindicated for strangulated hernias.

Grade of recommendation: B.

For inguinal hernias, Lichtenstein repair reduces recurrence rates as compared to tissue repairs, though there is some suggestion that a preperitoneal approach may better allow for bowel resection if needed.

Grade of recommendation: B.

Laparoscopic repair with mesh is not contraindicated for incarcerated and strangulated hernias and also suggests that the TAP approach is preferable for strangulated inguinal hernias, as it allows for good visualization of abdominal contents and bowel resection if needed.

Grade of recommendation: C.

56.1.3 What Are the Repair Options in the Face of Gastrointestinal Contamination or Infection?

The challenge of repairing abdominal wall defects in the face of significant gastrointestinal contamination or infection is formidable. Primary tissue repair avoids foreign body–based infections; however, subsequent recurrences are common [17, 18, 21] (Level IIB and IV evidence). Retrospective studies support the use of polypropylene mesh in selected settings, including patients who are immunosuppressed following solid organ transplantation, cases categorized as clean-contaminated or even contaminated, and in the setting of bowel resection without frank peritonitis [19, 29–33] (Level IIIB and IV evidence). These studies do not demonstrate any increased morbidity, mortality, or need for mesh removal in such cases. The use of biologic prostheses has become popular even though there are no long-term or randomized outcome studies concerning the use of biologic prostheses such as acellular dermis or reconstituted collagen in contaminated or infected settings. Retrospective reviews suggest imperfect but acceptable results in contaminated fields (CDC class I and II) with modest complication rates (infection and reoperation) equivalent between synthetic mesh and no mesh repairs regardless of the need for bowel resection. Recurrence was higher in the nonmesh group [34–40] (Level IIIB and IV evidence). The most current recommendation from the World Society of Emergency Surgery (WSES) for patients with gross contamination (CDC class III and IV) continues to suggest that biologic or absorbable mesh is preferred in these grossly contaminated settings [41, 42] (Level IIA evidence).

RECOMMENDATION

Primary repair is discouraged, as subsequent recurrence rates are higher. The use of synthetic prostheses for use in contaminated (CDC I and II) cases is safe and superior for reducing long-term recurrence.

Grade of recommendation: B.

The use of biologic prostheses is well described and is acceptable for use in high-risk and grossly contaminated (CDC III and IV) repairs.

Grade of recommendation: B.

Synthetic mesh is emerging as an acceptable alternative for hernia repair in the contaminated field.

Grade of recommendation: B.

56.1.4 What Are the Characteristics of Incarceration/Strangulation that Impact Mortality and Morbidity?

General features of risk stratification have been well worked out for emergency surgery. The APACHE classification assigns increasing risk for derangements of physiology, laboratory parameters, age greater than 55, and emergent surgery [43] (Level IIB evidence). The increased mortality noted in the large Swedish prospectively recorded database of nearly

108,000 hernia repairs highlights the increased risk of emergent surgery [44] (Level IIB evidence). A more recent large retrospective study by the same group, analyzing over 107,000 patients, confirms that emergency surgery increases mortality and additionally suggests that femoral hernias increase morality by 7-fold when compared to inguinal hernias and that mortality is increased 20-fold if bowel resection is undertaken. They also found that women overall had a higher mortality risk than men even when accounting for the higher proportion of femoral hernias and emergency surgery among women [45] (Level IIB evidence). Other retrospective series also generally suggest that increased mortality is most significantly influenced by the need for bowel resection, long duration of symptoms, delay to hospitalization, concomitant illness, and high American Society of Anesthesiologists (ASA) scores [46–50] (Level IV evidence). Retrospective studies by other groups also confirm the suggestion of worsened outcomes associated with femoral hernias, which are more common in women and are attributable to a higher risk of bowel resection in these patients [51, 52] (Level IIB and IIIB evidence).

Chung et al. reported the analysis of almost 4,300 cases of emergent abdominal wall surgery from the National Surgical Quality Improvement Program (NSQIP) database. They determined that several comorbid factors were correlated with increased short-term (30-day) mortality, including congestive heart failure, peripheral vascular disease, increased blood urea nitrogen (BUN), and elevated white blood cell count [53] (Level IIB evidence).

RECOMMENDATION

Emergent surgery for incarcerated hernias is associated with increased complications as compared to elective hernia repairs.

Grade of recommendation: B.

Specific risk factors associated with increased morbidity and mortality include long duration of symptoms, bowel resection, concomitant illness, high ASA scores, femoral hernia, and female gender.

Grade of recommendation: B.

56.1.5 What Are the Most Effective Intraoperative Evaluation Tools to Assess Bowel Viability?

Every abdominal surgeon has been faced with the need to evaluate an abnormally appearing bowel to determine its viability. In addition, there are circumstances where the reduction of an incarcerated hernia leaves a question of bowel viability unanswered. The surgical myth that "strangulated bowel will not reduce" has been disproven on many occasions. Several techniques have been offered to assess intestinal viability in trials currently. Most comparative studies were performed in preclinical settings. The most commonly evaluated modalities were clinical assessment, Doppler US, fluorescein dye administration, myoelectric activity, surface pulse oximetry, and noncontact laser Doppler blood flow assessment [46–56] (Level IIB and IIIB evidence). Preclinical comparative assessments

show mixed results when comparing pulse oximetry, Doppler US, and fluorescein, which are superior to clinical judgment alone. Laser Doppler may be superior when compared to fluorescein, and pulse oximetry and nonrandomized prospective evaluation demonstrated excellent predictive assessment when compared to clinical assessment [56–58] (Level IIIB evidence). Multiple accounts of the utility of laparoscopy or hernioscopy report clinical utility when assessing bowel liability in those cases where intestinal reduction occurs before clinical evaluation of intestinal viability [59–63] (Level IV evidence).

The use of indocyanine green (ICG) has gained popularity in the last several years in elective colorectal surgery to assess the viability of margins in minimally invasive colorectal resection and anastomosis. The use in the emergent setting is less well studied. Ruu et al. randomized patients to ICG or clinical evaluation only. The clinical evaluation–only group experienced a higher rate of bowel resection, suggesting that objective assessment with ICG is useful in this setting [64] (Level IIc evidence).

RECOMMENDATION

Objective techniques are superior to clinical evaluation alone when assessing intestinal ischemia. Laser Doppler flowmetry may be the most sensitive technique; however, Doppler US and/or fluorescein dye are likely to be more readily available.

Grade of recommendation: B.

Laparoscopy transabdominal or through the hernia sac is a useful technique for assessing intestinal viability in selected cases.

Grade of recommendation: C.

ICG is emerging as a common methodology for assessing bowel viability and can be utilized in open and minimally invasive settings.

Grade of recommendation: B.

56.1.6 Should Hernias Be Repaired to Prevent Incarceration and Strangulation?

Many authors recommend elective repair of inguinal hernia as a strategy to prevent complications and poorer outcomes associated with emergent repairs for incarcerated or strangulated hernias, particularly in elderly patients [11, 52, 65, 66] (Level IIB, IIIB, and IVB evidence). These studies show that approximately 5% of the hernia repairs reviewed were performed emergently. These cases were the source of most of the significant morbidity and mortality in the population studied. Comorbidities contributed significantly to poor outcomes in the emergent setting [11, 66]. Elective hernia repairs even in the very elderly population are safe, particularly when performed under local anesthesia [66, 68] (Level IIIB evidence).

Previously, the recommendation was to repair inguinal hernias, as they were discovered to prevent complications; however, this practice has been challenged. The prospective

Veterans Administration multicenter trial of immediate tension-free repair versus "watchful waiting" demonstrated a less than 1% risk of catastrophic events related to observation and study population [69] (Level IB evidence). The limitations of this initial study include a 30% rate of nonparticipation of the patients screened, a follow-up time of only 2 years, the exclusion of sicker patients, and that about only half the patients' hernias were detectable on cough impulse examination. This latter finding indicates a large proportion of very small, if real, hernias were included in the study. Nonetheless, this remains one of the best attempts to understand the natural history of modern hernias within the context of the severe limitations. A long-term follow-up to this study was published in 2013 which published findings after Fitzgibbons et al. continued to follow the men in the "watchful waiting" group for an additional 7 years [70] (Level IIB evidence). At the end of the initial study period, 32% of patients had crossed over and had their hernias repaired, and at the end of the additional follow-up period, this number had risen to 68%. The most common reason for repair was pain (54%), and men over 65 crossed over at a higher rate than those who were younger (79% vs. 62%). Only three patients required an emergency operation, and there were no mortalities. Thus, watchful waiting appears safe for healthy patients with minimally symptomatic hernias; however, patients should be counseled that

symptoms will likely progress and require eventual repair (grade B recommendation).

In an extensive literature analysis by van den Heuval et al., their team noted that the incarceration rate was about 4% (women somewhat higher than men) based on careful statistical analysis in Columbia. The predominant risk factors for incarceration were age >50 years, signs >3 months, and femoral hernia. When coupled with an ASA class greater than 2, the repair was recommended even for asymptomatic groin hernias [71] (Level IIC evidence).

RECOMMENDATION

The authors continue to cite the need for elective hernia repair to avoid morbidity and mortality; however, watchful waiting appears safe for younger healthy patients with minimally symptomatic hernias, though patients should be counseled that symptoms will likely progress and require eventual repair. Older patients with comorbidities should be considered for elective repair peremptorily.

Grade of recommendation: B.

TABLE 56.1

Evidence-Based Issues Concerning Incarcerated Hernia

Question	Answer	Grade of Recommendation	Level of Evidence	References
What are the appropriate physical examination and imaging evaluations necessary to diagnose an incarcerated hernia?	A thorough physical examination is mandatory and, except in rare cases, is acceptable for the diagnosis of most incarcerated hernias. Adjunctive imaging, usually CT or US, is acceptable in specific clinical scenarios where the diagnosis is difficult, such as Spigelian or obturator hernias, or if obesity limits physical examination, but routine imaging can lead to delay in surgical management.	B	IIB, IV, V	[3–13]
What are the technical considerations for treating incarcerated hernia that influence the choice of repair?	Repairing with mesh is not contraindicated for strangulated hernias.	B	IIB	[19–22]
	For inguinal hernias, Lichtenstein repair reduces recurrence rates as compared to tissue repairs, though there is some suggestion that a preperitoneal approach may better allow for bowel resection if needed.	B	2IIB	[18, 19, 21, 22]
	Laparoscopic repair with mesh is not contraindicated for incarcerated and strangulated hernias and also suggests that the TAP approach is preferable for strangulated inguinal hernias, as it allows for good visualization of abdominal contents and bowel resection if needed. The robotic approach is not contraindicated for incarcerated inguinal or incisional hernia repair.	C	IV	[24–31]

(Continued)

TABLE 56.1 (Continued)

Evidence-Based Issues Concerning Incarcerated Hernia

Question	Answer	Grade of Recommendation	Level of Evidence	References
What are the repair options in the face of GI contamination or infection?	Primary repair is discouraged, as subsequent recurrence rates are higher. The use of synthetic prostheses in contaminated cases (CDC I, II) is safe and superior for reducing long-term recurrence.	B	IIB, IIIB, IV	[19–22, 34–38, 42]
	The use of biologic prostheses is well described and is acceptable for use in high-risk and contaminated (CDC III and IV) repairs.	B	IIIB, IV	[39–41, 72–76]
What are the characteristics of incarceration/strangulation that impact mortality and morbidity?	Emergent surgery for incarcerated hernias is associated with increased complications as compared to elective hernia repairs.	B	IIB	[43, 44]
	Specific risk factors associated with increased morbidity and mortality include long duration of symptoms, bowel resection, concomitant illness, high ASA scores, CH,F PVD, elevated BUN/WBC, femoral hernia, and female gender.	B	IIB, IIIB, IV	[45–53]
What are the most effective intraoperative evaluation tools to assess bowel viability?	Objective techniques are superior to clinical evaluation alone when assessing intestinal ischemia. Laser Doppler flowmetry may be the most sensitive technique; however, Doppler ultrasound and/or fluorescein dye are more likely to be readily available.	B	IIB, IIIB	[54–58, 64, 77–84]
	Laparoscopy transabdominal or through the hernia sac is a useful technique for assessing intestinal viability in selected cases.	C	IV	[32, 33, 59–63]
Should hernias be repaired to prevent incarceration and strangulation?	The authors continue to cite the need for elective hernia repair to avoid morbidity and mortality; however, watchful waiting appears safe for healthy patients with minimally symptomatic hernias, though patients should be counseled that symptoms will likely progress and require eventual repair. Age >50, femoral location, signs >3 months, and elevated ASA are factors in favor of elective repair.	B	IB, IIB, IIIB, IV	[11, 52, 65, 66, 68, 69, 71]

Editor's Note

The management of incarcerated hernias has changed dramatically over the last half-century. Rather than perform a primary repair under tension, we evolved to utilize mesh to reduce recurrence rates. With little data, biologic meshes were touted as safer and more effective than synthetic mesh in the setting of contamination. These biologic meshes are hugely expensive (sometimes more than $50,000 for a single operation) compared to the cost of a few hundred dollars for most synthetic mesh products. How did these biologic meshes get approved by the FDA? The manufacturers of devices are only required to show that they resemble another product existing on the market. So once biologic mesh had been approved in the dark ages, all the others could join the melee. Soon, many biologic mesh products were available. My personal and my colleagues' experience was that these meshes seemed not to work, leading to more infections in the wound and simply dissolving, leaving the hernia defect unchanged. But for more than 40 years they continued to be touted as valuable and superior to synthetic mesh.

Why didn't we conduct a clinical trial to study this issue? The answer is, we tried. But if an investigator wants to do a randomized trial comparing two products (say biologic with synthetic mesh for abdominal wall hernias), they must provide both types of meshes free to the patient. They also must get FDA approval from the company to use their product in a clinical trial, something called an IDE (investigational device exemption). The astronomical cost of the biologic mesh made this too expensive for researchers to finance outside of a large federal grant. And, of course, the manufacturers were wary of performing such a study, as it might show that their cash cow was not effective. In the last couple of years, for the first time, randomized trials have been conducted and have proven that biological mesh is not as effective as plastic mesh. In my opinion, the use of biologic mesh has no place in the repair of hernias.

REFERENCES

1. Chen SC, Lee CC, Liu YP, et al. Ultrasound may decrease the emergency surgery rate of incarcerated inguinal hernia. *Scand J Gastroenterol.* 2005;*40*:721–724.

2. Ramseyer L, Abernethy EA, 3rd, McCune EA, Steffen HL. The role of CT in the diagnosis of small bowel obstruction: A case and literature review. *J Okla State Med Assoc.* 1998;*91*:103–106.

3. Buljevac M, Grgurevic I, Lackovic Z, Kujundzic M, Banic M. Duplex ultrasonography in diagnosis of spigelian hernia with incarcerated jejunal loop. *Acta Med Croat.* 2001;*55*:225–227.

4. van der Linden FM, Puylaert JB, De Vries BC. Ultrasound diagnosis of incarcerated obturator hernia. *Eur J Surg.* 1995;*161*:531–532.

5. Losanoff JE, Kjossev KT. Incarcerated Spigelian hernia in morbidly obese patients: The role of intraoperative ultrasonography for hernia localization. *Obes Surg.* 1997;*7*:211–214.

6. Avaro JP, Biance N, Savoie PH, et al. Incarcerated obturator hernia: Early diagnostic using helical computed tomography. *Hernia.* 2008;*12*:199–200.

7. Rodriguez-Hermosa JI, Codina-Cazador A, Maroto-Genover A, et al. Obturator hernia: Clinical analysis of 16 cases and algorithm for its diagnosis and treatment. *Hernia.* 2008;*12*:289–297.

8. Engin O, Cicek E, Oner SR, Yidirim M. Incarcerated femoral hernia containing the right uterine tube. A preoperative diagnosis is possible. *Ann Ital Chir.* 2011;*82*(5): 409–412.

9. Larson DW, Farley DR. Spigelian hernias: Repair and outcome for 81 patients. *World J Surg.* 2002;*26*:1277–1281.

10. Berney CR. Beware of spontaneous reduction "en masse" of inguinal hernia. *Hernia.* 2014.

11. Nilsson H, Nilsson E, Angeras U, Nordin P. Mortality after groin hernia surgery: Delay of treatment and cause of death. *Hernia.* 2011;*15*:301–307.

12. Russell KW, Mone MC, Scaife CL. Umbilical paracentesis for acute hernia reduction in cirrhotic patients. *BMJ Case Rep.* 2013 Oct 16;*2013*:bcr2013201304. doi: 10.1136/bcr-2013-201304. PMID: 24132449; PMCID: PMC3822191.

13. Takayama N, Omoto N, Tanaka A, Taniguchi N. Point-of-care ultrasonography for hernia reduction: A case of incarcerated umbilical hernia. *J Emerg Med.* 2019 Dec;*57*(6):848–851. doi: 10.1016/j.jemermed.2019.08.037. Epub 2019 Nov 7. PMID: 31708320.2

14. Mathes SJ, Steinwald PM, Foster RD, Hoffman WY, Anthony JP. Complex abdominal wall reconstruction: A comparison of flap and mesh closure. *Ann Surg.* 2000; *232*:586–596.

15. Luijendijk RW, Hop WC, van den Tol MP et al. A comparison of suture repair with mesh repair for incisional hernia. *N Engl J Med.* 2000;*343*:392–398.

16. Amid PK, Shulman AG, Lichtenstein IL. An analytic comparison of laparoscopic hernia repair with open "tension-free" hernioplasty. *Int Surg.* 1995;*80*:9–17.

17. Klaristenfeld DD, Mahoney E, Iannitti DA. Minimally invasive tension-free inguinal hernia repair. *Surg Technol Int.* 2005;*14*:157–163.

18. Karatepe O, Adas G, Battal M et al. The comparison of preperitoneal and Lichtenstein repair for incarcerated groin hernias: A prospective randomized study. *Int J Surg.* 2008;*6*:189–192.

19. Elsebae MM, Nasr M, Said M. Tension-free repair versus Bassini technique for strangulated inguinal hernia: A controlled randomized study. *Int J Surg.* 2008;*6*:302–305.

20. Abdel-Baki NA, Bessa SS, Abdel-Razek AH. Comparison of prosthetic mesh repair and tissue repair in the emergency management of incarcerated para-umbilical hernia: A prospective randomized study. *Hernia.* 2007;*11*:163–167.

21. Derici H, Unalp HR, Nazli O, et al. Prosthetic repair of incarcerated inguinal hernias: Is it a reliable method? *Langenbecks Arch Surg.* 2008;*395*:575–579.

22. Papaziogas B, Lazaridis C, Makris J, Koutelidakis J, Patsas A, Grigoriou M, Chatzimavroudis G, Psaralexis K, Atmatzidis K. Tenstion-free repair versus modified Bassini technique Andrews technique for strangulated inguinal hernia: A comparative study. *Hernia.* 2005;*9*:156–159.

23. Neumayer L, Giobbie-Hurder A, Jonasson O, et al. Open mesh versus laparoscopic mesh repair of inguinal hernia. *N Engl J Med.* 2004;*350*:1819–1827.

24. Landau O, Kyzer S. Emergent laparoscopic repair of incarcerated incisional and ventral hernia. *Surg Endosc.* 2004;*18*:1374–1376.

25. Shah RH, Sharma A, Khullar R, Soni V, Baijai M, Chowbey PK. Laparoscopic repair of incarcerated ventral abdominal wall hernias. *Hernia.* 2008;*12*:457–463.

26. Ferzli G, Shapiro K, Chaudry G, Patel S. Laparoscopic extraperitoneal approach to acutely incarcerated inguinal hernia. *Surg Endosc.* 2004;*18*:228–231.

27. Wysocki A, Pozniczek M, Krzywon J, Strzalka M. Lichtenstein repair for incarcerated groin hernias. *Eur J Surg.* 2002;*168*:452–454.

28. Yau KK, Siu WT, Cheung YS, Wong CH, Chung CC, Li KW. Laparoscopic management of acutely incarcerated femoral hernia. *J Laparoendosc Adv Surg Tech A.* 2007;*17*:759–762.

29. Yang S, Zhang G, Jin C, Cao J, Zhu Y, Shen Y, Wang M. Transabdominal preperitoneal laparoscopic approach for incarcerated inguinal hernia repair. *Medicine.* 2016;*95*(52): e5686. DOI: 10.1097/MD.0000000000005686.

30. Bou-Ayash N, Gokcal F, Kudsi OY. Robotic inguinal hernia repair for incarcerated hernias. *J Laparoendosc Adv Surg Tech A.* 2021 Aug;*31*(8):926–930. DOI: 10.1089/lap.2020.0607. Epub 2020 Oct 5. PMID: 33180657.

31. Kudsi OY, Bou-Ayash N, Chang K, Gokcal F. Perioperative and midterm outcomes of emergent robotic repair of incarcerated ventral and incisional hernia. *J Robot Surg.* 2021 Jun;*15*(3):473–481. DOI: 10.1007/s11701-020-01130-2. Epub 2020 Jul 28. PMID: 32725328.

32. Legnani GL, Rasini M, Pastori S, Sarli D. Laparoscopic trans-peritoneal hernioplasty (TAPP) for the acute management of strangulated inguino-crural hernias: A report of nine cases. *Hernia.* 2008;*12*:185–188.

33. Rebuffat C, Galli A, Scalambra MS, Balsamo F. Laparoscopic repair of strangulated hernias. *Surg Endosc.* 2006;*20*:131–134.

34. Antonopoulos IM, Nahas WC, Mazzucchi E, Piovesan AC, Birolini C, Lucon AM. Is polypropylene mesh safe and effective for repairing infected incisional hernia in renal transplant recipients? *Urology.* 2005;*66*:874–877.

35. Muller V, Lehner M, Klein P, Hohenberger W, Ott A. Incisional hernia repair after orthotopic liver transplantation: A technique employing an inlay/onlay polypropylene mesh. *Langenbecks Arch Surg.* 2003;*388*:167–173.

36. Kelly ME, Behrman SW. The safety and efficacy of prosthetic hernia repair in clean-contaminated and contaminated wounds. *Am Surg.* 2002;68:524–528; discussion 8–9.

37. Catena F, La Donna M, Gagliardi S, et al. Use of prosthetic mesh in complicated incisional hernias. *Minerva Chir.* 2002;57:363–369.

38. Geisler DJ, Reilly JC, Vaughan SG, Glennon EJ, Kondylis PD. Safety and outcome of use of nonabsorbable mesh for repair of fascial defects in the presence of open bowel. *Dis Colon Rectum.* 2003;46:1118–1123.

39. Bellows CF, Albo D, Berger DH, Awad SS. Abdominal wall repair using human acellular dermis. *Am J Surg.* 2007;194:192–198.

40. Bachman S, Ramshaw B. Prosthetic material in ventral hernia repair: How do I choose? *Surg Clin North Am.* 2008;88:101–112, ix.

41. Birindelli A, Sartelli M, Di Saverio S, et al. 2017 update of the WSES guidelines for emergency repair of complicated abdominal wall hernias. *World J Emerg Surg.* 2017;12:37. DOI: 10.1186/s13017-017-0149-y.

42. Morris MP, Mellia JA, Christopher AN, Basta MN, Patel V, Qiu K, Broach RB, Fischer JP. Ventral hernia repair with synthetic mesh in a contaminated field: A systematic review and meta-analysis. *Hernia.* 2021 Aug;25(4):1035–1050. DOI: 10.1007/s10029-020-02358-5. Epub 2021 Jan 19. PMID: 33464537.

43. Knaus WA, Wagner DP, Draper EA, et al. The APACHE III prognostic system. Risk prediction of hospital mortality for critically ill hospitalized adults. *Chest.* 1991;100: 1619–1636.

44. Nilsson E, Haapaniemi S, Gruber G, Sandblom G. Methods of repair and risk for reoperation in Swedish hernia surgery from 1992 to 1996. *Br J Surg.* 1998;85:1686–1691.

45. Nilsson H, Stylianidis G, Haapamaki M, Milsson E, Nordin P. Mortality after groin hernia surgery. *Ann Surg.* 2007;245:656–660.

46. Kulah B, Kulacoglu IH, Oruc MT, et al. Presentation and outcome of incarcerated external hernias in adults. *Am J Surg.* 2001;181:101–104.

47. Alvarez JA, Baldonedo RF, Bear IG, Solis JA, Alvarez P, Jorge JI. Incarcerated groin hernias in adults: Presentation and outcome. *Hernia.* 2004;8:121–126.

48. Kurt N, Oncel M, Ozkan Z, Bingul S. Risk and outcome of bowel resection in patients with incarcerated groin hernias: Retrospective study. *World J Surg.* 2003;27:741–743.

49. Alvarez-Perez JA, Baldonedo-Cernuda RF, Garcia-Bear I, Suarez-Solis JA, Alvarez-Martinez P, Jorge-Barreiro JI. Presentation and outcome of incarcerated external hernias in adults. *Cir Esp.* 2005;77:40–45.

50. Heydorn WH, Velanovich V. A five-year U.S. Army experience with 36,250 abdominal hernia repairs. *Am Surg.* 1990;56:596–600.

51. Corder AP. The diagnosis of femoral hernia. *Postgrad Med J.* 1992;68:26–28.

52. Koch A, Edwards A, Haapaniemi S, Nordin P, Kald A. Prospective evaluation of 6895 groin hernia repairs in women. *Br J Surg.* 2005;92:1553–1558.

53. Chung PJ, Lee JS, Tam S, Schwartzman A, Bernstein MO, Dresner L, Alfonso A, Sugiyama G. Predicting 30-day postoperative mortality for emergent anterior abdominal wall hernia repairs using the American College of Surgeons National Surgical Quality Improvement Program database.

Hernia. 2017 Jun;21(3):323–333. DOI: 10.1007/s10029-016-1538-y. Epub 2016 Sep 16. PMID: 27637187.

54. Johansson K, Ahn H, Kjellstrom C, Lindhagen J. Laser Doppler flowmetry in experimental mesenteric vascular occlusion. *Int J Microcirc Clin Exp.* 1989;8:183–190.

55. Orland PJ, Cazi GA, Semmlow JL, Reddell MT, Brolin RE. Determination of small bowel viability using quantitative myoelectric and color analysis. *J Surg Res.* 1993;55:581–587.

56. Ando M, Ito M, Nihei Z, Sugihara K. Assessment of intestinal viability using a non-contact laser tissue blood flowmeter. *Am J Surg.* 2000;180:176–180.

57. Redaelli CA, Schilling MK, Carrel TP. Intraoperative assessment of intestinal viability by laser Doppler flowmetry for surgery of ruptured abdominal aortic aneurysms. *World J Surg.* 1998;22:283–289.

58. Redaelli CA, Schilling MK, Buchler MW. Intraoperative laser Doppler flowmetry: A predictor of ischemic injury in acute mesenteric infarction. *Dig Surg.* 1998;15:55–59.

59. Lavonius MI, Ovaska J. Laparoscopy in the evaluation of the incarcerated mass in groin hernia. *Surg Endosc.* 2000;14:488–489.

60. Al-Naami MY, Al-Shawi JS. The use of laparoscopy to assess viability of slipped content in incarcerated inguinal hernia: A case report. *Surg Laparosc Endosc Percutan Tech.* 2003;13:292–294.

61. Guvenc BH, Tugay M. Laparoscopic evaluation in incarcerated groin hernia following spontaneous reduction. *Ulus Travma Acil Cerrahi Derg.* 2003;9:143–144.

62. Lin E, Wear K, Tiszenkel HI. Planned reduction of incarcerated groin hernias with hernia sac laparoscopy. *Surg Endosc.* 2002;16:936–938.

63. Morris-Stiff G, Hassn A. Hernioscopy: A useful technique for the evaluation of incarcerated hernias that retract under anaesthesia. *Hernia.* 2008;12:133–135.

64. Ryu S, Hara K, Goto K, Okamoto A, Kitagawa T, Marukuchi R, Ito R, Nakabayashi Y. Fluorescence angiography vs. direct palpation for bowel viability evaluation with strangulated bowel obstruction. *Langenbecks Arch Surg.* 2022 Mar;407(2):797–803. DOI: 10.1007/s00423-021-02358-8. Epub 2021 Oct 19. PMID: 34664121.

65. Nehme AE. Groin hernias in elderly patients. Management and prognosis. *Am J Surg.* 1983;146:257–260.

66. Alvarez Perez JA, Baldonedo RF, Bear IG, Solis JA, Alvarez P, Jorge JI. Emergency hernia repairs in elderly patients. *Int Surg.* 2003;88:231–237.

67. Kulah B, Duzgun AP, Moran M, Kulacoglu IH, Ozmen MM, Coskun F. Emergency hernia repairs in elderly patients. *Am J Surg.* 2001;182:455–459.

68. Rigberg D, Cole M, Hiyama D, McFadden D. Surgery in the nineties. *Am Surg.* 2000;66:813–816.

69. Fitzgibbons RJ, Jr., Giobbie-Harder A, Gibbs JO, et al. Watchful waiting vs repair of inguinal hernia in minimally symptomatic men: A randomized clinical trial. *JAMA.* 2006;295:285–292.

70. Fizgibbons RJ, Jr., Ramanan B, Arya S et al. Longterm results of a randomized controlled trial of a nonoperative strategy (watchful waiting) for men with minimally symptomatic inguinal hernias. *Ann Surg.* 2013;258:508–515.

71. van den Heuvel B, Dwars BJ, Klassen DR, Bonjer HJ. Is surgical repair of an asymptomatic groin hernia appropriate? A review. *Hernia.* 2011 Jun;15(3):251–259. DOI: 10.1007/s10029-011-0796-y. Epub 2011 Feb 5. PMID: 21298308.

72. Franklin ME, Jr., Trevino JM, Portillo G, Vela I, Glass JL, Gonzalez JJ. The use of porcine small intestinal submucosa as a prosthetic material for laparoscopic hernia repair in infected and potentially contaminated fields: Long-term follow-up. *Surg Endosc.* 2008;*22*:1941–1946.

73. Diaz JJ, Jr., Guy J, Berkes MB, Guillamondegui O, Miller RS. Acellular dermal allograft for ventral hernia repair in the compromised surgical field. *Am Surg.* 2006;*72*:1181–1187; discussion 7–8.

74. Gupta A, Zahriya K, Mullens PL, Salmassi S, Keshishian A. Ventral herniorrhaphy: Experience with two different biosynthetic mesh materials, Surgisis and Alloderm. *Hernia.* 2006;*10*:419–425.

75. Kim H, Bruen K, Vargo D. Acellular dermal matrix in the management of high-risk abdominal wall defects. *Am J Surg.* 2006;*192*:705–709.

76. Patton JH, Jr., Berry S, Kralovich KA. Use of human acellular dermal matrix in complex and contaminated abdominal wall reconstructions. *Am J Surg.* 2007;*193*:360–363; discussion 3.

77. Holmes NJ, Cazi G, Reddell MT, et al. Intraoperative assessment of bowel viability. *J Invest Surg.* 1993;*6*:211–221.

78. Horgan PG, Gorey TF. Operative assessment of intestinal viability. *Surg Clin North Am.* 1992;*72*:143–155.

79. Shah SD, Andersen CA. Prediction of small bowel viability using Doppler ultrasound. Clinical and experimental evaluation. *Ann Surg.* 1981;*194*:97–99.

80. Bergman RT, Gloviczki P, Welch TJ, et al. The role of intravenous fluorescein in the detection of colon ischemia during aortic reconstruction. *Ann Vasc Surg.* 1992;*6*:74–79.

81. Erikoglu M, Kaynak A, Beyatli EA, Toy H. Intraoperative determination of intestinal viability: A comparison with transserosal pulse oximetry and histopathological examination. *J Surg Res.* 2005;*128*:66–69.

82. Freeman DE, Gentile DG, Richardson DW, et al. Comparison of clinical judgment, Doppler ultrasound, and fluorescein fluorescence as methods for predicting intestinal viability in the pony. *Am J Vet Res.* 1988;*49*:895–900.

83. Tollefson DF, Wright DJ, Reddy DJ, Kintanar EB. Intraoperative determination of intestinal viability by pulse oximetry. *Ann Vasc Surg.* 1995;*9*:357–360.

84. Wright CB, Hobson RW, 2nd. Prediction of intestinal viability using Doppler ultrasound techniques. *Am J Surg.* 1975;*129*:642–645.

57

Surgical Endocrine Emergencies

Sara B. Edwards, Steven Brower, and Ki Won Kim

57.1 Endocrine Surgical Emergencies

Although endocrine surgical emergencies are uncommon, a surgeon should have a basic knowledge of the pathophysiology of these crises to properly diagnose, evaluate, and treat affected patients. Such disorders include central diabetes insipidus, carcinoid crisis, thyroid storm, hypercalcemic crisis, adrenal crisis, and hypertensive crisis secondary to pheochromocytoma.

57.2 Central Diabetes Insipidus

57.2.1 Introduction

Central diabetes insipidus (CDI) results from inadequate secretion of the hypothalamic polypeptide antidiuretic hormone (ADH). ADH originates in the supraoptic and paraventricular nuclei of the hypothalamus and is excreted by the posterior pituitary gland [1]. Hypovolemia or increased serum osmolality stimulates ADH secretion, which increases renal water reabsorption. Insufficient ADH secretion results in polyuria that can lead to severe hypovolemia, hypotension, and hypernatremia if unrecognized. With CDI, urine output exceeds 30 mL/kg in 24 hours despite fluid restriction [2]. The urine is dilute, with specific gravity below 1.005 and urine osmolality below 200 mOsm/kg. Plasma osmolality and serum sodium are increased as a result. Other causes of polyuria in the differential diagnosis include osmotic diuresis of diabetes mellitus (DM), psychogenic polydipsia, primary polydipsia from excessive water intake, and diuretic use. The osmotic diuresis of DM may be distinguished from CDI by the presence of glucosuria. With polydipsia, specific gravity and osmolality will increase with fluid restriction, and plasma vasopressin levels will increase with decreased water intake. This is in contrast to CDI, where the vasopressin levels remain low [1–3].

57.2.1.1 What Are the Causes of Central Diabetes Insipidus?

CDI most commonly occurs in the setting of traumatic brain injury (TBI), brain tumors, or following neurosurgery [2–4]. CDI has also been identified in thoracic spinal injury [5]. Injury to the hypothalamic osmoreceptors, supraoptic or paraventricular nuclei, or the supraopticohypophyseal tract halts ADH production and release, resulting in CDI [1–4]. Injury to the posterior pituitary gland, the site of storage and secretion of ADH, will often result in transient CDI. In the setting of such an injury, the hypothalamus may directly release ADH [1, 4].

> **RECOMMENDATION**
>
> Central diabetes insipidus is most commonly seen in TBI, brain tumors, or following neurosurgery.
>
> Grade of recommendation: C.

57.2.1.2 What Is the Optimal Treatment of Central Diabetes Insipidus?

> **RECOMMENDATION**
>
> Initial treatment of CDI involves the replacement of fluids with a hypotonic solution to match urine output and the replacement of ADH with a synthetic analog, d-DAVP or desmopressin [3, 6]. This medication can be delivered orally, intravenously, or as a nasal spray. The doses are titrated using urine and blood osmolality and sodium levels. Patients must be monitored closely, as overcorrection can lead to hemodilution and hyponatremia [6, 7].
>
> Grade of recommendation: B.

57.3 Carcinoid Crisis

57.3.1 Introduction

Carcinoid tumors are of neuroendocrine origin and are derived from enterochromaffin, or Kultschitzky cells. They may occur in sites of the developmental foregut, midgut, or hindgut, including the lungs, thymus, gastrointestinal tract, liver, pancreas, or genitourinary system. Primary tumors are most commonly present in the small intestine, and 30% of small intestinal tumors will metastasize [8]. Fifteen percent of patients present with metastatic disease to the liver [9]. Carcinoid tumors are rare, occurring in 2 of 100,000 people. Distribution is bimodal, with peak incidences in adolescence and the elderly. Although most carcinoid tumors occur spontaneously, 1% may be familial [9].

Carcinoid syndrome is caused by tumor secretion and systemic action of polypeptides, biogenic amines, and prostaglandins. The most significant carcinoid secretions are serotonin, histamine, tachykinins, kallikrein, and prostaglandins. These hormones are hepatically cleared. Tumor secretions must overwhelm or bypass the hepatic metabolism to produce symptoms. Therefore, carcinoid syndrome is limited to patients with metastatic disease to the liver, primary lung tumors, high tumor burden, or direct tumor manipulation [9, 10].

Carcinoid crisis is a severe sequela of carcinoid syndrome, characterized by excessive diarrhea and flushing. Fluid losses may result in dehydration, electrolyte abnormalities, arrhythmias, and hypovolemic or cardiogenic shock. Chronic exposure to serotonin and other tumor secretions may contribute to carcinoid heart disease (CHD) and severe fibrosis of the endocardium with resultant valvular and wall motion abnormalities [10]. Venous telangiectasia, bronchospasm, pellagra, and muscle wasting may also be present [9].

57.3.1.1 How Is a Carcinoid Tumor Diagnosed?

Patients with carcinoid tumors are definitively diagnosed with tissue biopsy. With carcinoid syndrome, serum platelet serotonin and urinary 5-HIAA, a metabolite of serotonin, will be elevated. Chromogranin A (CgA), a protein found on neuroendocrine cells, is not limited to serotonin-secreting tumors and can help identify the presence of inactive tumors. Imaging to localize the carcinoid primary and to evaluate the extent of disease includes CT, video enterography, endoscopy, and meta-iodobenzylguanidine (MIBG) scans. 18 F-fluorodeoxyglucose positron emission tomography (FDG PET) scans have poor utility, as carcinoid tumors display limited metabolic activity and are consequently not FDG avid. Octreotide scintigraphy scans may also aid in tumor localization [9, 11].

RECOMMENDATION

Carcinoid tumors are definitively diagnosed with tissue biopsy. Tumors may be difficult to identify on imaging, and multiple modalities may be needed for localization. Serum platelet serotonin, urinary 5-HIAA, and CgA levels are commonly elevated.

Grade of recommendation: B.

57.3.1.2 What Is the Optimal Treatment of Carcinoid Crisis?

Carcinoid crisis is treated with octreotide, a somatostatin analog with a prolonged half-life of 100 hours. Octreotide binds to somatostatin tumor receptors, limiting hormone and neurotransmitter release. An initial bolus of 25–500 mcg is administered, followed by a continuous infusion of 50–150 mcg/hour. Higher doses of octreotide may be required in patients with CHD or those previously treated with octreotide. Interferon-a has been used as an adjunct to octreotide, though efficacy has varied and the mechanism of action is poorly

understood [9, 11, 12]. The hypotension of carcinoid crisis results from diarrhea-induced hypovolemia and vasoactive peptide–induced vasodilatation. Vasopressors are often ineffective and may be deleterious, as they may exacerbate bronchospasm [12, 13]. To prevent a carcinoid crisis, patients with carcinoid syndrome should receive aggressive fluid resuscitation to prevent hypovolemia, with close monitoring of electrolytes. They may also benefit from antidiarrheals, such as loperamide [9–11, 14].

RECOMMENDATION

Carcinoid crisis is treated with intravenous fluids, electrolyte supplementation, and octreotide.

Grade of recommendation: C.

57.4 Thyroid Storm

57.4.1 Introduction

Thyroid storm (TS) is characterized by severe thyrotoxicosis and may result in multiorgan system failure [15]. TS is rare, occurring in only 1–2% of patients with thyrotoxicosis. It occurs primarily in the setting of Graves disease; rarely, it may be due to a solitary toxic adenoma, toxic multinodular goiter, subacute thyroiditis, thyroid hormone–secreting hormone (TSH)–secreting pituitary tumor, or amiodarone. TS may occur in patients with poorly controlled hyperthyroidism or be precipitated by stressors, and such inciting events include trauma, surgery, infection, cerebrovascular accidents, diabetic ketoacidosis, myocardial infarction, radioactive iodine, or pregnancy. Nonsteroidal antiinflammatory drugs, antidepressants, steroids, insulin, and thiazide diuretics may exacerbate thyrotoxicosis [16, 17]. As mortality approaches 15%, timely intervention is critical [15–17].

57.4.1.1 What Are the Symptoms and Signs of Thyroid Storm?

Thyroid hormones, prohormone thyroxine (T_4), and triiodothyronine (T_3) alter gene expression by systemically binding to mitochondrial and nuclear deoxyribonucleic acid (DNA)-binding proteins, promoting metabolism and growth. Symptoms and signs of TS include fever, palpitations, atrial fibrillation, tachypnea, congestive heart failure (CHF), diarrhea, vomiting, jaundice, delirium, seizures, and coma [16]. Serum T_4 and T_3 levels are markedly elevated. TSH is suppressed unless the source of hyperthyroidism is due to a TSH-secreting pituitary tumor [15]. Additional laboratory abnormalities may include leukocytosis, elevated liver enzymes, elevation in lactate dehydrogenase, metabolic acidosis, and hyperglycemia [16].

To aid in the differentiation of TS from simple thyrotoxicosis, Burch and Wartofsky, in 1993, developed a point system based on a history of hyperthyroidism, the presence of fever, altered mental status, gastrointestinal and hepatic manifestations (nausea, vomiting, diarrhea, lactic acidosis, liver failure), atrial fibrillation, and heart failure [18]. In a Japanese sampling modeled after Burch and Wartofsky, nausea, vomiting, and diarrhea were found to be nearly exclusive to TS. Atrial fibrillation and CHF were noted as common complications and were associated with increased mortality [17]. Intraoperative manifestation of TS may be difficult to distinguish from anesthesia-related malignant hypertension, and prompt supportive management is warranted.

RECOMMENDATION

TS presents in the setting of thyrotoxicosis and physiologic stress. Diagnostic criteria for TS require the presence of thyrotoxicosis (low TSH and elevated free T_4) and symptoms and signs, including fever, altered mental status, gastrointestinal and hepatic manifestations, atrial fibrillation, and CHF.

Grade of recommendation: C.

57.4.1.2 What Is the Appropriate Management of Thyroid Storm?

The management of TS is primarily pharmacologic. Medical treatment includes antithyroid agents, antihypertensive agents, glucocorticoids, anticoagulants, and antipyretic agents.

β-adrenergic blockade is given to treat hypertension and tachycardia associated with TS [15]. Propranolol is preferred over other β-blockers for its dual effect of β-blockade and the prevention of peripheral conversion of T_4 to T_3 [15, 16, 19]. Propranolol should not be administered in the setting of decompensated heart failure, as suppression of sympathetic stimulation may precipitate cardiovascular collapse [16].

The antithyroid medications propylthiouracil (PTU) and methimazole (MMI) are used in the treatment of thyrotoxicosis. Both inhibit the formation of thyroid hormones by reducing iodine organification. PTU also reduces peripheral deiodination of T_4 to T_3 and should be used preferentially in the setting of life-threatening thyrotoxicosis [15, 16, 20]. The indications for antithyroid agents are informed by side effect profiles. MMI should be avoided in the first trimester of pregnancy, as severe congenital abnormalities may occur. Hepatotoxicity, necessitating liver transplant, has occurred with the administration of PTU, and therefore, MMI is preferentially used for the initial treatment of non-TS hyperthyroidism. Monitoring of hepatic function has not been shown to improve outcomes in fulminant PTU-induced hepatotoxicity [19, 20].

Iodine, administered as sodium iodide or Lugol's solution (a mixture of elemental iodine and potassium iodide), can be used to treat TS by temporarily preventing the synthesis and release of thyroid hormone. Iodine solutions should be administered no sooner than 1 hour before antithyroid medications to avoid stimulation of hormone production. Lithium carbonate (Li_2CO_3) prevents the proteolysis of colloids and may also be used in the treatment of TS [15].

Glucocorticoids are used as adjuncts in the treatment of TS. Glucocorticoid stores are depleted in the hypermetabolic state of TS. Exogenous administration of glucocorticoids helps to stabilize blood pressure and inhibit peripheral deiodination of T_4 to T_3. They also serve as an antipyretic and promote vasomotor stability [15, 16, 21].

Circulating procoagulation factors are increased in TS while inhibitors, such as plasminogen and proteins C and S, are transiently reduced. Consequently, thromboembolic events may occur in TS and are responsible for up to 18% of thyrotoxic-related deaths [21]. Prophylactic anticoagulation should be administered. Patients with preexisting coagulation disorders or atrial fibrillation, present in 40% of TS cases, should be considered for therapeutic anticoagulation [15, 17].

In TS refractory to standard treatment, other agents may be considered. Reserpine, an inhibitor of norepinephrine transport, may successfully treat hypertension in patients who are refractory to β-blockade. Guanethidine, a norepinephrine antagonist, is a useful alternative to β-blockers or reserpine in the setting of asthma or bronchospasm. Cholestyramine can be used as a binding agent to lower thyroid hormone levels by facilitating intestinal excretion. L-carnitine inhibits cellular uptake of thyroid hormone. As a last resort, plasmapheresis, dialysis, or charcoal hemoperfusion may be used to temporarily reduce circulating T_3 and T_4 [15–17, 21]. Fever in thyrotoxicosis may exceed 38°C, resulting in increased cardiac output, vasodilation, tachyarrhythmias, lactic acidosis, tachypnea, coma, and even death. Salicylates should be avoided in TS, as they increase free T_3 and T_4 by inhibiting binding in serum to thyroxine-binding globulin (TBG). Therefore, acetaminophen is the preferred agent for fever. External cooling measures, including alcohol sponges, ice packs, and cooling blankets, may be necessary [15–17].

Insensible fluid losses in TS may lead to profound hypovolemia. Therefore, fluid resuscitation should begin early. Given the risk in TS for cardiac complications and CHF, administration of intravenous fluid (IVF) should be performed with close monitoring of intravascular volume status to avoid hypervolemia.

RECOMMENDATION

The management of TS is primarily treated with β-blockers, antithyroid agents, and glucocorticoids. Fluid resuscitation and thermoregulation are crucial. Underlying stressors leading to TS should be aggressively treated.

Grade of recommendation: B.

57.4.1.3 When in the Setting of Thyroid Storm Is Thyroidectomy Indicated?

Thyroidectomy may be required for cases refractory to medical management. Surgery has been recommended for patients who fail to improve after 12–24 hours of treatment, as mortality approaches 75% without surgery (vs. 10% with surgery) [19, 22–25]. Plasmapheresis or dialysis may be attempted to achieve temporary euthyroidism before surgery [23].

RECOMMENDATION

Surgical management during TS may be urgently required in patients who are refractory to medical management.

Grade of recommendation: C.

57.5 Hypercalcemic Crisis

57.5.1 Introduction

Hypercalcemic crisis most commonly arises as a consequence of primary hyperparathyroidism or malignancy; rarely, it can be due to parathyroid carcinoma or sarcoidosis. Hypercalcemic crisis generally occurs at levels above 14 mg/dL. Gastrointestinal symptoms are common and include nausea, vomiting, abdominal pain, and constipation. Changes in cognitive function range from fatigue to confusion, seizures, and coma. Hypovolemia, tetany, arrhythmias, heart block, cardiac arrest, pancreatitis, nephrolithiasis, nephrogenic diabetes insipidus, and renal failure may also occur [26].

57.5.1.1 What Are the Causes of Hypercalcemic Crisis?

Primary hyperparathyroidism and malignancy are the most common causes of hypercalcemic crisis. If due to primary hyperparathyroidism, a single parathyroid adenoma is the most common pathology [26]. Hypercalcemic crisis may also occur in the setting of malignancy, from either direct osteolysis by bony metastases or osteolysis from osteoclastic activity stimulated by parathyroid hormone-related protein (PTHrP) or proinflammatory mediators released by the tumor. Hypercalcemia due to malignancy most commonly occurs with breast, lung, and hematologic malignancies. The prognosis for patients with hypercalcemic crisis of malignancy is often dismal, with a median survival of 30 days [27].

Secondary hyperparathyroidism (SHPT) from end-stage renal disease (ESRD) results from inadequate renal activation of vitamin D, inadequate phosphate excretion, and low calcium levels, resulting in parathyroid gland hypertrophy. Although calcium levels typically do not exceed 11 mg/dL, hypercalcemia has been shown to correlate with increased mortality in dialysis patients [28]. The treatment of SHPT initially includes active vitamin D and phosphate binders. Cinacalcet, a calcimimetic, may be added if initial medical management fails to lower parathyroid hormone (PTH) and calcium levels. Patients with SHPT due to ESRD who fail medical management or who have persistent disease after renal transplant can be treated with subtotal parathyroidectomy [29].

RECOMMENDATION

Hypercalcemic crisis is most commonly caused by primary hyperparathyroidism or malignancy.

Grade of recommendation: B.

57.5.1.2 How Is Hypercalcemic Crisis Evaluated and Treated?

In the evaluation of patients with hypercalcemia, laboratory tests to be ordered include calcium, intact PTH, creatinine, 25-OH vitamin D, and PTHrP levels. In the setting of primary hyperparathyroidism, calcium and PTH will be elevated, while PTHrP is normal [27]. PTH levels will be suppressed in hypercalcemia of malignancy. Initial treatment of hypercalcemia involves the administration of IVF to restore intravascular volume and promote diuresis. A 1-liter bolus is given, followed by a continuous infusion, titrated to a urine output of 1–2 mL/kg/hour [27]. Loop diuretics may then be initiated to increase the renal excretion of calcium. Bisphosphonates may be administered to limit osteoclastic activity and prevent the release of calcium from bone [27]. Calcitonin, cinacalcet, and glucocorticoids may be given to patients refractory to initial medical therapy. In life-threatening hypercalcemia, as with arrhythmias or coma, hemodialysis may be used for rapid calcium clearance.

The underlying etiology of hypercalcemia should be identified. Once the patient is medically optimized and calcium has decreased with medical management to less than 12 mg/dL, primary hyperparathyroidism may be definitively treated with parathyroidectomy. When preoperative localization suggests a single adenoma, a focused surgical approach can be performed. While parathyroid cancer is exceedingly rare, consideration of this diagnosis is warranted with a hypercalcemic crisis, and surgical treatment includes parathyroidectomy, ipsilateral thyroidectomy, and central neck dissection.

RECOMMENDATION

Treatment of hypercalcemia includes aggressive fluid resuscitation, loop diuretics, and bisphosphonates. Calcitonin, glucocorticoids, and cinacalcet may be added for refractory cases. Hypercalcemia due to hyperparathyroidism is definitively treated with surgery.

Grade of recommendation: C.

57.6 Adrenal Crisis

57.6.1 Introduction

The adrenal gland is composed of the cortex, which produces steroid hormones, and the medulla, responsible for the secretion of catecholamines. An adrenal crisis occurs with disruption of the hypothalamic-pituitary-adrenal (HPA) axis, primarily resulting in acute mineralocorticoid deficiency. Common causes include Addison's disease, discontinuation of exogenous corticosteroids, hemorrhagic adrenalitis, adrenal infarction, or severe physiologic stress [30]. Adrenal crisis in the critically ill is likely caused by an exaggerated inflammatory response, tissue resistance to corticosteroids, and intrinsic adrenal gland deficiency [31].

57.6.1.1 What Signs and Symptoms Are Found in Patients with Adrenal Crisis?

Adrenal crisis presents with hypovolemic shock refractory to fluid resuscitation and vasopressors. A delay in diagnosis and treatment can be fatal. Other symptoms include nausea, vomiting, abdominal pain, fever, confusion, and lethargy. Close monitoring of electrolytes is required, as patients may develop hyponatremia and hyperkalemia. Adrenal insufficiency should be suspected in all septic patients unresponsive to fluids and vasopressors.

RECOMMENDATION

Symptoms of adrenal insufficiency include nausea, vomiting, abdominal pain, fever, and lethargy. Adrenal crisis is characterized by hypotension unresponsive to fluid resuscitation or vasopressors.

Grade of recommendation: B.

57.6.1.2 What Is the Appropriate Workup When Adrenal Insufficiency Is Suspected?

Adrenal insufficiency is defined by low serum cortisol levels (<10 mcg/dL) or failure of cortisol to rise (<9 mcg/dL) after attempted stimulation with corticotropin (adrenocorticotropic hormone [ACTH]) 250 mcg [31, 32]. Low-dose (1 mcg) corticotropin stimulation testing is more sensitive than high-dose testing [33]. In the septic patient, empiric treatment is recommended if adrenal insufficiency is suspected, and therefore, testing is not necessary.

RECOMMENDATION

Patients with adrenal insufficiency will commonly have decreased serum cortisol levels and will often fail low-dose corticotropin stimulation testing. However, as these tests are not 100% sensitive, critically ill patients unresponsive to IVFs and vasopressors should be empirically treated for adrenal insufficiency.

Grade of recommendation: B.

57.6.1.3 What Is the Optimal Treatment for Patients in Adrenal Crisis?

Patients suspected of having an adrenal crisis should be treated empirically, as mortality is considerable if left untreated. Hydrocortisone is the mainstay of treatment for its dual mineralocorticoid and glucocorticoid action. Patients require close hemodynamic monitoring during treatment. Fluid resuscitation and electrolyte repletion are essential. Patients with HPA axis disruption may have concurrent hypothyroidism. Precipitating factors, such as infection or myocardial ischemia, should be identified and treated [30, 34].

Empiric treatment of adrenal insufficiency with hydrocortisone should be considered in patients with septic shock who are unresponsive to fluid resuscitation and vasopressors [35]. Given the variability of corticosteroid levels during periods of septic shock, corticotropin stimulation testing may not accurately identify patients who require supplementation [35, 36].

RECOMMENDATION

A trial of corticosteroids should be instituted in patients in septic shock refractory to fluid resuscitation and vasopressors.

Grade of recommendation: B.

57.7 Hypertensive Crisis Due to Pheochromocytoma

57.7.1 Introduction

Paragangliomas (PGLs) occur within the adrenal gland (pheochromocytoma) or in an extraadrenal location, such as the neck, mediastinum, abdomen, pelvis, or the organ of Zuckerkandl. Nearly, half of all pheochromocytomas are identified incidentally, and most are sporadic [37]. They may also be associated with familial disorders, such as multiple endocrine neoplasia type 2A (MEN2A) and MEN2B, neurofibromatosis type 1, Von Hippel–Lindau syndrome, or succinate dehydrogenase B and D (SDHB, SDHD) gene mutations [37, 38].

57.7.1.1 What Are the Signs and Symptoms of Pheochromocytoma?

Pheochromocytomas are classically associated with a triad of headaches, palpitations, and diaphoresis. Other symptoms such as anxiety, dizziness, syncope, or flushing may occur [37]. Pheochromocytomas are responsible for 1% of all cases of hypertension and may result in a hypertensive emergency. As hypertension is often episodic, up to 50% of patients with pheochromocytomas may be normotensive at presentation [38]. In pregnancy, the hypertension of pheochromocytoma may be mistaken for preeclampsia. Mortality may be as high as 50% for the mother and fetus. Hypertension of pheochromocytoma may be distinguished from preeclampsia by the absence of proteinuria and an early trimester presentation [38].

RECOMMENDATION

Pheochromocytomas are associated with a triad of headaches, palpitations, and diaphoresis. Other symptoms may include anxiety, dizziness, syncope, or flushing.

Grade of recommendation: B.

57.7.1.2 How Are Pheochromocytomas Diagnosed?

Evaluation begins with the measurement of plasma or urinary metanephrines in symptomatic patients or those with an adrenal mass. The diagnosis is made biochemically. Metanephrine levels are typically elevated fourfold [39, 40]. CT or MRI is the initial imaging modality of choice to localize tumors. Pheochromocytomas will often appear hyperintense on a T2-weighted MRI and hypointense on T1-weighted images [41]. On CT, pheochromocytomas may be homogenous, heterogeneous, or cystic and typically have attenuation greater than 10 Hounsfield units (HU) on noncontrast CT. Functional imaging with ^{131}I-radiolabeled MIBG may be performed in the setting of a negative CT or MRI or in cases of suspected bilateral tumors or metastatic disease [42]. FDG-PET CT may also be used to assess the extent of disease in the setting of known malignant pheochromocytoma or when ^{131}I MIBG is negative.

RECOMMENDATION

Pheochromocytoma is diagnosed biochemically, with elevated plasma or urinary metanephrines. CT or MRI is the initial imaging modality of choice.

Grade of recommendation: B.

57.7.1.3 How Does a Pheochromocytoma Cause Hypertensive Crisis?

Hypertensive crisis in patients with pheochromocytoma is due to high levels of catecholamine production and release. Commonly, it occurs in cases of locally advanced or metastatic disease, or it may be precipitated by anesthesia induction or direct tumor manipulation. The release of catecholamines leads to vasoconstriction and tachycardia, resulting in hypertension. Complications of the hypertensive crisis include myocardial infarction, cerebrovascular accidents, seizures, cardiovascular collapse, and shock. Pheochromocytoma multisystem crisis (PMC) is characterized by hyperthermia, encephalopathy, and multiorgan system failure. Mortality rates may exceed 85% [30, 43].

RECOMMENDATION

Hypertensive crisis results from excess catecholamine release. Uncontrolled hypertension may lead to significant morbidity, including multiorgan failure and death.

Grade of recommendation: B.

57.7.1.4 What Is the Recommended Treatment for Hypertensive Crisis Due to Pheochromocytoma?

Treatment begins with an α-blocker; the agent of choice is phenoxybenzamine, a nonselective α-blocker. In all patients with pheochromocytoma, α-blockade should be administered for 10–14 days before operative intervention [38]. Dosing is titrated to orthostatic hypotension and blood pressure below 160/90 [43]. Alternatives to phenoxybenzamine include selective α-1 receptor blockers such as terazosin, prazosin, and doxazosin. Due to shorter half-lives, the incidence of postoperative reflex tachycardia and hypotension may be reduced with these agents.

β-Blockers are added to treat reflex tachycardia arising from α-blockade. Administration of β-blockers should occur only after α-blockade is initiated; otherwise, the patient will develop a hypertensive crisis through unopposed α-stimulation. During the α-blockade, the patient is encouraged to liberally consume salt and fluids to replenish intravascular volume. This is critical in preparation for adrenalectomy, as immediate loss of α-stimulation and vasoconstriction with tumor extirpation can result in significant hypotension if the patient is hypovolemic. Calcium channel antagonists (e.g., nicardipine) may also be used in the treatment of pheochromocytoma [30, 43]. In refractory cases, α-methyl tyrosine (metyrosine) may be administered to decrease catecholamine biosynthesis [30, 38, 43].

Intraoperative management of pheochromocytomas requires careful hemodynamic monitoring, with prompt treatment of hemodynamic instability. Nitroglycerine or nitroprusside may be delivered as a continuous infusion for hypertension. Magnesium sulfate may be administered to lower blood pressure, stabilize hyperdynamic myocardium, and prevent arrhythmias. Nicardipine, clevidipine, esmolol, and phentolamine are also used to lower blood pressure intraoperatively.

RECOMMENDATIONS

Initial management of patients with hypertensive crisis from a pheochromocytoma includes α-blockade, subsequent β-blockade, and intravascular volume repletion. Other agents, including calcium channel blockers or α-methyl tyrosine, may be required. Nitroglycerine or nitroprusside may be required intraoperatively for refractory cases.

Grade of recommendation: A.

57.7.1.5 How Are Pheochromocytomas Approached Surgically?

The definitive treatment for pheochromocytomas is adrenalectomy, after medical optimization with α-blockade, intravascular volume repletion, and hemodynamic stabilization. Most adrenalectomies can be performed with a minimally invasive approach, either laparoscopically (transabdominal) or retroperitoneoscopically. When compared to an open approach, the minimally invasive approach results in decreased blood loss and shorter recovery time, with no difference in intraoperative hemodynamics or operative length [44, 45]. Contraindications to a minimally invasive approach include suspected malignancy and large tumors (>8–10 cm), due to the risk of incomplete resection or seeding of the tumor bed [45, 46].

Emergency adrenalectomy for patients with PMC carries significant morbidity and mortality. However, surgery may be the only option for patients with multiorgan failure refractory to medical management [47, 48].

RECOMMENDATION

A minimally invasive approach is preferred to open adrenalectomy. Contraindications to minimally invasive surgery include suspected malignant disease or very large tumors. In patients with PMC, patients refractory to medical management may require emergency adrenalectomy (Tables 57.1 and 57.2).

Grade of recommendation: B.

TABLE 57.1

Question and Answer Summaries and Recommendations

Question	Answer	Levels of Evidence	Grade of Recommendation	References
What are the causes of CDI?	CDI is most commonly observed in traumatic brain injury (TBI), brain tumors, or following neurosurgery.	IIa, IIIa	C	[1–4]
What is the optimal treatment of CDI?	Initial treatment of CDI involves the replacement of fluids with a hypotonic solution to match urine output and the replacement of ADH with a synthetic analog, d-DAVP, or desmopressin. This medication can be delivered orally, intravenously, or as a nasal spray. The doses are titrated using urine and blood osmolality and sodium levels. Patients must be monitored closely, as overcorrection can lead to hemodilution and hyponatremia.	IIa, III	B	[3–7]
How is a carcinoid tumor diagnosed?	Carcinoid tumors are definitively diagnosed with tissue biopsy. Tumors may be difficult to identify on imaging, and multiple modalities may be needed for localization. Serum platelet serotonin, urinary 5-HIAA, and CgA levels are commonly elevated.	IIa, IIIb	B	[9, 11]
What is the optimal treatment for carcinoid crisis?	Carcinoid crisis is treated with intravenous fluids, electrolyte supplementation, and octreotide.	IIa, III	C	[9–14]
What are the symptoms and signs of thyroid storm?	Thyroid storm presents in the setting of thyrotoxicosis and physiologic stress. Diagnostic criteria for TS require the presence of thyrotoxicosis (low TSH and elevated free thyroxine) and symptoms and signs, including fever, altered mental status, gastrointestinal and hepatic manifestations, atrial fibrillation, and congestive heart failure.	IIIa	C	[16–18]
What is the appropriate management of thyroid storm?	The management of thyroid storm is primarily treated with β-blockers, antithyroid agents, and glucocorticoids. Fluid resuscitation and thermoregulation are crucial. Underlying stressors leading to thyroid storm should be aggressively treated.	IIa, IIIa	B	[15–21]
When in the setting of a thyroid storm is thyroidectomy indicated?	Surgical management during thyroid storm may be urgently required in patients who are refractory to medical management.	IIa, III	C	[19, 22–25]
What are the causes of hypercalcemic crisis?	Hypercalcemic crisis is most commonly caused by primary hyperparathyroidism or malignancy.	IIa, IIIa	B	[26–29]
How is a hypercalcemic crisis evaluated and treated?	Treatment of hypercalcemia includes aggressive fluid resuscitation, loop diuretics, and bisphosphonates. Calcitonin, glucocorticoids, and cinacalcet may be added for refractory cases. Hypercalcemia due to hyperparathyroidism is definitively treated with surgery.	IIIa	C	[27]

(Continued)

TABLE 57.1 (Continued)

Question and Answer Summaries and Recommendations

Question	Answer	Levels of Evidence	Grade of Recommendation	References
What signs and symptoms are found in patients with adrenal crisis?	Symptoms of adrenal insufficiency include nausea, vomiting, abdominal pain, fever, and lethargy. Adrenal crisis is characterized by hypotension unresponsive to fluid resuscitation or vasopressors.	III	B	[30–31]
What is the appropriate workup when adrenal insufficiency is suspected?	Patients with adrenal insufficiency will commonly have decreased serum cortisol levels and will often fail low-dose corticotropin stimulation testing. However, as these tests are not 100% sensitive, critically ill patients unresponsive to intravenous fluids and vasopressors should be empirically treated for adrenal insufficiency.	IIa, IIIa	B	[31–33]
What is the optimal treatment for patients with adrenal crisis?	A trial of corticosteroids should be instituted in patients in septic shock refractory to fluid resuscitation and vasopressors.	II	B	[30, 34–36]
What are the signs and symptoms of pheochromocytoma?	Pheochromocytomas are associated with a triad of headaches, palpitations, and diaphoresis. Other symptoms may include anxiety, dizziness, syncope, or flushing.	IIa	B	[37, 38]
How are pheochromocytomas diagnosed?	Pheochromocytoma is diagnosed biochemically, with elevated plasma or urinary metanephrines. CT or MRI is the initial imaging modality of choice.	II, IIIa	B	[39–41]
How does a pheochromocytoma cause a hypertensive crisis?	A hypertensive crisis results from excess catecholamine release. Uncontrolled hypertension may lead to significant morbidity, including multiorgan failure and death.	II	B	[30, 43]
What is the recommended treatment for hypertensive crisis due to pheochromocytoma?	Initial management of patients with hypertensive crisis from a pheochromocytoma includes α-blockade, subsequent β-blockade, and intravascular volume repletion. Other agents, including calcium channel blockers or α-methyl tyrosine, may be required. Nitroglycerine or nitroprusside may be required intraoperatively for refractory cases.	II	A	[30, 38, 40]
How are pheochromocytomas approached surgically?	A minimally invasive approach is preferred to open adrenalectomy. Contraindications to minimally invasive surgery include suspected malignant disease or very large tumors. In patients with PMC, patients refractory to medical management may require emergency adrenalectomy.	Ib, IIa, IIIb	B	[44–48]

TABLE 57.2

Review of References

Author (References)	Year	Level of Evidence	Groups	Design	Median Follow-up	Endpoint
Babey et al. [1]	2011	IIa	Patients with familial central diabetes insipidus	Review	N/A	Review of clinical presentation, treatment, and molecular characteristics
Schneider et al. [4]	2007	IIa	Patients with pituitary abnormalities due to traumatic brain injury or subarachnoid hemorrhage	Meta-analysis	3 months to 22 years (median not calculated)	Anterior hypopituitarism: Insulin level, insulin tolerance, GHRH, GH, TSH, LH/FSH, ACTH, arginine, and growth hormone releasing–peptide 6 levels Posterior hypopituitarism: Prevalence of DI
Vande Walle et al. [7]	2007	IIa	Patients treated with desmopressin for diabetes insipidus	Review of retrospective cohort studies and RCTs	NR	Resolution of symptoms or onset of complications

(Continued)

TABLE 57.2 (Continued)

Review of References

Author (References)	Year	Level of Evidence	Groups	Design	Median Follow-up	Endpoint
Zuetenhurst and Taal [9]	2005	IIC	Patients with carcinoid tumors	Review of the retrospective cohort, RCTs, and outcomes research	NR	Examine the epidemiology, current diagnostic criteria, treatments, and prognosis
Seymour and Sawh [11]	2013	IIA	Patients treated with high-dose octreotide for carcinoid crisis	Review of retrospective cohort studies and consensus statements	NR	Resolution of symptoms, side effects, mortality
Castillo et al. [12]	2012	IIIB	Carcinoid tumor–induced cardiac disease	Review of case series and retrospective cohort studies	NR	Patient optimization and octreotide dosing
Kinney et al. [14]	2001	IIB	Patients who underwent abdominal surgery for metastatic carcinoid tumors	Retrospective cohort study	30 days	Perioperative morbidity and mortality
Akamizu et al. [17]	2012	IIC	Japanese patients with thyrotoxicosis, with and without thyroid storm (TS)	Outcomes research	NR	The onset of TS, irreversible complications, death, resolution of TS
Burch and Wartofsky [18]	1993	IIA	Patients with TS	Review of retrospective cohort studies	NR	Resolution of symptoms, death
Bahn et al. [19]	2011	Grade B	Recommendations for the management of hyperthyroidism	Consensus statement (national task force)	NA	NA
Stagnaro-Green et al. [20]	2011	Grade B	Recommendations for the diagnosis and management of thyroid disease in pregnancy and the postpartum period	Consensus statement (national task force)	NA	NA
Klubo-Gwiezdzinska and Wartofsky [21]	2012	IIA	Recommendations for the management of hypothyroid and hyperthyroid emergencies	Review of retrospective cohort studies	N/A	N/A
Clines [27]	2011	IIA	Patients with hypercalcemia of malignancy	Retrospective cohort studies, RCTs	NA	NA
Fukagawa et al. [28]	2014	IIB	Patients with secondary hyperparathyroidism due to ESRD	Prospective case-cohort study	3 years	All-cause mortality
Tucci and Sokari [30]	2014	IIA	Patients with adrenal emergencies	Review of retrospective cohorts, RCTs	NA	NA
Marik et al. [31]	2008	Grade B	Recommendations for corticosteroid insufficiency	Consensus statement (international task force)	NA	NA
Annane et al. [32]	2006	IIB	Septic and nonseptic patients	Consecutive cohort study	NR	Baseline cortisol level, free cortisol level, and delta cortisol level after stimulation
Siraux et al. [33]	2005	IIB	Patients administered a low-dose (1 μg) corticotropin stimulation test vs. the standard (250 μg) test for the diagnosis of relative adrenal insufficiency	Consecutive cohort study	28 days	Cortisol levels, maximum cortisol levels, hemodynamic stability, length of ICU stay, ICU mortality, 28-day survival
Dellinger et al. [35]	2013	Grade B	Recommendations for the management of severe sepsis and septic shock	Consensus statement (international task force)	NA	NA
Briegel et al. [36]	2009	IIB	Patients in septic shock	Retrospective cohort study	NR	Cortisol level, diagnosis of corticosteroid insufficiency

(Continued)

TABLE 57.2 (Continued)

Review of References

Author (References)	Year	Level of Evidence	Groups	Design	Median Follow-up	Endpoint
Wachtel et al. [37]	2014	IIB	Adrenalectomy in patients with incidental or symptomatic pheochromocytoma	Retrospective cohort study	NR	Histologic evidence of malignant or benign disease
Chen et al. [38]	2010	Grade B	Recommendations for the diagnosis and management of neuroendocrine tumors	Consensus statement (international task force)	NA	NA
Kirshtein et al. [39]	2007	IIC	Adrenalectomy for adrenal incidentaloma	Outcomes research	NR	NA
Lenders et al. [40]	2002	IIB	Patients evaluated for pheochromocytoma (1994–2001)	Retrospective cohort study	NR	Sensitivities and specificities of the biochemical markers of pheochromocytoma
Bhatia et al. [42]	2005	IIB	Patients who underwent both preoperative [(123)I] MIBG and cross-sectional imaging for confirmed pheochromocytoma and paraganglioma	Retrospective analysis	NR	Sensitivity of MIBG vs. CT/MRI scans for the detection of adrenal and extraadrenal tumors
Tiberio et al. [44]	2008	IB	Comparison of laparoscopic vs. open adrenalectomy for pheochromocytoma	A prospective randomized controlled trial	NR	Operative time, hypertensive episodes, and long-term follow-up
Bentrem et al. [45]	2002	IIB	Laparoscopic, laparoscopic-assisted, and open adrenalectomies	Retrospective cohort study	6.5 days	Operative times, blood loss, length of stay
Phitayakorn and McHenry [46]	2008	IIB	Comparison of laparoscopic adrenalectomy to laparoscopic adrenalectomy converted to open	Retrospective cohort study	NR	Conversion to open procedure

Acknowledgments

We gratefully acknowledge Christopher Busken, MD, Rebecca Coefield, MD, and Robert Kelly, MD, who contributed to a prior version of this chapter [49].

Editor's Note

This chapter nicely describes the rare endocrine emergencies that an acute care surgeon might encounter. But it may be beneficial to focus on adrenal insufficiency, as this is one endocrine entity that is not rare today and often presents surreptitiously, absent an existing diagnosis from an endocrinologist. Many of our patients are receiving exogenous steroids or have received them in the previous year. These patients may require the administration of glucocorticoids to avoid becoming hypoadrenal. Individuals with adrenal insufficiency will not respond to volume resuscitation or vasopressors and thus may have refractory hypotension. Confirming the diagnosis can be difficult, and there are convincing data suggesting that corticotropin stimulation tests are inaccurate [50]. Therefore, when a patient may have adrenal suppression, we must administer exogenous steroids empirically. The low steroid doses required are not immunosuppressive and therefore do not increase the risk of complications.

REFERENCES

1. Babey M, Kopp P, Robertson GL. Familial forms of diabetes insipidus: Clinical and molecular characteristics. *Nat Rev Endocrinol*. 2011;*7(12)*:701–714.
2. Leroy C, Karrouz W, Douillard C, et al. Diabetes insipidus. *Ann Endocrinol (Paris)*. 2013;*74(5–6)*:496–507.
3. Devin JK. Hypopituitarism and central diabetes insipidus: Perioperative diagnosis and management. *Neurosurg Clin North Am*. 2012;*23(4)*:679–689.
4. Schneider HJ, Kreitschmann-Andermahr I, Ghigo E, et al. Hypothalamopituitary dysfunction following traumatic brain injury and aneurysmal subarachnoid hemorrhage: A systematic review. *JAMA*. 2007;*298(12)*:1429–1438.
5. Kuzeyli K, Cakir E, Baykal S, et al. Diabetes insipidus secondary to penetrating spinal cord trauma: Case report and literature review. *Spine* (Phila Pa 1976). 2001;*26(21)*: E510–E511.
6. Chanson P, Salenave S. Treatment of neurogenic diabetes insipidus. *Ann Endocrinol (Paris)*. 2011;*72(6)*:496–499.
7. Vande Walle J, Stockner M, Raes A, Nørgaard JP. Desmopressin 30 years in clinical use: A safety review. *Curr Drug Safety*. 2007;*2(3)*:232–238.
8. Modlin IM, Lye KD, Kidd M. A 5-decade analysis of 13,715 carcinoid tumors. *Cancer*. 2003;*97(4)*:934–959.
9. Zuetenhorst JM, Taal BG. Metastatic carcinoid tumors: A clinical review. *Oncologist*. 2005;*10(2)*:123–131.

10. Mehta AC, Rafanan AL, Bulkley R, et al. Coronary spasm and cardiac arrest from carcinoid crisis during laser bronchoscopy. *Chest.* 1999;*115(2)*:598–600.

11. Seymour N, Sawh SC. Mega-dose intravenous octreotide for the treatment of carcinoid crisis: A systematic review. *Can J Anaesth.* 2013;*60(5)*:492–499.

12. Castillo JG, Silvay G, Solis J. Current concepts in diagnosis and perioperative management of carcinoid heart disease. *Semin Cardiothorac Vasc Anesth.* 2013;*17(3)*:212–223.

13. Vaughan DJ, Brunner MD. Anesthesia for patients with carcinoid syndrome. *Int Anesthesiol Clin.* 1997;*35(4)*: 129–142.

14. Kinney MA, Warner ME, Nagorney DM, et al. Perianaesthetic risks and outcomes of abdominal surgery for metastatic carcinoid tumours. *Br J Anaesth.* 2001;*87(3)*:447–452.

15. Papi G, Corsello SM, Pontecorvi A. Clinical concepts on thyroid emergencies. *Front Endocrinol (Lausanne).* 2014; *5*:102.

16. Hampton J. Thyroid gland disorder emergencies: Thyroid storm and myxedema coma. *AACN Adv Crit Care.* 2013; *24(3)*:325–332.

17. Akamizu T, Satoh T, Isozaki O, et al. Diagnostic criteria, clinical features, and incidence of thyroid storm based on nationwide surveys. *Thyroid.* 2012;*22(7)*:661–679.

18. Burch HB, Wartofsky L. Life-threatening thyrotoxicosis. Thyroid storm. *Endocrinol Metab Clin North Am.* 1993;*22(2)*:263–277.

19. Bahn RS, Burch HB, Cooper DS, et al. Hyperthyroidism and other causes of thyrotoxicosis: Management guidelines of the American Thyroid Association and American Association of Clinical Endocrinologists. *Endocr Pract.* 2011;*17(3)*:456–520.

20. Stagnaro-Green A, Abalovich M, Alexander E, et al. Guidelines of the American Thyroid Association for the diagnosis and management of thyroid disease during pregnancy and postpartum. *Thyroid.* 2011;*21(10)*:1081–1125.

21. Klubo-Gwiezdzinska J, Wartofsky L. Thyroid emergencies. *Med Clin North Am.* 2012;*96(2)*:385–403.

22. Uchida N, Suda T, Ishiguro K. Thyroidectomy in a patient with thyroid storm: Report of a case. *Surg Today.* 2013;*45(1)*:110–114.

23. Yamamoto J, Dostmohamed H, Schacter I, et al. Preoperative therapeutic apheresis for severe medically refractory amiodarone-induced thyrotoxicosis: A case report. *J Clin Apher.* 2014;*29(3)*:168–170.

24. Scholz GHHE, Arkenau C, Engelmann L, Lamesch P, Schreiter D, Schoenfelder M, Olthoff D, Paschke R. Is there a place for thyroidectomy in older patients with thyrotoxic storm and cardiorespiratory failure? *Thyroid.* 2003;*13(10)*:933–940.

25. Reichmann I, Frilling A, Hormann R, et al. Early operation as a treatment measure in thyrotoxic crisis. *Chirurg.* 2001;*72(4)*:402–407.

26. Khan MA, Rafiq S, Lanitis S, et al. Surgical treatment of primary hyperparathyroidism: Description of techniques and advances in the field. *Indian J Surg.* 2014;*76(4)*: 308–315.

27. Clines GA. Mechanisms and treatment of hypercalcemia of malignancy. *Curr Opin Endocrinol Diabetes Obes.* 2011;*18(6)*:339–346.

28. Fukagawa M, Kido R, Komaba H, et al. Abnormal mineral metabolism and mortality in hemodialysis patients with secondary hyperparathyroidism: Evidence from marginal structural models used to adjust for time-dependent confounding. *Am J Kidney Dis.* 2014;*63(6)*:979–987.

29. Dewberry LK, Weber C, Sharma J. Near total parathyroidectomy is an effective therapy for tertiary hyperparathyroidism. *Am Surg.* 2014;*80(7)*:646–651.

30. Tucci V, Sokari T. The clinical manifestations, diagnosis, and treatment of adrenal emergencies. *Emerg Med Clin North Am.* 2014;*32(2)*:465–484.

31. Marik PE, Pastores SM, Annane D, et al. Recommendations for the diagnosis and management of corticosteroid insufficiency in critically ill adult patients: Consensus statements from an international task force by the American College of Critical Care Medicine. *Crit Care Med.* 2008;*36(6)*:1937–1949.

32. Annane D, Maxime V, Ibrahim F, et al. Diagnosis of adrenal insufficiency in severe sepsis and septic shock. *Am J Respir Crit Care Med.* 2006;*174(12)*:1319–1326.

33. Siraux V, De Backer D, Yalavatti G, et al. Relative adrenal insufficiency in patients with septic shock: Comparison of low-dose and conventional corticotropin tests. *Crit Care Med.* 2005;*33(11)*:2479–2486.

34. Bancos I, Hahner S, Tomlinson J, et al. Diagnosis and management of adrenal insufficiency. *Lancet Diabetes Endocrinol.* March 2014;*3(3)*:216–226.

35. Dellinger RP, Levy MM, Rhodes A, et al. Surviving Sepsis Campaign: International guidelines for the management of severe sepsis and septic shock, 2012. *Intensive Care Med.* 2013;*39(2)*:165–228.

36. Briegel J, Sprung CL, Annane D, et al. Multicenter comparison of cortisol as measured by different methods in samples of patients with septic shock. *Intensive Care Med.* 2009;*35(12)*:2151–2156.

37. Wachtel H, Cerullo I, Bartlett EK, et al. Characteristics of incidentally identified pheochromocytoma. *Ann Surg Oncol.* January 2015;*22(1)*:132–138.

38. Chen H, Sippel RS, O'Dorisio MS, et al. The North American Neuroendocrine Tumor Society consensus guideline for the diagnosis and management of neuroendocrine tumors: Pheochromocytoma, paraganglioma, and medullary thyroid cancer. *Pancreas.* 2010;*39(6)*:775–783.

39. Kirshtein B, Ragliarello G, Yelle JD, et al. Incidence of pheochromocytoma in trauma patients during the management of unrelated illness: A retrospective review. *Int J Surg.* 2007;*5(5)*:332–335.

40. Lenders JW, Eisenhofer G, Mannelli M, et al. Biochemical diagnosis of pheochromocytoma: Which test is best? *JAMA.* 2002;*287(11)*:1427–1434.

41. Mayo-Smith WW, Boland GW, Noto RB, et al. State-of-the-art adrenal imaging. *Radiographics.* 2001;*21(4)*:995–1012.

42. Bhatia KS, Ismail MM, Sahdev A, et al. 123I-metaiodobenzylguanidine (MIBG) scintigraphy for the detection of adrenal and extra-adrenal phaeochromocytomas: CT and MRI correlation. *Clin Endocrinol (Oxford).* 2008;*69(2)*:181–188.

43. Kinney MA, Narr BJ, Warner MA. Perioperative management of pheochromocytoma. *J Cardiothorac Vasc Anesth.* 2002;*16(3)*:359–369.

44. Tiberio GA, Baiocchi GL, Arru L, et al. Prospective randomized comparison of laparoscopic versus open adrenalectomy for sporadic pheochromocytoma. *Surg Endosc.* 2008; *22*(6):1435–1439.

45. Bentrem DJ, Pappas SG, Ahuja Y, et al. Contemporary surgical management of pheochromocytoma. *Am J Surg.* 2002;*184*(6):621–624; discussion 624–625.

46. Phitayakorn R, McHenry CR. Laparoscopic and selective open resection for adrenal and extraadrenal neuroendocrine tumors. *Am Surg.* 2008;*74*(*1*):37–42.

47. Bos JC, Toorians AWFT, van Mourik JC, et al. Emergency resection of an extra-adrenal phaeochromocytoma: Wrong or right? A case report and a review of the literature. *Neth J Med.* 2003;*61*(*8*):258–265.

48. Uchida N, Ishiguro K, Suda T, et al. Pheochromocytoma multisystem crisis successfully treated by emergency surgery: Report of a case. *Surg Today.* 2010;*40*(*10*):990–996.

49. Busken C, Kelly B. 2009. *Acute Care Surgery and Trauma: Evidence-Based Practice.* Boca Raton, FL: CRC Press, pp. 451–456.

50. Sprung Kim, K., Cohn, S. Hydrocortisone therapy for patients with septic shock. *N Engl J Med.* 2008 Jan 10;*358*(2): 111–124. doi: 10.1056/NEJMoa071366.

Index

Note: Locators in *italics* represent figures and **bold** indicate tables in the text.